Priorities in
Critical Care
Nursing

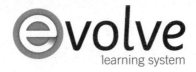
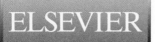

SIXTH EDITION

Priorities in Critical Care Nursing

Linda D. Urden, DNSc, RN, CNS, NE-BC, FAAN
Professor and Director, Master's and International Programs
Hahn School of Nursing and Health Science
University of San Diego
San Diego, California

Kathleen M. Stacy, PhD, RN, CNS, CCRN, PCCN, CCNS
Clinical Nurse Specialist–Intermediate Care Unit
Palomar Pomerado Health
Escondido, California
Adjunct Faculty Member
School of Nursing, College of Health and Human Services
San Diego State University
San Diego, California

Mary E. Lough, PhD, RN, CNS, CCRN, CNRN, CCNS
Critical Care Clinical Nurse Specialist
Stanford University Hospital and Clinics
Stanford, California
Clinical Professor
Department of Physiological Nursing
University of California, San Francisco
San Francisco, California

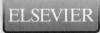

With approximately 180 Illustrations

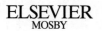

ELSEVIER
MOSBY

3251 Riverport Lane
St. Louis, Missouri 63043

PRIORITIES IN CRITICAL CARE NURSING   ISBN: 978-0-323-07461-2

Notice

Knowledge and best practice in this field are constantly changing. As new research and experience broaden our knowledge, changes in practice, treatment, and drug therapy may become necessary or appropriate. Readers are advised to check the most current information provided (i) on procedures featured or (ii) by the manufacturer of each product to be administered, to verify the recommended dose or formula, the method and duration of administration, and contraindications. It is the responsibility of the practitioner, relying on their own experience and knowledge of the patient, to make diagnoses, to determine dosages and the best treatment for each individual patient, and to take all appropriate safety precautions. To the fullest extent of the law, neither the Publisher nor the Authors assume any liability for any injury and/or damage to persons or property arising out or related to any use of the material contained in this book.

The Publisher

Nursing Diagnoses—Definitions and Classifications 2009–2011. Copyright © 2009, 2007, 2005, 2003, 2001, 1998, 1996, 1994 by NANDA International. Used by arrangement with Wiley-Blackwell Publishing, a company of John Wiley and Sons, Inc.

Library of Congress Cataloging-in-Publication Data or Control Number

Priorities in critical care nursing / [edited by] Linda D. Urden, Kathleen M. Stacy, Mary E. Lough.—6th ed.
       p. ; cm.
   Includes bibliographical references and index.
   ISBN 978-0-323-07461-2 (pbk. : alk. paper)
   I. Urden, Linda Diann.   II. Stacy, Kathleen M.   III. Lough, Mary E.
   [DNLM: 1. Critical Care.   2. Nursing Care.   3. Critical Illness–nursing. WY 154]
   LC classification not assigned
   616.02′8–dc23

                                                      2011034430

Senior Editor: Tamara Myers
Senior Developmental Editor: Linda Thomas
Publishing Services Manager: Deborah Vogel
Project Manager: Bridget Healy
Designer: Maggie Reid

Printed in the United States of America

Last digit is the print number: 9   8   7   6   5   4   3   2

Beverly Carlson, PhD, RN, CNS, CCRN
Lecturer, School of Nursing
San Diego State University
San Diego, California
*Chapter 26, Shock, Sepsis, and Multiple
Organ Dysfunction Syndrome*

Joni L. Dirks, MS, RN-BC, CCRN
Critical Care Educator
Adult ICU and Simulation
Providence Sacred Heart Medical Center
Spokane, Washington
*Chapter 13, Cardiovascular Therapeutic
Management*

**Lorraine Fitzsimmons, PhD, APRN,
FNP, ANP-BC**
Chair, Advanced Practice Nursing of Adults
and Elderly
Assistant Professor
School of Nursing
San Diego State University
San Diego, California
*Chapter 26, Shock, Sepsis, and Multiple
Organ Dysfunction Syndrome*

Céline Gélinas, PhD, RN
Assistant Professor
School of Nursing
McGill University
Montreal, Quebec, Canada
Chapter 8, Pain and Pain Management

Marian Grant, DNP, CRNP, ACHPN
Assistant Professor
School of Nursing
University of Maryland
Baltimore, Maryland
Chapter 10, End-of-Life Care

Annette Haynes, MS, RN, CCRN
Cardiology Clinical Nurse Specialist
Stanford University Hospital and Clinics
Stanford, California
Chapter 12, Cardiovascular Disorders

**Sheryl Leary, MS, RN, CCNS, CCRN,
PCCN**
Progressive Care Clinical Nurse Specialist
VA San Diego Healthcare System
San Diego, California
*Chapter 22, Gastrointestinal Disorders and
Therapeutic Management*

**Mary E. Lough, PhD, RN, CNS, CCRN,
CNRN, CCNS**
Critical Care Clinical Nurse Specialist
Stanford University Hospital and Clinics
Stanford, California
Clinical Professor
Department of Physiological Nursing
University of California, San Francisco
San Francisco, California
*Chapter 9, Sedation and Delirium
Management*
*Chapter 11, Cardiovascular Clinical
Assessment and Diagnostic Procedures*
*Chapter 20, Renal Disorders and
Therapeutic Management*
*Chapter 23, Endocrine Clinical Assessment
and Diagnostic Procedures*
*Chapter 24, Endocrine Disorders and
Therapeutic Management*

Jeanne M. Maiden, PhD, RN, CNS
Professor
School of Nursing
Point Loma Nazarene University
San Diego, California
*Chapter 14, Pulmonary Clinical Assessment
and Diagnostic Procedures*

Barbara Mayer, MS, PhD(c), RN-BC
Director of Professional Nursing Practice
St. Vincent Medical Center
Los Angeles, California
Chapter 3, Patient and Family Education
*Chapter 27, Hematological and Oncological
Emergencies*

**Mary Schira, PhD, RN, ACNP-BC,
CNN-NP**
Associate Dean and Chair
Department of Advanced Practice Nursing
College of Nursing
The University of Texas at Arlington
Arlington, Texas
*Chapter 19, Renal Clinical Assessment and
Diagnostic Procedures*

**Elizabeth Scruth, PhD(c), MN, RN,
MPH, CNS, CCRN**
Clinical Practice Consultant
Kaiser Permanente NCAL
Regional Quality and Regulatory Services
San Jose, California
Chapter 12, Cardiovascular Disorders

Kara Snyder, MS, RN, CCRN
Clinical Nurse Specialist
Surgical/Trauma Critical Care
University Medical Center
Tucson, Arizona
Chapter 25, Trauma

**Kathleen M. Stacy, PhD, RN, CNS,
CCRN, PCCN, CCNS**
Clinical Nurse Specialist–Intermediate
Care Unit
Palomar Pomerado Health
Escondido, California
Adjunct Faculty Member
School of Nursing, College of Health and
Human Services
San Diego State University
San Diego, California
*Chapter 14, Pulmonary Clinical Assessment
and Diagnostic Procedures*
Chapter 15, Pulmonary Disorders
*Chapter 16, Pulmonary Therapeutic
Management*
*Chapter 17, Neurological Clinical Assessment
and Diagnostic Procedures*
*Chapter 18, Neurological Disorders and
Therapeutic Management*
*Chapter 21, Gastrointestinal Clinical
Assessment and Diagnostic Procedures*

**Linda D. Urden, DNSc, RN, CNS,
NE-BC, FAAN**
Professor and Director
Master's and International Programs
Hahn School of Nursing and Health
Science
University of San Diego
San Diego, California
*Chapter 1, Caring for the Critically Ill
Patient*
Chapter 2, Ethical and Legal Issues
Chapter 4, Psychosocial Alterations
Chapter 5, Sleep Alterations
Chapter 6, Nutritional Alterations
Chapter 7, Gerontological Alterations

**Christopher Walker, MS, RN, NP, CNS,
CCRN**
Emergency Services
Sharp Memorial Hospital
San Diego, California
*Chapter 26, Shock, Sepsis, and Multiple
Organ Dysfunction Syndrome*

Mali M. Bartges, DNP, RN, CCRN
Associate Professor of Nursing
Northampton Community College
Bethlehem, Pennsylvania

Karen J. Brasel, MD, MPH
Professor
Surgery, Bioethics, and Medical
    Humanities
Medical College of Wisconsin
Milwaukee, Wisconsin

**Marylee Bressie, MSN, RN, CCRN,
CCNS, CEN**
RN/Doctoral Candidate
Providence Hospital/Samford University
Mobile, Alabama

**Nita Jane Carrington, EdD, RN, ANP,
MSN, MBA, MPA**
Associate Professor
College of Nursing and Health Sciences
Hawaii Pacific University
Kaneohe, Hawaii

**Reba Felks-McVay, MSN, RN, CNS-BC,
CCRN**
Administrative Director, Cardiovascular
    Services
Southern Maryland Hospital Center
Clinton, Maryland

**Joyce Foresman-Capuzzi, MSN, RN,
CCNS, CEN, CPN, CCRN, CTRN,
CPEN, SANE-A, EMT-P**
Clinical Nurse Educator, Emergency
    Department
Lankeanu Medical Center
Main Line Health Systems
Wynnewood, Pennsylvania

Susan K. Frazier, PhD, RN
Associate Professor
Co-director, RICH Heart Program
Web Editor, *The Journal of Cardiovascular
    Nursing*
College of Nursing
University of Kentucky
Lexington, Kentucky

Cheryl K. Kent, MS, RN
Instructor, Division of Nursing
Northwestern Oklahoma State University
Enid, Oklahoma

Dana M. Kyles, MS, RN
Nurse Manager
Nursing (Clinical Informatics)
Medical/Surgical/Telemetry and
    Transfusion Services
University of Washington
Seattle, Washington

Robert E. Lamb, PharmD
Principle, REL & Associates, LLC
Downingtown, Pennsylvania

Patricia Mullen, PhD, RN, CNE
Assistant Professor
Loretto Heights School of Nursing
Regis University
Denver, Colorado

Sandra O'Sullivan, MS, RN, CCRN
Instructor
School of Nursing
The Pennsylvania State University
Hershey, Pennsylvania

Michaelynn Paul, MS, RN, CCRN
Assistant Professor of Nursing
School of Nursing (Portland Campus)
Walla Walla University
Walla Walla, Washington

**Deanna L. Reising, PhD, RN, ACNS-BC,
ANEF RN**
Associate Professor/Research Clinical Nurse
    Specialist
Indiana University School of Nursing
Bloomington Hospital
Bloomington, Indiana

Connie Schroeder, MS, RN
Director, Nursing Education
School of Nursing
Danville Area Community College
Danville, Illinois

Sandra L. Siedlecki, PhD, RN
Assistant Professor and Senior Nurse
    Researcher
Department of Nursing
Ursuline College and Cleveland Clinic
Cleveland, Ohio

**Elizabeth Simon, PhD, RN, CCRN,
CEN, ANP-BC**
Professor and Director
School of Nursing
Nyack College
New York, New York

Sharon Souter, PhD, RN, CNE
Dean, Scott and White College of Nursing
University of Mary Hardin Baylor
Belton, Texas

Michelle Smeltzer, MSN, RN, CEN
Clinical Nurse Specialist, Emergency
    Services
Albert Einstein Medical Center
Philadelphia, Pennsylvania

**Deborah Tuggle, MN, APRN, CCNS,
FCCM**
Clinical Nurse Specialist, Critical Care
Kentucky and Central Baptist Hospital
Lexington, Kentucky

**Eric Watson, Lieutenant Colonel, US
Army, RN, CCRN, APN**
Director, Critical Care Nursing Course
Department of Nursing Sciences, Army
    Nurse Professional Branch
US Army Academy of Health Sciences
Fort Sam Houston, Texas

Lynn White, MSN, CNS, RN
Assistant Professor of Nursing
Augustana College
Simulation Specialist
Avera McKennan Hospital and University
    Health Center
Sioux Falls, South Dakota

ACKNOWLEDGMENTS

The talent, hard work, and inspiration of many people have produced the Sixth Edition of *Priorities in Critical Care Nursing*. We appreciate the assistance of the editorial teams that worked with us on this edition: Maureen Iannuzzi and Robin Richman at the beginning and Tamara Myers and Linda Thomas, who saw us through to publication. We are also grateful to our project manager, Bridget Healy, for her scrupulous attention to detail.

We are grateful to the many students, nurses, and educators who made the first five editions of *Priorities in Critical Care Nursing* successful. The emphasis continues to be on priorities for the critical care nurse. We believe that prioritizing conditions and issues will assist critical care nurses in quickly assessing and intervening in the most efficient and effective manner.

Organization

The book is comprised of nine major units, with two appendices. The chapter content of Unit One, *Foundations of Critical Care Nursing*, forms the basis of practice regardless of the physiologic alterations of the critically ill patient. Unit Two, *Common Problems in Critical Care*, examines potential critical care practice problems. Unit Three, *Cardiovascular Alterations*, and Unit Four, *Pulmonary Alterations*, are each organized according to the three-chapter format of Clinical Assessment and Diagnostic Procedures, Disorders, and Therapeutic Management. Unit Five, *Neurological Alterations*; Unit Six, *Renal Alterations*; Unit Seven, *Gastrointestinal Alterations*; and Unit Eight, *Endocrine Alterations*, are each organized according to the two-chapter format of Clinical Assessment and Diagnostic Procedures and Disorders and Therapeutic Management. Unit Nine, *Multisystem Alterations*, addresses disorders that affect multiple body systems and necessitate discussion as a separate category: Trauma; Shock Sepsis, and Multiple Organ Dysfunction Syndrome; and Hematological Disorders and Oncological Emergencies

Appendix A, *Nursing Management Plans of Care*, contains the core of critical care nursing practice in a nursing process format: signs and symptoms, nursing diagnosis, outcome criteria, and nursing interventions. The Nursing Management Plans of Care are referenced throughout the book within the *Nursing Diagnosis Priorities* boxes. Appendix B, *Physiological Formulas for Critical Care*, features common hemodynamic and oxygenation formulas and other calculations presented in easily understood terms.

Evidence-Based Practice and Research

The power of research-based critical care practice has been incorporated into nursing interventions. To foster critical thinking and decision making, a boxed menu of nursing diagnoses complete with specific etiologic or related factors accompanies each medical disorder and major medical treatment discussion and directs the learner to the section of the book where appropriate nursing management is detailed.

Sixth Edition Continuing Features

In keeping with the emphasis on priorities in critical care, *Nursing Diagnosis Priorities* boxes list the most urgent potential nursing diagnoses to be addressed. To facilitate student learning, the *Nursing Management Plans of Care* (Appendix A) incorporate nursing diagnoses, etiologic or related factors, clinical manifestations, and interventions with rationales.

These *Plans of Care* are cross-referenced throughout the book. *Patient Safety Priorities* boxes alert the nurse to special evidence-based considerations to specific practices and interventions that ensure safe patient care and best outcomes. *Concept Maps* appearing throughout the book link pathophysiological processes, clinical manifestations, and medical and nursing interventions. *Patient Education* boxes appear where key content is important for educating patients and families. *Collaborative Management* boxes contain key management tasks carried out by both nursing and medicine in a collaborative approach to treat certain conditions. *Evidence-Based Collaborative Practice* boxes present referenced recommendations put forth by various specialty healthcare organizations.

New to This Edition

New to this edition are *Case Studies* with critical thinking questions consisting of a brief patient history, clinical assessment, diagnostic procedures, and medical diagnosis(es), Questions follow that correspond with key points of the case. Another new feature new is the *Priority Medications* box, which describes drug class, priority nursing considerations, side effects and clinical assessment, and clinical examples of use of the medication.

Teaching and Learning Package

The Instructor Resources are located on the supplemental Evolve website. They include an Instructor's Manual with chapter outline and teaching strategies, a test bank with over 700 questions, answers to in-text *Case Studies,* an image collection, and a PowerPoint collection with audience-response questions.

The Student Resources, also located on the Evolve website, offer many new educational opportunities: New to this edition are review questions for NCLEX, CCRN, and PCCN. Fifteen procedures from *Mosby's Nursing Skills* are also included. Chapter summaries are provided to facilitate understanding of key chapter content. Animations, audio clips, a concept map creator, and sample concept maps also enhance student understanding of priority content. Open-book quizzes round out this substantial offering of review and reinforcement materials.

Priorities in Critical Care Nursing, Sixth Edition, represents our continued commitment to bringing you the best in all things a textbook can offer: the best and brightest in contributing and consulting authors; the latest in scientific research; a logical organizational format that exercises diagnostic reasoning skills; and artwork that enhances student learning. We pledge our continued commitment to excellence in critical care education.

Linda D. Urden
Kathleen M. Stacy
Mary E. Lough

UNIT 9 MULTISYSTEM ALTERATIONS

UNIT 1
Foundations in Critical Care Nursing

Caring for the Critically Ill Patient

Linda D. Urden

evolve WEBSITE

Be sure to check out the bonus material, including free self-assessment exercises, on the Evolve web site at
http://evolve.elsevier.com/Urden/priorities/.

OBJECTIVES

- Describe critical care nursing roles.
- Discuss the importance of holistic care for the critically ill patient and family.
- Compare and contrast interdisciplinary critical care management models and tools.

- Explain safety issues in the critical care environment.
- Discuss the six standards of a healthy work environment.

CRITICAL CARE NURSING ROLES

Nurses provide and contribute to the care of critically ill patients in a variety of roles. The most prominent role for the professional registered nurse (RN) is that of direct care provider. Other nurse clinicians also contribute to patient care, including patient educators, cardiac rehabilitation specialists, physician's office nurses, and infection control specialists. The specific types of expanded-role nursing positions are determined by individual organizational resources and needs.

Advanced-practice nurses (APNs) have met educational and clinical requirements beyond the basic nursing educational requirements for all nurses. The APNs in critical care areas are predominantly the clinical nurse specialist (CNS) and the acute care nurse practitioner (ACNP). APNs have a broad depth of knowledge and expertise in their specialty area and manage complex clinical and systems issues. The organizational system and existing resources of an institution determine what roles may be needed and how these roles function.

CNSs serve in specialty roles that require their clinical, teaching, research, leadership, and consultative abilities. In addition to providing education and mentoring to staff nurses, they work in direct clinical roles, systems or administrative roles, and in various other settings in the health care system. They may be organized by specialty, such as cardiovascular, or function, such as cardiac rehabilitation. CNSs also may be designated as case managers for specific patient populations.

Nurse Practitioners (NPs) and ACNPs manage clinical care of a group of patients and have various levels of prescriptive authority, depending on the state and practice area in which they work. They also provide care consistency, interact with families, plan for patient discharge, and provide teaching to patients, families, and other members of the heath care team.[1]

CRITICAL CARE NURSING STANDARDS

The American Association of Critical-Care Nurses (AACN) has established nursing standards to provide a framework for critical care nurses. The standards are authoritative statements that describe the level of care and performance by which the quality of nursing care can be judged.

Standards serve as descriptions of expected nursing roles and responsibilities.[2] The six AACN Standards of Care for Acute and Critical Care Nursing Practice are prescriptive of a competent level of nursing practice: assessment, diagnosis, outcomes identification, planning, implementation, and evaluation.

EVIDENCE-BASED NURSING PRACTICE

Much of early medical and nursing practice was based on nonscientific traditions that resulted in variable and haphazard patient outcomes.[3] These traditions and rituals, which were based on folklore, gut instinct, trial and error, and personal preference, were often passed down from one generation of practitioners to another.[3-5] Examples of nonscientific-based critical care nursing practice include suctioning artificial airways every two hours, using iced saline injectable when measuring cardiac output, always using lead II for cardiac monitoring, stripping chest tubes every two hours, and limiting visiting hours for all patients.[4]

The dramatic and multiple changes in health care and the ever-increasing presence of managed care in all geographic regions have placed greater emphasis on demonstrating the effectiveness of treatments and practices on outcomes.[6,7] In addition, emphasis is greater on efficiency, cost-effectiveness, quality of life, and patient satisfaction ratings.[8] It has become essential for nurses to use the best data available to make patient care decisions and carry out the appropriate nursing interventions.[8] By means of a scientific basis, with its ability to explain and predict, nurses are able to provide research-based interventions with consistent, positive outcomes. The content of this book is evidence based, with the most current, cutting-edge research abstracted and placed throughout the chapters as appropriate to topical discussions.

The increasingly complex and changing health care system presents multiple challenges for creating an evidence-based practice. Not only must appropriate research studies be designed to answer clinical questions, but also research findings must be used to make necessary changes for implementation in practice.[9] Multiple evidence-based practice and research utilization models exist to guide practitioners in the use of existing research findings. One such model is the Iowa Model of Evidence-Based Practice to Promote Quality Care, which incorporates both evidence and research as the basis for practice.[10] Inquisitive practitioners who strive for best practices using valid and reliable data will demonstrate quality outcomes-driven care and practices.[11]

Evidence-based nursing practice considers the best research evidence on the care topic, along with clinical expertise of the nurse, and patient preferences.[12] For instance, when determining the frequency of vital sign measurement, the nurse would use available research, nursing judgment (stability, complexity, predictability, vulnerability, and resilience of the patient),[13] along with the patient's preference for decreased interruptions and the ability to sleep for longer periods of time. At other times the nurse will implement an evidence-based protocol or procedure that is based on evidence, including research. An example of an evidence-based protocol is one in which the prevalence of indwelling catheterization and incidence of hospital-acquired catheter-associated urinary tract infections in the critical care unit can be decreased.[14]

The AACN has promulgated several practice summaries in the form of a "Practice Alert." These alerts are short directives that can be used as a quick reference for practice areas (e.g., oral care, noninvasive blood pressure monitoring, ST segment monitoring). They are succinct, supported by evidence, and address both nursing and multidisciplinary activities. Each alert includes the clinical information, followed by references that support the practice.[15]

HOLISTIC CARE

The high-technology–driven critical care environment is fast paced and directed toward monitoring and treating life-threatening changes in patient conditions. For this reason, attention is often focused on the technology and treatments necessary for maintaining stability in the physiological functioning of the patient. Great emphasis is placed on technical skills, professional competence, and responsiveness to critical emergencies. Concern has been voiced about the lesser emphasis on the caring component of nursing in this fast-paced, highly technological health care environment.[16,17] Nowhere is this more evident than in areas where critical care nursing is practiced. Keeping the care in nursing care is one of the greatest challenges.[17] The critical care nurse must be able to deliver high-quality care skillfully, using all applicable technologies, while incorporating psychosocial and other holistic approaches as appropriate to the time and the patient's condition.

The caring aspect is fundamental to the nurse-patient relationship and to the health care experience. Holistic care focuses on human integrity and stresses that the body, mind, and spirit are interdependent and inseparable. Thus all aspects need to be considered in planning and delivering care.[18,19]

Health care providers clearly understand that a patient's physical condition progresses in fairly predictable stages, depending on the presence or absence of comorbid conditions. Less clearly understood is the effect of psychosocial issues on the healing process. For this reason, special consideration must be given to determining the unique interventions that will positively impact each individual patient and help the patient progress toward desired outcomes.

An important aspect in the care delivery to—and recovery of—critically ill patients is the personal support of family members and significant others. The value of both patient-centered and family-centered care should not be underestimated.[20] It is important for families to be included in care decisions and to be encouraged to participate in the care of the patient as appropriate for the patient's level of needs and the family's level of ability.

Cultural diversity in health care is not a new topic but is gaining emphasis and importance as the world becomes more accessible to all as the result of increasing technologies and interfaces with places and peoples. Diversity includes not only ethnicity but also differences in lifestyles, opinions, values, and beliefs.

Unless cultural differences are taken into account, optimal health care cannot be provided. More attention has been directed recently at determining the physiological and disease development and progression differences among various ethnic groups. Mortality rates from cardiovascular disease are significantly higher for both black men and black women than for white men and white women. The prevalence of coronary heart disease is highest in black women, followed by Mexican American men.[21] Care providers must develop an increased sensitivity to the health care needs and vulnerabilities of all groups.

Cultural competence is one way to ensure that individual differences related to culture are incorporated into the plan of care.[22,23] Nurses must possess knowledge about biocultural, psychosocial, and linguistic differences in diverse populations to make accurate assessments.

Interventions must then be tailored to address the uniqueness of each patient and family.

Spirituality can become more important as people search for meaning and guidance in critical, emergent, and unexpected tragic circumstances.[24] Likewise, many health care practitioners turn to their own spirituality to manage stress and find answers to the health care issues that they face on a daily basis. Spiritual practices consist of meditation, prayer, and spiritual materials and are based on personal values and beliefs. Holt-Ashley[24] describes how to incorporate prayer into the critical care unit, concentrating on patients and families and the nurse. The author also offers strategies for creating an environment that is conducive to spiritual well-being for both patients and staff.

NURSING'S UNIQUE ROLE IN CRITICAL CARE

Researchers have studied critical care nurses to better understand their clinical judgment and interventions and the link between the two. They identified two major categories of thought and action and nine categories of practice that illustrate clinical judgment and the clinical knowledge development of critical care nurses. These major categories[25] are delineated in Box 1-1.

Critical care nurses are essential in facilitating communication among all health care providers, patients, and their families. They must be confident and assertive when talking with care providers, communicating essential information and advocating for patients. Communication skills are as important as clinical skills to ensure that the appropriate actions and interventions are done. Nurses also must be knowledgeable about the latest evidence to support their practice and share this and mentor others on the team. The critical care nurse plays a crucial team role in formulating patient care goals.[26]

BOX 1-1 CATEGORIES OF CRITICAL CARE NURSING THOUGHT, ACTION, AND PRACTICE

Thought and Action
- Clinical grasp and clinical inquiry: problem identification and clinical problem solving
- Clinical forethought: anticipating and preventing potential problems

Practice
- Diagnosing and managing life-sustaining physiological functions in unstable patients
- Managing a crisis by using skilled know-how
- Providing comfort measures for the critically ill
- Caring for patients' families
- Preventing hazards in a technological environment
- Facing death: end-of-life care and decision making
- Communicating and negotiating multiple perspectives
- Monitoring quality and managing breakdown
- Exhibiting the skilled know-how of clinical leadership and the coaching and mentoring of others

---

INTERDISCIPLINARY CRITICAL CARE MANAGEMENT

The managed care environment has placed emphasis on examining methods of care delivery and processes of care by all health care professionals. Partnerships have been formed or strengthened, with a focus on increasing quality of care and services while containing or decreasing costs. Coordination of care in critical care units has been demonstrated to influence patient outcomes significantly.[27]

Thornby[28] discussed the importance of skilled communication as essential to excellent patient care and a climate of safety. Ineffective nurse-physician communication has been related to adverse patient events, and nurse burnout and turnover.[29] Gerardi and Fontaine[30] described a model of true collaboration that could be used to improve interdisciplinary communications and ultimately to have a positive impact on patient outcomes. In this model, there is a continuum of collaboration that has seven components: self-awareness, information sharing, negotiation, feedback, conflict engagement, conflict resolution, and forgiveness and reconciliation. Successfully working through these stages will result in a collaborative environment.

Case Management

Case management is the process of overseeing the care of patients and organizing services in collaboration with the patient's physician or primary health care provider. The case manager may be a nurse, allied health care provider, or the patient's primary care provider. Case managers are usually assigned to a specific population group, and they facilitate effective coordination of care services as patients move in and out of different settings. Ideally, the case manager oversees the care of the patient across the continuum of care.

Outcomes Management

Outcomes management refers to a model aimed at managing the outcomes of care by the use of various tools, quality improvement processes, and interdisciplinary team involvement and action. Specifically, emphasis is placed on consistent standards of care, measurement of disease-specific clinical outcomes, patient functioning and well-being, and assessment of clinical and outcome data for the specific conditions.[31] Outcomes management also takes place in multiple settings across the continuum of care. Professional nurse outcomes managers ensure that variances from the plan of care are addressed in a timely manner. They also examine aggregate information with the team for quality improvement in the interdisciplinary plan of care.

Care Management Tools

Many quality improvement tools are available to providers for care management.

Algorithm

An algorithm is a stepwise decision-making flowchart for a specific care process or processes. Algorithms are more focused than clinical pathways and guide the clinician through the "if, then" decision-making process, addressing patient responses to particular treatments. Well-known examples of algorithms are the advanced cardiac life support (ACLS) algorithms published by the American Heart Association.

Practice Guideline

A practice guideline is usually developed and written by a team of experts representing professional organizations (e.g., AACN, Society of Critical Care Medicine, American College of Cardiology) or a governmental agency to provide recommendations to care providers. Recommendations are given for managing care and treatments for specific diseases and are based on research or expert opinions.[32] Practice guidelines are generally written in text prose, rather than in the flowchart format of algorithms. Practice guidelines are used as resources in formulating the pathway or algorithm. An example is a ventilator-associated pneumonia clinical practice guideline that was developed with major implications for nursing practice: head-of-bed elevation, hand hygiene, oral care, glove use, and ventilator tubing condensate removal.[33]

Protocol

A protocol is a common tool in research studies. Protocols are more directive and rigid than pathways or guidelines, and providers should not vary from a protocol. Patients are screened carefully for specific entry criteria before being started on a protocol. The many national research protocols include those for cancer and chemotherapy studies. Protocols are helpful when built-in alerts signal the provider to potentially serious problems. Computerization of protocols assists providers in being more proactive regarding dangerous drug interactions, abnormal laboratory values, and other untoward effects that are preprogrammed into the computer.

QUALITY, SAFETY, AND REGULATORY ISSUES IN CRITICAL CARE

Patient safety has become a major focus of attention for health care consumers, as well as providers of care and administrators of health care institutions. The Institute of Medicine publication *Crossing the Quality Chasm: A New Health System for the 21st Century* has been the impetus for debate and actions to improve the safety of health care environments. In this report, information and details were given indicating that health care harms patients too frequently and routinely fails to deliver its potential benefits.[34] Oftentimes, the definitions of medical errors and approaches to resolving patient safety issues differ among nurses, physicians, administrators, and other health care providers.[35]

Patient safety has been described as an ethical imperative, and one that is inherent in health care professionals' actions and interpersonal processes.[36] In critical care units errors may occur because of the hectic, complex environment, where there is little room for error and safety is essential.[37] In this environment, patients are particularly vulnerable because of their compromised physiological status, multiple technological and pharmacological interventions, and multiple care providers who frequently work at a fast pace. It is essential that care delivery processes that minimize the opportunity for errors are designed and that a "safety culture" rather than a "blame culture" is created.[38,39] When an injury or inappropriate care occurs, it is crucial that health care professionals promptly give an explanation of how the injury or mistake occurred and the short- or long-term effects to the patient and family. They should be informed that the factors involved in the injury will be investigated so that steps can be taken to reduce or prevent the likelihood of similar injury to other patients.

The Joint Commission has approved 2010 National Patient Safety Goals (NPSGs)[40] that are to be implemented in health care organizations (Box 1-2).

The Safe Medical Device Act (SMDA) requires that hospitals report serious or potentially serious device-related injuries or illness of patients and/or employees to the manufacturer of the device, and if death is involved, to the U.S. Food and Drug Administration (FDA). In addition, implantable devices must be documented and tracked.[41] This reporting serves as

---

BOX 1-2   2011 PATIENT SAFETY GOALS – HOSPITALS

1. Identify patients correctly.
2. Improve staff communication.
3. Use medicines safely.
4. Prevent infection.
5. Identify patient safety risks.
6. Prevent mistakes in surgery.

From *2011 Hospital National Patient Safety Goals;* The Joint Commission (website). http://www.jointcommission.org/patientsafety/nationalpatientsafetygoals/. Accessed August 8, 2011.

an early warning system so that the FDA can obtain information on device problems. Failure to comply with the act will result in civil action.

It has been shown that intimidating and disruptive clinician behaviors can lead to errors and preventable adverse patient outcomes. Verbal outbursts, physical threats, and more passive behaviors such as refusing to carry out a task or procedure are all under this category. Unfortunately, these types of behavior are not rare in health care organizations, with as many as 40% of clinicians having said that they were involved in such interactions. If these behaviors go unaddressed, it can lead to extreme dissatisfaction, depression, and turnover. There are also systems issues that lead to or perpetuate these situations, such as push for increased productivity, financial constraints, fear of litigation, and embedded hierarchies in the organization.[43]

Technologies are both a solution to error-prone procedures and functions, and another potential cause for error. Consider bar-code medication administration procedures, multiple bedside testing devices, computerized medical records, bedside monitoring, computerized physician order entry (CPOE), and many others now in development. Each in itself can be a great assistance to the clinician, but must be monitored for effectiveness and accuracy to ensure the best in outcomes as intended for specific use.[44]

Medication administration continues to be one of the most error-prone nursing interventions for the critical care nurse. Many medication errors are related to system failures, specifically distraction as a major factor. Various interventions have been created in an attempt to decrease medication errors. Most recently, a published study reported establishing a "no interruption zone" for medication safety in an intensive care unit. In this pilot study, there was a 40% decrease in interruptions from the baseline measurement. Although researchers questioned the feasibility of sustaining this decrease in interruptions in the future,[45] this is an example of an approach to increase medication safety in the critical care unit.

PRIVACY AND CONFIDENTIALITY

A landmark law was passed to provide consumers with greater access to health care insurance, promote more standardization and efficiency in the health care industry, and protect the privacy of health care data.[42] The Health Insurance Portability and Accountability Act of 1996 (HIPAA) has created additional challenges for health care organizations and providers because of the stringent requirements and additional resources needed to meet the requirements of the law. Most specific to critical care clinicians is the privacy and confidentiality related to protection of health care data. This has implications when interacting with family members and others, and the oftentimes very close work environment, tight working spaces, and emergency situations. Clinicians are referred to their organizational policies and procedures for specific procedures for their organizations.

HEALTHY WORK ENVIRONMENT

The health care environment is stressful, and increasing challenges in the areas of financial constraints, regulatory requirements, consumer scrutiny, quickly changing technologies and treatment regimens, and workforce diversity contribute to conflicts and difficulties on a daily basis. In this environment, it is essential to offer support for health care providers that can mitigate these challenges and ensure a healthy place to work.

There is an increasing amount of evidence that unhealthy work environments lead to medical errors, suboptimal safety monitoring, ineffective communication among health care providers, and increased conflict and stress among care providers. Synthesis of research in the area of work environment has demonstrated that a combination of leadership styles and characteristics contributes to the development and sustainability of healthy work environments.[46]

The AACN has formulated standards for establishing and sustaining healthy work environments (HWE). The intent of the standards is to promote creation of environments that will have a positive impact on nursing and patient outcomes. Evidence-based and relationship-centered principles were used to create the standards of professional performance. A summary of the six standards is provided in Box 1-3. Figure 1-1 illustrates the interdependence of each standard, and the ultimate impact on optimal patient outcomes and clinical excellence.

BOX 1-3　HEALTHY WORK ENVIRONMENT STANDARDS

Standard I: Skilled Communication
Nurses must be as proficient in communication skills as they are in clinical skills.

Standard II: True Collaboration
Nurses must be relentless in pursuing and fostering true collaboration.

Standard III: Effective Decision Making
Nurses must be valued and committed partners in making policy, directing and evaluating clinical care, and leading organizational operations.

Standard IV: Appropriate Staffing
Staffing must ensure the effective match between patient needs and nurse competencies.

Standard V: Meaningful Recognition
Nurses must be recognized and must recognize others for the value each brings to the work of the organization.

Standard VI: Authentic Leadership
Nurse leaders must fully embrace the imperative of a healthy work environment, authentically live it, and engage others in its achievement.

From American Association of Critical-Care Nurses (AACN): *Standards for establishing and sustaining healthy work environments*, Aliso Viejo, Calif., 2005, AACN.

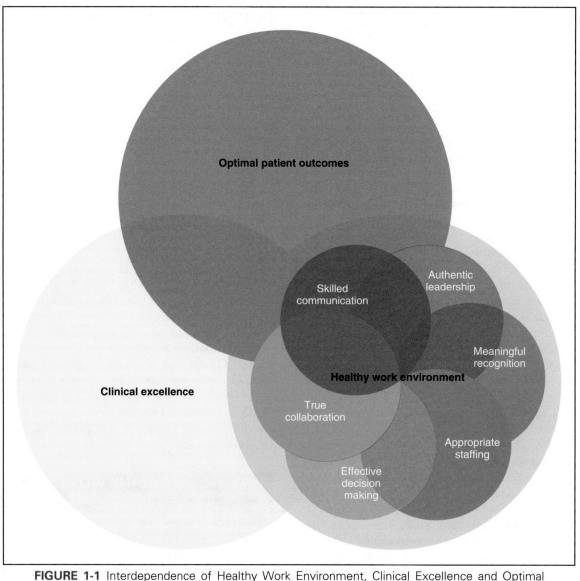

FIGURE 1-1 Interdependence of Healthy Work Environment, Clinical Excellence and Optimal Patient Outcomes. (From American Association of Critical-Care Nurses (AACN): *Standards for establishing and sustaining healthy work environments*, Aliso Viejo, Calif., 2005, AACN.)

Everyone has a role in creating and sustaining a healthy work environment. Although the manager has a major role in establishing the culture, it is the staff who greatly impact the culture by mentoring new staff, role modeling behaviors, and leading interdisciplinary teams. It is this peer pressure that has the most impact on all other staff.[47] Bylone discussed her experience of talking with many staff members about how they think that they can influence the work unit culture. She recommends asking themselves how they influence each of the HWE standards, thus making it a personal experience and journey in achieving the HWE.[48] Kupperschmidt and colleagues posed a five-factor model for becoming a skilled communicator: 1) becoming aware of self-deception; 2) becoming authentic; 3) becoming candid; 4) becoming mindful; and 5) becoming reflective; all of which leads to being a skilled communicator, thus creating a healthy work environment.[49]

REFERENCES

1. Kleinpell R: Reports of role descriptions of acute care nurse practitioners, *AACN Clin Issues* 9(2):290, 1998.
2. American Association of Critical-Care Nurses: *Practice resources* (website). www.aacn.org.
3. Omery A, Williams RP: An appraisal of research utilization across the United States, *J Nurs Adm* 29(12):50, 1999.
4. Wojner AW: Why do we do the things we do? Stop the carnage of nursing research, *AACN News* 17(4):2, 2000.
5. Mick D: Folklore, personal preference, or research-based practice, *Am J Crit Care* 9(1):6, 2000.
6. Rosswurm MA, Larrabee JH: A model for change to evidence-based practice, *Image J Nurs Sch* 31(4):317, 1999.
7. Fineout-Overholt E, Melnyk B: Building a culture of best practice, *Nurse Leader* 3(6):26, 2005.

8. McPheeters M, Lohr KN: Evidence-based practice and nursing: commentary, *Outcomes Manag Nurs Pract* 3(3):99, 1999.

9. Newhouse RP: Examining the support for evidence-based practice, *J Nurs Adm* 36(7/8):337, 2006.

10. Titler MG, et al: The Iowa model of evidence-based practice to promote quality care, *Crit Care Nurs Clin North Am* 13(4):497, 2001.

11. Hopp L: Talk to me about evidence-based practice! *AACN Adv Crit Care* 17(23):250, 2006.

12. Marshall M: Strategies for success: bringing evidence-based practice to the bedside, *Clin Nurse Spec* 20(3):124, 2006.

13. Schulman CS, Staul L: Standards for frequency of measurement and documentation of vital signs and physical assessments, *Crit Care Nurse* 30(3):74, 2010.

14. Gray M: Reducing catheter-associated urinary tract infection in the critical care unit, *AACN Adv Crit Care* 21(3):247, 2010.

15. American Association of Critical-Care Nurses: *Practice alert* (website). http://www.aacn.org/wd/practice/content/practicealerts.pcms?menu=practice, accessed April 7, 2007.

16. Panting K: Intensive care/intensive cure: the future of critical care? *Crit Care Nurse* 15(12):100, 1995.

17. Miller KL: Keeping the care in nursing care: our biggest challenge, *J Nurs Adm* 25(11):29, 1995.

18. Mariano C: Holistic ethics, *Am J Nurs* 101(1):24A, 2001.

19. Bishop LC, Griffin C: Holistic healing methods positively advance patient care, *Nurs Manage* 37(7):30, 2006.

20. Powers PH, et al: The value of patient- and family-centered care, *Am J Nurs* 100(5):84, 2000.

21. Alspach G: Time for sensitivity training: cultural diversity in cardiovascular disease, *Crit Care Nurse* 20(3):14, 2000.

22. Gonzales RI, Gooden MB, Porter CP: Eliminating racial and ethnic disparities in health care, *Am J Nurs* 100(3):56, 2000.

23. Leonard B, Plotnikoff GA: Awareness: the heart of cultural competence, *AACN Clin Issues* 11(1):51, 2000.

24. Holt-Ashley M: Nurses pray: use of prayer and spirituality as a complementary therapy in the intensive care setting, *AACN Clin Issues* 11(1):60, 2000.

25. Benner P, et al: Clinical wisdom and interventions in critical care, Philadelphia, 1999, Saunders.

26. Martin B, Koesel N: Nurses' role in clarifying goals in the intensive care unit, *Critical Care Nurse* 30(3):64-73, 2010.

27. Knaus W, et al: An evaluation of outcome from intensive care in major medical centers, *Ann Intern Med* 104(3):410, 1986.

28. Thornby D: Beginning the journey to skilled communication, *AACN Adv Crit Care* 17(3):266, 2006.

29. Arford PH: Nurse-physician communication: an organizational accountability, *Nurs Econ* 23(2):72, 2005.

30. Gerardi D, Fontaine DK: True collaboration: envisioning new ways of working together, *AACN Adv Crit Care* 18(1):10, 2007.

31. Wojner A: Outcomes management: an interdisciplinary search for best practice, *AACN Clin Issues* 7(1):133, 1996.

32. Hedges C: Show me the guidelines, *AACN Adv Crit Care* 18(1):88, 2007.

33. Abbott CA, et al: Adoption of a ventilator-associated pneumonia clinical practice guideline, *Worldviews Evid Based Nurs* 3(4):139, 2006.

34. Institute of Medicine: Crossing the quality chasm: a new health system for the 21st century, Washington, D.C., 2001, National Academy Press.

35. Cook A, et al: An error by any other name, *Am J Nurs* 104(6):32, 2004.

36. White GB: Patient safety: an ethical imperative, *Nurs Econ* 20(4):195, 2002.

37. Benner P: Creating a culture of safety and improvement: a key to reducing medical error, *Am J Crit Care* 10(4):281, 2001.

38. Smith AP: In search of safety: an interview with Gina Pugliese, *Nurs Econ* 20(1):6, 2002.

39. Kalisch BJ, Aebersold M: Overcoming barriers to patient safety, *Nurs Econ* 24(3):143, 2006.

40. The Joint Commission: National patient safety goals, http://www.jointcommission.org/standards_information/npsgs.aspx, accessed April 7, 2007.

41. Jensen JR: FDA's safe medical device act, *Risk Manag Rep* 1(2):1, 1997.

42. Centers for Medicare & Medicaid Services: Health Insurance Portability and Accountability Act (HIPAA) – administrative simplification, www.cms.gov.

43. The Joint Commission: Behaviors that undermine a culture of safety, *Sentinel Event Alert* Issue 40, July 9, 2008, http://www.jointcommission.org/sentinel_event.aspx, accessed September 19, 2010.

44. Henneman EA: Patient safety and technology, *AACN Adv Crit Care* 20(2):128, 2009.

45. Anthony K, et al: No interruptions please: impact of a no interruption zone on medication safety in intensive care units, *Crit Care Nurse* 30(3):21, 2010.

46. Pearson A, et al: Comprehensive systematic review of evidence on developing and sustaining nursing leadership that fosters a healthy work environment in healthcare, *Int J Evid Based Healthc* 5:208, 2007.

47. Bylone M: Healthy work environments: whose job is it anyway? *AACN Adv Crit Care* 20(4):325, 2009.

48. Bylone M: "I think they are talking about me!!" *AACN Adv Crit Care* 20(2):137, 2009.

49. Kupperschmidt B, et al: A healthy work environment: it begins with you, *The Online Journal of Issues in Nursing* 15(1) manuscript 3, 2010. http://nursingworld.org/mainmenucategories/ANAMarketplace/ANAPeioidicals/OJIN/ accessed February 17, 2010.

2

Ethical and Legal Issues

Linda D. Urden

⊖volve WEBSITE

Be sure to check out the bonus material, including free self-assessment exercises, on the Evolve web site at
http://evolve.elsevier.com/Urden/priorities/.

OBJECTIVES

- Discuss ethical principles as they relate to critical care patients.
- Discuss strategies to address moral distress in critical care nursing.
- Discuss the concept of medical futility.
- Describe what constitutes an ethical dilemma.
- List steps for making ethical decisions.

- Identify legal and professional obligations of critical care nurses.
- Describe the elements of certain torts that may result from critical care nursing practice.
- Identify and discuss specific legal issues in critical care nursing practice.

MORALS AND ETHICS

Morals are the "shoulds," "should nots," "oughts," and "ought nots" of actions and behaviors and have been related closely to sexual mores and behaviors in Western society. Religious and cultural values and beliefs largely mold a person's moral thoughts and actions. Morals form the basis for action and provide a framework for evaluation of behavior.

Ethics is concerned with the "why" of the action rather than with whether the action is right or wrong, good or bad. Ethics implies that an evaluation is being made and is theoretically based on or derived from a set of standards.

MORAL DISTRESS

Moral distress is a serious problem for nurses. It occurs when one knows the ethically appropriate action to take but cannot act upon it. It also presents when one acts in a manner contrary to personal and professional values. There can be an internal conflict when one's ethical framework clashes with the ethical beliefs of the patient.[1,2] As a result, there can be significant emotional and physical stress that leads to feelings of loss of personal integrity and dissatisfaction with the work environment.[3] Relationships with both co-workers and patients are affected and can negatively impact the quality of care. There is also a great impact on personal relationships

and family life. It is therefore important that nurses recognize moral distress and actively seek strategies to address the issue through institutional, personal, and professional organizational resources. Knowledge and application of ethical principles and guidelines will assist the nurse in daily practice when ethical dilemmas occur. The American Association of Critical-Care Nurses (AACN) has written a position statement on moral distress that describes the phenomenon and lists actions for individual nurses and employers to address moral distress. Refer to Box 2-1. The AACN[3,4] has created a framework to support those nurses who are experiencing moral distress (Figure 2-1).

ETHICAL PRINCIPLES

Certain ethical principles were derived from classic ethical theories that are used in health care decision making. *Principles* are general guidelines that govern conduct, provide a basis for reasoning, and direct actions. The six ethical principles discussed here are autonomy, beneficence, nonmaleficence, veracity, fidelity, and justice (Box 2-2).

Autonomy

The concept of autonomy appears in all ancient writings and early Greek philosophy. In health care, autonomy can be viewed as the freedom to make decisions about one's own

BOX 2-1 MORAL DISTRESS

Issue

Moral distress is a serious problem in nursing. It results in significant physical and emotional stress, which contributes to nurses' feelings of loss of integrity and dissatisfaction with their work environment. Studies demonstrate that moral distress is a major contributor to nurses leaving the work setting and profession. It affects relationships with patients and others and can affect the quality, quantity, and cost of nursing care.

Definition

Moral distress occurs when:
- You know the ethically appropriate action to take, but are unable to act upon it.
- You act in a manner contrary to your personal and professional values, which undermines your integrity and authenticity.

From AACN Public Policy. Position Statement: Moral Distress. Aliso Viejo, Calif. August 2008.

body without the coercion or interference of others. Autonomy is a freedom of choice or a self-determination that is a basic human right. It can be experienced in all human life events. Involving the patient and family in decision making is also an indication of respect and family-centered care.[5]

The critical care nurse is often "caught in the middle" in ethical situations, and promoting autonomous decision making is one of those situations. As the nurse works closely with patients and families to promote autonomous decision making, another crucial element becomes clear. Patients and families must have all the information about a particular situation before they can make a decision that is best for them. They not only should be given all the pertinent information and facts but also must have a clear understanding of what was presented.[6] In this situation the nurse assumes one of the most important roles of the health care team, that is, as *patient advocate*, providing more information as needed, clarifying points, reinforcing information, and providing support during the decision-making process.

Beneficence

The concept of doing good and preventing harm to patients is a sine qua non for the nursing profession. However, the ethical principle of beneficence, which requires that one *promote* the well-being of patients, indicates the importance of this duty for the health care professional. The principle of beneficence presupposes that harms and benefits are balanced, leading to positive or beneficial outcomes.

In approaching issues related to beneficence, conflict with the principle of autonomy is common. Paternalism exists when the nurse or physician makes a decision for the patient without consulting the patient.

Traditional health care has been based on a paternalistic approach to patients. Many patients are still more comfortable in deferring all decisions about care and treatment to their health care provider. Active involvement by various organizations and agencies in regard to health care has demonstrated a trend toward the public's need and desire for more information about health care in general, as well as more about alternative treatments and providers. Paternalism, or *maternalism* in the case of female providers, may always be a possibility in the health care setting, but enlightened consumers are causing a change in this practice of health care professionals.

Nonmaleficence

The ethical principle of nonmaleficence, which dictates that one prevent harm and correct harmful situations, is a prima facie duty for the nurse. Thoughtfulness and care are necessary, as is balancing risks and benefits. Beneficence and nonmaleficence are on two ends of a continuum and are often adhered to differently, depending on the views of the practitioner.

Veracity

Veracity, or truth telling, is an important ethical principle that underlies the nurse-patient relationship. Communication trust, or the trust of disclosure, is rooted in respect and based on veracity.[7]

Veracity is important when soliciting informed consent because the patient needs to be aware of all potential risks of and benefits to be derived from specific treatments or alternative therapies.[8-10] Again, the critical care nurse may be in the middle of a situation where all the facts and information about a particular treatment option are not disclosed. Sometimes information has been given accurately to the patient and family but has been delivered with bias or in a misleading way. Veracity must guide all areas of practice for the nurse, that is, in colleague relationships and employee relationships, as well as in the nurse-patient relationship.

Fidelity

Fidelity, or faithfulness and promise keeping to patients, is also a sine qua non for nursing. It forms a bond between individuals and is the basis of all relationships, both professional and personal. Regardless of the amount of autonomy that patients have in the critical care areas, they still depend on the nurse for many types of physical care and emotional support. A trusting relationship that establishes and maintains an open atmosphere is positive for all involved.[11] Making a promise to a patient is voluntary for the nurse, whereas having respect for a patient's decision making is a moral obligation.[12]

Fidelity extends to the family of the critical care patient. When a promise is made to the family that they will be called if an emergency arises or that they will be informed of any other special events concerning the patient, the nurse must make every effort to follow through on the promise. Fidelity not only will uphold the nurse-family relationship but also will reflect positively on the nursing profession as a whole and on the institution where the nurse is employed.

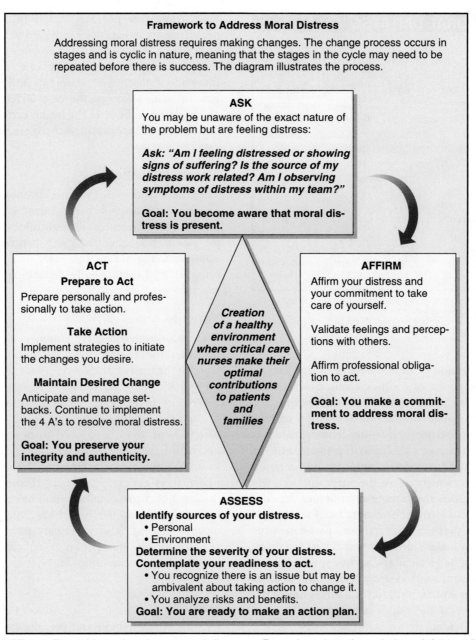

Framework to Address Moral Distress

Addressing moral distress requires making changes. The change process occurs in stages and is cyclic in nature, meaning that the stages in the cycle may need to be repeated before there is success. The diagram illustrates the process.

ASK

You may be unaware of the exact nature of the problem but are feeling distress:

Ask: "Am I feeling distressed or showing signs of suffering? Is the source of my distress work related? Am I observing symptoms of distress within my team?"

Goal: You become aware that moral distress is present.

ACT

Prepare to Act

Prepare personally and professionally to take action.

Take Action

Implement strategies to initiate the changes you desire.

Maintain Desired Change

Anticipate and manage setbacks. Continue to implement the 4 A's to resolve moral distress.

Goal: You preserve your integrity and authenticity.

Creation of a healthy environment where critical care nurses make their optimal contributions to patients and families

AFFIRM

Affirm your distress and your commitment to take care of yourself.

Validate feelings and perceptions with others.

Affirm professional obligation to act.

Goal: You make a commitment to address moral distress.

ASSESS

Identify sources of your distress.
- Personal
- Environment

Determine the severity of your distress.
Contemplate your readiness to act.
- You recognize there is an issue but may be ambivalent about taking action to change it.
- You analyze risks and benefits.

Goal: You are ready to make an action plan.

FIGURE 2-1 The 4A's to rise above moral distress. (From American Association of Critical-Care Nurses, Aliso Viejo, Calif., 2004.)

BOX 2-2   ETHICAL PRINCIPLES IN CRITICAL CARE

- Autonomy
- Beneficence
- Nonmaleficence
- Veracity
- Fidelity
  - Confidentiality
  - Privacy
- Justice/allocation of resources

Confidentiality is one element of fidelity that is based on traditional health care professional ethics. Confidentiality is described as a right whereby patient information can be shared only with those involved in the care of the patient. An exception to this guideline might be when the welfare of others will be put at risk by keeping patient information confidential. Again in this situation, the nurse must balance ethical principles and weigh risks with benefits. Special circumstances, such as the existence of mandatory reporting laws, will guide the nurse in certain situations.

Privacy also has been described as being inherent in the principle of fidelity. Privacy may be closely aligned with confidentiality of patient information and a patient's right to privacy of his or her person, such as maintaining privacy for the patient by pulling the curtains around the bed or making sure that the patient is adequately covered.

Justice

The principle of justice is often used synonymously with the concept of allocation of scarce resources. With escalating health care costs, expanded technologies, an aging population with their own special health care needs, and in some cases a scarcity of health care personnel, the question of how to allocate health care becomes even more complex. With the recent passage of landmark legislation that will lead to major changes in health care, numerous questions are presently unanswered about the impact on our citizens.[13]

The application of the justice principle in health care is concerned primarily with divided or portioned allocation of goods and services, which is termed distributive justice. As health care resources become increasingly scarce, allocation of resources to certain programs and rationing of resources within certain programs will become more evident.

MEDICAL FUTILITY

The concept of medical futility has resulted in various discussions and proposed criteria and formulas to predict outcomes of care.[14-16] Medical futility has both a qualitative and a quantitative basis and can be defined as "any effort to achieve a result that is possible but that reasoning or experience suggests is highly improbable and that cannot be systematically reproduced."[17]

Therapy or treatment that achieves its predictable outcome and desired effect is, by definition, effective. Effect must be distinguished from benefit, however; although predictable and desired, the effect is nonetheless futile if it is of no benefit to the patient.

ETHICAL FOUNDATION FOR NURSING PRACTICE

Traditional theories of professions include a code of ethics upon which the practice of the profession is based. It is by adherence to a code of ethics that the professional fulfills an obligation to provide quality practice to society.

A professional ethic forms the framework for any profession[18] and is based on three elements: (1) the professional code of ethics, (2) the purpose of the profession, and (3) the standards of practice of the professional. The code of ethics developed by the profession is the delineation of its values and relationships with and among members of the profession and society. The need for the profession and its inherent promise to provide certain duties form a contract between nursing and society. The professional standards describe specifics of practice in a variety of settings and subspecialties. Nursing professionals must stay consistent with their values

BOX 2-3	CODE OF ETHICS FOR NURSES

1. The nurse, in all professional relationships, practices with compassion and respect for the inherent dignity, worth, and uniqueness of every individual, unrestricted by considerations of social or economic status, personal attributes, or the nature of health problems.
2. The nurse's primary commitment is to the patient, whether an individual, family group, or community.
3. The nurse promotes, advocates for, and strives to protect the health, safety, and rights of the patient.
4. The nurse is responsible and accountable for individual nursing practice and determines the appropriate delegation of tasks consistent with the nurse's obligation to provide optimum patient care.
5. The nurse owes the same duties to self as to others, including the responsibility to preserve integrity and safety, to maintain competence, and to continue personal and professional growth.
6. The nurse participates in establishing, maintaining, and improving health care environments and conditions of employment conducive to the provision of quality health care and consistent with the values of the profession through individual and collective action.
7. The nurse participates in the advancement of the profession through contributions to practice, education, administration, and knowledge development.
8. The nurse collaborates with other health care professionals and the public in promoting community, national, and international efforts to meet health needs.
9. The profession of nursing, as represented by associations and their members, is responsible for articulating nursing values, for maintaining the integrity of the profession and its practice, and for shaping social policy.

From American Nurses Association: *Code of ethics for nurses with interpretive statements*, Washington, D.C., 2002, ANA.

and ethics, and ensure that the ethical environment is maintained wherever nursing care and services are performed.[19,20] Each element is dynamic, and ongoing evaluations are necessary as societal expectations change, technologies increase, and the profession evolves.

Nursing Code of Ethics

The American Nurses Association (ANA) provides the major source of ethical guidance for the nursing profession. The *Code of Ethics for Nurses* serves as the basis for nurses in analyzing ethical issues and decision making (Box 2-3).[21]

What Is An Ethical Dilemma?

In general, ethical cases are not always clear-cut or "black and white." The most common ethical dilemmas encountered in critical care are forgoing treatment and allocating the scarce resources of critical care. Before the application of any decision model is made, it must be determined whether a true ethical dilemma exists. Thompson and Thompson[22] delineate the following three criteria for defining moral and ethical dilemmas in clinical practice:

BOX 2-4	STEPS IN ETHICAL DECISION MAKING

1. Identify the health problem.
2. Define the ethical issue.
3. Gather additional information.
4. Delineate the decision maker.
5. Examine ethical and moral principles.
6. Explore alternative options.
7. Implement decisions.
8. Evaluate and modify actions.

1. An awareness of the different options
2. An issue that has different options
3. Two or more options with true or "good" aspects, with the choice of one option over the other compromising the option not chosen

One must pause, expand group consciousness about the issue, validate assumptions, look for patterns of thoughts or behaviors, and facilitate reflection and inquiry prior to making any decision.[23]

Steps in Ethical Decision Making

To facilitate the ethical decision-making process, a model or framework must be used so that all parties involved will consistently and clearly examine the multiple ethical issues that arise in critical care. There are various ethical decision-making models in the literature.[24,25] Box 2-4 lists steps in a model that will be briefly discussed in this chapter.

Step One

First, the major aspects of the medical and health problems must be identified. In other words, the scientific basis of the problem, potential sequelae, prognosis, and all data relevant to the health status must be examined.

Step Two

The ethical problem must be clearly delineated from other types of problems. *Systems problems* result from failures and inadequacies in the health care facility's organization and operation or in the health care system as a whole and are often misinterpreted as ethical issues. *Social problems* arising from conditions in the community, state, or country as a whole also are occasionally confused with ethical issues. Social problems can lead to *systemic problems*, which can constrain responses to ethical problems.

Step Three

Although categories of necessary additional information will vary, whatever is missing in the initial problem presentation should be obtained. If not already known, the health prognosis and potential sequelae should be clarified. Usual demographic data (e.g., age, ethnicity, religious preferences, educational/economic status) may be considered in the decision-making process. The role of the family or extended family and other support systems needs to be examined. Any

desires that the patient may have expressed about the treatment decision, either in writing or in conversation, must be obtained.

Step Four

The patient is the primary decision maker and autonomously makes these decisions after receiving information about the alternatives and sequelae of treatments or lack of treatment. In many ethical dilemmas the patient is not competent to make a decision, however, as when the patient is comatose or otherwise physically or mentally unable to make a decision. In these cases, surrogates are designated or court appointed because the urgency of the situation requires a quick decision.

Others who are involved in the decision also need to be identified at this time, such as family, nurse, physician, social worker, clergy, and members of other disciplines in close contact with the patient. The role of the nurse must be examined. It may not be necessary for the nurse to make a decision at all; rather, the nurse's role may be simply to provide additional information and support to the decision maker.

Step Five

Personal values, beliefs, and moral convictions of all persons involved in the decision-making process need to be known. Whether actually achieved through a group meeting or through personal introspection, values clarification facilitates the decision-making process.

General ethical principles also need to be examined in regard to the case at hand. For example, are veracity, informed consent, and autonomy being promoted? Beneficence and nonmaleficence will be analyzed as they relate to a patient's condition and desires. Close examination of these principles will reveal any compromise of ethical or moral principles for either the patient or the health care provider and will assist in decision making.

Step Six

After the identification of alternative options, the outcome of each action must be predicted. This analysis helps the person select the option with the best "fit" for the specific situation or problem. Both short- and long-range consequences of each action must be examined, and new or creative actions must be encouraged. Consideration also must be given to the "no action" option, which is another choice.

Step Seven

When a decision has been reached, it is usually after much thought and consideration.

Step Eight

Evaluation of an ethical decision serves both to assess the decision at hand and to provide a basis for future ethical decisions. If outcomes are not as predicted, it may be possible to modify the plan or to use an alternative that was not originally chosen.

LEGAL RELATIONSHIPS

When a professional nurse commences employment in a critical care facility, three legal relationships are formed. First, on accepting employment, the relationship between the nurse and the *employer* is formed. Second, on assuming the care of a patient, a relationship is created between the *patient* and nurse. Third, every state has a law that mandates the entry-level educational requirements that must be met for a person to become licensed to practice nursing. The act of licensing creates a legal relationship between the nurse and the *state*.

These relationships impose legal obligations. The nurse owes a patient the duty of reasonable and prudent care under the circumstances. The nurse owes the employer the duty of competency and the ability to follow policies and procedures; other contractual duties may exist as well. The nurse owes the state and public the duty of safe, competent practice as legally defined by practice standards.

The critical care nurse's legal duties are enforceable, and the nurse can be held legally accountable for breach or violation through a variety of laws and legal processes. Nurses, hospitals, patients, and other health care providers can be involved in a variety of legal disputes, including negligence and professional malpractice, incompetence, unauthorized practice, unprofessional or illegal conduct, workers' compensation, and contract and labor disputes.

Tort Liability

The area of civil law is divided into many categories, two of which are contracts and torts. The law of contracts contains a set of rules governing the creation and enforcement of an agreement between two or more parties (entities or individuals). For example, contract law may apply to a dispute between the nurse, as employee, and an institution, as employer. In contrast, a *tort* is a type of civil wrong or injury that results from a breach of a legal duty. Tort law is generally divided into intentional and unintentional torts, strict liability, and specific torts (Box 2-5).

Intentional torts involve (1) a mind-set indicative of purpose and (2) an act. Intent exists when the person forms a mental design to achieve a particular outcome and consequence. Assault, battery, false imprisonment, trespass, and intentional infliction of emotional distress are all examples of intentional torts. In each of these torts, a specific act is required, and there is purposeful interference with a person or property.

In assault the act is a behavior that places the plaintiff (person being wronged who later sues) in fear or apprehension of offensive physical contact; in civil law the defendant is the person being sued for wronging another. Battery is the unlawful or offensive touching of or contact with the plaintiff or something attached to the plaintiff. False imprisonment is detaining, confining, or restraining another against the person's will. The two types of trespass involve (1) a person's land and (2) an individual's personal property. These acts are defined as "unauthorized entry onto land of another" or "unauthorized handling of another's personal property." In

BOX 2-5 CLASSIFICATION OF TORTS
Intentional Torts
Assault
Battery
False imprisonment
Trespass
Infliction of mental or emotional distress
Specific Torts
Defamation
Slander
Libel
Invasion of privacy
Unintentional Torts
Negligence
Medical/nursing treatment torts
Professional malpractice
Abandonment
Strict Liability
Product liability

addition, the law protects a person's interest in peace of mind through the tort claim of infliction of mental or emotional distress. The act in this case, however, must involve extreme misconduct or outrageous behavior.

Unintentional torts involve failures or breach of nursing duties that lead to harm, including negligence, malpractice, and abandonment. Negligence is the failure to meet an ordinary standard of care, resulting in injury to the patient or plaintiff. Malpractice is a type of professional liability based on negligence and includes professional misconduct, breach of a duty or standard of care, illegal or immoral conduct, or failure to exercise reasonable skill, all of which lead to harm (see later discussion). Abandonment is a type of negligence in which a duty to give care exists, is ignored, and results in harm to a patient. It is the absence of care and the failure to respond to a patient that may give rise to an allegation of abandonment.

Specific torts involve privacy and reputation interests and include invasion of privacy and defamation. Defamation is composed of two torts: slander (oral defamation) and libel (written defamation). Defamation is not the mere statement or writing of words that injures a person's reputation or good name; the words also must be communicated to another. If the words are true, this may provide a defense against a defamation claim. Invasion of privacy involves the violation of a person's right to privacy. Nurses can invade another's privacy by revealing confidential information without authorization or by failing to follow the patient's health care decisions.

Nurses can avoid allegations of these specific claims by (1) making statements about another's reputation only when necessary and substantiated by fact and (2) respecting another's privacy and autonomy and maintaining a confidential relationship with the patient.

Administrative Law and Licensing Statutes

A second type of law and legal process in which nurses are involved is administrative law and the regulatory process. This area of law governs the nurse's relationship with the *government*, either state or federal. Administrative law involves the rules of the government's activities in regulating health care delivery and practice; the rules of investigation, procedure, and evidence differ from those of civil and criminal law. Several government health care agencies are involved in such regulation.

A state has the power to regulate nursing because the state is responsible for the health, safety, and welfare of its citizens. Therefore, establishing minimal entry-level requirements, standards of nursing practice, and educational requirements are acceptable state actions. State legislatures create laws governing nursing practice, generally termed nurse practice acts, and a unit of the state government within the executive branch is responsible for the enforcement of nursing laws. This unit is often called the *State Board of Nursing* or *Board of Nurse Examiners*; however, the name varies by state. Standards also vary by state, which is another important reason that nurses should seek advice from counsel licensed to practice law in their own state. Because law is the minimum expected behavior, the profession oftentimes sets a higher standard. Additional methods to ensure competency are continuing education for renewal of license, work-based orientation programs, and certification in specialty practice areas. Self-reflection and assessment of one's current competencies and level of technical knowledge can serve to elevate practice.[26]

Negligence and Malpractice

As defined earlier, negligence is an unintentional tort involving a breach of duty or failure (through an act or an omission) to meet a standard of care, causing personal harm. Malpractice is a type of professional liability based on negligence in which the defendant is held accountable for breach of a duty of care involving special knowledge and skill. These torts have several elements, all of which the plaintiff has the burden of proving.

The law recognizes four elements of negligence and malpractice. The first element, a duty, or legal obligation, requires the person ("actor") to conform to a certain standard of conduct for the protection of others against unreasonable risks. The critical care nurse's legal duty is to act in a reasonable and prudent manner, as any other critical care nurse would act under similar circumstances. The standard is that of a critical care nurse, a professional with special knowledge and skill in critical care. The standard is that owed at the time the incident or injury occurred, not at the time of litigation. In most jurisdictions the standard of care is a national standard, as opposed to a local or community standard. General critical care nursing duties are implied by statute and administrative rules and regulations and are stated explicitly in judicial decisions (Box 2-6).

BOX 2-6   LEGAL DUTIES OF CRITICAL CARE NURSES

- Observe.
- Assess.
- Conduct ongoing observations and assessments.
- Recognize significance of information.
- Report.
- Plan, implement, and evaluate care.
- Respond to changes.
- Interpret and carry out orders.
- Take reasonable measures to ensure patient safety.
- Exercise professional judgment.
- Properly perform procedures.
- Follow hospital policies and procedures.
- Record and document.

The second element, breach of duty, involves a failure on the actor's part to conform to the standard required. Causation, the third element, involves proving that the actor's breach was reasonably close or causally connected to the resulting injury. This is also referred to as *proximate cause*. The fourth element, injury or damages, must involve an actual loss or damage to the plaintiff or his or her interest. A plaintiff may claim different types of damages, such as compensatory and punitive. Patient injury can range in value, depending on what happened to the patient. The plaintiff must produce evidence of the damages and their value. If the nurse breaches a standard of care that leads to injury, the plaintiff must show what amount of money will compensate for his or her injuries. The goal of the compensation is to provide the amount of money that will return the plaintiff to the position that existed before the injury occurred.

Res ipsa loquitur, "the thing speaks for itself," is a rule of evidence used by plaintiffs in negligence or malpractice litigation. It is a rebuttable presumption or inference of negligence by the defendant, which arises on the plaintiff's proof that (1) the injury is one that ordinarily does not happen in the absence of negligence and (2) the instrumentality causing the injury was in the defendant's exclusive management and control. The burden then shifts to the defendant to prove absence of negligence. For example, negligence can be inferred when muscle ischemia and necrosis occur as a result of improper body positioning and the application of splints or restraints. Negligence can also be inferred from a foreign object left in a patient's body cavity after surgery.

Because critical care nurses deal with life-threatening situations, any patient injury is potentially severe or may result in death. Should the injury occur as a result of alleged negligence, the nurse may be held liable for the patient's death and also for the resulting loss to surviving family members. All states have "wrongful death" acts, and a number of states have both "death" acts and "survival" acts, which are prosecuted concurrently. With the two causes of action, the expenses, pain and suffering, and loss of earnings of the decedent up to the time of death are allocated to the survival action, and

BOX 2-7 SELECT CRITICAL CARE NURSING ACTIONS IN NEGLIGENCE LAWSUITS

General
- Failure to advise physician/supervisor of change in patient's health status
- Failure to monitor patients at requisite intervals
- Failure to adhere to established institutional protocols
- Failure to assess patients' clinical status adequately
- Failure to respond to alarms
- Failure to maintain accurate, timely, and complete medical records
- Failure to carry out treatment and evaluate treatment results properly
- Failure to use safe, functional equipment

Specific
- Failure to provide supplemental oxygen when the ventilator cannot be promptly reattached
- Failure to use intravenous (IV) infusion equipment properly, causing extensive fluid extravasation
- Failure to monitor IV infusions, recognize infiltration, and discontinue IV therapy
- Failure to recognize signs of intracranial bleeding
- Failure to investigate patient's complaint of pain and discover hematoma under blood pressure cuff

BOX 2-8 SIX GENERAL CATEGORIES OF NURSING NEGLIGENCE

1. Improper administration of treatments
2. Improper administration of medications
3. Inadequate or false written and verbal communication
4. Insufficient supervision of patients
5. Improper postoperative treatment and wound care
6. Incorrect perioperative instrument and sponge counts

loss of benefits to the survivors is allocated to the wrongful death action.

Specific critical care nursing actions have resulted in litigation (Box 2-7). In such cases the nurse's action is central to the lawsuit. However, nurses are named as sole defendant or codefendant in a comparatively small percentage of cases. Although this pattern is changing, physicians and hospitals are generally named as defendants.

Typically, nursing negligence cases involve breach or failure in six general categories (Box 2-8). The first category includes the use of defective equipment or the failure to perform safety and maintenance assessments. Nurses have made errors in drug identification, administration, and dosages. Nurses have failed to report changes in patient status to physicians in a timely manner. Nurses have not communicated to supervisors a physician's failure to respond to the nurse's communication. Failure to supervise and assist patients who subsequently fall is also a source of nursing negligence. Improper wound care with resulting infection

and incorrect instrument and sponge counts in the surgical setting have also led to patient injury and lawsuits.

It is important to report and document any adverse event or unexpected outcome in an honest and genuine manner. Disclosure should take place as soon as possible after the event has been identified. This information needs to be orally discussed with the patient and family and documented. Documentation, also upon identification of the issue, needs to include the date, time, place, and all individuals involved, including the discussion with the patient and family. Document the discussion with the patient and family (use quotations of any key statements of anyone involved), the follow-up plan, and any subsequent discussions. The documentation must be accurate and concise with no admission of guilt or negligence.[27]

Legal Doctrines and Theories of Liability

In tort law the nurse's action may be examined and legal duties defined according to the following theories of liability:

- Personal liability
- Vicarious liability: respondeat superior
- Corporate liability
- Other liability doctrines (e.g., temporary or borrowed servant, captain of the ship)

Under the theory of personal liability, each individual is responsible for his or her own actions, including the critical care nurse, supervisor, physician, hospital, and patient. Each has responsibilities that are uniquely his or her own. In contrast to personal liability, the individual may be afforded the protection of personal immunity.

Vicarious liability is indirect responsibility, such as the liability of an employer for the acts of the employee. Under the doctrine of *respondeat superior*, a "master" is liable for certain wrongful acts of a "servant," as is a principal for those of an agent. An employer may be liable for an employee's acts that are performed within the legitimate scope of employment. In critical care the nurse typically is an employee of a hospital. However, nurses may be independent contractors with the hospital through critical care nursing agencies or businesses. If the latter is the case, the nurse is not an employee of the hospital, and the hospital is not vicariously liable for the nurse's action.

Corporate liability is the liability attached to the corporate entity (e.g., the hospital) for its own corporate activities and decisions.

Other doctrines, such as temporary servant or borrowed servant and captain of the ship, may apply to the critical care nurse and the critical care unit. These doctrines are used when the plaintiff argues that the physician is responsible for the nurse's actions, even though the nurse is an employee of the hospital, not of the physician. If it can be shown that the nurse acted under the direction and control of the physician, the physician may be accountable for the nurse's actions. However, these doctrines are becoming increasingly uncommon. What viability remains is typically found in cases involving nurse anesthetists and operating room nurses.

NURSE PRACTICE ACTS

The practice of nursing is regulated by the state. As a general rule, the state's police power to regulate prevails, as long as the state's actions are not arbitrary or capricious. All nurses must be licensed to practice under their individual state's licensure statutes. Licensure authorizes (1) the right to practice and (2) access to employment. Therefore licensure is a property right that is constitutionally protected. Every state has legislation that defines the legal scope of nursing practice and defines unprofessional and illegal conduct that may lead to investigation and disciplinary action by the state and sanctions on the right to practice. The state nurse practice act establishes entry requirements, definitions of practice, and criteria for discipline. Although licensure is mandatory for registered nurses (RNs), statutory content varies among the states.

Generally, state law contains two definitions of nursing: one for the RN (or professional nurse) and one for the licensed practical (or vocational or technical) nurse. These definitions determine titles that may be used by nurses, the scope of nursing practice, and requirements for entering the nursing profession. In some states, advanced RN practice, prescriptive authority for certain nurses, and third-party reimbursement are also defined by statute.

Mandatory continuing education requirements are also defined by statute in most states. The state authorizes its board of nursing to monitor practice, implement standards of care, enforce rules and regulations, and issue sanctions. Sanctions include additional education, restricted practice, supervised practice, license suspension, and license revocation. Some form of disciplinary action generally occurs as a result of unauthorized practice, negligence or malpractice, incompetence, chemical or other impairment, criminal acts, or violations of specific nurse practice act provisions.

The scope of medical practice is also statutorily defined, and in most states a physician is given broad discretion to delegate tasks to others. Physicians may delegate to critical care nurses through written protocols or standing orders, which must be written, dated, and signed by the physician; standing orders and protocols must be updated regularly. The nurse must be adequately prepared to follow the protocol and perform with a reasonable degree of skill, care, and diligence as performed by similar nurses under similar circumstances. Protocol and standing orders should identify unambiguously the corresponding roles of hospital administrators, nurses, and physicians. Within a state's jurisdiction, however, the scope of medical practice and the scope of nursing practice often overlap because each practice may authorize the same functions. Such overlapping creates problems at the regulatory level and will expand as the role of nursing continues to evolve.

Chemical impairment is a common reason for disciplinary action. In some states the impaired nurse may avoid serious sanctions by voluntarily suspending practice and entering a rehabilitation program. This must be done with the advice of counsel (the nurse's own lawyer). Generally, this option is available as long as no patient has been harmed because of the nurse's impairment.

SPECIFIC PATIENT CARE ISSUES

Myriad legal issues and controversies exist in the field of critical care. Concerns often arise in the areas of (1) informed consent and authorization for treatment and (2) the patient's right to accept or refuse medical treatment.

Informed Consent and Authorization for Treatment

There are two types of consent: express and implied. Express consent may be written or verbal and is the consent given specifically for nonroutine procedures. Implied consent may be implied in fact, an assumption based on patient behavior (e.g., patient extending arm for venipuncture or nodding approval), or may be implied in law (e.g., unconscious, hemorrhaging patient in emergency department). This discussion summarizes the elements of valid informed consent, the adequacy of consent and negligent nondisclosure, and exceptions to consent requirements and the duty to disclose.

Valid consent must be (1) voluntary, (2) obtained, and (3) informed. Although consent can be verbal or written, most hospital policies require that informed, voluntary consent to nonroutine procedures be obtained and confirmed in writing, as signed and dated by the patient, physician, and witness (if required). Most informed consent statutes provide that a consent in writing to a medical or surgical procedure that meets the consent and disclosure requirements of the statute creates a legal presumption that informed consent was given. Research has shown that participant comprehension of the informed consent process continues to be deficient in how much the persons who sign consents actually know and/or understand.[28]

In the vast majority of jurisdictions the decision maker (person giving consent) must be a legally competent adult (i.e., having reached age of majority, or age 18 years in most states). Competence is a legal judgment, and as a general rule, there is a legal presumption of patient competence.[29] A person is mentally incompetent (thereby rendering a consent invalid) if adjudicated incompetent. A person must likewise have the capacity (a medical and nursing judgment) to give consent. The patient must be oriented and understand what he or she has been told, and current medications must be documented. For adults legally adjudicated incompetent, the guardian may give consent if the guardian has been given this authority.

Minors are legally incompetent, and consent is obtained from the parent or guardian. In many jurisdictions, however, there are two important exceptions to this rule: (1) mature minors may consent to treatment for substance abuse, sexually transmitted disease, and matters involving contraception and reproduction; and (2) emancipated minors may consent to treatment in general. Minors are considered "emancipated" if married or divorced before the age of majority, if in the military service, or if living independently with parental consent.

Consent must also be informed and timely. The physician has a duty to disclose the diagnosis, condition, prognosis, material risks/benefits associated with the treatment or procedure, explanation of the treatment, providers of the treatment (who is performing, supervising, and assisting in procedure), material risks and benefits of alternative therapy, and the probable outcome (including material risks/benefits) if the patient refuses the treatment or procedure. Failure to disclose such information or inadequate disclosure with resultant injury may constitute negligence and give rise to tort claims of malpractice, battery, negligent nondisclosure, and abandonment. Consent is generally valid for 7 to 30 days. However, the time at which consent expires must be explicitly stated in the institutional policy and procedure manual.

There are many exceptions to consent requirements and the duty to disclose, and clearly the exceptions vary according to jurisdiction. Emergencies constitute one exception, unless the patient refuses treatment or has previously made a competent and informed refusal. States vary significantly in the following treatment situations: endangered fetal viability, alcohol or other drug detoxification, emergency blood transfusion, cesarean birth, and substance abuse during pregnancy. Jurisdictions also vary on the issue of sources of consent (informal directives) for the incompetent patient or the patient in an emergency who has no legal guardian. Alternatives include consensus from as many next of kin as possible, with evidence that (1) the treatment is reasonable and necessary and (2) the family's decision would not be contrary to the patient's wishes, known as *substituted judgment* (made by a surrogate decision maker). Another alternative is a court order for treatment. In the absence of substituted judgment, many courts use the "best interests" standard.

RIGHT TO ACCEPT OR REFUSE MEDICAL TREATMENT

The right to consent and informed consent includes the right to refuse treatment. In most cases a competent adult's decision to refuse even life-sustaining treatment is honored.[30-34] The underlying rationale is that the patient's right to withdraw or withhold treatment is not outweighed by the state's interest in preserving life. The right to refuse treatment is *not* honored in some situations, including (but not limited to) the following:

1. The treatment relates to a contagious illness that threatens the health of the public.
2. Innocent third parties will suffer (e.g., parent's wish to refuse blood transfusion to child most likely would be overruled to save child's life).
3. The refusal violates ethical standards.
4. Treatment must be instituted to prevent suicide and to preserve life.

When patients refuse treatment, complex ethical, legal, and practical problems arise. Hospitals should have specific policies to guide nurses in these areas, and nurses' participation in hospital or institutional ethics committees is strongly advised.

Withholding and Withdrawing Treatment

As stated, an adult has the right to refuse treatment, even treatment that sustains life. This right means that the critical care nurse may participate in the withholding or withdrawing of treatment. Historically, the distinction between withholding and withdrawing treatment was considered the issue of importance, but this is no longer the case. Health care decisions become most complex when patients lose competency and capacity to make their own decisions personally.

Advance Directives

The U.S. Congress passed landmark legislation known as the Patient Self-Determination Act/Omnibus Budget Reconciliation Act (OBRA) of 1990.[35-44] The statute requires that all adults must be provided written information on an individual's rights under state law to make medical decisions, including the right to refuse treatment and the right to formulate advance directives.

The law mandates that providers of health care services under Medicare and Medicaid must comply with requirements relating to patient advance directives, which are written instructions recognized under state law for provisions of care when persons are incapacitated. Providers may not be reimbursed for the care they provide unless the requirements of this provision are met. Despite various methods to inform patients about the importance of having advance directives, there are still persons seeking health care who do not have completed advanced health care directives in place.[45]

Providers must have written policies and procedures (1) to inform all adult patients at initiation of treatment of their right to execute an advance directive and of the provider's policies on the implementation of that right, (2) to document in the medical record whether an individual has executed an advance directive, (3) *not* to condition care and treatment or otherwise discriminate on the basis of whether a patient has executed an advance directive, (4) to comply with state laws on advance directives, and (5) to provide information and education to staff and the community on advance directives.

Patients themselves can provide clear direction by preparing in advance written documents that specify their wishes.[46] These documents are termed advance directives and include the living will and durable power of attorney for health care. To be effective in a jurisdiction, both these directives must be statutorily or judicially recognized. The living will specifies that if certain circumstances occur, such as terminal illness, the patient will decline specific treatment, such as cardiopulmonary resuscitation and mechanical ventilation. The living will does not cover all treatment; in some states, for example, nutritional support may not be declined through a living will. The durable power of attorney for health care is a directive through which a patient designates an "agent," someone who will make decisions for the patient if the patient becomes unable to do so. Critical care nurses whose patients have executed advance directives must follow state law provisions and the hospital's policies and require education regarding advance directives and their important role in patient advocacy.[47]

Orders Not To Resuscitate

Hospital policies that address orders to withhold or withdraw treatment should exist in all critical care units. For example, orders not to resuscitate, typically referred to as do-not-resuscitate (DNR) orders, should be governed by written policies, including (but not limited to) the following:

1. DNR orders should be entered in the patient's record with full documentation by the responsible physician about the patient's prognosis and the patient's agreement (if he or she is capable) or, alternatively, the family's consensus.
2. DNR orders should have the concurrence of another physician designated in the policy.
3. Policies should specify that orders are reviewed periodically (some policies require daily review).
4. Patients with capacity must give their informed consent.

5. For patients without capacity, that incapacity must be thoroughly documented, along with the diagnosis, prognosis, and family consensus.
6. Judicial intervention before writing a DNR order is usually indicated when the patient's family does not agree or there is uncertainty or disagreement about the patient's prognosis or mental status. As a general rule, however, in the absence of conflict or disagreement, DNR orders are legal in a majority of jurisdictions if executed clearly and properly.
7. Policies should specify who is to be contacted and notified within the hospital administration.

Other orders to withhold or withdraw treatment may involve mechanical ventilation, dialysis, nutritional support, hydration, and medications such as antibiotics. The legal and ethical implications of these orders for each patient must be carefully considered. Hospitals should have written policies on all orders to withhold and withdraw treatment. Policies must cover how decisions will be made, who will decide, and what roles the patient, family, health care providers, and the institution will play. Policies must be developed that consider state laws and judicial opinions.

REFERENCES

1. Angelucci P, Carefoot S: Working through moral anguish, *Nurs Manage* 38(9):10, 2007.
2. Nelson WA: Ethical uncertainty and staff stress, *Healthc Exec* 24(4):38, 2009.
3. American Association of Critical-Care Nurses: *Position statement: moral distress*, Calif., July 8, 2004, Aliso Viejo, AACN.
4. Rushton CH, American Association of Critical-Care Nurses: Defining and addressing moral distress, *AACN Adv Crit Care* 17(6):4, 2000.
5. Rushton CH: Respect in critical care – a foundational ethical principle, *AACN Adv Crit Care* 18(2):149, 2007.
6. Correll N: The power of one: identifying patient's needs helps with ethical dilemmas, *AACN News* 17(6):4, 2000.
7. Rushton CH, Reina ML, Reina DS: Building trustworthy relationships with critically ill patients and families, *AACN Adv Crit Care* 18(1):19, 2007.
8. Dennis BP: The origin and nature of informed consent: experiences among vulnerable groups, *J Prof Nurs* 15(5):285, 1999.
9. Crow KG, Matheson L, Steed A: Informed consent and truth telling: cultural direction of healthcare providers, *J Nurs Adm* 30(3):148, 2000.
10. Michael JE: Stay in-the-know regarding informed consent, *Nurs Manage* 33(5):22, 2002.
11. Washington G: Trust: a critical element in critical care nursing, *Focus Crit Care* 17(5):418, 1990.
12. Aroskar M: Fidelity and veracity: questions of promise keeping, truth telling and loyalty. In Foweler M, Levine-Ariff J, editors: *Ethics at the bedside*, Philadelphia, 1987, Lippincott.
13. Day L: Health care reform, health, and social justice, *Am J Crit Care* 19(5):459, 2010.
14. Ewer MS: The definition of medical futility: are we trying to define the wrong term? *Heart Lung* 30(1):3, 2001.

15. Angelucci PA: Grasping the concept of medical futility, *Nurs Manage* 37(2):12, 2006.
16. Pfeifer GM: Understanding medical futility, *Am J Nurs* 106(5):25, 2006.
17. Schneiderman LJ, Jecker NS, Jonsen AR: Medical futility: its meaning and ethical implications, *Ann Intern Med* 112(12):949, 1990.
18. Lachman VD: Practical use of the nursing code of ethics: part I, *Medsurg Nurs* 18(1):55, 2009.
19. Curtin L: Ethics for nurses in everyday practice, *American Nurse Today* 5(2), 2010.
20. Murray JS: Creating ethical environments in nursing, *American Nurse Today* 2(10):48, 2007.
21. American Nurses Association: *Code of ethics for nurses with interpretive statements*, Washington, D.C., 2002, ANA.
22. Thompson J, Thompson H: *Bioethical decision-making for nurses*, Norwalk, Conn., 1985, Appleton-Century-Crofts.
23. Rushton CH: Ethical discernment and action: the art of pause, *AACN Adv Crit Care* 20(1):108, 2009.
24. Rushton CH, Penticuff JH: A framework for analysis of ethical dilemmas in critical care nursing, *AACN Adv Crit Care* 18(3):323, 2007.
25. Clark AP: A model for ethical decision making in cases of patient futility, *Clin Nurse Spec* 24(4):189, 2010.
26. Ludwick R: Ethical thoughtfulness and nursing competency, *Online J Issues Nurs* 18(3) (serial online): www.nursingworld.org/MainMenuCategories/ANAMarketplace/ANAPeriodicals/OJIN/Columns/Ethics/EthicalThoughtfulnessandNursingCompetency.aspx. Accessed January 3, 2011.
27. Monson MS: Disclosing adverse events: you said it, now write it, *Nurs Manage* 37(8):16, 2006.
28. Cohn E, Larson E: Improving participant comprehension in the informed consent process, *J Nurs Scholarsh* 39(3):273, 2007.
29. Northrop CE, Kelly ME: *Legal issues in nursing*, St Louis, 1987, Mosby.

30. *Bouvia v Superior Court*, 225 Cal Rptr 297; 179 C.A.3d 1127, review denied (Cal App 1986).
31. *In re Farrell*, 529 A.2d 404 (N.J. 1987).
32. McKay v *Bergstedt*, 801 P.2d 617 (Nev. 1990).
33. *State v McAfee*, 385 S.E.2d 651 (Ga. 1989).
34. Wilson-Clayton ML, Clayton MA: Two steps forward, one step back: *McKay v Bergstedt, Whittier Law Rev* 12:439, 1991.
35. Advance directives for health care: deciding today about your care in the future, Des Moines, 1991, Iowa Hospital Association, Iowa Medical Society, Iowa State Bar Association.
36. Put it in writing: a guide to promoting advance directives, Chicago, 1991, American Hospital Association.
37. Cate FH, Gill BA: *The Patient Self-Determination Act: implementation issues and opportunities*, Washington, D.C., 1991, Annenberg Washington Program.
38. Advance directive protocols and the Patient Self-Determination Act: a resource manual for the development of *institutional protocols*, New York, 1991, Choice in Dying (212-366-5540; formerly Society for the Right to Die/Concern for Dying).
39. Emanuel L, Emanuel E: The medical directive: a new comprehensive advance care document, *JAMA* 261(22):3288, 1989.
40. The Patient Self-Determination Act of 1990: implementation in Iowa hospitals, Des Moines, 1991, Iowa Hospital Association (515-288-1955).
41. Advance medical directives, Arlington, Va., 1991, National Hospice Organization (703-243-5900).
42. The patient self-determination directory & resource guide, Washington, D.C., 1991, National Health Lawyers Association (202-833-1100).
43. Patient Self-Determination Act/Omnibus Budget Reconciliation Act of 1990, Pub L No 101-508, Sec 4206, 42 USC Sec 1395cc(a)(1) (1990).
44. Advance directives, Des Moines, 1991, Unisys (800-776-6045).
45. Durbin CR, et al: Systematic review of educational interventions for improving advance directive completion, *J Nurs Scholarsh* 42(3):234, 2010.
46. Douglas R, Brown HN: Patients' attitudes toward advance directives, *J Nurs Scholarsh* 34(1):61, 2002.
47. Ryan CJ, et al: Perceptions about advance directives by nurses in a community hospital, *Clin Nurse Spec* 15(6):246, 2001.

Patient and Family Education

Barbara Mayer

evolve WEBSITE

Be sure to check out the bonus material, including free self-assessment exercises, on the Evolve web site at
http://evolve.elsevier.com/Urden/priorities/.

OBJECTIVES

- Adapt and apply teaching-learning theory to the critical care setting.
- Perform a learning needs assessment.
- Construct a teaching plan for patients in the critical care unit.

- Discuss four methods of instruction and the appropriateness of each to the critical care setting.
- Describe informational needs of families of critically ill patients.

ADULT LEARNING PRINCIPLES

Central to successful implementation of an education plan in the critical care and telemetry environment is the incorporation of the principles of adult learning theory.[1] Adults must be ready to learn, having moved from one developmental or educational task to the next. They need to know why it is important to learn something before they can actually learn it. Inherent in their attitudes is a responsibility for their own decisions. Consequently, they may resent when others try to force different beliefs on them. Adults bring a wealth of experience to the learning environment that must be recognized and promoted in educational techniques. Because their orientation to learning is life centered, the tasks being taught should focus on current problem resolution. Finally, motivation for the adult learner arises out of internal pressures such as self-esteem and quality of life.

TEACHING-LEARNING PROCESS

The teaching-learning process is a dynamic, continuous activity (Box 3-1). Teaching is not just the passing of facts and information from one person to another. Learning is both growth and development. It is an active process that occurs internally over time and cannot be forced. Learning involves altering behavior to produce changes in one or more of the three learning domains: knowledge, attitudes, and skills.[2]

Assessment

Assessment is the gathering of information for the purpose of identifying actual or potential learning needs. It identifies gaps in the knowledge, attitudes, and skills the patient or family has regarding the illness, environment, or lifestyle (Box 3-2). Knowing this information will allow the nurse to develop a collaborative, individualized, need-targeted education plan of care. The assessment process does not stop after the completion of the admission assessment; it is continuous and ongoing.

Patients and families may be so overwhelmed by what they see or have already been told that they may be unable to identify their own learning needs. The bedside nurse is responsible for involving both the patient and the family in the assessment process and discovering what they want and need to know. Involving patients and families in this needs assessment process gives value to their needs and assists them in gaining some control over a situation in which they may feel powerless. Active participation and control stimulate the motivation to receive information, as well as make the overall education process more satisfying; in essence, the patient/family will learn more.

Assessing ability, willingness, and readiness to learn is an essential part of developing and implementing an education plan of care. Readiness to learn is the motivation to try out new concepts and behaviors.[3] The ability to learn is the capacity of the learner to understand, pay attention, and

BOX 3-1	STEPS IN THE EDUCATION PROCESS

Step 1: Assessment: Information Gathering
Patient/family: culture, age-specific considerations
Actual and potential learning needs
Possible barriers to the teaching-learning process

Step 2: Education Plan Development
Identify needs and write expected outcomes
Design interventions: information to be taught, removal of barriers
Mobilize resources as needed to remove barriers and enhance communication of information

Step 3: Implementation
Implement interventions for information sharing, learner participation in education process
Use written plan to structure the teaching encounter, cover essential information, and communicate outcomes between practitioners

Step 4: Evaluation
Evaluate learner response to the encounter, any need for follow-up teaching to attain goals
Evaluate learner comfort level with information: coping and adaptation

Step 5: Documentation
Document interventions used, resources used, information taught, and outcome of teaching encounter

BOX 3-2	ASSESSMENT QUESTIONS FOR THE CRITICALLY ILL PATIENT AND FAMILY

- What brings you to the hospital? Can you tell me what happened? Can you tell me more?
- What have you been told so far about your (your family member's) condition and plan of care?
- What is the most important thing for you to know right now?
- What would you like to know? What information can I give you right now?
- Who are your main support people?
- Has anything like this ever happened to you (your family) before?
- Have you (your family) ever been in an intensive care unit or hospital before?
- Do you have any special concerns that we need to address right now?

Modified from Reeder J: *AACN Clin Issues* 2(2):188, 1991.

comprehend the material being taught. Willingness to learn describes the learner's openness to new ideas and concepts. Several factors affect ability, willingness, and readiness to learn as well as the ability to cope and adapt to the current situation. These factors include physiological, psychological, sociocultural, financial, and environmental aspects.[2-4]

BOX 3-3	ESSENTIAL CRITICAL CARE INFORMATION FOR THE PATIENT/FAMILY

- Orientation to the various care providers and the services they deliver
- Orientation to the unit environment (e.g., call light, bed controls)
- Orientation to unit routines and plan of care: visiting hours, frequency of monitoring and nurse assessments, venipuncture to obtain blood specimens, daily weights, special shift routines
- Explanations regarding reasons for equipment, monitors, and associated alarms (e.g., cardiac monitor, ventilator, intravenous [IV] lines, IV pumps, pacemaker, pulse oximeter)
- Explanation of all procedures and expected sensations/discomforts both in and off the unit
- Medications given: drug name, reason for receiving, side effects to report to nurse/others
- Immediate plan of care
- Transition to next level of care: reason for transfer, environment, staffing, availability of care providers
- Discharge plan: medications, diet, activity, pathophysiology of disease, symptom management, special procedures and associated equipment, when to call health care provider, available community resources

Development of Education Plan

The education plan must be ongoing, interactive, and consistent with the patient's plan of care and education level (Box 3-3). Information gathered from the assessment must be analyzed and used to prioritize educational needs, formulate a nursing diagnosis, and develop an education plan of care. The nurse also must consider the patient's clinical and emotional status when setting education priorities. **The education plan should include (1) expected outcomes, (2) objectives, (3) content to be taught, (4) interventions, (5) available educational materials, and (6) appropriate teaching strategies. Refer to the Nursing Management Plan for Deficient Knowledge (Appendix A, p. A-15).**

Establish Education Phases and Priorities

It can be a difficult task to prioritize the multitude of learning needs that practitioners are required to address during a period in acute care. Learning needs in the intensive care unit (ICU), the progressive care, or the telemetry setting can be separated into six different categories to help set teaching priorities in each phase of the hospitalization (Table 3-1). Learning needs during the initial contact or first hours of hospitalization can be predicted. Education during this time frame should be directed toward the reduction of immediate stress, anxiety, and fear rather than future lifestyle alterations or rehabilitation needs. The plan should focus on survival skills, orientation to the environment and equipment, communication of prognosis, procedure explanations, and the immediate plan of care.

TABLE 3-1	EDUCATION PHASES AND PRIORITIES
PHASE	**EDUCATION PRIORITIES**
Initial contact/first visit Focus on immediate needs	Preparation for the visit: patient representatives or nurses can prepare the family and patient for the first visit • What to expect in the environment • How long the visit will last • What the patient may look like (e.g., tubes, IV lines) Orientation to unit/environment: call light, bed controls, waiting rooms, unit contact numbers Orientation to unit policies/hospital policies • HIPAA, advance directives, visitation policies Equipment orientation: monitors, IV pumps, pulse oximetry, pacemakers, ventilators Medications: rationale, effects, side effects What to do during the visit: talk to the patient, hold patient's hand, length of visits (if applicable) Patient status: stable or unstable and what that terminology means What treatments and interventions are being done for the patient Upcoming procedures When the doctor visited or is expected to visit Disciplines involved in care and the services they provide Immediate plan of care (next 24 hours) Mobilization of resources for crisis intervention
Continuous care	Day-to-day routine: meals, laboratory visits, doctor visits, frequency of monitoring (VS), nursing assessments, daily weights, and shift routines Explanation of any procedures: expected sensations or discomforts (e.g., chest tube removal, arterial sheath removal) Plan of care: treatments, progress, patient accomplishments (e.g., extubation) Medications: name, why the patient is receiving them, side effects to report to the nurse or health care team Disease process: what it is and how it will affect life, symptoms to report to health care team How to mobilize resources to assist the patient/family in coping with stress and crisis: pastoral care, social workers, case managers, victim assistance, domestic violence Gifts: When a loved one is ill, it is traditional to send flowers, balloons, or cards; if your unit has any restrictions on gifts, make the family aware Begin teaching self-management skills and discuss aftercare information
Transfer to a different level of care	*Sending Unit* Acknowledge positive move out of critical care When the transfer will occur Why the transfer is occurring What to expect in the different unit Name of the new caregiver Availability of care provider Visiting hours Directions, how to get there; the new room number and phone number *Receiving Unit* Orientation to environment, visitation policies, visitors Unit routine, meals, shift changes, doctor visits Expectations about patient self-care; ADLs Medication and diagnostic testing routine times
Planning for aftercare, discharge planning	Self-care management: symptom management, medication administration, diet, activity, durable medical equipment, tasks or procedures What to do for an emergency What constitutes an emergency or when to call the physician How to care for incisions or procedure sites
Completed throughout the hospital stay	Return appointment: name of physician practice, practice phone numbers and contacts Obtaining medications: prescriptions, pharmacy, special drug ordering information Required lifestyle changes: mobility and safety issues for the paraplegic or stroke victim, activities of daily living issues relative to medications or symptoms Potential risk modifications: smoking cessation, diet modifications, exercise Resources: cardiac rehabilitation, support groups, home health care agencies End-of-life care: participation in care, services available, mobilizing resources Palliative care Hospice

HIPAA, Health Insurance Portability and Accountability Act of 1996; *IV,* intravenous; *VS,* vital signs; *ADLs,* activities of daily living.

As the hospital length of stay increases, patients and families begin to adapt to the situation and learning needs change. The patient/family develops positive feelings of relief and happiness in the fact that survival has been achieved. Because lower-level, physiological needs are met, the patient's efforts can be concentrated on modifying behavior to meet higher-level needs such as self-concept and self-actualization. Teaching during the continuous phase of nursing care is aimed at answering patient or family questions about the treatment plan or how the acute illness will impact their day-to-day lives. Education on lifestyle modification and self-management skills should be presented during this phase of nursing care. Discharge planning is also part of the education process and should start with admission to the hospital. Instructions for home health care, also known as aftercare, should be provided before the day of discharge to avoid decreased retention of education that occurs with information overload.

Teaching Methods

There are three basic methods of teaching: lecture, discussion, and demonstration. The selection of the methods will be determined by various factors, including patient clinical status, readiness to learn, cognitive abilities, learning style, instructional time, and availability of teaching materials and resources. In addition, innovative methods of teaching and presentation of educational materials must be developed and used efficiently to maximize existing resources.[5]

Lecture. Lecture is the presentation of information in a highly structured format to a group. In this method the teacher provides a great deal of material but may not provide ample opportunities for teacher-learner interaction. This style of teaching is inappropriate for acutely ill patients in the critical care unit, although it may be useful in the telemetry unit. Optimally, the group size should be arranged to enable the learners to ask questions and receive appropriate feedback on content presented.

Discussion. Discussion is less structured than lecturing and allows an exchange and feedback between the teacher and learner. The teacher can adapt the material to meet the needs of the individual or group. Discussion groups can be effective with hospitalized patients when a group with similar problems and at similar stages of adaptation can be gathered. Individual discussion with patients/families is appropriate and valuable during the acute phase of illness because it allows them to express their feelings and interpretations.

Demonstration and Practice. Demonstration involves acting out a procedure while giving appropriate explanations to provide the learner with a clear idea of how to perform a task. Patients can then practice the skill and can be given feedback about their performance. This method is often used in the acute care setting, as when coughing/deep breathing or taking one's own pulse is taught.

Other Methods of Instruction. In addition to the three basic methods, several other approaches are available to deliver or augment information in a patient teaching program. These methods include commercially prepared or custom-designed printed materials, bedside videotape programs, and computer-assisted patient education programs.

Written Materials. Written materials can be very useful tools in patient/family education. These materials allow repetition and reinforcement of content and provide basic information in printed form for reference later. To be useful, however, the content must be accurate and current, and the patient/family must be able to read and understand it.

Low literacy levels are considered to be a barrier to successful patient/family education and the teaching-learning process.[6] Typical patient education materials are written at or above the eighth-grade or ninth-grade reading level and may be out of reach for many people.[3,7] Almost 20% of the U.S. adult population has low literacy skills and reads at or below the fifth-grade reading level.[8] To help overcome the problem of low literacy and improve health literacy, it is recommended that patient education materials be written at or below the fifth-grade reading level[7,9] (Box 3-4).

Audiovisual Media. Using media devices can be an excellent method of instruction. Use of overhead projectors, slides, pictures, videos, and closed-circuit patient education TV channels are the most frequently used audiovisual media strategies. These methods entertain the learners and provide them with important information they should know. This type of media can provide "nice to know" information as well as "need to know" information. Viewing a video alone does not ensure retention of material or knowledge acquisition. Patient education channels and videos should not replace nurse interaction and should be used jointly. The nurse must review with the learner the content presented to reiterate key points and evaluate the outcome.

Closed-circuit television (CCTV) is a common service in many health care settings. CCTV is best used as one component of a comprehensive educational program and is not intended to be used alone. CCTV allows for viewing of the session at a time that best suits the patient/family and can be stopped, restarted, or repeated as necessary.

BOX 3-4 EXAMPLE OF DIFFERENT READING LEVELS IN CRITICAL CARE EDUCATION

College Reading Level
Consult your physician immediately with the onset of chest discomfort, shortness of breath, or increased perspiration.

Twelfth-Grade Reading Level
Call your physician immediately if you experience chest discomfort, shortness of breath, or increased sweatiness.

Eighth-Grade Reading Level
Call your doctor immediately if you start having chest pain or shortness of breath or feel sweaty.

Fourth-Grade Reading Level
Call your doctor right away if you start having chest pain, can't breathe, or feel sweaty.

Computer-Assisted   Instruction. Computer-assisted instruction (CAI) is new in the patient/family education arena. Although personal computers are now commonplace, this learning medium may not be suitable for some individuals because comfort levels with technical aspects of the computer vary. The learner must pay attention to the material being presented and must not be preoccupied with learning how to use the computer mouse. Many computer systems available to the general public for learning purposes have touch screens that are easy to use and do not depend on the learner being familiar with computers. These CAI programs are generally easy to use, self-directed, and presented in a pleasant, colorful format.

Internet Websites. Patients and families often use Internet websites to research information regarding the illness or condition of concern. Websites contain a wealth of information, but not all the information is accurate. The nurse can and should play a role in assisting patients in selecting websites and evaluating the content they contain. Strategies may include explaining the difference between commercially supported sites versus sites maintained by the government or professional organizations; asking the patient to print out and bring in such material so that it can be discussed; or simply asking the patient what they may have learned through the Internet and ensuring the information is accurate.[10]

Implementation of Education Plan

Patients in the critical care environment are educated in many informal interactions with the nurse, and the knowledge gained fosters patient understanding and well-being. Educational opportunities can be present during various nursing care activities, such as bathing and administration of medication. Each encounter with the patient/family must be viewed as a teachable moment. At times during the hospitalization, however, more formal or structured educational experiences may be required.

Learning Environment

As discussed, patient barriers to learning are related to physiological, emotional, and motivational factors. To structure a successful teaching-learning experience in a critical care area, the nurse must also carefully assess the environmental and iatrogenic barriers that affect the interaction. Bright lights, unpleasant odors, unfamiliar noises, and untidy surroundings can distract patients and add to cognitive impairment. Control of these factors can facilitate the learning process. Factors that cannot be controlled must be explained to the patient to alleviate anxiety and facilitate a trusting relationship between patient and nurse.

Keys to Successful Patient Education

Clinical practice today is characterized by increasing patient acuity and a focus on decreasing length of stay, leaving little time for providing patient education. The nurse may only have a few days to provide education for a patient/family about the patient's illness and ongoing care, therefore it is imperative to use every learning opportunity efficiently and effectively. Several strategies can enhance the education process.[11]

Get the Patient's Attention. The nurse must ensure that the information presented is perceived by the patient as important and necessary to know, relevant, and valuable to recovery from illness. Whether using a teachable moment, creating a written teaching tool, or using a visual aid, the topic should be clearly stated at the very beginning. The importance of the information being presented can be communicated to the patient by varying the tone of voice used to emphasize key points. Using assorted teaching tools—discussion, demonstration, pictures or diagrams—will help focus the patient on essential information. Finally, turning abstract theory into meaningful information can be accomplished by using examples familiar to the patient.

Stick to the Basics. Use simple, everyday language when teaching. Avoid the use of medical terms. Avoid trying to teach everything all at once. Identify three or four key points the patient needs to know and focus on those. The nurse can always reinforce teaching by providing supplemental material the patient can review when their condition improves.

Make the Most of Your Time. Teachable moments occur throughout daily patient care—while bathing, administering medications, or taking vital signs. If the family is present in the room, involving them in the teaching process can be beneficial in reinforcing content. Verbal teaching can be supplemented with printed or recorded materials that can be reviewed by the patient and family later.

Reinforce Learning. Provide positive rewards when the patient demonstrates understanding. Be sure to provide documentation when the patient is transferred so that education supplied can be reinforced as the patient progresses.

Evaluation
What to Evaluate

The evaluation process helps the nurse determine the effectiveness of patient/family education interventions. The nurse must decide how well the learner has met the expected outcomes and objectives. Evaluation should be done as each intervention is carried out to allow the nurse to give feedback to the patient/family and revise the education plan of care to accommodate continued learning needs. It is also important to assess the patient/family's response to the process. The response to the teaching-learning interaction includes the level of interest, willingness to learn, and level of participation.

How to Evaluate

There are several ways to determine the effectiveness of the teaching-learning process. Evaluating knowledge can be done through verbal questioning or written testing on the topic. Questioning provides an interactive avenue for the nurse to assess whether the learner has retained the information taught. Verbal questioning should occur not only immediately after the teaching event but also later to assess knowledge retention. Some CAI programs include a posttest that provides participants with immediate feedback on their learning. Written tests may also be administered to assess knowledge retention but are infrequently used in the critical care setting.

Observation and return demonstration represent the evaluation of choice for the skills-learning domain. For the patient/family to be "checked off" on a particular skill, they should be able to perform it independently, using the nurse only as a resource for questions. Endotracheal suctioning, placing condom catheters, and performing dressing changes are common tasks that patients and families may be asked to learn. Because of the increasingly complex care patients now require at home after discharge, these skills may be the entire focus of teaching before discharge.

It is important to remember that not every teaching moment is a success, and the nurse should not have feelings of guilt or failure when the learner has not achieved the desired objective. Revisiting and revising the goals and objectives during the teaching-learning session may be necessary to meet the ever-changing needs of the patient or family.

Documentation

Documentation of the teaching-learning process is multifaceted and should reflect each component in the education plan of care. Whenever a teaching-learning encounter has been completed, the interaction, material taught, and learner response must be recorded.[12] The assessment documentation should include assessment of patient/family learning needs, abilities, preferences, and readiness to learn as well as potential barriers to learning. The remainder of the documentation should include the expected outcome/goals, objectives, interventions, who was taught, what was taught, materials used, patient/family response to teaching, and any follow-up education or materials needed.

SPECIAL CONSIDERATIONS

The Older Adult

As individuals age, cognitive, physiological, and psychological changes occur that must be considered when planning and implementing a teaching plan. It is the nurse's responsibility to understand the effects of aging and adjust teaching strategies to accommodate them.[13]

Cognitive Effects of Aging

Cognitive effects include processing information more slowly, a decrease in the ability to take in multiple messages, and difficulty understanding the abstract. When teaching the older adult, nurses should provide information slowly and deliberately to allow the patient time to process each concept. Information should be presented in two to three essential points and reviewed frequently. Nurses should avoid using vague terms such as "several times a day" or "until better". Instead, they must be very specific with amounts, times, and frequencies.

Physical Effects of Aging

Presbyopia, cataracts, glaucoma, and macular degeneration affect the vision of many older adults. Although additional lighting is necessary, it is also necessary to avoid direct sunlight, harsh lights, and using glossy paper. Colors in the blue end of the spectrum are difficult for the older adult to distinguish because of yellowing of the lens of the eye. When using written instructions or color-coded dosing, blues, greens, and purples should not be used.

High-pitched tones become more difficult to hear as an individual ages. Female nurses will need to make an effort to modulate their voices into the lower register so the older adult can hear better. In addition, careful enunciation of words containing higher-pitched sounds like "f", "s", "k", and "sh" may be necessary. Providing audio and video recordings will help reinforce learning.

Aging and associated co-morbidities may result in fatigue, joint pain, or decreased dexterity. Learning can be facilitated by scheduling teaching sessions early in the day, keeping sessions short, and managing pain prior to learning.

Psychological Effects of Aging

Older adults often suffer from depression. Learning can be enhanced by selecting content that holds value and relevance to the individual. Nurses should choose content that is perceived by the learner as important in maintaining quality of life, and should try to relate what they are teaching to the individual's previous life experiences.

Sedated and Unconscious Patients

Patient education should not be reserved for the conscious and coherent patient only; it should be provided to the unconscious or sedated patient as well. Addressing the learning needs of this critically ill population of patients is challenging. These patients cannot communicate their educational needs, nor can they interact and participate in the learning process. Although it is truly not known what the unconscious or sedated patient hears or remembers, it is known that some sedated patients undergoing surgery remember discussions that took place among physicians and staff during the procedure. Therefore, one should not ignore unconscious or sedated patients during the education process. These patients may not be able to respond or participate, and the effectiveness of the teaching process cannot be evaluated, but providing information regarding environment, procedures, sensations, and time of day is benevolent and may help to decrease immediate physiological stress.

The Illiterate Patient

Illiteracy affects 44 million people in the United States and may be difficult to diagnose.[14] The nurse must be aware of the subtle signs, such as avoiding reading or asking others to read and complete forms, or becoming defensive when handed written materials during teaching. If the patient is illiterate, using simple language, providing frequent examples and using teach-back or return demonstration can be useful

---

BOX 3-5   CONTRIBUTING FACTORS TO NONCOMPLIANCE

- Limited English Proficiency (LEP)
- Lack of education
- Cultural or ethnic beliefs
- Financial constraints
- Lack of adequate tools or supplies
- Lack of family support

BOX 3-6   TIPS FOR USING AN INTERPRETER

- Speak directly to the patient, not the interpreter.
- Position yourself so that you can maintain eye contact with the patient.
- Introduce the interpreter and clarify roles of others in the room.
- Nothing should be said that the patient shouldn't hear.
- Pause after each complete thought to give interpreter time to translate.
- Plan ahead, let the interpreter know exactly the content and purpose of the session.
- Use the teach-back method to evaluate learning.
- Listen to the interpreter, who may identify cultural practice or norms that impede understanding.

From Patient Education Management. July, 77: 2007.

---

in providing patient education. Pictures, diagrams, and audio or videotapes can also be useful for these patients.

The Noncompliant Patient

Noncompliance, or an unwillingness to learn, does not necessarily mean that the patient is consciously choosing not to participate in their care or follow medical instructions. There are many other issues that can lead to noncompliance. The nurse must be alert for barriers that may prevent a willing patient from being compliant. Box 3-5 lists factors that may contribute to noncompliance or unwillingness to learn.[15]

Using an Interpreter

The patient/family with Limited English Proficiency (LEP) presents a challenge for the nurse in providing education. In addition to the basics already presented, more preparation is required to ensure a productive teaching session. Box 3-6 describes helpful techniques when using an interpreter for patient education.[16]

INFORMATIONAL NEEDS OF FAMILIES IN CRITICAL CARE

Family members and significant others of critically ill patients are integral to the recovery of their loved ones. When planning for the overall care of patients, nurses and other caregivers need to consider the informational and emotional support needs of this group.[17] Families of critically ill patients report their greatest need is for information.[17] Flexible visiting hours and informational booklets regarding the critical care experience are recommended to meet this need.[18]

PREPARATION OF PATIENT/FAMILY FOR TRANSFER FROM CRITICAL CARE

When patients are more stable, requiring less hemodynamic monitoring and close observation, they are frequently transferred to another level of care in a different geographic hospital setting. They may be transferred to an intermediate care unit (also called step-down, intermediate care area, or telemetry). While on these units, patients receive optimal care to their level of requirement, a lower nurse-to-patient ratio, and less expensive technological monitoring in a quieter environment.[19,20]

Being transferred from the critical care unit to a step-down unit may cause the patient anxiety and stress. By this time, patients and families have become dependent on the monitors, equipment, constant nursing attention, and abundant information received while in the critical care unit. The patient has become secure knowing that immediate physiological and emotional needs are being met. A strong bond has often developed between the staff and the family. Many patients and families are reluctant to give up that bond and believe that their needs will not be met as well on a step-down unit. To avoid anxiety and provide the patient and family with some control over the event, nurses need to prepare them for the transfer process.

Preparation for transfer should start after the patient has been stabilized and the life-threatening event that resulted in hospitalization has subsided. The stressor at this point is not the now-familiar critical care environment but the unfamiliar step-down environment. Information such as where the patient will be transferred, the reason for transfer, and the name of the nurse who will be providing care should be given as soon as known. Before transfer, information about changes in care, expectations for self-care, and visiting hours should be provided to the patient/family. Family members should also be contacted concerning exactly when the patient will be transferred so they can be present during the transfer or made aware of the patient's new location.

The education plan of care and tips learned by the critical care staff about that particular patient and family should be communicated to the step-down unit staff. Most of the patient transfers made from the critical care unit to a step-down unit are planned events. At times, however, unplanned or unexpected transfers occur, usually when the critical care unit requires bed space for a more seriously ill patient. In this situation the transfer occurs quickly, either during the day or often at night. Families may be present in the hospital or may have gone home for the evening. This sudden need to transfer the patient can produce as much anxiety as the initial event, primarily because the patient/family may not feel ready for the transfer or may think they have lost control of the situation. Providing the patient/family with concrete evidence of improvement, such as more favorable vital signs or the need for fewer medications or tubes, can assure them of improvement in the patient's condition before unplanned transfers occur. Increased communication and providing consistent information to patients and families also increases satisfaction with care and services.[21,22]

REFERENCES

1. Hansen M, Fisher JC: Patient-centered teaching from theory to practice, *Am J Nurs* 98(1):56, 1998.
2. Phillips LD: Patient education: understanding the process to maximize time and outcomes, *J Intraven Nurs* 22(1):19, 1999.
3. Rankin S, Stallings K: *Patient education: issues, principles, practices*, ed 3, Philadelphia, 1996, Lippincott.
4. Ruzicki D: Realistically meeting the educational needs of hospitalized acute and short-stay patients, *Nurs Clin North Am* 24(3):629, 1989.
5. Barnes LP: The illiterate client: strategies in patient teaching, *MCN Am J Matern Child Nurs* 17(3):127, 1992.
6. Quirk P: Screening for literacy and readability: implications for the advanced practice nurse, *Clin Nurse Spec* 14(1):26, 2000.
7. Doak C, Doak L, Root J: *Teaching patients with low literacy skills*, ed 2, Philadelphia, 1996, Lippincott.
8. Doak C et al: Improving comprehension for cancer patients with low literacy skills: strategies for clinicians, *CA Cancer J Clin* 48(3):151, 1998.
9. Klingbeil C, Speece M, Schubiner H: Readability of pediatric patient education materials, *Clin Pediatr (Phila)* 34(2):96, 1995.
10. Kuhns K: Do you know what your patients are learning online? *Pa Nurse* 64(1):4, 2009.
11. Katz J: Back to Basics: Providing effective patient education, *Am J Nurs* 97(5):33, 1997.
12. Casey F: Documenting patient education: a literature review, *J Contin Educ Nurs* 26(6):257, 1995.
13. Speros C: More than words: Promoting health literacy in older adults, *Online J Issues Nurs* 14(3), 2009.
14. Smith L: Help! My patient's illiterate, *Nursing* 33(11):32hn6, 2003.
15. Thomas M, editor: Lack of compliance may mean patients don't understand, *Case Management Advisor* 20(8):85, 2009.
16. Techniques for educating with the aid of an interpreter, *Patient Educ Manag* July:77, 2007.
17. Doering LV, McGuire AW, Rourke D: Recovering from cardiac surgery: what patients want to know, *Am J Crit Care* 11(4):333, 2002.
18. Henneman EA, McKenzie JB, Dewa CS: An evaluation of interventions for meeting the information needs of families of critically ill patients, *Am J Crit Care* 1(3):85, 1993.
19. Miracle VA, Hovenkamp G: Needs of families of patients undergoing invasive cardiac procedures, *Am J Crit Care* 3(3):155, 1994.
20. White SK, Edwards RJ: Visitation guidelines promote safe, satisfying environments, *Nurs Manage* 37(8):21, 2006.
21. Radtke A: Telemetry monitoring: a preferred solution for intermediate care, *Nurs Manage* 37(12):52A, 2006.
22. Mages ME: Helping patients, helping families, *Healthc Exec* 11(4):40, 2006.

CHAPTER

4

Psychosocial Alterations

Linda D. Urden

⊖volve WEBSITE

Be sure to check out the bonus material, including free self-assessment exercises, on the Evolve web site at
http://evolve.elsevier.com/Urden/priorities/.

OBJECTIVES

- Explain the following coping strategies as they relate to critically ill patients: suppression, denial, hope, trust, family support, and spiritual practices.
- Describe the needs and coping mechanisms of families of critically ill patients.

- Explain interventions and nursing management for patients with coping alterations.
- Compare and contrast hopelessness with powerlessness.

Patients who require critical care must cope with a variety of stressors. A patient's response to these stressors depends on individual differences, such as age, gender, social support, cultural background, medical diagnosis, current hospital course, and prognosis. A person's perceptions of self and relationships with others, of spiritual values, and of self-competency in social roles also play a major role in how he or she responds to stress and illness. The purpose of this chapter is to provide a theoretical basis for understanding these various issues and to provide the nurse with additional insight into implementing holistic nursing care.

The selected diagnoses presented relate to the major concerns and problems that are common to the critical care setting. Customary responses to stress, such as anxiety, are described, as well as the risks for spiritual distress, powerlessness, hopelessness, and self-directed violence (suicide). Ways to enhance patient coping mechanisms and support family and friends with an attitude of care, openness, and warmth are presented. These interpersonal skills lead to effective interventions.

EFFECTS OF STRESS ON MIND-BODY INTERACTIONS

Stress of any type—whether positive or negative, biological, psychological, or social—elicits the same physical responses.[1] Extensive literature exists describing the relationship between mind-body interactions and the immune response to stress. All personal resources can be depleted by exposure to severe or prolonged stress. Several studies have shown the effects of life events such as an acute illness that is perceived to be a threat to personal integrity.[2-4] The effects of an illness that requires hospitalization can be further compounded if admission to an intensive care unit (ICU) becomes necessary.

The ICU environment can be frightening. Technological equipment can control one's breathing and prevent speaking. Invasive procedures, abrupt or continual noises, loss of privacy, sleep interruptions, pain, medications, isolation, and minimal contact with significant support people all create feelings of powerlessness and loss of control. Disorientation, which is common for patients in the ICU, is influenced by several factors, including the severity of the physical problem,

BOX 4-1 STRESSORS IN THE CRITICAL CARE SETTING

Although the experience of critical illness and care varies, each patient must cope with at least some of the following stressors:

- Threat of death
- Threat of survival with significant residual problems related to the illness or injury
- Pain or discomfort
- Lack of sleep
- Loss of autonomy over most aspects of life and daily functioning
- Loss of control over one's environment, such as loss of privacy and exposure to light, noise, and general activity of the critical care unit, including the care of other patients
- Daily hassles or common frustrations
- Loss of usual role and, with that, the arena in which usual coping mechanisms serve the patient
- Separation from family and friends
- Loss of dignity
- Boredom broken only by brief visits, threatening stimuli, and frightening thoughts
- Loss of ability to express oneself verbally when intubated

Effects of and responses to stressors depend on the individual's perception of the intensity of the stress and the following factors:

- Acute and chronic duration of stressors
- Cumulative effect of simultaneous stressors
- Sequence of stressors
- Individual's previous experience with stressors and coping effectiveness
- Amount of social support

chemical imbalances, sensory overload or deprivation, and previous experiences with the health care system. In addition to these factors are personal variables such as biological factors, social roles, and the individual's emotional responses of anxiety, confusion, or depression.[1-3] However, for some people, the ICU is perceived as a safe environment where life-saving procedures are immediately at hand and administered by highly competent caregivers.

Precipitating stressors may arise from the individual's internal or external environment; adaptation may depend on the number of stressors and the timing of their occurrence, as well as the degree of change that is represented. See Box 4-1 for a listing of stressors in the critical care unit. The accumulation of daily hassles can often influence a person's response to a major stressor. Personal characteristics that facilitate constructive adaptation to stress include hardiness, resilience, hope, a positive self-concept and internal locus of control, a sense of belonging, and the presence of social support.[5-7] Use of maladaptive or destructive measures may temporarily minimize anxiety but do not resolve the personal conflicts. There are four stages of nursing activities: (1) stabilizing the patient in a time of crisis, (2) providing symptomatic relief and assessment of the patient's coping responses, (3) reinforcing adaptive behaviors and improved patient functioning, and (4) implementing strategies for health promotion and optimal quality of life.

ANXIETY AS A RESPONSE TO STRESS

Anxiety is a normal subjective human response to a perceived or actual threat to self-integrity, which can range from a vague, generalized feeling of discomfort to a state of panic and loss of control. Anxiety is the most common of all mental illnesses.[8] Symptoms of anxiety closely parallel the biological stress responses described earlier. The initial emotional responses of excitement and heightened awareness diminish as anxiety levels increase, the individual's perceptual field narrows, and problem-solving and coping skills are lost. Prolonged stress can exhaust available resources.

ANXIETY AND PAIN

A cyclic relationship exists between levels of anxiety and perceptions and tolerance of pain. This relationship varies according to whether pain is produced by disease processes or invasive procedures, is acute or chronic, or is anticipatory. Pain affects the whole person. It has been defined as "an unpleasant sensory and emotional experience associated with actual and potential damage, or described in terms of such damage."[9] Pain is also multidimensional in nature, necessitating comprehensive assessment and management. In conditions of high acuity, pain can be caused by a variety of factors, such as injured tissues, imposed immobility, intubation, lighting, noise, and interrupted sleep.

When an illness or pain is severe enough, the person experiencing it is forced to conserve all energies and focus inward to gain control of anxiety feelings. He or she may startle easily, become irritable, display anger and rage, be vigilant and wary of caregivers, or be demanding. There is a tendency to blame others, to be confused, and to be indecisive. The patient may withdraw from interpersonal contact and may indicate that the situation is overwhelming.[8,10] It is crucial for the nurse to identify the cause of the patient's pain, validate observations with the patient, and identify a plan for pain management. (For detailed information on pain management, see Chapter 8.)

Once pain management has been addressed, the nurse evaluates for ongoing anxiety. Again, the nurse needs to identify the cause of a patient's anxiety and to validate observations with the patient. Medications frequently administered in the ICU can contribute to feelings of anxiety; they include theophylline, anticholinergics, dopamine, levodopa, salicylates, and steroids.[8,9,11] Whether the causes of anxiety are biochemically induced, related to genetic factors, or secondary to a threat imposed in an emergency or a crisis situation, the nurse must take all factors into consideration for interventions to be effective. Panic attacks (outcomes of severe anxiety), which are frequent occurrences in the ICU, can also produce physiological symptoms such as tachycardia, hyperventilation, and dyspnea.[10]

POWERLESSNESS

Powerlessness, as a nursing diagnosis, is defined as the perception of the individual that his or her own actions will not significantly affect an outcome.[12] Unrelieved powerlessness may result in hopelessness, which is discussed in the next section.

The causes of powerlessness include factors in the health care environment, interpersonal interactions, cultural and religious beliefs, illness-related regimen, and a lifestyle of helplessness. The range in levels of powerlessness varies and depends on the person's perceived sense of control, the amount of loss experienced, and the availability of social support. Powerlessness can be manifested by delayed decision making or refusal to make decisions or by expressions of self-doubt in role performance. Frustration, anger, and resentment over being dependent on others often occur and are exhibited as verbal expressions regarding dissatisfaction with care.[13]

Individuals vary in the amount of control they prefer.[14] The routines of the critical care unit may oppose or preclude any control by the patient. The person for whom control is important should be helped to continue to control as many areas of his or her life as possible. On the other hand, a patient must be given the opportunity to choose not to control.

Critically ill patients generally have experienced a rapid onset of illness without having had time to acquire the illness role. If control is defined as the ability to determine the use of time, space, and resources, admission to a critical care unit strips away this power. On admission, persons lose their independent status. They become patients. Choice of clothing and use of other personal belongings are usually restricted in a critical care unit. Patients cannot decide who enters the room, who provides personal care, or who intrudes with painful treatments. Hospital rules are usually not open to modification. Patients may feel anxious because they are separated from a familiar environment and have restrictions on who may visit them.

Poor interactions with health care providers can make the situation worse. Patients may react aggressively, may try bargaining, or may refuse to comply with diagnostic and treatment regimens. They may resent the close scrutiny of the nurses and physicians and the invasion of their privacy. By virtue of their experiences with critical illness and care, people may lose sight of areas of influence they still do retain over themselves because so much control has been taken from them. Nurses can emphasize the patient's influence or control and thereby help to preserve it.[13,15]

HOPELESSNESS

Hopelessness is a subjective state in which an individual sees limited or no alternatives or personal choices available and is unable to mobilize energy on his or her own behalf.[12] To help clarify hopelessness, the following definition of hope is included: a feeling that provides comfort while enduring life threats and personal challenges; a feeling that what is wanted will happen; a desire that is accompanied by anticipation or expectation. Most people agree that an element of hope must

be maintained, no matter how hopeless things appear. Hope is a force that helps one survive.[16,17] An interdisciplinary concept analysis of hope and hopelessness in the literature from theology, medicine, nursing, and psychology revealed that absolute hopelessness is viewed as incompatible with life. Hope often arises in the presence of crisis and instills vigorous resistance to giving up. The help of others in the situation supports the patient's belief.[5,15] Hope wards off despair, mental anguish, disorganization, and helplessness.[17] When people expect something to happen, they usually act in ways that increase the likelihood that the expectation will be met.[18] The expectation, whether positive or negative, becomes stronger the more times the "reinforcing circle" occurs. This process is defined as a *self-fulfilling prophecy.*

The critically ill patient is a multiproblem patient. Nurses and physicians are tempted to focus on the crisis and the use of technical equipment and to overlook the patient in his or her totality. The health care team may stereotype patients and underestimate their individual strengths.[19,20] The very nature of the critical care unit is frightening and increases a patient's sense of vulnerability and fear of death. Therefore, it is important to foster a realistic sense of hope in the patient.[12,21] The critical care nurse can project an attitude of hope; identify some aspect of the situation in which hope is warranted, no matter how grave the situation; and attempt to channel feelings toward some positive outcome.

When the situation moves from hopeful to hopeless in the critical care unit, the decision to write a do-not-resuscitate order must be carefully considered.[22,23] It must be recognized that members of the health care team and the family may reach this decision at varying times.[24,25] However, it is important to not avoid difficult conversations and to keep patients and families informed. Careful medical and nursing assessments, use of family and team conferences to foster communication, and enlisting the assistance of a spiritual counselor can make these situations less frustrating for all concerned.

Families also need hope. Nursing strategies for supporting the family include clarifying any distorted thinking, providing opportunities for the family to be with the patient, presenting realistic patient outcome expectations, and expanding the coping repertoire of the family.[22-24,26] See Box 4-2 for additional strategies.

SPIRITUAL DISTRESS

Spiritual distress has been defined as a disruption in the life principle that pervades a person's entire being and that integrates and transcends one's biological and psychosocial nature.[12] Adherence to a particular philosophical, psychological, sociological, or political belief may provide a sense of one's value and of life's meaning. Threats imposed by any physiological or psychological illness or prolonged pain and suffering can challenge a person's spirituality.[27] Life-threatening illness causes a person to face his or her own mortality. The provision of holistic nursing care is not limited to meeting a patient's religious needs; it also encompasses all that provides meaning to life.

BOX 4-2 STRATEGIES TO INSPIRE HOPE IN FAMILIES OF CRITICALLY ILL PATIENTS

Responding to Family Concerns

- Explore one's own feelings about interacting with families of critically ill patients and end-of-life issues.
- Use active listening, therapeutic communication skills, and touch (when appropriate); allow the family to share concerns; avoid giving messages that convey false hope.
- Establish mutually trusting relationships with the patient and family.
- Provide comfort and pain relief care to the patient; demonstrate a caring attitude.
- Provide adequate and appropriate information regarding the patient's condition and progress; clarify misinformation.
- Express empathy; consider the impact of the patient's illness on roles within the family; respect membership in nontraditional family structures.
- Assess ability to cope; recognize that family members may use defense mechanisms to cope with anxiety or a crisis situation; accept individual responses to stress (which typically are not characteristic of usual behavior).
- Be sensitive to reactions to adverse changes in the patient's condition; observe for expressions of anticipatory grief, helplessness, hopelessness, and depression.
- Address spiritual needs through facilitating contacts with a chaplain or spiritual counselor; notify the family about areas available for privacy or meditation.
- Support processes that are meaningful to the family and congruent with their cultural beliefs and values.

Responding to the Family's Physical Needs

- Encourage family members to attend to their own health and physical needs—nutrition, rest, and sleep.
- Provide information about available community resources for personal needs.

Family Participation

- Prepare the family regarding the patient's condition and behaviors; instruct them about the environment of the intensive care unit before their first visit; monitor family interactions with the patient; discourage confrontations; remove overemotional persons from the unit, and provide support until they can gain control of their emotions.
- Involve the family in decision making and in participation in basic patient care activities (they can be a patient's major support system).
- If possible, have the family select one person to serve as liaison at interdisciplinary team planning sessions and to be the contact for scheduling visits and receiving updates of information to decrease uncertainties the family may have.
- Use the expertise of the interdisciplinary team to provide social support, explore the meaning of the crisis, expand the coping repertoire, and help maintain caring relationships among family members.

Data from Wheeler RW: Helping families cope with death and dying, *Nursing* 26(7):25, 1996; Czerwiec M: When a loved one is dying: families talk about nursing care, *Am J Nurs* 96(5):32, 1996; Durham E: How patients die, *Am J Nurs* 97(12):41, 1997; Powers P, et al: The value of patient- and family-centered care, *Am J Nurs* 100(5):84, 2000; and Barry P: *Psychosocial nursing: assessment and intervention in care of the physically ill,* ed 3, Philadelphia, 1996, JB Lippincott.

An individual who is in spiritual distress may question the meaning of suffering and death in relation to his or her personal belief system. Anger toward God or a supreme being, feelings of self-blame, or regret over inability to practice belief rituals may be expressed. Individuals may even question the necessity for the therapeutic regimen. Spiritual care has been described as health-promoting interventions to relieve responses to stress that affect the spiritual perspectives of individuals or groups.[12] Creating an environment of compassion in which patients feel that their emotional and spiritual needs are met is at the heart of holistic care.[28] Listening to the patient's concerns, offering support, and enlisting the support of a spiritual counselor can promote the healing process.

MAJOR DEPRESSIVE EPISODE

A major depressive episode is a mood disorder of at least two weeks' duration that is characterized by depressed mood, diminished interest or pleasure in usual activities, insomnia, poor appetite, psychomotor retardation or agitation, and loss of energy. Patients with this disorder also may report feelings of hopelessness, worthlessness, and guilt. Recurrent thoughts of death, loss of interest in life, and recurrent suicidal ideation

may be present.[29] Major depression may complicate a patient's underlying physical illnesses; for example, asthma, headaches, ulcers, arthritis, or coronary heart disease may be exacerbated to the point of a life-threatening situation.[10,29] Depression deepens and suicide ideation frequently resurfaces after surgery if a life-threatening diagnosis is confirmed.

The nurse can listen empathetically and convey to the patient that recovery from the depression is expected, while understanding that the patient's depression cannot be overcome by cheerfulness or reassurance. If the patient is on suicide precautions, the nurse safeguards the patient according to department policy and procedure and alerts all members of the health care team and the family. The nurse also informs the patient that precaution measures are being taken as a safeguard until his or her mood improves. Requesting a comprehensive mental health assessment by a mental health professional would provide the means for giving proper attention to the patient's mind-body experience.

SUICIDE ATTEMPT

Depression is a causal factor in 30% to 70% of suicide attempts among the high-risk groups of youth (ages 15 to 24 years), the elderly population (>65 years), and individuals with psychiatric disorders. Suicide has been described as a self-destructive response to a stimulus resulting from an undesirable, unacceptable, or overwhelming event; as a response to overcome high anxiety feelings about abandonment by God or significant others; as a hostility toward self; and as the only solution for ending a helpless or hopeless situation. Nurses in high acuity and emergency settings will be challenged by patients who have attempted suicide or are at risk for doing so. Persons with cognitive impairment resulting from delirium effects of medications, fluid and electrolyte imbalances, anoxia, surgery, or trauma are at greatest risk for attempting suicide. Hallucinations may compel their self-destructive behavior.[30] A primary focus for care of the person with self-destructive behavior is protection from harm.[10,30,31] Nurses also must consider their own responses to patients' self-destructive behaviors, which can enhance or inhibit their interactions with patients. Interventions may include removal of harmful objects; consistent supervision; active listening; contracting with the individual to cease harmful activities; promoting the person's self-esteem and self-control in regulating emotions and behaviors, which frequently includes administering anxiolytic medications and mobilizing social support systems; and providing mental health education.

COPING

Patients who require critical care must cope with a variety of stressors (Box 4-1). Each patient's response to these stressors is unique and depends on a variety of environmental factors and individual differences. The nurse's knowledge of assessment, diagnosis, and effective coping strategies also affects how well the patient copes. The uncomfortable effects of a situation (e.g., anxiety, grief, loss of control) can lessen the effectiveness of coping mechanisms when people are faced with serious problems that they cannot overcome using familiar behaviors.

Coping is a dynamic process involving cognitive and behavioral efforts to manage specific internal or external demands that are perceived to exceed the person's resources.[32,33] Aguilera[34] states that coping activities encompass all the diverse behaviors that people use to meet actual or potential demands. The available coping mechanisms are those behaviors that a person draws on that have been found to be effective in the past. The key to effective coping is using the best strategy or mix of strategies in a given situation.

Coping Mechanisms

When a patient copes effectively, what he or she is doing to cope often goes unnoticed. Emotionally, the patient seems relatively comfortable, is a cooperative recipient of care, and exhibits nonproblematic behavior. The patient may be using multiple appropriate coping mechanisms that help to manage a problem or a stressful situation. The following discussion covers several coping mechanisms that may or may not be effective, depending on the degree to which they are used. Some authors differentiate between coping mechanisms

that relate to adjusting, adapting, and successfully meeting a challenge and defense mechanisms that are automatic self-protective measures developed in response to an internal or external stressor.[2,20,35] Examples of the latter include denial, acting-out behavior, avoidance, hypochondriasis, passive-aggressive behavior, and projection.

Suppression

Suppression is a conscious, intentional process in which patients push ideas, problems, or desires out of their conscious thoughts.[35] Patients often use suppression when their problems are overwhelming and they are in no position to resolve them. For example, before becoming ill, an individual might have been struggling to meet financial obligations, but she or he now uses suppression to postpone dealing with this concern until further along in the recovery phase.

Denial

Patients may deny various aspects of their illness. Some deny the probable medical significance of symptoms, as in the case of the 55-year-old cardiologist who interprets severe substernal chest pain as indigestion or the quadriplegic who cheerfully insists that he will be back on his feet in no time. Other patients cannot recognize signs of illness that are obvious to others, as in the case of the patient who cannot "see" the gangrenous foot requiring amputation.[36] Other people cannot readily influence the beliefs of a patient who is using denial. For example, the patient who is denying a myocardial infarction will not be convinced of its occurrence by being shown the cardiogram interpretation or laboratory reports. This patient is best served by a nurse who recognizes the patient's need to deny at the present time but who watches for cues from the patient that indicate readiness to accept the reality of the medical diagnosis. A patient with a tracheostomy may refuse to look at her body, avoid mirrors, and fear rejection by others because of her appearance. Forcing her to look at herself before she is ready can be extremely detrimental.

Trust

Trust manifests itself in the critical care patient as a belief that the staff will get him or her through the illness, managing any untoward event that might occur. Trust is an unconscious process in which the patient transfers the trust learned in early significant relationships onto caregivers in the present.[10,37] For example, a patient with severe burns must learn to trust caregivers. Intense fear of pain or of falling when being moved from a stretcher to a Hubbard tank can affect other coping skills as well.

Hope

Although hope has long been recognized as a significant factor in patient recovery and survival, the phenomenon receives little attention until the patient comes to feel hopeless. Hope is the expectation that a desire will be fulfilled. It can exist even in the face of a realistic appraisal of a grim situation.[38] Hope supports the patient and helps the patient endure the physical and psychological insults that are a part of the daily experience. Hope is central to resilience and spiritual strength.[39]

Spiritual Beliefs and Practices

Spiritual beliefs and practices may provide the patient with some measure of acceptance of an illness, a sense of mastery and control, a source of hope and trust beyond the limits of what the staff can provide, and strength to endure the current stress. A patient may discuss personal beliefs and concerns openly or may view the subject as a private and personal matter.[40-46]

Use of Family Support

The patient can use the presence of a supportive family to cope with critical illness. The patient with a supportive family knows that family members share a past and hope for a future with the patient. Family members love the patient as a person and as a member of the family. The patient also realizes that family members know him or her in ways the staff cannot. With family, the patient may know that his or her experience is truly understood, even when little is said. Family members can be involved in the patient's personal care and can attend to practical problems the patient cannot take care of, such as managing finances.[47] Family members can help the nurse to understand and know the patient, especially patients who are unable to communicate.

Sharing Concerns

Sharing concerns with a caring and understanding listener can relieve some of the patient's spiritual and emotional distress. The patient is consoled knowing that he or she is not alone and that someone knows and cares about what is being experienced (as mentioned earlier in the discussion of suicidal ideation).[19,20,48] Although the patient may share concerns with family members, she or he may be reluctant to upset loved ones further or may have a family among whom such communication is not the norm. A patient who relies on this coping mechanism will benefit from a nurse who recognizes when the patient needs to talk and who knows how to listen.

Coping Assessment

Ineffective coping may be suggested by patient behaviors. Overt hostility, severe regression, or noncompliance with treatment may suggest ineffective coping. The patient may also report such problems as severe anxiety, despondence, or despair. The nurse who suspects that coping is ineffective should consider a number of factors before questioning the patient directly.[20] It is not always clear whether the patient's coping is truly ineffective or whether intervention by the nurse is indicated. Witnessing problematic behavior can be very uncomfortable, especially when that behavior is directed at the caregiver. Careful evaluation of one's reaction to the behavior is needed to discover whether patient care can continue to be provided objectively by the nurse alone or whether consultation with others on the team is needed to alleviate the problem.[13,19]

Enhancing the Coping Process
Supporting the Patient

Attention to the total patient is an ultimate goal of nursing care. Nightingale believed that it was "unthinkable to consider sick humans as mere bodies who could be treated in isolation from their minds and spirits."[44] Essential techniques for effective interventions include an attitude of caring; openness and warmth; and withholding judgment until you know the patient (have an understanding of the individual's self-perception), the current illness or problem, and the type of social support available. Assessment skills are essential, as is a willingness to become involved when the potential or actual use of ineffective coping mechanisms exists.

Teaching the patient new coping skills may be impossible, because individuals have a repertoire of conscious and unconscious defense and coping mechanisms that automatically come into play when they are facing a stressful situation. A person who is experiencing extreme psychological stress cannot learn new methods to manage these defense mechanisms. However, the nurse may help to reduce the level of anxiety by employing active listening, by encouraging support from family members and other caregivers, and by introducing changes in the environment as appropriate. In doing so, the nurse can facilitate the changes the patient must make. It is extremely important that the patient express an interest in learning and recognize a personal need for help.[10,46]

A patient's trust in the nurse's competence in the physical and technical aspects of care aids in the patient's participation. Hope is instilled when the nurse and other caregivers display a sense of realistic optimism regarding the patient's progress. It is essential that patients receive honest feedback, as patients are keen observers of their caregivers and read them well. Trust and hope are easily lessened when inappropriate information is given.

Supporting Family Members

Patient-centered care is also family-centered care. Consideration of nonbiological or nonlegal partners of the patient as members of the patient's support system is also necessary in providing holistic care. The nurse's support of family members at the bedside can enhance the value of the visits for the patient. Patients often look to the family for love, understanding, support, and for care of matters to which they cannot attend themselves. The nurse can observe the quality of the patient-family interaction and formulate interventions that will aid the family in supporting the patient.[19,49,50]

Illness of a family member can be a hardship on the whole family. The illness (or death) of a patient can affect the health of other family members—particularly an elderly spouse.[22,47] Reactions to the stress are similar to the emotions experienced by the patient. The extended waiting time between visits with the patient, lack of information or misinterpretation of information, disruption in family roles and routines, being in an unfamiliar and challenging environment, and worry over outcomes, finances, and additional responsibilities can be overwhelming. Disorganization and emotional turmoil may result. Sleep deprivation is a frequent experience leading to confusion and inability to make decisions.

Family members also may react to the crisis with expressions of anger and hostility toward the patient or staff, or they may be immobilized.[23,40] The family member may be at a loss for what to say or do during visits with the patient. The nurse might find some words to put the family member at ease and offer a suggestion for what to say to his or her loved one.

If the family member is so upset that he or she completely loses composure, a brief attempt at supporting this family member away from the bedside may be an adequate intervention. In doing so, the nurse may determine that the family member needs the assistance of a consistent outside source of support and therefore may consult with another member of the health care team, such as a psychiatric nurse consultant, pastor or chaplain, or social worker.

Communication between family members and the health care team is crucial, especially when patients are critically ill. Satisfaction and understanding the events and course of treatment in critical care by patients and their families are increasingly recognized as indicators of care quality for the critical care experiences.[51] Family members have their own issues to deal with when their loved ones are critically ill. Oftentimes family members are overwhelmed, and may be at higher risk for depression, thus diminishing the support that they can offer to their loved one.[52]

Family members use a variety of coping mechanisms. Various factors impact how family members cope, including previous experience with critical care, uncertainty of treatment outcomes, suddenness of the critical event, and availability of support for themselves.[53] Another population of patients often found in critical care or a progressive unit are those who have a chronic critical illness. This condition introduces a whole other phenomenon for family members to deal with while supporting their loved ones. The uncertainness and lack of stability with the patient who has a chronic yet critical illness can lead to anxiety, depression, and posttraumatic stress disorder. Therefore, there needs to be support and early and ongoing screening for symptoms of psychological distress in family members.[54]

Families often must deal with the impending death of a loved one when the patient's condition deteriorates despite all efforts. Anticipatory grief is a process that is filled with emotional upheaval and can be as intense as when the loved one actually dies.[55-57] At such times, family members are particularly sensitive to the nurse's words and actions and may misinterpret them as signs of indifference. This may be particularly true for nontraditional family members. It is essential that the health care team conveys understanding and acceptance of the patient and his or her family. Some interventions that are meaningful to the family are reassurance that the patient is receiving adequate pain medication, telling the family what to expect as the dying process progresses, and helping them to comfort the patient with their presence. After the death, family members should be allowed to spend some time alone with the patient; be supportive of them as they work through their grief. Recognizing cultural and religious factors and incorporating them into the plan of care is also beneficial to the family.[24,38]

Supporting Spiritual Care

Spiritual needs assessment is often inadequate when patients are asked only about their religious affiliation. If no affiliation is mentioned, no further questions are asked of the patient regarding spiritual matters. Spirituality is a basic human phenomenon that helps create meaning in the world and can be experienced before any awareness of religious beliefs.[39,58] Separation from philosophical and religious rituals and ties, together with intense suffering, can induce spiritual distress for patients and their families. Some individuals may question their very existence and may even display anger toward religious representatives. Others may view their illness as fate or just punishment and resist help, give up, and wait to die.[59] Philosophical belief practices can directly affect caregiving practices such as diet, hygiene, and rituals surrounding birth, death, and medical interventions. The nurse should have a basic understanding of the various religious tenets of Eastern and Western philosophies and how they may affect a patient's plan of care.[10,43,44] Patients can easily succumb to feelings of helplessness and powerlessness in the technological, impersonalized environment of the ICU.

Including a pastor or chaplain on the health care team is also an important aspect of holistic care. The chaplain may be the best person to assess spiritual needs and to assist patients and their families in coping with the crisis. Providing access to religious rituals, prayer, scriptures, and readings is a meaningful strategy to help alleviate stress for patients and their families. The patient, with the help of the agency chaplain, pastor, or counselor, can identify inner resources of strength, meaning, and purpose to help cope with the crisis event. The spiritual leader is also valuable in ethical decisions such as termination of life support. Moreover, the spiritual advisor can be of great assistance to the health care team as their own personal resources are drained as a result of the sustained or cumulative assistance they have provided to others in crisis.[44]

Spiritual health has been found to be associated with hardiness, a composite measure composed of commitment, challenge, a sense of control, and a mark of psychological health.[24,44,58] Spiritual well-being also can refer to one's valuing of goodness, love, and relatedness to others or a general feeling of having a purposeful and fulfilled life.

Supporting Complementary Therapies

The field of complementary therapies is evolving. The purpose of these therapies and practices is to help maintain wellness and, when necessary, to facilitate the body's own healing responses to restore balance and harmony. Integrative health care implies blending conventional health care with complementary therapies, accompanied by open communications among practitioners and conscious recognition of the possible synergy. Integrative health care, like nursing, holds a holistic philosophy.

Interest in complementary therapies has increased dramatically in the past decade, and the national demand for these services has reached unprecedented levels. Time trends have been examined, revealing that almost 70% of adults in the United States had used at least one complementary therapy in their lifetime.[60] The number of hospitals providing complementary therapies is also growing. Nursing, in turn, is returning to those holistic roots with an increased awareness and integration of complementary therapies. Today, nursing combines biomedical understanding of disease and treatment with the caring behaviors and treatments that have been part of holistic nursing practice throughout history.[61]

REFERENCES

1. Selye H: *Stress in health and disease*, Boston, 1976, Butterworth.
2. Bauer S: *Psychological and immunological correlates of surviving breast cancer dissertation*, Chicago, 1997, Rush University.
3. Motzer SA, et al: Natural killer cell function and psychological distress in women with and without irritable bowel syndrome, *Biol Res Nurs* 4(1):31, 2002.
4. Dropkin MJ: Anxiety, coping strategies, and coping behaviors in patients undergoing head and neck cancer surgery, *Cancer Nurs* 24(2):143, 2001.
5. Morse J, Penrod J: Linking concepts of enduring, uncertainty, suffering, and hope, *Image J Nurs Sch* 31(2):145, 1999.
6. Tusaie K, Dyer J: Resilience: a historical review of the construct, *Holist Nurs Pract* 18(1):3, 2004.
7. Wagnild G, Young H: Development of psychometric evaluation of the resilience scale, *J Nurs Meas* 1(2):165, 1993.
8. Doenges ME, Moorhouse MF: *Nurse's pocket guide: diagnoses, interventions, and rationales*, ed 7, Philadelphia, 2004, FA Davis.
9. Porth C: *Pathophysiology: concepts of altered health states*, ed 5, Philadelphia, 1998, JB Lippincott.
10. Stuart G: A stress adaptation model of psychiatric nursing care. In Stuart GW, editor: *Principles and practices of psychiatric nursing*, ed 6, St Louis, 2004, Mosby.
11. O'Leary A, et al: Stress and immune function. In Miller T, editor: *Clinical disorders and stressful life events*, Madison, Conn., 1997, International Universities.
12. McFarland G, McFarland E: *Nursing diagnosis and interventions*, ed 3, St Louis, 1997, Mosby.
13. Nield-Anderson L, et al: Responding to 'difficult' patients, *Am J Nurs* 99(12):27, 1999.
14. Hollinger-Smith L: Growth and development across the life span. In Fortinash K, Holoday-Worret P, editors: *Psychiatric mental health nursing*, ed 3, St Louis, 2004, Mosby.
15. Radwin LE, Alster K: Individualized nursing care: an empirically generated definition, *Int Nurs Rev* 49(1):54, 2002.
16. Morse J: Responding to threats to integrity of self, *ANS Adv Nurs Sci* 19(4):21, 1999.
17. Herth K: Abbreviated instrument to measure hope: development and psychometric evaluation, *J Adv Nurs* 17(10):1251, 1992.
18. Stein K: Schema model of the self-concept, *Image J Nurs Sch* 27(3):187, 1995.
19. Snyder M, et al: Use of presence in the critical care unit, *AACN Clin Issues* 11(1):27, 2000.
20. Minarik P: Psychosocial intervention with ineffective coping responses to physical illness: depression-related. In Barry P, editor: *Psychosocial nursing*, ed 3, Philadelphia, 1996, JB Lippincott.
21. Morse J, Doberneck B: Delineating the concept of hope, *Image J Nurs Sch* 27(4):277, 1995.
22. Wheeler RW: Helping families cope with death and dying, *Nursing* 26(7):25, 1996.
23. Czerwiec M: When a loved one is dying: families talk about nursing care, *Am J Nurs* 96(5):32, 1996.
24. Spector R: *Cultural diversity in health and illness*, ed 6, Upper Saddle River, N.J., 2003, Prentice-Hall Health.
25. Durham E, Weiss L: How patients die, *Am J Nurs* 97(12):41, 1997.
26. Powers P, et al: The value of patient- and family-centered care, *Am J Nurs* 100(5):84, 2000.
27. Pettie D, Triolo A: Illness as evolution: the search for identity and meaning in the recovery process, *Psychiatr Rehabil J* 22(3):255, 1999.
28. Nussbaum GB: Spirituality in critical care: patient comfort and satisfaction, *Crit Care Nurs Q* 26(3):214, 2003.
29. Hagerty B, Patusky KL: Mood disorders: depression and mania. In Fortinash K, Holoday-Worret P, editors: *Psychiatric mental health nursing*, ed 3, St. Louis, 2004, Mosby.
30. Badger JM, et al: Reaching out to the suicidal patient, *Am J Nurs* 95(3):24, 1995.
31. Robie D, et al: Suicide prevention protocol, *Am J Nurs* 99(12):53, 1999.
32. Lazarus R, Lazarus B: *Passion and reason: making sense of emotions*, New York, 1994, Oxford University.
33. Neurnberger P: *Freedom from stress: a holistic approach*, Honesdale, Pa., 1981, Himalayan International Institute of Yoga Science and Philosophy.
34. Aguilera DC: *Crisis intervention: theory and methodology*, ed 7, St Louis, 1998, Mosby.
35. Holoday-Worret P: Foundations of psychiatric mental health nursing. In Fortinash K, Holoday-Worret P, editors: *Psychiatric mental health nursing*, ed 3, St Louis, 2004, Mosby.
36. Beyers M: The new reality, *J Nurs Adm* 26(6):5, 1996.
37. Beyea S: Collaboration in health practice. In Blais K, et al: *Professional nursing practice: concepts and perspectives*, ed 4, Menlo Park, Calif., 2001, Addison Wesley.
38. Czerwiec M: When a loved one is dying: families talk about nursing care, *Am J Nurs* 96(5):32, 1996.
39. O'Neill D, Kenny E: Spirituality and chronic illness, *Image J Nurs Sch* 30(3):275, 1998.
40. In Phillips S, Benner P, editors: *The crisis of care: affirming and restoring caring practices in helping professions*, Washington, D.C., 1994, Georgetown University.
41. Sumner C: Recognizing and responding to spiritual distress, *Am J Nurs* 98(1):26, 1998.
42. Armentrout D: Heart cry: a biblical model of depression, *Journal of Psychology & Theology* 14(2):101, 1995.
43. Dossey B, Dossey L: Holistic modalities and healing moments, *Am J Nurs* 98(6):44, 1998.
44. Gillman J: Religious perspectives on organ donation, *Crit Care Nurs Q* 22(3):19, 1999.

45. Holt-Ashley M: Nurses pray: use of prayer and spirituality as complementary therapy in the intensive care setting, *AACN Clin Issues* 11(1):60, 2000.

46. Lövgren G, et al: A care policy and its implementation, *Int J Nurs Pract* 7(2):92, 2001.

47. Johnson S, et al: Perceived changes in adult family members' roles and responsibilities during critical illness, *Image J Nurs Res* 27(3):238, 1995.

48. Marcus P: Suicide. In Fortinash K, Holoday-Worret P, editors: *Psychiatric mental health nursing*, ed 3, St Louis, 2004, Mosby.

49. Johnson C, et al: Racial and gender differences in quality of life following kidney transplantation, *Image J Nurs Sch* 30(2):125, 1998.

50. Carroll RG: Psychosocial foundations. In Black JM, Hawks JH, editors: *Medical-Surgical nursing*, ed 8, St Louis, 2009, Saunders.

51. Jacobowski NL, et al: Communication in critical care: family rounds in the intensive care unit, *Am J Crit Care* 19(5):421, 2010.

52. Hickman RL, et al: Informational coping style and depressive symptoms in family decision makers, *Am J Crit Care* 19(5):410, 2010.

53. Casarini KA, Gorayeb R, Basile Filho A: Coping by relatives of critical care patients, *Heart Lung* 38(3):217, 2009.

54. Hickman RL, Douglas SL: Impact of chronic critical illness on the psychological outcomes of family members, *AACN Adv Crit Care* 21(1):80, 2010.

55. Wheeler RW: Helping families cope with death and dying, *Nursing* 26(7):25, 1996.

56. Durham E: How patients die, *Am J Nurs* 97(12):41, 1997.

57. Buchanan H, et al: Trauma bereavement program: review of development and implementation, *Crit Care Nurs Q* 19(1):35, 1996.

58. Frankl V: *Man's search for meaning*, New York, 1959, Washington Square Press.

59. Shelly J: *Spiritual care: a guide for caregivers*, Downers Grove, Ill., 2000, InterVarsity Press.

60. Kessler R, et al: Long-term trends in the use of complementary and alternative medical therapies in the United States, *Ann Intern Med* 135(4):262, 2001.

61. Libster M: *Demonstrating care: the art of integrative nursing*, Independence, Ky., 2001, Thompson Delmar Learning.

Sleep Alterations

Linda D. Urden

OBJECTIVES

- Define the stages of sleep.
- Explain the physiological effects that occur during rapid eye movement (REM) sleep.
- Describe changes in sleep resulting from the aging process.
- Name three commonly prescribed critical care medications that decrease REM sleep.
- Describe evidence-based practice methods for promoting sleep in critical care.
- Compare and contrast obstructive sleep apnea with central sleep apnea.

Nurses who have an appreciation of the importance of sleep place a priority on protection of patients' sleep.[1] Health care providers may interrupt a patient's sleep for assessment or treatments; in addition, sleep can be disturbed by pain, anxiety, or environmental noise.[2] A recent study indicated that critical care nurses "group" nursing care activities together and attempt to limit interruptions, especially during the night. The use of light among nurses during the nighttime in surgical intensive care units appears to be individualized. Sleep interruptions occur most frequently at the beginning and end of the nursing shifts.[3] Although prioritizing care is essential, the consequence of sleep interruptions is not merely sleep-deprived patients; alterations in sleep patterns can delay physical and mental healing.[1] To facilitate sleep and healing, critical care nurses need to understand the essentials of sleep and chronobiology, the effect of pharmacological therapy on sleep, and the consequences of disrupted sleep. The purpose of this chapter is to acquaint nurses with the characteristics of normal human sleep, changes in sleep associated with aging and pharmacological treatment, and abnormal sleep patterns that may affect critically ill patients. Evidence-based nursing care for critically ill patients with sleep disturbances is discussed.

NORMAL HUMAN SLEEP

Sleep Physiology

Humans spend about one third of their lives engaged in a process known as *sleep*. Although little is now known about the physiological process or the depths to which it affects us, researchers are learning more about sleep every day. The behavioral definition of sleep is a reversible behavioral state of perceptual disengagement from and unresponsiveness to the environment.[4] Sleep is a basic human need, just as food and water are. For patients to regain and maintain their optimal physical and emotional health, they must be able to get adequate amounts of quality sleep. To help patients obtain their optimal amount of sleep, a nurse must first understand what constitutes normal sleep and how the nursing plan of care can contribute to accomplishing this goal.

Polysomnography (PSG) is the collection of multiple channels of physiological data to assess sleep and its disorders using various electrodes.[5] Electroencephalographic (EEG) electrodes are attached to the patient's scalp to measure brain waves. Changes in the EEG frequency (number of waveforms) and amplitude (height of waveform) over the course of the study allow the sleep to be scored into stages. Sleep stages are distinguished primarily by the EEG waveforms they produce. Sleep is scored by each 30-second epoch or segment of the tracing. The criteria for scoring sleep in infants differ from those used for adults.

Electrooculography (EOG) measures eye movement activity. The study can help to determine when the patient is in rapid eye movement (REM) sleep; it also can establish when sleep onset occurs as reflected by slow, rolling eye movements. Electromyography (EMG) involves leads placed over various muscle groups. When placed over the chin, the leads can help detect muscle atonia associated with REM sleep. Intercostal leads detect respiratory effort, whereas leads over the anterior tibialis detect leg movements that may be causing the patient to arouse. The electrocardiogram (ECG) shows any cardiac abnormalities, oximetry monitors the oxygen saturation levels, and piezoelastic bands around the chest and abdomen detect respiratory disorders such as apnea. Thermocouples are used to monitor airflow through the nose and mouth.

SLEEP STAGES

Non-Rapid Eye Movement Sleep

Humans experience three states of sleep. They are awake, in REM sleep, or in non-rapid eye movement (NREM) sleep. NREM sleep can be further divided into stages 1 through 4, with each stage being a progressively deeper sleep state. Adults usually enter sleep through NREM stage 1 sleep, which is a transitional, lighter sleep state from which the patient can be easily aroused by light touch or by someone softly calling his or her name. Stage 1 comprises 2% to 5% of a night's sleep and is demonstrated by an EEG pattern of low-voltage, mixed-frequency waveforms with vertex sharp waves. The EOG during stage 1 may demonstrate slow, side-to-side eye movements. A patient with severely disrupted sleep may experience an increase in the length of stage 1 sleep throughout the sleep cycle. As a patient makes the transition from awake to asleep, a brief memory impairment may occur.[6] As a result, the patient may not remember educational or care instructions given by the nurse during the transition between sleep and wake states. Patients sometimes may experience muscle jerks and recall vivid images on awakening. This is called hypnic myoclonia; although not pathological, it can cause the patient to awaken feeling frightened.

Stage 2 NREM sleep occupies about 45% to 55% of the night, with sleep deepening and a higher arousal threshold being required to awaken the patient. Changes seen in the EEG pattern include sleep spindles and K complexes. As stage 2 continues, high-voltage, slow-wave activity begins to appear. When these slow waves represent 20% of the EEG activity per page, the criteria are met for stage 3 sleep, which constitutes 3% to 8% of the cycle. In stage 3 NREM sleep, slow waves continue to develop until 50% of the EEG waveforms are slow wave; this is called stage 4 sleep. Stage 4 comprises 10% to 15% of the cycle. Stages 3 and 4 often are combined and referred to as *slow-wave sleep,* or *delta sleep.* Delta sleep has the highest arousal threshold. NREM sleep usually occupies

70% to 75% of the sleep cycle, with REM sleep comprising 20% to 25%.

NREM sleep is dominated by the parasympathetic nervous system. The body tries to maintain a homeostatic regulation, and this causes a decreased level of energy expenditure. Blood pressure, heart and respiratory rates, and the metabolic rate return to basal levels. EMG levels are lower in NREM as opposed to wake states, but not as low as in REM sleep. Sweating or shivering that a patient may experience with temperature extremes occurs during NREM sleep, but this ceases during REM sleep.[4]

During slow-wave sleep, 80% of the total daily growth-stimulating hormone is released, which works to stimulate protein synthesis while sparing catabolic breakdown. The release of other hormones, such as prolactin and testosterone, suggests that anabolism is occurring during slow-wave sleep. Cortisol release peaks during early morning hours, whereas melatonin is released only during darkness, and thyroid-stimulating hormone is inhibited during sleep. The activities associated with stage 4 NREM sleep include protein synthesis and tissue repair, such as the repair of epithelial cells and specialized cells of the brain, skin, bone marrow, and gastric mucosa.[7] Some theorize that NREM sleep is a restorative period that relieves the stresses of waking activities, whereas REM sleep serves to refuel creative brain stores.

Rapid Eye Movement Sleep

REM sleep occupies about 20% to 25% of the night in healthy young adults and is sometimes known as the *dream stage.* However, dreaming is not the exclusive property of any one stage. REM can be viewed as a highly active brain in a paralyzed body and is frequently referred to as a *paradoxical sleep.* The paradox is that some areas of the brain remain very active, whereas others are suppressed. EEG waveforms are relatively slow voltage, and sawtooth waves are present. Increased cortical activity occurs, with the EEG pattern resembling those of the wake state. Synchronized bursts of rapid, side-to-side eye movements with suppressed EMG activity (muscle atonia) are seen, indicating functional paralysis of the skeletal muscles. Infants enter sleep onset through REM and spend about 50% of their night in REM sleep.

The sympathetic nervous system predominates during REM sleep.[7] Oxygen consumption increases and blood pressure, cardiac output, and respiratory and heart rates become variable. The body's response to decreased oxygen levels and increased carbon dioxide levels is lowest during REM sleep. Cardiac efferent vagus nerve tone is generally suppressed during REM sleep, and irregular breathing patterns can lead to oxygen reduction, particularly in patients with pulmonary or cardiac disease. An increase in premature ventricular contractions and tachydysrhythmias may be associated with respiratory pauses during REM sleep.[7] Arterial pressure surges and increases in heart rate, coronary arterial tone, and blood viscosity may cause the combination of plaque rupture and hypercoagulability in persons with cardiac disease.[8]

Sleep Cycles

NREM and REM sleep cycles alternate throughout the night. Sleep onset usually occurs in stage 1 sleep, progressing through stages 2 to 4, and then going back to stage 2, at which time the person usually enters REM. This first cycle typically takes about 70 to 100 minutes, with later cycles lasting 90 to 120 minutes. Four to five cycles are completed during normal adult sleep. NREM sleep predominates during the first third of the night, whereas REM is more prominent during the last third. Brief episodes of wakefulness (usually less than 5%) tend to intrude later into the night and are usually not remembered the next morning.

The amount of sleep required is uncertain. No set number of hours has been established, and sleep length may be determined by many factors, including genetic predisposition. A sufficient amount of sleep has been achieved when one awakens without external stimuli and gets through the day without feeling sleepy.

SLEEP CHANGES IN AGING

Important changes in sleep occur with aging, and critical care nurses must consider these changes when planning care for older patients. Assessment for sleep disturbances in the older adult is essential, because lack of sleep can compromise daytime function, thereby lowering quality of life.[9]

Older adults most commonly complain about excessive sleepiness or insomnia, and current research offers justification for both of these complaints.[10] Sleep pattern changes in older adults include fewer episodes of stages 3 and 4 NREM and REM sleep.[11] Older adults also report that they do not sleep as soundly or feel as rested after awakening.[12] One reason for this may be that older adults do not consolidate their sleep into one session. They may go to bed, awake 4 hours later, stay awake for an extended period, and then go back to sleep, resulting in fragmented sleep patterns.[9] Many of the diseases associated with aging may contribute to these nocturnal arousals, including diabetes, nocturia, cardiovascular symptoms, chronic pain, and depression.[9,13,14] Sleep-related respiratory disorders and increased incidence of periodic leg movements in older adults may further disrupt their sleep.[15] Increasing age brings many physical and social changes with which older adults must cope. Assessment of older patients must always include sleep history as an indicator of mental health, because depression is a common struggle for older adults.[16]

In critical care areas, nurses need to identify these altered sleep patterns as well as other impediments to adequate rest and methods to minimize acute disruption of sleep while accommodating age-related changes in sleep patterns. Authorities on sleep[17] recommend the use of nonpharmacological means to promote sleep, such as control of environmental noise and light, use of white noise, music, massage, and allowing specified blocks of time for sleep. It is also important for nurses to educate patients about the changes in sleep that result from aging and to teach sleep hygiene practices such as adhering to regular bedtimes and rising times and avoiding napping.

PHARMACOLOGY AND SLEEP

Many drugs essential to treatment of critically ill patients impact sleep quality (Table 5-1).[18-21] It is important to understand the relationship between various medications and the sleep of patients in the critical care unit. Pathophysiology and age may profoundly affect not only medication absorption and elimination but also how patients cope with their illness and their ability to maintain health.

ABNORMAL SLEEP

Sleep Apnea Syndrome

Sleep apnea syndrome, sometimes called *sleep-disordered breathing*, occurs when airflow is absent or reduced. Apnea during sleep can be divided into three types: (1) obstructive, (2) central, and (3) mixed. In obstructive apnea, the absence of airflow is caused by an obstruction in the upper airway. Complete obstruction lasting 10 seconds or longer is referred to as an obstructive apnea, whereas a partial obstruction is known as a hypopnea. In central apnea, airflow is absent because of lack of ventilatory muscle effort. The third type of sleep apnea syndrome, mixed apnea, occurs when a combination of obstructive and central patterns occurs in a single apneic event. An apnea-hypopnea index (the number of apneas and hypopneas per hour divided by the hours of sleep) of 5 or greater is diagnostic of sleep apnea syndrome. With new understandings of alterations in ventilatory effort, researchers have developed the respiratory distress index (RDI). To calculate the index, the total number of apneas and hypopneas plus the number of respiratory effort-related arousals (RERAs) or other respiratory events is divided by the hours of sleep. An RDI greater than 5 in addition to reports of daytime sleepiness supports a diagnosis of sleep apnea.[22]

All types of sleep apnea syndrome are accompanied by arterial desaturation and potentially by hypoxemia, which may cause pulmonary vasoconstriction and an increased systemic vascular resistance. However, desaturation and hypoxemia are most severe in the obstructive type. Although the pathophysiology of OSA is unclear, research findings indicate that the various types of sleep apnea are all part of a disease continuum. Failure of the central respiratory rhythm control center to generate a stable rhythm is thought to be the basic defect responsible for sleep apnea syndrome. Cyclic oscillations occur with greater frequency at night and are further exacerbated by mouth breathing.[23]

Obstructive Sleep Apnea
Definition, Etiology, and Pathophysiology

OSA syndrome occurs when at least five apnea or hypopnea events per hour of sleep occur as the result of an obstruction in the upper airway. In the general population, between 3% and 7% of people have severe OSA.[24] The incidence of OSA

TABLE 5-1	PHARMACOLOGICAL MANAGEMENT: DRUGS THAT AFFECT SLEEP AND WAKEFULNESS		
MEDICATION CLASS AND DRUG GROUP	**EXAMPLES**	**EFFECTS**	**COMMENTS**
Hypnotics[18]			
Benzodiazepines		↓ SWS, ↑ TST, ↓ WASO, ↓ stage 1 sleep, mild REM suppression	↑ Apnea, ↑ daytime residual sedation, mild respiratory depression, ↓ psychomotor function
Immediate-acting	Quazepam	Half-life of 20-120 hr	
	Temazepam	Half-life of 8-20 hr	
Long-acting	Flurazepam, HCl	Half-life of 40-250 hr	
Rapid-acting	Triazolam	Half-life of 2-6 hr	Rebound insomnia
	Estazolam	Half-life of 8-24 hr	
Nonbenzodiazepines		No effect on REM or SWS	
Rapid-acting	Zolpidem	Half-life of 1 hr	
	Zaleplon	Half-life of 1 hr	No cognitive or performance impairment; ↓ abuse potential; may be taken in middle of night
Intermediate-acting	Eszopiclone	Half-life of 5-7 hr	May cause impairment of activities the next day
Wake-Promoting Medications[19]			
Nicotine		↑ SL, ↓ TST, ↓ REM	
Amphetamines		↓ REM, ↓ SWS, ↓ TST, ↑ WASO	Less daytime fatigue
Nonsympathomimetics	Xanthine derivatives: coffee, chocolate, tea; scopolamine; strychnine; pentylenetetrazol; modafinil	↓ TST, ↓ REM, ↓ SWS, ↑ SL, ↑ WASO	
Direct sympathomimetics	Isoproterenol, epinephrine, norepinephrine, phenylephrine, phenylpropanolamine, apomorphine	↑ Wakefulness, ↑ REM onset, ↓ fatigue, ↓ sleepiness	↑ Blood pressure, ↓ heart rate
Indirect sympathomimetics	Amphetamine, methamphetamine, cocaine, piperacillin (Pipradrol), methylphenidate, tyramine	↑ WASO, ↑ daytime SL, ↓ sleepiness	Narcolepsy treatment, ↑ cognitive tasks
	Pemoline		Possible liver damage
Antihypertensives[20]			
β-Antagonists	Propranolol, metoprolol	↑ Wakefulness, TWT, SL, ↓ REM	Insomnia, nightmares
α₂-Agonists	Atenolol, clonidine	↓ REM, ↓ TST in hypertensives, ↑ TST in normal subjects	Nightmares, sedation, ↓ concentration, mental slowing
Methyldopa		↑ REM, ↑ TST	Sedation, insomnia, nightmares
Diuretics	Hydrochlorothiazide, chlorthalidone, indapamide	No data	CNS effects unlikely
Vasodilators	Hydralazine	No data	Depression, insomnia, anxiety
Catecholamine depletors	Reserpine	↑ REM and stage shifts	
Calcium antagonists	Verapamil, nifedipine, diltiazem, amlodipine, felodipine, nisoldipine	No data	Insomnia, nightmares, depression, sedation, difficulty concentrating

TABLE 5-1 PHARMACOLOGICAL MANAGEMENT: DRUGS THAT AFFECT SLEEP AND WAKEFULNESS—cont'd

MEDICATION CLASS AND DRUG GROUP	EXAMPLES	EFFECTS	COMMENTS
Antihistamines[20]			
H₁ antihistamines (chem. class: selective histamine H₁-receptor antagonist)	Diphenhydramine, hydroxyzine, triprolidine	↑ Drowsiness, ↓ SL	Impaired daytime performance
H₁ antihistamines (chem. class: ethanolamine derivative H₁-receptor antagonist)	Loratadine, terfenadine	No sedation effects	
H₂ antagonists	Cimetidine, ranitidine	May cause insomnia or somnolence	Drowsiness in patients; renal impairment
Antidepressants[20]			
Tricyclic antidepressants	Amitriptyline, doxepin, imipramine (Trimipramine), clomipramine, desipramine, nortriptyline, protriptyline	↑ TST, ↓ wakefulness	↓ Psychomotor and cognitive performance and daytime drowsiness
Selective serotonin reuptake inhibitors	Fluoxetine	↑ TST, ↑ wakefulness, ↑ stage 1, ↑ SEM	Mild ↑ in psychomotor performance
	Paroxetine	↑ Wakefulness, ↓ TST, ↑ stage 1, ↑ SL	
	Sertraline	No data	Insomnia 7-16%
	Fluvoxamine	↓ TST, ↑ wakefulness, ↑ stage 1, ↑ SL	
	Citalopram	No change	Insomnia, no impairment in performance
	Trazodone	Variable, may ↑ TST, ↓ SL	↓ Cognitive performance in elderly
Monoamine oxidase inhibitors	Phenelzine, tranylcypromine, moclobemide, brofaromine	↑ Daytime sleepiness because of ↓ TST, ↑ wakefulness	Some improved psychomotor performance
Other Compounds Used for Insomnia[21]			
Melatonin (hormone)		↓ SL, ↑ TST	Study results are mixed, nonaddictive
Valerian (plant extract)		↓ SL, ↓ WASO	Side effects include headache and rare morning drowsiness

REM, Rapid eye movement; *SEM*, slow eye movement; *SL*, sleep latency; *SWS*, slow-wave sleep; *TST*, total sleep time; *TWT*, total wakefulness time; *WASO*, wakefulness after sleep onset.

is believed to increase with age. Consequences include chronic hypoventilation syndrome; arousals that fragment sleep; cardiovascular changes such as hypertension, stroke, ischemic heart disease, insulin resistance, ventricular hypertrophy; and nocturnal angina.[25] Because of the cardiovascular complications and accidents caused by sleepiness, such as motor vehicle accidents, job related injuries, falls, and other nonintentional accidents related to lack of concentration, OSA is a significant condition that should be effectively evaluated.

The cause of OSA is not entirely understood; however, upper airway structure, hormonal balance, and neural control are implicated. Factors that contribute to OSA are (1) anatomic narrowing of the upper airway, (2) increased compliance of the upper airway tissue, (3) reflexes affecting upper airway caliber, and (4) pharyngeal inspiratory muscle

function.[26] Computed tomographic studies of awake subjects have shown that patients with OSA have narrower airways than normal subjects do. The narrower the airway, the more easily it may become obstructed (Figure 5-1).

Upper airway patency is also affected by upper airway function, which is under the control of the respiratory motor neurons. During sleep, this control varies and causes decreased neural activity, thereby narrowing the airway. This effect is especially prevalent during REM sleep, when the motor neurons are hypotonic. Unstable control of the respiratory nerves of the diaphragmatic, intercostal, and upper airway muscles can cause sleep apneas.[23] Hypothyroidism can alter respiratory controls and thereby contribute to OSA. Other contributing disorders are exogenous obesity, kyphoscoliosis, and autonomic dysfunction.

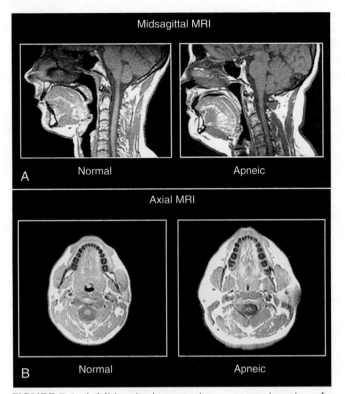

Midsagittal MRI

A   Normal   Apneic

Axial MRI

B   Normal   Apneic

FIGURE 5-1 *A,* Midsagittal magnetic resonance imaging of a normal subject *(left)* and a subject with sleep apnea *(right).* Notice the narrowing of the trachea and the elongated soft palate. *B,* Axial image of a normal subject *(left)* and a subject with sleep apnea *(right).* Notice the diameter of the trachea in the subject with sleep apnea. (From Kryger MH et al, editors: *Principles and practice of sleep medicine,* ed 4, p. 990, Philadelphia, 2005, Saunders.)

The patient with OSA develops cycles of hypoxemia, hypercapnia, and acidosis with each episode of apnea until he or she is aroused and airflow resumes. Alveolar hypoventilation accompanies each episode of apnea and results in hypercapnia. Between episodes, alveolar ventilation improves so that overall there is no retention of carbon dioxide (CO_2).

With obstruction, inspiratory subatmospheric intrathoracic pressures are abnormally elevated. This leads to a tendency for airways to collapse, resulting in hemodynamic and electrocardiographic changes. The extremely elevated pressures that occur in individuals with OSA who have apneic episodes in REM and NREM stages cause systemic and pulmonary hypertension. Systemic pressures of 200/120 mm Hg (awake control: 130/80 mm Hg) and pulmonary artery pressures of 80/54 mm Hg (awake control: 30/20 mm Hg) have been reported.[27] Cardiac dysrhythmias associated with obstructive apnea include bradycardias, sinus arrest, and occasionally, second-degree heart blocks. After resumption of airflow, tachycardias commonly occur. Bradycardia-tachycardia syndrome is associated with OSA.[28]

Assessment and Diagnosis

Careful monitoring of oxygen saturation and breathing patterns can help the critical care nurse identify patients with this syndrome and assist in its diagnosis and treatment. Patients at risk for OSA may have the following symptoms: snoring; obesity; short, thick neck circumference; cardiovascular disease; systemic hypertension; pulmonary hypertension; sleep fragmentation; gastroesophageal reflux; and an impaired quality of life. Apneas may occur in people whose throats are abnormally small or collapsible. Muscles that would normally hold the throat open relax while the patient is asleep. Snoring is caused when those soft tissues in the throat vibrate. Snoring often precedes the complaint of daytime sleepiness, and the intensity increases with weight gain and alcohol ingestion.[26] Men with a collar size of 17 or greater and women with a size 16 or greater are thought to have an increased incidence of apnea. Friedman and others showed a clinical correlation between modified Mallampati grade (MMP), tonsil size, body mass index, and the severity of apnea. These assessments are used by anesthesiologists to determine intubation difficulty.[26] There is an increased incidence of sleep apnea among African Americans as well as Mexican Americans, and an increased incidence is observed among those with metabolic syndrome.

OSA episodes frequently end in brief EEG arousals. Patients may experience hundreds of arousals and not even realize they awaken hundreds of times during the night. These arousals cause sleep fragmentation and daytime sleepiness, which can lead to irritability, poor job performance, troubled relationships, depression, and impaired quality of life.

The definitive diagnosis of OSA syndrome is made with PSG during an overnight sleep study. PSG is used to determine the number and length of apnea episodes and sleep stages, number of arousals, airflow, respiratory effort, and oxygen desaturation.

Medical Management

For patients with mild OSA (apnea-hypopnea index of 5 to 10), weight loss, sleeping on the side if apneas are associated with sleeping on the back, avoidance of sedative medications and alcohol before bedtime, and avoidance of sleep deprivation may be all that is necessary. Oral appliances may be prescribed to stabilize the jaw or retain the tongue. These devices must be fitted by a dentist and are not always as effective as continuous positive airway pressure (CPAP). Moderate to severe levels of apnea may be treated with mechanical, surgical, or pharmacological therapy. Treatment can vary depending on the type and severity of illness.

CPAP via nasal mask is the treatment of choice. CPAP machines are simply pressure generators with the effective pressure being determined during the titration part of the PSG. This holds the airway open and prevents collapse. The patient wears a small, triangle-shaped mask over the nose or uses nasal pillows if the mask is not tolerated. CPAP treats the obstruction and the snoring, choking, and gasping that accompany it, and it provides cardiovascular benefits. Although CPAP is the treatment of choice, it is effective only if the patient is compliant with therapy. Regular attendance at CPAP clinics can improve patient compliance.[29] If a patient

- Make sure that the mask fits snugly.
- Maintain the prescribed airway pressure.
- Ensure that air is not leaking, especially to the eye area.
- Monitor skin integrity under the mask.
- Make sure that the patient does not experience gastric insufflation.
- Encourage compliance at home.

cannot tolerate the continuous pressure of CPAP, bimodal positive airway pressure (BiPAP), which provides separate pressures for inspiration and expiration, may be tried. Refer to Box 5-1 for nursing care of the patient using CPAP.

Various surgical interventions are available for the treatment of apnea and snoring. Patients with mild OSA or snoring alone may undergo an outpatient procedure called laser uvulopalatopharyngoplasty (LAUP), which uses lasers to remove excess tissue at the soft palate level. For patients who snore but do not have apnea, somnoplasty may provide relief. Somnoplasty involves inserting a small electrode into the soft palate and heating the tissue, causing the area to shrink and tighten.[30]

Uvulopalatopharyngoplasty (UPPP) was one of the earlier surgeries used to treat OSA. Essentially, a large tonsillectomy is performed and all redundant tissue is removed (Figure 5-2). Reports of success from UPPP vary widely, with 40% to 80% of patients experiencing sleep apnea improvement.[30,31] Complications include speech impairment, inability to eat, postoperative bleeding, and infection. Severe pain after UPPP is documented and may continue well into the postoperative period.[31] Although tracheostomy was the original surgical procedure used to treat OSA, it is now used only in the most severe cases of apnea that do not respond to other treatments. Bariatric surgery is an effective means to facilitate weight loss and subsequent improvement in OSA.[32]

Treatment of OSA with medication is usually a last resort and has proved to be very disappointing. Protriptyline has been shown to decrease apnea and reduce excessive daytime sleepiness by decreasing sleep apnea frequency that increases during REM sleep. Oxygen may be used to lower hypoxemia and nocturnal desaturations.

Nursing Management

The nurse's role in the management of sleep apnea includes educating the patient and family about the syndrome and the consequences of nonadherence with treatment regimens. This education may also include preoperative teaching for any surgical procedures such as UPPP. Monitoring of patients with OSA while in critical care should include assessment of the breathing patterns, hours of sleep, and pulse oximetry. Cautious administration of narcotics to patients with sleep apnea is suggested because of the potential for respiratory depression, although the concern regarding adequate pain relief is not well studied.

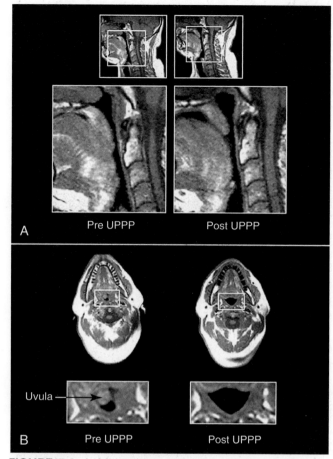

FIGURE 5-2 *A,* Midsagittal images of a patient before and after uvulopalatopharyngoplasty (UPPP). Notice the shortened uvula. Because the soft palate was not resected, the tracheal lumen remains narrow. *B,* Axial images at the level of the uvula; notice the significant increase in the diameter of the airway. (From Kryger MH et al, editors: *Principles and practice of sleep medicine,* ed 4, p. 996, Philadelphia, 2005, Saunders.)

Nasal CPAP is most effective when patients are properly fitted with the nasal mask and have clear instructions regarding its use. Several types and sizes of masks are available, including one type called a *nasal pillow,* which does not cover the nose but instead fits into the nostrils. If patients are admitted to the critical care unit with a history of OSA, they need to use their home CPAP mask and equipment as part of their regular sleep routine. The nurse can enhance compliance with the CPAP system. Nursing care includes ensuring proper fit of the CPAP mask, with no air blowing into the patient's eyes, correct airway pressure, no pressure sores from the mask, and no gastric insufflation.

UPPP patients are not usually admitted to critical care areas because the postoperative recovery does not require intensive care.[33] Postoperative monitoring after UPPP includes risk of aspiration, pain management, anxiety relief, patient education, and monitoring for respiratory complications, hemorrhage, infection, impaired speech, nutritional concerns, and sleep disturbance.

Central Sleep Apnea

Definition, Etiology, and Pathophysiology

Central sleep apnea (CSA) can be seen on PSG as an absence of airflow and respiratory effort for at least 10 seconds. A complete loss of electromyographic activity by the respiratory muscles would be expected since CSA is defined as a pause in respiration without ventilatory effort.[34]

A chemoreceptor sensitive to the levels of CO_2 resides within the brain. When CO_2 levels become excessive, ventilatory efforts are increased to blow off the excess CO_2. This negative-feedback loop exists to provide a homeostatic balance in the carbon dioxide and oxygen levels of the body. Whereas OSA results from an obstructed or collapsed airway, patients with CSA suffer from a lack of ventilatory effort. This can be observed in patients with cardiopulmonary disease (e.g., COPD) or heart failure, because their chemoreceptors have become adjusted to an increased CO_2 level. It is not uncommon for a patient who experiences CSA to also have some obstructive events.

CSA may result from many physiological or pathophysiological events.[35] Possible causes of nonhypercapnic CSA include periodic breathing at high altitude, renal or metabolic disturbances, and idiopathic central apnea seen at sea level. Hypercapnic CSA can occur in many neuromuscular conditions such as spinal cord or brain injury, encephalitis, brainstem neoplasm or infarcts, muscular dystrophy, myasthenia gravis, bulbar poliomyelitis, and postpolio syndrome.

Assessment and Diagnosis

Clinical characteristics of hypercapnic CSA include respiratory failure, cor pulmonale, peripheral edema, polycythemia, daytime sleepiness, and snoring. Patients with nonhypercapnic CSA have clinical features very similar to those of OSA. Nonhypercapnic CSA characteristics include daytime sleepiness, insomnia or poor sleep, mild or intermittent snoring, and awakenings accompanied by choking or feeling short of breath; frequently, the patients are of normal body weight. Diagnosis is made by overnight PSG or sleep study, which will determine the respiratory and sleep patterns of the patient.

Medical Management

Because there are two types of CSA, there are two therapeutic approaches depending on the cause of the apnea. The hypercapnic patient who has worsening hypoventilation during sleep is best served by nocturnal ventilation. Most such patients experience some respiratory muscle failure. One treatment for nonhypercapnic or heart failure patients is nasal CPAP, which also may provide a beneficial cardiovascular effect. Nocturnal oxygen supplementation may be effective as well. If CPAP is not tolerated, pharmacologic management may be tried. Medroxyprogesterone, a respiratory stimulant, may improve ventilation in selected patients.[34] Acetazolamide, a carbonic anhydrase inhibitor that can result in metabolic acidosis, also may decrease the frequency of apneic episodes.

Nursing Management

For the nurse caring for a patient with CSA, patient and family education about the patient's condition and treatment regimen can help to ensure patient compliance. The nurse needs to address any fear or anxiety about going to sleep. Nurses also need to caution patients to avoid alcohol and sedative medications. Weight loss is recommended if the patient is obese. The nurse needs to carefully monitor and assess the respiratory status of the patient.

REFERENCES

1. Evans JC, French DG: Sleep and healing in intensive care settings, *Dimens Crit Care Nurs* 14(4):189, 1995.
2. Celik S, et al: Sleep disturbance: the patient care activities applied at the night shift in the intensive care unit, *J Clin Nurs* 14(1):102, 2005.
3. Dunn H, Anderson MA, Hill PD: Nighttime lighting in intensive care units, *Crit Care Nurse* 30(3):31, 2010.
4. Carskadon MA, Dement WC: Normal human sleep: an overview. In Kryger MH, et al, editors: *Principles and practice of sleep medicine*, ed 4, Philadelphia, 2005, Saunders.
5. Rechtschaffen A, Kales A: *A manual of standardized terminology, techniques, and scoring system for sleep stages of human subjects*, Bethesda, Md., 1968, U.S. Department of Health, Education, and Welfare.
6. Douglas NJ: Respiratory physiology: control of ventilation. In Kryger MH, et al, editors: *Principles and practice of sleep medicine*, ed 4, Philadelphia, 2005, Saunders.
7. Davidhizar RE, et al: What nurses need to know about sleep, *J Nurs Sci* 1:61, 1995.
8. Krachman SL, et al: Sleep in the intensive care unit, *Chest* 107(6):1713, 1995.
9. Vitiello MV: Normal versus pathological sleep changes in aging humans. In Kuna ST, editor: *Sleep and respiration in aging*, St Louis, 1991, Mosby.
10. Ancoli-Israel S, et al: Identification and treatment of sleep problems in the elderly, *Sleep Med Rev* 1(1):3, 1997.
11. Ancoli-Israel S: Sleep problems in older adults: putting myths to bed, *Geriatrics* 52(1):20, 1997.
12. Buysse DJ, et al: Napping and 24-hour sleep/wake patterns in healthy elderly and young adults, *J Am Geriatr Soc* 40(8):779, 1992.
13. Bliwise DL: Normal aging. In Kryger MH, et al, editors: *Principles and practice of sleep medicine*, ed 4, Philadelphia, 2005, Saunders.
14. Bliwise DL, et al: Habitual sleep durations and health in a 50-65 year old population, *J Clin Epidemiol* 47(1):35, 1994.
15. Sloan E, Flint A: Circadian rhythms and psychiatric disorders in the elderly, *J Geriatr Psychiatry Neurol* 9(4):164, 1996.
16. Arbelaez JJ, et al: Depressive symptoms, inflammation, and ischemic stroke in older adults: a prospective analysis in the cardiovascular health study, *J Am Geriatr Soc* 55(11):1825, 2007.
17. Richards KC: Sleep promotion, *Crit Care Nurs Clin North Am* 8(1):39, 1996.

18. Mendelson WB: Hypnotic medications: Mechanisms of action and pharmacologic effects. In Kryger MH, et al, editors: *Principles and practice of sleep medicine*, ed 4, Philadelphia, 2005, Saunders.

19. Mitler MM, O'Malley MB: Wake-promoting medications: efficacy and adverse effects. In Kryger MH, et al, editors: *Principles and practice of sleep medicine*, ed 4, Philadelphia, 2005, Saunders.

20. Schweitzer PK: Drugs that disturb sleep and wakefulness. In Kryger MH, et al, editors: *Principles and practice of sleep medicine*, ed 4, Philadelphia, 2005, Saunders.

21. Buysse DJ, et al: Clinical pharmacology of other drugs used as hypnotics. In Kryger MH, et al, editors: *Principles and practice of sleep medicine*, ed 4, Philadelphia, 2005, Saunders.

22. Guilleminault C, Bassiri A: Clinical features and evaluation of obstructive sleep apnea-hypopnea syndrome and upper airway resistance syndrome. In Kryger MH, et al, editors: *Principles and practice of sleep medicine*, ed 4, Philadelphia, 2005, Saunders.

23. Hudgel DW: Mechanisms of obstructive sleep apnea, *Chest* 101(2):541, 1992.

24. Punjabi NM: The epidemiology of adult obstructive sleep apnea, *Proc Am Thorac Soc* 5(2):136, 2008.

25. Krieger S, Caples SM: Obstructive sleep apnea and cardiovascular disease: implications for clinical practice, *Cleve Clin J Med* 74(12):853, 2007.

26. Friedman M, et al: Clinical predictors of obstructive sleep apnea, *Sleep (Abstract Supplement #2)* 23:A268, 2000.

27. Young T, Javaheri S: Systemic and pulmonary hypertension in obstructive sleep apnea. In Kryger MH, et al, editors: *Principles and practice of sleep medicine*, ed 4, Philadelphia, 2005, Saunders.

28. Somers VK, Javaheri S: Cardiovascular effects of sleep-related breathing disorders. In Kryger MH, et al, editors: *Principles and practice of sleep medicine*, ed 4, Philadelphia, 2005, Saunders.

29. Neumeyer DA, et al: Compliance of CPAP in patients with obstructive sleep apnea who are enrolled in a CPAP clinic, *Sleep (Abstract Supplement #2)* 23:A257, 2000.

30. Krug P: Snoring and obstructive sleep apnea, *AORN J* 69(4):792, 1999.

31. Carpenter JM, LaMear WR: Uvulopalatopharyngoplasty: results of a patient questionnaire, *Ann Otol Rhinol Laryngol* 117(1):24, 2008.

32. Buchwald H, et al: Bariatric surgery: a systematic review and meta-analysis, *JAMA* 292(14):1724, 2004.

33. Mickelson SA, Hakim I: Is postoperative intensive care monitoring necessary after uvulopalatopharyngoplasty? *Otolaryngol Head Neck Surg* 119(4):352, 1998.

34. White DP: Central sleep apnea. In Kryger MH, et al, editors: *Principles and practice of sleep medicine*, ed 4, Philadelphia, 2005, Saunders.

35. Ekhert DJ, et al: Central sleep apnea: Pathophysiology and treatment, *Chest* 131(2):595, 2007.

Nutritional Alterations

Linda D. Urden

ⓔvolve WEBSITE

Be sure to check out the bonus material, including free self-assessment exercises, on the Evolve web site at *http://evolve.elsevier.com/Urden/priorities/*.

OBJECTIVES

- Describe the adverse effects of nutritional impairments on critically ill patients.
- Assess the nutritional status of critically ill patients with cardiovascular, pulmonary, neurological, renal, gastrointestinal, and endocrine alterations.
- Recognize nutritional alterations associated with cardiovascular, pulmonary, neurological, renal, gastrointestinal, and endocrine alterations.

- Collaborate with a multidisciplinary team in designing a nutrition program for critically ill patients.
- Identify complications of nutrition support and nursing interventions for prevention and management of these complications.

IMPLICATIONS OF UNDERNUTRITION FOR THE SICK OR STRESSED PATIENT

Although illness or injury is the major factor contributing to development of malnutrition, other possible contributing factors are lack of communication among the nurses, physicians, and dietitians responsible for the care of these patients; frequent diagnostic testing and procedures, which lead to interruption in feeding; medications and other therapies that cause anorexia, nausea, or vomiting and thereby interfere with food intake; insufficient monitoring of nutrient intake; and inadequate use of supplements, tube feedings, or total parenteral nutrition (TPN) to maintain the nutritional status of these patients.

Nutritional status tends to deteriorate during hospitalization unless appropriate nutrition support is started early and continually reassessed. Malnutrition in hospitalized patients is associated with a wide variety of adverse outcomes. Wound dehiscence, pressure ulcers, sepsis, infections, respiratory failure requiring ventilation, longer hospital stays, and death are more common among malnourished patients.[1-3] Decline in nutritional status during hospitalization is associated with higher incidences of complications, increased mortality rates, increased length of stay, and higher hospital costs.

ASSESSING NUTRITIONAL STATUS

A nutrition screening should be conducted on every patient. A brief questionnaire to be completed by the patient or significant other, the nursing admission form, or the physician's admission note usually provides enough information to determine whether the patient is at nutritional risk (Box 6-1). Any patient judged to be nutritionally at risk needs a more thorough nutrition assessment.

Nutrition support is the provision of specially formulated or delivered oral, enteral, or parenteral nutrients to maintain or restore optimal nutrition status.[4] The nutrition assessment can be performed by or under the supervision of a registered dietitian or by a nutrition care specialist (e.g., nurse with specialized expertise in nutrition). Figure 6-1 shows the route of administration of specialized nutrition support.

Biochemical Data

A wide range of laboratory tests can provide information about nutritional status. Those most often used in the clinical setting are described in Table 6-1. No diagnostic tests for evaluation of nutrition are perfect, and care must be taken in interpreting the results of the tests.[5]

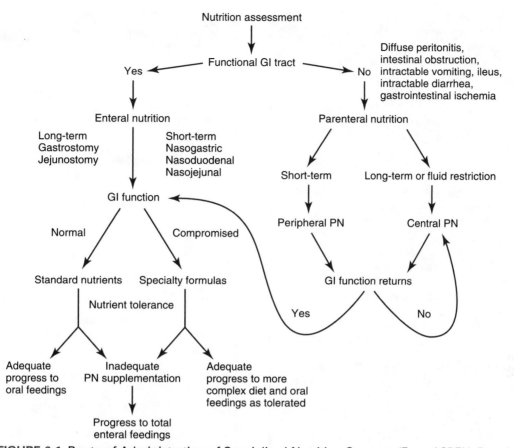

FIGURE 6-1 Route of Administration of Specialized Nutrition Support. (From ASPEN, Board of Directors, and the Clinical Guidelines Task Force: *JPEN J Parenter Enteral Nutr* 26[suppl 1]: 8SA, 2002.)

BOX 6-1	**PATIENTS AT RISK FOR MALNUTRITION**

- Involuntary loss or gain of a significant amount of weight (>10% of usual body weight in 6 months, >5% in 1 month), even if the weight achieved by loss or gain is appropriate for height
- Chronic disease
- Chronic use of a modified diet
- Increased metabolic requirements
- Illness or surgery that may interfere with nutritional intake
- Inadequate nutrient intake for >7 days
- Regular use of three or more medications
- Poverty

Clinical or Physical Manifestations

A thorough physical examination is an essential part of nutrition assessment. Box 6-2 lists some of the more common findings that may indicate an altered nutritional state. It is especially important for the nurse to check for signs of muscle wasting, loss of subcutaneous fat, skin or hair changes, and impairment of wound healing.

TABLE 6-1	**COMMON BLOOD AND URINE TESTS USED IN NUTRITION ASSESSMENT**

TEST	COMMENTS/LIMITATIONS
Serum Proteins Albumin or prealbumin	Levels decrease with protein deficiency but also in liver failure; albumin levels are slow to change in response to malnutrition and repletion; prealbumin levels fall in response to trauma and infection
Hematologic Values Anemia	
Normocytic (normal MCV, MCHC)	Common with protein deficiency
Microcytic (decreased MCV, MCH, MCHC)	Indicative of iron deficiency (can be from blood loss)
Macrocytic (increased MCV)	Common in folate and vitamin B_{12} deficiency
Lymphocytopenia	Common in protein deficiency

MCV, mean corpuscular volume; *MCHC,* mean corpuscular hemoglobin concentration; *MCH,* mean corpuscular hemoglobin.

BOX 6-2   CLINICAL MANIFESTATIONS OF NUTRITIONAL ALTERATIONS

Manifestations That May Indicate Protein-Calorie Malnutrition
- Hair loss; dull, dry, brittle hair; loss of hair pigment
- Loss of subcutaneous tissue; muscle wasting
- Poor wound healing; decubitus ulcer
- Hepatomegaly
- Edema

Manifestations Often Present in Vitamin Deficiencies
- Conjunctival and corneal dryness (vitamin A)
- Dry, scaly skin; follicular hyperkeratosis, in which the skin appears to have gooseflesh continually (vitamin A)
- Gingivitis; poor wound healing (vitamin C)
- Petechiae; ecchymoses (vitamin C or K)
- Inflamed tongue, cracking at the corners of the mouth (riboflavin [vitamin B_2], niacin, folic acid, vitamin B_{12}, or other B vitamins)
- Edema; heart failure (thiamine [vitamin B_1])
- Confusion; confabulation (thiamine [vitamin B_1])

Manifestations Often Present in Mineral Deficiencies
- Blue sclerae; pale mucous membranes; spoon-shaped nails (iron)
- Hypogeusia, or poor sense of taste; dysgeusia, or bad taste; eczema; poor wound healing (zinc)

Manifestations Often Observed with Excessive Vitamin Intake
- Hair loss; dry skin; hepatomegaly (vitamin A)

BOX 6-3   NUTRITION HISTORY INFORMATION

Inadequate Intake of Nutrients
- Alcohol abuse
- Anorexia, severe or prolonged nausea or vomiting
- Confusion, coma
- Poor dentition
- Poverty

Inadequate Digestion or Absorption of Nutrients
- Previous gastrointestinal surgeries, especially gastrectomy, jejunoileal bypass, and ileal resection
- Certain medications, especially antacids and histamine H_2-receptor antagonists (reduce upper small bowel acidity), cholestyramine (binds fat-soluble nutrients), and anticonvulsants

Increased Nutrient Losses
- Blood loss
- Severe diarrhea
- Fistulae, draining abscesses, wounds, decubitus ulcers
- Peritoneal dialysis or hemodialysis
- Corticosteroid therapy (increased tissue catabolism)

Increased Nutrient Requirements
- Fever
- Surgery, trauma, burns, infection
- Cancer (some types)
- Physiologic demands (pregnancy, lactation, growth)

Diet and Health History

Information about dietary intake and significant variations in weight is a vital part of the history. Dietary intake can be evaluated in several ways, including a diet record, a 24-hour recall, and a diet history. Other information to include in a nutrition history is listed in Box 6-3.

Evaluating Nutrition Assessment Findings

It is rare for a patient to exhibit a lack of only one nutrient. Nutritional deficiencies usually are combined, with the patient lacking adequate amounts of protein, calories, and possibly vitamins and minerals. A common form of combined nutritional deficit among hospitalized patients is protein calorie malnutrition (PCM). Two types of PCM are kwashiorkor and marasmus.

Kwashiorkor results in low levels of the serum proteins *albumin, transferrin,* and *prealbumin*; low total lymphocyte count; impaired immunity; loss of hair or hair pigment; edema resulting from low plasma oncotic pressure caused by a loss of plasma proteins; and an enlarged, fatty liver. Marasmus is recognizable by weight loss, loss of subcutaneous fat, and muscle wasting. In the marasmic person, creatinine excretion in the urine is low, an indication of reduced muscle mass. Because PCM weakens muscles, increases vulnerability to infection, and can prolong hospital stays, the health care team should diagnose this serious disorder as quickly as possible so that an appropriate nutrition intervention can be implemented.

Determining Nutritional Needs

Calorie and protein needs of patients are often estimated using formulas that provide allowances for increased nutrient use associated with injury and healing. Although indirect calorimetry is considered the most accurate method to determine energy expenditure, estimates using formulas have demonstrated reasonable accuracy.[6,7] Some rules of thumb are available to provide a rough estimate of caloric needs so that nurses and other caregivers can quickly determine if patients are being seriously overfed or underfed (Table 6-2).

The goal of nutrition assessment is to obtain the most accurate estimate of nutritional requirements. Underfeeding and overfeeding must be avoided during critical illness. Overfeeding results in excessive production of carbon dioxide, which can be a burden in the person with pulmonary compromise. Overfeeding increases fat stores, which can contribute to insulin resistance and hyperglycemia. Hyperglycemia increases the risk of postoperative infections in diabetic and nondiabetic individuals.[8-10] Hyperglycemia is a complication to be avoided if possible.

TABLE 6-2	ESTIMATING ENERGY NEEDS		
CATEGORY	**DESCRIPTION**	**CALORIES/KG**	**CALORIES/LB**
Obese	More than 40% over ideal body weight or BMI >30	21	9.5
Sedentary	Relatively inactive individual without regular aerobic exercise; hospitalized patient without severe injury or sepsis	25-30	11-13.5
Moderate activity or injury	Individual obtaining regular aerobic exercise plus routine activities; patient with trauma or sepsis	30-35	13.5-16
Very active or severe injury	Manual laborer or athlete in very active training; patient with major burns or trauma	40	18

NUTRITION AND CARDIOVASCULAR ALTERATIONS

Diet and cardiovascular disease may interact in a variety of ways. On the one hand, excessive nutrient intake, manifested by overweight or obesity and a diet rich in cholesterol and saturated fat, is a risk factor for development of arteriosclerotic heart disease. On the other hand, the consequences of chronic myocardial insufficiency may include malnutrition.

Nutrition Assessment in Cardiovascular Alterations

A nutrition assessment provides the nurse and other members of the health care team the information necessary to plan the patient's nutrition care and education. Common findings in the nutrition assessment of the cardiovascular patient are summarized in Box 6-4. The major nutritional concerns relate to appropriateness of body weight and the levels of serum lipids and blood pressure.

Nutrition Intervention in Cardiovascular Alterations
Myocardial Infarction
The following guidelines will assist the nurse in providing appropriate nutritional care for the patient in the immediate post-myocardial infarction period:

- Limit meal size for the patient with severe myocardial compromise or postprandial angina.
- Monitor the effect of caffeine on the patient, if caffeine is included in the diet.
- Use caution in serving foods at temperature extremes.

Hypertension

A substantial number of individuals with hypertension are "salt sensitive," with their disorder improving when sodium intake is limited. Therefore restriction of sodium intake, usually to 2.5 g/day or less, is often advised to help control hypertension.[11] One teaspoon of salt provides about 2.3 g of sodium. Most salt substitutes contain potassium chloride and may be used with the physician's approval by the patient who has no renal impairment. A diet rich in fruits, vegetables, and low-fat dairy products (the DASH, or Dietary Approaches to Stopping Hypertension, diet) combined with a sodium

BOX 6-4	COMMON FINDINGS IN PATIENTS WITH CARDIOVASCULAR DISEASE

- Overweight/obesity, underweight (cardiac cachexia)
- Abdominal fat; increased risk of cardiovascular disease with waist measurement >102 cm (>40 inches) for men and >88 cm (>35 inches) for women
- Elevated total serum cholesterol, LDL cholesterol, and triglycerides
- Wasting of muscle and subcutaneous fat (cardiac cachexia)
- Sedentary lifestyle
- Excessive intake of saturated fat, cholesterol, salt, and alcohol
- Angina, respiratory difficulty, fatigue during eating
- Medications that impair appetite (e.g., digitalis preparations, quinidine)

LDL, low-density lipoprotein.

restriction is often more effective than sodium restriction alone.[12]

Heart Failure

Nutrition intervention for the patient with heart failure is designed to reduce fluid retained within the body and thus reduce the preload. Because fluid accompanies sodium, limitation of sodium is necessary to reduce fluid retention. Specific interventions include limiting salt intake, usually to 5 g/day or less, and limiting fluid intake as appropriate. If fluid is restricted, the daily fluid allowance is usually 1.5 to 2 L/day, to include both fluids in the diet and those given with medications and for other purposes.

Cardiac Cachexia

The severely malnourished cardiac patient often develops heart failure. Therefore sodium and fluid restriction, as previously described, is appropriate. It is important to concentrate nutrients into as small a volume as possible and to serve small amounts frequently, rather than three large meals daily. The individual should be encouraged to consume calorie-dense foods and supplements. Good choices include meats and poultry, cheeses, yogurt, frozen yogurt, and ice cream.

Because the patient is likely to tire quickly and to suffer from anorexia, enteral tube feeding may be necessary. Typical tube feeding formulas provide 1 calorie per milliliter (cal/ml), but more concentrated products are available to provide adequate nutrients in a smaller volume. The nurse must monitor the fluid status of these patients carefully when they are receiving nutrition support. Assessing breath sounds and observing for presence and severity of peripheral edema and changes in body weight are performed daily or more frequently. A consistent weight gain of more than 0.11 to 0.22 kg (0.25 to 0.5 lb) per day usually indicates fluid retention rather than gain of fat and muscle mass.

Nutrition and Pulmonary Alterations

Malnutrition has extremely adverse effects on respiratory function, decreasing surfactant production, diaphragmatic mass, vital capacity, and immunocompetence. Patients with acute respiratory disorders find it difficult to consume adequate oral nutrients and can rapidly become malnourished. Individuals who have an acute illness superimposed on chronic respiratory problems are also at high risk. Almost three fourths of patients with chronic obstructive pulmonary disease (COPD) have had weight loss. Patients with undernutrition and end-stage COPD, however, often cannot tolerate the increase in metabolic demand that occurs during refeeding. In addition, they are at significant risk for development of cor pulmonale and may fail to tolerate the fluid required for delivery of enteral or parenteral nutrition support. Prevention of severe nutritional deficits, rather than correction of deficits once they have occurred, is important in nutritional management of these patients.

NUTRITION ASSESSMENT IN PULMONARY ALTERATIONS

Common findings in nutrition assessment related to pulmonary alterations are summarized in Box 6-5. The patient with respiratory compromise is especially vulnerable to the effects of fluid volume excess and must be assessed continually for this complication, particularly during enteral and parenteral feeding.

BOX 6-5   COMMON FINDINGS IN PATIENTS WITH PULMONARY DISEASE

- Underweight
- Elevated carbon dioxide partial pressure related to overfeeding
- Edema, dyspnea, signs of pulmonary edema related to fluid volume excess
- Poor food intake related to dyspnea
- Unpleasant taste in mouth from sputum production or bronchodilator therapy
- Endotracheal intubation preventing oral intake

Nutrition Intervention in Pulmonary Alterations
Prevent or Correct Undernutrition/Underweight

The nurse and dietitian work together to encourage oral intake in the undernourished or potentially undernourished patient who is capable of eating. Small, frequent feedings are especially important because a very full stomach can interfere with diaphragmatic movement. Mouth care should be provided before meals and snacks to clear the palate of the taste of sputum and medications. Administering bronchodilators with food can help to reduce the gastric irritation caused by these medications.

Because of anorexia, dyspnea, debilitation, or need for ventilatory support, however, many patients will require enteral tube feeding or TPN. It is especially important for the nurse to be alert to the risk of pulmonary aspiration in the patient with an artificial airway. To reduce the risk of pulmonary aspiration during enteral tube feeding, the nurse should (1) keep the patient's head elevated at least 45 degrees during feedings, unless contraindicated; (2) discontinue feedings 30 to 60 minutes before any procedures that require lowering the head; (3) keep the cuff of the artificial airway inflated during feeding, if possible; (4) monitor the patient for increasing abdominal distention; and (5) check tube placement before each feeding (if intermittent) or at least every 4 to 8 hours if feedings are continuous.

Avoid Overfeeding

Overfeeding increases the production of carbon dioxide (CO_2). This is unlikely to be significant in the patient who is eating foods. Instead, it is an iatrogenic complication of TPN or enteral feeding. Arterial CO_2 tension ($Paco_2$) may rise sufficiently to make it difficult to wean a patient from the ventilator. A balanced regimen with both lipids and carbohydrates providing the nonprotein calories is optimal for the patient with respiratory compromise, and the patient needs to be reassessed continually to ensure that caloric intake is not excessive.

Prevent Fluid Volume Excess

Pulmonary edema and failure of the right side of the heart, which may be precipitated by fluid volume excess, further worsen the status of the patient with respiratory compromise. Maintaining careful intake and output records allows for accurate assessment of fluid balance. Usually the patient requires no more than 35 to 40 ml/kg/day of fluid. For the patient receiving nutrition support, fluid intake can be reduced by (1) using 20% or 30% lipid emulsions as a source of calories, (2) using tube feeding formulas providing at least 2 cal/ml (the dietitian can recommend appropriate formulas), and (3) choosing oral supplements that are low in fluid.

NUTRITION AND NEUROLOGIC ALTERATIONS

Because neurological disorders such as stroke and closed head injury tend to be long-term problems, these patients require good nutritional care to prevent nutritional deficits and promote well-being.

Nutrition Assessment in Neurological Alterations

Nutrition-related assessment findings vary widely in the patient with neurological alterations, depending on the type of disorder present (Box 6-6).

Nutrition Intervention in Neurological Alterations: Prevent or Correct Nutrition Deficits

Oral Feedings

Patients with dysphagia or weakness of the swallowing musculature often experience the greatest difficulty in swallowing dry foods and thin liquids (e.g., water) that are difficult to control.

Tube Feedings and Total Parenteral Nutrition

Patients who are unconscious or unable to eat because of severe dysphagia, weakness, ileus, or other reasons require tube feedings or TPN. Prompt initiation of nutrition support must be a priority in the patient with neurological impairment. Needs for protein and calories are increased by infection and fever, as in the patient with encephalitis or meningitis. Needs for protein, calories, zinc, and vitamin C are increased during wound healing, as in trauma patients and those with pressure ulcers.

Patients with neurological deficits have an increased risk of certain complications (particularly pulmonary aspiration) during tube feeding and therefore require especially careful nursing management. Patients of most concern are (1) those with an impaired gag reflex, such as some patients with cerebrovascular accident (stroke); (2) those with delayed gastric emptying, such as patients in the early period after spinal cord injury and patients with head injury treated with barbiturate coma; and (3) those likely to experience seizures. To help prevent pulmonary aspiration, the patient's head is kept elevated, if not contraindicated; when elevation of the head is not possible, administering feedings with the patient in the prone or lateral position will allow free drainage of emesis from the mouth and decrease the risk of aspiration.

Administering phenytoin with enteral formulas decreases the absorption of the drug and the peak serum level achieved and thus may increase the risk of seizures. The phenytoin dosage must be adjusted appropriately. Phenytoin levels should be monitored carefully in patients receiving enteral feedings.[13]

Hyperglycemia is a common complication in patients receiving corticosteroids. Regular monitoring of blood glucose is an important part of their care. They may require insulin to control the hyperglycemia.

Prompt use of nutrition support is especially important for patients with head injuries because head injury causes marked catabolism, even in patients who receive barbiturates, which should decrease metabolic demands. Head-injured patients rapidly exhaust glycogen stores and begin to use body proteins to meet energy needs, a process that can quickly lead to PCM. The catabolic response is partly a result of corticosteroid therapy in head-injured patients. However, the hypermetabolism and hypercatabolism are also caused by dramatic hormonal responses to this type of injury.[14] Levels of cortisol, epinephrine, and norepinephrine increase as much as seven times normal. These hormones increase the metabolic rate and caloric demands, causing mobilization of body fat and proteins to meet the increased energy needs. Furthermore, head-injured patients undergo an inflammatory response and may be febrile, creating increased needs for protein and calories. Improvement in outcome and reduction in complications have been observed in head-injured patients who receive adequate nutrition support early in the hospital course.[15]

NUTRITION AND RENAL ALTERATIONS

Providing adequate nutrition care for the patient with renal disease can be extremely challenging. Although renal disturbances and their treatments can greatly increase needs for nutrients, necessary restrictions in intake of fluid, protein, phosphorus, and potassium make delivery of adequate calories, vitamins, and minerals difficult. Thorough nutrition assessment provides the basis for successful nutrition management in patients with renal disease.

Nutrition Assessment in Renal Alterations

Some common assessment findings in individuals with renal disease are listed in Box 6-7.

Nutrition Intervention in Renal Alterations

The goal of nutrition intervention is to administer adequate nutrients, including calories, protein, vitamins, and minerals, while avoiding excesses of protein, fluid, electrolytes, and other nutrients with potential toxicity.

Protein

The kidney is responsible for excreting nitrogen from amino acids or proteins in the form of *urea*. Thus, when urinary excretion of urea is impaired in renal failure, blood levels of urea rise. Excessive protein intake may worsen uremia.

BOX 6-7 **COMMON FINDINGS IN THE PATIENT WITH RENAL FAILURE**

- Underweight (may be masked by edema)
- Electrolyte imbalances
- Hypoalbuminemia related to protein restriction and amino acid losses in dialysis
- Anemia related to inadequate erythropoietin production and blood loss with hemodialysis
- Hypertriglyceridemia related to use of glucose as osmotic agent in dialysis and use of carbohydrates to supply needed calories
- Wasting of muscle and subcutaneous tissue (may be masked by edema)
- Poor dietary intake related to protein and electrolyte restrictions

---

However, the patient with renal failure often has (1) other physiological stresses that actually increase protein/amino acid needs; (2) losses from dialysis, wounds, and fistulae; (3) use of corticosteroid drugs that exert a catabolic effect; (4) increased endogenous secretion of catecholamines, corticosteroids, and glucagon, all of which can cause or aggravate catabolism; (5) metabolic acidosis, which stimulates protein breakdown; and (6) catabolic conditions (e.g., trauma, surgery, sepsis). Therefore patients with acute renal failure need adequate amounts of protein to avoid catabolism of body tissues. Approximately 1.5 to 1.7 g/kg/day has successfully maintained adequate protein nutrition in these patients.[16,17]

During hemodialysis and arteriovenous hemofiltration, amino acids are freely filtered and lost, but proteins such as albumin and immunoglobulin are not lost. Both proteins and amino acids are removed during peritoneal dialysis, creating a greater nutritional requirement for protein. Protein needs are estimated at approximately 1.0 to 1.2 g/kg/day for stable patients receiving hemodialysis or hemofiltration and 1.2 to 1.3 g/kg/day for those receiving peritoneal dialysis.[18,19] Patients in the process of wound healing and those with ongoing protein losses have greater needs.

Fluids

The patient with renal insufficiency usually does not require a fluid restriction until urine output begins to diminish. Patients receiving hemodialysis are limited to a fluid intake resulting in a gain of no more than 0.45 kg (1 lb) per day on the days between dialysis. This generally means a daily intake of 500 to 750 ml plus the volume lost in urine. With the use of continuous peritoneal dialysis, hemofiltration, or hemodialysis, the fluid intake can be liberalized.[20] This more liberal fluid allowance permits more adequate nutrient delivery, whether by oral, tube, or parenteral feedings. Enteral formulas containing 1.5 to 2.0 cal/ml or more provide a concentrated source of calories for tube-fed patients who require fluid restriction. Intravenous lipids, particularly 20%

emulsions, can be used to supply concentrated calories for the TPN patient. Intradialytic TPN can be used to supply an additional source of nutrients at a time when the fluid can be rapidly removed in dialysis.[21,22]

Energy (Calories)

Energy needs are not increased by renal failure, but adequate calories must be provided to avoid catabolism.[16] It is essential that the renal patient receive an adequate number of calories to prevent catabolism of body tissues to meet energy needs. Catabolism not only reduces the mass of muscle and other functional body tissues but also releases nitrogen that must be excreted by the kidney. Adults with renal insufficiency need about 30 to 35 cal/kg/day, compared with the 25 to 30 cal/kg/day needed by healthy adults, to prevent catabolism and ensure that all protein consumed is used for anabolism rather than to meet energy needs.[19] After renal transplantation, when the patient initially receives large doses of corticosteroids, it is especially important to ensure that caloric intake is adequate (usually 25 to 35 cal/kg/day) to prevent undue catabolism.

Hypertriglyceridemia is found in a substantial number of patients with renal disorders. This condition is worsened by excessive intake of simple refined sugars, such as sucrose (table sugar) or glucose. Glucose in the peritoneal dialysate may be a significant calorie source and a contributing factor in hypertriglyceridemia. Approximately 70% of the glucose instilled during peritoneal dialysis to serve as an osmotic agent may be absorbed, and this must be considered part of the patient's carbohydrate intake. The glucose monohydrate used in intravenous and dialysate solutions supplies 3.4 cal/g. Thus, if a patient receives 4.25% glucose (4.25 g glucose per 100 ml solution) in the dialysate, the patient receives the following:

$$42.5 \text{ g/L} \times 70\% \times 3.4 \text{ cal/g} = 101 \text{ cal/L of dialysate}$$

To help control hypertriglyceridemia, only about 30% to 35% of the patient's calories should come from carbohydrates, including glucose from the dialysate, with the major portion of dietary carbohydrate coming from complex carbohydrates (starches and fibers).

NUTRITION AND GASTROINTESTINAL ALTERATIONS

Because the gastrointestinal (GI) tract is so inherently related to nutrition, it is not surprising that impairment of the GI tract and its accessory organs has a major impact on nutrition. Two of the most serious GI-related illnesses seen among critical care patients are hepatic failure and pancreatitis.

Nutrition Assessment in Gastrointestinal Alterations

Common assessment findings in patients with GI disease are listed in Box 6-8.

Nutrition Intervention in Gastrointestinal Alterations

Hepatic Failure

Because the diseased liver has impaired ability to deactivate hormones, levels of circulating glucagon, epinephrine, and cortisol are elevated. These hormones promote catabolism of body tissues and cause glycogen stores to be exhausted. Release of lipids from their storage depots is accelerated, but the liver has decreased ability to metabolize them for energy. Furthermore, inadequate production of bile salts by the liver results in malabsorption of fat from the diet. Therefore body proteins are used for energy sources, producing tissue wasting.

The *branched-chain amino acids* (BCAAs)—leucine, isoleucine, and valine—are especially well used for energy, and their levels in the blood decline. Conversely, levels of the *aromatic amino acids* (AAAs)—phenylalanine, tyrosine, and tryptophan—rise as a result of tissue catabolism and impaired ability of the liver to clear them from the blood. The AAAs are precursors for neurotransmitters in the central nervous system (serotonin and dopamine). Rising levels of AAAs may alter nerve activity within the brain, leading to symptoms of encephalopathy. In addition, the damaged liver cannot clear ammonia from the circulation adequately, and ammonia accumulates in the brain. The ammonia may contribute to the encephalopathic symptoms and also to brain edema.[23,24]

Monitoring Fluid and Electrolyte Status. Ascites and edema occur because of a combination of factors. There is decreased colloid osmotic pressure in the plasma, because of the reduction of production of albumin and other plasma proteins by the diseased liver, increased portal pressure caused by obstruction, and renal sodium retention from secondary hyperaldosteronism. To control the fluid retention, restriction of sodium (usually 2000 mg) and fluid (1500 ml or less daily) is generally necessary, in conjunction with administration of diuretics. Patients are weighed daily to evaluate the success of treatment. Physical status and laboratory data must be closely monitored for deficiencies of potassium, phosphorus, and vitamins A, D, E, and K, and zinc.[25]

Provision of a Nutritious Diet and Evaluation of Response to Dietary Protein. PCM and nutritional deficiencies are common in hepatic failure. The causes of malnutrition are complex and usually related to decreased intake, malabsorption, maldigestion, and abnormal nutrient metabolism. Nutrition intervention is individualized and based on these metabolic changes. A diet with adequate protein helps to suppress catabolism and promote liver regeneration. Stable patients with cirrhosis usually tolerate 0.8 to 1 g protein/kg/day. Patients with severe stress or nutritional deficits have increased needs—as much as 1.2 to 2 g/kg/day.[26] Aggressive treatment with medications, including lactulose, neomycin, or metronidazole, is considered first-line therapy in the management of acute hepatic encephalopathy. In a minority of patients, pharmacotherapy may not be effective, and protein restriction to as little as 0.5 g/kg/day or less may be necessary for brief periods. Chronic protein restriction is not recommended as a long-term management strategy for patients with liver disease.[25,26]

Anorexia may interfere with oral intake, and the nurse may need to provide much encouragement to the patient to ensure intake of an adequate diet. Prospective calorie counts may need to be instituted to provide objective evidence of oral intake. Small, frequent feedings are usually better tolerated by the anorexic patient than are three large meals daily. Soft foods are preferred because the patient may have esophageal varices that might be irritated by high-fiber foods. If patients are unable to meet their caloric needs, they may require oral supplements or enteral feeding. Small-bore nasoenteric feeding tubes can be used safely without increasing risk of variceal bleeding.[26] TPN should be reserved only for patients who are absolutely unable to tolerate enteral feeding.[25] Diarrhea from concurrent administration of lactulose should not be confused with feeding intolerance.

A diet adequate in calories (at least 30 cal/kg daily) is provided to help prevent catabolism and to prevent the use of dietary protein for energy needs.[27] In cases of malabsorption, medium-chain triglycerides (MCTs) may be used to meet caloric needs. Pancreatic enzymes may also be considered for malabsorption problems.

BCAA-enriched products have been developed for enteral and parenteral nutrition of patients with hepatic disease. These products may be used in patients with acute hepatic encephalopathy who do not tolerate standard diets or enteral formulas, or who are unresponsive to lactulose. However, no substantial evidence exists showing BCAAs are superior to standard formulas in regard to nitrogen balance or as treatment for encephalopathy.[25,26] The patient who undergoes successful liver transplantation is usually able to tolerate a regular diet with few restrictions. Intake during the postoperative period must be adequate to support nutritional repletion and healing; 1 to 1.2 g protein/kg/day and approximately 30 cal/kg/day are usually sufficient. Immunosuppressant therapy (corticosteroids and cyclosporine or tacrolimus) contributes to glucose intolerance. Dietary measures to control glucose intolerance include (1) obtaining approximately 30% of dietary calories from fat, (2) emphasizing complex sources of carbohydrates, and (3) eating several small meals daily. Moderate exercise often helps to improve glucose tolerance.

Pancreatitis

The pancreas is an exocrine and endocrine gland required for normal digestion and metabolism of proteins, carbohydrates, and fats. Acute pancreatitis is an inflammatory process that occurs as a result of autodigestion of the pancreas by enzymes normally secreted by that organ. Food intake stimulates pancreatic secretion and thus increases the damage to the pancreas and the pain associated with the disorder. Patients usually present with abdominal pain and tenderness and elevations of pancreatic enzymes. A mild form of acute pancreatitis occurs in 80% of patients requiring hospitalization, and severe acute pancreatitis occurs in the other 20%.[28] Patients with the mild form of acute pancreatitis do not require nutrition support and generally resume oral feeding within 7 days. Chronic pancreatitis may develop and is characterized by fibrosis of pancreatic cells. This results in loss of exocrine and endocrine function because of the destruction of acinar and islet cells. The loss of exocrine function leads to malabsorption and steatorrhea. In chronic pancreatitis, the loss of endocrine function results in impaired glucose tolerance.[28]

Prevention of Further Damage to the Pancreas and Preventing Nutritional Deficits. Effective nutritional management is a key treatment for patients with acute pancreatitis or exacerbations of chronic pancreatitis. The concern that feeding may stimulate the production of digestive enzymes and perpetuate tissue damage has led to the widespread use of TPN and bowel rest. Recent data suggest that enteral nutrition infused into the distal jejunum bypasses the stimulatory effect of feeding on pancreatic secretion and is associated with fewer infectious and metabolic complications compared to TPN.[29,30]

The results of randomized studies comparing TPN with total enteral nutrition (TEN, or enteral tube feeding) indicate that TEN is preferable to TPN in patients with severe acute pancreatitis, reducing costs and the risk of sepsis and improving clinical outcome.[29-31] Patients unable to tolerate TEN should receive TPN, and some patients may require a combination of TEN and TPN to meet nutritional requirements.[32,33] Low-fat enteral formulas and those with fat provided by MCTs are more readily absorbed than formulas that are high in long-chain triglycerides (e.g., corn or sunflower oil).

When oral intake is possible, small frequent feedings of low-fat foods are least likely to cause discomfort.[30] Alcohol intake should be avoided because it worsens the tissue damage and the pain associated with pancreatitis. Guidelines for treatment of diabetes (see following sections) are appropriate for the care of the person with glucose intolerance or diabetes related to pancreatitis.

NUTRITION AND ENDOCRINE ALTERATIONS

Endocrine alterations have far-reaching effects on all body systems and thus affect nutritional status in a variety of ways. One of the most common endocrine problems, both in

---

BOX 6-9	COMMON FINDINGS IN PATIENTS WITH ENDOCRINE DISEASE

- Hyperglycemia related to poor diabetic control, infection, trauma/burns, or glucocorticoid use
- Elevated hemoglobin A_{1c} related to chronic poor diabetic control
- Hypoglycemia related to vomiting or poor food intake without adjustment of the dosage of insulin or oral hypoglycemic agents

---

the general population and among critically ill patients, is diabetes mellitus.

Nutrition Assessment in Endocrine Alterations

Common assessment findings in individuals with endocrine alterations are listed in Box 6-9. Because of the prevalence of patients with non-insulin-dependent (type 2) diabetes mellitus among the hospitalized population, the acute nutritional problems most often noted in patients with endocrine alterations are related to glycemic control.

Nutrition Intervention in Endocrine Alterations
Nutrition Support and Blood Glucose Control

Patients with insulin-dependent (type 1) diabetes mellitus or endocrine dysfunction caused by pancreatitis often have weight loss and malnutrition as a result of tissue catabolism because they cannot use dietary carbohydrates to meet energy needs. Although patients with type 2 diabetes are more likely to be overweight than underweight, they too may become malnourished as a result of chronic or acute infections, trauma, major surgery, or other illnesses. Nutrition support should not be neglected simply because a patient is obese, because PCM develops even in these patients. When a patient is not expected to be able to eat for at least 5 to 7 days or when inadequate intake persists for that period, initiation of tube feedings or TPN is indicated. No disease process benefits from starvation, and development or progression of nutritional deficits may contribute to complications such as pressure ulcers, pulmonary or urinary tract infections, and sepsis, which prolong hospitalization, increase the costs of care, and may even result in death.

Blood glucose control is especially important in the care of surgical patients. Hyperglycemia in the early postoperative period is associated with increased rates of hospital-acquired infection. To maintain tight control of blood glucose, glucose levels are monitored regularly, usually several times a day until the patient is stable. Regular insulin added to the solution is the most common method of managing hyperglycemia in the patient receiving TPN. Multiple injections of regular insulin may be used to maintain tight control of blood glucose in the enterally fed patient.

In patients receiving enteral tube feedings, the postpyloric route (via nasoduodenal, nasojejunal, or jejunostomy tube) may be the most effective, because gastroparesis may limit tolerance of intragastric tube feedings.[34] Postpyloric feedings are given continuously because dumping syndrome and poor absorption may occur if feedings are given rapidly into the small bowel. Continuous enteral infusions are associated with improved control of blood glucose. Fiber-enriched formulas may slow the absorption of the carbohydrate, producing a more delayed and sustained glycemic response. Most standard formulas contain balanced proportions of carbohydrate, protein, and fats appropriate for diabetic patients. Specialized diabetic formulas have not shown improved outcomes compared to standard formulas.[35]

Severe Vomiting or Diarrhea in the Patient with Type 1 Diabetes Mellitus. When insulin-dependent patients experience vomiting and diarrhea severe enough to interfere significantly with oral intake or result in excessive fluid and electrolyte losses, adequate carbohydrates and fluids must be supplied. Nausea and vomiting should be treated with antiemetic medication.[34] Delayed gastric emptying is common in diabetes and may improve with administration of prokinetic agents.[34] Small amounts of food or liquids taken every 15 to 20 minutes are generally the best tolerated by the patient with nausea and vomiting. Foods and beverages containing approximately 15 g of carbohydrate include ½ cup regular gelatin, ½ cup custard, ¾ cup regular ginger ale, ½ cup regular soft drink, and ½ cup orange or apple juice. Blood glucose levels should be monitored at least every 2 to 4 hours.

ADMINISTERING NUTRITION SUPPORT

Enteral Nutrition

Whenever possible, the enteral route is the preferred method of feeding. Patients with abdominal trauma in particular have lower morbidity and mortality rates if fed enterally rather than parenterally.

There are a variety of commercial enteral feeding products, some of which are designed to meet the specialized needs of the critically ill. Products designed for the stressed patient with trauma or sepsis are usually rich in glutamine, arginine, and antioxidant nutrients (e.g., vitamins C, E, and A; selenium). The antioxidants help to reduce oxidative injury to the tissues (e.g., from reperfusion injury). Some products can be consumed orally, but it can be difficult for the critically ill patient to consume enough orally to meet the increased needs associated with stress. Refer to Table 6-3 for enteral formulas.

Oral Supplementation

Oral supplementation may be necessary for patients who can eat and have normal digestion and absorption but simply cannot consume enough regular foods to meet caloric and protein needs. Patients with mild to moderate anorexia, burns, or trauma may be included in this category.

Tube Feeding

Tube feedings are used for patients who have at least some digestive and absorptive capability but are unwilling or unable to consume enough by mouth. Patients with profound anorexia and those experiencing severe stress (e.g., major burns, trauma) that greatly increases their nutritional needs often benefit from tube feedings. Individuals who require elemental formulas because of impaired digestion or absorption or specialized formulas for altered metabolic conditions such as renal or hepatic failure usually require tube feeding because the unpleasant flavors of the free amino acids, peptides, or protein hydrolysates used in these formulas are very difficult to mask.

Location and Type of Feeding Tube

Nasal intubation is the simplest and most common route for gaining access to the GI tract; this method allows access to the stomach, duodenum, or jejunum. Tube enterostomy—a gastrostomy or jejunostomy—is used primarily for long-term feedings (6 to 12 weeks or more) and when obstruction makes the nasoenteral route inaccessible. Tube enterostomies may also be used for the patient who is at risk for tube dislodgment because of severe agitation or confusion. A conventional gastrostomy or jejunostomy is often performed at the time of other abdominal surgery. The percutaneous endoscopic gastrostomy (PEG) tube has become extremely popular because it can be inserted without the use of general anesthetics. Percutaneous endoscopic jejunostomy (PEJ) tubes are also used.

Transpyloric feedings via nasoduodenal, nasojejunal, or jejunostomy tubes are typically used when there is a risk of pulmonary aspiration, because theoretically the pyloric sphincter provides a barrier that lessens the risk of regurgitation and aspiration. If nasogastric tubes are used, choosing the smallest possible tube diameter reduces the risk of gastroesophageal reflux and pulmonary aspiration. Transpyloric feedings have an advantage over intragastric feedings for patients with delayed gastric emptying, such as those with head injury, gastroparesis associated with uremia or diabetes, or postoperative ileus. Small bowel motility returns more quickly than gastric motility after surgery, and thus it is often possible to deliver transpyloric feedings within a few hours of injury or surgery.[36] Promotility agents such as metoclopramide may improve feeding tolerance.[37] See Figure 6-2 for location of tube feeding sites.

Nursing Management

The nurse's role in delivery of tube feedings usually includes (1) insertion of the tube, if a temporary tube is used; (2) maintenance of the tube; (3) administration of the feedings; (4) prevention and detection of complications associated with this form of therapy; and (5) participation in assessment of the patient's response to tube feedings.

Tube Placement. Critical care nurses are usually familiar with tube insertion, and therefore this topic is not discussed here. However, it is well to remember that if transpyloric positioning is desirable, administration of metoclopramide or erythromycin before tube insertion increases the likelihood of tube passage through the pylorus.[38]

Correct tube placement must be confirmed before initiation of feedings and regularly throughout the course of

TABLE 6-3   ENTERAL FORMULAS

FORMULA TYPE	NUTRITIONAL USES	CLINICAL EXAMPLES	EXAMPLES OF COMMERCIAL PRODUCTS (MANUFACTURER)
Formulas Used When GI Tract Is Fully Functional			
Polymeric (standard): Contains whole proteins (10%-15% of calories), long-chain triglycerides (25%-40% of calories), and glucose polymers or oligosaccharides (50%-60% of calories); most provide 1 calorie/mL	Inability to ingest food Inability to consume enough to meet needs	Oral or esophageal cancer Coma, stroke Anorexia resulting from chronic illness Burns or trauma	Ensure (Ross) NuBasics (Nestlé) IsoSource (Novartis) PediaSure (Ross), for children 1-10 years old Boost (Mead Johnson)
High-nitrogen: Same as polymeric except protein provides >15% of calories	Same as polymeric plus mild catabolism and protein deficits	Trauma or burns Sepsis	IsoSource HN (Novartis) Osmolite HN (Ross) Ultracal (Mead Johnson)
Concentrated: Same as polymeric except concentrated to 2 calorie/mL	Same as polymeric but fluid restriction needed	Heart failure Neurosurgery COPD Liver disease	Deliver 2.0 (Mean Johnson) TwoCal HN (Ross) Nutren 2.0 (Nestlé)
Formulas Used When GI Function Is Impaired			
Elemental or predigested: Contains hydrolyzed (partially digested) protein, peptides (short chains of amino acids), and/or amino acids, little fat (<10% of calories) or high MCT, and glucose polymers or oligosaccharides; most provide 1 calorie/mL	Impaired digestion and/or absorption	Short bowel syndrome Radiation enteritis Inflammatory bowel disease	Criticare HN (Mead Johnson) Vital High Nitrogen (Ross) Reabilan HN (Nestlé)
Diets for Specific Disease States*			
Renal failure: Concentrated in calories; low sodium, potassium, magnesium, phosphorus, and vitamins A and D; low protein for renal insufficiency; higher protein formulas for dialyzed patients	Renal insufficiency Dialysis	Predialysis Hemodialysis or peritoneal dialysis	Suplena (Ross) Renalcal (Nestlé) Nepro (Ross) Magnacal Renal (Mead Johnson)
Hepatic failure: Enriched in BCAA; low sodium	Protein intolerance	Hepatic encephalopathy	NutriHep (Nestlé) Hepatic-Aid II (B Braun/McGaw)
Pulmonary dysfunction: Low carbohydrate, high fat, concentrated in calories	Respiratory insufficiency	Ventilator dependence	NutriVent (Nestlé) Pulmocare (Ross)
Glucose intolerance: High fat, low carbohydrate (most contain fiber and fructose)	Glucose intolerance	Individuals with diabetes mellitus whose blood sugar is poorly controlled with standard formulas	Glucerna (Ross) Choice DM (Mead Johnson) Diabetisource (Novartis) Glytrol (Nestlé)
Critical care, wound healing: High protein; most contain MCT to improve fat absorption; some have increased zinc and vitamin C for wound healing; some are high in antioxidants (vitamin E, betacarotene); some are enriched with arginine, glutamine, and/or omega-3 fatty acids	Critical illness	Severe trauma or burns Sepsis	Immun-Aid (B Braun/McGaw) Impact (Novartis) Perative (Ross) Crucial (Nestlé) TraumaCal (Mead Johnson)

GI, gastrointestinal; *COPD*, chronic obstructive pulmonary disease; *MCT*, medium-chain triglyceride; *BCAA*, branched-chain enriched amino acid. *These diets may be beneficial for selected patients; costs and benefits must be considered. (From Urden LD, Stacy KM, Lough ME: *Critical care nursing: Diagnosis and management*, ed 6, St. Louis, 2010, Mosby.)

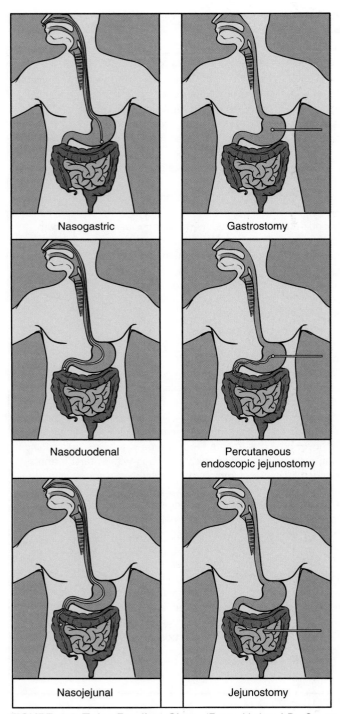

FIGURE 6-2 Tube Feeding Sites. (From Urden LD, Stacy KM, Lough ME: *Critical care nursing: Diagnosis and management,* ed. 6, St. Louis, 2010, Mosby.)

enteral feedings. Radiographs are the most accurate way of assessing tube placement, but repeated radiographs are costly and can expose the patient to excessive radiation. An inexpensive and relatively accurate alternative method involves assessing the pH of fluid removed from the feeding tube; some tubes are equipped with pH monitoring systems.

If the pH is less than 4.0 in patients not receiving gastric acid inhibitors, or less than 5.5 in patients who are receiving acid inhibitors, the tube tip is likely to be in the stomach.[39]

Intestinal secretions usually have a pH greater than 6.0, and respiratory tract fluids usually have a pH greater than 5.5. The esophagus may have an acid pH, which may cause confusion between esophageal and gastric placement. However, other clues can help in identifying a tube that has its distal tip in the esophagus: it may be especially difficult to aspirate fluid out of the tube; a large portion of the tube may extend out of the body (although a tube inserted to the proper length could be coiled in the esophagus); and belching often occurs immediately after air is injected into the tube.[39]

Assessing both the pH and the *bilirubin* concentration of fluid aspirated from the feeding tube is a promising new method for confirming tube placement.[40] The bilirubin concentration in tracheobronchial and pleural fluid and in the stomach is approximately 90% less than in the intestine. Therefore the nurse who obtains fluid with a pH greater than 5.0 and a low bilirubin concentration from a feeding tube can be relatively sure that the distal tip of the tube is in the pulmonary system.[40] Measurement of end-tidal CO_2 also shows promise for confirming tube placement in ventilated patients.

Formula Delivery. Careful attention to administration of tube feedings can prevent many complications. Very clean or aseptic technique in the handling and administration of the formula can help prevent bacterial contamination and a resultant infection. The optimal schedule for delivery of feedings also is important. Tube feedings may be administered intermittently or continuously.

Bolus feedings, which are intermittent feedings delivered rapidly into the stomach or small bowel, are likely to cause distention, vomiting, and dumping syndrome with diarrhea. Instead of using bolus feedings, nurses can gradually drip intermittent feedings, with each feeding lasting 20 to 30 minutes or longer, to promote optimal assimilation. The question of which feeding schedule—continuous or intermittent—is superior in critically ill patients remains unanswered.

Prevent or Correct Complications. Some of the more common complications of tube feeding are pulmonary aspiration, diarrhea, constipation, tube occlusion, and gastric retention (Table 6-4).

Total Parenteral Nutrition

Total parenteral nutrition (TPN) refers to the delivery of all nutrients by the intravenous (IV) route. TPN is used when the GI tract is not functional or when nutritional needs cannot be met solely via the GI tract. Likely candidates for TPN include patients who have a severely impaired absorption (as in short bowel syndrome, collagen-vascular diseases, and radiation enteritis), intestinal obstruction, peritonitis, and prolonged ileus. In addition, some postoperative, trauma, and burn patients may need TPN to supplement the nutrient intake they are able to tolerate via the enteral route.

Types of Parenteral Nutrition

TPN involves administration of highly concentrated dextrose that ranges from 25% to 70%, providing a rich source of calories. Such highly concentrated dextrose solutions are

TABLE 6-4	MANAGEMENT OF TUBE FEEDING COMPLICATIONS	
COMPLICATION	**POSSIBLE CAUSE**	**SUGGESTED INTERVENTION**
Pulmonary aspiration*	Feeding tube in esophagus or respiratory tract	Confirm proper placement of tube before administering any feeding; check placement at least every 4-8 hrs during continuous feedings.
	Regurgitation of formula	Consider giving feeding into small bowel rather than stomach; keep head elevated 30-45 degrees during feedings; stop feedings temporarily during treatments such as chest physiotherapy.
Diarrhea	Antibiotic therapy	Antidiarrheal medications may be ordered if the possibility of infection with *Clostridium difficile* has been ruled out; *Lactobacillus* or *Saccharomyces boulardii* are sometimes given enterally in an effort to establish benign gut flora.
	Hypertonic medications (e.g., KCl or medications containing sorbitol)	Dilute enteral medications well; evaluate sorbitol content of medications.
	Malnutrition/hypoalbuminemia	Use continuous rather than bolus feedings; consider a formula with MCT and/or soluble fiber.
	Bacterial contamination	Use scrupulously clean formula preparation and administration techniques; refrigerate home-prepared, reconstituted, or opened cans of formula until ready to use, and use all such products within 24 hrs.
	Predisposing illness (e.g., short bowel syndrome, inflammatory bowel disease, AIDS)	Use continuous feedings; consider a formula with MCT and/or soluble fiber.
	Lactose intolerance	Use a lactose-free formula.
	Fecal impaction	Perform digital examination to rule out fecal impaction with seepage of liquid stool around the obstruction.
	Intestinal mucosal atrophy	Consider use of formula containing soluble fiber and MCT.
Constipation	Lack of fiber	Consider fiber-containing formula; ensure that fluid intake is adequate; stool softeners may be ordered.
Tube occlusion	Administration of medications via tube	Avoid crushing tablets; administer medications in elixir or suspension form whenever possible; irrigate feeding tube with water before and after giving medications; never mix medication with enteral formulas because this may cause clumping of formula.
	Sedimentation of formula	Irrigate tube with water [†] every 4-8 hrs during continuous feedings and after every intermittent feeding; irrigate tubes well if gastric residuals are measured, as gastric juices left in the tube may cause precipitation of formula in the tube; instilling pancreatic enzyme into the tube may clear some occlusions.
Delayed gastric emptying	Serious illness, diabetic gastroparesis, prematurity, surgery, high-fat content of formula, hyperglycemia	Consult with physician regarding whether feedings can be administered into the small bowel, a lower-fat formula can be used, or metoclopramide can be administered to stimulate gastric emptying; improve glycemic control if hyperglycemia exists.
Hyperglycemia	Excessive glucose in feedings/fluids, glucose intolerance due to stress/sepsis, concomitant disease (e.g., diabetes), drug therapy (e.g., corticosteroids)	Monitor serum glucose several times daily until stable and regularly thereafter; correct underlying illness if possible; reduce enteral or parenteral feedings if excessive; consider use of insulin; consider higher fat/lower carbohydrate formula.

From Moore MC: *Pocket Guide to Nutritional Assessment and Care*, ed 5, St Louis, 2005, Mosby.
MCT, medium-chain triglyceride.
*Signs and symptoms of pulmonary aspiration include tachypnea, shortness of breath, hypoxia, and infiltrate on chest radiographs.
[†]Fluids such as cranberry juice or Coca-Cola are sometimes used as irrigants, in the belief that they are better than water at preventing tube occlusion. However, research has shown cranberry juice to be inferior to and Coca-Cola no better than water.

hyperosmolar, as much as 1800 mOsm/L, and therefore must be delivered through a central vein.[41] Peripheral parenteral nutrition (PPN) has a glucose concentration of 5% to 10% and may be delivered safely through a peripheral vein. PPN solution delivers nutrition support in a large volume that cannot be tolerated by patients who require fluid restriction.

It provides short-term nutrition support for a few days to less than 2 weeks.

Regardless of the route of administration, both PPN and TPN provide glucose, fat, protein, electrolytes, vitamins, and trace elements. Although dextro-amino acid solutions are commonly thought of as good growth media for microorganisms, they actually suppress the growth of most organisms usually associated with catheter-related sepsis, except yeasts. However, because the many manipulations required to prepare solutions increase the possibility of contamination, TPN solutions are best used with caution. They should be prepared under laminar flow conditions in the pharmacy, with avoidance of additions on the nursing unit. Solution containers need to be inspected for cracks or leaks before hanging, and solutions must be discarded within 24 hours of hanging. An in-line 0.22-micron filter, which eliminates all microorganisms but not endotoxins, may be used in administration of solutions. Use of the filter, however, cannot be substituted for good aseptic technique.

Nursing Management of Potential Complications

Nursing management of the patient receiving TPN includes catheter care, administration of solutions, prevention or correction of complications, and evaluation of patient responses to IV feedings. Refer to Table 6-5 for nursing management of TPN complications.

Because TPN requires an indwelling catheter in a central vein, it carries an increased risk of sepsis as well as potential insertion-related complications such as pneumothorax and hemothorax. Air embolism is also more likely with central vein TPN. Patients requiring multiple IV therapies and frequent blood sampling usually have multilumen central venous catheters, and TPN is often infused via these catheters.

Some clinical studies have reported that catheter-related sepsis is higher with multilumen catheters; others have found no difference compared with single-lumen catheters.[42] Clearly, patients requiring multilumen catheters are likely to be very ill and immunocompromised, and scrupulous aseptic technique is essential in maintaining multilumen catheters. The manipulation involved in frequent changes of IV fluid and obtaining blood specimens through these catheters increases the risk of catheter contamination. Peripherally inserted central catheters (PICCs) allow central venous access through long catheters inserted in peripheral sites. This reduces the risk of complications associated with percutaneous cannulation of the subclavian vein and provides an alternative to PPN.[43]

The indwelling central venous catheter provides an excellent nidus for infection. Catheter-related infections arise from endogenous skin flora, contamination of the catheter hub, seeding of the catheter by organisms carried in the bloodstream from another site, or contamination of the infusate. Good hand hygiene and scrupulous aseptic technique in all aspects of catheter care and TPN delivery are the primary steps for prevention of catheter-related infections. Other measures to reduce the incidence of catheter-related infections include using maximal barrier precautions (i.e., cap, mask, sterile gloves, sterile drape) at the time of insertion, tunneling the catheter underneath the skin, use of a 2% chlorhexidine preparation for skin cleansing, no routine replacement of the central venous catheter for prevention of infection, and use of antiseptic/antibiotic-impregnated central venous catheters.[44]

Metabolic complications associated with parenteral nutrition include glucose intolerance and electrolyte imbalance. Slow advancement of the rate of TPN (25 ml/hr) to goal rate will allow pancreatic adjustment to the dextrose load. Capillary blood glucose should be monitored every 4 to 6 hours. Insulin can be added to the TPN solution or can be infused as a separate drip to control glucose levels. Rapid cessation of TPN may not lead to hypoglycemia; however, tapering the infusion over 2 to 4 hours is recommended.[45]

Serum electrolyte levels are obtained upon starting TPN. During critical illness, levels should be monitored and corrected daily, and then weekly or twice weekly once the patient is more stable. The refeeding syndrome is a potentially lethal condition characterized by generalized fluid and electrolyte imbalance. It occurs as a potential complication after initiation of oral, enteral, or parenteral nutrition in malnourished patients. During chronic starvation, several compensatory metabolic changes occur. The reintroduction of carbohydrates and amino acids leads to increased insulin production. This creates an anabolic environment that increases intracellular demand for phosphorus, potassium, magnesium, vitamins, and minerals.[46] These metabolic demands result in severe shifts from the extracellular compartment. Increased insulin levels also result in fluid retention. Severe hypophosphatemia, hypokalemia, and hypomagnesemia result in altered cardiac, gastrointestinal, and neurologic function. In particular, hypophosphatemia causes a decrease in 2,3-diphosphosoglycerate (2,3 DPG) and also limits the many reactions that require ATP. As a result, hypophosphatemia and other electrolyte deficiencies may lead to respiratory failure, congestive heart failure, and dysrhythmias.

It is important to anticipate refeeding syndrome in patients who may be at risk. Patients with chronic malnutrition or underfeeding, chronic alcoholism, or anorexia nervosa, or those maintained NPO for several days with evidence of stress are at risk for refeeding syndrome.[47] In high-risk patients, nutrition support should be started cautiously at 25% to 50% of required calories and slowly advanced over 3 to 4 days as tolerated. Close monitoring of serum electrolyte levels before and during feeding is essential. Normal values do not always reflect total body stores. Correction of preexisting electrolyte imbalances is necessary before initiation of feeding. Continued monitoring and supplementation with electrolytes and vitamins is necessary throughout the first week of nutrition support.[47]

Lipid Emulsion

Lipids or intravenous fat emulsions (IVFE) provide calories for energy and prevent essential fatty acid depletion. In contrast to dextro-amino acid solutions, IVFE provide a rich environment for the growth of bacteria and fungi including *Candida albicans*. Furthermore, IVFE cannot be filtered through an in-line 0.22-μm filter, because some particles in the emulsions have larger diameters than this. Lipids may be infused into the TPN line downstream from

TABLE 6-5	NURSING MANAGEMENT OF TPN COMPLICATIONS	
COMPLICATION	**SIGNS/SYMPTOMS**	**PREVENTION/INTERVENTION**
Catheter site infection	Erythema, warmth, inflammation, and pus at the catheter insertion site	Insert catheter with maximal barrier precautions (gown, mask, gloves, drapes) and strict aseptic technique; use aseptic technique in maintaining the insertion site; monitor insertion site regularly; culture site and administer antibiotics as appropriate if infection is apparent.
Catheter-related sepsis	Fever, chills, glucose intolerance, positive blood culture; bacterial colony counts in blood from the catheter 5-10 times higher than in blood obtained from a peripheral site	Insert catheter with maximal barrier precautions (gown, mask, gloves, drapes) and strict aseptic technique; maintain an intact dressing; change if contaminated by vomitus, sputum, etc.; use aseptic technique whenever handling catheter, IV tubing, and TPN solutions; hang a single bottle of TPN no longer than 24 hrs and lipid emulsion no longer than 12 hrs; use a 0.22 μm filter with solutions that contain lipids; avoid using single-lumen nontunneled catheter for blood sampling and infusion of non-TPN solutions if possible.
Air embolism	Dyspnea, cyanosis, tachycardia hypotension, possibly death	Use Luer lock system or secure all connections well; Groshong catheter, which has valve at tip, may reduce risk of air embolism; use an in-line 0.22 μm air-eliminating filter if solutions do not contain lipids or 1.2 μm or larger if solutions contain lipids; have patient perform Valsalva's maneuver during tubing changes; if air embolism is suggested, place patient in left lateral decubitus position and administer oxygen; immediately notify physician, who may attempt to aspirate air from the heart.
Central venous thrombosis	Unilateral edema of neck, shoulder, and arm; development of collateral circulation on chest; pain in insertion site	Follow measures to prevent sepsis; repeated or traumatic catheterizations are most likely to result in thrombosis; treatment usually includes anticoagulation; if symptoms are not too severe, thrombolytic therapy may be attempted, but catheter removal is usually necessary.
Catheter occlusion or semiocclusion	No flow or sluggish flow through the catheter; or infusion through the catheter possible, but blood cannot be aspirated from the catheter	Flush catheter with heparinized saline if infusion is stopped temporarily; if catheter appears to be occluded, attempt to aspirate the clot; thrombolytic agent may restore patency if clotted or occluded by fibrin sheath; hydrochloric acid, 0.1 N, has been used to clear drug precipitates and 70% ethanol to clear lipid precipitates.
Hypoglycemia	Diaphoresis, shakiness, confusion, loss of consciousness	Do not discontinue TPN abruptly, taper rate over several hrs; use pump to regulate infusion so that it remains ±10% of ordered rate; if hypoglycemia is suggested, then administer oral carbohydrate; if oral intake is contraindicated or patient is unconscious, a bolus of IV dextrose may be used.
Hyperglycemia	Thirst, headache, lethargy, increased urination	Monitor blood glucose frequently until stable; TPN is usually initiated at a slow rate or with a low dextrose concentration and increased over 2-3 days to avoid hyperglycemia; the patient may require insulin added to the TPN if the problem is severe.
Hypertriglyceridemia	Serum triglyceride concentrations elevated (especially serious if >400 mg/dL); serum may appear turbid	Monitor serum triglycerides after each increase in rate and at least 3 times weekly until stable in patients receiving lipid emulsions; reduce lipid infusion rate or administer low-dose heparin with lipid emulsions if elevated levels are observed.

From Moore MC: *Pocket Guide to Nutritional Assessment and Care*, ed 5, St Louis, 2005, Mosby.

the filter. No other drugs should be infused into a line containing lipids or TPN. Lipid emulsions are handled with strict asepsis, and they must be discarded within 12 to 24 hours of hanging. There is a trend toward mixing lipid emulsions with dextro-amino acid TPN solutions; these are called 3-in-1 solutions or total nutrient admixtures (TNA). Consolidating the nutrients in one container is more economical and saves nursing time, although TNA solutions may be less stable.[41]

EVALUATING RESPONSE TO NUTRITION SUPPORT

A multidisciplinary approach is required in evaluating the effects of nutrition support on clinical outcomes. Assessment of response to nutrition support is an ongoing process that involves anthropometric measurements, physical examination, and biochemical evaluation. Daily monitoring of nutritional intake is an important aspect of critical care and is a key element in preventing problems associated with underfeeding and overfeeding. Daily weights and the maintenance of accurate intake-and-output records are crucial for evaluating nutritional progress and the state of hydration in the patient receiving nutrition support. A variety of metabolic complications (hypernatremia and hyponatremia, hyperkalemia and hypokalemia, hypercalcemia and hypocalcemia, hyperphosphatemia and hypophosphatemia, etc.) as well as deficiencies of vitamins and minerals occur in patients receiving enteral and parenteral nutrition. For this reason, adequacy of electrolytes, calcium, phosphate, magnesium, zinc, and other nutrients must be assessed regularly (frequently during the early stages, less frequently in stable long-term patients) for the duration of nutrition support. Serum levels of electrolytes, calcium, phosphorus, and magnesium serve as a guide to the amount of these nutrients that has to be supplied; blood urea nitrogen and creatinine levels reflect the adequacy of renal function to handle nutrition support; blood glucose is an indicator of the patient's tolerance of the carbohydrate; prealbumin is an indicator of the adequacy of nutrition support; and serum triglyceride concentrations (in patients receiving intravenous lipid emulsions) reflect the ability of the tissues to metabolize the lipids.

Recently, the Society of Critical Care Medicine (SCCM) and the American Society for Parenteral and Enteral Nutrition (A.S.P.E.N.) published *The Guidelines for the Provision and Assessment of Nutrition Support Therapy in the Adult Critically Ill Patient*. The publication is based on an extensive review of 307 articles and is intended for the care of critically ill adults who require a stay of greater than three days in the critical care area. All practitioners who care for this target population are encouraged to become familiar with these evidence-based guidelines.[48]

It is within the scope of practice for critical care nurses to calculate caloric requirements and analyze daily caloric delivery, advocate for early nutrition support, and minimize feeding interruptions through careful patient assessment and interruption analysis. In addition to monitoring changes in weight and laboratory values, the nurse is the health care team member who has the most constant contact with the patient and who is therefore uniquely qualified to evaluate feeding tolerance and adequacy of delivery.

REFERENCES

1. Braunschweig C, et al: Impact of declines in nutritional status on outcomes in adult patients hospitalized for more than 7 days, *J Am Diet Assoc* 100(11):1316, 2000.
2. Mathus-Vliegen EMH: Nutritional status, nutrition and pressure ulcers, *Nutr Clin Pract* 16(5):286, 2001.
3. Rubinson L, et al: Low caloric intake is associated with nosocomial bloodstream infections in patients in the medical intensive care unit, *Crit Care Med* 32(2):350, 2004.
4. August D, et al: Guidelines for the use of parenteral and enteral nutrition in adult and pediatric patients, *JPEN J Parenter Enteral Nutr* 26(suppl 1):1SA, 2002.
5. Raguso C, et al: The role of visceral proteins in the nutritional assessment of intensive care unit patients, *Curr Opin Nutr Metab Care* 6(2):211, 2003.
6. Cheng CH, et al: Measured versus estimated energy expenditure in mechanically ventilated critically ill patients, *Clin Nutr* 21(2):165, 2002.
7. Alberda CL, et al: Energy requirements in critically ill patients: how close are our estimates? *Nutr Clin Pract* 17(1):38, 2002.
8. Van den Berghe G, et al: Intensive insulin therapy in critically ill patients, *N Engl J Med* 345(19):1359, 2001.
9. Rassias AJ, et al: Insulin increases neutrophil count and phagocytic capacity after cardiac surgery, *Anesth Analg* 94(5):1113, 2002.
10. Clement S, et al: Management of diabetes and hyperglycemia in hospitals, *Diabetes Care* 27(2):553, 2004.
11. National Education Programs Working Group report on the management of patients with hypertension and high blood cholesterol, *Ann Intern Med* 114(3):224, 1991.
12. Vollmer WM, et al: Effects of diet and sodium intake on blood pressure: subgroup analysis of the DASH-sodium trial, *Ann Intern Med* 135(12):1019, 2001.
13. Yeung SC, Ensom MH: Phenytoin and enteral feedings: does evidence support an interaction? *Ann Pharmacother* 34(7-8): 895, 2000.
14. Wilson RF, Tyburski JG: Metabolic responses and nutritional therapy in patients with severe head injuries, *J Head Trauma Rehabil* 13(1):11, 1998.
15. Taylor SJ, et al: Prospective, randomized, controlled trial to determine the effect of early enhanced enteral nutrition on clinical outcome in mechanically ventilated patients suffering head injury, *Crit Care Med* 27(11):2525, 1999.
16. Kierdorf HP: The nutritional management of acute renal failure in the intensive care unit, *New Horiz* 3(4):699, 1995.
17. Bellomo R, et al: A prospective comparative study of moderate versus high protein intake for critically ill patients with acute renal failure, *Ren Fail* 19(1):111, 1997.
18. Mitch WE, Maroni BJ: Factors causing malnutrition in patients with chronic uremia, *Am J Kidney Dis* 33(1):176, 1999.
19. Kopple J: Therapeutic approaches to malnutrition in chronic dialysis patients: the different modalities of nutritional support, *Am J Kidney Dis* 33(1):180, 1999.
20. Riella MC: Nutrition in acute renal failure, *Ren Fail* 19(2):237, 1997.
21. Brewer ED: Pediatric experience with intradialytic parenteral nutrition and supplemental tube feeding, *Am J Kidney Dis* 33(1):205, 1999.
22. Cato Y: Intradialytic parenteral nutrition therapy for the malnourished hemodialysis patient, *J Intraven Nurs* 20(3):130, 1997.
23. Hazell AS, Butterworth RF: Hepatic encephalopathy: an update of pathophysiologic mechanisms, *Proc Soc Exp Biol Med* 222(2):99, 1999.
24. Albrecht J, Jones EA: Hepatic encephalopathy: molecular mechanisms underlying the clinical syndrome, *J Neurol Sci* 170(2):138, 1999.
25. August D, et al: Guidelines for the use of parenteral and enteral nutrition in adult and pediatric patients, *JPEN J Parenter Enteral Nutr* 26(suppl 1):18SA, 2002.
26. Patton KM, Aranda-Michel J: Nutritional aspects in liver disease and liver transplantation, *Nutr Clin Pract* 17(6):332, 2002.

27. Florez DA, Aranda-Michel J: Nutritional management of acute and chronic liver disease, *Semin Gastrointest Dis* 13(3): 169, 2002.

28. Khokhar AS, Seidner DL: The pathophysiology of pancreatitis, *Nutr Clin Pract* 19(1):5, 2004.

29. Avgerinos C, et al: Nutritional support in acute pancreatitis, *Dig Dis* 21(3):214, 2003.

30. Russell MK: Acute pancreatitis: a review of pathophysiology and nutrition management, *Nutr Clin Pract* 19(1):16, 2004.

31. Al-Omran M, Groof A, Wilke D: Enteral versus parenteral nutrition for acute pancreatitis, *Cochrane Database Syst Rev* 1:1, 2003.

32. Dejong CH, Greve JW, Soeters PB: Nutrition in patients with acute pancreatitis, *Curr Opin Crit Care* 7(4):251, 2001.

33. Abou-Assi S, O'Keefe SJ: Nutrition support during acute pancreatitis, *Nutrition* 18(11-12):938, 2002.

34. Jones MP: Management of diabetic gastroparesis, *Nutr Clin Pract* 19(2):145, 2004.

35. Charney P, Hertzler SR: Management of blood glucose and diabetes in the critically ill patient receiving enteral feeding, *Nutr Clin Pract* 19(2):129, 2004.

36. Braga M, et al: Artificial nutrition after major abdominal surgery: impact of route of administration and composition of the diet, *Crit Care Med* 26(1):24, 1998.

37. Booth CM, Heyland DK, Paterson WG: Gastrointestinal promotility drugs in the critical care setting: a systematic review of the evidence, *Crit Care Med* 30(7):1429, 2002.

38. Lord LM, et al: Comparison of weighted vs. unweighted enteral feeding tubes for efficacy of transpyloric intubation, *JPEN J Parenter Enteral Nutr* 17(3):71, 1993.

39. Metheny NA, et al: pH testing of feeding-tube aspirates to determine placement, *Nutr Clin Pract* 9(5):185, 1994.

40. Metheny NA, et al: pH and concentration of bilirubin in feeding tube aspirates as predictors of tube placement, *Nurs Res* 48(4):189, 1999.

41. Worthington P, Gilbert KA, Wagner BA: Parenteral nutrition for the acutely ill, *AACN Clin Issues* 11(4):559, 2000.

42. Dobbins BM, et al: Each lumen is a potential source of central venous catheter-related bloodstream infection, *Crit Care Med* 31(6):1688, 2003.

43. Orr ME: The peripherally inserted central catheter: what are the current indications for its use? *Nutr Clin Pract* 17(2):99, 2002.

44. O'Grady NP, et al: Guidelines for the prevention of intravascular catheter-related infections, *Infect Control Hosp Epidemiol* 23(12):759, 2002.

45. Speerhas R, et al: Maintaining normal blood glucose concentrations with total parenteral nutrition: is it necessary to taper total parenteral nutrition? *Nutr Clin Pract* 18(5):414, 2003.

46. Crook MA, Hally V, Panteli JV: The importance of the refeeding syndrome, *Nutrition* 17(7-8):632, 2001.

47. Hearing SD: Refeeding syndrome, *BMJ* 328(7445):908, 2004.

48. McClave SA, et al. Society of Critical Care Medicine (SCCM) and American Society for Parenteral and Enteral Nutrition (A.S.P.E.N.): Guidelines for the provision and assessment of nutrition support therapy in the adult critically ill patient, Sage Journals Online, 2009. http://pen.sagepub.com/content/22/277.full. Accessed 10/2/2010.

Gerontological Alterations

Linda Urden

OBJECTIVES

- Describe the age-associated physiological changes that occur in the cardiovascular, respiratory, renal, gastrointestinal, hepatic, integumentary, immune, and central nervous systems.
- State the clinical significance of age-related physiological changes and the expected nursing considerations or interventions used in caring for older critical care patients.
- Relate the age-related changes in hepatic function and the accompanying pharmacokinetic changes to the administration of various cardiovascular medications.

Patients in critical care units include an increasing number of older adults. According to a U.S. Department of Health and Human Services report, the United States population older than 65 years reached 35.6 million, accounting for 12.3% of the overall population. Those in the 65- to 74-year age group numbered 18.3 million, 75- to 84-year-olds accounted for 12.7 million, and those in the 85-year or older age group numbered 6 million. This latter group is expected to reach 9.6 million by 2030.[1] In 2001 a 65-year-old woman had a life expectancy of 19.4 more years, whereas men could expect to live another 16.4 years.[1]

The process of senescence (growing old) is characterized by tissue and organ changes. This, in combination with the prevalence of chronic conditions in the older adult, contributes to increased morbidity and mortality in the critical care unit. Aging is accompanied by physiological changes in the cardiovascular, respiratory, renal, gastrointestinal (GI), hepatic, integumentary, immune, and central nervous systems. With advancing age the incidence of disease increases, with cardiovascular and neoplastic diseases being the most common causes of death.[2] However, although physiological decline and disease processes influence each other, physiological decline occurs independently of disease and is responsible for the development of symptoms at an earlier stage of disease in older adults than in their younger counterparts.[2] Therefore changes in physiological function are important to consider when caring for the older adult patient (Table 7-1, Figure 7-1, Box 7-1).

CARDIOVASCULAR SYSTEM

Advancing age has many effects on the cardiovascular system. With advancing age both the myocardium and the vascular system undergo a multitude of anatomic and cellular changes that alter the function of both the myocardium and peripheral vascular system.[3] These changes in cardiovascular function significantly impact critical illness in the older adult because of the age-related effects on cardiovascular structure and function. In addition, because age is a major risk factor for cardiovascular disease in the older adult, this high-risk population will encounter more cardiovascular events when admitted for noncardiac problems to the critical care unit.[4]

Age-Related Changes in Myocardial Structure and Function

Myocardial collagen content increases with age.[5,6] Collagen is the principal noncontractile protein occupying the cardiac interstitium.[7] Increased myocardial collagen content renders the myocardium less compliant; therefore a decrease in myocardial compliance can adversely affect diastolic filling (through decreased distensibility and dilation) and myocardial relaxation. Consequently, the left ventricle must develop

TABLE 7-1 SUMMARY OF AGE-RELATED PHYSIOLOGICAL CHANGES AND RELATED CLINICAL CONSIDERATIONS

AGE-RELATED EFFECT	CLINICAL CONSIDERATIONS
Cardiovascular System	
↓ Inotropic and chronotropic response of myocardium to catecholamine stimulation	The increase in cardiac output during stress or exercise is achieved by an increase in diastolic filling (increased dependence on Starling's law of the heart)
↑ Myocardial collagen content	Leads to a decrease in the compliance of the ventricle (higher filling pressures are needed to maintain stroke volume)
↓ Baroreceptor sensitivity	↑ Tendency for orthostatic hypotension after prolonged bed rest or if patient is taking antihypertensive medication or has systolic hypertension
Prolonged rate of relaxation	May predispose the elderly patient to hemodynamic derangements in the presence of tachydysrhythmias, hypertension, or ischemic heart disease
↓ Compliance of blood vessels	↑ Peripheral vascular resistance and blood pressure
Respiratory System	
↓ Strength of the respiratory muscles, recoil of lungs, chest wall compliance, and efficiency and number of cilia in airways	↑ Susceptibility to aspiration, atelectasis, and pulmonary infection Patient may require more frequent deep breathing, coughing, and position change
↓ Pao_2 level	↓ Ventilatory response to hypoxia and hypercapnia ↑ Sensitivity to narcotics
Renal System	
↓ Glomerular filtration rate	Careful observation of patient when administering aminoglycosides, antibiotics, and contrast dyes
↓ Ability to concentrate and conserve water	May predispose patient to development of dehydration and hypernatremia, especially if patient is fluid-restricted and insensible losses are high (e.g., during mechanical ventilation or fever)
↓ Ability to excrete salt and water loads, as well as urea, ammonia, and drugs	Observe for clinical manifestations of fluid overload and drug reactions
↓ Response to an acid load	After an acid load (i.e., metabolic acidosis), the older patient may be in a state of uncompensated metabolic acidosis for a longer period
Liver	
↓ Total liver blood flow	Adverse drug reactions, especially with polypharmacy
Gastrointestinal System	
Diminished ability to swallow Impaired esophageal motility Delayed emptying of liquids	May predispose older patient to aspiration pneumonia Assess for proper fit of dentures and ability to chew Flex head forward 45 degrees Develop awareness for complaints of food or medications "sticking in throat" Assess for complaints of heartburn or epigastric discomfort Avoid prolonged supine position
↓ Stool weight and transit time	Examine abdomen for distention Investigate complaints of anorexia Obtain thorough bowel history and note routine use of laxative Increase intake of dietary fiber and assess for fecal incontinence and impaction
Neurological System	
↑ Cranial dead space	Older persons may sustain a significant amount of hemorrhage before symptoms are apparent
↓ Number of neurons and dendrites and length of dendrite spines	Delayed or impaired processing of sensory and motor information
Delay in the rate of synaptogenesis Changes in neurotransmitter turnover	May cause desynchronization of neurotransmission

Modified from Rebenson-Piano M: The physiologic changes that occur with aging. *Crit Care Q* 12(1):1, 1989.
CO, Cardiac output; *GFR,* glomerular filtration rate.

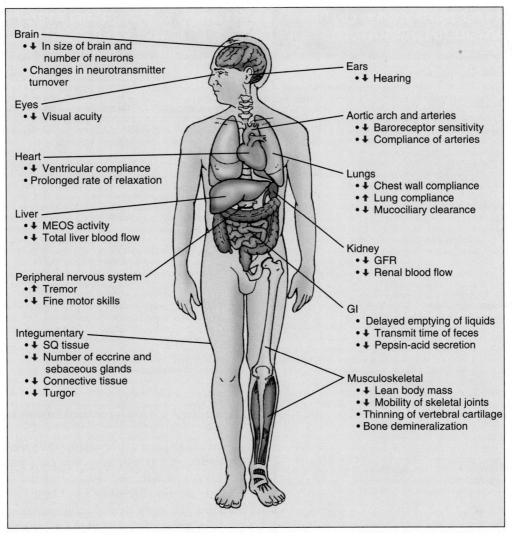

FIGURE 7-1 Summary of physiological changes that occur in all systems and that the critical care nurse must consider in caring for older patients in the critical care unit. *MEOS,* Microsomal enzyme oxidative system; *GFR,* glomerular filtration rate; *GI,* gastrointestinal; *Sub-Q,* subcutaneous. (From Urden LD, Stacy KM, Lough ME: *Critical care nursing: Diagnosis and management,* ed 6, St. Louis, 2010, Mosby.)

a higher filling pressure for a given increase in ventricular volume. Decreased left ventricular compliance may be evident in the older adult by the presence of an S_4 heart sound.[8]

The functional consequence of these changes could be an increase in myocardial oxygen consumption. Under normal physiological conditions, an increase in myocardial oxygen demand is met with a corresponding increase in coronary artery blood flow. However, in the presence of coronary artery disease, coronary artery blood flow can be limited because of atherosclerotic-mediated narrowing of the coronary arteries. Hence the older patient is at risk for developing myocardial ischemia and/or infarction. Clinical manifestations of myocardial ischemia include electrocardiographic (ECG) changes and chest pain. However, the sensation of chest pain may be altered in the older adult. Atypical symptoms, such as dyspnea, confusion, and failure to thrive are frequently the only symptoms associated with myocardial infarction in this high-risk population.[9]

The aging heart also undergoes a modest degree of hypertrophy that is similar to pressure overload-induced hypertrophy. Such hypertrophy entails a thickening of the left ventricular wall without appreciable changes in left ventricular cavity size.[10] However, increases in left ventricular cavity size associated with aging occur only in men.[9] The increase in left ventricular wall thickness is a result primarily of an increase in muscle cell size. In older individuals the myocardial hypertrophy may be caused by corresponding increases in aortic impedance and systemic vascular resistance.[11]

Myocardial contractility depends on numerous factors. However, the most important determinants of myocardial contraction are the intracellular level of free calcium and the sensitivity of the contractile proteins for calcium.[11,12] Because peak contractile force in the senescent myocardium is unaltered, this suggests that neither the amount of intracellular free calcium during systole nor the sensitivity of the contractile proteins for calcium is altered. The prolonged duration

BOX 7-1 EFFECTS OF AGING ON VARIOUS LABORATORY VALUES

Values that Do Not Change with Age
Red blood cells
White blood cells total
Prothrombin time
Partial thromboplastin time
Platelets
Sodium
Potassium
Chloride
High-density lipoprotein (HDL)
Acid phosphatase
Creatinine kinase
pH (arterial)
$PaCO_2$ (arterial)
HCO_3 (arterial)

Values that Change with Age
↓ Hemoglobin/Hematocrit
↑ Uric acid
↓ Calcium
↓ Phosphorus
↑ Amylase
↓ Albumin
↑ Blood urea nitrogen
↓ Creatinine
↑ Alkaline phosphatase
↓ Thyroxine (T_4)
↓ Triiodothyronine (T_3)
↓ O_2 saturation (arterial)
↓ Magnesium
↑ Fasting glucose
↓ Cholesterol (total)
↑ Low-density lipoprotein (LDL)
↓ PaO_2 (arterial)

Adapted from Pagana KD, Pagana TJ: *Diagnostic and laboratory test reference*, ed. 6, Mosby, St. Louis, 2003; and Pagana KD, Pagana TJ: Manual of diagnostic and laboratory tests, ed. 2, Mosby, St. Louis, 2004.
↔, No change; ↓, decreased; ↑, increased.

TABLE 7-2 AGE-RELATED CHANGES IN ELECTROCARDIOGRAPHIC VARIABLES

ECG VARIABLE	AGE (YEARS)			
	YOUNGER THAN 30	30-39	40-49	OLDER THAN 49
R wave amplitude (mm)	10.43	10.53	9.01	9.25
S wave amplitude (mm)	15.21	14.21	12.22	12.42
Frontal plane axis (degrees)	48.93	48.13	36.50	38.83
PR duration (ms)	15.89	16.23	16.04	16.25
QRS duration (ms)	7.64	7.51	7.36	8.00
QT duration (ms)	37.83	37.50	37.99	39.58
T-wave amplitude (ms)	5.21	4.57	4.31	4.42

Data from Bachman S, Sparrow D, Smith LK: Effect of aging on the electrocardiogram. *Am J Cardiol* 48(3):513, 1981.
ECG, Electrocardiogram.

during exercise, the older person's capacity for exercise may be limited.

Resting CO and stroke volume (SV) are not changed with advancing age. At rest, left ventricular end-diastolic volume (LVEDV, preload), end-systolic volume, and the ejection fraction are not affected by age.[15] In the older human myocardium, the early diastolic filling period and isovolumic phase of myocardial relaxation are prolonged.[15-17] However, these changes, although suggestive of diastolic dysfunction, do not translate into decreases in end-diastolic volume or stroke volume.[16,17] Finally, aging is associated with a moderate increase in pulmonary artery pressure.[18]

Advancing age produces changes in the ECG. R-wave and S-wave amplitude significantly decrease in persons older than 49 years, whereas QT duration increases[19] (Table 7-2). The incidence of asymptomatic cardiac dysrhythmias increases in older patients.[20] The most common dysrhythmia occurring in older individuals is the premature ventricular contraction (PVC). Carom et al[21] and Fleg and Kennedy[22] report that 70% to 80% of all patients older than 60 years experience PVCs. Other common types of dysrhythmias are sinus node dysfunction (atrial fibrillation, atrial flutter, or paroxysmal supraventricular tachycardia) and atrioventricular conduction disturbances.[15,19,20] Because the majority of patients are asymptomatic, the use of antidysrhythmics is generally not recommended. The side effects and toxic effects of antidysrhythmics impose more of a risk, as compared with the risk of mortality or morbidity related to the dysrhythmia.[20,23] In contrast, for patients who are symptomatic and have malignant ventricular dysrhythmias (sustained ventricular tachycardia and/or fibrillation), pharmacological therapy is warranted.[20,23]

of contraction (systole) is caused in part by a slowed or delayed rate of myocardial relaxation, which may be an adaptive mechanism to preserve contractile function compromised by age-related increases in afterload.[3,12]

Age-Associated Changes in Hemodynamics and the Electrocardiogram

Resting (supine) heart rate decreases with age.[13,14] Cinelli et al[13] reported a decrease in the resting heart rate from 78.8 beats/min in young adults to 62.3 beats/min in older adults. Heart rate is an important determinant of cardiac output (CO), and the normal resting heart beats approximately 70 times a minute. At rest or with minimal activity, the older adult probably will not experience any untoward cardiovascular effect (i.e., a decrease in CO) with a heart rate of 62 beats/min. However, if the heart rate response is attenuated

Age-Related Changes in Baroreceptor Function

Baroreceptor reflex function is altered with aging.[24] Baroreceptors, located at the bifurcation of the common carotid artery and aortic arch, are mechanoreceptors that respond to stretch and other changes in the blood vessel wall.[25] Impulses arising in the baroreceptor region project to the vasomotor center (nucleus of tractus solitarius) in the medulla. Abrupt changes in blood pressure caused by increases in peripheral resistance, CO, or blood volume are sensed by the baroreceptors, resulting in an increase in the impulse frequency to the vasomotor center within the medulla. This increase inhibits vasoconstrictor impulses arising from the vasoconstrictor region within the medulla.[25] The result is a decrease in heart rate (HR) and peripheral vasodilation; both these effects return the blood pressure to within normal limits.

Postural hypotension was once thought to occur more frequently in older persons and to be related to age. However, recent studies have shown that the prevalence of postural hypotension is quite low in older persons.[26,27] The prevalence of orthostatic hypotension is greater in institutionalized older patients who are receiving antihypertensive medications.[28]

Left Ventricular Function

In most individuals, aging is associated with a decline in exercise performance. The thickening of the left ventricular wall along with stiffening of the aortic and mitral valves makes the aging heart less able to provide adequate contractile strength.[29] With advancing age the maximal HR achieved during exercise is attenuated; however, the decreased HR response is accompanied by an increase in LVEDV and SV. This augmentation in LVEDV and SV offsets the attenuated HR response and maintains CO in exercise.

Healthy older persons have no age-associated decline in CO during exercise, but other factors (e.g., neural functioning, skeletal/joint functioning, pulmonary function) may limit an older individual's ability to exercise.

Peripheral Vascular System

The effects of aging on the peripheral vascular system are reflected in the gradual but linear rise in systolic blood pressure.[30,31] Diastolic blood pressure is less affected by age and generally remains the same or decreases.[31]

Important determinants of systolic blood pressure include the compliance of the vasculature and the blood volume within the vascular system. Similar to the heart, the compliance of the vasculature is determined by its cell type and tissue composition. With advancing age the intimal layer thickens, principally because of an increase in smooth muscle cells that have migrated from the medial layer, and the amount of connective tissue (collagen, elastic tissue) increases.[30] These changes occur in the intima of the large and distal arteries. This gradual decrease in arterial compliance, or "stiffening of the arteries," is known as arteriosclerosis. Arteriosclerotic and atherosclerotic processes cause the arteries to become progressively less distensible, altering the vascular pressure-volume relationship. These changes are clinically significant because small changes in intravascular volume are accompanied by disproportionate increases in systolic blood pressure. The decrease in arterial compliance and disproportionate increase in systolic blood pressure may lead to an increase in afterload and the development of concentric (pressure-induced) ventricular hypertrophy in the elderly patient.[32]

Arterial pressure is also governed by the amount of blood volume, which in turn is regulated by plasma levels of sodium and water and the activity of the renin-angiotensin system.[33] Plasma renin activity declines with age, and aging per se has no appreciable effect on sodium and water homeostasis.[34,35] As noted later, however, age-related changes occur in renal tubular function, and the glomerular filtration rate (GFR) decreases, both of which can affect overall sodium and water homeostasis. Circulating levels of sodium-regulating hormones, such as natriuretic hormone, aldosterone, and antidiuretic hormone (ADH), are not appreciably altered by advancing age.[35,36] However, a delayed natriuretic response after sodium loading and plasma volume expansion and a diminished renal response to ADH secretion have been reported in older persons.[36]

PULMONARY SYSTEM

Many of the changes in the pulmonary system that occur with aging are reflected in pulmonary function tests and include changes in thoracic wall expansion and respiratory muscle strength, morphology of alveolar parenchyma, and decreases in arterial oxygen tension (Pao_2)[37] (Table 7-3). These changes occur progressively as age advances and should not alter the older person's ability to breathe effortlessly. However, factors such as repeated exposure to environmental pollutants, cigarette smoking, and frequent pulmonary infections can accelerate age-related changes, thereby making it difficult to identify the age-associated changes in pulmonary function.

Thoracic Wall and Respiratory Muscles

Upper airway changes include weakening support of upper and lower cartilage, predisposing older persons to obstructive changes. Submucosal glands decrease production of mucus,

TABLE 7-3	PROGRESSIVE CHANGES IN ARTERIAL OXYGEN TENSION (Pao_2) AND CARBON DIOXIDE TENSION ($Paco_2$)	
AGE-GROUP (YEARS)	**Pao_2 (MM HG)**	**$Paco_2$ (MM HG)**
≤30	94	39
31-40	87	38
41-50	84	40
51-60	81	39
>60	74	40

Modified from Sorbini CA, et al: Arterial oxygen tension in relation to age in healthy subjects. *Respiration* 25(1):3, 1968.

leading to dryness and thickened secretions.[38] With advancing age the chest wall (thoracic skeleton) and vertebrae undergo a small degree of osteoporosis, and at the same time the costal cartilages that connect the rib cage together become calcified and stiff. These changes may produce kyphosis and reduce chest wall compliance, respectively.[37,39,40] The functional effect is a decrease in thoracic wall excursion. Other factors, such as an increase in abdominal girth and change in posture, also decrease thoracic excursion. These anatomic changes are reflected by an increase in residual volume and decrease in vital capacity.

The strength of the respiratory muscles (diaphragm, external/internal intercostal muscles) gradually decreases. Respiratory muscle weakness begins as early as age 55.[41] During aging, skeletal muscle progressively atrophies and its energy metabolism decreases, which may partially explain the declining strength of the respiratory muscles.[42,43] In addition, an age-associated decrease occurs in the effectiveness of the cough reflex, possibly caused by a decrease in ciliary responsiveness and motion.[44]

Alveolar Parenchyma

With advancing age a diminished recoil (or increased compliance) of the lung occurs.[45] The reduced recoil results from the increase in the ratio of elastin to collagen content that occurs with advancing age.[46] Collagen, elastin, and reticulin are the primary connective tissue proteins of the lung tissue.[47,48] They are responsible for the elasticity and performance of the airways of the lung. Whereas total lung collagen remains unaltered, the amount of elastin increases with age in the interlobular septa and pleura and possibly within the bronchi and their vessels. These anatomic changes are reflected by an increase in residual volume and a decrease in forced expiratory volume. With changes in cartilage the trachea and bronchi become stiffer and less compliant.[38] Also, the size of the alveolar ducts increases after age 40.[37] The bronchial enlargement displaces inhaled air volume away from the alveoli that line the alveolar ducts (Figure 7-2).

Ventilation and oxygen/carbon dioxide exchange (diffusion) depend on numerous factors, including the surface area

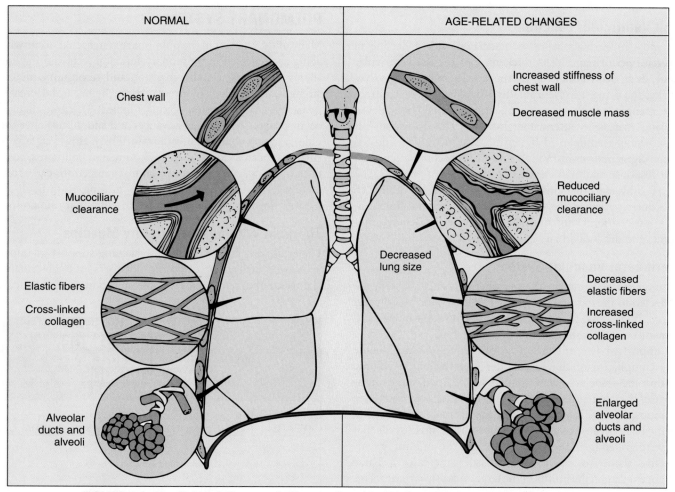

FIGURE 7-2 Age-Related Changes in Human Respiratory System. With advancing age, compliance of the chest wall and lung tissue changes, with reduced clearance of mucus by cilia that line the pulmonary tree and enlargement of alveolar ducts and alveoli. (From Urden LD, Stacy KM, Lough ME: *Critical care nursing: Diagnosis and management,* ed 6, St. Louis, 2010, Mosby.)

available for diffusion. A displacement of inhaled air volume away from the alveoli limits the surface area available for gas exchange. This may partly explain the progressive and linear decrease in the pulmonary diffusion capacity, which depends on both surface area and capillary blood volume. Capillary blood volume and surface area have been reported to decrease with advancing age.[49]

Pulmonary Gas Exchange

The arterial oxygen tension (Pao_2) decreases with age, such that the median Pao_2 for healthy persons older than 60 years is 74.3 mm Hg, as compared with 94 mm Hg for younger adults.[50] In contrast, arterial carbon dioxide ($Paco_2$) does not change with advancing age (see Table 7-2).[50] The decrease in Pao_2 may be the result of an increase of air trapping as the result of a ventilation/perfusion mismatch.[51,52] Consequently, dependent lung zones may be ventilated intermittently, leading to regional differences in ventilation. It is possible that alterations in blood volume and vascular resistance within the pulmonary circulation may also contribute to ventilation/perfusion (V/Q) mismatching. Other factors, such as smoking and pulmonary disease, also have an impact on the level of arterial oxygenation.

Lung Volumes and Capacities

With advancing age, total lung capacity and tidal volume do not change.[39] Residual volume (RV) increases with age, paralleling the decrease in chest wall compliance and reduced strength of the respiratory muscles. The increase in RV may also add to the diminished strength of the inspiratory muscles by stretching the diaphragm and altering the tension-length relationship.

RENAL SYSTEM

Aging produces changes in renal structure and function, many of which begin at approximately 30 to 40 years of age.[53,54] One of the prominent changes is a decrease in the number and size of the nephrons, which begins in the cortical regions and progresses toward the medullary portions of the kidney.[55] The decrease in the number of nephrons corresponds to a 20% decrease in the weight of the kidney between 40 and 80 years of age.[55] Initially this loss of nephrons does not appreciably alter renal function because of the large renal reserve: the kidney contains approximately 2 million to 3 million nephrons, all of which are not needed to maintain adequate fluid and acid-base homeostasis. However, with time the geriatric patient also loses this renal reserve.[55] Nephron loss is caused by a gradual reduction in blood flow to the glomerular capillary tuft.[56] Total renal blood flow declines after the fourth decade of life[53] because of hyaline arteriosclerosis.[56,57] The etiology of this vascular lesion within the glomerular tuft is unknown. By the eighth decade of life, 50% of the glomeruli are lost as a result of this arteriolar hyalinization.[55]

Fluid Filtration

GFR decreases with advancing age.[58,59] In older persons the decrease in GFR is most likely caused by the decrease in nephron number as well as decreased renal blood flow.[58]

Even though the remaining nephrons adapt to the loss of nephrons by glomerular hyperfiltration and increased solute load per nephron, the reduced GFR predisposes the elderly patient to adverse drug reactions and drug-induced renal failure. Some drugs are excreted unchanged in the urine, whereas other drugs have active or nephrotoxic metabolites that are excreted in the urine. In addition, the senescent kidney is more susceptible to injury by hypotensive episodes because of the age-related decrease in renal blood flow and reduced pressure gradient across the afferent arteriole.[60]

Age-related changes also occur in tubular function. The age-related changes in tubular function become apparent when extreme changes occur in the body fluid composition or acid-base balance. For example, with systemic acidosis the rate and amount of total acid excretion (bicarbonate, titratable acid, ammonium) are reduced.[58,60] This predisposes the older patient to metabolic acidosis, volume depletion, and hyperchloremia. At a normal pH level, however, the kidney of an older person can maintain acid-base homeostasis.

The senescent kidney has diminished capability to excrete a free water load, conserve water during periods of dehydration, and conserve sodium during periods of low salt intake.[58] Older persons are at high risk for dehydration because of these renal changes, along with decreased overall total body water, decreased concentrating ability, and decreased thirst perception.[61] Age-related changes also occur in extrarenal mechanisms, such as the decreased activity and responsiveness of the senescent kidney to the sympathetic nervous system and renin-angiotensin-aldosterone system, which are important in integrating overall fluid homeostasis and maintaining blood pressure in response to changes in body position.[34]

GASTROINTESTINAL SYSTEM

Age-related gastrointestinal changes occur in the processes of swallowing, motility, and absorption.[62,63] Swallowing may be difficult for the older person because of incomplete mastication of food.[63] Deteriorating dentition, diminished lubrication (secondary to salivary dysfunction), and poorly fitting dentures result in insufficient mastication of food within the oral cavity, predisposing the older patient to aspiration.[62] In addition, the number and velocity of the peristaltic contractions of the older person's esophagus decrease, and the number of nonperistaltic contractions increases.[63]

These changes in esophageal motility are referred to as presbyesophagus. These changes may predispose the patient to erosion of the esophageal wall (recurrent esophagitis) because food remains in the esophagus longer. In addition, bed rest and reclining in a supine position for a prolonged period can cause esophageal reflux, which also can lead to esophagitis.

The aging process produces thinning of the smooth muscle within the gastric mucosa.[64] The epithelial layer of the gastric mucosa, which contains the chief and parietal cells, undergoes a modest degree of atrophy, resulting in the hyposecretion of pepsin and acid, respectively.[65]

Mucin secretion from the mucous cells decreases, thereby altering the protective function of the gastric mucosal (bicarbonate) barrier. Because of this, the stomach wall is more susceptible to acid injury, thus increasing the incidence of gastric ulcerations.[66] Aging does not appreciably alter gastric emptying of solid foods. Alterations within the small intestine include a decrease in intestinal weight after age 50 and a flattening and shortening of jejunal villi.[67] Age produces no change in the small intestine's absorption of fats and proteins; however, decreased carbohydrate absorption has been reported.[68,69] There is essentially no change in vitamin or mineral absorption, except for a decrease in calcium absorption from the aged duodenum.[63]

Liver

With advancing age, both hepatocyte number and liver weight decrease.[70] Total liver blood flow decreases by 50% between 25 and 65 years of age.[70-72] The liver has many complex functions, including carbohydrate storage, ketone body formation, reduction/conjugation of adrenal and gonadal steroid hormones, synthesis of plasma proteins, deamination of amino acids, storage of cholesterol, urea formation, and detoxification of toxins and drugs. Despite changes in hepatocyte number and blood flow, however, liver function is not appreciably altered.[72] Several liver function tests, including serum bilirubin, alkaline phosphatase, and aspartate aminotransferase (AST) levels, are not altered with advancing age. However, because of the decrease in total liver blood flow, first-pass clearance of drugs is somewhat reduced. The most important age-related change in liver function is the decrease in the liver's capacity to metabolize drugs.[73,74] Although liver function tests do not reflect this change in metabolism, it is well recognized that drug side effects and toxic effects occur more frequently in older adults than in young adults.[74]

CENTRAL NERVOUS SYSTEM

Cognitive Functioning

Cognitive functioning involves the process of transforming, synthesizing, storing, and retrieving sensory input. Additional components include perception, attention, thinking, memory, and problem solving. For the aging individual, cognition is altered by the speed at which information is processed and retrieved.[75] Performance on timed tests declines slowly after age 20. Intelligence remains fairly stable after age 30 until the mid-80s. Although the rate at which complex tasks are completed may be diminished, these age-related changes are not synonymous with cognitive impairment.

Marked deterioration of any component of cognitive functioning is not a normal expectation of the aging process.[76] Cognitive impairment in older adults more often results from acute and chronic etiologies. Acute problems such as infection, electrolyte imbalance, and pharmacological toxicity are generally reversible once identified. Long-term chronic impairment develops from more organic causations, such as multi-infarct dementia or Alzheimer's disease.[77]

Changes in Structure and Morphology

The brain decreases approximately 20% in size between 25 and 95 years of age (Figure 7-3).[78] The reduced brain weight may be related in part to the overall decrease in the number of neurons that occurs with advancing age. Neurons are lost from the hippocampus, amygdala, and cerebellum and from areas of the brainstem such as the locus ceruleus, dorsal motor nucleus of vagus nerve, and substantia nigra.[75] In contrast, very few neurons disappear with advancing age in areas such as the hypothalamus.[77] In addition, portions of the cerebral cortex atrophy, principally the frontal (superior frontal gyrus) and temporal (superior temporal gyrus) cortical association areas.[78]

The cerebral ventricles enlarge and develop an asymmetric appearance. Cerebrospinal fluid (CSF) also accumulates in the ventricles, although total brain CSF is not increased.[79] Accompanying the loss of neurons are changes in the ultrastructure and intracellular structures of the neuron.[80] Also, neuron shrinkage and degenerative changes in the cell bodies and axons of certain acetylcholine-secreting neurons have been reported. There are also increases in norepinephrine and dopamine synthesis.[81] These changes may explain alterations in processing and receiving information.[77]

In the senescent brain, synaptogenesis (synaptic regeneration) still occurs after partial nerve degeneration. After a nerve fiber is damaged, neighboring undamaged neurons often sprout new fibers and form new connections. However, synaptogenesis occurs at a slower rate in the older brain.[80]

Cerebral Metabolism and Blood Flow

Cerebral blood flow decreases with advancing age. This decrease parallels the decrease in brain weight and is most likely caused by the reduction in neuron number and metabolic needs of the cerebral tissue.[82]

IMMUNE SYSTEM

Several changes in immune function render the older adult more susceptible to infections.[83-88] Infections in the geriatric population are associated with higher rates of mortality.[88] Common infections in the older adult include bacterial pneumonia, urinary tract infection, intraabdominal infections, gram-negative bacteremia, and decubitus ulcers.[88] The reasons for the increased susceptibility are multifactorial and include changes in cell- and humoral-mediated immunity; breakdown in physical barriers, such as the skin and oral mucosa; and changes in nutrition.

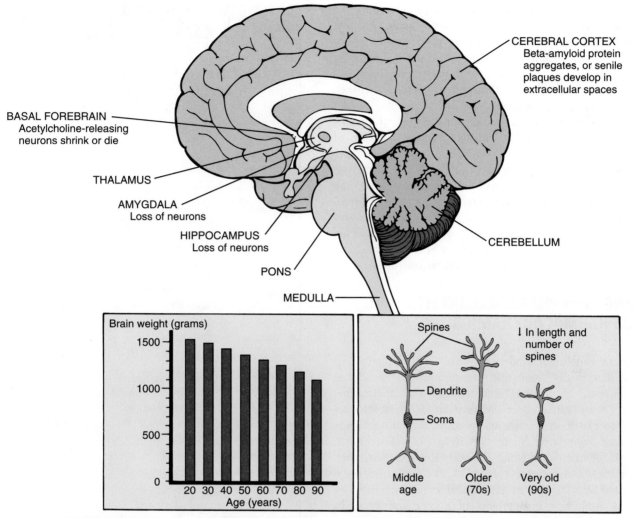

FIGURE 7-3 Summary of Age-Related Changes in the Brain. (From Selkoe DJ: Aging brain, aging mind. *Sci Am* 267(3):134-42, 1992.)

Cell-Mediated and Humoral-Mediated Immunity

Immune system function depends on many cell types with distinct functions. T cells are the primary effector of cell-mediated immunity, whereas bone marrow-derived B cells produce antibodies that are the effector cells of humoral-mediated immunity.[83,85,87] With aging, cell-mediated immunity declines. Even though the total number of T cells remains unchanged with advancing age, T-cell function decreases.[85,87] For example, there is a decrease in T-cell production of interleukin-2 (IL-2) and in differentiation of T cells into effector cells. IL-2 is essential for activating B cells, which eventually differentiate into antibody-secreting cells. Subsets of T cells mature into cytotoxic cells, whereas other T cells activate B cells and stimulate B-cell proliferation. Changes in B-lymphocyte function are not as well understood, even though with age the ability of B cells to produce antibodies into new antigens declines.[83,85]

Furthermore, inadequate emptying of urine secondary to bed rest, obstruction, or side effects from anticholinergic medications can result in stagnation of urine and recurrent urinary tract infections. Long-term placement of urinary catheters is a significant source of bacteriuria. However, treatment with antibiotic therapy is not indicated unless the patient becomes symptomatic with anorexia or cognitive impairment or has a history of a chronic illness such as diabetes or chronic obstructive pulmonary disease.[83,88]

INTEGUMENTARY AND MUSCULOSKELETAL SYSTEMS

The loss of elastic and connective tissue causes the skin to wrinkle; both skin wrinkles and sagging may be found over many areas of the body. Underlying structures, such as the veins and muscles, are more visible because of the transparency of the skin.

Multiple ecchymotic areas may result from decreased protective subcutaneous tissue layers, increased capillary fragility, and flattening of the capillary bed, all of which predispose elderly persons to developing ecchymosis.[89-92] In conjunction with frequent aspirin use, these physiological factors result in increased bleeding tendencies and the appearance of ecchymotic areas. However, areas of unexplained ecchymosis may also indicate elder abuse.

Changes that occur in the musculoskeletal system are a decrease in lean body mass, compression of the spinal column resulting from the thinning of cartilage between vertebra, and a decrease in the mobility of skeletal joints.[93] Muscle rigidity increases, especially in the neck, shoulders, hips, and knees,[94] possibly causing changes in range of motion.

Bone demineralization affects both men and women as they age but occurs four times more often in women than men. Bone demineralization refers to an increase in osteoblast and osteoclast activity, which decreases calcium absorption into the bone.[93] Osteoporosis produces bones that are more "porous" or fragile. With extensive bone demineralization, an older patient may sustain multiple fractures.

CHANGES IN PHARMACOKINETICS AND PHARMACODYNAMICS

The many benefits of modern advancements in pharmacological therapy are frequently counterbalanced by adverse drug effects, medication interactions, and therapeutic failure.[84] Adverse drug effects and medication interactions are related to pharmacokinetics and pharmacodynamics. There are many age-related changes in drug pharmacokinetics, which is the manner in which the body absorbs, distributes, metabolizes, and excretes a drug.[95,96] The aging process is associated with changes in gastric acid secretion, which can alter the ionization or solubility of a drug and hence its absorption[95,96] (Table 7-4).

Drug distribution depends on body composition, as well as the physiochemical properties of the drug. With advancing age, fat content increases, lean body mass decreases, and total body water decreases, which can alter the drug disposition.[96] For example, because of the increase in the ratio of body fat content to body weight, lipophilic drugs have a greater volume of distribution per body weight in older adults as compared with younger adults. Other age-related factors[95,97] affecting drug disposition are listed in Table 7-4.

As noted, the senescent liver and kidneys are less able to metabolize and excrete drugs, which also affects clinical outcomes. For example, the rate of absorption, time to peak plasma concentration, and clearance of loop diuretics is reduced in older adults, which may necessitate high dosing regimens in order to facilitate diuresis.[98,99] This poses an increased risk of metabolic acidosis, because the higher diuretic dose increases competition for the organic acid transport pathway at the proximal tubule. Using the example of diuretics, bioavailability between agents may also be variable. For instance, bumetanide has a fairly consistent bioavailability in advanced age, whereas that of furosemide varies from 20% to 80%.[99]

Similarly, other drugs associated with management of common disorders seen in critically ill patients—such as

TABLE 7-4   AGE-RELATED CHANGES IN PHARMACOKINETICS

ACTION	DEFINITION	CHANGES
Absorption	Receptor-coupled or diffusional uptake of drug into tissue	Decreased absorptive surface area of small intestine Decreased splanchnic blood flow Increased gastric acid pH Decreased gastrointestinal motility
Distribution	Theoretic space (tissue) or body compartment into which free form of drug distributes	Decreased lean body mass and total body water Increased total body fat Decreased serum albumin level Increased α_1-acid glycoprotein
Metabolism	Chemical change in drug that renders it active or inactive	Decreased liver mass Decreased activity of microsomal drug-metabolizing enzyme system Decreased total liver blood flow
Excretion	Removal of drug through an eliminating organ, often the kidney; some drugs are excreted in bile or feces, in saliva, or through the lungs	Decreased renal blood flow and glomerular filtration rate Decreased distal renal tubular secretory function

Data from Gilman AG, et al, editors: *Goodman and Gilman's the pharmacological basis of therapeutics*, ed 8, London, 1990, Pergamon; and Vestal RE, Cusack BJ: In Schneider EL, Rowe JW, editors: *Handbook of the biology of aging*, San Diego, 1990, Academic Press.

digoxin, angiotensin II-converting enzyme (ACE) inhibitors, and angiotensin II-receptor blockers (ARBs)[97]—have delayed excretion, increased serum concentration, and more prolonged duration of action because their excretion parallels GFR (which decreases with age).[97] See Table 7-4 for age-related changes in drug pharmacokinetics.

Age-related changes in pharmacodynamics have also been reported. Pharmacodynamics refers to the pharmacological or physiological response to a drug that occurs after the drug interacts with its receptor on the plasma membrane. The chronotropic and inotropic effects of b-adrenergic agonists reportedly decrease in older patients.[98,99] There also are reports that age produces no change in heparin-stimulated increases in partial thromboplastin time, whereas the effects of warfarin (Coumadin) are very susceptible to medication interactions.

The use of multiple medications in the presence of multiple comorbidities has been associated with an increase in adverse drug reactions. Although this is not always avoidable, it is important to avoid choosing an agent for its side effect profile (e.g., diphenhydramine for sedative effects) and monitor the effects of the chosen agent. A major cause of therapeutic failure is the underuse or inappropriate use of drug therapy that is indicated for the treatment of a particular problem. It is not uncommon for delirium not associated with a withdrawal syndrome to be treated with benzodiazepines in critical care. However, this frequently makes agitation worse, once the sedative effects are gone, in comparison to a low-dose antipsychotic agent.[100,101].

REFERENCES

1. Administration on Aging, US Department of Health and Human Services: A Profile of Older Americans: 2003. www.aoa.gov/AoAroot/Aging_Statistics/Profile/2003/index.aspx. Accessed April 5, 2011.

2. Resnick NM: Geriatric medicine. In Braunwald E, et al, editors: Harrison's principles of internal medicine, ed 15, New York, 2001, McGraw Hill.

3. Levine BS, Craven RF: Physiologic adaptations with aging. In Woods SL, et al, editors: Cardiac nursing, ed 5, Philadelphia, 2005, Lippincott Williams & Wilkins.

4. Polanczyk C, et al: Impact of age on perioperative complications and length of stay in patients undergoing noncardiac surgery, Ann Intern Med 134(8):637, 2001.

5. Eghbali M, et al: Collagen accumulation in heart ventricles as a function of growth and aging, Cardiovasc Res 23(8):723, 1989.

6. Wegelius O, von Knorring J: The hydroxyproline and hexosamine content in human myocardium at different ages, Acta Med Scand 412(Suppl):233, 1964.

7. Katz AM: Heart failure. In Fozzard HA, et al, editors: The heart and cardiovascular system, New York, 1991, Raven.

8. Eaton L: Cardiovascular function. In Lueckenotte AG, editor: Gerontologic nursing, ed 2, St Louis, 2000, Mosby.

9. Lakatta EG, Schulman SP, Gerstenblith G: Cardiovascular aging in health and therapeutic considerations in older patients with cardiovascular diseases. In Fuster V, et al, editors: Hurst's the heart, ed 10, New York, 2001, McGraw-Hill.

10. Gerstenblith G, et al: Echocardiographic assessment of normal adult aging population, Circulation 56(2):273, 1977.

11. Opie LH: The physiology of the heart and metabolism, New York, 1991, Raven.

12. Lakatta EG, et al: Prolonged contraction duration in aged myocardium, J Clin Invest 55(1):61, 1975.

13. Cinelli P, et al: Effect of age on mean heart rate and heart rate variability, Age 10(4):146, 1987.

14. Ribera JM, et al: Cardiac rate and hyperkinetic rhythm disorders in healthy elderly subjects: evaluation by ambulatory electrocardiographic monitoring, Gerontology 35(2-3):158, 1989.

15. Aronow WS: Effects of aging on the heart. In Tallis RC, Fillit HM, editors: Brocklehurst's textbook of geriatric medicine and gerontology, ed 6, London, 2003, Churchill Livingstone.

16. Bonow RO, et al: Effects of aging on asynchronous left ventricular regional function and global ventricular filling in normal human subjects, J Am Coll Cardiol 11(1):50, 1988.

17. Miller TR, et al: Left ventricular diastolic filling and its association with age, Am J Cardiol 58(6):531, 1986.

18. Davidson WR, Fee EC: Influence of aging on pulmonary hemodynamics in a population free of coronary artery disease, Am J Cardiol 65(22):1454, 1990.

19. Bachman S, Sparrow D, Smith LK: Effect of aging on the electrocardiogram, Am J Cardiol 48(3):513, 1981.

20. Horowitz LN, Lynch RA: Managing geriatric arrhythmias, I: General considerations, Geriatrics 46(3):31, 1991.

21. Camm AJ, et al: The rhythm of the heart in active elderly subjects, Am Heart J 99(5):598, 1980.

22. Fleg JL, Kennedy HL: Cardiac arrhythmias in a healthy elderly population: detection by a 24-hour ambulatory electrocardiography, Chest 81(3):302, 1982.

23. Aronow WS: Cardiac arrhythmias. In Tallis RC, Fillit HM, editors: Brocklehurst's textbook of geriatric medicine and gerontology, ed 6, London, 2003, Churchill Livingstone.

24. Docherty JR: Cardiovascular responses in ageing: a review, Pharmacol Rev 42(2):103, 1990.

25. Opie LH: The physiology of the heart and metabolism, New York, 1991, Raven.

26. Smith JJ, et al: The effect of age on hemodynamic response to graded postural stress in normal men, J Gerontol 42(4):406, 1987.

27. Dambrink JH, Wieling W: Circulatory response to postural change in healthy male subjects in relation to age, Clin Sci 72(3):335, 1987.

28. Applegate WB, et al: Prevalence of postural hypotension at baseline in the Systolic Hypertension in the Elderly Program (SHEP) cohort, J Am Geriatr Soc 39(11):1057, 1991.

29. Stanley M: Congestive heart failure in the elderly, Geriatr Nurs 20(4):180, 1999.

30. Bierman EL: Arteriosclerosis and aging. In Finch CE, Schneider EL, editors: Handbook of the biology of aging, New York, 1985, Van Nostrand Reinhold.

31. Schoenberger JA: Epidemiology of systolic and diastolic systemic blood pressure elevation in the elderly, Am J Cardiol 57(5):45C, 1986.

32. Rowe JW: Clinical consequences of age-related impairments in vascular compliance, Am J Cardiol 60(12):68G, 1987.

33. Rose BD: Clinical physiology of acid-base and electrolyte disorders, New York, 1989, McGraw-Hill.

34. Hall JE, Coleman TG, Guyton AC: The renin-angiotensin system. Normal physiology and changes in older hypertensives, J Am Geriatr Soc 37(8):801, 1989.

35. Crane MG, Harris JJ: Effect of aging on renin activity and aldosterone excretion, J Lab Clin Med 87(6):947, 1976.

36. Sica DA, Harford A: Sodium and water disorders in the elderly. In Zawada ET, Sica DA, editors: Geriatric nephrology and urology, Littleton, Mass, 1985, PSG.

37. Webster JR, Kadah H: Unique aspects of respiratory disease in the aged, Geriatrics 46(7):31, 1991.

38. Sheahan SL, Musialowski R: Clinical implications of respiratory system changes in aging, J Gerontol Nurs 27(5):26, 2001.

39. Levitzky MG: Effects of aging on the respiratory system, *Physiologist* 27(2):102, 1984.

40. Mittman C, et al: Relationship between chest wall and pulmonary compliance and age, *J Appl Physiol* 20(6):1211, 1965.

41. Anderson WM, Tockman MS: Aging and the lungs. In Beers MH, Berkow R, editors: *Merck manual of geriatrics*, www.merck.com/pubs/mm_geriatrics.

42. Rizzato G, Marazzini L: Thoracoabdominal mechanics in elderly men, *J Appl Physiol* 28(4):457, 1970.

43. Gutmann E, Hanzlíková V: Fast and slow motor units in ageing, *Gerontology* 22(4):280, 1976.

44. Pontoppidan H, Beecher HK: Progressive loss of protective reflexes in the airway with advance of age, *JAMA* 174:2209, 1960.

45. Knudson RJ, et al: Changes in the normal maximal expiratory flow-volume curve with growth and aging, *Am Rev Respir Dis* 127(6):725, 1983.

46. Turner JM, Mead J, Wohl ME: Elasticity of human lungs in relation to age, *J Appl Physiol* 25(6):664, 1968.

47. Pierce JA, Hocott JB: Studies on the collagen and elastin content of the human lung, *J Clin Invest* 39:8, 1960.

48. Pierce JA, Ebert RV: Fibrous network of the lung and its change with age, *Thorax* 20(5):469, 1965.

49. Semmens M: The pulmonary artery in the normal aged lung, *Br J Dis Chest* 64(2):65, 1970.

50. Sorbini CA, et al: Arterial oxygen tension in relation to age in healthy subjects, *Respiration* 25(1):3, 1968.

51. Leblanc P, Ruff F, Milic-Emili J: Effects of age and body position on "airway closure" in man, *J Appl Physiol* 28(4):448, 1970.

52. Holland J, et al: Regional distribution of pulmonary ventilation and perfusion in elderly subjects, *J Clin Invest* 47(1):81, 1968.

53. Weder AB: The renally compromised older hypertensive: therapeutic considerations, *Geriatrics* 46(2):36, 1991.

54. Maddox DA, Alavi FK, Zawada ET: The kidney and aging. In Massry SG, Glassock RJ, editors: *Textbook of nephrology*, ed 4, Philadelphia, 2001, Lippincott Williams & Wilkins.

55. Gilbert BR, Vaughan ED: Pathophysiology of the aging kidney, *Clin Geriatric Med* 6(1):13, 1990.

56. Kasiske BL: Relationship between vascular disease and age-associated changes in the human kidney, *Kidney Int* 31(5):1153, 1987.

57. Anderson S, Brenner BM: Effects of aging on the renal glomerulus, *Am J Med* 80(3):435, 1986.

58. Weder AB: The renally compromised older hypertensive: therapeutic considerations, *Geriatrics* 46(2):36, 1991.

59. Gilbert BR, Vaughan ED: Pathophysiology of the aging kidney, *Clin Geriatr Med* 6(1):13, 1990.

60. Watters JM, McClaran JC: The elderly surgical patient. In Wilmore DW, et al, editors: *Care of the surgical patient*, vol 7, Special problems, New York, 1990, Scientific American.

61. Bennett JA: Dehydration: Hazards and benefits, *Geriatr Nurs* 21(2):84, 2000.

62. Brandt LJ: Gastrointestinal disorders in the elderly. In Rossman I, editor: *Clinical geriatrics*, ed 3, Philadelphia, 1986, Lippincott.

63. Williams SA, Fogel RP: Common gastrointestinal problems in the elderly, *J KY Med Assoc* 87(1):29, 1989.

64. Altman DF: Changes in gastrointestinal, pancreatic, biliary and hepatic function with aging, *Gastroenterol Clin North Am* 19(2):227, 1990.

65. Thomson AB, Keelan M: The aging gut, *Can J Physiol Pharmacol* 64(1):30, 1986.

66. Bansal SK, et al: Upper gastrointestinal haemorrhage in the elderly: a record of 92 patients in a joint geriatric/surgical unit, *Age Aging* 16(5):279, 1987.

67. Schuster MM: Disorders of the aging GI system, *Hosp Prac* 11(9):95, 1976.

68. Curran J: Overview of geriatric nutrition, *Dysphagia* 5(2):72, 1990.

69. Ausman LM, Russell RM: Nutrition and aging. In Schneider EL, Rowe JW, editors: *Handbook of the biology of aging*, San Diego, 1990, Academic Press.

70. Sato TG, Miwa T, Tauchi H: Age changes in the human liver of the different races, *Gerontologia* 16(6):368, 1970.

71. Bach B, et al: Disposition of antipyrine and phenytoin correlated with age and liver volume in man, *Clin Pharmacokinet* 6(5):389, 1981.

72. Kampmann JP, Sinding J, Moller-Jorgensen I: Effect of age on liver function, *Geriatrics* 30(8):91, 1975.

73. Schmucker DL, Wang RK: Age-related changes in liver drug metabolism: structure vs function, *Proc Soc Exp Biol Med* 165(2):178, 1980.

74. Vestal RE, Cusack BJ: Pharmacology and aging. In Schneider EL, Rowe JW, editors: *Handbook of the biology of aging*, San Diego, 1990, Academic Press.

75. Katzman R: Human nervous system. In Masoro EJ, editor: *Handbook of physiology: aging*, New York, 1995, Oxford University Press.

76. Foreman MD, Grabowski R: Diagnostic dilemma: cognitive impairment in the elderly, *J Gerontol Nurs* 18(9):5, 1992.

77. Arriagada P, et al: Neurofibrillary tangles but not senile plaques parallel duration and severity of Alzheimer's disease, *Neurology* 42(3):631, 1992.

78. Selkoe DJ: Aging brain, aging mind, *Sci Am* 267(3):134, 1992.

79. Morris JC, McManus DQ: The neurology of aging: normal versus pathologic change, *Geriatrics* 46(8):47, 1991.

80. Lytle LD, Altar A: Diet, central nervous system, and aging, *Fed Proc* 38(6):2017, 1979.

81. Stuart-Hamilton IA: Normal cognitive aging. In Tallis RC, Fillit HM, editors: *Brocklehurst's textbook of geriatric medicine and gerontology*, ed 6, London, 2003, Churchill Livingstone.

82. Gottstein U, Held K: Effects of aging on cerebral circulation and metabolism in man, *Acta Neurol Scand Suppl* 72:54, 1979.

83. Gravenstein S, Fillit HM, Ershler WB: Clinical immunology of aging. In Tallis RC, Fillit HM, editors: *Brocklehurst's textbook of geriatric medicine and gerontology*, ed 6, London, 2003, Churchill Livingstone.

84. Hanlon JT, et al: Geriatric pharmacotherapy. In Tallis RC, Fillit HM, editors: *Brocklehurst's textbook of geriatric medicine and gerontology*, ed 6, London, 2003, Churchill Livingstone.

85. Miller RA: Immune system. In Masoro EJ, editor: *Handbook of physiology: aging*, New York, 1995, Oxford University Press.

86. Terpenning MS, Bradley SF: Why aging leads to increased susceptibility to infection, *Geriatrics* 46(2):77, 1991.

87. Miller RA: The aging immune system: primer and prospectus, *Science* 273(5271):70, 1996.

88. Rajagopalan S, Moran D: Infectious disease emergencies in older adults, *Clin Geriatr* 9:1, 2001, http://www.mmhc.com/engine.pl?station=mmhc&template=cgfull.html&id=1003.

89. Jones PL, Millman A: Wound healing and the aged patient, *Nurs Clin North Am* 25(1):263, 1990.

90. Kelley L, Mobily PR: Iatrogenesis in the elderly: Impaired skin integrity, *J Gerontol Nurs* 17(9):24, 1991.

91. Shenefelt PD, Fenske NA: Aging and the skin: recognizing and managing common disorders, *Geriatrics* 45(10):57, 1990.

92. Wenger NK: Cardiovascular disease in the elderly, *Curr Probl Cardiol* 17(10):609, 1992.

93. Kalu DN: Bone. In Masoro EJ, editor: *Handbook of physiology: aging*, New York, 1995, Oxford University Press.

94. Exton-Smith AN: Mineral metabolism. In Finch CE, Schneider EL, editors: *Handbook of the biology of aging*, New York, 1985, Van Nostrand Reinhold.

95. Guay DRP, et al: The pharmacology of aging. In Tallis RC, Fillit HM, editors: *Brocklehurst's textbook of geriatric medicine and gerontology*, ed 6, London, 2003, Churchill Livingstone.

96. Yuen GJ: Altered pharmacokinetics in the elderly, *Clin Geriatric Med* 6(2):257, 1990.

97. Schwertz DW, Buschmann MT: Pharmacogeriatics, *Crit Care Nurs Q* 12(1):26, 1989.

98. Bertel O, et al: Decreased beta-adrenoreceptor responsiveness as related to age, blood pressure and plasma catecholamines in patients with essential hypertension, *Hypertension* 2(2):130, 1980.

99. Kendall MJ, et al: Responsiveness to beta-adrenergic receptor stimulation: the effects of age are cardioselective, *Br J Clin Pharmacol* 14(6):821, 1982.

100. Pompei P: Delirium. In Tallis RC, Fillit HM, editors: *Brocklehurst's textbook of geriatric medicine and gerontology*, ed 6, London, 2003, Churchill Livingstone.

101. Litton KA: Delirium in the critical care patient: what the professional staff needs to know, *Crit Care Nurs Q* 26(3):208, 2003.

8

Pain and Pain Management

Céline Gélinas

evolve WEBSITE

Be sure to check out the bonus material, including free self-assessment exercises, on the Evolve web site at *http://evolve.elsevier.com/Urden/priorities/*.

OBJECTIVES

- Explain the physiology of pain.
- Discuss how to perform a pain assessment in the critically ill patient.
- Identify patient and health care professional barriers to a pain assessment.
- Describe the pharmacological and nonpharmacological interventions for pain management.
- Describe nursing interventions that are essential in the treatment of acute pain.

Despite national and international efforts, guidelines, standards of practice, position statements, and many important discoveries in the field of pain management in the past three decades, pain remains a major stressor for patients in critical care settings.[1] Because many sources of pain are present in critical care settings, such as acute illness, surgery, trauma, invasive equipment, and nursing and medical interventions,[2,3] it is not surprising that more than 50% of critically ill patients experience moderate to severe pain.[4-6] In a large, international study involving 5957 critically ill adults, the Thunder Project II sponsored by the American Association of Critical-Care Nurses (AACN), turning, drain removal, wound care, and endotracheal suctioning were described as painful procedures of moderate to severe intensity.[5] Despite these findings, pain remains undertreated in most critically ill patients.[4,6-9] In the Thunder Project II, less than 20% of critically ill adults received opiates before and during painful procedures.[9] Poor treatment of acute pain may lead to the development of serious complications[10,11] and chronic pain syndromes,[12,13] which may seriously impact the patient's functioning, quality of life, and well-being.

IMPORTANCE OF PAIN ASSESSMENT

To detect pain, it must be adequately assessed. Because pain is recognized as a subjective experience,[14] the patient's self-report is the most valid measure for pain. Unfortunately in critical care, many factors alter verbal communication with patients: the administration of sedative agents, mechanical ventilation, and the patient's change in level of consciousness.[2,3,15] Nevertheless, except for being unable to speak, many mechanically ventilated patients can communicate that they are in pain by using head nodding, grimacing, hand motions, or by seeking attention with other movements.[4,16]

Pain scales have been used with postoperative mechanically ventilated patients who were asked to point on the pain intensity scale to communicate their pain.[5,17,18] However, in a study of mechanically ventilated adults with various diagnoses (trauma, surgical, or medical), only one third of mechanically ventilated patients were able to use a pain intensity scale.[19] With a greater degree of critical illness, providing a pain intensity self-report becomes more difficult because it requires concentration and energy. When the patient is unable to express himself or herself in any way, observable, clustered behavioral and physiological indicators become unique indices for pain assessment and are part of clinical guidelines and recommendations developed in North America.[20-23] Many health care agencies have increased their vigilance regarding patients' pain and its management, including designating pain assessment as the fifth vital sign, as stated by the American Pain Society.

DEFINITION AND DESCRIPTION OF PAIN

Pain is described as an unpleasant sensory and emotional experience associated with actual or potential tissue damage.[14] This definition emphasizes its subjective and multidimensional nature. Its subjective characteristic implies that pain is whatever the person experiencing it says it is and that pain exists whenever he or she says it does.[24] This definition implies that the patient is able to self-report. In the critical care context, many patients are unable to self-report.[25]

Infants represent a unique group of vulnerable patients who cannot self-report their pain and therefore communicate by behaviors. Clinicians must be attuned to infant's behaviors for pain-related clinical assessment.[25] This same principle applies to any nonverbal population, for whom behavioral alterations caused by pain are valuable forms of self-report and should be considered as alternative measures of pain.[25] Based on this idea, pain assessment must be designed to conform to the patient's communication capabilities, and this is consistent with the fact that pain is multidimensional.

Components of Pain

The experience of pain includes sensory, affective, cognitive, behavioral, and physiological components:[26,27]

- *Sensory component*: Perception of pain characteristics, such as intensity, location, and quality.
- *Affective component*: Negative emotions, such as unpleasantness, anxiety, and fear associated with the experience of pain.
- *Cognitive component*: Interpretation of pain by the person who experiences it.
- *Behavioral component*: Behaviors or coping strategies used by the person to express, avoid, or control pain.
- *Physiological component*: Nociception and the stress response.

Types of Pain

Pain can be acute or chronic, with different sensations related to the origin of the pain.

Acute Pain

Acute pain has a short duration, represents tissue damage from an identifiable cause, and corresponds to the healing process (30 days). Undertreated prolonged acute pain can become chronic pain.[12,13]

Chronic Pain

Chronic pain persists for longer than 3 to 6 months after the healing process from the original injury.[28,29] It develops when the healing process is incomplete or with permanent damage to the nervous system. It has also been associated with a prolonged stress response.[27] Acute and chronic types of pain can have a nociceptive or neuropathic origin.[30]

Nociceptive Pain

Nociceptive pain refers to the nociception mechanism, and can be somatic or visceral. Somatic pain involves superficial tissues, including skin, muscles, joints, and bones; the location is well defined; and it may be described as tender, burning, shooting or throbbing. Visceral pain involves organs including the heart, stomach, and liver; location is diffuse, and it is usually described as aching or cramping.

Neuropathic Pain

Neuropathic or deafferentation pain is described as an abnormal sensory process caused by changes in the excitability of nerve cells.[31] These changes are associated with the acute inflammatory process or with nerve damage that can be caused by surgery or an illness process.[32-34] The origin of the pain may be peripheral or central.

Pain in Critical Care

Pain in the critical care setting is a subjective and multidimensional experience. Its components are sensory, affective, cognitive, behavioral, and physiological. Pain experienced by critical care patients is mostly acute with multiple origins. An understanding of pain physiology provides the foundation for assessment and treatment.

PHYSIOLOGY OF PAIN

Nociception

Nociception represents the neural and brain activity that is necessary, but not sufficient, for pain. Pain is the conscious experience that emerges from nociception, especially from brain activity.[35] Four processes are involved in nociception:[30]

1. Transduction
2. Transmission
3. Perception
4. Modulation

These four processes are shown in Figure 8-1 and Figure 8-2, which integrates pain assessment with nociception.

Transduction

Transduction refers to mechanical (e.g., surgical incision), thermal (e.g., burn), or chemical (e.g., toxic substance) stimuli that damage tissues. These stimuli activate the liberation of chemical substances, such as prostaglandins, bradykinin, serotonin, histamine, glutamate, and substance P, which stimulate peripheral nociceptive receptors and initiate nociceptive transmission.

Transmission

As a result of transduction, an action potential is produced and transmitted by nociceptive nerve fibers in the spinal cord that reach higher centers of the brain. This is called transmission, and it represents the second process of nociception. The principal nociceptive fibers are the Aδ and C fibers. These fibers synapse with two spinothalamic pathways: *neospinothalamic* (NS) and *paleospinothalamic* (PS) pathways. Generally, the Aδ fibers transmit the pain sensation to the brain within the NS pathway, and the C fibers use the PS pathway.[36]

Through synapsing of nociceptive fibers with motor fibers in the spinal cord, muscle rigidity can appear because of a reflex activity.[10] Muscle rigidity can be a behavioral indicator associated with pain. It can contribute to immobility and decrease diaphragmatic excursion. This can lead to hypoventilation and hypoxemia. Hypoxemia can be detected by a pulse oximeter (SpO_2) and by oxygen arterial pressure (PaO_2)

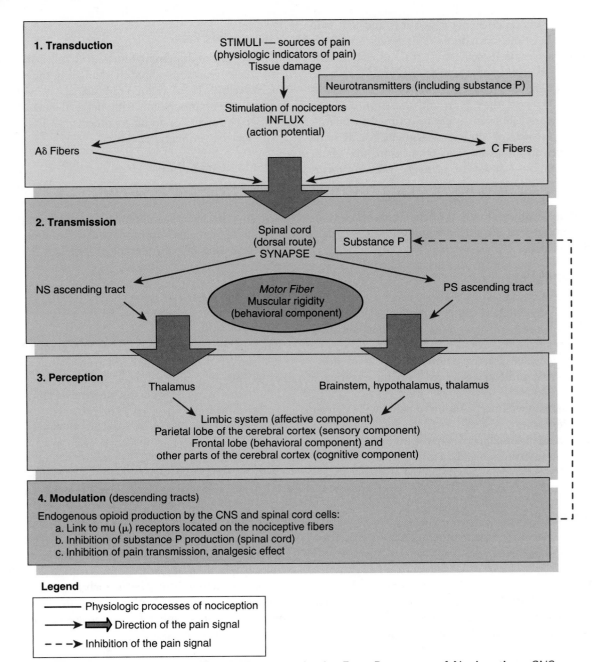

Legend

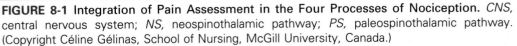

——— Physiologic processes of nociception

———➤ ▭➤ Direction of the pain signal

– – –➤ Inhibition of the pain signal

FIGURE 8-1 Integration of Pain Assessment in the Four Processes of Nociception. *CNS,* central nervous system; *NS,* neospinothalamic pathway; *PS,* paleospinothalamic pathway. (Copyright Céline Gélinas, School of Nursing, McGill University, Canada.)

monitoring. A ventilated patient's interaction with the machine (e.g., activation of alarms, fighting the ventilator) also may indicate the presence of pain.[37]

Perception

The pain message is transmitted via the spinothalamic pathways to centers in the brain where pain is initially perceived. Pain sensation transmitted by the NS pathway reaches the thalamus, and the pain sensation transmitted by the PS pathway reaches brainstem, hypothalamus, and thalamus.[36] Projections to the limbic system and the frontal cortex allow

expression of the affective component of pain.[38-40] Projections to the sensory cortex located in the parietal lobe allow the patient to describe the sensory characteristics of his or her pain, such as location, intensity, and quality.[38-42] The cognitive component of pain involves many parts of the cerebral cortex and is complex. These three components (affective, sensory, and cognitive) represent the subjective interpretation of pain. Parallel to this subjective process, certain facial expressions and body movements are behavioral indicators of pain occurring as a result of pain fiber projections to the motor cortex in the frontal lobe.

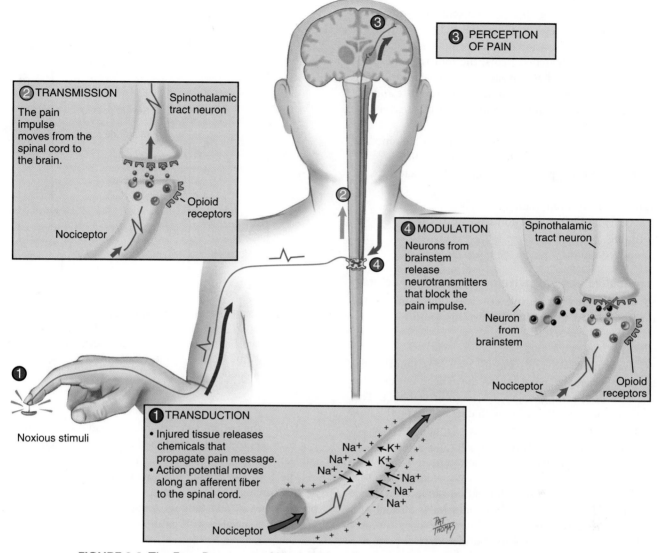

FIGURE 8-2 The Four Processes of Nociception. (From Jarvis C: *Physical examination & health assessment*, ed 6, St. Louis, 2011, Saunders. Illustration by Pat Thomas, CMI.)

Modulation

Modulation is the liberation of endogenous opioids, such as β-endorphins, enkephalins, and dynorphins, by the CNS. Through the descending pathways endogenous opioids inhibit the transmission of pain sensation in the spinal cord and produce analgesia. These substances link to mu (μ) receptors located on nociceptive fibers, inhibiting the liberation of substance P and blocking the transmission of the pain sensation.

PAIN ASSESSMENT

Pain assessment is a vital part of nursing care. It is a prerequisite for adequate pain control and relief. Pain is a subjective, multidimensional concept that requires complex assessment. Pain assessment has two major components: nonobservable/subjective and observable/objective.

Pain Assessment: The Subjective Component

Pain is an entirely subjective experience.[14,47-49] The subjective component of pain assessment refers to the patient's self-report of pain. Because it is the most valid measure, the patient's self-report must be obtained whenever possible.[21] A simple yes or no (presence versus absence of pain) is considered a valid self-report. Mechanical ventilation should not be a barrier to document patients' self-reports of pain. Many mechanically ventilated patients can communicate that they have pain or can use pain scales by pointing to numbers or symbols on the scale.[4,5,17-19] Before concluding that a patient is unable to self-report, three attempts to ask the patient about pain are recommended.[3] Sufficient time should be allowed for the patient to respond with each attempt.

If sedation and cognition levels allow the patient to give more information about pain, a multidimensional assessment can be documented. Multidimensional pain assessment tools, including the sensorial, emotional, and cognitive components, are available (e.g., Brief Pain Inventory,[50] Initial Pain Assessment Tool,[30] Short-Form McGill Pain Questionnaire[51]). Because of the administration of sedative and analgesic agents in mechanically ventilated patients, the tool must be short enough to be completed. For instance, the short-form McGill Pain Questionnaire takes 2 to 3 minutes to complete and has been used to assess mechanically ventilated patients who were in stable condition.[5,17,18]

The patient's self-report of pain can also be obtained by questioning the patient using the mnemonic PQRSTU:[52]
- **P:** provocative and palliative or aggravating factors
- **Q:** quality
- **R:** region or location, radiation
- **S:** severity and other symptoms
- **T:** timing
- **U:** understanding

P: Provocative and Palliative or Aggravating Factors

The **P** investigates what provokes or causes the pain, and the moderating factors that reduce pain or discomfort.

Q: Quality

The **Q** in the mnemonic refers to the pain sensation that the patient is experiencing. For instance, the patient may describe the pain as dull, aching, sharp, burning, or stabbing. This information provides the nurse with data regarding the type of pain the patient is experiencing (i.e., somatic or visceral). The differentiation between types of pain may contribute to the determination of cause and management. A patient who has had open-heart surgery may complain of chest pain that is shooting or burning.[4] This information can lead the nurse to investigate for cutaneous or bone injuries as a result of a sternotomy. Another patient may describe a sharp thoracic pain that may lead the nurse to consider visceral pain as a result of pulmonary embolism. A verbal description of pain is important because it provides a baseline account, allowing the critical care nurse to monitor changes in the type of pain, which may indicate a change in the underlying pathology.

R: Region or Location, Radiation

R usually is easy for the patient to identify, although visceral pain is more difficult for the patient to localize.[30] If the patient has difficulty naming the location or is mechanically ventilated, ask that the patient to point to the location on himself or herself or on a simple anatomic drawing.[53]

S: Severity and Other Symptoms

S denotes pain severity or intensity. Many visual analog scales are available, as are the descriptive and numeric pain rating scales used in critical care (Figure 8-3). Numeric and descriptive pain rating scales have been used to assess pain in mechanically ventilated patients.[5,19,46] The Faces Pain Rating Scale was identified as the easiest pain intensity scale by adults in acute and critical care settings.[54,55] To have a faces scale more specific to adults, Gélinas[56] developed and validated the Faces Pain Thermometer (FPT) for critically ill patients.

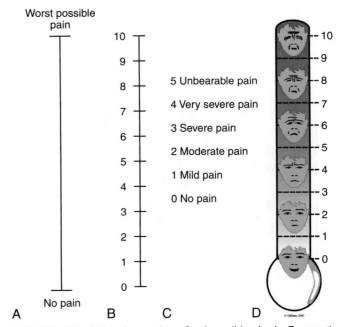

FIGURE 8-3 Pain Intensity Scales (Vertical Format). *A,* Visual analog scale (VAS). *B,* Numeric Rating Scale (NRS). *C,* Descriptive Rating Scale (DRS). *D,* Faces Pain Thermometer. (Copyright Céline Gélinas, School of Nursing, McGill University, Canada.)

Asking the patient to grade the pain on a scale of 0 to 10 is a consistent method and aids the nurse in objectifying the subjective nature of the patient's pain.

The **S** in the mnemonic also refers to other symptoms accompanying the pain experience, such as shortness of breath, nausea, and fatigue. Anxiety and fear are common emotions associated with pain.

T: Timing

The **T** refers to documenting the onset, duration, and frequency of pain. This information can help determine whether the pain is acute or chronic. Duration of pain can indicate the severity of the problem.

U: Understanding

The **U** in the mnemonic is the patient's perception of the problem or cognitive experience of pain.

Nurses should start by asking, "Do you have pain?" The use of a simple yes or no question allows the patient to answer verbally or indicate a response by a nod of the head or other signs.[3] Pain intensity and location also are necessary for the initial assessment of pain.[53]

Pain Assessment: The Observable or Objective Component

When the patient's self-report is impossible to obtain, nurses can rely on observation of behavioral and physiological indicators that are strongly recommended for pain management in nonverbal patients.[20-22] Pain-related behaviors have received attention in critical care and were also studied in the AACN

Thunder Project II.[57] Patients who experienced pain during nociceptive procedures were three to ten times more likely to have increased behavioral responses such as facial expressions, body movement responses, and verbal responses than patients without pain. Similar observations were found in a study of 257 mechanically ventilated adults in critical care. Patients who experienced pain during turning showed more intense facial expressions (e.g., grimacing), muscle rigidity, and ventilator dyssynchrony compared with patients without pain.[58]

Behavioral indicators are strongly recommended for pain assessment in nonverbal patients,[21,25] and several tools have been developed and tested in critically ill adults: *Behavioral Pain Scale* (BPS),[43-45] *Critical-Care Pain Observation Tool* (CPOT),[59] *Post Anesthesia Care Unit Behavioral Pain Rating Scale* (PACU-BPRS),[60] *Pain Behavioral Assessment Tool* (PBAT),[57] and *Pain Assessment and Intervention Notation* (PAIN) algorithm.[46] The BPS and the CPOT are supported by experts as appropriate for use with uncommunicative critically ill adults[61,62] and by the clinical practice recommendations of a task force of the American Society for Pain Management Nursing (ASPMN).[21] The implementation of pain assessment tools is essential so that health care teams can establish a common language of communication. This facilitates inter-professional collaboration and benefits patients.

Behavioral Pain Scale

The BPS shown in Table 8-1 was mainly tested in mechanically ventilated, unconscious patients.[43,45,63,64] Its validity was supported with significantly higher BPS scores during nociceptive procedures (e.g., turning, endotracheal suctioning) compared with rest or nonnociceptive procedures (e.g., central venous catheter dressing change, compression stocking applications, eye care). Most clinicians were satisfied with

TABLE 8-1	BEHAVIORAL PAIN SCALE (BPS)	
ITEM	**DESCRIPTION**	**SCORE**
Facial expression	Relaxed	1
	Partially tightened (e.g., brow lowering)	2
	Fully tightened (e.g., eyelid closing)	3
	Grimacing	4
Upper limbs	No movement	1
	Partially bent	2
	Fully bent with finger flexion	3
	Permanently retracted	4
Compliance with ventilation	Tolerating movement	1
	Coughing but tolerating ventilation for most of the time	2
	Fighting ventilator	3
	Unable to control ventilation	4
Total		3 to 12

From Payen JF, et al: Assessing pain in the critically ill sedated patients by using a behavioral pain scale, *Crit Care Med* 29(12):2258, 2001.

its ease of use, but some expressed concerns about its relative complexity.[45] For instance, scores of 3 and 4 for compliance with the ventilator may be ambiguous, and movements with upper limbs may be confused with muscle tension.[61]

Critical-Care Pain Observation Tool

The CPOT shown in Table 8-2 was tested in verbal and nonverbal critically ill adult patients.[19,59] Content validity was supported by ICU expert clinicians, including nurses and physicians.[65] Validity of the CPOT was supported with significantly higher CPOT scores during a nociceptive procedure (e.g., turning with or without other care) compared with rest or a nonnociceptive procedure (e.g., taking blood pressure). Significant positive associations were also found between the CPOT scores and the patient's self-report of pain (the gold standard).[66] Feasibility of the CPOT was positively evaluated by ICU nurses.[67] Nurses agreed that the CPOT was quick enough to be used in the ICU, simple to understand, easy to complete, and helpful for nursing practice. The CPOT identifies patients with severe pain very well. For patients with moderate to severe pain, the cutoff seems to be between 2 and 3, depending on the patient's condition.[68] Head injury patients seemed to react differently to the nociceptive procedure.[19] They were less likely to show frowning, brow lowering, and grimacing. Compared with other patients, a higher proportion of head injury patients showed tearing and open eyes when exposed to the nociceptive procedure.[58]

Behaviors represent valid information for pain assessment in the critically ill patient, but they present some limitations. They are impossible to monitor in paralyzed patients receiving neuromuscular blocking agents, and their presence may be blurred by the use of high doses of sedative agents such as propofol or midazolam.[19] Minimal behavioral responses to painful procedures were found in unconscious mechanically ventilated ICU adults who were more heavily sedated compared with conscious patients.[58] Similar results were found in previous studies in which patients who received a higher dose of midazolam obtained a lower score on the BPS.[45,64] In those difficult situations, the only possible clues left for the detection of pain are physiological indicators.

Physiological Indicators

Physiological vital signs as indicators of pain have received little attention in critically ill adults. Although vital sign values generally increase during painful procedures,[19,45,58,64] they are not consistently related to the patient's self-report of pain, nor are they predictive of pain.[19,58] None of the monitored vital signs (heart rate, mean arterial pressure [MAP], respiratory rate, transcutaneous oxygen saturation [Spo_2], or end-tidal CO_2) predicted the presence of pain in ICU patients.[58]

The ASPMN recommendations emphasize that vital signs should not be considered as primary indicators of pain because they can be attributed to other distress conditions, homeostatic changes, and medications.[21] Changes in vital signs should rather be considered a cue to begin further assessment of pain or other stressors.

TABLE 8-2 CRITICAL CARE PAIN OBSERVATION TOOL (CPOT)

INDICATOR	SCORE		DESCRIPTION
Facial expression	Relaxed, neutral	0	No muscle tension observed
	Tense	1	Frowning, brow lowering, orbit tightening, and levator contraction or any other change (e.g., opening eyes or tearing during nociceptive procedures)
	Grimacing	2	All previous facial movements plus eyelids tightly closed (the patient may present with mouth open or biting the endotracheal tube)

Relaxed, neutral — 0 Tense — 1 Grimace — 2

INDICATOR	SCORE		DESCRIPTION
Body movements	Absence of movements or normal position	0	Does not move at all (does not necessarily mean absence of pain) or normal position (movements not aimed toward the pain site or not made for the purpose of protection)
	Protection	1	Slow, cautious movements, touching or rubbing the pain site, seeking attention through movements
	Restlessness	2	Pulling the tube, attempting to sit up, moving limbs or thrashing, not following commands, striking at staff, trying to climb out of bed
Compliance with the ventilator (mechanically ventilated patients)	Tolerating ventilator or movement	0	Alarms not activated, easy ventilation
	Coughing but tolerating	1	Coughing, alarms may be activated but stop spontaneously
	Fighting ventilator	2	Asynchrony; blocking ventilation, alarms frequently activated
or Vocalization (nonventilated patients)	Talking in normal tone or no sound	0	Talking in normal tone or no sound
	Sighing, moaning	1	Sighing, moaning
	Crying out, sobbing	2	Crying out, sobbing
Muscle tension Evaluation by passive flexion and extension of upper limbs when patient is at rest or evaluation when patient is being turned	Relaxed	0	No resistance to passive movements
	Tense, rigid	1	Resistance to passive movements
	Very tense or rigid	2	Strong resistance to passive movements, incapacity to complete them
TOTAL		0-8	

Directions for Using the CPOT

1 The patient is observed at rest for 1 minute to obtain a baseline value of the CPOT.

2 The patient is observed during nociceptive procedures (e.g., turning, endotracheal suctioning, wound dressing) to detect any changes in the patient's behavioral responses to pain.

3 The patient is evaluated before and at the peak effect of an analgesic agent to assess whether the treatment was effective in relieving pain.

4 For the rating of the CPOT, the patient should be given the highest score observed during the assessment period.

5 Muscle tension is evaluated last, especially when the patient is at rest, because the stimulation of touch (passive flexion and extension of the arm) may lead to behavioral reactions.

6 The patient is given a score for each behavior included in the CPOT.

Modified from Gélinas C, et al: Validation of the Critical-Care Pain Observation Tool in Adult Patients, *Am J Crit Care*, 15(4):420, 2006. Figure courtesy Caroline Arbour, RN, BSc, PhD-student, McGill University, Canada.

Fifth Vital Sign

Because pain is considered the fifth vital sign, including pain assessment with other routinely documented vital signs ensures that pain level is assessed in all patients on a regular basis. This approach can ensure that pain is detected and treatment implemented before the patient develops complications associated with unrelieved pain. The use of a pain flow sheet incorporated into the critical care documentation allows for visible and ongoing pain assessment before and after an intervention for pain that is accessible to all clinicians involved in the assessment and management of pain.[69,70]

PATIENT BARRIERS TO PAIN ASSESSMENT AND MANAGEMENT

Communication

The most obvious patient barrier to the assessment of pain in the critical care population is the inability to communicate. Patients who are mechanically ventilated cannot verbalize their pain. If the patient can communicate by head nodding or pointing, pain can be reported in that manner. If writing is possible, the patient may be able to describe the pain. With nonverbal patients, the nurse relies on behavioral clues to assess pain.

The patient's family can contribute significantly in the assessment of pain. The family is intimately familiar with the patient's normal responses to pain and can assist the nurse in identifying clues. A family member's impression of a patient's pain should be considered in the pain assessment process of the critically ill patient.[21]

Altered Level of Consciousness

The unconscious patient presents a dilemma for all clinicians. Because pain relies on cortical response to provide recognition, the belief may persist that the patient without higher cortical function has no perception of pain. Interviews by Lawrence[71] with 100 patients, who recalled their experiences from a time when they were unconscious in critical care, revealed that they could hear, understand, and respond emotionally to what was being said. Experts recommend assuming that unconscious patients have pain and treating them the same way as conscious patients are treated when they are exposed to sources of pain.[21]

Studies[19,45] have demonstrated that behavioral and physiological indicators of pain can be observed in reaction to a painful procedure in critically ill patients, no matter what their level of consciousness. Knowing this, the critical care nurse can initiate a discussion with the other members of the health care team to formulate a plan of care for the patient's comfort.

Older Patients

Many older patients do not complain about pain. Some misconceptions, such as believing that pain is a normal consequence of aging or being afraid to disturb the health care team, are barriers to pain expression for the older adult.[30] Cognitive deficits or delirium present additional pain assessment barriers. Many older patients with mild to moderate cognitive impairments and even some with severe impairment are able to use pain intensity scales.[72,73] Vertical pain intensity scales are more easily understood by this group of patients and are recommended[74] (see Figure 8-3). Older patients with cognitive deficits should receive repeated instructions and be given sufficient time to respond.[28] When the self-report of pain is impossible to obtain, direct observation of pain-related behaviors is highly recommended in this population.[21,73] More than 24 behavioral tools have been developed for older patients with cognitive deficits.[72,75,76] The *Pain Assessment Checklist for Seniors with Limited Ability to Communicate* (PACSLAC)[77] and *Doloplus-2*[78,79] are promising tools for use with older adults.[73,75,76]

Delirium is a form of transient cognitive impairment that is highly prevalent among older patients in the ICU.[80] A major challenge with delirium is that there is overlap between delirium behaviors and pain-related behaviors. Pain is recognized as a potentially modifiable contributor to delirium management.[81]

Cultural Influences

Cultural influences are compounded when the patient speaks a language other than that of the health team members.[82] Additionally, differences in pain reporting may exist. To facilitate communication, the use of a pain intensity scale in the patient's language is vital. The 0 to 10 numeric pain scales have been translated into many different languages.[30]

Some cultures believe that God's test or punishment takes the form of pain. Persons with these cultural backgrounds do not necessarily believe that the pain should be relieved. Other cultures perceive pain as being associated with an imbalance in life. Persons from these cultures believe they need to manipulate the environment to restore balance to control pain.[82]

Lack of Knowledge

A relatively overlooked patient barrier to accurate pain assessment is the public knowledge deficit regarding pain and pain management. Many patients and their families are frightened by the risk of addiction to pain medication. They fear that addiction will occur if the patient is medicated frequently or with sufficient amounts of opiates necessary to relieve the pain. This concern is so powerful for some that they will deny or deliberately underreport the frequency or intensity of pain. Another misconception is the expectation that unrelieved pain is simply part of a critical illness or procedure.[83] Many patients have no memory of receiving an explanation of a pain management plan.[84] With this in mind, it is important to teach the family and the patient about the importance of pain control and the use of opioids in treating pain in critical illness.

Health Professional Barriers to Pain Assessment and Management

The health professional's beliefs and attitudes about pain and pain management are frequently a barrier to accurate and adequate pain assessment. Misconceptions or lack of knowledge regarding addiction, physiological dependence, drug tolerance, and respiratory depression remain.

Addiction and Tolerance

Addiction is defined by a pattern of compulsive drug use that is characterized by an incessant longing for an opioid and the need to use it for effects other than pain relief.

Tolerance is defined as a diminution of opioid effects over time. Physical dependence and tolerance to opioids may develop if the drug is given over a long period. Physical dependence is manifested by withdrawal symptoms when the opioid is abruptly stopped. If this is an anticipated problem, withdrawal may be avoided by weaning the patient from the opioid slowly to allow the brain to reestablish neurochemical balance in the absence of the opioid.[30]

Respiratory Depression

Another concern for health care professionals is the fear that aggressive management of pain with opioids causes respiratory depression. The incidence of respiratory depression in the critically ill is less than 2%.[85]

PAIN MANAGEMENT

The management of pain in the critically ill patient is as multidimensional as the assessment. It is a multidisciplinary task. The control of pain can be pharmacological, nonpharmacological, and ideally a combination of the two therapies.

Pharmacological Control of Pain

Pharmacological management of pain has infinite variety in the critical care unit. Pain pharmacology is divided into three categories of action: opioid agonists (morphine, fentanyl, hydromorphone, meperidine, codeine, methadone, and more potent drugs), nonopioids (acetaminophen, nonsteroidal antiinflammatory drugs [NSAIDs]), and adjuvants such as anticonvulsants, antidepressants, and local anesthetics. Elements of the 2002 clinical guidelines[22] of the Society of Critical Care Medicine (SCCM) for pharmacological interventions in the critically ill adult are presented for each opiate discussed (updates to these guidelines are in the process of revision). The algorithm from the current SCCM guidelines for sedation and analgesia management is shown in Figure 10-1 in Chapter 10. How pain is approached and managed is a progression or combination of the available agents, the type of pain, and the patient response to the therapy. Figure 8-4 illustrates the analgesic action sites in relation to nociception.

Opioid Analgesics

The opioids most commonly used and recommended as first-line analgesics are the agonists. These opioids bind to mu (μ)

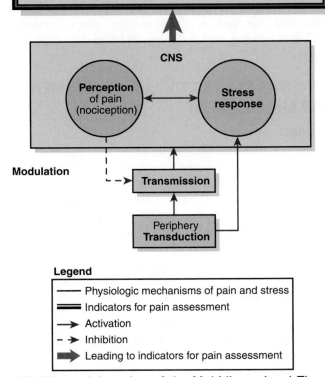

Legend
— Physiologic mechanisms of pain and stress
≡ Indicators for pain assessment
→ Activation
- → Inhibition
⇒ Leading to indicators for pain assessment

FIGURE 8-4 Adaptation of the Multidimensional Theory of Melzack. *CNS,* central nervous system. (From Melzack R: Pain and stress: a new perspective. In Gatchel RJ, Turk DC, editors: *Psychological factors in pain,* p 98, New York, 1999, Guilford Press.)

receptors (transmission process; Figure 8-5), which appear to be responsible for pain relief. Additional pharmacological information is presented in Table 8-3 and Box 8-1. In the SCCM guidelines, scheduled opioid doses or a continuous infusion is preferred over an as-needed regimen to ensure consistent analgesia in critically ill patients.[22]

Morphine. Morphine is the most commonly prescribed opioid in the critical care unit. Because of its water solubility, morphine has a slower onset of action and a longer duration compared with lipid-soluble opioids (e.g., fentanyl). This makes morphine and hydromorphone the preferred opioids for intermittent therapy in the SCCM guidelines.[22] Morphine has two main metabolites: morphine-3-glucuronide (M3G, inactive) and morphine-6-glucuronide (M6G, active). M6G is responsible for the analgesic effect but may accumulate and cause excessive sedation in patients with kidney failure or liver failure.[86] Morphine is available in a variety of delivery methods. It is the standard by which all other opioids are

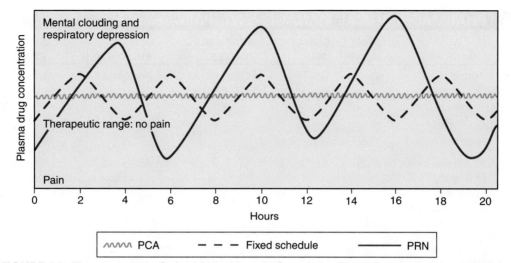

FIGURE 8-5 Fluctuations in Opioid Blood Levels Seen With Three Dosing Procedures. *PCA,* patient-controlled analgesia; *PRN,* as required. (From Lehne RA: *Pharmacology for nursing care,* ed 5, St Louis, 2004, Saunders.)

TABLE 8-3	PHARMACOLOGICAL MANAGEMENT: PAIN					
DRUG	DOSAGE	ONSET (MIN)	DURATION (HR)	AVAILABLE ROUTES	PROPERTIES	SIDE EFFECTS AND COMMENTS
Morphine	1-5 mg IV bolus 1-10 mg IV infusion	5-10	3-4	PO, SL, R, IV, IM, SC, EA, IA	Analgesia, antianxiety	Standard for comparison Side effects: sedation, respiratory depression, euphoria or dysphoria, hypotension, nausea, vomiting, pruritus, constipation, urinary retention M6G can accumulate in renal failure or hepatic dysfunction patients
Fentanyl	25-100 mcg IV bolus 25-200 mcg IV infusion	1-5	0.5-4	OTFC, IV, IM, TD, EA, IA	Analgesia, antianxiety	Same side effects as morphine Rigidity with high doses
Hydromorphone (Dilaudid)	0.2-1 mg IV bolus 0.2-2 mg IV infusion	5	3-4	PO, R, IV, IM, SC, EA, IA	Analgesia, antianxiety	Same side effects as morphine
Codeine	15-30 mg IM, SC	10-20	3-4	PO, IM, SC	Analgesia (mild to moderate pain)	Lacks potency (unpredictable absorption; not all patients convert it to an active form to achieve analgesia) Most common side effects: light-headedness, dizziness, shortness of breath, sedation, nausea, and vomiting

TABLE 8-3 **PHARMACOLOGICAL MANAGEMENT: PAIN—cont'd**

DRUG	DOSAGE	ONSET (MIN)	DURATION (HR)	AVAILABLE ROUTES	PROPERTIES	SIDE EFFECTS AND COMMENTS
Methadone (Dolophine)	5-10 mg IV	10	4-8	PO, SL, R, IV, SC, IM, EA, IA	Analgesia	Usually less sedating than morphine, but repeated doses can result in accumulation and can cause serious sedation (2-5 days)
Acetaminophen	650 mg maximum of 4 g/day; 3 g/day if history of alcohol abuse or malnutrition; 2 g/day in older patients	20-30	4-6	PO, R	Analgesia, antipyretic	Rare side effects Hepatotoxicity
Ketorolac (Toradol)	15-30 mg IV	<10	6-8	PO, IM, IV	Analgesia, minimum antiinflammatory effect	Short-term use (<5 days) Side effects: gastric ulceration, bleeding, exacerbation of kidney failure Use with care in older adults and kidney failure

EA, epidural analgesia; *IA,* intrathecal analgesia; *IM,* intramuscular; *IV,* intravenous; *M6G,* morphine-6-glucuronide; *OTFC,* oral transmucosal fentanyl citrate; *PO,* oral; *R,* rectal; *SC,* subcutaneous; *SL,* sublingual; *TD,* transdermal.

BOX 8-1 **A GUIDE TO USING EQUIANALGESIC CHARTS**

- Equianalgesic means approximately the same pain relief.
- The equianalgesic chart is a guideline. Doses and intervals between doses are titrated according to the individual's response.
- The equianalgesic chart is helpful when switching from one drug to another or when switching from one route of administration to another.
- Dosages in the equianalgesic chart for moderate to severe pain are not necessarily starting doses. The doses suggest a ratio for comparing the analgesia of one drug with another.
- For older patients, initially reduce the recommended adult opioid dose for moderate to severe pain by 25% to 50%.
- The longer the patient has been receiving opioids, the more conservative the starting dose of a new opioid.

measured. It is also the agent that most closely mimics the endogenous opioids in the human pain modification system.

Morphine is indicated for severe pain. It has additional actions that are helpful for managing other symptoms. Morphine dilates peripheral veins and arteries, making it useful in reducing myocardial workload. Morphine is also viewed as an anti-anxiety agent because of the calming effect it produces.

Many side effects have been reported with the use of morphine (see Table 8-3 and Morphine Priority Medications

Box). The hypotensive effect can be particularly problematic in the hypovolemic patient. The vasodilation effect is potentiated in the volume-depleted patient, and the hemodynamic status must be carefully monitored. Volume resuscitation restores blood pressure in the event of a prolonged hypotensive response.

PRIORITY MEDICATIONS
Morphine Sulfate

Drug Class: Opiate
Drug Action: Analgesia

Drug Delivery and Drug Dosage
Morphine is administered in many ways. In critical care usual routes are IV bolus, IV continuous infusion, and PCA; also administered PO in tablet or liquid form (see Table 8-3). In hemodynamically stable patients for acute pain management 0.01-0.15 mg/kg every 1-2 hours IV bolus is recommended until pain is controlled per SCCM guidelines (see Figure 9-1).[22] Morphine may also be administered via continuous IV infusion. Dosage requirements vary widely between individuals depending on whether morphine is used to treat acute pain or chronic pain. Dosage requirements are generally higher in chronic pain related to pain severity and development of drug tolerance over time. Consultation with a medical pain service to effectively manage chronic pain and enable the transition from IV to oral morphine is often helpful. Morphine is the standard opiate used for opiate comparison and conversion in equianalgesic dosing (see Table 8-4).

💊 PRIORITY MEDICATIONS—cont'd
Morphine Sulfate

Priority Nursing Considerations
The goal is to alleviate pain while minimizing side effects. Morphine has many secondary effects that are unpleasant. The experience of unwanted secondary effects is not the same for everyone. In order of occurrence secondary symptoms include: dry mouth, sedation, constipation, anxiety, confusion, nausea, sadness, myoclonus, difficulty urinating, hallucination, and vomiting. Nursing interventions to alleviate unpleasant symptoms include oral care to relieve dry mouth, use of an antiemetic to relieve nausea and vomiting, use of a stool softener and mobility as tolerated to decrease constipation, dosage adjustments or switching opiates to alleviate symptoms of sedation, confusion, hallucination, and myoclonus. If the patient does not have a urinary drainage catheter (Foley) inserted, assess ability to voluntarily void urine. The risk of respiratory depression is a concern in the non-intubated patient. Monitoring of the respiratory rate, depth, and SpO_2 level to detect hypoventilation and respiratory depression is an essential nursing responsibility.

Clinical Examples
Morphine is used in a variety of clinical situations in critical care. It is successfully used to treat acute pain postoperatively. It is used to manage chronic pain such as severe cancer pain. Morphine is also used to alleviate symptoms of dyspnea and provide comfort at end of life (see Chapter 10). In each case the dose and delivery mechanism can differ. In each situation, the nurse must know the reason the drug is being given; continuously assess for side effects, and re-assess the efficacy of pain control.

A more serious side effect requiring diligent monitoring is the respiratory depressant effect. Opioids may cause this complication because they reduce the responsiveness of carbon dioxide chemoreceptors in the respiratory center located in the medulla in the brainstem.[87] Although infrequent, this effect can have significant sequelae for the critically ill patient. A subset of patients is at greater risk for respiratory depression after opioid administration. This subset includes newborns (younger than 6 months), older patients with chronic obstructive pulmonary disease (COPD) or known obstructive sleep apnea syndrome, patients who are opiate naïve (receiving opiates for less than a week), and patients with kidney failure.[85] Critical care nurses must monitor these patients intensively to prevent this complication. Monitoring of patients receiving opioid analgesics is discussed in more detail later in this chapter. In addition to side effects common to all opioids, morphine may stimulate histamine release from mast cells, resulting in cardiac instability and allergic reactions.

Fentanyl. Fentanyl is a synthetic opioid preferred for critically ill patients with hemodynamic instability or morphine allergy. It is a lipid-soluble agent that has a more rapid onset than morphine and a shorter duration.[86] The metabolites of fentanyl are largely inactive and nontoxic, which makes it an effective and safe opioid. However, repeated doses may cause accumulation and prolonged effects of the drug. The use of fentanyl in the critical care unit is growing in popularity, and it is the preferred agent for acutely distressed patients, hemodynamically unstable patients, and for those with impaired kidney function[22] (see Table 8-3 and Fentanyl Priority Medications Box). Fentanyl is available in intravenous, intraspinal, and transdermal forms. The transdermal form is commonly referred to as the Duragesic patch or the 72-hour patch.

💊 PRIORITY MEDICATIONS
Fentanyl

Drug Class: Opiate
Drug Action: Analgesia

Drug Delivery and Dosage
Fentanyl is administered via IV bolus (0.35-1.5 mcg/kg every 0.5-1 hour) until pain is relieved in hemodynamically unstable patients per SCCM guidelines (see Figure 9-1).[22] A fentanyl IV bolus is high-potency, short-acting, and takes effect within 15 minutes. If pain is not relieved, the dose is repeated until the pain is controlled. Following pain control, continuous infusion or scheduled doses are administered to manage pain.

Priority Nursing Considerations
Fentanyl is lipid-soluble. It is classified as a short-acting opioid with a short half-life, but this depends on how the drug is administered. When given as an IV bolus, it provides rapid relief of pain, but the analgesic effect wears off quickly. This makes IV fentanyl a good choice to treat breakthrough pain, while a longer-acting opioid is taking effect in the background. If fentanyl is delivered by continuous IV infusion over several days, it can accumulate in the fat tissues over time, and the half-life is prolonged. Fentanyl accumulates in the tissues because it is lipid-soluble. In general the side effects are similar to those of morphine, including risk of respiratory depression and hypotension related to vasodilation in hypovolemic patients. Muscle rigidity is an uncommon side effect associated with fentanyl. As with other opioids, the goal of treatment is to alleviate pain while minimizing or avoiding opiate-related side effects.

Clinical Examples
Fentanyl is frequently used to control postoperative pain either as a continuous infusion or with IV bolus dosing in critical care. In a recent survey of sedation practices in mechanically ventilated patients in the United States, fentanyl and morphine were the most frequently administered continuous opiate infusions. In mechanically ventilated patients, use of an opiate infusion alone was uncommon; opiates were usually administered in combination with continuous sedatives. This practice follows the recommendations of the SCCM guidelines (see Figure 9-1).

Because the side effects of fentanyl are similar to those of morphine, the nurse must monitor carefully the hemodynamic and respiratory responses. When fentanyl is given by rapid administration and at higher doses, it has been associated with the additional hazard of bradycardia and rigidity in the chest wall muscles.[22,86] The use of transdermal fentanyl is indicated rarely in the acutely critically ill patient. The customary use of the "fentanyl patch" is for those experiencing chronic pain or cancer pain, and in critical care it is used for patients who require extended pain control. Transdermal delivery requires 12 to 16 hours for onset of action, and the patch duration is 72 hours.[30] If the transdermal delivery method is used, the patient will require concurrent opioid management until the fentanyl patch takes effect.

Hydromorphone. Hydromorphone is a semisynthetic opioid that has an onset of action and duration similar to those of morphine.[86] It is an effective opioid with multiple routes of delivery. It is more potent than morphine. Hydromorphone is a safe choice in patients with kidney failure as it lacks active metabolites.[22] Also, it has been shown that some side effects (e.g., pruritus, sedation, nausea, vomiting) may occur less with hydromorphone than morphine[87] (see Table 8-3).

Meperidine. Meperidine (Demerol) is a less potent opioid with agonist effects similar to those of morphine. It is considered the weakest of the opioids, and it must be administered in large doses to be equivalent in action to morphine. Because the duration of action is short, dosing is frequent. A major concern with this drug is the metabolite normeperidine, which is a CNS neurotoxic agent. At high doses in patients with kidney failure or liver dysfunction or in older patients, it may induce CNS toxicities, including irritability, muscle spasticity, tremors, agitation, and seizures.[30] Research has shown that meperidine can cause delirium in postoperative patients of all ages.[88] Although meperidine is useful in short-term specific conditions (e.g., treating postoperative shivering), it should be avoided in patients who require longer periods of analgesia and is not recommended for repetitive use.[22]

Codeine. Codeine has limited use in the management of severe pain. It is rarely used in the critical care unit. It provides analgesia for mild to moderate pain. It is usually compounded with a nonopioid (e.g., acetaminophen). To be active, codeine must be metabolized in the liver to morphine.[30] Codeine is available only through oral, intramuscular, and subcutaneous routes, and its absorption can be reduced in the critical care patient by altered gastrointestinal motility and decreased tissue perfusion.[89]

Methadone. Methadone is a synthetic opioid with morphine-like properties that causes less sedation. It is longer acting than morphine and has a long half-life. This makes it difficult to titrate in the critical care patient. Methadone lacks active metabolites, and routes other than the kidney eliminate 60% of the drug. This means that methadone does not accumulate in patients with kidney failure.[90] Methadone is recommended as a second-line opioid analgesic.[91] It may be a good alternative for the patient who has a long recovery ahead with an anticipated prolonged weaning from mechanical ventilation.[86]

More Potent Opioids: Remifentanil and Sufentanil. Remifentanil and sufentanil are agonist opioids. The use of these potent drugs has been studied in critically ill patients.

Remifentanil is 250 times more potent than morphine, and it has a rapid onset and predictable offset of action. For this reason, it allows a rapid emergence from sedation, facilitating the evaluation of the neurological state of the patient after stopping the infusion.[92,93]

Sufentanil is 7 to 13 times more potent than fentanyl and 500 to 1000 times more potent than morphine. It has more pronounced sedation properties than fentanyl and other opioids. Patients under sufentanil require minimal sedative agent doses to achieve an adequate sedation level. It has a rapid distribution and a high clearance rate, preventing accumulation when given for a long period.[94] Sufentanil has a longer emergence from sedation compared with remifentanil, but it allows a longer analgesic effect after stopping its administration.[93]

Preventing and Treating Respiratory Depression

Respiratory depression is the most life-threatening opioid side effect. The risk of respiratory depression increases when other drugs with CNS depressant effects (e.g., benzodiazepines, antiemetics, neuroleptics, antihistamines) are concomitantly administered to the patient.[86] Respiratory depression is defined as a decrease in the rate or depth of respirations, not necessarily a specific number of respirations per minute. Respiratory rates less than 8 or 10 require rapid assessment. A change in the patient's level of consciousness or an increase in sedation normally precedes respiratory depression.

Monitoring. Patients should be monitored before the administration of the opioid agent and at its peak effect. Monitoring for the following parameters at least every 1 to 2 hours for the first 24 hours and every 4 hours thereafter in stable patients[95,96] is recommended to prevent respiratory depression:

- Pain intensity, using a valid pain scale
- Respiratory rate and depth
- Sedation level, using a valid sedation scale (see Chapter 9, Table 9-1)

Monitoring oxygen saturation (SpO_2) is recommended to detect deterioration in respiratory condition.[97] The use of capnography, which is available in many critical care settings, should be considered for non-intubated high-risk patients receiving opiate parenteral therapy.[96]

Opioid Reversal. Critical respiratory depression can be readily reversed with the administration of the opiate antagonist naloxone (Narcan). The usual dose is 0.4 mg, mixed with 10 mL of normal saline[98] (for a concentration of 0.04 mg/mL). Naloxone is administered intravenously (IV), very slowly, and can be discontinued as soon as the patient is responsive to physical stimulation and able to take deep breaths. Because the duration of naloxone is shorter than most opioids, another dose of naloxone may be needed as early as 30 minutes after the first dose. The nurse monitors sedation and respiratory status and frequently reminds the patient to breathe deeply. The benefits of reversing respiratory depression with naloxone must be weighed against the risk of sudden onset of pain and the difficulty of achieving pain relief. To prevent this from occurring, it is important to provide a nonopioid medication for pain management.[98] Moreover, the use of naloxone is not recommended after prolonged analgesia, because it can induce withdrawal and may cause nausea and cardiovascular complications (e.g., dysrhythmias).[22]

Nonopioid Analgesics

In the SCCM guidelines, the use of nonopioids in combination with an opioid is recommended in selected critical care patients.[22] The goal is to reduce opioid requirements and provide greater analgesic effect through peripheral and central levels.[23] Pharmacological information is presented in Table 8-3.

Delivery Methods

The most common route for drug administration is IV by means of continuous infusion, bolus administration, or patient-controlled analgesia (PCA). Traditionally, the choice has been IV bolus administration. The benefits of this method are the rapid onset of action and the ease of titration. The major disadvantage is the rise and fall of the serum level of the opioid, leading to periods of pain control with periods of breakthrough pain[99] (see Figure 8-5).

Patient-Controlled Analgesia. Patient-controlled analgesia (PCA) is a method of drug delivery that uses the intravenous route and an infusion pump. It allows the patient to self-administer small doses of analgesics. Different opioids can be used, but the most extensively used is morphine.[99] This method of medication delivery allows self-administration of a medication bolus the moment the pain begins (see Figure 8-5). Naloxone must be readily available to reverse adverse opiate respiratory effects. Ideally, the patient undergoing an elective procedure requiring opioid analgesia postoperatively is instructed in the use of PCA during preoperative teaching. This allows the patient to become comfortable with the concept of self-medication before use.

Intraspinal anesthesia uses the concept that the spinal cord is the primary link in nociceptive transmission. The goal is to mimic the body's endogenous opioid pain modification system by interfering with the transmission of pain and providing an opiate receptor-binding agent directly into the spinal cord. The benefits of the intraspinal route include good to excellent pain control with typically lower doses of opioids, increased patient mobility, minimal sedation, and increased patient satisfaction.[100] The hemodynamic status of the patient changes very little.

Intraspinal anesthesia is particularly appropriate for pain in the thorax, upper abdomen, and lower extremities. The two intraspinal routes are intrathecal and epidural. Regardless of the route, the effects of the opioid agonist used are the same, and assessment parameters are the same as those used for other routes.

Intrathecal Analgesia. Intrathecal (subarachnoid) opioids are placed directly into the cerebral spinal fluid and attach to spinal cord receptor sites. Opioids introduced at this site act quickly at the dorsal horn. The dural sheath is punctured, eliminating the barrier for pathogens between the environment and the cerebral spinal fluid. This creates the risk of serious infections. The intrathecal route is usually reserved for intraoperative use. Single-bolus dosing provides short-term relief for pain that is short lived (the pain of labor and delivery is well managed using this regimen. Side effects of intrathecal pain control include postdural puncture headache and infection.[101]

Epidural Analgesia. Epidural analgesia is commonly used in the critical care unit after major abdominal surgery, nephrectomy, thoracotomy, and major orthopedic procedures. Certain conditions preclude the use of this pain control method: systemic infection, anticoagulation, and increased intracranial pressure. Epidural delivery of opiates provides longer-lasting pain relief with less dosing of opiates. When delivered into the epidural space, 5 mg of morphine may be effective for 6 to 24 hours, compared with 3 to 4 hours when delivered intravenously. Opioids infused in the epidural space are more unpredictable than those administered intrathecally. The epidural space is filled with fatty tissue and is external to the dura mater. The fatty tissue interferes with uptake, and the dura acts as a barrier to diffusion, making diffusion rate difficult to predict.

The type of drug used determines the rapidity of drug diffusion. Drugs are *hydrophilic* or *lipophilic*. Hydrophilic drugs like morphine are water-soluble and penetrate the dura slowly, giving them a longer onset and duration of action. Lipophilic drugs including fentanyl are lipid-soluble; they penetrate the dura rapidly and therefore have a rapid onset of action and a shorter duration of action.

The dura acts as a physical barrier and causes delay in diffusion of the drug. Compared with the intrathecal route, it allows more of the drug to be absorbed in the systemic circulation, requiring greater doses for pain relief.[100] Drugs delivered epidurally may be administered by bolus or continuous infusion. Epidural analgesia is being used more often in the critical care environment, and it requires careful monitoring.

The nurse must assess the patient for respiratory depression. This phenomenon may occur early in the therapy or as late as 24 hours after initiation. The epidural catheter also puts the patient at risk for infection. The efficiency of this pain control method, and the patient's increased mobility, do not diminish the nurse's responsibility to monitor and evaluate the outcomes of the pain-management protocol in use.

Equianalgesia

When a change of opioid is considered, the nurse must be aware of equianalgesic dosages. In doing any conversion, the goal is to provide equal analgesic effects with the new agents. This concept is referred to as equianalgesia. Morphine is the standard for the conversion of opioids. Prescribed dosages must take into account the patient's age and health status.[30] Because of the variety of agents and routes, the professional pain organizations have developed equianalgesia charts for use by health care professionals. All critical care units need a chart posted for easy referral. Table 8-4 provides the equianalgesia dose for different drugs used in clinical practice.

TABLE 8-4	EQUIANALGESIC CHART: APPROXIMATE EQUIVALENT DOSES OF OPIOIDS FOR MODERATE-TO-SEVERE PAIN		
ANALGESIC	PARENTERAL (IM, SC, IV) ROUTE[1,2] (MG)	PO ROUTE[1] (MG)	COMMENTS
Mu Opioid Agonists			
Morphine	10	30	Standard for comparison; multiple routes of administration; available in immediate-release and controlled-release formulations; active metabolite M6G can accumulate with repeated dosing in kidney failure
Codeine	130	200 NR	IM has unpredictable absorption and high side-effect profile; used PO for mild-to-moderate pain; usually compounded with nonopioid (e.g., Tylenol No. 3)
Fentanyl	100 mcg/hr parenterally and transdermally ≅4 mg/hr morphine parenterally; 1 mcg/hr transdermally ≅2 mg/24 hr morphine PO	–	Short half-life, but at steady state, slow elimination from tissues can lead to a prolonged half-life (up to 12 hr); start opioid-naïve patients on no more than 25 mcg/hr transdermally; transdermal fentanyl NR for acute pain management; available by oral transmucosal route
Hydromorphone (Dilaudid)	1.5	7.5	Useful alternative to morphine; no evidence that metabolites are clinically relevant; shorter duration than morphine; available in high-potency parenteral formulation (10 mg/mL) useful for SC infusion; 3 mg rectal ≅ 650 mg aspirin PO; with repeated dosing (e.g., PCA), it is more likely than 2-3 mg parenteral hydromorphone = 10 mg parenteral morphine
Levorphanol (Levo-Dromoran)	2	4	Longer-acting than morphine when given repeatedly; long half-life can lead to accumulation within 2-3 days of repeated dosing
Meperidine	75	300 NR	No longer preferred as a first-line opioid for the management of acute or chronic pain due to potential toxicity from accumulation of metabolite, normeperidine; normeperidine has 15-20 hr half-life and is not reversed by naloxone; NR in older patients or patients with impaired kidney function; NR by continuous IV infusion
Methadone (Dolophine)	10	20	Longer-acting than morphine when given repeatedly; long half-life can lead to delayed toxicity from accumulation within 3-5 days; start PO dosing on PRN schedule; in opioid-tolerant patients converted to methadone, start with 10%-25% of equianalgesic dose
Oxycodone	–	20	Used for moderate pain when combined with a nonopioid (e.g., Percocet, Tylox); available as single entity in immediate-release and controlled-release formulations (e.g., OxyContin); can be used like PO morphine for severe pain
Oxymorphone (Numorphan)	1	10 rectal	Used for moderate to severe pain; no PO formulation

| TABLE 8-4 | EQUIANALGESIC CHART: APPROXIMATE EQUIVALENT DOSES OF OPIOIDS FOR MODERATE-TO-SEVERE PAIN—cont'd | | |

ANALGESIC	PARENTERAL (IM, SC, IV) ROUTE[1,2] (MG)	PO ROUTE[1] (MG)	COMMENTS
Agonist-Antagonist Opioids: Not recommended for severe, escalating pain. If used in combination with mu agonists, may reverse analgesia and precipitate withdrawal in opioid-dependent patients.			
Buprenorphine (Buprenex)	0.4	–	Not readily reversed by naloxone; NR for laboring patients
Butorphanol (Stadol)	2	–	Available in nasal spray
Dezocine (Dalgan)	10	–	
Nalbuphine (Nubain)	10	–	
Pentazocine (Talwin)	30	50	

Data from Pasero, C., & McCaffery, M (2010). *Pain assessment and pharmacologic management.* Mosby Elsevier: St Louis. Selected references for more information: American Pain Society (APS): *Principles of analgesic use in the treatment of acute and cancer pain*, ed 3, Glenview, Ill., 1992, APS; Lawlor P, et al: Dose ratio between morphine and hydromorphone in patients with cancer pain: a retrospective study, *Pain* 72(1-2):79, 1997; Manfredi PL, et al: Intravenous methadone for cancer pain unrelieved by morphine and hydromorphone: clinical observations, *Pain* 70(1):99, 1997; Portenoy RK: Opioid analgesics. In Portenoy RK, Kanner RM, editors: *Pain management: theory and practice*, Philadelphia, 1996, FA Davis.

[1]Duration of analgesia is dose dependent; the higher the dose, usually the longer the duration.

[2]IV boluses may be used to produce analgesia that lasts approximately as long as IM or SC doses. However, of all routes of administration, IV produces the highest peak concentration of the drug, and the peak concentration is associated with the highest level of toxicity (e.g., sedation). To decrease the peak effect and lower the level of toxicity, IV boluses may be administered more slowly (e.g., 10 mg of morphine over a 15-minute period), or smaller doses may be administered more often (e.g., 5 mg of morphine every 1-1.5 hours).

IM, intramuscular; *IV*, intravenous; *M6G*, morphine-6-glucuronide; *MCG*, micrograms; *MG*, milligrams; *NR*, not recommended; *PCA*, patient-controlled analgesia; *PO*, by mouth; *PRN*, pro re nata (as needed); *SC*, subcutaneous.

Nonpharmacological Methods of Pain Management

Although numerous methods of pain management other than drugs appear in critical care literature,[102] very few studies have been done to provide evidence of their effectiveness in the critical care settings. Nonpharmacological methods can be used to supplement analgesic treatment, but they are not intended to replace analgesics.[103] In most instances, these therapies may augment and enhance the pharmacological management of the patient's pain. Critical care nurses identify many barriers to use of nonpharmacological methods for pain management, including lack of knowledge, training, and time.[104]

Cognitive Techniques

Cognitive techniques include patient teaching, relaxation, distraction, guided imagery, and music therapy.

Relaxation. Relaxation is a well-documented method for reducing the distress associated with pain. Although not a substitute for pharmacology, relaxation is an excellent adjunct for controlling pain.[105,106] Relaxation decreases oxygen consumption and muscle tone, and it can decrease heart rate and blood pressure. Relaxation can give the patient a sense of control over the pain and reduce muscle tension and anxiety. Not all patients are interested in relaxation therapy. For those patients, deep-breathing exercises may be helpful, and they frequently lead to relaxation.[107] Excellent references for techniques in relaxation therapy are available.[30]

Guided Imagery. Guided imagery uses the imagination to provide control over pain. It can be used to distract or relax. Guiding a patient to a place that is pain free and relaxing takes a considerable time commitment on the part of the nurse. Although this may be difficult in the critical care environment, guiding patients to a place in their imagination that is free from pain may be beneficial.[102]

Music Therapy. Music therapy is a commonly used intervention for relaxation. Music that is pleasing to the patient may have soothing effects, but its effects on reducing pain are controversial.[108] Ideally, the music should be supplied by a small set of headphones. It is important to educate the patient and family regarding the role of music in relaxation and pain control and to provide music of the patient's choice. The patient and family may also provide information about sources of distraction for the patient. Some persons are distracted by television; for others, television may increase anxiety.

The key to success with pain management in critically ill patients is a comprehensive understanding of effective pain assessment methods and drug mechanisms of action so that the therapy matches the needs of the patient. In addition, when used effectively, nonpharmacological options such as relaxation and music therapy may assist with pain management in critical illness.

CASE STUDY   PATIENT WITH PAIN

Answers to the Case Study Questions can be found on the Evolve web site at http://evolve.elsevier.com/Urden/priorities/.

Brief Patient History

Ms. X is a woman with type 2 diabetes mellitus and peripheral arterial occlusive disease with neuropathy. Ms. X is disabled because of limited mobility and chronic pain associated with lower extremity claudication and neuropathic pain. She has been admitted for an elective right femoral to distal tibial bypass. Ms. X's chronic pain has been effectively managed with gabapentin (600 mg three times daily) and a 75-mcg fentanyl patch every third day. Ms. X reports that her pain patch is due to be changed the next day. Her diabetes mellitus has been effectively managed with diet and a combination of oral agents. Postoperatively, orders for pain management include her home regimen of gabapentin and fentanyl patch and an order for morphine for breakthrough pain.

Clinical Assessment

Ms. X is admitted to the intensive care unit from the perianesthesia recovery room after an 8-hour surgical revascularization of the right lower extremity. She is awake, alert, and oriented to person, time, place, and situation. Ms. X is breathing through her mouth and taking shallow breaths. She complains of right lower extremity and bilateral foot pain. Her skin is warm and dry. Ms. X is able to move her toes on command, and lower extremity sensation to touch is intact; however, she is complaining of severe burning in both feet.

Diagnostic Procedures

Ms. X reports that her pain is a 10 on the NRS. The Riker Sedation-Agitation Scale score is 5.

Medical Diagnosis

The diagnosis is acute postoperative incisional pain superimposed on chronic neuropathic pain involving both lower extremities. Neuropathic pain is likely worsened because of missed doses of gabapentin.

Questions

1. What major outcomes do you expect to achieve for this patient?
2. What problems or risks must be managed to achieve these outcomes?
3. What interventions must be initiated to monitor, prevent, manage, or eliminate the problems and risks identified?
4. What interventions should be initiated to promote optimal functioning, safety, and well-being of the patient?
5. What possible learning needs do you anticipate for this patient?
6. What cultural and age-related factors may have a bearing on the patient's plan of care?

REFERENCES

1. Rotondi AJ, et al: Patients' recollections of stressful experiences while receiving prolonged mechanical ventilation in an intensive care unit, *Crit Care Med* 30(4):746, 2002.
2. Hamill-Ruth RJ, Marohn L: Evaluation of pain in the critically ill patient, *Crit Care Clin* 15(1):35, 1999.
3. Kwekkeboom KL, Herr K: Assessment of pain in the critically ill, *Crit Care Nurs Clin North Am* 13(2):181, 2001.
4. Gélinas C: Management of pain in cardiac surgery ICU patients: have we improved over time? *Intensive Crit Care Nurs* 23(5):298, 2007.
5. Puntillo KA, et al: Patients' perceptions and responses to procedural pain: results from Thunder Project II, *Am J Crit Care* 10(4):238, 2001.
6. Stanik-Hutt J, et al: Pain experiences of traumatically injured patients in a critical care setting, *Am J Crit Care* 10(4):252, 2001.
7. Desbiens NA, et al: Pain and satisfaction with pain control in seriously ill hospitalized adults: findings from the SUPPORT research investigations, *Crit Care Med* 24(12):1953, 1996.
8. Gélinas C, et al: Pain assessment and management in critically ill intubated patients: a retrospective study, *Am J Crit Care* 13(2):126, 2004.
9. Puntillo KA, et al: Practices and predictors of analgesic interventions for adults undergoing painful procedures, *Am J Crit Care* 11(5):415, 2002.
10. Carr DB, Goudas LC: Acute pain, *Lancet* 353(9169):2051, 1999.
11. Kehlet H: Surgical stress and postoperative outcome – from here to where? *Reg Anesth Pain Med* 31(1):47, 2006.
12. Joshi GP, Ogunnaike BO: Consequences of inadequate postoperative pain relief and chronic persistent postoperative pain, *Anesthesiol Clin North Am* 23(1):21, 2005.
13. Kehlet H, et al: Persistent postsurgical pain: risk factors and prevention, *Lancet* 367(9522):1618, 2006.
14. International Association for the Study of Pain (IASP) Subcommittee on Taxonomy: Pain terms: a list with definitions and notes on usage, *Pain* 6(3):249, 1979.
15. Shannon K, Bucknall T: Pain assessment in critical care: what have we learnt from research, *Intensive Crit Care Nurs* 19(3):154, 2003.
16. Puntillo KA: Pain experiences of intensive care unit patients, *Heart Lung* 19(5 part 1):526, 1990.
17. Puntillo KA: Dimensions of procedural pain and its analgesic management in critically ill surgical patients, *Am J Crit Care* 3(2):116, 1994.
18. Puntillo KA, Weiss SJ: Pain: its mediators and associated morbidity in critically ill cardiovascular surgical patients, *Nurs Res* 43(1):31, 1994.
19. Gélinas C, Johnston C: Pain assessment in the critically ill ventilated adult: validation of the Critical-Care Pain Observation Tool and physiologic indicators, *Clin J Pain* 23(6):497, 2007.
20. Gordon DB, et al; American Pain Society recommendations for improving the quality of acute and cancer pain management. *Archives of Internal Medicine*, 165:1574, 2005.
21. Herr K, et al: Pain assessment in the nonverbal patient: Position statement with clinical practice recommendations, *Pain Manag Nurs* 7(2):44, 2006.

22. Jacobi J, et al: Clinical practice guidelines for the sustained use of sedatives and analgesics in the critically ill adult, *Crit Care Med* 30(1):119, 2002.

23. Joint Commission on Accreditation of Healthcare Organizations (JCAHO): *Pain: current understanding of assessment, management, and treatments*, Oakbrook Terrace, Ill., 2001, JCAHO.

24. McCaffery M: *Nursing management of the patient with pain*, ed 2, Philadelphia, 1979, JB Lippincott.

25. Puntillo K, et al: Evaluation of pain in ICU patients, *Chest* 135(4):1069, 2009.

26. McGuire D: Comprehensive and multidimensional assessment and measurement of pain, *J Pain Symptom Manage* 7(5):312, 1992.

27. Melzack R: Pain and stress: a new perspective. In Gatchel RJ, Turk DC, editors: *Psychological factors in pain*, New York, 1999, Guilford Press.

28. American Geriatrics Society (AGS) Panel on Persistent Pain in Older Persons: The management of persistent pain in older persons, *J Am Geriatr Soc* 50(Suppl 6):S205, 2002.

29. International Association for the Study of Pain (IASP) Task Force on Taxonomy: *Classification of chronic pain*, Seattle, 1994, IASP Press.

30. McCaffery M, Pasero C: *Pain: clinical manual for nursing practice*, ed 2, St Louis, 1999, CV Mosby.

31. Dworkin RH, et al: Advances in neuropathic pain: diagnosis, mechanisms, and treatment recommendations, *Arch Neurol* 60(11):1524, 2003.

32. Hayes C, Molloy AR: Neuropathic pain in the perioperative period, *Int Anesthesiol Clin* 35(2):67, 1997.

33. Siddall PJ, Cousins MJ: Neurobiology of pain, *Int Anesthesiol Clin* 35(2):1, 1997.

34. Woolf CJ, Mannion RJ: Neuropathic pain: aetiology, symptoms, mechanisms, and management, *Lancet* 353(9168):1959, 1999.

35. Charlton JE: *Core curriculum for professional education in pain*, ed 3, Seattle, 2005, IASP Press.

36. Melzack R, Wall PD: *The challenge of pain*, ed 2, London, 1996, Penguin Books.

37. Gélinas C, et al: Les indicateurs de la douleur en soins critiques [Pain indicators in critical care], *Perspect Infirm* 2(4):12, 2005.

38. Hofbauer RK, et al: Cortical representation of the sensory dimension of pain, *J Neurophysiol* 86(1):402, 2001.

39. Rainville P: Brain mechanisms of pain affect and pain modulation, *Curr Opin Neurobiol* 12(2):195, 2002.

40. Rainville P, et al: Pain affect encoded in human anterior cingulate but not somatosensory cortex, *Science* 277(5328):968, 1997.

41. Derbyshire SW, Osborn J: Modeling pain circuits: how imaging may modify perception, *Neuroimaging Clin N Am* 17(4):485, 2007.

42. Treede RD, et al: The cortical representation of pain, *Pain* 79(2-3):105, 1999.

43. Payen JF, et al: Assessing pain in the critically ill sedated patients by using a behavioral pain scale, *Crit Care Med* 29(12):2258, 2001.

44. Chanques G, et al: Assessing pain in non-intubated critically ill patients unable to self report: an adaptation of the Behavioral Pain Scale, *Intensive Care Med* 35(12):2060-2067, 2009.

45. Ahlers S, et al: Comparison of different pain scoring systems in critically ill patients in a general ICU Critical Care 12:R15. Can be accessed online at: http://ccforum.com/content/12/1/R15.

46. Puntillo KA, et al: Relationship between behavioral and physiological indicators of pain, critical care patients' self-reports of pain, and opioid administration, *Crit Care Med* 2(7)5:1159, 1997.

47. Asian FE, et al: Patients' experience of pain after cardiac surgery, *Contemp Nurse* 34(1):48-54, 2009.

48. Arbour C, Gélinas C: Are vital signs valid indicators for the assessment of pain in postoperative cardiac surgery ICU adults, *Intensive Crit Care Nurs* 26(2):83-90, 2010.

49. Rose L, et al: Survey of assessment and management of pain for critically ill adults, *Intensive Crit Care Nurs* 27(3):121-128, 2011.

50. Daut RL, Cleeland CS: The prevalence and severity of pain in cancer, *Cancer* 50(9):1913, 1982.

51. Melzack R: The short form McGill Pain Questionnaire, *Pain* 30(2):191, 1987.

52. Jarvis C: *Physical examination & health assessment*, ed 5, Philadelphia, 2008, Saunders.

53. Puntillo KA: Pain management. In Schell HM, Puntillo KA, editors: *Critical care nursing secrets*, ed 2, Philadelphia, 2006, Hanley & Belfus.

54. Carey SJ, et al: Improving pain management in an acute care setting: the Crawford Long Hospital of Emory University Experience, *Orthop Nurs* 16(4):29, 1997.

55. Stuppy DJ: The Faces Pain Scale: reliability and validity with mature adults, *Appl Nurs Res* 11(2):84, 1998.

56. Gélinas C: Le thermomètre d'intensité de douleur: un nouvel outil pour les patients adultes en soins critiques [The Faces Pain Thermometer: a new tool for critically ill adults], *Perspect Infirm* 4(4):12, 2007.

57. Puntillo KA, et al: Pain behaviors observed during six common procedures: results from Thunder Project II, *Crit Care Med* 32(2):421, 2004.

58. Gélinas C, Arbour C: Behavioral and physiological indicators during a nociceptive procedure in conscious and unconscious mechanically ventilated adults: similar or different? *J Crit Care* 24(4):628, 2009.

59. Gélinas C, et al: Validation of the Critical-Care Pain Observation Tool in adult patients, *Am J Crit Care* 15(4):420, 2006.

60. Mateo OM, Krenzischek DA: A pilot study to assess the relationship between behavioral manifestations and self-report of pain in postanesthesia care unit patients, *J Post Anesth Nurs* 7(1):15, 1992.

61. Li D, et al: A review of objective pain measures for use with critical care adult patients unable to self-report, *J Pain* 9(1):2, 2008.

62. Sessler CN, et al: Evaluating and monitoring analgesia and sedation in the intensive care unit, *Crit Care* 12(suppl 3):S2, 2008.

63. Aïssaoui Y, et al: Validation of a behavioral pain scale in critically ill, sedated, and mechanically ventilated patients, *Anesth Analg* 101(5):1470, 2005.

64. Young J, et al: Use of a Behavioural Pain Scale to assess pain in ventilated, unconscious and/or sedated patients, *Intensive Crit Care Nurs* 22(1):32, 2006.

65. Gélinas C, et al: Item selection and content validity of the Critical-Care Pain Observation Tool for non-verbal adults, *J Adv Nurs* 65(1):203, 2009.

66. Gélinas C, et al: Theoretical, psychometric, and pragmatic issues in pain measurement, *Pain Manag Nurs* 9(3):120, 2008.

67. Gélinas C: Nurses' evaluations of the feasibility and the clinical utility of the Critical-Care Pain Observation Tool, *Pain Manag Nurs* 11(12):115, 2010.

68. Gélinas C, et al: Sensitivity and specificity of the Critical-Care Pain Observation Tool for the detection of pain in intubated adults after cardiac surgery, *J Pain Symptom Manage* 37(1):58, 2009.

69. Gordon DB, et al: American Pain recommendations for improving the quality of acute and cancer pain management, *Arch Intern Med* 165(14):1574, 2005.

70. Miaskowski C, et al: *Guidelines for the management of cancer pain in adults and children*, Clinical Practice Guidelines Series, no 3, Glenview, Ill., 2005, American Pain Society.

71. Lawrence M: The unconscious experience, *Am J Crit Care* 4(3):227, 1995.

72. Bjoro K, Herr K: Assessment of pain in the nonverbal or cognitively impaired older adult, *Clin Geriatr Med* 24(2):237, 2008.

73. Hadjistavropoulos T, et al: An interdisciplinary expert consensus statement on assessment of pain in older persons, *Clin J Pain* 23(1 supp):S1, 2007.

74. Herr KA, Mobily PR: Comparison of selected pain assessment tools for use with the elderly, *Appl Nurs Res* 6(1):39, 1993.

75. Aubin M, et al: L'évaluation systématique des instruments pour mesurer la douleur chez les personnes âgées ayant des capacités réduites à communiquer, *Pain Res Manag* 12(3):195, 2007.

76. Zwakhalen SM, et al: Pain in elderly people with severe dementia: a systematic review of behavioural pain assessment tools, *BMC Geriatr* 6(3), 2006.

77. Fuchs-Lacelle S, Hadjistavropoulos T: Development and preliminary validation of the Pain Assessment Checklist for Seniors with Limited Ability to Communicate (PACSLAC), *Pain Manag Nurs* 5(1):37, 2004.

78. Wary B, Doloplus C: Doloplus-2, a scale for pain measurement, *Soins Gerontol* 19:25, 1999.

79. Wary B, et al: Doloplus 2: validation d'une échelle d'évaluation comportementale de la douleur chez la personne âgée, *Douleurs* 1:35, 2001.

80. McNicoll L, et al: Delirium in the intensive care unit: occurrence and clinical course in older patients, *J Am Geriatr Soc* 51(5):591, 2003.

81. Graf C, Puntillo KA: Pain in the older adult in the intensive care unit, *Crit Care Clin* 19(4):749, 2003.

82. Bozeman M: Cultural aspects of pain management. In Salerno E, Willens J, editors: *Pain management handbook: an interdisciplinary approach*, St Louis, 1996, Mosby.

83. Ulmer J: Identifying and preventing pain mismanagement. In Salerno E, Willens J, editors: *Pain management handbook: an interdisciplinary approach*, St Louis, 1996, Mosby.

84. Carroll KC, et al: Pain assessment and management in critically ill postoperative and trauma patients: a multisite study, *Am J Crit Care* 8(2):105, 1999.

85. Smith LH: Opioid safety: is your patient at risk for respiratory depression? *Clin J Oncol Nurs* 11(2):293, 2007.

86. Liu LL, Gropper MA: Postoperative analgesia and sedation in the adult intensive care unit: a guide to drug selection, *Drugs* 63(8):755, 2003.

87. Sarhill N, et al: Hydromorphone: pharmacology and clinical applications in cancer patients, *Support Care Cancer* 9(2):84, 2001.

88. Marcantonio ER, et al: The relationship of postoperative delirium with psychoactive medications, *JAMA* 272(19):1518, 1994.

89. McGory R: Pharmacokinetic and pharmacodynamic concerns in the critically ill. In Hamill RJ, Rowlingson RC, editors: *Handbook of critical care pain management*, New York, 1994, McGraw-Hill.

90. Davis MP, Walsh D: Methadone for relief of cancer pain: a review of pharmacokinetics, pharmacodynamics, drug interactions and protocols of administration, *Support Care Cancer* 9(2):73, 2001.

91. World Health Organization (WHO): *Cancer pain relief*, Geneva, 1986, WHO.

92. Cavaliere F, et al: A low-dose remifentanil infusion is well tolerated for sedation in mechanically ventilated, critically-ill patients, *Can J Anaesth* 49(10):1088, 2002.

93. Soltész S, et al: Recovery after remifentanil and sufentanil for analgesia and sedation of mechanically ventilated patients after trauma or major surgery, *Br J Anaesth* 86(6):763, 2001.

94. Ethuin F, et al: Pharmacokinetics of long-term sufentanil infusion for sedation in ICU patients, *Intensive Care Med* 29(11):1916, 2003.

95. Pasero CL, McCaffery M: Avoiding opioid-induced respiratory depression, *Am J Nurs* 94(4):24, 1994.

96. Pasero C, et al: PAIN Control: IV opioid range orders for acute pain management, *Am J Nurs* 107(2):62, 2007.

97. Yantis MA: Obstructive sleep apnea syndrome, *Am J Nurs* 102(6):83, 2002.

98. Pasero C, McCaffery M: Reversing respiratory depression with naloxone. *Am J Nurs* 100(2):26, 2000.

99. Lehne RA: *Pharmacology for nursing care*, ed 6, Philadelphia, 2007, Saunders.

100. Dyble K: Epidural and intrathecal methods of analgesia in the critically ill. In Puntillo K, editor: *Pain in the critically ill: assessment and management*, Gaithersburg, MD, 1991, Aspen.

101. Deer TR, et al: Consensus guidelines for the selection and implantation of patients with noncancer pain for intrathecal drug delivery, *Pain Physician* 13:E175, 2010.

102. Gujol M: A survey of pain assessment and management practices among critical care nurses, *Am J Crit Care* 3(2):123, 1994.

103. Pasero C, et al: Postoperative pain management in the older adult. In Gibson D, Weiner D, editors: *Pain in older persons. Progress in pain research and management*, vol 35, Seattle, 2005, IASP Press.

104. Tracy MF, et al: Nurse attitudes towards the use of complementary and alternative therapies in critical care, *Heart Lung* 32(3):197, 2003.

105. Houston S, Jesurum J: The quick relaxation technique: effect on pain associated with chest tube removal, *Appl Nurs Res* 12(4):196, 1999.

106. Miller KM, Perry PA: Relaxation technique and postoperative pain in patients undergoing cardiac surgery, *Heart Lung* 19(2):136, 1990.

107. Good M, et al: Relief of postoperative pain with jaw relaxation, music and their combination, *Pain* 81(1-2):163, 1999.

108. Biley FC: The effects on patient well-being of music listening as a nursing intervention: a review of the literature, *J Clin Nurs* 9(5):668, 2000.

Sedation and Delirium Management

Mary E. Lough

OBJECTIVES

- Explain the differences among light, moderate, and deep levels of sedation.
- Describe the role of standardized assessment tools to determine sedation requirements.
- Compare and contrast the pharmacological agents used to provide sedation.

- List the risk factors for development of delirium in critical illness.
- Describe the management of delirium tremens in critical illness.

One of the challenges facing clinicians is how to provide a therapeutic healing environment for patients in the alarm-filled, emergency-focused critical care unit. Many critical care patients demonstrate some degree of agitation and discomfort caused by painful procedures, invasive tubes, sleep deprivation, fear, anxiety, and physiological stress.

Clinical practice guidelines were developed by the Society of Critical Care Medicine (SCCM) to increase awareness of these issues in the critically ill.[1] The goal is to find a balance between providing compassionate patient care and avoiding the perils of oversedation.

SEDATION

SEDATION SCALES

The use of scoring systems to assess and record levels of sedation and agitation is now strongly recommended.[1] Four frequently used scales are the Ramsay Scale,[2] the Riker Sedation-Agitation Scale (SAS),[3] the Motor Activity Assessment Scale (MAAS),[4] and the Richmond Agitation-Sedation Scale (RASS)[5,6] (Table 9-1). Because individuals do not metabolize sedative medications at the same rate, the use of a standardized scale can ensure that continuous infusions of sedatives such as propofol or lorazepam are titrated to a

specific goal. Collaboratively, the critical care team must determine which level of sedation is most appropriate for each individual patient.[1]

The first step in assessing the agitated patient is to rule out any sensations of pain.[1] Clinical assessment is more challenging when the patient is obtunded or has an artificial airway in place. If the patient can communicate, the verbal pain scale of 0 to 10 is very useful. If the patient is intubated and cannot vocalize, pain assessment becomes considerably more complex. After medication for pain has been provided, the next step is to determine the minimum level of sedation required (Box 9-1). The SCCM guidelines recommend that all critically ill, intubated, mechanically ventilated patients have stated goals for analgesia and sedation[1] (Figure 9-1). The use of validated assessment scales is advised (see Table 9-1).

COMPLICATIONS OF SEDATION

Oversedation is recognized as a state of unintended patient unresponsiveness in which the patient resides in a state of suspended animation resembling general anesthesia. Prolonged deep sedation is associated with significant complications of immobility, including pressure ulcers, thromboemboli, gastric ileus, nosocomial pneumonia, and delayed weaning from mechanical ventilation.

TABLE 9-1	SEDATION SCALES	
SCORE	**DESCRIPTION**	**DEFINITION**
Riker Sedation-Agitation Scale (SAS)[*]		
7	Dangerously agitated	Pulls at endotracheal tube (ETT), tries to remove catheters, climbs over bed rail, strikes at staff, thrashes side to side
6	Very agitated	Does not calm despite frequent verbal reminding of limits, requires physical restraints, bites ETT
5	Agitated	Anxious or mildly agitated, attempts to sit up, calms down to verbal instructions
4	Calm and cooperative	Calm, awakens easily, follows commands
3	Sedated	Difficult to arouse, awakens to verbal stimuli or gentle shaking but drifts off again; follows simple commands
2	Very sedated	Arouses to physical stimuli but does not communicate or follow commands; may move spontaneously
1	Unarousable	Minimal or no response to noxious stimuli; does not communicate or follow commands
Motor Activity Assessment Scale (MAAS)[†]		
6	Dangerously agitated	No external stimulus required to elicit movement; is uncooperative, pulls at tubes or catheters, thrashes side to side, strikes at staff, tries to climb out of bed, does not calm down when asked
5	Agitated	No external stimulus required to elicit movement; attempts to sit up or move limbs out of bed, does not consistently follow commands (e.g., will lie down when asked but soon reverts back to attempts)
4	Restless and cooperative	No external stimulus required to elicit movement; picks at sheets or tubes or uncovers self; follows commands
3	Calm and cooperative	No external stimulus required to elicit movement; adjusts sheets or clothes purposefully; follows commands
2	Responsive to touch or name	Opens eyes, raises eyebrows, or turns head toward stimulus; or, moves limbs when touched or when name loudly spoken
1	Responsive only to noxious stimulus	Opens eyes, raises eyebrows, or turns head toward stimulus; or, moves limbs with noxious stimulus
0	Unresponsive	Does not move with noxious stimulus
Ramsey Scale[‡]		
1	Awake	Anxious; agitated and/or restless
2		Cooperative, oriented, and tranquil
3		Responds only to commands
4	Asleep	Brisk response to light glabellar tap or loud auditory stimulus
5		Sluggish response to light glabellar tap or loud auditory stimulus
6		No response to light glabellar tap or loud auditory stimulus
Richmond Agitation-Sedation Scale (RASS)[§],[¶]		
+4	Combative	Overtly combative, violent, immediate danger to staff
+3	Very agitated	Pulls or removes tube(s) or catheter(s); aggressive
+2	Agitated	Frequent nonpurposeful movement, fights ventilator
+1	Restless	Anxious but movements not aggressive or vigorous
0	Alert and calm	
−1	Drowsy	Not fully alert, but has sustained awakening (eye-opening/eye contact) to *voice* (**≥10 seconds**) ⎤
−2	Light sedation	Briefly awakens with eye contact to *voice* (**<10 seconds**) ⎥ Verbal Stimulation
−3	Moderate sedation	Movement or eye opening to voice (but no eye contact) ⎦
−4	Deep sedation	No response to voice, but movement or eye opening to physical stimulation ⎤ Physical Stimulation
−5	Unresponsive	No response to voice or physical stimulation ⎦

[*]Riker RR, et al: Prospective evaluation of the Sedation-Agitation Scale for adult critically ill patients, *Crit Care Med* 27(7):1325, 1999.
[†]Devlin JW, et al: Motor Activity Assessment Scale: a valid and reliable sedation scale for use with mechanically ventilated patients in an adult surgical intensive care unit, *Crit Care Med* 27(7):1271, 1999.
[‡]Ramsay MA, et al: Controlled sedation with alphaxalone-alphadolone, *Br Med J* 2(5920):656, 1974.
[§]Sessler CN, et al: The Richmond Agitation-Sedation Scale: validity and reliability in adult intensive care unit patients, *Am J Respir Crit Care Med* 166(10):1338, 2002.
[¶]Ely EW, et al: Monitoring sedation status over time in ICU patients: reliability and validity of the Richmond Agitation-Sedation Scale (RASS), *JAMA* 289(22):2983-2991, 2003.

BOX 9-1   LEVELS OF SEDATION

Light Sedation (Minimal Sedation, Anxiolysis)

Drug-induced state during which patients respond normally to verbal commands. Although cognitive function and coordination may be impaired, ventilatory and cardiovascular functions are unaffected.

Moderate Sedation with Analgesia (Conscious Sedation, Procedural Sedation)

Drug-induced depression of consciousness during which patients respond purposefully to verbal commands, alone or accompanied by light tactile stimulation. No interventions are required to maintain a patent airway, and spontaneous ventilation is adequate. Cardiovascular function is usually maintained.

Deep Sedation and Analgesia

Drug-induced depression of consciousness during which patients cannot be easily aroused but respond purposefully after repeated or painful stimulation. The ability to maintain ventilatory function independently is impaired. Patients require assistance in maintaining a patent airway, and spontaneous ventilation may be inadequate. Cardiovascular function is usually maintained.

General Anesthesia

Drug-induced loss of consciousness during which patients are not arousable, even by painful stimulation. The ability to maintain ventilatory function independently is impaired, and assistance to maintain a patent airway is required. Positive-pressure ventilation may be required because of depressed spontaneous ventilation or drug-induced depression of neuromuscular function. Cardiovascular function may be impaired.

Data from Joint Commission on Accreditation of Healthcare Organizations: *Comprehensive accreditation manual for hospitals*, Oakbrook Terrace, Ill., 2000, The Joint Commission; and Jacobi J, et al: Clinical practice guidelines for the sustained use of sedatives and analgesics in the critically ill adult, *Crit Care Med* 30(1):119, 2002.

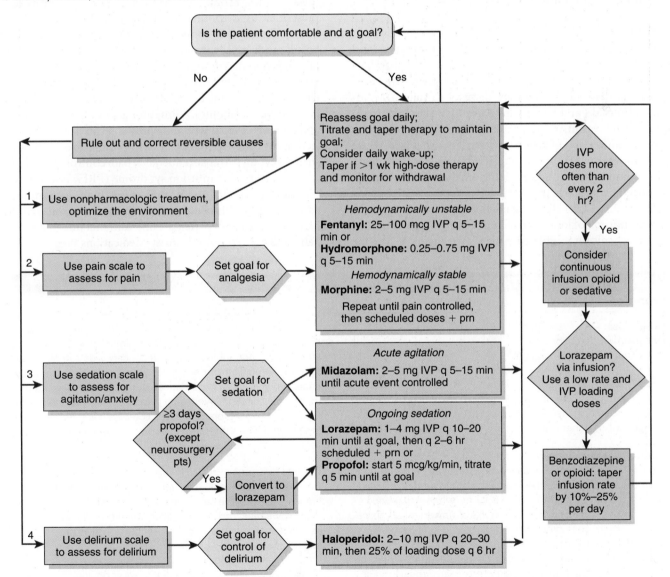

FIGURE 9-1 The algorithm provides guidelines for the use of analgesics and sedatives in mechanically ventilated patients. The text describes clinical and pharmacological issues that dictate optimal drug selection, recommended assessment scales, and precautions for patient monitoring. Doses are approximate for a 70-kg (154-pound) adult. *IVP*, intravenous push; *Q*, every; *PRN*, pro re nata (as needed). (From Jacobi J, et al: Clinical practice guidelines for the sustained use of sedatives and analgesics in the critically ill adult, *Crit Care Med* 30(1):119, 2002.)

Too little sedation is equally hazardous. Most nurses have experienced the challenge of caring for a patient who unexpectedly removes the endotracheal or nasogastric tube. Unplanned extubation in restless, anxious, agitated patients occurs in 8% to 10% of intubated patients after an average of 3.5 days in the critical care unit. Six percent of self-extubation events cause significant complications, including aspiration, dysrhythmias, bronchospasm, and bradycardia.[7]

PHARMACOLOGICAL MANAGEMENT OF SEDATION

Several categories of sedatives are available. If the patient is experiencing pain, analgesia must be administered in addition to any sedative agents. Sedative agents include the benzodiazepines, sedative-hypnotic agents such as propofol, and the central alpha agonists (Table 9-2).[1]

Benzodiazepines

Benzodiazepines have powerful amnesic properties that inhibit reception of new sensory information.[1,7] Benzodiazepines do not confer analgesia. The most frequently used critical care benzodiazepines are diazepam (Valium), midazolam (Versed), and lorazepam (Ativan). Midazolam is recommended for control of acute short-term agitation because its intravenous onset of action is within 3 minutes (see Figure 9-1.) However, when midazolam is administered for longer than 24 hours as a continuous infusion, the sedative effect is prolonged by its active metabolites.[1]

The 2002 SCCM clinical guidelines[1] recommend a continuous infusion of lorazepam if long-term sedation is needed for a mechanically ventilated patient (see Figure 9-1). One advantage of lorazepam is that it does not have active metabolites that contribute to the overall sedative effect. Disadvantages to use of lorazepam include more days on the ventilator and an increased risk of delirium.[8-10]

The major unwanted side effects associated with the benzodiazepines are dose-related respiratory depression and hypotension. If needed, flumazenil (Romazicon) is the antidote used to reverse benzodiazepine overdose in symptomatic patients.[7] Flumazenil should be avoided in patients with benzodiazepine dependence, because rapid withdrawal can induce seizures.[7,11]

Sedative-Hypnotic Agents

Propofol is classified as a sedative-hypnotic. It is also used as an intravenous general anesthetic agent. At high doses, propofol is intended to produce a state of general anesthesia in the operating room.[12] In the critical care unit, propofol is prescribed as a continuous infusion at lower doses (5 to 80 mcg/kg/min)[1] to induce a state of deep sedation in intubated, mechanically ventilated patients.[12] The clinical advantage of propofol is its rapid onset of action (about 30 seconds), very short half-life with initial use (2 to 4 minutes), and rapid elimination from the body (30 to 60 minutes).[12,13] It does not have active metabolites.[13] Propofol is not a reliable amnesic, and patients sedated with only propofol can have vivid recollections of their experiences. It is important to add an opiate, such as fentanyl, to ensure adequate pain control and amnesia.

Propofol related infusion syndrome (PRIS) is a rare complication associated with prolonged high-dose propofol administration.[14] It occurs more commonly in children than in adult critically ill patients. For additional information, see Table 9-2 and Propofol Priority Medications Box.

⬭ PRIORITY MEDICATIONS BOX

Propofol

Drug Class: Sedative-Hypnotic
Drug Action: Sedation
Drug Delivery: Intravenous (IV)

Drug Dosage
Expected doses in critical care range from 5-80 mcg/kg/min IV.[1] Higher doses are used short-term in the operating room as a component of general anesthesia.

Priority Nursing Considerations
Propofol is a powerful sedative and respiratory depressant used for sedation in mechanically ventilated patients in critical care. It is immediately identifiable by its white milky appearance, always in a glass container. Risks of unwanted complications increase when propofol is administered long-term at high doses (>66 mcg/kg/min for longer than 48 hours).[1] Propofol is delivered in a fat-based emulsion, and side effects may be related to disruption of fatty acid metabolism, muscle injury, and release of toxic intracellular contents. Various complications have been collectively grouped under the term Propofol Related Infusion Syndrome (PRIS), including metabolic acidosis, muscular weakness, rhabdomyolysis, myoglobinuria, acute kidney injury, and cardiovascular dysrhythmia. PRIS affects about 1% of all patients who receive propofol; almost one third of those affected will not survive. Other secondary side effects related to the fat-emulsion carrier include hyperlipidemia, hypertriglyceridemia, and acute pancreatitis. Nursing vigilance is required to monitor sedation levels, and also to be alert for the rare but significant risk of propofol-related complications. Serum triglycerides should be measured on all patients who receive propofol for longer than 48 hours.

Clinical Examples
Because propofol is lipid-soluble, it quickly crosses cell membranes, including the cells that comprise the blood-brain barrier. This allows rapid onset of sedation with immediate loss of consciousness. For this reason a protected airway is mandatory. In addition, when used short-term, propofol is rapidly metabolized. When the propofol infusion is stopped, patients can be awakened in minutes for a sedation vacation and spontaneous breathing trial (SBT), or for a neurological status assessment. This feature makes propofol an ideal drug to manage rapid ventilator weaning post-surgery. Propofol is both clinically effective and cost effective because it shortens time to extubation.

TABLE 9-2	PHARMACOLOGICAL MANAGEMENT: SEDATION		
DRUGS	**DOSAGE**	**ACTIONS**	**SPECIAL CONSIDERATIONS**
Benzodiazepines			
Diazepam	0.03-0.1 mg/kg every 0.5-6 hr (slow IV intermittent doses)	Anxiolysis Amnesia Sedation	*Onset:* 2-5 min after IV administration *Side effects:* hypotension, respiratory depression *Half-life of parent compound:* long (20-120 hr); active sedative metabolites also contribute to prolonged sedative effect *Drug tolerance:* physical tolerance develops with prolonged use, and higher dosage is required to achieve the same effect over time; slow wean required from diazepam after continuous prolonged use Phlebitis can occur with peripheral IV administration.
Lorazepam	0.02-0.06 mg/kg every 2-6 hr (slow IV intermittent doses) 0.01-0.1 mg/kg/hr (continuous infusion)	Anxiolysis Amnesia Sedation	*Onset:* 5-20 min after IV administration *Side effects:* hypotension, respiratory depression *Half-life of parent compound:* relatively long (8-15 hr); sedative effect is also prolonged *Drug tolerance:* physical tolerance develops with use, and higher drug dosage is required to achieve the same effect over time; slow wean required from lorazepam after continuous prolonged use Solvent-related acidosis and kidney failure can occur at high doses
Midazolam	0.02-0.08 mg/kg every 0.5-2 hr (slow IV intermittent doses) 0.04-0.2 mg/kg/hr (continuous infusion)	Anxiolysis Amnesia Sedation	*Onset:* 2-5 min after IV administration *Side effects:* hypotension, respiratory depression *Half-life of parent compound:* 3-11 hr; sedative effect is prolonged when midazolam infusion has continued for many days, due to presence of active sedative metabolites; sedative effect is also prolonged in renal failure *Drug tolerance:* physical tolerance develops with prolonged use, and higher drug dosage is required to achieve the same effect over time; slow wean required from midazolam after prolonged use
Sedative-Hypnotics			
Propofol	5-80 mcg/kg/min (continuous infusion)	Anxiolysis Amnesia Sedation	*Onset:* very rapid onset (1-2 min) after IV administration *Side effects:* hypotension, respiratory depression (patient must be intubated and mechanically ventilated to eliminate this complication) *Half-life of parent compound:* 2-8 min when used as a short-term agent *Sedative effect:* range of 26-32 hr with prolonged continuous IV infusion; effective short-term anesthetic agent, useful for rapid "wake-up" of patients for assessment; if continuous infusion is used for many days, emergence from sedation can take hours or days; sedative effect depends on dose administered, depth of sedation, and length of time sedated Change IV infusion tubing every 12 hr Requires a dedicated IV catheter and tubing (do not mix with other drugs) Monitor serum triglyceride levels
Neuroleptic Agents			
Haloperidol	0.03-0.15 mg/kg every 0.5-6 hr (IV intermittent doses) 0.04-0.15 mg/kg/hr (continuous infusion)	Antipsychotic Antidelirium	*Onset:* 3-20 min after IV administration *Half-life of parent compound:* 18-54 hr Used in management of delirium; sedation is an unintended side effect Measure QT interval at baseline and routinely during haloperidol infusion. Active metabolites may cause extrapyramidal symptoms (EPS); anticholinergic agent may be administered if EPS occur

TABLE 9-2	PHARMACOLOGICAL MANAGEMENT: SEDATION—cont'd		
DRUGS	**DOSAGE**	**ACTIONS**	**SPECIAL CONSIDERATIONS**
Central α-Adrenergic Receptor Agonists			
Dexmedetomidine	1 mcg/kg initial loading dose over 10 min	Anxiolysis Analgesia Sedation	*Half-life:* ≈6 mins; clearance from the body in about 2 hrs Duration of infusion is up to 24 hr Intermittent bolus dosing is not recommended
	0.2-0.7 mcg/kg/hr (continuous infusion for ICU sedation), and 0.2 -1.0 mcg/kg/hr for procedural sedation		Maintenance infusion is adjusted within parameters to achieve desired level of sedation *Side effects:* bradycardia and hypotension may occur in presence of volume depletion

Data from: Jacobi J, et al: Clinical practice guidelines for the sustained use of sedatives and analgesics in the critically ill adult, *Crit Care Med* 30(1):119, 2002. http://www.precedex.com/safety-information/. Accessed 2/2/2011.

Central Alpha Agonists

Two central α-adrenergic agonists with sedative properties are available. Dexmedetomidine (Precedex) is an intravenous α$_2$-agonist that is approved for continuous infusion as a short-term sedative (<24 hours) in mechanically ventilated patients. Dexmedetomidine confers sedation and analgesic effects without respiratory depression.[15] This has made it useful in weaning patients from short-term ventilation after cardiac surgery.[16] Dexmedetomidine has also been used for patients on noninvasive mask ventilation.[17]

Dexmedetomidine is prescribed with a loading dose of 1.0 mcg/kg over 10 minutes, followed by a continuous infusion of 0.4 mcg/kg (range 0.2 to 0.7 mcg/kg/hr).[15] Dexmedetomidine has a short half-life (6 minutes) and is eliminated from the body in about 2 hours.[15] Elimination from the body is dramatically slowed if the patient has liver failure. For additional information, see Table 9-2 and Dexmedetomidine Priority Medications Box. Clonidine (Catapres) is an older α$_2$-agonist, that may be administered as a transdermal patch, as adjunctive therapy, for patients with alcohol use disorder; it is not used for sedation.

The choice of sedative is highly specific to the patient and the situation. If the need is for *short-term* sedation (<24 hours), the most frequently used sedatives are midazolam or

PRIORITY MEDICATIONS BOX

Dexmedetomidine

Drug Class: Central alpha-2 agonist
Drug Action: Sedative with anxiolysis and analgesic effect
Drug Delivery: IV

Drug Dosage
Initial IV loading dose of 1 mcg/kg over 10 minutes. The maintenance IV dose range is from 0.2-0.7 mcg/kg/hr[15] (see Table 9-2). Titrate maintenance dose to achieve targeted sedation level. Dosage can be reduced for patients older than 65 years, with liver failure, or kidney failure. This regimen is for sedation in the ICU; other dose ranges may apply in different clinical settings. Note that this medication is administered in mcg/kg/hr and NOT in mcg/kg/min; errors in programming of the infusion pump rate can produce a 60-fold overdose.[15]

After the loading dose and initiation of maintenance infusion, sedative effects may take 10 to 15 minutes to start to work. Frequently critical care patients also receive additional sedative and opiate agents that confer a sedative effect.

Priority Nursing Considerations
Dexmedetomidine is a central alpha-2 agonist; sedation occurs when the drug activates post-synaptic alpha-2 receptors in the central nervous system in the brain. This activation inhibits norepinephrine release and blocks sympathetic nervous system (SNS) fight-or-flight functions, leading to sedation. SNS inhibition also causes hypotension and bradydysrhythmias, both well-known side effects of dexmedetomidine. Analgesic effects occur because dexmedetomidine binds to alpha-2 receptors in the spinal cord. These unique mechanisms of action allow patients to be sedated but still arousable, which is associated with a shorter time to extubation compared with traditional sedative regimens. Many patients will have other sedatives or opiates infusing in addition to dexmedetomidine, and the combination may potentiate the overall sedative effect. Monitoring of sedation level, blood pressure, heart rate, respiratory rate, and pulse oximetry is mandatory.

Clinical Examples
Dexmedetomidine has less respiratory depressant effect than other sedatives. Consequently patients can be extubated while still on a dexmedetomidine infusion. This can be helpful for patients who are anxious during ventilator weaning.

propofol.[1] Both drugs may be combined with a short-acting opioid analgesic (e.g., fentanyl). If the need is for *intermediate-term* sedation (1 to 3 days), the most frequently prescribed drugs again are propofol and midazolam, plus an opiate. If the need is for *long-term* sedation, the recommended agent is lorazepam.[1]

Preventing Sedative Dependence and Withdrawal

The question of which drugs to use for prolonged sedation is complex. Some critically ill patients are mechanically ventilated and seriously ill for weeks or months. Sedation and analgesia are administered to aid the patient in tolerating the ventilator and other procedures. Over time patients become physically and psychologically dependent; when the drug dosage is reduced, they may become physically agitated (Table 9-3).

Physical signs of sedative withdrawal may include agitation with increased heart rate, blood pressure, and respiratory rate. Other notable symptoms are lack of self-awareness, unawareness of surroundings, very short-term memory for information, irritability, anxiety, confusion, delirium, and even seizures.[1] Patients may pull at the tubes, attempt to climb out of bed, and represent a danger to themselves, the nurse, and family visitors.

Sedation Vacation. One innovative strategy to avoid the pitfalls of sedative dependence and withdrawal is a planned strategy to turn off the sedative infusions once each day. This intervention has been given several names, including *drug holiday, sedation vacation,* and *spontaneous awakening*

TABLE 9-3	SIGNS AND SYMPTOMS OF SEDATIVE OR ANALGESIC DRUG WITHDRAWAL*	
SYSTEM	OPIATE WITHDRAWAL	BENZODIAZEPINE WITHDRAWAL†
Neurological	Delirium, tremors, seizures	Agitation, anxiety, delirium, tremors, myoclonus, headache, seizures, fatigue, paresthesia, sleep disturbances
Sensory	Dilation of pupils, teary eyes, irritability, increased sensitivity to pain, sweating, yawning	Increased sensitivity to light/sound, sweating
Musculoskeletal	Cramps, muscle aches	Muscle cramps
Gastrointestinal	Vomiting, diarrhea	Nausea, diarrhea
Respiratory	Tachypnea	Tachypnea

*Data on propofol is limited, but withdrawal symptoms after prolonged use are similar to those of the benzodiazepines.[3]
†Not all symptoms are seen in all patients.[3]

trial. When the patient is hemodynamically stable without contraindications to ventilator weaning, sedation interruption has been shown to shorten time to extubation.[18-20] At a scheduled time, all sedative drugs are stopped. Sometimes analgesic drugs are also stopped, depending on the hospital's protocol. The patient is allowed to regain consciousness for clinical assessment using a standardized instrument such as the RASS (see Table 9-1).[18-20] The patient is carefully monitored, and when awareness is attained, an assessment of level of consciousness and neurological function is performed. If the patient becomes agitated, it is essential that a protocol be in place for the nurse to restart the sedatives, plus opiates if applicable. One protocol scheduled the daily interruption of sedatives in the morning and recommended, after a full assessment, restarting the sedative and opiate infusions at 50% of the previous morning dose and adjusting upward until the patient was comfortable.[19]

An important nursing responsibility is ongoing assessment of patients' level of consciousness to avert complications during sedative or analgesic drug withdrawal (Table 9-3). If the patient is seriously agitated, it is vital to consult with the physician and pharmacist to establish an effective treatment plan that will allow safe weaning from sedative drugs (see Table 9-1).

DELIRIUM

Delirium represents a global impairment of cognitive processes, usually of sudden onset, coupled with disorientation, impaired short-term memory, altered sensory perceptions (i.e., hallucinations), abnormal thought processes, and inappropriate behavior. Delirium is more prevalent than generally recognized; it is difficult to diagnose in the critically ill patient and represents acute brain dysfunction caused by sepsis, critical illness, or dysfunction of other vital organs (Box 9-2). The incidence of delirium ranges from 60% to 85% among mechanically ventilated patients.[21] Delirium increases hospital stay and mortality rates for patients who are mechanically ventilated.[22] The increased mortality remains even after controlling for associated variables such as coma and administration of sedatives and analgesics.[22]

When patients are agitated, restless, and pulling at tubes and lines, they are often identified as being delirious. In this scenario, delirium may be described as "ICU psychosis" or "sundowner syndrome." However, the delirious patient is not always agitated, and it is much more difficult to detect delirium when the patient is physically calm.[1,23] Provision of adequate analgesia is an essential component of delirium prevention.[1]

Specific scoring instruments are available to assess delirium, and two have been validated for use with mechanically ventilated critical care patients.[24] They are the Confusion Assessment Method for the Intensive Care Unit (CAM-ICU) (Figure 9-2),[25-27] and the Intensive Care Delirium Screening Checklist (ICDSC).[28,29] Both instruments are used in tandem with the RASS to exclude patients in coma, and identify

BOX 9-2   CAUSES OF DELIRIUM IN CRITICALLY ILL PATIENTS

Metabolic Causes
- Acid-base disturbance
- Electrolyte imbalance
- Hypoglycemia

Intracranial Causes
- Epidural or subdural hematoma
- Intracranial hemorrhage
- Meningitis
- Encephalitis
- Cerebral abscess
- Tumor

Endocrine Causes
- Hyperthyroidism or hypothyroidism
- Addison's disease
- Hyperparathyroidism
- Cushing's syndrome

Organ Failure
- Liver encephalopathy
- Uremic encephalopathy
- Septic shock

Respiratory Causes
- Hypoxemia
- Hypercarbia

Drug-Related Causes
- Alcohol withdrawal syndrome
- Benzodiazepines
- Heavy metal poisoning

Modified from Szokol JW, Vender JS: Anxiety, delirium, and pain in the intensive care unit, *Crit Care Clin* 17(4):821-842, 2001.

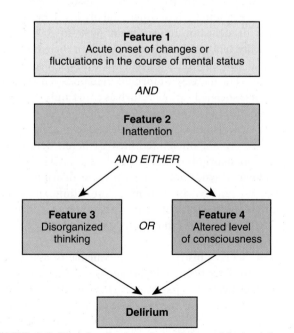

FIGURE 9-2 The Confusion Assessment Method for the ICU (CAM-ICU).

hyperactive delirium (see Table 9-1). Both instruments provide a structured format to evaluate delirium for verbal patients and for nonverbal and mechanically ventilated patients.

PHARMACOLOGICAL MANAGEMENT OF AGITATION AND DELIRIUM

Selecting medications that provide sedation but avoid withdrawal-associated agitation is a priority. The neuroleptic drug haloperidol (Haldol) is administered to treat hyperactive delirium.[30] This antipsychotic agent stabilizes cerebral function by blocking dopamine-mediated neurotransmission at the cerebral synapses and in the basal ganglia. Electrocardiographic (ECG) monitoring is recommended, because haloperidol prolongs the QTc-interval, increasing the risk of ventricular dysrhythmias.

NONPHARMACOLOGICAL INTERVENTIONS TO PREVENT DELIRIUM

Hyperactive delirium is frequently associated with critical illness.[1] The nonpharmacological strategies used to prevent agitation and delirium are similar to those used as adjuncts to minimize pain.[1] These methods include back massage, music therapy, noise reduction, decreasing lights at night to promote sleep, clustering nursing care interventions to provide some uninterrupted rest, and speaking in a calm and gentle voice. Some preexisting conditions increase the likelihood that a patient will experience delirium, including dementia, alcohol use disorder, and prior sedative/opiate dependence.

ALCOHOL WITHDRAWAL SYNDROME AND DELIRIUM TREMENS

Critically ill patients who are alcohol-dependent, and were drinking prior to hospital admission, are at risk of alcohol withdrawal syndrome (AWS).[31] AWS is associated with an increased risk of delirium, hallucinations, seizures, increased need for mechanical ventilation, and death. When hyperactive agitated delirium is caused by alcohol withdrawal, it is termed delirium tremens, often called DTs.[31] Following hospital admission, as the alcohol-dependent patient's blood-alcohol concentration (BAC) falls, about 50% of patients will have AWS-related symptoms.[32] Fewer than 5% will experience severe complications such as delirium tremens or a seizure.[31,32] Screening tools to identify alcohol dependence, such as the Alcohol Use Disorders Identification Test (AUDIT) shown in Table 25-1 in the Trauma chapter (25), are very helpful. Management of alcohol withdrawal involves close monitoring of AWS-related agitation and administration of IV benzodiazepines, generally diazepam (Valium) or lorazepam (Ativan). Diazepam has the advantage of a longer half-life and high lipid solubility.[31] Lipid-soluble medications quickly cross the blood-brain barrier and enter the central nervous system to rapidly produce a sedative effect.[31,33]

Benzodiazepines should be administered in response to increased signs of agitation associated with DTs, with dosage guided by a clinical protocol. This is described as an AWS symptom-triggered approach.[31] The severity of alcohol withdrawal can be assessed with a scale such as the Clinical Institute Withdrawal Assessment of Alcohol Scale (revised) (CIWA-Ar).[31,33] Multivitamins, including thiamine (vitamin B_1), are administered prophylactically to prevent additional neurological sequelae.[31-34] Delirium related to alcohol withdrawal is pharmacologically managed very differently from delirium from other causes. Long-acting benzodiazepines are the drugs of choice in AWS.[31] In contrast, benzodiazepines are contraindicated for treatment of delirium from non-alcohol-related causes.[35]

COLLABORATIVE MANAGEMENT

Collaborative management of anxiety, agitation, sedation, and delirium is a responsibility shared by all members of the health care team, as seen in the Evidence-Based Collaborative Practice box on Sedation in the Critically Ill). Recognition of the problem is the first step toward a solution to establish a more effective standard of patient care in sedation, analgesia, and delirium management.

EVIDENCE-BASED COLLABORATIVE PRACTICE
Sedation in the Critically Ill

The key recommendations from the clinical practice guideline for the sustained use of sedatives and analgesia in the critically ill adult, based on research and expert panel opinion, are as follows.

Assessment, Communication, and Documentation
1. Frequent assessment of critically ill patients is mandated to determine whether sedation and analgesia are required and appropriate as part of the plan of care.
2. A sedation goal or end-point should be established for each patient at the beginning of therapy; for example, "a calm patient that can be easily aroused with maintenance of the normal sleep-wake cycle." Some patients may require deep sedation to facilitate synchrony with mechanical ventilation.
3. Need for sedation should be re-evaluated on a frequent basis as the clinical condition of the patient changes.
4. Sedation regimens should be written with the flexibility to allow titration to the desired end-point, anticipating fluctuations in sedation requirements throughout the day.
5. Use of a validated sedation assessment scale to standardize assessment among clinicians and document the patient's level of sedation and response to sedatives is recommended. Vital signs such as blood pressure or heart rate are not sufficiently specific or sensitive to serve as indicators of sedation effectiveness.
6. Sedation and analgesia goals must be communicated to all caregivers and to the patient and family.
7. Because of insufficient research, use of sedation monitors that interpret EEG data is not endorsed for monitoring of critical care patients.

Agitation
8. Sedation of agitated critically ill patients should be started only after adequate analgesia and treatment for reversible physiological causes of agitation have been provided.
9. Cautious use of sedatives is warranted for patients who are not yet intubated, because of the risk of respiratory depression.

Drug Therapy
10. Midazolam or diazepam should be used for rapid sedation of acutely agitated patients.
11. Propofol is the preferred sedative when rapid awakening for neurological assessment or extubation is important.
12. Midazolam is recommended for short-term use only, because it provokes unpredictable awakening and time to extubation when infusions continue longer than 48 to 72 hours.
13. Lorazepam is the recommended sedative when prolonged mechanical ventilation is required and is given by intermittent intravenous administration or continuous infusion.

Avoidance of Complications
14. Titration of the sedative dose to a defined end-point is recommended, with systematic tapering of the dose or daily interruption with re-titration to minimize prolonged sedative effects.
15. Triglyceride concentrations should be monitored after 2 days of propofol infusion, and the total caloric intake from lipids should be included in the nutrition support prescription.
16. The potential for opioid, benzodiazepine, and propofol withdrawal should be considered after high doses of more than approximately 7 days of continuous therapy. Doses should be tapered systematically to prevent withdrawal symptoms.

Delirium
17. Routine assessment for the presence of delirium is recommended. The CAM-ICU is a promising assessment tool for delirium assessment.
18. Haloperidol is the preferred agent for the treatment of delirium in critically ill patients.
19. ECG monitoring for detection of potential QT interval prolongation and dysrhythmias is recommended when haloperidol is administered.

Sleep
20. Sleep promotion should include optimization of the environment and nonpharmacological methods to promote relaxation with adjunctive use of hypnotics.

CAM-ICU, Confusion Assessment Method-ICU instrument; ECG, electrocardiogram; EEG, electroencephalogram.
Data from Jacobi J, et al: Clinical practice guidelines for the sustained use of sedatives and analgesics in the critically ill adult, *Crit Care Med* 30(1):119, 2002.

CASE STUDY   PATIENT WITH DELIRIUM

Answers to the Case Study Questions can be found on the Evolve web site at http://evolve.elsevier.com/Urden/priorities/.

Brief Patient History

Mr. K is a 42-year-old, Asian, out-of-town businessman in your city. He is transported to your facility from his hotel because of a witnessed grand mal seizure. Paramedics administered lorazepam in the field. Mr. K's wife reports by phone that he is in good health and that she is not aware that he takes any medications regularly. However, she states that he recently quit drinking alcohol because of pressure from the family. She also comments that she thinks he takes alprazolam to calm his nerves once in a while.

Clinical Assessment

Mr. K is admitted to the intensive care unit from the emergency department with hypertension, restlessness, mental confusion, paranoid ideations with rambling speech, and visual and auditory hallucinations. Mr. K's skin is warm and moist. Intravenous administration of thiamine, folic acid, multivitamins, and magnesium was begun in the emergency department. Physician orders were written for lorazepam every 6 hours and clonidine every 4 hours as needed for delirium-related symptoms.

Diagnostic Procedures

Mr. K's baseline vital signs are as follows: blood pressure of 190/92 mm Hg, heart rate of 130 beats/min (sinus tachycardia), respiratory rate of 26 breaths/min, and temperature of 98.8° F.

Pulse oximetry O_2 saturation is 90% on 4 L/min oxygen using a nasal cannula. Confusion Assessment Method indicates presence of acute and fluctuating change in mental status, inattention, and disorganized thinking. The Riker Sedation-Agitation Scale score is 5. Serum and urine toxicology studies are negative for ethyl alcohol, cannabis, and opioids; urine is strongly positive for benzodiazepines. The sodium level is 135 mmol/L, potassium level is 4.3 mmol/L, chloride level is 84 mmol/L, carbon dioxide level is 26 mEq/L, calcium level is 8 mg/dL; magnesium level is 2.0 mg/dL, and γ-glutamyl transpeptidase (GGT) level is 80 IU/L.

Medical Diagnosis

Mr. K is diagnosed with delirium tremens caused by alcohol and benzodiazepine withdrawal.

Questions

1. What major outcomes do you expect to achieve for this patient?
2. What problems or risks must be managed to achieve these outcomes?
3. What interventions must be initiated to monitor, prevent, manage, or eliminate the problems and risks identified?
4. What interventions should be initiated to promote optimal functioning, safety, and well-being of the patient?
5. What possible learning needs do you anticipate for this patient?
6. What cultural and age-related factors may have a bearing on the patient's plan of care?

REFERENCES

1. Jacobi J, et al: Clinical practice guidelines for the sustained use of sedatives and analgesics in the critically ill adult, *Crit Care Med* 30(1):119, 2002.
2. Ramsay MA, et al: Controlled sedation with alphaxalone-alphadolone, *Br Med J* 2(5920):656, 1974.
3. Riker RR, et al: Prospective evaluation of the Sedation-Agitation Scale for adult critically ill patients, *Crit Care Med* 27(7):1325, 1999.
4. Devlin JW, et al: Motor Activity Assessment Scale: a valid and reliable sedation scale for use with mechanically ventilated patients in an adult surgical intensive care unit, *Crit Care Med* 27(7):1271, 1999.
5. Ely EW, et al: Monitoring sedation status over time in ICU patients: reliability and validity of the Richmond Agitation-Sedation Scale (RASS), *JAMA* 289(22):2983, 2003.
6. Sessler CN, et al: The Richmond Agitation-Sedation Scale: validity and reliability in adult intensive care unit patients, *Am J Respir Crit Care Med* 166(10):1338, 2002.
7. Young CC, Prielipp RC: Benzodiazepines in the intensive care unit, *Crit Care Clin* 17(4):843, 2001.
8. Fong JJ, et al: Propofol associated with a shorter duration of mechanical ventilation than scheduled intermittent lorazepam: a database analysis using Project IMPACT, *Ann Pharmacother* 41(12):1986, 2007.
9. Pandharipande P, et al: Lorazepam is an independent risk factor for transitioning to delirium in intensive care unit patients, *Anesthesiology* 104(1):21, 2006.
10. Pandharipande P, et al: Effect of sedation with dexmedetomidine vs lorazepam on acute brain dysfunction in mechanically ventilated patients: the MENDS randomized controlled trial, *JAMA* 298(22):2644, 2007.
11. Betten DP, et al: Antidote use in the critically ill poisoned patient, *J Intensive Care Med* 21(5):255, 2006.
12. Whitcomb JJ, et al: The use of propofol in the mechanically ventilated medical/surgical intensive care patient: is it the right choice? *Dimens Crit Care Nurs* 22(2):60, 2003.
13. Zaccheo MM, Bucher DH: Propofol infusion syndrome: a rare complication with potentially fatal results, *Crit Care Nurse* 28(3):18, 2008.
14. Corbett SM, et al: Propofol-related infusion syndrome in intensive care patients, *Pharmacotherapy* 28(2):250, 2008.
15. Lam SW, Alexander E: Dexmedetomidine use in critical care, *AACN Adv Crit Care* 19(2):113, 2008.
16. Dasta JF, et al: Addition of dexmedetomidine to standard sedation regimens after cardiac surgery: an outcomes analysis, *Pharmacotherapy* 26(6):798, 2006.
17. Akada S, et al: The efficacy of dexmedetomidine in patients with noninvasive ventilation: a preliminary study, *Anesth Analg* 107(1):167, 2008.

18. Kress JP, et al: The long-term psychological effects of daily sedative interruption on critically ill patients, *Am J Respir Crit Care Med* 168(12):1457, 2005.

19. Kress JP, et al: Daily interruption of sedative infusions in critically ill patients undergoing mechanical ventilation, *N Engl J Med* 342(20):1471, 2000.

20. Girard TD, et al: Efficacy and safety of a paired sedation and ventilator weaning protocol for mechanically ventilated patients in intensive care (Awakening and Breathing Controlled trial): a randomised controlled trial, *Lancet* 371(9607):126, 2008.

21. Pun BT, Ely EW: The importance of diagnosing and managing ICU delirium, *Chest* 132(2):624, 2007.

22. Ely EW, et al: Delirium as a predictor of mortality in mechanically ventilated patients in the intensive care unit, *JAMA* 291(14):1753, 2004.

23. Roberts BL, et al: Patients' dreams in ICU: recall at two years post discharge and comparison to delirium status during ICU admission. A multicentre cohort study, *Intensive Crit Care Nurs* 22(5):264, 2006.

24. Plaschke K, et al: Comparison of the confusion assessment method for the intensive care unit (CAM-ICU) with the Intensive Care Delirium Screening Checklist (ICDSC) for delirium in critical care patients gives high agreement rate(s), *Intensive Care Med* 34(3):431, 2008.

25. Ely EW, et al: Evaluation of delirium in critically ill patients: validation of the Confusion Assessment Method for the Intensive Care Unit (CAM-ICU), *Crit Care Med* 29(7):1370, 2001.

26. Ely EW, et al: Delirium in mechanically ventilated patients: validity and reliability of the confusion assessment method for the intensive care unit (CAM-ICU), *JAMA* 286(21):2703, 2001.

27. Pun BT, et al: Large-scale implementation of sedation and delirium monitoring in the intensive care unit: a report from two medical centers, *Crit Care Med* 33(6):1199, 2005.

28. Bergeron N, et al: Intensive Care Delirium Screening Checklist: evaluation of a new screening tool, *Intensive Care Med* 27(5):859, 2001.

29. Ouimet S, et al: Subsyndromal delirium in the ICU: evidence for a disease spectrum, *Intensive Care Med* 33(6): 1007, 2007.

30. Milbrandt EB, et al: Haloperidol use is associated with lower hospital mortality in mechanically ventilated patients, *Crit Care Med* 33(1):226, 2005.

31. Sarff M, Gold JA: Alcohol withdrawal syndromes in the intensive care unit, *Crit Care Med* 38(Suppl 9), S494, 2010.

32. Schuckit MA: Alcohol-use disorders, *Lancet* 373(9662):492, 2009.

33. Amato L, et al: Benzodiazepines for alcohol withdrawal, *Cochrane Database Syst Rev* 3:CD005063, 2010.

34. Repper-DeLisi J, et al: Successful implementation of an alcohol-withdrawal pathway in a general hospital, *Psychosomatics* 49(4):292, 2008.

35. Lonergan E, et al: Benzodiazepines for delirium, *Cochrane Database Syst Rev* 4:CD006379, 2009.

CHAPTER 10

End-of-Life Care

Marian Grant

evolve WEBSITE

Be sure to check out the bonus material, including free self-assessment exercises, on the Evolve web site at
http://evolve.elsevier.com/Urden/priorities/.

OBJECTIVES

- Describe the impact of advance directives and advance care planning on provision of end-of-life care in critical care.
- Discuss the concepts of patient- and family-centered communication and decision making.
- Explain the need for symptom assessment and management during end-of-life care in the critical care unit, especially related to withdrawal of life support.
- Discuss professional issues and end-of-life care in critical care units.

The aging of the population and increasing acuity of hospital patients has made end of life an important clinical topic in critical care, although requisite improvements in end-of-life care have been slow to follow. Because the primary purpose of admission of patients to a critical care unit is, typically, to provide life-saving care, the death of a patient may be perceived as a failure. The critical care culture emphasizes saving lives, and the language that describes the end of life often employs negative terms, such as forgoing life-sustaining treatments, do not resuscitate (DNR), and withdrawal of life support.

Lately, more attention is being given to the quality of the end-of-life experience of the critically ill, with recognition of the increasing numbers of patients who die in critical care units. This chapter focuses on the evidence available for the care nurses render to dying critical care patients, and their families.

END-OF-LIFE EXPERIENCE IN CRITICAL CARE

Attention to the end of life of hospitalized patients began with the publication of the landmark Study to Understand Prognoses and Preferences for Outcomes and Risks of Treatments (SUPPORT).[1] In this major report, more than 9000 seriously ill patients in five medical centers were studied. Despite an intervention to improve communication, shortcomings were found, aggressive treatment was common, and only one half of physicians knew their patients' preferences

to avoid cardiopulmonary resuscitation (CPR).[1] More than one third of patients who died spent at least 10 days in a critical care unit, and for 50% of conscious patients, family members reported moderate to severe pain at least one half of the time.[1]

Following closely after the publication of the SUPPORT study, the Institute of Medicine (IOM) released a report, *Approaching Death: Improving Care at the End of Life*, which detailed deficiencies in care and gave seven recommendations to improve care:[2]

1. Patients with fatal illnesses and their family should receive reliable, skillful, and supportive care.
2. Health professionals should improve care for the dying.
3. Policymakers and consumers should work with health professionals to improve quality and financing of care.
4. Health profession education should include end-of-life content.
5. Palliative care should be developed, possibly as a medical specialty.
6. Research on end of life should be funded.
7. The public should communicate more about the experience of dying and options available.

In SUPPORT and the IOM report, critical care patients were not distinguished from other hospitalized patients, preventing distinctions between types of units. To describe the number of deaths in critical care units, hospital discharge records from six states and the National Death Index were reviewed.[3] Of the more than 500,000 deaths studied, 38.3%

were in hospitals, and 22% (59% of all hospital deaths) occurred after admission to the critical care unit. Terminal admissions associated with critical care accounted for 80% of all terminal hospitalization costs.[3] The likelihood of dying in the hospital increased with age, with the likelihood of dying after critical care unit admission at 25% of all deaths for each age category. Although 90% of people would prefer to die in their own homes,[2] more than 20% of those who died received high-tech, aggressive care in an intensive care unit (ICU) before death.[3]

PLANNING FOR THE END OF LIFE

Advance Directives

The Patient Self-Determination Act supports the patient's right to control future treatment in the event the individual cannot speak for himself or herself. Advance directives, typically comprised of a living will and a health care power of attorney, are intended to ensure that patients receive the care they desire at end of life, but their actual contribution has been less than desired. Like other preventive measures, advance directives are underused, even though they are inexpensive and potentially effective. Most patients have expressed a desire to avoid "general life support" if dying or permanently unconscious, but few have confirmed preferences regarding specific life-sustaining treatments.[4]

Advance Care Planning

Cultural influences in the United States discourage discussion of death. Planning for decisions to be made at a later date when one is deemed incompetent is difficult, but knowledge about patient preferences helps family members make difficult treatment choices. In this case, the term *family* means whomever the patient states is the family.

Advance care planning for those with chronic illness is advantageous for all involved.[5] When surrogate decision makers know the patient's wishes for end-of-life care, they can be more congruent and knowledgeable about those wishes in future decision making. If these wishes have not been put in writing by the patient as an advance directive, they may at least have been discussed with the surrogate decision maker. Families and care providers should be informed if patients decline aggressive care, so they will not be left with difficult decisions in emergency situations. Critical care nurses can help facilitate such discussions.

Ethical and Legal Issues in Advance Care Planning

Legal and ethical principles guide many of our decisions in caring for the dying patient and the family. The patient is respected as autonomous and able to make his or her own decisions. When the patient is unable to make decisions, as is often the case in critical care, the same respect should be accorded to the patient's surrogate decision makers.

Withholding and withdrawing care are considered to be morally and legally equivalent.[6] However, because families experience more stress in withdrawing treatments than in

withholding them,[7] treatments should not be started that the patient would not want, or that offer no benefit.

The goal of withdrawal of life-sustaining treatments is to remove treatments that are not beneficial and may be uncomfortable. Any treatment in this circumstance may be withheld or withdrawn. Treatments that cause discomfort should not be continued. When disagreements arise, ethics consultations can help to resolve conflicts regarding inappropriately prolonged, nonbeneficial, or unwanted treatments.[8]

Forgoing life-sustaining treatments is not the same as active euthanasia or assisted suicide. Allowing a person to die by withholding or withdrawing life-sustaining treatment fosters a more natural death after an incurable illness or trauma.[9]

Critical Care Issues in Advance Planning

Cardiopulmonary Resuscitation. CPR is a key issue when discussing advance care planning with patients and families. The benefits of resuscitation may be overestimated for survival and for the more relevant outcome of returning to baseline functional status. In a meta-analysis of 51 studies, the rate of overall survival to discharge after in-hospital CPR was 13.4%.[10] Poorer outcomes occurred among those patients with sepsis the day before resuscitation, metastatic cancer, dementia, coronary artery disease, and for those resuscitated in the ICU. A Norwegian study reported that only 17% of patients older than 75 years survived resuscitation to return home.[11]

As important as survival is the functional status outcome following resuscitation.[12] Functional status among almost half of the survivors of in-hospital CPR had deteriorated compared with their condition 2 months before the event.[12] Six months after resuscitation, 30% of those patients had died, and two thirds continued to lose function.[12] Despite these dismal statistics, CPR is often offered as an option without fully informing patients or families of the low possibility of surviving CPR, or the potential for decline in functional status.

One evolving aspect of CPR is the presence of family members in the room during resuscitation. The American Association of Critical-Care Nurses (AACN)[13] and the Emergency Nurses Association (ENA)[14] have issued position statements recommending that families be present during CPR and invasive procedures. Family presence is a significant source of support for the patient, and may benefit the family. Observing the resuscitation can aid in the grieving process, especially when resuscitation is not successful. The family will know that everything was done that could have been done.

Misunderstandings Around Do-Not-Resuscitate Orders. Even as a patient's condition deteriorates, there is often reluctance to consider a DNR order.[15] A DNR order is intended to prevent the initiation of life-sustaining measures such as endotracheal intubation or CPR. However, some providers equate DNR with "do not treat." Sadly, this means that patients with a DNR order sometimes receive less care[16] and some treatments are withheld.[17] Families should be assured that patients will continue to receive nursing and medical care, including pain and symptom management, but that aggressive measures to extend life will not be employed. DNR orders should be written before withdrawal of life support is initiated; this documentation ensures that the patient is not subjected to unwanted interventions during the period between initiation of withdrawal and death.

Prognostication and Uncertainty. It is often challenging to identify which patients will survive an ICU stay and which will not. This is because prognostication on an individual basis can be very difficult. Evidence shows that physicians' ability to prognosticate the length of time before death is limited[18,19] and that the time to death usually is overestimated. Patients' treatment wishes usually are not known, may be vague,[20] or change over the course of an illness.[21] Because of uncertainty, and because a few patients who were thought not likely to survive actually return to visit a critical care unit, professionals are often not confident about issues of survivability. This, combined with the fact that many families cling to small hopes of survival and recovery, results in generally overly optimistic prognoses.

DECISION MAKING AND COMMUNICATION

Patients and families prefer to share decision making with health professionals in cases of life and death. However, shared decision making about end-of-life treatment choices in physician-family conferences are often incomplete.[22] Higher levels of shared decision making are associated with greater family satisfaction. Families go through a process in their decision making in which they consider the personal domain (rallying support and evaluating quality of life), the ICU environment domain (chasing the doctors and relating to the health care team), and the decision domain (arriving at a new belief and making and communicating the decision).[23] Improving ICU communication when patients are dying reduces lengths of stay and resource use.[24] This is because improved communication identifies those patients for whom critical care is either not desired, given patient or family goals of care, or medically inappropriate given the patient's prognosis.

Critical Care Recommendations to Improve Family Interactions

A consensus statement from the Society of Critical Care Medicine (SCCM) recommends focusing on and supporting the families of ICU patients.[25] Forty-three recommendations are presented, including an endorsement of a shared decision-making model; family care conferencing; culturally appropriate requests for truth-telling and informed refusal; spiritual support; staff education and debriefing; family presence at rounds and resuscitation; open and flexible visitation; family-friendly signage; and family support before, during, and after a death. One use of this guideline is to assess the level of family support for each ICU so that the most deficient areas could be addressed with quality-improvement actions. The categories used in this guideline are for general support of ICU families, as seen in the Evidence-Based Collaborative

Practice: End-of-Life Care box. The needs of a family with a dying patient include decision-making support; spiritual and cultural support; emotional and practical support, including visitation and family preparation for death; and continuity of care.[26]

EVIDENCE-BASED COLLABORATIVE PRACTICE

End-of-Life Care

The key topics of the guidelines for end-of-life care in the intensive care unit, based on research and expert panel review, are categorized.

Patient- and Family-Centered Care and Decision Making: The Comprehensive Ideal for End-of-Life Care
- Use the legal standards for decision making
- Resolve conflict
- Communicate with families

Ethical Principles Related to Withdrawal of Life-Sustaining Treatment
- Withholding versus withdrawing
- Killing versus allowing to die
- Intended versus merely foreseen consequences

Practical Aspects of Withdrawing Life-Sustaining Treatments in the Intensive Care Unit
- The procedure
- Specific issues
- Use of paralytics

Symptom Management in End-of-Life Care
- Pain and dyspnea
- Delirium
- Medications used

Considerations at the Time of Death
- Notification of death
- Brain death
- Organ donation
- Bereavement and support
- Needs of the interdisciplinary team

Research, Quality Improvement, and Education
- Develop interventions likely to improve the quality of care
- Develop education programs

Data from Truog RD, et al: Recommendations for end-of-life care in the intensive care unit: a consensus statement by the American College of Critical Care Medicine, *Crit Care Med* 36(3):953, 2008.

Cultural and Religious Influences

Cultural and religious influences on attitudes and beliefs about death and dying differ dramatically. A cultural and religious assessment is warranted in all situations, because cultural or religious affiliation does not imply that patients or families follow all of the tenets of that group. The cultures of the predominant religions commonly seen in the surrounding community should be familiar to the local health care team. These differences may affect how the health care team is viewed, how decisions are made, whether aggressive treatment is preferred, how death is met, and how grieving will occur.[27] Satisfaction with ICU care has been associated with the extent to which the family is satisfied with their spiritual care, especially when the patient is near death.[28] Use of hospital chaplains or other spiritual resources is highly encouraged. Staff members' own attitudes about the specific practices of a culture should be carefully assessed[29] and tempered with respect and humility. Interpreters are necessary when the patient or the family members do not speak English. In order to ensure accurate translation of any important information, family members should not be used as interpreters.

Discussing Prognosis

Discussions about the potential for impending death are never held early enough. Often, the first discussions with the patient or family occur in conjunction with the topic of discontinuation of life support. This is frequently some time after the health care team has concluded the prognosis is poor and there is a need to stop life support. That gap in time is often why the family lags the team in understanding and accepting what is happening medically. The late timing of the first discussion is also an issue for those families who may come to terms with withdrawal before physicians.[30] It is important to give families time to adjust to this information, and make preparations by early and regular discussions about prognosis, goals of therapy, and the patient's wishes.[31]

Conflict and Staff Distress

Nurses and doctors frequently disagree about the futility of interventions. Sometimes, nurses consider withdrawal before physicians and patients do, and they then feel the care they are giving is unnecessary and possibly harmful. Nurses in one study were found to be more pessimistic, yet more often correct than physicians about the prognoses of dying patients. However, the nurses also proposed treatment withdrawal for some very sick patients who survived.[32] This issue is a serious one for critical care nurses, because concerns over providing futile care can led to emotional and ethical distress and, ultimately, to burnout.[33]

COMFORT CARE AND SYMPTOM MANAGEMENT

Many patients die an undignified death with uncontrolled symptoms. This is particularly likely in critical care, where the shift from the traditional intensive rescue approach to one of comfort care of the dying is difficult and dramatic.[34]

Steps Toward Comfort Care

Comfort care is a broad term with different meanings depending on the patient and the ICU. Typically, it refers to removing any treatments that are no longer providing a medical benefit and/or may be causing discomfort to the patient. It is important to educate families as to the physiological reasons for

discontinuing treatments, so that they understand that the benefits of such treatments are usually outweighed by the discomfort they can cause dying patients. In addition, comfort care recognizes that certain symptoms, like pain or agitation, which were perhaps lower priorities while seeking aggressive curative treatment, may now instead be the most important issues to be addressed.

Withdrawal of specific treatments can also have effects necessitating symptom management. If a series of interventions is to be withdrawn, there tends to be a typical sequence of withdrawal. First, dialysis usually is discontinued along with diagnostic tests and vasopressors. This can cause fluid issues and dyspnea and may necessitate the use of opioids or diuretics. Next, intravenous fluids, monitoring, laboratory tests, and antibiotics are typically stopped.[34] This results in a more natural death, but with accompanying symptoms from dehydration or infection that must be managed. Efforts to discontinue artificial feeding may be met with concern from the family, because offering food has great social significance. However, fluids or food are usually physically burdensome to the dying patient and should only be continued if the patient wants or can tolerate them.

Palliative Care

Patients in the last stages of their illness require aggressive symptom management. The most relevant clinical goal is to manage or *palliate* these unpleasant situations by assessing and implementing appropriate interventions.[9] Palliative care guidelines may provide guidance when the usual first-line treatments do not promote comfort for critically ill patients.[35] Palliative care is a medical and nursing specialty that focuses on quality of life for patients and families dealing with serious illness. More and more hospitals have palliative care consultant teams to help provide such care. Unfortunately, palliative care has been thought of as desirable only when the patient nears death or when several interventions have been unsuccessful for symptom management. However, palliative care guidelines[35] and the IOM report *Improving Palliative Care for Cancer*[36] confirm that palliative care ideally begins at the time of diagnosis of a life-threatening illness and continues through cure or until death and into the family's bereavement period.

Hospice

Hospice is the form of palliative care that focuses on patients with a prognosis of six or fewer months. It is a Medicare-provided service that usually requires patients to forgo life-prolonging treatment. Patients and families often consider this method of care only in the last days or weeks of end-stage illness and may view hospice care as "giving up." Health professionals can assist patients and families by providing information about the hospice benefit and stressing the support it provides. The focus on quality of life can be helpful to patients and families. Palliative care teams often provide "hospice" care in the hospital, which can include symptom management, and social, spiritual, and bereavement support for families.

Pain Management

Because many critical care patients are not conscious, assessment of pain and other symptoms is difficult. Nonverbal pain assessment scales[37] that use facial expressions, body movements, and ventilator dyssynchrony are described in Chapter 8. The World Health Organization advocates a three-step approach to pain management starting with nonopioid medications for mild pain and moving up to opioids for severe pain. In critical care units, opioids are frequently used because of the pain intensity.[38]

Opioids can cause respiratory depression and hypotension, but usually not when they are titrated carefully. They are particularly beneficial for the ventilated patient because in addition to helping treat dyspnea, they provide sedation, anxiolysis, and analgesia. Morphine is often the drug of choice, although hydromorphone and fentanyl are also used, and there is no upper limit in dosing.[9] The SCCM guideline[39] for the sustained use of sedatives and analgesia in critical care is an additional resource described in Chapter 9.

Non-Pain Symptom Management

The following symptoms often occur in the dying patient:[9] dyspnea, nausea and vomiting, fever and infection, edema and pulmonary edema, anxiety, delirium, metabolic derangements, skin integrity, anemia, and hemorrhage.[9]

Dyspnea

Patients who are near death are frequently unable to self-report dyspnea.[40] Dyspnea is best managed with close evaluation of the patient and the use of opioids, diuretics, sedatives, and nonpharmacological interventions (oxygen, positioning, and increased ambient air flow). Opioids can reduce muscle tension and increase pulmonary vasodilatation. Benzodiazepines may be used in patients for whom anxiety is a key contributor to respiratory discomfort. Benzodiazepines and opioids should be titrated to effect. Treatment efforts are aimed at the patient's expression of dyspnea rather than at respiratory rates or oxygen levels.[41]

Nausea and Vomiting

Nausea and vomiting are common and are treated with antiemetics. The cause of nausea and vomiting may be intestinal obstruction. However, treatment for decompression such as nasogastric tubes may be uncomfortable in dying patients, and their use should be weighed using a benefit-to-burden perspective.

Fever and Infection

Fever and infection necessitate assessment of the benefits of continuing antibiotics so as not to prolong the dying process.[9] Management of the fever with antipyretics may be appropriate for the patient's comfort, but other methods such as cooling baths, ice, or hypothermia blankets should be balanced against the amount of discomfort the patient may experience.

Edema

Edema can cause discomfort, and diuretics may be effective if kidney function is intact. Dialysis is not warranted at the end of life. The use of fluids may contribute to edema when kidney function is impaired and bodily functions are slowing. In a Database of Abstracts of Reviews of Effects (DARE) report,[42] little relationship was found between thirst and fluid therapy or fluid status. Instead, excellent oral care is the best way to address the discomfort of dry mouth.

Anxiety

Anxiety should be assessed verbally, if possible, or by changes in vital signs or restlessness. Benzodiazepines, especially midazolam with its rapid onset and short half-life, are frequently used. Existential distress can cause anxiety at the end of life, so spiritual or social work resources may also be helpful if the patient verbalizes anxiety.

Delirium

Delirium is commonly observed in the critically ill and in those approaching death. Haloperidol is recommended and restraints should be avoided.

Metabolic Derangement

Treatments for metabolic derangements are tempered with concerns for the patient's comfort. Only interventions promoting comfort are performed. Patients do not necessarily feel better "when the laboratory values are right."

Skin Integrity

While always a consideration in a critical care nursing, wounds and other skin issues can be a source of patient discomfort at the end of life. However, aggressive turning regimens and wound care may be counter-productive if the patient has only days or hours to live. Unit protocols may need to be adjusted in favor of comfort for such situations. Families may also want to assist with some aspects of skin care and should be given appropriate tasks, such as applying lotion, if they request.

Anemia

This can be a common problem at the end of life with cancer and other debilitating illnesses. Anemia is treated only when a transfusion could increase the patient's quality of life, such as providing the energy to participate with family. Routine blood draws to determine blood counts should be stopped since values will likely be abnormal.

Hemorrhage

This can occur with illnesses such as liver failure, and families should be educated about the risks. Again, if the goals of care are comfort, and to allow a natural death, then transfusions to address bleeding are likely not appropriate. As part of enrolling family in the treatment plan, transfusions should be discussed and agreement reached in advance.

PROVIDING COMFORT

The nursing interventions at end of life focus on the provision of comfort care as an active, desirable, and important service. Unnecessary verification of vital signs, laboratory work, and any treatment that does not promote comfort is avoided. Positioning the patient who is actively dying has as its purpose only comfort, not the schedule to promote skin integrity. Coordinating this care with the many members of the critical care team is important to ensure consistency across disciplines. When symptom management is not successful in ensuring comfort, the services of the pain team or the palliative care service may be required.

Near-Death Awareness

Two hospice nurses have described the phenomenon of patient behaviors and near-death awareness.[43] The same behaviors may be seen in critical care patients near death. Having an awareness of the phenomenon enables more careful assessment of behaviors that may be interpreted as delirium, acid-base imbalance, or other metabolic derangements. Patient behaviors include communicating with someone who is not alive, preparing for travel, describing a place they can see, or even knowing when death will occur.[44] Family members may find these behaviors disturbing but find comfort in understanding the phenomenon and in sharing these experiences with their loved one.

WITHDRAWING LIFE SUPPORT

Family Meetings

Although family meetings should ideally be held within 72 hours of any ICU admission,[45] they are frequently only held to formulate a decision to withdraw life support. One clinical practice study showed that earlier meetings led to shorter medical ICU stays, and earlier access to palliative care for patients who eventually died.[46]

Preparing to Withdraw Life Support

Typically a time to initiate withdrawal is established with the family and health care team. This allows the family to prepare and for all necessary resources to be present. For example, a distant family member may need to arrive, and then the procedure will occur. It is helpful if other staff members are alerted to the fact that a withdrawal is occurring. A neutral sign hung on the door or use of a special room may caution staff to avoid loud conversations and laughter, which can be upsetting to grieving families.

After the decision to remove life support is made and the family is gathered, the family should be told what the impending death may be like. When the patient is totally dependent on ventilatory support or vasopressors and that support is removed, death typically follows in minutes. The patient appears as if asleep, and the usual signs of color and skin temperature changes will not be seen before death. The opposite is true if the patient is not ventilator dependent. Providing information to families for the experience of withdrawal

alerts them to what the patient may exhibit as death approaches, reducing the distress families feel during the withdrawal process.[47]

Implantable cardioverter-defibrillators should be turned off to prevent patient distress from their firing and to avoid interfering with the pronouncement of death. Neuromuscular blocking agents should be discontinued, because paralysis precludes both assessment of the patient's discomfort and the means to communicate with loved ones. Time for clearance of the medication should be carefully considered in planning the withdrawal process.[34]

The removal of monitors is usually recommended but families should be given this choice.[48] Physicians and nurses may use the monitor to assess the distress of the patient during the withdrawal process and to adjust the amount of medication needed for symptom management. Families may glance at the monitor to verify that electrical activity has ceased, because the appearance of death may be too subtle to detect. One option is to turn the monitor off in the patient's room but leave the leads on so that vital signs can be monitored from the nurses' station.

Opioids and Sedatives

Opioids and benzodiazepines are the most commonly administered pre-withdrawal medications because dyspnea and anxiety are the usual symptoms related to ventilator withdrawal.[49] A bolus dose of morphine (2 to 10 mg IV) and a continuous morphine infusion at 50% of the bolus dose per hour is recommended as a starting point.[50] A midazolam bolus (1 to 2 mg IV) followed by an infusion at 1 mg/hr is also recommended.[50] The intent is to provide good symptom control with a respiratory rate below 30 breaths per minute without grimacing or agitation;[50] dosages accelerate until the patient's comfort is achieved. In one study, the use of opiates or benzodiazepines to treat discomfort after withdrawal of life support did not hasten death in critically ill patients.[51]

Ventilator Withdrawal

There are two methods for discontinuing ventilator support: extubation and terminal weaning. Both involve premedicating the patient to provide comfort. In the first, extubation, the endotracheal tube is withdrawn at the beginning of the process and the patient is on room air, a nasal cannula, or a T-piece. When this method is used, the family should be prepared for respiratory noises and deeper, faster respirations. Some providers do a trial of reduced ventilatory support before extubation to ensure the patient has been appropriately medicated and will be comfortable. One benefit of extubation is that withdrawing the endotracheal tube can remove the discomfort some patients' experiences. Extubation also leaves the patient with a more natural appearance.

In the other option, terminal weaning, the endotracheal tube is removed at the end of the withdrawal process. In this case, the patient's comfort is also monitored and, once achieved, ventilator settings are reduced. Positive end-expiratory pressure (PEEP) is reduced to normal, and then the mode is set to patient control. Next, the FIO_2 is reduced to 0.21 (21%). All of these steps are taken slowly while observing the patient for distress or anxiety. An experienced physician, a respiratory therapist, and a nurse should be present during this time. Ventilator alarms are turned off. The terminal wean offers the most control over secretions, respiratory noises, and gasping. Patients who survive for some time after ventilator withdrawal should ideally be transferred to a private room so family can visit as much as possible in the remaining hours to days.

PROFESSIONAL ISSUES REGARDING END OF LIFE IN THE ICU

Health Care Providers

Some interventions have been found helpful for health professionals in improving patient care at the end of life. A standardized order form for withdrawal was found to increase the amount of medications nurses administered for sedation, although it did not improve nurses' assessment of patients' dying experience.[52] Death rounds for ICU residents where cases were discussed post-mortem were well received and recommended to be included in future rotations.[53]

Emotional Support for the Nurse

Nurses who care for the dying patient need to have their expertise valued as highly as other high-technology interventions in critical care. Critical care units usually have several nurses who are looked to by other staff to provide end-of-life care, or to assist with withdrawal of life support. When several deaths occur close together, those nurses may be called on frequently. Some consideration in assignment should be given when a nurse has more than one death in a shift or a week. Taking a new admission is also difficult immediately after a death, and it can occur before the family has left the unit. Nurse administrators can provide some additional resources, debriefing, or time off when the burden has been high. Hearing supportive words from colleagues has been reported by critical care nurses as helpful in coping with the death of a patient.[54]

Nurses experience moral distress when aggressive care is offered to patients who are not expected to benefit from it. These levels of distress are high and have implications for retention of highly skilled nurses.[55] Nurses had a number of suggestions when questioned about what could be done to improve end-of-life care, such as facilitating dying with dignity, having someone with patients who are dying, managing patients' symptoms, knowing and then following patients' wishes for end-of-life care, and promoting earlier cessation of treatment or not initiating aggressive treatment at all.[56]

Organ Donation

The Social Security Act Section 1138 requires that hospitals have written protocols for the identification of potential organ donors.[57] The Joint Commission also has a standard on organ donation.[58] Although an impending death marks a difficult time for family members, the nurse notifies the organ procurement official to approach the family with a donation request. These individuals have training to make a supportive request. If the patient's disease precludes donation, the family is not approached.

Death may be pronounced when the patient meets a list of neurological criteria. However, there are differences among hospital policies for certification of brain death, which can result in varying circumstances under which patients can be pronounced dead.[59] Families may not understand the meaning of brain death, and they are less likely to donate organs when they believe the patient will not be dead until the ventilator is turned off and the heart stops.[60] How these conversations are held will determine families' understanding and positively affect donation. Clinicians should not suggest that the organs are alive while the brain is dead, but rather that the organs are functioning as a result of the machines used.[9]

Family Care

Families look for the good news in any message received from health professionals and are often surprised when told that death is the only outcome possible.[54] Families need assistance in forming their expectations about outcomes. Ongoing communication about the patient's progress is preferable to waiting until the patient is near death and then communicating with the family.

One intervention used with families at the end of life is a grieving cart. In one ICU,[61] the cart has a top drawer with English and Spanish versions of the Bible, Koran, and Book of Mormon, and pamphlets about grief and bereavement. The lower portion of the cart holds paper cups, napkins, and condiments. Fresh coffee and tea are brewed on the unit and served with muffins and cookies from the cafeteria. Family responses have been positive because they are reluctant to leave the bedside at such a time.

Delivering Bad News

Patients and families do not come to the critical care unit with the expectation of death. Even those who have had previous admissions expect to be "saved." They tend to listen to imparted information looking for good news; even when bad news is given, they may initially deny it or have great difficulty taking it in.[62] Having this in mind while talking to families may assist professionals in interpreting families' responses.

Preparing families for changes in the patient as the health condition deteriorates helps them to make plans. They need to know if other family members should be called, if someone should spend the night, or if financial arrangements should be changed before an impending death (e.g., to enable a surviving spouse to have access to funds). Anticipated physical changes can be described to help prepare families.

Families may refuse to forgo life-supporting treatments and want "everything done" because of mistrust of health professionals, poor communication, survivor guilt, or religious or cultural reasons.[30] Effective communication throughout the hospitalization and information provided throughout the stay predispose the family to better acceptance of news as the patient deteriorates. Family satisfaction is increased when they feel supported during their decision making and hear more empathic statements from physicians.[63]

Family Responses to Bad News

Families may experience a sense of crisis as emergencies occur or as the patient deteriorates and dies. Responses to the news of the death vary. Family members may show anger or be quiet, exhibit emotions or stoicism. Culture or religious beliefs may affect their response to news. It is helpful to ask if they would like to see a chaplain or a social worker. Quiet, calm, some privacy, and support are always appreciated.

Multidisciplinary family meetings in the ICU consistently have been shown to help families and health care providers arrive at a common understanding of the patient's prognosis and goals for future care. An analysis of the amount of opportunity families had to speak in these meetings revealed that when families had greater opportunity to talk, their satisfaction with physician communication increased and their ratings of conflict with the physician decreased. After the patient's death, greater family satisfaction with withdrawal of life support was associated with the following measures:[64]

- The process of withdrawal of life support being well explained
- Withdrawal of life support proceeding as expected
- Patient appearing comfortable
- Family and friends being prepared
- Appropriate person initiating discussion
- Adequate privacy during withdrawal of life support
- A chance to voice concerns

These meetings provide the opportunity to listen to family; to acknowledge and address emotions; and to pursue key tenets of palliative care, such as patient preferences, surrogate decision making, and nonabandonment.[65]

Policies Regarding Family Presence during Cardiopulmonary Resuscitation

Critical care nurses and emergency nurses have taken family members to the bedside for resuscitation or invasive procedures, but most hospitals do not have written policies for the family's presence.[66] Development and implementation of such policies benefit both staff and families.[13] Witnessing the steps of resuscitation may help family accept the patient's death.

Visiting Hours

Visiting in the ICU continues to be restricted,[67] despite national calls for increases in patient or family control over the care. Restricting visiting for dying ICU patients is unconscionable. Providing the visiting time to help family members say good-bye is an important function. Family members may have difficulty in seeing the person they knew among all the tubes. Coaching can be provided about how to approach the patient and about how the patient may still be able to hear despite appearing to be nonresponsive. Children, unless they represent a significant source of infection, should be allowed to say good-bye, but they may need adult assistance in understanding the situation. Families may have religious or cultural ceremonies that are important for them to perform before the patient dies or experiences withdrawal of life support. These practices are to be encouraged and facilitated as much as possible.

Continuity of Nursing Care

Continuity of care by the same nurse is important as patients near death. When possible, and agreeable to staff and families, the same nurse can be assigned over consecutive shifts to maintain continuity. Nurses have sometimes stayed with the family after the end of a shift when death was imminent so the family would not need to adjust to another person at this difficult time.[54]

After Death

After the death, the family may wish to spend time at the bedside. They need adequate room to sit and their time with the body should be unhurried and private. They can be asked if they need assistance or resources or whether they wish to be alone or have someone nearby. Nurses need to be aware of their own judgment on what is an appropriate response, because individuals respond differently to the same news, even within the same family. Frequently, the bed is needed for another patient, and juggling is required to ensure that the family has sufficient time even as another patient needs to be admitted. This is another reason to try to transfer patients earlier out of the unit to a private room elsewhere in the hospital. Supporting families after a death involves immediate bereavement support, information on what to do about the death, bereavement support for the future, contact with the family after death, and assessment of the quality of care the patient experienced.[68] Having material already prepared with the necessary after-death information is quite helpful at this time.

COLLABORATIVE CARE

The ability to provide collaborative, compassionate end-of-life care is the responsibility of all clinicians who work with the critically ill. Interdisciplinary collaborative efforts are associated with improvement in care. In 2008 the SCCM published a revised guideline, "Recommendations for End-of-Life Care in the Intensive Care Unit," to provide guidance for end-of-life care for the team.[69] The Evidence-Based Practice box on End-of-Life Care provides a summary of the topics included. The Robert Wood Johnson Foundation (RWJF) Critical Care End-of-Life Peer Workgroup[70] identified seven end-of-life care domains for use in the ICU:

1. Patient- and family-centered decision making
2. Communication

3. Continuity of care
4. Emotional and practical support
5. Symptom management and comfort care
6. Spiritual support
7. Emotional and organizational support for ICU clinicians

Individuals[71] and groups[72] have developed websites for online tools to improve end-of-life care. The same attention should be placed on improving end-of-life care that is placed on skills of electrocardiogram interpretation or hemodynamic monitoring.

CASE STUDY PATIENT AT THE END OF LIFE

Answers to the Case Study Questions can be found on the Evolve web site at http://evolve.elsevier.com/Urden/ priorities/.

Brief Patient History

Mr. C is a 17-year-old, African-American man who was involved in a motor vehicle accident. He sustained a cervical fracture at the level of C2 that transected his spinal column and both vertebral arteries. Rescue breathing was begun in the field by bystanders, and he was intubated by paramedics en route to the hospital. Mr. C's parents state that they want everything possible done and that they have faith that God will heal their son.

Clinical Assessment

Mr. C is admitted to the critical care unit from the emergency department. He is ventilator dependent. His skin is warm and dry. He is unresponsive to verbal or painful stimuli, and there is no physical movement. Mr. C's family remains at the bedside 24 hours each day throughout the week. They converse with Mr. C, speaking about all the things they are going to do when he gets home.

Diagnostic Procedures

Mr. C's vital signs are as follows: blood pressure of 120/72 mm Hg, heart rate of 120 beats/min (sinus tachycardia),

no spontaneous respiration, temperature of 97.8° F, and Glasgow Coma Scale score of 3. Computed tomography of the head showed a global ischemic infarct involving both ventricles, and electroencephalography revealed no detectable cortical activity.

Medical Diagnosis

Mr. C is diagnosed with brain death.

Questions

1. What major outcomes do you expect to achieve for this patient?
2. What problems or risks must be managed to achieve these outcomes?
3. What interventions must be initiated to monitor, prevent, manage, or eliminate the problems and risks identified?
4. What interventions should be initiated to promote optimal functioning, safety, and well-being of the patient?
5. What possible learning needs do you anticipate for this patient?
6. What cultural and age-related factors may have a bearing on the patient's plan of care?

REFERENCES

1. SUPPORT Principal Investigators: A controlled trial to improve care for seriously ill hospitalized patients. The study to understand prognoses and preferences for outcomes and risks of treatments (SUPPORT), *JAMA* 274(20):1591, 1995.
2. Field MJ, Cassell CK, editors: *Approaching death: improving care at the end of life*, Washington, D.C., 1997, National Academy Press.
3. Angus DC, et al: Use of intensive care at the end of life in the United States: an epidemiologic study, *Crit Care Med* 32(3):638-643, 2004.
4. Nishimura A, et al: Patients who complete advance directives and what they prefer, *Mayo Clin Proc* 82(12):1480, 2007.
5. Briggs LA, et al: Patient-centered advance care planning in special patient populations: a pilot study, *J Prof Nurs* 20(1): 47, 2004.
6. Rubenfeld GD: Principles and practice of withdrawing life-sustaining treatments, *Crit Care Clin* 20(3):435, 2004.
7. Tilden V, et al: Family decision-making to withdraw life-sustaining treatments from hospitalized patients, *Nurs Res* 50(2):105, 2001.
8. Gilmer T, et al: The costs of nonbeneficial treatment in the intensive care setting, *Health Aff (Millwood)* 24(4):961, 2005.
9. Campbell ML: *Forgoing life-sustaining therapy: how to care for the patient who is near death*, Aliso Viejo, Calif., 1998, AACN.

10. Ebell MH, et al: Survival after in-hospital cardiopulmonary resuscitation: a meta-analysis, *J Gen Intern Med* 13(12):805, 1998.
11. Elshove-Bolk J, et al: In-hospital resuscitation of the elderly: characteristics and outcome, *Resuscitation* 74(2):372, 2007.
12. FitzGerald JD, et al: Functional status among survivors of in-hospital cardiopulmonary resuscitation. SUPPORT investigators study to understand progress and preferences for outcomes and risks of treatment, *Arch Intern Med* 157(1):72, 1997.
13. American Association of Critical-Care Nurses: Family presence during CPR and invasive procedures 2004 (website). www.aacn.org/WD/Practice/Docs/Family_Presence_During_ CPR_11-2004.pdf (accessed January 2011).
14. Emergency Nurses Association: Family presence at the bedside during invasive procedures and cardiopulmonary resuscitation, 2005. Available at http://www.ena.org/ SiteCollectionDocuments/Position%20Statements/Family_ Presence_-_ENA_PS.pdf (accessed August 2010).
15. Covinsky KE, et al: Communication and decision-making in seriously ill patients: findings of the SUPPORT project. The Study to Understand Prognoses and Preferences for Outcomes and Risks of Treatments, *J Am Geriatr Soc* 48(suppl 5):S187, 2000.
16. Burns JP, et al: Do-not-resuscitate order after 25 years, *Crit Care Med* 31(5):1543, 2003.

17. Keenan CH, Kish SK: The influence of do-not-resuscitate orders on care provided for patients in the surgical intensive care unit of a cancer center, *Crit Care Nurs Clin North Am* 12(3):385, 2000.

18. Christakis NA, Lamont EB: Extent and determinants of error in doctors' prognoses in terminally ill patients: prospective cohort study, *BMJ* 320(7233):469, 2000.

19. Lynn J, et al: Prognoses of seriously ill hospitalized patients on the days before death: implications for patient care and public policy, *New Horiz* 5(1):56, 1997.

20. McDonald DD, et al: Communicating end-of-life preferences, *West J Nurs Res* 25(6):652; discussion 667, 2003.

21. Fried TR, Bradley EH: What matters to seriously ill older persons making end-of-life treatment decisions? A qualitative study, *J Palliat Med* 6(2):237, 2003.

22. White DB, et al: Toward shared decision making at the end of life in intensive care units: opportunities for improvement, *Arch Intern Med* 167(5):461, 2007.

23. Limerick MH: The process used by surrogate decision makers to withhold and withdraw life-sustaining measures in an intensive care environment, *Oncol Nurs Forum* 34(2):331, 2007.

24. Ahrens T, et al: Improving family communications at the end of life: implications for length of stay in the intensive care unit and resource use, *Am J Crit Care* 12(4):317; discussion 324, 2003.

25. Davidson JE, et al: Clinical practice guidelines for support of the family in the patient-centered intensive care unit: American College of Critical Care Medicine Task Force 2004-2005, *Crit Care Med* 35(2):605, 2007.

26. Kirchhoff KT, Faas AI: Family support at end of life, *AACN Adv Crit Care* 18(4):426, 2007.

27. Degenholtz HB, et al: Race and the intensive care unit: disparities and preferences for end-of-life care, *Crit Care Med* 31(suppl 5):S373, 2003.

28. Wall RJ, et al: Spiritual care of families in the intensive care unit, *Crit Care Med* 35(4):1084, 2007.

29. Crawley LM: Racial, cultural, and ethnic factors influencing end-of-life care, *J Palliat Med* 8(suppl 1):S58, 2005.

30. Prendergast TJ, Puntillo KA: Withdrawal of life support: intensive caring at the end of life, *JAMA* 288(21):2732, 2002.

31. Curtis JR, Rubenfeld GD, editors: *Managing death in the intensive care unit: the transition from cure to comfort*, New York, 2001, Oxford University Press.

32. Frick S, et al: Medical futility: predicting outcome of intensive care unit patients by nurses and doctors – a prospective comparative study, *Crit Care Med* 31(2):456, 2003.

33. Meltzer LS, Huckabay LM: Critical care nurses' perceptions of futile care and its effect on burnout, *Am J Crit Care* 13(3):202, 2004.

34. Faber-Langendoen K, Lanken PN: Dying patients in the intensive care unit: forgoing treatment, maintaining care, *Ann Intern Med* 133(11):886, 2000.

35. National Consensus Project: Clinical practice guidelines for quality palliative care, ed 2, Pittsburgh, 2004, National Consensus for Quality Palliative Care. (website) www.nationalconsensusproject.org/guideline.pdf. Accessed January 2011.

36. Institute of Medicine: Improving palliative care for cancer: summary and recommendations, Washington, D.C., 2001, National Academy Press.

37. Gélinas C, et al: Pain assessment and management in critically ill intubated patients: a retrospective study, *Am J Crit Care* 13(2):126, 2004.

38. Foley KM: Pain and symptom control in the dying ICU patient. In Curtis JR, Rubenfeld GD, editors: *Managing death in the intensive care unit: the transition from cure to comfort*, New York, 2001, Oxford University Press.

39. Jacobi J, et al: Clinical practice guidelines for the sustained use of sedatives and analgesics in the critically ill adult, *Crit Care Med* 30(1):119, 2002.

40. Campbell ML, et al: Patients who are near death are frequently unable to self-report dyspnea, *J Palliat Med* 12(10):881, 2009.

41. Fabbro ED, et al: Symptom control in palliative care-part III: dyspnea and delirium, *J Palliat Med* 9(2):422, 2006.

42. Viola RA, et al: The effects of fluid status and fluid therapy on the dying: a systematic review, *J Palliat Care* 13(4):41, 1997.

43. Callanan M, Kelley P: Final gifts: understanding the special awareness, needs, and communications of the dying, New York, 1997, Bantam Books.

44. Marchand L: Near death awareness, *Fast Facts and Concepts* 118, 2004. (website) www.eperc.mcw.edu/fastFact/ff_118.htm (accessed January 2011).

45. Lilly CM, et al: An intensive communication intervention for the critically ill, *Am J Med* 109(6):469, 2000.

46. Lilly CM, et al: Intensive communication: four-year follow-up from a clinical practice study, *Crit Care Med* 31(suppl 5):S394, 2003.

47. Kirchhoff KT, et al: Preparing families of intensive care patients for withdrawal of life support: a pilot study, *Am J Crit Care* 17(2):113, 2008.

48. Rubenfeld GD, Crawford SW: Withdrawal of life-sustaining treatment. In Curtis JR, Rubenfeld GD, editors: *Managing death in the intensive care unit: the transition from cure to comfort*, New York, 2001, Oxford University Press.

49. Campbell ML: How to withdraw mechanical ventilation: a systematic review of the literature, *AACN Adv Crit Care* 18(4):397, 2007.

50. von Gunten C, Weissman DE: Symptom control for ventilator withdrawal in the dying patient, ed 2, *Fast Facts and Concepts* 34, 2005. (website) www.mcw.edu/fastFact/ff_34.htm (accessed January 2011).

51. Chan JD, et al: Narcotic and benzodiazepine use after withdrawal of life support: Association with time to death? *Chest* 126(1):286, 2004.

52. Treece PD, et al: Evaluation of a standardized order form for the withdrawal of life support in the intensive care unit, *Crit Care Med* 32(5):1141, 2004.

53. Hough CL, et al: Death rounds: End-of-life discussions among medical residents in the intensive care unit, *J Crit Care* 20(1):20, 2005.

54. Kirchhoff KT, et al: Intensive care nurses' experiences with end-of-life care, *Am J Crit Care* 9(1):36, 2000.

55. Elpern EH, et al: Moral distress of staff nurses in a medical intensive care unit, *Am J Crit Care* 14(6):523, 2005.

56. Beckstrand RL, et al: Providing a "good death": critical care nurses' suggestions for improving end-of-life care, *Am J Crit Care* 15(1):38, 2006.

57. Social Security Administration: Hospital protocols for organ procurement and standards for organ procurement agencies, 2004: compilation of the Social Security laws. (website) www.ssa.gov/OP_Home/ssact/title11/1138.htm (accessed January 2011).

58. Joint Commission on Accreditation of Healthcare Organizations: Approved: revisions to Standard LD.3.1.10, Element of Performance 12, for critical access hospitals and hospitals, *Jt Comm Perspect* 27(6):14, 2007.

59. Powner DJ, et al: Variability among hospital policies for determining brain death in adults, *Crit Care Med* 32(6):1284, 2004.

60. Siminoff LA, et al: Families' understanding of brain death, *Prog Transplant* 13(3):218, 2003.

61. Whitmer M, et al: Caring in the curing environment. *J Hosp Palliat Nurs* 9(6):329, 2007.

62. Kirchhoff KT, et al: The vortex: families' experiences with death in the intensive care unit, *Am J Crit Care* 11(3):200, 2002.

63. Selph RB, et al: Empathy and life support decisions in intensive care units, *J Gen Intern Med* 23(9):1311, 2008.

64. Keenan SP, et al: Withdrawal of life support: how the family feels, and why, *J Palliat Care* 16(suppl):S40, 2000.

65. Curtis JR, et al: Missed opportunities during family conferences about end-of-life care in the intensive care unit, *Am J Respir Crit Care Med* 171(8):844, 2005.

66. MacLean SL, et al: Family presence during cardiopulmonary resuscitation and invasive procedures: practices of critical care and emergency nurses, *Am J Crit Care* 12(3):246, 2003.

67. Kirchhoff KT, Dahl N: American Association of Critical-Care Nurses' national survey of facilities and units providing critical care, *Am J Crit Care* 15(1):13, 2006.

68. Shannon S: Helping families cope with death in the ICU. In Curtis JR, Rubenfeld GD, editors: *Managing death in the intensive care unit: the transition from cure to comfort*, New York, 2001, Oxford University Press.

69. Truog RD, et al: Recommendations for end-of-life care in the intensive care unit: a consensus statement by the American College of Critical Care Medicine, *Crit Care Med* 36(3):953, 2008.

70. Clarke EB, et al: Quality indicators for end-of-life care in the intensive care unit, *Crit Care Med* 31(9):2255, 2003.

71. Curtis JR: End of life care research program (website), 2008. Available at depts.washington.edu/eolcare/currentprojects/ (accessed January 2010).

72. Promoting Excellence in End of Life Care: Innovative models and approaches for palliative care (website). www.promotingexcellence.org (accessed January 2011).

CHAPTER

11

Cardiovascular Clinical Assessment and Diagnostic Procedures

Mary E. Lough

℮volve WEBSITE

Be sure to check out the bonus material, including free self-assessment exercises, on the Evolve web site at
http://evolve.elsevier.com/Urden/priorities/.

OBJECTIVES

- Identify the components of a cardiovascular history.
- Describe inspection, palpation, percussion, and auscultation of the patient with cardiovascular dysfunction.
- Describe the use of arterial, central venous, and pulmonary artery catheters for bedside hemodynamic monitoring.
- Compare and contrast options for measuring cardiac output: invasive versus noninvasive or minimally invasive methods.
- Outline the steps to interpret a change in $Scvo_2/Svo_2$ values.
- Illustrate the correct placement of the electrodes for accurate bedside electrocardiographic (ECG) monitoring.

- Outline the steps in analyzing an ECG rhythm strip.
- Explain the significance of normal and abnormal ECG findings.
- Describe nursing actions for management of significant atrial, ventricular, and junctional dysrhythmias.
- Discuss the clinical significance of selected laboratory tests used in the assessment of cardiovascular disorders.
- Describe key diagnostic procedures used in assessment of the patient with cardiovascular dysfunction.
- Discuss the different purposes of three cardiovascular diagnostic procedures.

Physical assessment of the cardiovascular patient is a skill that must not be lost amid the technology of the critical care setting. Data collected from a thorough, thoughtful history and examination contribute to both the nursing and the medical decisions for therapeutic interventions.

HISTORY

The patient history is important because it provides data that contribute to the cardiovascular diagnosis and treatment plan. For a patient in acute distress, the history is curtailed to just a few questions about the patient's chief complaint, the precipitating events, and current medications. For a patient

without obvious distress, the history focuses on the following four areas:
1. Review of the patient's present illness.
2. Overview of the patient's general cardiovascular status, including previous cardiac diagnostic studies, interventional procedures, cardiac surgeries, and current medications (i.e., cardiac, noncardiac, and over-the-counter drugs).
3. Examination of the patient's general health status, including family history of coronary artery disease (CAD), hypertension, diabetes, peripheral arterial disease, or stroke.
4. Survey of the patient's lifestyle, including risk factors for CAD.

One of the unique challenges in cardiovascular assessment is identifying when "chest pain" is of cardiac origin and when it is not. The following safety information should always be considered:

- If there is any evidence of CAD or risk of heart disease, assume that the chest pain is caused by myocardial ischemia until proven otherwise.
- Questions to elicit the nature of the chest pain cover five basic areas: quality, location, duration of pain, factors that provoke the pain, and factors that relieve the pain.
- There may be little correlation between the severity of chest discomfort and the gravity of its cause. This is a result of the subjective nature of pain and the unique presentation of ischemic disease in women, older patients, and individuals with diabetes.
- Subjective descriptors vary greatly among individuals. Not all patients use the word "pain"; some may describe "pressure," "heaviness," "discomfort," or "indigestion."
- There is not always a correlation between the location of chest discomfort and its source because of *referred pain*. For example, in patients with gastroesophageal reflux disease (GERD), esophageal spasm can cause visceral substernal chest pain that radiates to the left arm and jaw, described by patients as "heartburn."[1,2]
- Other nonpainful symptoms that may signal cardiac dysfunction are dyspnea, palpitations, cough, fatigue, edema, ischemic leg pain, nocturia, syncope, and cyanosis.

In a meta-analysis of the evaluation of stable, intermittent chest pain, a patient's description of chest pain was found to be the most important predictor of underlying coronary disease.[3] In the evaluation of acute chest pain, the 12-lead electrocardiogram was the most useful bedside predictor for a diagnosis of ST-elevation myocardial infarction (STEMI).[3]

PHYSICAL EXAMINATION

A comprehensive physical assessment is fundamental to the achievement of an accurate diagnosis. The nurse who has developed the skills of inspection, palpation, and auscultation can be confident when assessing patients with cardiovascular disease. Percussion is not employed when assessing the cardiovascular system.

Inspection

The priorities for inspection of the patient with cardiovascular dysfunction are: (1) assessing the general appearance; (2) examining the extremities; (3) estimating jugular venous distention; and (4) observing the apical impulse.

Assessing General Appearance

The face is observed for the color of the skin (i.e., cyanotic, pale, or jaundiced) and for apprehensive or painful expressions. The skin, lips, tongue, and mucous membranes are inspected for pallor or cyanosis. *Central cyanosis* is a bluish discoloration of the tongue and sublingual area. Multiracial studies indicate that the tongue is the most sensitive site for observation of central cyanosis, which must be recognized

and treated as a medical emergency. Pulse oximetry, arterial blood gas analysis, and treatment with 100% oxygen must be instituted immediately.

The anterior thorax and posterior thorax are inspected for skeletal deformities that may displace the heart and cause cardiac compromise. The skin on the chest wall and abdomen is inspected for scars, bruises, wounds, and bulges associated with pacemaker or defibrillator implants. Respiratory rate, pattern, and effort are also observed and recorded. The abdomen is assessed for signs of distention or ascites that may be associated with right-sided heart failure. Abdominal adiposity is a known risk factor for CAD.

Body posture can indicate the amount of effort it takes to breathe. For example, sitting upright to breathe may be necessary for the patient with acute heart failure, and leaning forward may be the least painful position for the patient with pericarditis. The patient is observed for signs of confusion or lethargy that may indicate hypotension, low cardiac output (CO), or hypoxemia.

Examining the Extremities

The legs are inspected for signs of peripheral arterial or venous vascular disease. The visible signs of arterial vascular disease include pale, shiny legs with sparse hair growth. Venous disease creates an edematous limb with deep red rubor, brown discoloration, and, frequently, leg ulceration. A comparison of arterial and venous disease is presented in Table 11-1.

The nail beds are inspected for signs of discoloration or cyanosis. *Clubbing* in the nail bed is a sign associated with long-standing central cyanotic heart disease or pulmonary disease with hypoxemia.[4] Clubbing describes a nail that has lost the normal angle between the finger and the nail root; the nail becomes wide and convex. The terminal phalanx of the finger also becomes bulbous and swollen, sometimes described as *drumstick fingers*.[5] Clubbing is rare. It denotes long-standing severe central cyanosis (Figure 11-1). Platelet-derived vascular endothelial growth factor is thought to play a key role in the development of clubbing.[6]

Peripheral cyanosis, a bluish discoloration of the nail bed, is more commonly seen. Peripheral cyanosis results from a reduction in the quantity of oxygen in the peripheral extremities from arterial disease or decreased CO. Clubbing never occurs as a result of peripheral cyanosis.

Estimating Jugular Venous Distention

The jugular veins of the neck are inspected for a noninvasive estimate of intravascular volume and pressure. The internal jugular veins are observed for *jugular vein distention* (JVD) (Figure 11-2 and Box 11-1). JVD is caused by an elevated central venous pressure (CVP).[7] This occurs with fluid volume overload and right ventricular dysfunction, which elevates right atrial pressure.[8] The right internal jugular vein can be used for measurement of CVP in centimeters of water (Figure 11-3 and Box 11-2).[9-11]

The abdominojugular reflux sign can assist with the diagnosis of right ventricular failure. This noninvasive test is used in conjunction with measurement of JVD. The procedure for

TABLE 11-1	INSPECTION AND PALPATION OF EXTREMITIES: COMPARISON OF ARTERIAL AND VENOUS DISEASE	
CHARACTERISTIC	**ARTERIAL DISEASE**	**VENOUS DISEASE**
Hair loss	Present	Absent
Skin texture	Thin, shiny, dry	Flaking, stasis, dermatitis, mottled
Ulceration	Located at pressure points; painful, pale, dry with little drainage; well-demarcated with eschar or dried; surrounded by fibrous tissue; granulation tissue scant and pale	Usually at the ankles; painless, pink, moist with large amount of drainage; irregular, dry, and scaly; surrounded by dermatitis; granulation tissue healthy
Skin color	Elevational pallor, dependent rubor	Brown patches, rubor, mottled cyanotic color when dependent
Nails	Thick, brittle	Normal
Varicose veins	Absent	Present
Temperature	Cool	Warm
Capillary refill	Greater than 3 seconds	Less than 3 seconds
Edema	None or mild, usually unilateral	Usually present foot to calf, unilateral or bilateral
Pulses	Weak or absent (0 to 1+)	Normal, strong, and symmetric

Modified from Krenzer ME: Peripheral vascular assessment: finding your way through arteries and veins, *AACN Clin Issues* 6(4):631, 1995.

Clubbing of Nail Beds

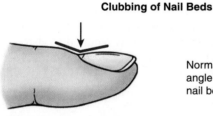

Normal Finger and Nail Bed

Normal nail shows a slight angle between root of nail bed and finger.

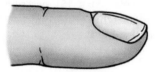

Early Clubbing

Early clubbing shows loss of angle at root of nail bed. Finger tip is of normal size.

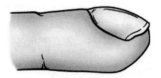

Moderate Clubbing

Moderate clubbing shows bulging of angle at root of nail bed. Distal finger/toe is enlarged.

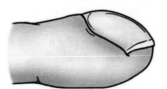

Advanced Clubbing

Advanced clubbing shows bulging and widening of nail bed. Distal finger/toe is bulbous.

FIGURE 11-1 Clubbing of the nail beds.

assessing abdominojugular reflux is described in Box 11-3. A positive abdominojugular reflux sign is an increase in the jugular venous pressure (CVP equivalent) of 4 cm or more sustained for at least 15 seconds.[12]

Observing the Apical Impulse

The thoracic cage is divided with imaginary vertical lines (sternal, midclavicular, axillary, vertebral, and scapular), and the intercostal spaces are divided with horizontal lines to serve as reference points in locating or describing cardiac findings (Figure 11-4). The anterior thorax is inspected for the *apical impulse,* sometimes referred to as the *point of maximal impulse* (PMI). The apical impulse occurs as the left ventricle contracts during systole and rotates forward, causing the left ventricular apex of the heart to hit the chest wall. The apical impulse is a quick, localized, outward movement normally located just lateral to the left midclavicular line at the fifth intercostal space in the adult patient (Figure 11-5). The apical impulse is the only normal pulsation visualized on the chest wall. In the patient without cardiac disease, PMI may not be noticeable (see Figure 11-5).

Palpation

The priorities for palpation of the patient with cardiovascular dysfunction are: (1) assessing arterial pulses; (2) evaluating capillary refill; (3) estimating edema; and (4) assessing for signs of deep vein thrombosis.

Assessing Arterial Pulses

Seven pairs of bilateral arterial pulses are palpated. The examination incorporates bilateral assessment of the carotid, brachial, radial, ulnar, popliteal, dorsalis pedis, and posterior tibial arteries. The pulses are palpated separately and compared bilaterally to check for consistency. Pulse volume is

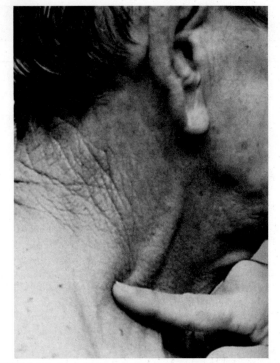

FIGURE 11-2 Assessment of jugular vein distention (JVD). Applying light finger pressure over the sternocleidomastoid muscle, parallel to the clavicle, helps identify the external jugular vein by occluding flow and distending it. The finger pressure is released, and the patient is observed for true distention. If the patient's trunk is elevated to 30 degrees or more, JVD should not be present.

BOX 11-1	PROCEDURE FOR ASSESSING JUGULAR VEIN DISTENTION

1. Patient reclines at a 30- to 45-degree angle.
2. The examiner stands on the patient's right side and turns the patient's head slightly toward the left.
3. If the jugular vein is not visible, light finger pressure is applied across the sternocleidomastoid muscle just above and parallel to the clavicle. This pressure fills the external jugular vein by obstructing flow.
4. After the location of the vein has been identified, the pressure is released, and the presence of jugular vein distention (JVD) is assessed.
5. Because inhalation decreases venous pressure, JVD should be assessed at end-exhalation.
6. Any fullness in the vein extending more than 3 cm above the sternal angle is evidence of increased venous pressure. Generally, the higher the sitting angle of the patient when JVD is visualized, the higher the central venous pressure.
7. Documentation: JVD is reported by including the angle of the head of the bed at the time JVD was evaluated (e.g., "presence of JVD with the head of the bed elevated to 45 degrees").

graded on a scale of 0 to 3+ (Box 11-4). The abdominal aortic pulse can also be palpated. If a distal pulse cannot be palpated using light finger pressure, a Doppler ultrasound stethoscope can increase diagnostic accuracy.[13] It is important to mark the location of the audible signal with an indelible ink marker pen for future evaluation of pulse quality. The radial and ulnar arterial pulses must be evaluated for collateral flow before an arterial line is inserted; this test, known as the *Allen test*, is described in Box 11-5.

Evaluating Capillary Refill

Capillary refill assessment is a maneuver that uses the patient's nail beds to evaluate arterial circulation to the extremity and overall perfusion. The nail bed is compressed to produce blanching, after which release of the pressure should result in a return of blood flow and baseline nail color within 2 seconds.[14] The severity of arterial insufficiency is directly proportional to the amount of time required to reestablish baseline flow and color.

Estimating Edema

Edema is fluid accumulation in the extravascular spaces of the body. The dependent tissues within the legs and sacrum are particularly susceptible. The nurse should observe whether the edema is dependent, unilateral or bilateral, pitting or nonpitting. The amount of edema is quantified by measuring the circumference of the limb or by pressing the skin of the feet, ankles, and shins against the underlying bone. Edema is a symptom associated with several diseases, and further diagnostic evaluation is required to determine the cause. Although no universal scale for pitting edema exists, one example is a 0 to 4+ system (Table 11-2).

Auscultation

The priorities for auscultation of the patient with cardiovascular dysfunction are: (1) measuring blood pressure; (2) detecting orthostatic hypotension; (3) measuring pulse pressure (4) detecting pulsus paradoxus; (5) assessing normal heart sounds; and (6) identifying abnormal heart sounds, murmurs, and pericardial rubs.

Measuring Blood Pressure

Blood pressure measurement is an essential component of every complete physical examination. Hypertension is diagnosed as a systolic blood pressure (SBP) of 140 mm Hg or higher, or a diastolic blood pressure (DBP) of 90 mm Hg or above.[15] Prehypertension is defined as an SBP in the range of 120 to 139 mm Hg in association with a DBP between 80 to 89 mm Hg.[15,16] The incidence of hypertension in the United States has increased dramatically as a result of an aging population and an increasing prevalence of obesity. During the period from 1999 to 2000, 65 million adults in the United States were hypertensive, compared with 50 million in 1988 through 1994—an increase of 30%.[17] Risk of hypertension increases with older age. More than 90% of people who have a normal blood pressure at 55 years of age eventually develop hypertension, according to findings from the Framingham Heart Study.[16]

In the critical care setting, systemic blood pressure can be measured directly or indirectly. Arterial monitoring devices that directly measure arterial pressure by means of an invasive

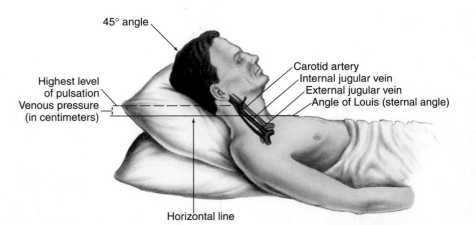

FIGURE 11-3 Position of internal and external jugular veins. Pulsation in the internal jugular vein can be used to estimate central venous pressure. (Modified from Thompson JM, et al: *Mosby's clinical nursing*, ed 5, St Louis, 2002, Mosby.)

BOX 11-2   PROCEDURE FOR ASSESSING CENTRAL VENOUS PRESSURE

1. The patient reclines in the bed. The highest point of pulsation in the internal jugular vein is observed during exhalation.
2. The vertical distance between this pulsation (top of the fluid level) and the sternal angle is estimated or measured in centimeters.
3. This number is then added to 5 cm for an estimation of CVP. The 5 cm is the approximate distance of the sternal angle above the level of the right atrium (see Figure 11-3).
4. Documentation: The degree of elevation of the patient is included in the report (e.g., "CVP estimated at 13 cm, using internal jugular vein pulsation, with the head of the bed elevated 45 degrees").

BOX 11-3   PROCEDURE FOR ASSESSING ABDOMINOJUGULAR REFLUX

1. Ask the patient to relax and breathe normally through an open mouth.
2. Measure the jugular vein distention (JVD) in the patient's right internal jugular vein, following the procedure described in Box 11-1.
3. Apply firm pressure of approximately 20 to 35 mm Hg to the patient's mid-abdomen for 15 to 30 seconds, and remeasure the JVD during the compression.
4. Measure the right JVD a third time after the compression is released.
5. Ask the patient not to tense or hold the breath during the test (doing so increases venous return to the heart and may produce a falsely positive result).
6. A positive abdominojugular reflux (AJR) is identified when abdominal compression causes a sustained JVD increase of 4 cm or more. This sign is indicative of right-sided heart failure.
7. A normal AJR is reported if there is no rise in JVD, a transient (<10 seconds) rise in JVD, or a rise in JVD less than or equal to 3 cm sustained throughout compression.

---

catheter technique are considered the gold standard.[18] Accurate use of a stethoscope and sphygmomanometer or electronic measuring devices can produce indirect blood pressure values that closely reflect direct measurements.[19]

Detecting Orthostatic Hypotension

When a healthy person stands, 10% to 15% of the blood volume is pooled in the legs; this reduces venous return to the right side of the heart, which decreases CO and lowers arterial blood pressure.[20] The fall in blood pressure activates baroreceptors; the subsequent reflex increase in sympathetic outflow and parasympathetic inhibition leads to peripheral vasoconstriction, with increased heart rate and contractility.[20] Postural (orthostatic) hypotension occurs when the SBP drops 10 to 20 mm Hg or the diastolic BP drops 5 mm Hg after a change from the supine to the upright posture.[20,21] It is usually accompanied by complaints of dizziness, lightheadedness, or syncope. If a patient experiences these symptoms, it is important to complete a full set of postural vital signs before increasing the patient's activity level (Box 11-6).

Orthostatic hypotension can have many causes. The three most common causes of orthostatic vital sign changes (i.e., drop in blood pressure and rise in heart rate) observed in critical care are:

1. Intravascular volume depletion or fluid loss caused by bleeding, excessive diuresis, or fever
2. Inadequate vascular vasoconstrictor mechanisms to constrict the arterial bed, which can occur in older patients after prolonged immobility[21] or as a result of spinal cord injury
3. Autonomic insufficiency caused by administration of pharmacological agents such as beta-blockers, angiotensin-converting enzyme (ACE) inhibitors, and calcium channel blockers

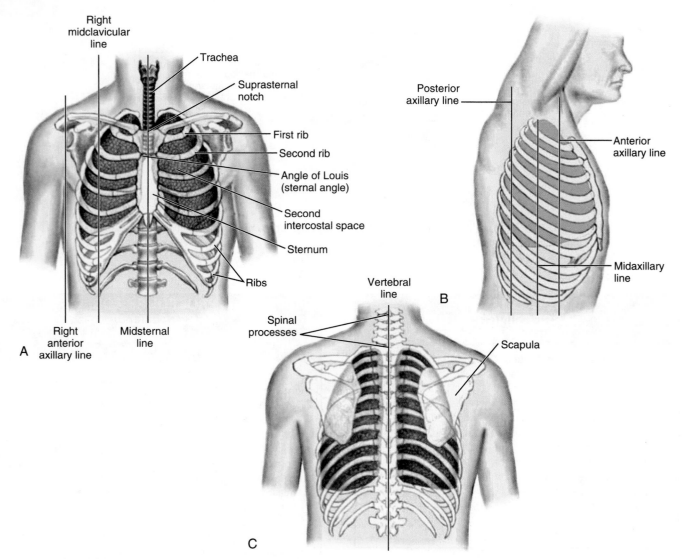

FIGURE 11-4 Thoracic landmarks. **A,** Anterior thorax. **B,** Right lateral thorax. **C,** Posterior thorax.

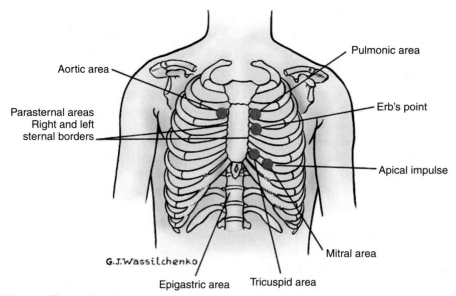

FIGURE 11-5 Thoracic palpation and auscultation points: Apical impulse position is shown.

BOX 11-4   PULSE PALPATION SCALE

0	Not palpable
1+	Faintly palpable (weak and thready)
2+	Palpable (normal pulse)
3+	Bounding (hyperdynamic pulse)

BOX 11-5   PROCEDURE FOR ASSESSMENT OF ARTERIAL BLOOD SUPPLY TO THE HAND: THE ALLEN TEST

Before a radial artery is punctured or cannulated, the Allen test is performed to assess blood flow to the hand and ensure that it is adequate.

Allen Test by Visual Inspection

1. If the patient is alert and cooperative, he or she is asked to repeatedly make a tight fist to squeeze the blood out of the hand.
2. The radial artery is compressed with firm thumb pressure by the examiner.
3. The patient is requested to open the hand, palm side up, while the radial artery is still occluded.
4. Pressure is released, and the time it takes for the color to return to the hand is noted.

If the ulnar artery is patent, the color will return within 3 seconds. The patient may describe a tingling in the palm as blood flow returns. Delayed color return (a "failed" Allen test) implies that the ulnar artery is inadequate; the radial artery is the only source of blood flow to the hand and must not be punctured or cannulated.

Allen Test with Pulse Oximetry

1. If the patient is unable to cooperate to make a fist, an alternative approach is to use a pulse oximeter that displays a pulse waveform.
2. Place the pulse oximeter on the middle finger and establish an adequate pulse amplitude display on the monitor.
3. Simultaneously compress the radial and ulnar arteries until the waveform clearly decreases or vanishes.
4. Release pressure off the ulnar artery only. If the ulnar artery is patent, the pulse amplitude recovers its normal appearance.
5. Repeat the procedure with the radial artery.
6. Only if there is adequate blood supply to the hand can arterial catheterization of the radial artery be accomplished safely.

Measuring Pulse Pressure

Pulse pressure describes the difference between the systolic and diastolic blood pressure values. The normal pulse pressure is 40 mm Hg (i.e., the difference between an SBP of 120 mm Hg and a DBP of 80 mm Hg). In the critically ill patient, a low blood pressure is frequently associated with a narrow pulse pressure. For example, a patient with a blood pressure of 90/72 mm Hg has a pulse pressure of 18 mm Hg. The narrowed pulse pressure is a temporary compensatory mechanism caused by arterial vasoconstriction resulting

BOX 11-6   MEASUREMENT OF POSTURAL (ORTHOSTATIC) VITAL SIGNS

Guidelines

1. Record blood pressure (BP) and heart rate (HR) in each position.
2. Do not remove cuff between measurements.
3. Record all associated signs and symptoms.
4. Clearly document patient position.

Lying	Sitting	Standing

Technique

1. Keep patient as flat as possible for 10 minutes before the initial assessment.
2. Patient supine: Obtain initial BP and HR measurements.
3. Patient sitting with legs hanging: Measure immediately and after 2 minutes.
4. Patient standing: Measure immediately and after 2 minutes. If BP and HR are stable but orthostasis is suspected, BP and HR can be repeated every 2 minutes. Note that this is rarely practical for the critically ill patient.

Results

Normal Changes

HR increases by 5 to 20 beats/min (transiently).
  Systolic BP drops 10 mm Hg.
  Diastolic BP drops 5 mm Hg.

Positive Orthostasis

Drop in systolic BP by more than 20 mm Hg.
  Drop in diastolic BP by more than 10 mm Hg within 3 minutes.

TABLE 11-2   PITTING EDEMA SCALE INDENTATION DEPTH

SCALE	EDEMA	ENGLISH UNITS	METRIC UNITS	TIME TO BASELINE
0	None	0	0	
1+	Trace	0-0.25 inch	<6.5 mm	Rapid
2+	Mild	0.25-0.5 inch	6.5-12.5 mm	6.5-12.5 mm
3+	Moderate	0.5-1 inch	12.5 mm-2.5 cm	1-2 min
4+	Severe	>1 inch	>2.5 cm	2-5 min

from volume depletion or heart failure. The narrow pulse pressure ensures that the MAP (78 mm Hg in this example) remains in a therapeutic range to provide adequate organ perfusion.

In contrast, a hypotensive septic patient who exhibits vasodilation will have a wide pulse pressure and inadequate organ perfusion. If the blood pressure is 90/36 mm Hg, the pulse pressure is 54 mm Hg, and the MAP calculates to an inadequate 54 mm Hg. In both of these examples, the SBP is the same (90 mm Hg); the difference in pulse pressure is a function of intravascular volume and vascular tone.

Detecting Pulsus Paradoxus

In normal physiology, the strength of the pulse fluctuates throughout the respiratory cycle. When the "pulse" is measured using the SBP, the pressure is observed to decrease slightly during inspiration and to rise slightly during respiratory exhalation. The normal difference is 2 to 4 mm Hg.[8] One exception is cardiac tamponade, where the blood pressure decline is abnormally large during inspiration. In general, an inspiratory decline of SBP greater than 10 mm Hg is considered diagnostic of pulsus paradoxus.[22-24] The traditional technique for measuring pulsus paradoxus using a sphygmomanometer and a blood pressure cuff[18] and pulse oximetry[22-24] is described in Box 11-7.[18] If the patient is hypotensive, pulsus paradoxus is more accurately assessed in the critical care unit by monitoring a pulse oximetry waveform or an indwelling arterial catheter waveform.[22-24]

Assessing Normal Heart Sounds

Auscultation of the heart is the most challenging part of the cardiac physical examination, and, in an era of increasing technological demands, it is daunting to new clinicians.[25] To summarize the advice given by most experts, the examiner must do the following:

1. Auscultate systematically across the precordium.[26]
2. Visualize the cardiac anatomy under each point of auscultation, expecting to hear the physiologically-associated sounds.[26]
3. Memorize the cardiac cycle to enhance the ability to hear abnormal sounds.[26]
4. Practice, practice, practice.[27]

First and Second Heart Sounds. Normal heart sounds are referred to as the first heart sound (S_1) and the second heart sound (S_2). S_1 is the sound associated with mitral and tricuspid valve closure and is heard most clearly in the mitral and tricuspid areas. S_2 (aortic and pulmonic closure) can be heard best at the second intercostal space to the right and left of the sternum (see Figure 11-5). Both sounds are high-pitched and heard best with the diaphragm of the stethoscope (Box 11-8). Each sound is loudest in an auscultation area located downstream from the actual valvular component of the sound, as shown in Figure 11-6.

Pathological Splitting of S_1 and S_2. A variety of abnormalities can alter the intensity and timing of split heart sounds. For example, during auscultation in the pulmonic area, a pathological split is audible with a stethoscope if the

---

BOX 11-7 **PROCEDURE FOR MEASURING PULSUS PARADOXUS**

Measurement with a Sphygmomanometer

1. The patient should be lying supine in a comfortable position.
2. The breathing pattern should be of normal depth and rate to avoid excessive respiratory interference.
3. Blood pressure is measured following standard procedures (see Boxes 11-6 and 11-7). The sphygmomanometer cuff is inflated to a pressure greater than the systolic blood pressure (SBP), and Korotkoff sounds are auscultated over the brachial artery while the cuff is deflated at rate of approximately 2 to 3 mm Hg per heartbeat.
4. The peak SBP during expiration (i.e., the pressure at which Korotkoff sounds are heard only during expiration) should be identified and then reconfirmed.
5. The cuff is then deflated slowly to establish the SBP at which Korotkoff sounds become audible during both inspiration and expiration.
6. If the auscultated difference between these two SBP values exceeds 10 mm Hg during quiet respiration, a paradoxical pulse is present.

Measurement by Waveform Analysis

1. A pulse oximetry sensor with a visible pulse waveform can be used as an additional measurement device.
2. In the critical care unit, an arterial waveform from an indwelling arterial catheter (if present) can be used to measure the difference in SBP between expiration and inspiration.

BOX 11-8 **CHARACTERISTICS OF THE FIRST AND SECOND HEART SOUNDS**

FIRST HEART SOUND (S_1)	SECOND HEART SOUND (S_2)
High-pitched	High-pitched
Loudest in mitral area (apex)	Loudest in aortic area (base)

SPLIT S_1	SPLIT S_2
Normal split less than 20 msec	Normal split less than 30 msec
Split heard best in tricuspid area	Split heard best in pulmonic area
Important to differentiate between split S_1 and S_4	↑ Split with inhalation
Occurs immediately before carotid upstroke	↓ Split with exhalation

↑, increased; ↓, decreased.

pulmonic valve closure occurs after the aortic valve closure. Pathological splitting of S_1 and S_2 is associated with specific cardiovascular conditions such as pulmonary hypertension, pulmonic stenosis, right ventricular failure, and with electrical conduction disturbances such as right bundle branch block and premature ventricular contractions.

Identifying Abnormal Heart Sounds, Murmurs, and Pericardial Rubs

Third and Fourth Heart Sounds. The abnormal heart sounds are known as the third heart sound (S_3) and the fourth heart sound (S_4); they are referred to as gallops when auscultated during an episode of tachycardia. These low-pitched sounds occur during diastole and are best heard with the bell of the stethoscope positioned lightly over the apical impulse. The characteristics of S_3 and S_4 are detailed in Box 11-9. The presence of S_3 may be normal in children, young adults, and pregnant women because of rapid filling of the ventricle in a young, healthy heart.[28] However, an S_3 in the presence of cardiac symptoms is an indicator of heart failure in a noncompliant ventricle with fluid overload.[29] Not unexpectedly, the development of an S_3 heart sound is strongly associated with elevated levels of brain natriuretic peptide (BNP).[29,30]

Auscultation of an S_4 also leads the examiner to suspect heart failure and decreased ventricular compliance. An S_4, also referred to as an atrial gallop, occurs at the end of diastole (just before S_1), when the ventricle is full. The sound is associated with atrial contraction, also called atrial kick.

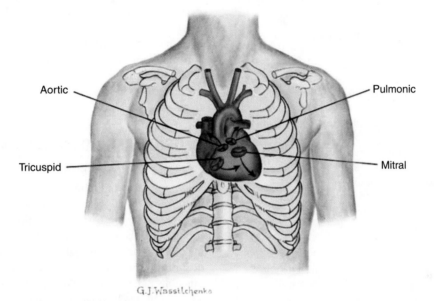

Aortic

Pulmonic

Tricuspid

Mitral

G.J.Wassilchenko

FIGURE 11-6 Transmission of heart sounds to the thorax and their relationship to the anatomic position of the heart valves.

BOX 11-9 CHARACTERISTICS OF THE THIRD AND FOURTH HEART SOUNDS

Third Heart Sound (S_3)

Physiological Causes
- Related to diastolic motion and rapid filling of ventricles in early diastole
- Can be normal in children and young adults (<40 yr)

Pathological Causes
- Ventricular dysfunction with an increase in end-systolic volume (MI, heart failure, valvular disease
- Systemic or pulmonary hypertension)
- Hyperdynamic states (anemia, thyrotoxicosis, mitral or tricuspid regurgitation)

Rhythmic Word Association
- Kentucky: S_1, S_2, S_3

Synonyms
- Ventricular gallop
- Protodiastolic gallop

Fourth Heart Sound (S_4)
- Related to diastolic motion and ventricular dilation with atrial contraction in late diastole
- May occur with or without cardiac decompensation
- Ventricular hypertrophy with a decrease in ventricular compliance (CAD, systemic hypertension, cardiomyopathy, aortic or pulmonary stenosis, increase in intensity with acute MI or angina)
- Hyperkinetic states (anemia, thyrotoxicosis, arteriovenous fistula)
- Acute valvular regurgitation

Rhythmic Word Association
- Tennessee: S_4, S_1, S_2

Synonyms
- Atrial gallop
- Presystolic gallop

CAD, coronary artery disease; *MI,* myocardial infarction.

BOX 11-10	TECHNIQUE OF AUSCULTATION OF HEART SOUNDS AND MURMURS

1. Stethoscope
   - Diaphragm
     Larger surface area
     Brings out higher frequency and filters out low frequency
     Use for listening to S_1/S_2 (split S_1/S_2), loud murmurs, pericardial friction rubs
   - Bell
     Smaller surface area
     Filters out high-frequency sounds and accentuates low-frequency sounds
     Rest lightly on area (or else it becomes a diaphragm)
2. Location: heart sounds auscultated at APTM
   A: aortic area (second right ICS along sternal border)
   P: pulmonic area (second left ICS along sternal border)
   T: tricuspid area (fourth left ICS along sternal border)
   M: mitral area (fifth ICS at MCL)
3. "Know your bases"
   - Base of the heart refers to the right and left second ICS beside the sternum S_2 where the aortic or pulmonic sounds are auscultated
   - Apex or left ventricular area refers to the fifth ICS along the MCL
     Most commonly referred to as the PMI
     Also referred to as the mitral area
     S_1 and mitral sounds are loudest here
   - Erb's point: second aortic area (third left ICS along sternal border); pericardial friction rubs are heard best here
4. Palpation
   - Location
   - Palpate carotid pulse (or watch ECG to identify S_1 and S_2)
5. Be quiet and patient!
   - Listen for S_1 and S_2 first, ignoring all other sounds
   - Inching technique
   - After you are sure which is S_1 or S_2, try to determine when the other sound comes in
   - Is it systolic or diastolic?
   - S_3 and S_4 are best heard with patient in left lateral decubitus position. Notice the location (suggests origin of sound)
   - Notice the timing (S_4 comes just before S_1, and S_3 comes just after S_2)
6. Interpret the sounds based on the clinical condition

ECG, electrocardiogram; *ICS,* intercostal space; *MCL,* midclavicular line; *PMI,* point of maximal impulse.

Heart Murmurs. *Heart valve murmurs* are prolonged extra sounds that occur during systole or diastole. Murmurs are produced by turbulent blood flow through the chambers of the heart, which results in vibrations that occur during systole or diastole. Most murmurs are caused by structural cardiac changes. The steps to effectively and accurately auscultate for cardiac murmurs are listed in Box 11-10. Murmurs are characterized by specific criteria:

- *Timing:* place in the cardiac cycle (systole/diastole)
- *Location:* where it is auscultated on the chest wall (mitral/aortic area)
- *Radiation:* how far the sound spreads across chest wall
- *Quality:* whether the murmur is blowing, grating, or harsh
- *Pitch:* whether the tone is high or low
- *Intensity:* the loudness is graded on a scale of 1 through 6; the higher the number, the louder the murmur.

Pericardial Friction Rub. A pericardial friction rub is a sound that can occur within 2 to 7 days after a myocardial infarction. The friction rub results from pericardial inflammation (pericarditis). Classically, a pericardia friction rub is a grating or scratching sound that is both systolic and diastolic, corresponding with cardiac motion within the pericardial sac. It is often associated with chest pain, which can be aggravated by deep inspiration, coughing, swallowing, and changing position. It is important to differentiate pericarditis from acute myocardial ischemia, and the detection of a pericardial friction rub through auscultation can assist in this differentiation, leading to effective diagnosis and treatment.

BEDSIDE HEMODYNAMIC MONITORING

Hemodynamic monitoring is at a critical juncture. The technology that launched invasive hemodynamic monitoring is more than 30 years old, and the search to find viable replacement monitoring technologies that are minimal or noninvasive is intense. This has created a new challenge in critical care. Although the use of invasive therapies is declining, they are still employed for hemodynamically unstable patients. Critical care nurses must be knowledgeable about traditional hemodynamic monitoring methods and be able to apply established physiological principles in new situations. As the technology evolves, the critical care nurse will apply the same physiological principles to the new methods to ensure safety and optimal outcomes for each patient.

Equipment

A traditional hemodynamic monitoring system has four component parts, as shown in Figure 11-7 and described in the following list:

1. An invasive catheter and high-pressure tubing connect the patient to the transducer.
2. The transducer receives the physiological signal from the catheter and tubing and converts it into electrical energy.
3. The flush system maintains patency of the fluid-filled system and catheter.
4. The bedside monitor contains the amplifier with recorder, which increases the volume of the electrical signal and displays it on an oscilloscope and on a digital scale in millimeters of mercury (mm Hg).

Although many different types of invasive catheters can be inserted to monitor hemodynamic pressures, all such

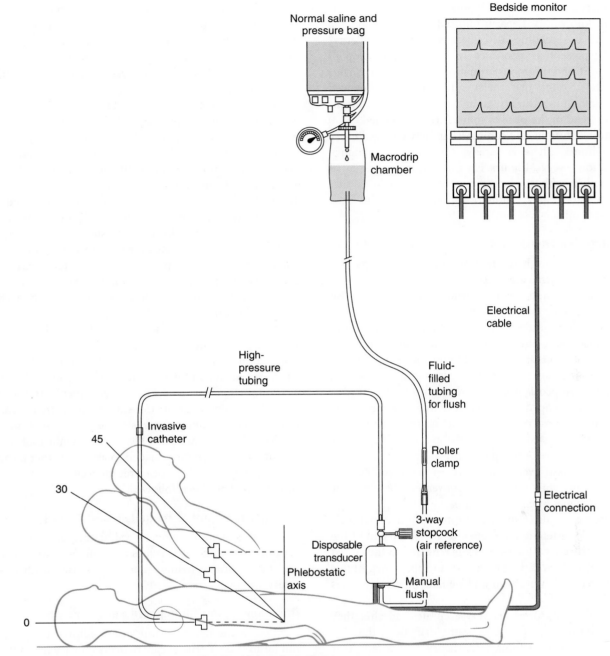

FIGURE 11-7 The four parts of hemodynamic monitoring include an invasive catheter attached to high-pressure tubing to connect to the transducer; a transducer; a flush system, including a manual flush; and a bedside monitor.

catheters are connected to similar equipment (see Figure 11-7). Even so, there remains considerable variation in the way different hospitals configure their hemodynamic systems. The basic setup consists of the following:

- A bag of 0.9% sodium chloride (normal saline) is used as a flush solution. In some hospitals heparin is added as an anticoagulant. A pressure infusion cuff covers the bag of flush solution and is inflated to 300 mm Hg.
- The system contains intravenous tubing, three-way stopcocks, and an in-line flow device attached for continuous fluid infusion and manual flush. High-pressure tubing

must be used to connect the invasive catheter to the transducer to prevent damping (flattening) of the waveform.
- A pressure transducer is used. Modern transducers are disposable, use a silicon chip, and are highly accurate.

Heparin

The use of the anticoagulant heparin added to the normal saline (NS) flush setup to maintain catheter patency remains controversial. A systematic review of the literature showed that a heparinized flush solution is associated with a longer duration of catheter patency.[31] Other units do not use heparin because of concern about development of the autoimmune condition known as heparin-induced thrombocytopenia (HIT). This is sometimes described as a "heparin allergy" and, when present, is associated with a dramatic drop in platelet count, and thrombus formation. Some trials have not found platelet counts or catheter duration to be influenced by heparin.[32,33] If heparin is used in the flush infusion, monitoring the trend in the platelet count is recommended.[34]

The flush solutions and tubing are usually changed every 72 to 96 hours. There is variety; some hospitals change flush solutions every 24 hours. For this reason, it is essential to be familiar with the specific written procedures that concern hemodynamic monitoring equipment in each critical care unit.

Calibrating Hemodynamic Monitoring Equipment

To ensure accuracy of hemodynamic pressure readings, two baseline measurements are necessary:

1. Calibration of the system to atmospheric pressure, also known as *zeroing the transducer*
2. Determination of the phlebostatic axis for transducer height placement, also called *leveling the transducer*[35]

Zeroing the Transducer. To calibrate the equipment to atmospheric pressure, referred to as zeroing the transducer, the three-way stopcock nearest to the transducer is turned simultaneously to open the transducer to air (atmospheric pressure) and to close it to the patient and the flush system. The monitor is adjusted so that "0" is displayed, which equals atmospheric pressure. Atmospheric pressure is not zero; it is 760 mm Hg at sea level. Using zero to represent current atmospheric pressure provides a convenient baseline for hemodynamic measurement purposes.

Some monitors also require calibration of the upper scale limit while the system remains open to air. At the end of the calibration procedure, the stopcock is returned to the closed position and a closed cap is placed over the open port. At this point, the patient's waveform and hemodynamic pressures are displayed.

Disposable transducers are very accurate, and after they are calibrated to atmospheric pressure, drift from the zero baseline is minimal. Although in theory this means that repeated calibration is unnecessary, clinical protocols in most units require the nurse to calibrate the transducer at the beginning of each shift for quality assurance.

Phlebostatic Axis. The phlebostatic axis is an external physical reference point on the chest that is used to ensure consistent transducer height placement. To obtain the axis, a theoretic line is drawn from the fourth intercostal space (ICS), where it joins the sternum to a midaxillary line on the side of the chest. The midaxillary line is one half of the anteroposterior (AP) depth of the lateral chest wall.[35] This line approximates the level of the atria, as shown in Figure 11-7. The phlebostatic axis is used as the reference mark for central venous pressure (CVP) and pulmonary artery catheter transducers. The level of the transducer approximates the level of the tip of an invasive hemodynamic monitoring catheter within the chest.

Leveling the Transducer. Leveling the transducer is different from zeroing. This process aligns the transducer with the level of the left atrium. The purpose is to line up the air-fluid interface with the left atrium to correct for changes in hydrostatic pressure in blood vessels above and below the level of the heart.[35]

A carpenter's level or laser-light level can be used to ensure that the transducer is parallel with the phlebostatic axis reference point. When there is a change in the patient's position, the transducer must be leveled again to ensure accurate hemodynamic pressure measurements are obtained.[35] Errors in measurement can occur if the transducer is placed above or below the phlebostatic axis.[36] If the transducer is placed below this level, the fluid in the system weighs on the transducer, creating additional hydrostatic pressure, to produce a falsely high reading. For every inch the transducer is below the tip of the catheter, the fluid pressure in the system increases the measurement by 1.87 mm Hg. For example, if the transducer is positioned 6 inches below the tip of the catheter, this falsely elevates the displayed pressure by 11 mm Hg.

If the transducer is placed above this atrial level, gravity and lack of fluid pressure will give an erroneously low reading. For every inch the transducer is positioned above the catheter tip, the measurement is 1.87 mm Hg less than the true value. If several clinicians are taking measurements, the reference point can be marked on the side of the patient's chest to ensure accurate measurements.[35] The American Association of Critical-Care Nurses (AACN) has an audit tool on their website that can be downloaded to assess whether all appropriate quality assurance measures for accurate hemodynamic monitoring have been followed.[37]

Recognizing Normal Hemodynamic Values

Once the system is correctly calibrated, the clinical team uses the known normal values as a reference when evaluating the patient's hemodynamic response to therapeutic interventions.

Accommodating Changes in Patient Position

Position of the hemodynamically monitored patient would not be an issue if critical care patients only lay flat in the bed. However, lying flat is not always a comfortable position, especially if the patient is alert or if the head of the bed needs to be elevated to decrease the work of breathing.

Head-of-Bed Position. Nurse researchers have determined that the CVP, pulmonary artery pressure (PAP), and pulmonary artery occlusion pressure (PAOP, also called pulmonary artery wedge pressure [PAWP]) can be reliably measured at head-of-bed positions from 0 (flat) to 60 degrees if the patient is lying on his or her back (supine).[35] If the patient is normovolemic and hemodynamically stable, raising the head of the bed usually does not affect hemodynamic pressure measurements. If the patient is so hemodynamically unstable or hypovolemic that raising the angle of the head of the bed negatively affects intravascular volume distribution, the first priority is to correct the hemodynamic instability and leave the patient in a supine position. In summary, most patients do not need the head of the bed to be lowered to 0 degrees (flat) to obtain accurate CVP, PAP, or PAOP readings.

Lateral Position. The landmarks for leveling the transducer are different if the patient is turned to the side. Researchers have evaluated hemodynamic pressure measurement readings with patients positioned in 30- and 90-degree lateral positions, with the head of the bed flat. The following transducer landmarks are recommended to achieve reliable measurements:[35]

- 30-degree lateral position: level the transducer at one half of the distance from the surface of the bed to the left sternal border.[35]
- 90-degree <u>right</u>-lateral position: level the transducer at the fourth ICS at the mid-sternum.[35]
- 90-degree <u>left</u>-lateral position: level the transducer at the fourth ICS at the left parasternal border (beside the sternum).[35]

It is important to know that measurements can be recorded in lateral positions, because critically ill patients must be turned to prevent development of pressure ulcers and other complications of immobility.

Establishing Safe Monitor Alarm Limits

All bedside hemodynamic monitoring systems have alarm limits that are preset to ensure patient safety. The alarms must be sufficiently distinctive and audible to be heard over the noise of a typical critical care unit. Patient safety guidelines are designed to promote clinical alarm goals. Some clinical situations create special challenges with respect to alarm safety. Nursing care actions that cause the patient to move in the bed will often trigger the alarms. Temporarily silencing the sound for 1 to 3 minutes while continuing to observe the bedside monitor is appropriate. The real challenge occurs when a patient is restless or fidgeting with IV tubing or electrodes, resulting in the alarms bring constantly triggered because the monitor is unable to evaluate the ECG rhythms and hemodynamic waveforms effectively. It is tempting to silence these "nuisance alarms" permanently. The alarms should not be turned off, however, because the patient is left in a vulnerable position if a dysrhythmia or hemodynamic complication arises. Clinical interventions to ameliorate the root cause of the problem (e.g., restlessness) are more appropriate. Education of nurses about the risk of becoming desensitized to the sound of beside alarms is also important.[38] Key issues concerning monitor alarms are presented in the Patient Safety Priorities box on Clinical Alarms.

Solving Hemodynamic Equipment Problems

Typical problems with bedside monitoring equipment and nursing measures to ensure patient safety and troubleshoot equipment problems are addressed in Table 11-3.

⚡ PATIENT SAFETY PRIORITIES

Clinical Alarms

Clinical Alarm System Effectiveness
1. Implement regular preventive maintenance and testing of alarm systems.
2. Ensure that alarms are activated with appropriate settings and are sufficiently audible with respect to distances and competing noise within the unit.

Clinical Alarm Safety
Alarm Identification
1. Audible and visual indication should be present for any condition that poses a risk to the patient. Indicators should be visible from at least 10 feet (3 m).
2. Cause of the alarm must be easily identifiable by the health care practitioner.
3. Life-threatening conditions should be clearly differentiated from noncritical alarm situations.
4. High-priority alarms should override low-priority alarms.
5. Alarm must be sufficiently loud or distinctive to be heard over the environmental noise of a busy critical care unit.
6. It should never be possible to turn the volume control off.

Disabling and Silencing Alarms
1. Alarm silence must have visual indicator to clearly show it is disabled.
2. Critical alarms should not be permanently overridden (turned off).
3. New, life-threatening alarm conditions should override a silenced alarm.

Power
Battery units should initiate an alarm before a unit stops working effectively.

Alarm Limits
1. Alarm limits can be adjusted to meet the clinical needs of a patient. The system should default to standard settings between patients.
2. It is preferable for alarm limits to be displayed on the monitor.

Data from www.jointcommission.org/ and Critical alarms and patient safety; ECRI's guide to developing effective alarm strategies and responding to JCAHO's alarm-safety goal, *Health Devices* 31(11):397–412, 2002; O'Grady NP, et al: Guidelines for the prevention of intravascular catheter-related infections, *Am J Infect Control* 30(8):476, 2002; Boyce JM, et al: Guideline for Hand Hygiene in Health-Care Settings. Recommendations of the Healthcare Infection Control Practices Advisory Committee and the HIPAC/SHEA/APIC/IDSA Hand Hygiene Task Force, *Am J Infect Control* 30(8):S1, 2002. Institute for Healthcare Improvement (IHI) Implement the Central Line Bundle (website) www.ihi.org/IHI/Topics/CriticalCare/IntensiveCare/Changes/ImplementtheCentralLineBundle.htm (accessed January 2011).

TABLE 11-3 **NURSING MEASURES TO ENSURE PATIENT SAFETY AND TO TROUBLESHOOT PROBLEMS WITH HEMODYNAMIC MONITORING EQUIPMENT**

PROBLEM	PREVENTION	RATIONALE	TROUBLESHOOTING
Overdamping of waveform	Provide continuous infusion of solution containing heparin through an in-line flush device (1 unit of heparin for each 1 mL of flush solution).	Ensure that recorded pressures and waveform are accurate because a damped waveform gives inaccurate readings.	Before insertion, completely flush the line and/or catheter. In a line attached to a patient, back flush through the system to clear bubbles from tubing or transducer.
Underdamping ("overshoot" or "fling")	Use short lengths of noncompliant tubing. Use fast-flush square wave test to demonstrate optimal system damping. Verify arterial waveform accuracy with the cuff blood pressure.	If the monitoring system is underdamped, the systolic and diastolic values will be overestimated by the waveform and the digital values. False high systolic values may lead to clinical decisions based on erroneous data.	Perform the fast-flush square wave test to verify optimal damping of the monitoring system.
Clot formation at end of the catheter	Provide continuous infusion of solution containing heparin through an in-line flush device (1 unit of heparin for each 1 mL of flush solution).	Any foreign object placed in the body can cause local activation of the patient's coagulation system as a normal defense mechanism. The clots that are formed may be dangerous if they break off and travel to other parts of the body.	If a clot in the catheter is suspected because of a damped waveform or resistance to forward flush of the system, gently aspirate the line using a small syringe inserted into the proximal stopcock. Flush the line again after the clot is removed, and inspect the waveform. It should return to a normal pattern.
Hemorrhage	Use Luer-lock (screw) connections in line setup. Close and cap stopcocks when not in use. Ensure that the catheter is sutured or securely taped in position.	A loose connection or open stopcock creates a low-pressure sump effect, causing blood to back into the line and into the open air. If a catheter is accidentally removed, the vessel can bleed profusely, especially with an arterial line or if the patient has abnormal coagulation factors (resulting from heparin in the line) or has hypertension.	After a blood leak is recognized, tighten all connections, flush the line, and estimate blood loss. If the catheter has been inadvertently removed, put pressure on the cannulation site. When bleeding has stopped, apply a sterile dressing, estimate blood loss, and inform the physician. If the patient is restless, an arm board may protect lines inserted in the arm.
Air emboli	Ensure that all air bubbles are purged from a new line setup before attachment to an indwelling catheter. Ensure that the drip chamber from the bag of flush solution is more than one-half full before using the in-line, fast-flush system. Some sources recommend removing all air from the bag of flush solution before assembling the system.	Air can be introduced at several times, including when central venous pressure (CVP) tubing comes apart, when a new line setup is attached, or when a new CVP or pulmonary artery (PA) line is inserted. During insertion of a CVP or PA line, the patient may be asked to hold his or her breath at specific times to prevent drawing air into the chest during inhalation. The in-line, fast-flush devices are designed to permit clearing of blood from the line after withdrawal of blood samples. If the chamber of the intravenous tubing is too low or empty, the rapid flow of fluid will create turbulence and cause flushing of air bubbles into the system and into the bloodstream.	Because it is impossible to get the air back after it has been introduced into the bloodstream, prevention is the best cure. If air bubbles occur, they must be vented through the in-line stopcocks and the drip chamber must be filled. The left atrial pressure (LAP) line setup is the only system that includes an air filter specifically to prevent air emboli.

TABLE 11-3	NURSING MEASURES TO ENSURE PATIENT SAFETY AND TO TROUBLESHOOT PROBLEMS WITH HEMODYNAMIC MONITORING EQUIPMENT—cont'd		
PROBLEM	**PREVENTION**	**RATIONALE**	**TROUBLESHOOTING**
Normal waveform with *low* digital pressure	Ensure that the system is calibrated to atmospheric pressure. Ensure that the transducer is placed at the level of the phlebostatic axis.	To provide a 0 baseline relative to atmospheric pressure. If the transducer has been placed *higher* than the phlebostatic level, gravity and the lack of hydrostatic pressure will produce a false *low* reading.	Recalibrate the equipment if transducer drift has occurred. Reposition the transducer at the level of the phlebostatic axis. Misplacement can occur if the patient moves from the bed to the chair or if the bed is placed in a Trendelenburg position.
Normal waveform with *high* digital pressure	Ensure that the system is calibrated to atmospheric pressure. Ensure that the transducer is placed at the level of the phlebostatic axis.	To provide a 0 baseline relative to atmospheric pressure. If the transducer has been placed *lower* than the phlebostatic level, the weight of hydrostatic pressure on the transducer will produce a false *high* reading.	Recalibrate the equipment if transducer drift has occurred. Reposition the transducer at the level of the phlebostatic axis. This situation can occur if the head of the bed was raised and the transducer was not repositioned. Some centers require attachment of the transducer to the patient's chest to avoid this problem.
Loss of waveform	Always have the hemodynamic waveform monitored so that changes or loss can be quickly noted.	The catheter may be kinked, or a stopcock may be turned off.	Check the line setup to ensure that all stopcocks are turned in the correct position and that the tubing is not kinked. Sometimes, the catheter migrates against a vessel wall, and having the patient change position restores the waveform.

Intraarterial Blood Pressure Monitoring

Indications

Intraarterial blood pressure monitoring is indicated for any major medical or surgical condition that compromises cardiac output (CO), tissue perfusion, or fluid volume status. The system is designed for continuous measurement of three blood pressure parameters: systole, diastole, and mean arterial blood pressure (MAP). The direct arterial access is helpful in the management of patients with acute respiratory failure who require frequent arterial blood gas measurements.

Catheters

The size of the catheter used is proportionate to the diameter of the cannulated artery. In small arteries—such as the radial and dorsalis pedis—a 20-gauge, 3.8-cm to 5.1-cm, nontapered catheter is used most often. If the larger femoral or axillary arteries are used, a 19- or 20-gauge, 16-cm catheter is used.

The catheter insertion is usually percutaneous, although the technique varies with vessel size. Catheters are most often inserted in the smaller arteries, using a "catheter-over-needle" unit in which the needle is used as a temporary guide for catheter placement. With this method, after the unit has been inserted into the artery, the needle is withdrawn, leaving the supple plastic catheter in place. Insertion of a catheter into a larger artery typically uses the Seldinger technique, which involves the following steps:

1. Entry into the artery using a needle
2. Passage of a supple guidewire through the needle into the artery
3. Removal of the needle
4. Passage of the catheter over the guidewire
5. Removal of the guidewire, leaving the catheter in the artery

Insertion and Allen Test. Several major peripheral arteries are suitable for receiving a catheter and for long-term hemodynamic monitoring. The most frequently used site is the radial artery. The femoral artery is a larger vessel that is also frequently cannulated. Other smaller arterials such as the dorsalis-pedis, axillary, or brachial arteries are avoided if possible, and only used when other arterial access is unavailable.

The major advantage of the radial artery is the supply of collateral circulation to the hand provided by the ulnar artery through the palmar arch, in most of the population. Before radial artery cannulation, collateral circulation must be assessed by using Doppler flow or by the Allen test, according to institutional protocol.[39-41] In the Allen test the radial and ulnar arteries are compressed simultaneously. The patient is asked to clench and unclench the hand until it blanches.

One of the arteries is then released, and the hand should immediately flush from that side. The same procedure is repeated for the remaining artery. Bedside ultrasound is increasingly used to increase the accuracy of catheter placement. If the catheter is placed on the first pass, this is both safer and more comfortable for the patient. The use of ultrasound to identify the radial artery prior to cannulation has been shown to increase first-pass placement accuracy.[42]

Nursing Management

Nursing priorities for the patient with intraarterial monitoring focus on (1) assessing arterial perfusion pressures, (2) interpreting the accuracy of the arterial pressure waveform, and (3) troubleshooting arterial waveform problems.

Intraarterial blood pressure monitoring is designed for continuous assessment of arterial perfusion to the major organ systems of the body. MAP is the clinical parameter most often used to assess perfusion, because MAP represents perfusion pressure throughout the cardiac cycle. Because one third of the cardiac cycle is spent in systole and two thirds in diastole, the MAP calculation must reflect the greater amount of time spent in diastole. This MAP formula can be calculated by hand or with a calculator, where diastole times 2 plus systole is divided by 3 as shown in the formula below:

$$(Diastole \times 2) + (Systole \times 1) \div 3 = MAP$$

A blood pressure of 120/60 mm Hg produces a MAP of 80 mm Hg. However, the bedside hemodynamic monitor may show a slightly different digital number because most computers calculate the area under the curve of the arterial line tracing (normal values listed in Table 11-4). The MAP represents an estimate of organ perfusion pressure.[43]

Assessing Arterial Perfusion Pressures. A MAP greater than 60 mm Hg is necessary to perfuse the coronary arteries. A higher MAP may be required to perfuse the brain and the kidneys. A MAP between 70 and 90 mm Hg is ideal for the cardiac patient to decrease left ventricular (LV) workload. After a carotid endarterectomy or neurosurgery, a MAP of 90 to 110 mm Hg may be more appropriate to increase cerebral perfusion pressure. Systolic and diastolic pressures are monitored in conjunction with the MAP as a further guide to the accuracy of perfusion. If CO decreases, the body compensates by constricting peripheral vessels to maintain the blood pressure. In this situation, the MAP may remain constant but the pulse pressure (difference between systolic and diastolic pressures) narrows. The following examples explain this point:

Mr. A: BP, 90/70 mm Hg; MAP, 76 mm Hg
Mr. B: BP, 150/40 mm Hg; MAP, 76 mm Hg

Both patients have a perfusion pressure of 76 mm Hg, but they are clinically very different. Mr. A is peripherally vasoconstricted, as is demonstrated by the narrow pulse pressure (90/70 mm Hg). His skin is cool to the touch, and he has weak peripheral pulses. Mr. B has a wide pulse pressure (150/40 mm Hg), warm skin, and palpable peripheral pulses.

Nursing assessment of the patient with an arterial line includes comparison of clinical findings with arterial line readings, including perfusion pressure and MAP.

Interpreting Arterial Pressure Waveforms. As the aortic valve opens, blood is ejected from the left ventricle and is recorded as an increase of pressure in the arterial system. The highest point recorded is called systole. After peak ejection (systole), the ejection force decreases, and the pressure decreases as a result, as seen on the waveform. A notch (dicrotic notch) may be visible on the downstroke of the arterial waveform, representing closure of the aortic valve. The dicrotic notch signifies the beginning of diastole. The remainder of the downstroke represents diastolic runoff of blood flow into the arterial tree. The lowest point recorded is called diastole. A normal arterial pressure tracing is shown in Figure 11-8. Time is measured from left to right on the waveform tracing. Notice that electrical stimulation (QRS) always comes first, and that the arterial pressure tracing follows the initiating QRS. If the arterial line becomes unreliable or dislodged, a cuff pressure can be used as a reserve system.[44]

Troubleshooting Arterial Pressure Monitoring Problems. Major complications associated with arterial pressure monitoring are rare. The most life-threatening risk is exsanguination if the Luer-Lock connections are not tight or if an in-line stopcock is inadvertently opened to air. Pressure monitor alarms must always be on, with alarm limits (high and low) set at a safe, audible warning range for each patient. When the arterial monitor displays a low blood pressure digital reading, it is a nursing responsibility to determine whether this is a true patient problem, or a problem with the monitoring equipment. A damped waveform occurs when communication from the artery to the transducer is interrupted and produces false values on the monitor and oscilloscope. Troubleshooting techniques are used to find the origin of the problem and to remove the cause of damping (see Table 11-3).

Fast-Flush Square Waveform Test. The monitoring system's dynamic response can be verified for accuracy at the bedside by the *fast-flush square waveform test,* also called the *dynamic frequency response test.*[35] The nurse performs this test to ensure that the patient pressures and waveform shown on the bedside monitor are accurate.[35] The test makes use of the manual flush system on the transducer. Normally, the flush device allows only 3 mL of fluid/hr. With the normal waveform displayed, the manual fast-flush procedure is used to generate a rapid increase in pressure, which is displayed on the monitor oscilloscope. As shown in Figure 11-9, the normal dynamic response waveform shows a square pattern with one or two oscillations before the return of the arterial waveform. If the system is overdamped, a sloped (rather than square) pattern is seen. If the system is underdamped, additional oscillations—or vibrations—are seen on the fast-flush square wave test. This test can be performed with any hemodynamic monitoring system. If air bubbles, clots, or kinks are in the system, the waveform becomes damped, or flattened, and this is reflected in the square waveform result.

TABLE 11-4 HEMODYNAMIC PRESSURES AND CALCULATED HEMODYNAMIC VALUES

HEMODYNAMIC PRESSURE	DEFINITION AND EXPLANATION	NORMAL RANGE
Mean arterial pressure (MAP)	Average perfusion pressure created by arterial blood pressure during the cardiac cycle. The normal cardiac cycle is one third systole and two thirds diastole. These three components are divided by 3 to obtain the average perfusion pressure for the whole cardiac cycle.	70-100 mm Hg
Central venous pressure (CVP)	Pressure created by volume in the right side of the heart. When the tricuspid valve is open, the CVP reflects filling pressures in the right ventricle. Clinically, the CVP is often used as a guide to overall fluid balance.	2-5 mm Hg 3-8 cm water (H_2O)
Left atrial pressure (LAP)	Pressure created by the volume in the left side of the heart. When the mitral valve is open, the LAP reflects filling pressures in the left ventricle. Clinically, the LAP is used after cardiac surgery to determine how well the left ventricle is ejecting its volume. In general, the higher the LAP, the lower the ejection fraction from the left ventricle.	5-12 mm Hg
Pulmonary artery pressure (PAP) PA systolic (PAS) PA diastolic (PAD) PAP mean (PAP_M)	Pulsatile pressure in the pulmonary artery measured by an indwelling catheter.	PAS 20-30 mm Hg PAD 5-10 mm Hg PAP_M 10-15 mm Hg
Pulmonary artery occlusion pressure (PAOP)*	Pressure created by the volume in the left side of the heart. When the mitral valve is open, the PAOP reflects filling pressures in the pulmonary vasculature, and pressures in the left side of the heart are transmitted back to the catheter "wedged" into a small pulmonary arteriole.	5-12 mm Hg
Cardiac output (CO)	Amount of blood pumped out by a ventricle. Clinically, it can be measured using the thermodilution CO method, which calculates CO in liters per minute (L/min).	4-6 L/min (at rest)
Cardiac index (CI)	CO divided by the body surface area (BSA), with tailoring of CO to individual body size. A BSA conversion chart is necessary to calculate CI, which is considered more accurate than CO because it is individualized to height and weight. CI is measured in liters per minute per square meter of BSA (L/min/m²).	2.2-4.0 L/min/m²
Stroke volume (SV)	Amount of blood ejected by the ventricle with each heartbeat. Hemodynamic monitoring systems calculate SV by dividing cardiac output (CO in L/min) by the heart rate (HR) and then multiplying the answer by 1000 to change liters to milliliters (mL).	60-70 mL
Stroke volume index (SI)	SV indexed to the BSA.	40-50 mL/m2
Systemic vascular resistance (SVR)	Mean pressure difference across the systemic vascular bed divided by blood flow. Clinically, SVR represents the resistance against which the left ventricle must pump to eject its volume. This resistance is created by the systemic arteries and arterioles. As SVR increases, CO falls. SVR is measured in Wood units or dyn·sec·cm⁻⁵. If the number of Wood units is multiplied by 80, the value is converted to dyn·sec·cm⁻⁵.	10-18 Wood units or 100-250 dyn·sec·cm⁻⁵
Systemic vascular resistance index (SVRI)	SVR indexed to BSA.	2000-2400 dyn·sec·cm⁻⁵
Pulmonary vascular resistance (PVR)	Mean pressure difference across pulmonary vascular bed divided by blood flow. Clinically, PVR represents the resistance against which the right ventricle must pump to eject its volume. This resistance is created by the pulmonary arteries and arterioles. As PVR increases, the output from the right ventricle decreases. PVR is measured in Wood units or dyn·sec·cm⁻⁵. PVR is normally one sixth of SVR.	1.2-3.0 Wood units or 100-250 dyn·sec·cm⁻⁵
Pulmonary vascular resistance index (PVRI)	PVR indexed to BSA.	225-315 dyn·sec·cm⁻⁵/m²

*Pulmonary artery occlusion pressure (PAOP) was formerly called pulmonary capillary wedge pressure (PCW or PCWP) or pulmonary arterial wedge pressure (PAWP).

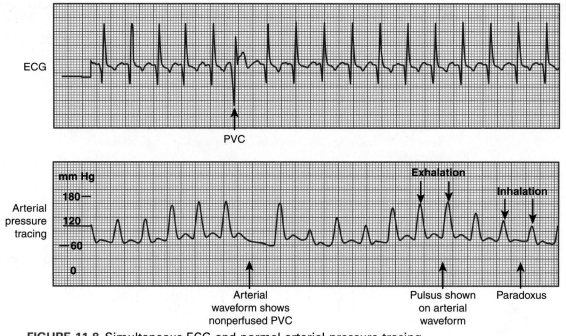

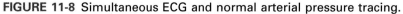

FIGURE 11-8 Simultaneous ECG and normal arterial pressure tracing.

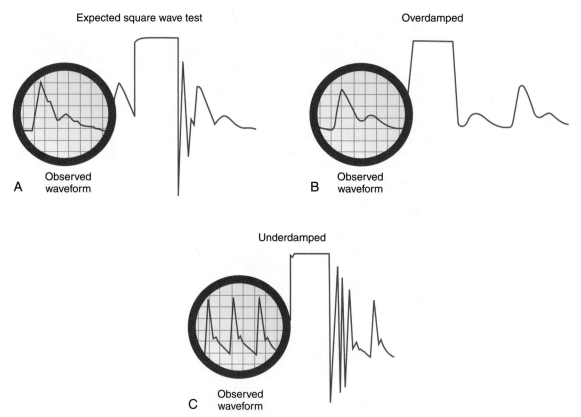

FIGURE 11-9 Square wave test. *A,* Expected square wave test result. *B,* Overdamped. *C,* Underdamped. (From Darovic GO: *Hemodynamic monitoring: invasive and noninvasive clinical application,* ed 3, Philadelphia, 2002, WB Saunders.)

This is an easy test to perform, and it should be incorporated into nursing care procedures at the bedside when the hemodynamic system is first set up, at least once per shift, after opening the system for any reason, and when there is concern about the accuracy of the waveform.[35] If the pressure waveform is distorted or the digital display is inaccurate, the troubleshooting methods described in Table 11-3 can be implemented. The nurse caring for the patient with an arterial line must be able to assess whether a low MAP or narrowed perfusion pressure represents decreased arterial perfusion or equipment malfunction. Assessment of the arterial waveform on the oscilloscope, in combination with clinical assessment and use of the square waveform test, will yield the answer.

Central Venous Pressure Monitoring

CVP monitoring is indicated whenever a patient has significant alteration in fluid volume. The CVP can be used as a guide in fluid volume replacement in hypovolemia and to assess the impact of diuresis after diuretic administration in the case of fluid overload. When a major intravenous line is required for volume replacement, a central venous catheter (CVC) is a good choice because large volumes of fluid can easily be delivered.

A range of CVC options are available as single-, double-, triple-, and quad-lumen infusion catheters, depending on the specific needs of the patient. CVCs are made from a variety of materials ranging from polyurethane to silicone; most are soft and flexible. Many catheters incorporate an antimicrobial coating to reduce the risk of bloodstream infections.[45]

Insertion

The large veins of the upper thorax—subclavian (SC) and internal jugular (IJ)—are most commonly used for percutaneous CVC line insertion. The femoral vein in the groin is used when the thoracic veins are not accessible. All three major sites have advantages and disadvantages.

Internal Jugular Vein. The IJ vein is the most frequently used access site for CVC insertion. Compared with the other thoracic veins, it is the easiest to canalize. If the IJ vein is not available, the external jugular (EJ) vein may be accessed, although blood flow is significantly higher in the IJ vein, making it the preferred site. Another advantage of the IJ vein is that the risk of creating an iatrogenic pneumothorax is small. Disadvantages to the IJ vein are patient discomfort from the indwelling catheter when moving the head or neck and contamination of the IJ vein site from oral or tracheal secretions, especially if the patient is intubated or has a tracheostomy. This may be the reason why catheter-related infections are higher in the IJ than the SC position for indwelling catheters left in place for more than 4 days.[46,47]

Subclavian Vein. If the anticipated CVC dwelling time is prolonged more than 5 days, the SC site is preferred. The SC position has the lowest infection rate and produces the least patient discomfort from the catheter. The disadvantages are that the SC vein is more difficult to access and carries a higher risk of iatrogenic pneumothorax or hemothorax, although the risk varies greatly, depending on the experience and skill of the physician inserting the catheter.

Femoral Vein. The femoral vein is considered the easiest cannulation site because there are no curves in the insertion route. The large diameter of the femoral vein carries a high blood flow that is advantageous for specialized procedures such as continuous renal replacement therapy (CRRT) or plasmapheresis. Disadvantages are that the patient cannot bend at the hip, because this interrupts blood flow through the catheter and may lead to thrombus formation; risk of retroperitoneal bleed; and a higher rate of nosocomial infections, probably due to site location near the groin area.[46]

During insertion of a catheter in the SC or IJ vein, the patient may be placed in a Trendelenburg position. Placing the head in a dependent position causes the IJ veins in the neck to become more prominent, facilitating line placement. To minimize the risk of air embolus during the procedure, the patient may be asked to "take a deep breath and hold it" any time the needle or catheter is open to air. The tip of the catheter is designed to remain in the vena cava and should not migrate into the right atrium. If the IJ or SC veins are not available, the femoral veins can be used for CVC access. The femoral veins are farther away from the heart; for accurate CVP measurements, the tip of the catheter must be advanced into the inferior vena cava near the right atrium. Because many patients are awake and alert when a CVC is inserted, a brief explanation about the procedure can minimize patient anxiety and result in cooperation during the insertion. This cooperation is important, because CVC insertion is a sterile procedure and because the supine or Trendelenburg position may not be comfortable for many patients. The electrocardiogram (ECG) should be monitored during CVC insertion because of the associated risk of dysrhythmias.

All central catheters are designed for placement by percutaneous injection after skin preparation and administration of a local anesthetic. A prepackaged CVC kit typically is used for the procedure. The standard CVC kit contains sterile towels, chlorhexidine and alcohol for skin preparation, a needle introducer, a syringe, guidewire, and a catheter. The Seldinger technique, in which the vein is located by using a "seeking" needle and syringe, is the preferred method of placement. A guidewire is passed through the needle, the needle is removed, and the catheter is passed over the guidewire. After the catheter is correctly placed in the vena cava, the guidewire is removed. A sterile intravenous tubing and solution is attached, and the catheter is sutured in place.

An important development in central venous catheter management is adherence to the Centers for Disease Control (CDC) and Institute for Healthcare Improvement (IHI) bundle approach to prevent blood stream infections. The CVC bundle places a strong emphasis upon infection control during insertion, to protect the patient. The IHI recommends meticulous hand hygiene, 2% chlorhexidine gluconate in 70% isopropyl patient skin preparation, full-barrier precautions for each CVC insertion, and optimal catheter site selection. In many hospitals the nurse is authorized to stop the procedure if these insertion infection control guidelines are not followed. A daily review to determine whether the catheter is still required is recommended to ensure CVCs are removed promptly when no longer needed.

After thoracic CVC placement, a chest radiograph is obtained to verify placement and the absence of an iatrogenic hemothorax or pneumothorax, especially if the SC vein was accessed. The use of Doppler ultrasound guidance to find the vein and guide insertion may reduce the incidence of iatrogenic complications.[46] In the very rare case when it is not possible to insert a CVC percutaneously, a surgical cutdown may be performed.

Nursing Management

Nursing priorities for the patient with CVP monitoring focus on (1) preventing central venous catheter-associated complications, (2) assessing fluid volume status, (3) accommodating changes in patient position, and (4) accurately interpreting the CVP waveforms and pressures.

Preventing Central Venous Catheter-Associated Complications. The CVC is an essential tool in care of the critically ill patient, but it is associated with some risks, and it is the responsibility of all clinicians to be informed about these hazards and to follow hospital procedures to avoid iatrogenic complications. CVC complications include air embolus, catheter-associated thrombus formation, and infection.

Air Embolus. The risk of air embolus, although uncommon, is always present for the patient with a central venous line in place. Air can enter during insertion[48] through a disconnected or broken catheter by means of an open stopcock,[49] or air can enter along the path of a removed CVC.[50] This is more likely if the patient is in an upright position, because air can be pulled into the venous system with the increase in negative intrathoracic pressure during inhalation. If a large volume of air is infused rapidly, it may become trapped in the right ventricular outflow tract, stopping blood flow from the right side of the heart to the lungs. Based on animal studies, this volume is approximately 4 mL/kg.[51] If the air embolus is large, the patient will experience respiratory distress and cardiovascular collapse. An auscultatory clinical sign specifically associated with a large venous air embolism is a mill wheel murmur.[49-51] A mill wheel murmur is a loud, churning sound heard over the middle chest, caused by the obstruction to right ventricular outflow. Treatment involves administering 100% oxygen and placing the patient on the left side with the head downward (left lateral Trendelenburg position).[49] This position displaces the air from the right ventricular outflow tract to the apex of the heart, where the air may be aspirated by catheter intervention or gradually absorbed by the bloodstream as the patient remains in the left lateral Trendelenburg position. Precautions to prevent an air embolism in a CVP line include using only screw (Luer-Lock) connections, avoiding long loops of intravenous tubing, and using closed-top screw caps on the three-way stopcock.

Thrombus Formation. Clot formation (thrombus) at the CVC site is unfortunately common. Ultrasound studies have found asymptomatic thrombus formation to be in the range of 33% to 67% when the catheter is in place for more than 7 days.[46] Symptomatic thrombi are reported in 0% to 5% of those cases.[46,47] Thrombus formation is not uniform; it may involve development of a fibrin sleeve around the catheter, or the thrombus may be attached directly to the vessel wall. Other factors that promote clot formation include rupture of vascular endothelium, interruption of laminar blood flow, and physical presence of the catheter, all of which activate the coagulation cascade. The risk of thrombus formation is higher if insertion was difficult or if there were multiple needlesticks.[46] Gradual thrombus formation may lead to "sudden" CVC occlusion. Usually, the CVC becomes more difficult to withdraw blood from, or the CVP waveform becomes intermittently damped over a period of hours or even 1 to 2 days and is reported as "needing frequent flushes" to remain patent. This situation is caused by the continued lengthening of a fibrin sleeve that extends along the catheter length from the insertion site past the catheter tip.[46,47] Some catheters are heparin coated to reduce the risk of thrombus formation, although the risk of HIT, reported to be 0.4% with indwelling CVC, does not make this a benign option.[47] Sometimes, CVC complications are additive; for example, the risk of catheter-related infection is increased in the presence of thrombi. The thrombus likely serves as a culture medium for bacterial growth.[47]

Infection. Infection related to the use of CVCs is a major problem. Risk factors for catheter-related infections include extremes of age, impaired host defense mechanisms, severe illness, malnutrition, and presence of other invasive lines. It is estimated that more than 50,000 infections related to CVC use occur annually in the United States, with associated mortality rates between 10% and 20%.[47]

The incidence of infection strongly correlates with the length of time the CVC has been inserted.[52] Catheters that are in place up to 3 days rarely lead to infection, provided that standard insertion and management procedures are followed. If the CVC remains between 3 and 7 days, the infection rate is 3% to 5%. Catheters remaining in one site more than 7 days have an infection rate of 5% to 10%.[47]

CVC-related infection is identified at the catheter insertion site or as a bloodstream infection (septicemia). Systemic manifestations of infection can be present without inflammation at the catheter site. In order to determine whether a suspect catheter is contaminated, after removal the tip may be placed in a sterile container and cultured. No decrease in infections was found when catheters were routinely changed to prevent infection, and this practice is no longer recommended.[53] A suspect CVC changed over a guidewire risks a higher rate of infection.[52,53] Prevention is the best defense against complications resulting from infections. Most infections are transmitted from the skin, and infection prevention begins prior to insertion of the CVC. Insertion guidelines state that the physician must use effective hand-washing procedures, clean the insertion site with 2% chlorhexidine gluconate in 70% isopropyl, use sterile technique during catheter insertion, and maintain maximal sterile barrier precautions (Patient Safety Priorities box on Prevention of Central Venous Catheter-Related Bloodstream Infections).[53]

⚡ PATIENT SAFETY PRIORITIES

Prevention of Central Venous Catheter-Related Bloodstream Infections

1. Education, Training, and Staffing
   a. Nurses and other health care providers should receive education about indications for central venous catheter (CVC) use, maintenance, and infection prevention.
   b. Only trained personnel should insert and maintain CVCs.
   c. Adequate staffing levels in ICUs are associated with fewer catheter related blood stream infections (CRBSI).
2. Selection of Catheters and Sites
   a. Use subclavian site rather than jugular or femoral insertion sites to minimize infection risk.
   b. Use ultrasound guidance to place CVCs.
   c. Remove any catheter that is no longer essential.
   d. If a CVC was placed in a medical emergency when aseptic technique was not assured, replace CVC within 48 hours.
3. Hand Hygiene and Aseptic Technique
   a. Perform hand hygiene procedures by washing hands with soap and water or alcohol-based hand rubs (ABHR) before and after palpating the CVC site, dressing the site or any other intervention.
   b. New sterile gloves must be worn by the professional inserting the CVC.
   c. New sterile gloves must be donned before touching a new catheter for CVC exchange over guidewire.
   d. Wear clean or sterile gloves when changing the catheter dressing.
4. Maximal Sterile Barrier Precautions
   a. For insertion, use maximal sterile barrier precautions including cap, mask, sterile gown, sterile gloves, and a full-body drape.
5. Skin Preparation
   a. Prepare clean skin with >0.5 chlorhexidine preparation with alcohol before CVC insertion.
   b. Antiseptics should be allowed to dry according to the manufacturer's recommendation before CVC insertion.
6. Catheter Site Dressing Regimens
   a. Transparent, semi-permeable polyurethane dressings permit continuous visualization of the CVC insertion site.
   b. Replace transparent dressings on CVC sites at least every 7 days.
   c. Monitor the site when changing the dressing or by palpation through an intact dressing.
   d. Replace catheter site dressing whenever the dressing becomes damp, loose, or soiled.
   e. Do not use topical antibiotic ointment or creams on insertion sites (except for dialysis catheters) because of increased fungal infection risk.
   f. Use a chlorhexidine-impregnated sponge dressing at CVC site if CRBSI rate is not decreasing by other means (no recommendation for other types of chlorhexidine dressings).
7. Patient Cleansing
   a. Use 2% chlorhexidine wash for daily skin cleaning to reduce CRBSI.
8. Catheter Securement Device
   a. Use a sutureless catheter securement device to reduce catheter movement, which may reduce infection risk.
9. Antimicrobial Strategies
   a. Use an antimicrobial impregnated CVC when catheters are expected to remain in place for longer than 5 days.
   b. Do not administer systemic antimicrobial prophylaxis to prevent CRBSI.
   c. Do not routinely use anticoagulant therapy to prevent CRBSI.
10. No Routine CVC Replacement
    a. Do not routinely replace CVCs.
    b. Do not replace CVCs on the basis of fever alone.

Data from: O'Grady P., et al. Guidelines for the prevention of intravascular catheter-related infections, *Am J Infect Control* 39 (4):S1-S34, 2011.

All clinicians must use good hand-washing technique and follow aseptic procedures during site care and any time the CVC system is entered to withdraw blood, give medications, or change tubing.[53,54] The infusion of high-dextrose solutions such as total parental nutrition (TPN) may be associated with an increased risk of infection. Methods to lower TPN-related complications include use of a single-lumen CVC that is not accessed for other medications or laboratory samples.

Incidence of infection is higher with use of occlusive site dressings that do not allow removal of moisture. Transparent, breathable dressings that allow removal of skin moisture are recommended. The use of chlorhexidine gluconate-impregnated dressings to cover the insertion site has recently been shown to reduce CVC-related bloodstream infections.[55] Additional improvements in catheter design may further reduce central line infection rates. Some catheters are impregnated with an antimicrobial substance[53] or have a silver-impregnated, tissue-barrier cuff attached to the catheter. These catheters are designed to lower the rate of CVC infection.

Assessing Fluid Volume Status. In the critically ill patient, the CVC is used to monitor CVP and waveform. The CVP catheter is used to measure the filling pressures of the right side of the heart. During diastole, when the tricuspid valve is open and blood is flowing from the right atrium to the right ventricle, the CVP accurately reflects right ventricular end-diastolic pressure (RVEDP). The normal CVP is 2 to 5 mm Hg (3 to 8 cm H_2O).

Low Central Venous Pressure. A low CVP often occurs in the hypovolemic patient and suggests that insufficient blood volume is in the ventricle at end-diastole to produce an adequate stroke volume. To maintain normal CO, the heart rate (HR) must increase. This HR increase produces the tachycardia often observed in hypovolemic states and increases myocardial oxygen demand.

The CVP is used in combination with the MAP and other clinical parameters to assess hemodynamic stability. In the hypovolemic patient, the CVP falls before a significant fall in MAP occurs, because peripheral vasoconstriction keeps the MAP normal. The CVP is an excellent early-warning system for the patient who is bleeding, vasodilating, receiving diuretics, or being rewarmed after cardiac surgery.

High Central Venous Pressure. An elevated CVP occurs in cases of fluid overload. To circulate the excess blood volume, the heart must greatly increase its contractile force to move the large volume of blood. This increases the cardiac workload and increases myocardial oxygen consumption. The critical care nurse follows the trend of the CVP measurements to determine subsequent interventions for optimal fluid volume management.

Central Venous Pressure Limitations. The CVP is not a reliable indicator of left ventricular dysfunction. LV dysfunction, which can occur after an acute myocardial infarction (MI), increases filling pressures on the left side of the heart. The CVP, because it measures RVEDP, remains normal until the increase in pressure from the left side of the heart is reflected back through the pulmonary vasculature to the right ventricle. In this situation, a pulmonary artery catheter that measures pressures on the left side of the heart is the monitoring method of choice. More information on PAP monitoring is provided later in this chapter.

Accommodating Changes in Patient Position. To achieve accurate CVP measurements, the phlebostatic axis is used as a reference point on the body, and the transducer or water manometer zero must be level with this point. If the phlebostatic axis is used and the transducer or water manometer is correctly aligned, any head-of-bed position of up to 60 degrees may be used for CVP accurate readings for most patients.[35] Elevating the head of the bed is especially helpful for the patient with respiratory or cardiac problems who cannot tolerate a flat position.

Interpreting the CVP Waveform. The normal right atrial (CVP) waveform has three positive deflections—a, c, and v waves—that correspond to specific atrial events in the cardiac cycle (Figure 11-10). The a wave reflects atrial contraction and follows the P wave seen on the ECG. The downslope of this wave is called the x descent and represents atrial relaxation. The c wave reflects the bulging of the closed tricuspid valve into the right atrium during ventricular contraction; this wave is small and not always visible, but corresponds to the QRS-T interval on the ECG. The v wave represents atrial filling and increased pressure against the closed tricuspid valve in early diastole. The downslope of the v wave is named the y descent and represents the fall in pressure as the tricuspid valve opens and blood flows from the right atrium to the right ventricle.

Cannon Waves. Dysrhythmias can change the pattern of the CVP waveform. In a junctional rhythm or following a PVC, the atria are depolarized after the ventricles. When retrograde conduction to the atria occurs, this produces a retrograde P wave on the ECG and a large combined *ac* or *cannon wave* on the CVP waveform (Figure 11-11). Cannon waves are clearly visible as large pulses in the jugular veins, and correspond to the cannon waves on the CVP tracing.

Specialized Central Venous Oximetry Catheters. A CVC that incorporates a fiberoptic sensor to continuously measure central venous oxygen saturation ($Scvo_2$) can be used as a traditional CVC and additionally can be used to follow the trend of venous oxygen saturation.[56,57] The physiology underlying use of this fiberoptic technology is discussed later in sections on monitoring mixed venous oxygen saturation (Svo_2) and $Scvo_2$.

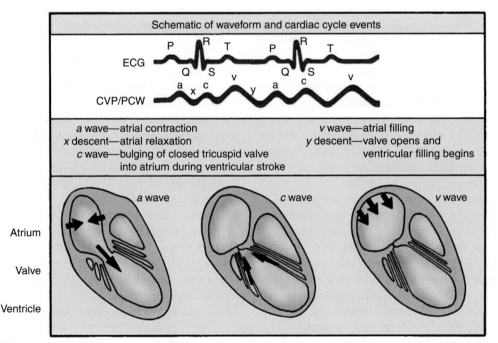

FIGURE 11-10 Cardiac events that produce the CVP waveform with *a, c,* and *v* waves. The *a* wave represents atrial contraction. The *x* descent represents atrial relaxation. The *c* wave represents the bulging of the closed tricuspid valve into the right atrium during ventricular systole. The *v* wave represents atrial filling. The *y* descent represents opening of the tricuspid valve and filling of the ventricle.

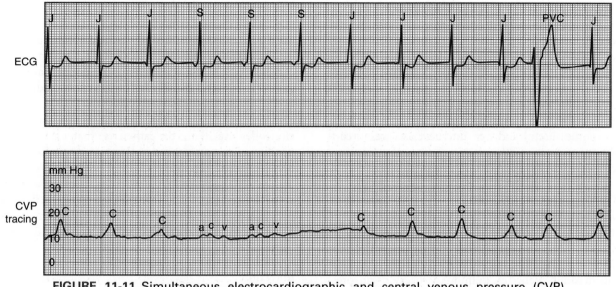

FIGURE 11-11 Simultaneous electrocardiographic and central venous pressure (CVP) tracings. The CVP waveform shows large cannon waves (*c* waves) corresponding to the junctional beats or premature ventricular contractions *(bottom strip)*. As the patient converts to sinus rhythm, the CVP waveform has a normal configuration. ac, normal right atrial pressure tracing; c, cannon waves on CVP tracing; J, junctional rhythm followed by cannon waves on CVP waveform; PVC, premature ventricular contraction followed by cannon wave on CVP; S, sinus rhythm followed by normal CVP tracing with *a*, *c*, and *v* waves.

Pulmonary Artery Pressure Monitoring

The pulmonary artery (PA) catheter is the most invasive of the critical care monitoring catheters. It is also known as a *right heart catheter* or *Swan-Ganz catheter* (named after the catheter's inventors). The practice of routinely using PA catheters has been called into question and is highly controversial. Several randomized, controlled trials of critically ill patients have not demonstrated a benefit to use of the PA catheter. A randomized, controlled trial of 676 critical care patients with acute respiratory distress syndrome (ARDS) in France reported no difference in mortality rates for patients when treatment was guided by PA catheter and for patients without this information.[58] A randomized, controlled trial of 1000 patients with acute lung injury in the United States found no difference in mortality rates for patients when treatment was guided by a PA catheter and those for whom diagnostic information was obtained from a CVP.[59]

The impact of PA catheterization on mortality rates for patients with acute heart failure has also been examined. A randomized, controlled trial of 433 patients with acute heart failure in the United States reported no difference in mortality based on whether fluid volume management was guided by PA catheter insertion or not.[60] Similar results were reported from a British multicenter trial enrolling more than 1000 critical care patients; there were no differences in mortality or in length of stay.[61,62] No survival benefit was found in a randomized, controlled trial enrolling older high-risk surgical patients who required critical care monitoring whether treatment was guided by PA catheter diagnostics or not.[63] Systematic reviews and meta-analysis of studies of PA catheter use have reached similar conclusions—that insertion of a PA catheter is neutral, it neither conferred a benefit nor increased risk to the patient. There was no increase in mortality or increase in the number of days in the critical care unit or the hospital.[64,65]

These findings have raised concerns about routine use of PA catheters for critically ill patients. The PA catheter is invasive. It previously seemed intuitive that the diagnostic information provided would confer a survival advantage over less invasive methods, but research has shown this is not the case. In 2000 the number of PA catheters used in the United States was reported as 1.5 million annually; 30% were used in cardiac surgery units, 30% in cardiac catheterization laboratories and coronary care units, 25% in high-risk surgery and trauma units, and 15% in medical intensive care units.[66] As a result of studies that document the failure of the PA catheter to lower mortality, the use of PA catheters has declined considerably. A study of PA catheterization between 1993 and 2004 reported a decline of 65% in PA catheter use in critically ill patients.[67] Although PA catheter use has declined in critical care units, right heart catheterization remains a useful diagnostic tool in the cardiac catheterization laboratory. While the PA catheter has not been associated with increased harm, the lack of clear benefit mandates that its importance in patient care management will continue to decline. In many critical care units, the PA catheter is reserved only for patients who are refractory to conventional treatment,[68] and increasingly, it will be replaced by less invasive technologies.

Pulmonary Artery Catheter Educational Resources

Clinicians who do not frequently work with PA catheters are less knowledgeable about waveform analysis and interpretation of data. With the decline in PA catheterization, this issue has become even more important. As a response to this concern, several professional organizations, including the American Association of Critical-Care Nurses (AACN), the Society of Critical Care Medicine (SCCM), and the American College of Chest Physicians (ACCP), endorse the Internet-based Pulmonary Artery Catheter Education Project (PACEP).[69] This website (www.pacep.org)[69] is free and is designed to provide education about PA hemodynamic monitoring. Another useful and free Internet-based resource is the Pulmonary Artery Catheter Primer from the American Thoracic Society.[70]

Indications

The thermodilution PA catheter is used for diagnosis and evaluation of heart disease, shock states, ARDS, and medical conditions that compromise CO or fluid volume status. The PA catheter can simultaneously assess pulmonary artery systolic and diastolic pressures, pulmonary artery mean pressure, and PAOP (wedge pressure). The PA catheter is used to measure CO, determine mixed-venous oxygen saturation, and calculate additional hemodynamic parameters.

Pulmonary Artery Catheters

The traditional PA catheter, invented by Swan and Ganz, has four lumens for measurement of right atrial pressure (RAP) or CVP, PA pressures, PAOP, and CO (Figure 11-12, *A*). Multifunction catheters may have additional lumens, which can be used for intravenous infusion (Figure 11-12, *B*) and to measure continuous mixed venous oxygen saturation (SvO_2), right ventricular volume, and continuous CO (Figure 11-12, *C*). Other PA catheters include transvenous pacing electrodes to pace the heart if needed.

The PA flow-directed catheter is 110 cm long. The most commonly used size is 7.5 or 8.0 Fr, although 5.0 and 7.0 Fr sizes are available. Each of the four lumens exits into the heart or pulmonary artery at a different point, graduated along the catheter length (see Figure 11-12, *A*).

Right Atrial Lumen. The proximal lumen is situated in the right atrium and is used for intravenous infusion, CVP measurement, withdrawal of venous blood samples, and injection of fluid for CO determinations. This port is often described as the right atrial port, also called the CVP port.

Pulmonary Artery Lumen. The distal PA lumen is located at the tip of the PA catheter and is situated in the pulmonary artery. It is used to record pulmonary artery pressures and can be used for withdrawal of blood samples to measure mixed-venous blood gases (e.g., SvO_2).

Balloon Lumen. The third lumen opens into a balloon at the end of the catheter that can be inflated with 0.8 mL (7 Fr) to 1.5 mL (7.5 Fr) of air. The balloon is inflated during catheter insertion after the catheter reaches the right atrium to assist in forward flow of the catheter and to minimize right ventricular ectopy from the catheter tip. The balloon is also inflated to obtain the PAOP measurements when the PA catheter is correctly positioned in the pulmonary artery.

Thermistor Lumen. The fourth lumen is a thermistor (temperature sensor) used to measure changes in blood temperature. It is located 4 cm from the catheter tip and is used to measure thermodilution CO. The connector end of the lumen is attached directly to the CO computer.

Additional Features. If continuous SvO_2 is measured, the catheter has an additional fiberoptic lumen that exits at the tip of the catheter (see Figure 11-12, *C*). If cardiac pacing is used, two PA catheter methods are available. One type of catheter has three atrial (A) and two ventricular (V) pacing electrodes attached to the catheter so that when it is properly positioned, the patient can be connected to a pacemaker and be AV paced. The other catheter method uses a specific transvenous pacing wire that is passed through an additional catheter lumen and exits into the right ventricle if ventricular pacing is required. A right ventricular volumetric PA catheter is available that measures stroke volume in the right ventricle.

Insertion

If a PA catheter is to be inserted into a patient who is awake, some brief explanations about the procedure are helpful to ensure that the patient understands what is going to happen. The initial insertion techniques used for placement of a PA catheter are similar to those described for CVC insertion. Because the PA catheter is positioned within the heart chambers and pulmonary artery on the right side of the heart, catheter passage is monitored using fluoroscopy or waveform analysis on the bedside monitor (Figures 11-1 and 11-13).

Before inserting the catheter into the vein, the physician—using sterile technique—tests the balloon for inflation and flushes the catheter with normal saline solution to remove any air. The PA catheter is then attached to the bedside hemodynamic line setup and monitor so that the waveforms can be visualized while the catheter is advanced through the right side of the heart (see Figure 11-13). A larger introducer sheath (8.5 Fr)—which has the tip positioned in the vena cava and has an additional intravenous side-port lumen—is often used to cannulate the vein first.[69] This introducer sheath is known by several different names in clinical practice, including sheath, cordis, introducer, or side port. This introducer sheath remains in place, and the supple PA catheter is threaded through it into the vena cava and into the right side of the heart.

Nursing Management

Nursing priorities for the patient with PA catheter monitoring focus on (1) accurately interpreting PA waveforms, (2) accommodating changes in patient position, (3) recognizing the effects of respiratory variation, (4) preventing PA catheter-related complications, (5) measuring cardiac output, and (6) evaluating hemodynamic performance.

Accurately Interpreting Pulmonary Artery Waveforms. Each chamber of the heart has a distinctive waveform with recognizable characteristics. It is the responsibility of the critical care nurse to recognize each waveform displayed on the bedside monitor when the catheter enters the corresponding chamber during insertion and during routine monitoring.[71]

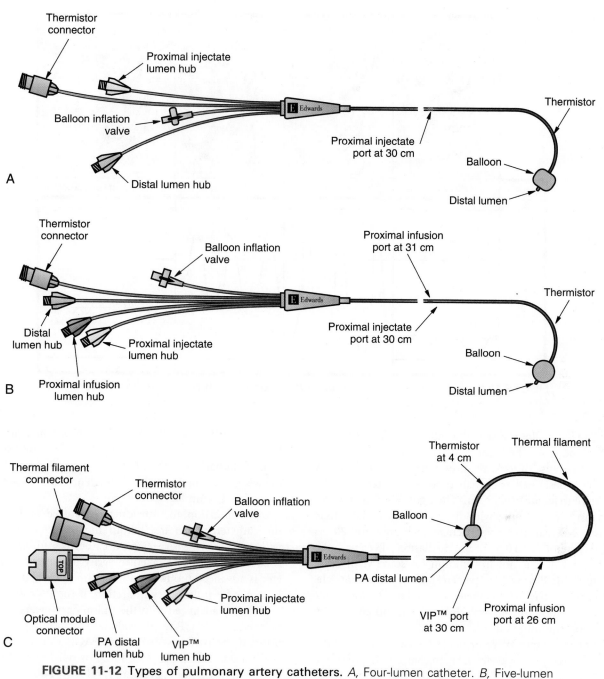

FIGURE 11-12 Types of pulmonary artery catheters. *A,* Four-lumen catheter. *B,* Five-lumen catheter that includes an additional venous infusion port (VIP) into the right atrium. *C,* Seven-lumen catheter that includes a VIP port and two additional lumens for continuous cardiac output (CCO) and a thermal filament and for continuous mixed venous oxygen saturation (SvO$_2$) monitoring (i.e., optical module connector). An additional option is to combine the use of the CCO filament and the thermistor response time to calculate continuous end-diastolic volume (CEDV). (©2001 Edwards Lifesciences LLC. All rights reserved. Reprinted with permission of Edwards Lifesciences, Swan-Ganz is a trademark of Edwards Lifesciences Corporation, registered with the U.S. Patent and Trademark Office.)

Right Atrial Waveform. As the PA catheter is advanced into the right atrium during insertion, a right atrial waveform must be visible on the monitor, with recognizable a, c, and v waves (see Figure 11-13). The normal mean pressure in the right atrium is 2 to 5 mm Hg. Before passage through the tricuspid valve, the balloon at the tip of the catheter is inflated for two reasons. First, it cushions the pointed tip of the PA catheter so that if the tip comes into contact with the right ventricular wall, it will cause less myocardial irritability and, consequently, fewer ventricular dysrhythmias. Second,

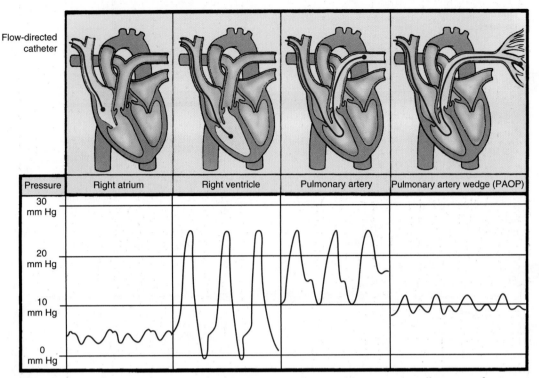

Pressure	Right atrium	Right ventricle	Pulmonary artery	Pulmonary artery wedge (PAOP)

Flow-directed catheter

30 mm Hg
20 mm Hg
10 mm Hg
0 mm Hg

FIGURE 11-13 Pulmonary artery (PA) catheter insertion with corresponding waveforms.

inflation of the balloon assists the catheter to float with the flow of blood from the right ventricle into the pulmonary artery. It is because of these features and the balloon that PA catheters are described as flow-directional catheters.

Right Ventricular Waveform. The right ventricular waveform is distinctly pulsatile, with distinct systolic and diastolic pressures. Normal right ventricular pressures are 20 to 30 mm Hg systolic and 0 to 5 mm Hg diastolic. Even with the balloon inflated, it is not uncommon for some ventricular ectopy to occur during passage through the right ventricle. All patients who have a PA catheter inserted must have simultaneous ECG monitoring, with defibrillator and emergency resuscitation equipment nearby.

Pulmonary Artery Waveform. As the catheter enters the pulmonary artery, the waveform again changes. The diastolic pressure rises. Normal PA pressures range from 20 to 30 mm Hg systolic over 10 mm Hg diastolic. A dicrotic notch, visible on the downslope of the waveform, represents closure of the pulmonic valve.

Pulmonary Artery Occlusion Waveform (Wedge). While the balloon remains inflated, the catheter is advanced into the wedge position. This maneuver produces the PAOP. The waveform decreases in size and is nonpulsatile, reflecting a normal left atrial tracing with a and v wave deflections. This is known as a wedge tracing, because the balloon is "wedged" into a small pulmonary vessel, but it is technically described as the PAOP (see Figure 11-13). The balloon occludes a small pulmonary vessel so that the PA catheter tip and lumen are protected from the pulsatile influence of the pulmonary artery, and are exposed only to the left ventricular end-diastolic pressure (LVEDP). The relationship of the PA

catheter tip to the left ventricle is shown in Figure 11-14. When the balloon is deflated, the catheter should spontaneously float back into the PA. When the balloon is reinflated, the wedge tracing should be visible. The normal PAOP ranges from 5 to 12 mm Hg.

After insertion, the introducer is sutured to the skin, and the catheter, which lies within the introducer, is secured with tape or with a specialized catheter securement device. A chest radiograph is taken to verify placement. If the catheter is advanced too far into the pulmonary bed, the patient is at risk for pulmonary infarction. If the PA catheter is not sufficiently advanced into the pulmonary artery, it will not be useful for PAOP readings. However, in many critical care units, if the patient's PADP and PAOP values approximate (within 0 to 3 mm Hg), the PADP is reliably used to follow the trend of LV filling pressure (preload). This prevents possible trauma from frequent balloon inflation; in such a situation, the PA catheter is consciously pulled back into the pulmonary artery, so that it is impossible to achieve an occlusion (wedged) tracing.

After insertion of the catheter, the chest radiograph or fluoroscopy is used to verify the PA catheter position to make sure that it is not looped or knotted in the right ventricle and to rule out pneumothorax or hemorrhagic complications. A thin plastic cuff can be placed on the outside of the catheter when it is inserted to maintain sterility of the part of the PA catheter that exits from the patient. If the PA catheter is not in the desired position or if it migrates out of position, it can be repositioned. The plastic cuff is designed to keep the external catheter sterile for a short period after insertion.

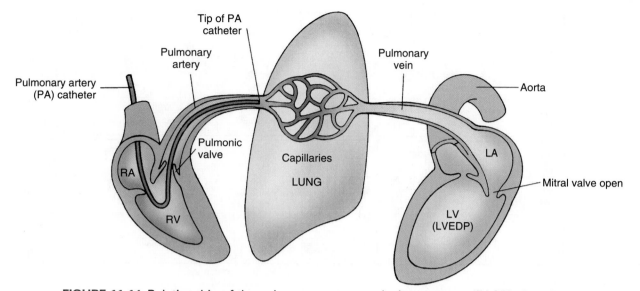

FIGURE 11-14 Relationship of the pulmonary artery occlusion pressure (PAOP), described as the "wedge pressure" to the left ventricular end-diastolic pressure (LVEDP). In most clinical situations, the PAOP accurately reflects the LVEDP. During diastole, when the mitral valve is open, there are no other valves or other obstructions between the tip of the catheter and the left ventricle (LV). The pressure exerted by the volume in the LV is reflected through the left atrium (LA), through the pulmonary veins, and to the pulmonary capillaries. *PA*, pulmonary artery; *RA*, right atrium; *RV*, right ventricle.

Accommodating Changes in Patient Position. The patient does not need to be flat for accurate pressure readings to be obtained. In the supine position, when the transducer is placed at the level of the phlebostatic axis, a head-of-bed position from flat up to 60 degrees is appropriate for most patients.[35] It is important to know that PADP and PAOP measurements in the lateral position may be significantly different from those taken when the patient is lying supine. If there is concern about the validity of pressure readings in a particular patient, it is more reliable to take measurements with the patient on his or her back, with the head of the bed elevated from flat to 60 degrees as tolerated. After a patient changes position, a stabilization period of 5 minutes is recommended before taking pressure readings if the patient has a healthy heart (normal left ventricle), and a stabilization period of 15 minutes is recommended if the patient has LV dysfunction.[72]

Recognizing the Effects of Respiratory Variation. All PADP and PAOP (wedge) tracings are subject to respiratory interference, especially when the patient is on a positive-pressure, volume-cycled ventilator.[35,71] During the positive-pressure inhalation phase, the increase in intrathoracic pressure may "push up" the pulmonary artery tracing, producing an artificially high reading (Figure 11-15, *A*). During inhalation with spontaneous breaths, negative intrathoracic pressure "pulls down" the waveform, producing an erroneously low measurement (see Figure 11-15, *B*). To minimize the impact of respiratory variation, the PADP is read at end-expiration, which is the most stable point in the respiratory cycle when intrapleural pressures are close to zero.[71] If the digital number fluctuates with respiration, a printed readout

on paper can be obtained to verify true PADP. In some clinical settings, ECG signals or airway pressure and flow are recorded simultaneously with the PADP/PAOP tracing to identify end-expiration.[35,73]

Positive End-Expiratory Pressure. Some clinical diagnoses, such as ARDS, require the use of high levels of PEEP set with the ventilator to treat refractory hypoxemia. If a PEEP of greater than 10 cm H_2O is used, PAOP (wedge) and pulmonary artery pressures will be artificially elevated, and CO may be negatively affected.[74,75] Because of this impact of PEEP, in the past, patients in some critical care units were taken off the ventilator to record pulmonary artery pressure measurements. It has since been shown that this practice closes alveoli, decreases the patient's oxygenation level, and may result in persistent hypoxemia.

Because patients remain on PEEP for treatment, they remain on it during measurement of pulmonary artery pressures. In this situation, the trend of pulmonary artery readings is more important than one individual measurement. The most important factor is not one individual measurement or the absolute number obtained; it is instead the trend of the measurements being used as a basis for clinical interventions to support and improve cardiopulmonary function in the critically ill.

Preventing PA Catheter-Related Complications. Potential cardiac complications include ventricular dysrhythmias, endocarditis, valvular damage, cardiac rupture, and cardiac tamponade. Potential pulmonary complications include rupture of a pulmonary artery, pulmonary artery thrombosis, embolism or hemorrhage, and infarction of a segment of lung. The PA catheter tracing is continuously monitored to

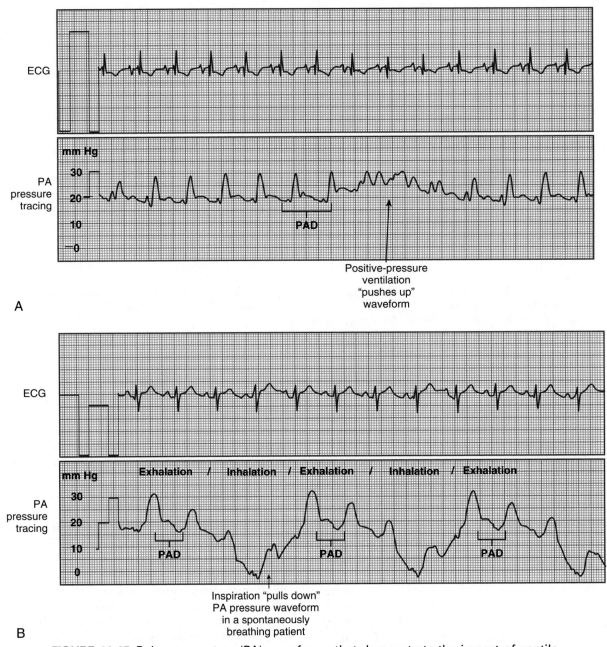

FIGURE 11-15 Pulmonary artery (PA) waveforms that demonstrate the impact of ventilation on PA pressure readings. For accuracy, PA pressures are read at the end of exhalation. *A,* In positive-pressure ventilation, the increase in intrathoracic pressure during inhalation "pushes up" the PA pressure waveform, creating a falsely high reading. *B,* In spontaneous breathing, the decrease in intrathoracic pressure during normal inhalation "pulls down" the PA waveform, creating a falsely low reading.

ensure that the catheter does not migrate forward into a spontaneous wedge or PAOP position. A segment of lung can suffer infarction if the wedged catheter occludes an arteriole for a prolonged period. If the catheter is spontaneously wedged, the critical care nurse can gently pull the catheter back out of the wedge position if the institutional policy allows.[76]

Infection is always a risk with a PA catheter. The risks are similar to those discussed in the section on CVCs (Patient Safety Priorities box on Prevention of Central Venous Catheter-Related Bloodstream Infections on page 137).

Removal of the Pulmonary Artery Catheter. PA catheters can be safely removed from the patient by critical care nurses competent in this procedure.[35,76,77] Removal is not usually associated with major complications. The most common incidents are PVCs in about 2% of patients as the catheter is pulled through the right ventricle.[35,77,78]

Monitoring Cardiac Output. Cardiac output (CO) is the product of heart rate (HR) multiplied by stroke volume (SV). Stroke volume is the volume of blood ejected by the heart during each beat (reported in milliliters).

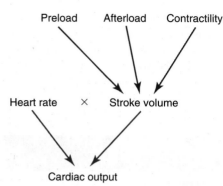

FIGURE 11-16 Preload, afterload, and contractility contribute to the heart's stroke volume. Stroke volume × Heart rate = Cardiac output.

$$HR \times SV = CO$$

The normal adult stroke volume is 60 to 70 mL. The clinical factors that contribute to the heart's stroke volume are *preload*, *afterload*, and *contractility* (Figure 11-16). Preload and afterload are assessed using data from the PA catheter. Heart rate is recorded from the ECG leads.

The PA catheter measures CO using an intermittent (bolus) or a continuous CO method.

Thermodilution Cardiac Output Bolus Method. The bolus thermodilution method is performed at the bedside and results in CO calculated in liters per minute. Three CO values that are within a 10% mean range are obtained at one time and are averaged to calculate CO. A known amount (5 mL) of iced or, more typically, 10 mL of room-temperature normal saline solution is injected into the proximal lumen of the PA catheter. The injectate exits into the right atrium and travels with the flow of blood past the thermistor (temperature sensor) located at the distal end of the catheter in the pulmonary artery. The injectate can be delivered by hand injection using individual syringes of saline. Frequently, a closed in-line system attached to a 500-mL bag of normal saline is used as a reservoir to deliver the individual injections.[79]

Sometimes, the right atrial (proximal) port is clotted and not usable. If another right atrial port is available, it can be substituted. However, if a usable port is not available, to ensure accurate CO data, a new pulmonary artery catheter is inserted.

Cardiac Output Curve Interpretation. The thermodilution CO method uses the indicator-dilution method, in which a known temperature is the indicator. It is based on the principle that the change in temperature over time is inversely proportional to blood flow. Blood flow can be diagrammatically represented as a CO curve on which temperature is plotted against time (Figure 11-17). Most hemodynamic monitors display this CO curve, which must then be interpreted to determine whether the CO injection is valid. The normal curve has a smooth upstroke, with a rounded peak and a gradually tapering downslope. If the curve has an uneven pattern, it may indicate faulty injection technique,

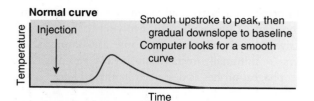
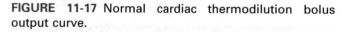

FIGURE 11-17 Normal cardiac thermodilution bolus output curve.

and the CO measurement must be repeated. Patient movement or coughing also alters the CO measurement.

Injectate Temperature. If the CO is within the normal range, and the patient has a normal body temperature, both iced and room temperature injectate are equally accurate.[80] To ensure accurate CO values, the difference between injectate temperature and body temperature must be at least 10° C.[81] If the patient is hypothermic, iced injectate may be needed to achieve this 10 degree difference. The injectate must be delivered within 4 seconds, with minimal handling of the syringe to prevent warming of the solution. With all delivery systems, the injectate is delivered at the same point in the respiratory cycle, usually end-exhalation.

Patient Position and Cardiac Output. In the normovolemic, stable patient, reliable CO measurements can be obtained in a supine position (patient lying on his or her back) with the head of the bed elevated up to 45 degrees.[82] If the patient is hypovolemic or unstable, leaving the head of the bed in a flat position or only slightly elevated is the most clinically appropriate choice. CO measurements performed when the patient is turned to the side are not considered as accurate as those performed with the patient in the supine position.

Clinical Conditions That Alter Cardiac Output. Two clinical conditions produce errors in the thermodilution CO measurement: tricuspid valve regurgitation and ventricular septal rupture. If the patient has tricuspid valve regurgitation, the expected flow of blood from the right atrium to the pulmonary artery is disrupted by backflow from the right ventricle to the right atrium. This creates a lower CO measurement than the patient's actual output. If the person has an intracardiac left-to-right shunt, as occurs after ventricular septal rupture, the thermodilution CO measures the large pulmonary volume and records a higher CO than the patient's true systemic output.

Continuous Cardiac Output Measurement Using the PA Catheter. The bolus thermodilution method is reliable but performed intermittently. Continuous CO monitoring using a PA catheter is also frequently used in clinical practice. One method employs a thermal filament on the PA catheter to emit small energy signals (the indicator) into the bloodstream. These signals are then detected by the thermistor near the tip of the PA catheter. The equivalent of an indicator curve is created, and a CO value is calculated from this data.

Noninvasive and Minimally Invasive Measurement of Cardiac Output. As a result of concerns over use of the pulmonary artery thermodilution catheter, combined with studies that have not shown improved outcomes with routine monitoring, there is tremendous interest in using less-invasive methods of CO measurement. Evolving techniques are less invasive than the PA catheter, some are noninvasive, and others are minimally invasive and involve vascular catheters or esophageal probes as described in Table 11-5.

Evaluating Hemodynamic Profiles. For the patient with a thermodilution PA catheter in place, additional hemodynamic information can be calculated using routine vital signs, CO, and body surface area (BSA). These measurements are calculated using specific formulas that are indexed to a

TABLE 11-5	NONINVASIVE AND MINIMALLY INVASIVE CARDIAC OUTPUT MEASUREMENT TECHNIQUES			
DEVICE NAME	**PROBE PLACEMENT**	**METHOD**	**CARDIAC OUTPUT CALCULATION**	**CLINICAL ISSUES**
Noninvasive Methods				
Bioimpedance	External electrodes placed on the neck and chest	Thoracic electric bioimpedance	1. A small alternating current is applied across the chest by skin electrodes. 2. Pulsatile changes in thoracic blood volume result in changes in electrical impedance. The rate of change of impedance during systole is measured and used to calculate CO.	Noninvasive Less accurate with low body temperature.
Minimally Invasive Methods				
Pulse Contour Waveform Methods				
LiDCO (LiDCO Ltd., Cambridge, United Kingdom)	Requires a venous access catheter (central or peripheral) and an arterial catheter with a lithium-monitoring sensor attached	Pulse contour waveform analysis method (calibrated)	Independent calibration with a lithium dilution technique is initially required: 1. A small, subtherapeutic dose of isotonic lithium chloride is injected through the venous catheter. 2. The lithium is detected at the arterial sensor (femoral artery), where a fixed flow pump ensures constant flow. 3. A concentration-time curve is produced for lithium before recirculation. 4. CO is calculated based on the lithium dose given and the measurement of area under the curve.	Easy to set up, uses conventional venous and arterial catheters; can measure extravascular lung water for patients in pulmonary edema. CO measurement is affected by artifact on arterial waveform and by irregular and damped arterial waveforms; can be used in conscious and in unresponsive patients. Requires calibration at least every 8 hours to maintain accuracy; cannot be used in patients on lithium therapy because this interferes with the calibration.
PiCCO (Pulsion Medical Systems, Munich, Germany)	Requires a central venous access catheter and uses a specialized arterial thermistor-tipped catheter in the femoral artery	Pulse contour waveform analysis method that uses transpulmonary thermodilution	1. A set volume of cold saline is injected through the central venous catheter. The arterial thermistor-tipped catheter detects the blood temperature change. 2. Continuous CO measurements are achieved by analyzing the systolic component of the arterial waveform.	CO measurement is affected by artifact on arterial waveform and irregular arterial waveforms. Three calibrations are required initially, and frequent recalibration is required to maintain accuracy.

TABLE 11-5	**NONINVASIVE AND MINIMALLY INVASIVE CARDIAC OUTPUT MEASUREMENT TECHNIQUES—cont'd**			
DEVICE NAME	**PROBE PLACEMENT**	**METHOD**	**CARDIAC OUTPUT CALCULATION**	**CLINICAL ISSUES**
Vigileo (Edwards Lifesciences, Irvine, CA)	Requires a functional arterial catheter	Pulse contour waveform analysis method (does not require calibration)	1. Calculates CO by use of the arterial pressure waveform analysis in conjunction with patient data (age, sex, height, weight). 2. Uses an internal proprietary algorithm based on the principle that pulse pressure (difference between systolic and diastolic pressure) is proportional to stroke volume and inversely proportional to aortic compliance. 3. Aortic pressure is sampled at 100 Hz and is updated every 20 seconds.	Does not require external calibration but requires zeroing of the transducer. Lack of calibration procedures is controversial.
Esophageal Probe Methods				
Esophageal Doppler	Ultrasound probe placed in the lower esophagus	Stroke volume is calculated by measurement of the aortic blood velocity in the descending thoracic aorta (by continuous wave Doppler) plus calculation of the cross-sectional area of the aorta; these values are used to calculate the CO.	1. Measurement of the aorta cross-sectional area, measured using M-mode ultrasound, and multiplying this value by blood velocity to calculate flow or CO. 2. The value of total CO is derived from a nomogram using aortic blood velocity, height, weight, and age.	Useful in the operating room or with deeply sedated patients. Probe is stiff, and placement is not well tolerated by conscious patients.
Transesophageal echocardiography (TEE)	Ultrasound probe placed in the esophagus	Probe placement allows imaging of the left ventricular outflow tract. Stroke volume is measured by Doppler.	1. The left ventricular (LV) outflow tract area is measured; this value is squared and multiplied by the velocity time interval of blood flow and heart rate. 2. LV stroke volume can be measured, as can heart rate to use the SV × HR = CO formula.	Useful in the operating room or with deeply sedated patients. Probe is stiff, and placement is not well tolerated by conscious patients. Requires skill to accurately position probe to visualize the LV outflow tract.

TABLE 11-5	NONINVASIVE AND MINIMALLY INVASIVE CARDIAC OUTPUT MEASUREMENT TECHNIQUES—cont'd			
DEVICE NAME	**PROBE PLACEMENT**	**METHOD**	**CARDIAC OUTPUT CALCULATION**	**CLINICAL ISSUES**
Partial CO_2 Rebreathing Method				
NICO 2 (Philips, Respironics)	Addition of a partial CO_2 rebreathing circuit to ventilator	Partial CO_2 rebreathing method	CO measurement is based on changes in respiratory CO_2 concentration obtained from a short period of rebreathing. CO_2 elimination is calculated by sensors that measure flow, airway pressure, and CO_2 concentration. These variables are used in the Fick partial rebreathing formula to calculate CO.	Can only be used in intubated and ventilated patients. Specialized additional tubing setup on ventilator. Cannot be used in patients who cannot tolerate hypercapnia (elevated CO_2). CO measurement is altered by intrapulmonary shunt.

CO, cardiac output; *CO_2,* carbon dioxide; *HR,* heart rate; *LV,* left ventricle; *SV,* stroke volume.

patient's body size. The BSA is calculated when the height and weight are entered into the hemodynamic bedside monitor.

Continuous Monitoring of Venous Oxygen Saturation

Indications

Continuous monitoring of venous oxygen saturation is indicated for the critically ill patient who has the potential to develop an imbalance between oxygen supply and metabolic tissue demand. This includes patients after high-risk surgery,[57] and in severe sepsis or septic shock.[83,84]

Continuous venous oxygen monitoring permits a calculation of the balance achieved between arterial oxygen supply (SaO2) and oxygen demand at the tissue level by sampling desaturated venous blood from the pulmonary artery catheter distal tip. This sample is called mixed venous oxygen saturation (SvO2) because it is a mixture of all of the venous blood drained from many body tissues. The same fiberoptic technology has been used in combination with a fiberoptic triple-lumen CVC. In this situation, the venous blood is sampled from the superior vena cava, just above the right atrium, and the central venous oxygen saturation (ScvO2) is measured.

Under normal conditions, the cardiopulmonary system achieves a balance between oxygen supply and demand. Four factors contribute to this balance:
1. Cardiac output (CO)
2. Hemoglobin (Hgb)
3. Arterial oxygen saturation (SaO2)
4. Tissue oxygen metabolism (VO2)

Three of these factors (CO, Hgb, and SaO2) contribute to the supply of oxygen to the tissues. Tissue metabolism (VO2) determines oxygen consumption or the quantity of oxygen extracted at tissue level that creates the demand for oxygen. The relationships of these factors are illustrated in Figure 11-18.

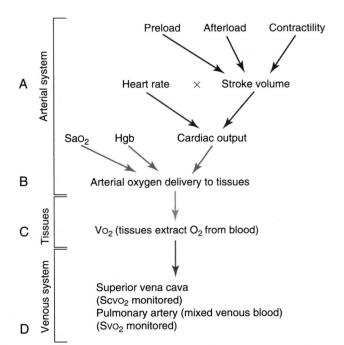

FIGURE 11-18 Several factors contribute to the mixed venous oxygen saturation (SvO2) value. *A,* Cardiac output (CO) is determined by heart rate (central venous oxygen saturation [ScvO2] HR) × stroke volume (SV). *B,* The oxygen saturation (SaO2), hemoglobin (Hgb) level, and CO contribute to arterial oxygen delivery at the tissue level. *C,* Tissues extract and use the oxygen carried in the blood. This process of cellular oxygen consumption is VO2. *D,* Blood returns to the superior vena cava (recorded as ScvO2) and then to the pulmonary artery, where the mixed venous blood is recorded as SvO2.

In addition to measurement of venous oxygen saturation, it is possible to calculate the quantity of oxygen (in mL/min) that is provided to the tissues by the cardiopulmonary system and to assess the amount of oxygen consumed by the body tissues. These calculations rely on principles of oxygen transport physiology and are the basis for calculation of Svo_2. These formulas are listed in Appendix B.

Catheters

The type of catheter used to measure venous oxygen saturation is defined by where the fiberoptic tip is located, either at the tip of a CVC or on the distal tip of a PA catheter.

Svo_2 Catheter. The pulmonary arterial Svo_2 catheter has the traditional four lumens plus a lumen containing two or three optical fibers. The fiberoptics are attached to an optical module that is connected to a small bedside computer. The optical module transmits a narrow band of light down one optical fiber. This light is reflected off the hemoglobin in the blood and returns to the optical module through the receiving fiberoptic. The Svo_2 signal is recorded on a continuous display.

$Scvo_2$ Catheter. The central venous $Scvo_2$ technology is incorporated into a multi-lumen CVC. The fiberoptic catheter tip is positioned in a central vein, such as the superior vena cava. The technology used to measure the venous saturation is identical in both types of catheters, and the same continuous display module is used for both catheters.

The $Scvo_2$ catheter has been used successfully to guide hemodynamic fluid resuscitation in septic patients.[83,84] The relationship between the values obtained from the traditional PA (Svo_2) catheter and the central venous ($Scvo_2$) catheter are very similar, although the $Scvo_2$ values are slightly higher. The trend of parallel measurements (up or down as patient condition changes) is in the same direction in about 90% of cases.

Svo_2 or $Scvo_2$ Catheter Calibration. The catheter is calibrated before insertion into the patient through a standardized color reference system, which is part of the catheter package. Insertion technique and sites are identical to those used for placement of conventional PA or CVC catheters. Waveform analysis or venous saturation measurement, or both, can be used for accurate placement. After the catheter is inserted, recalibration is unnecessary unless the catheter becomes disconnected from the optical module.

To recalibrate the fiberoptic module to verify accuracy when the catheter is already inserted in a patient, a mixed venous blood sample (Svo_2) or central venous sample ($Scvo_2$) must be withdrawn from the appropriate catheter tip and sent to the laboratory for oxygen saturation analysis. In many critical care units, this is a standard daily procedure to ensure that readings used to guide patient care remain accurate.[85]

Nursing Management

Nursing priorities for the patient with a catheter that monitors venous oxygenation include: (1) assessing the accuracy of the Svo_2/$Scvo_2$ values, and (2) incorporating the Svo_2/$Scvo_2$ values into the hemodynamic assessment.

Assessing the Accuracy of the Svo_2 or $Scvo_2$ Values. Svo_2 monitoring provides a continuous assessment of the balance of oxygen supply and demand for an individual patient. Nursing assessment includes evaluation of the Svo_2 or $Scvo_2$ value and evaluation of the four factors that maintain the oxygen supply-demand balance. These factors are: arterial oxygen saturation (Sao_2, or Spo_2), cardiac output (CO), hemoglobin (Hgb), and tissue oxygenation (VO_2), to maintain the oxygen supply-demand balance.

Normal Svo_2 Values. Normal Svo_2 is approximately 75% in the healthy individual (range, 60% to 80%). In critically ill patients, an Svo_2 value between 60% and 80% is evidence of adequate balance between oxygen supply and demand.

Normal $Scvo_2$ Values. The normal values for the $Scvo_2$ catheter are slightly higher,[56] because the reading is taken before the blood enters the right heart chambers, where the cardiac sinus (vein) delivers venous blood drained from the myocardium into the right atrium. The heavily desaturated myocardial blood decreases the oxygen saturation slightly. For this reason, Svo_2 values are always slightly lower than $Scvo_2$ readings in the same patient.[56]

If Svo_2 or $Scvo_2$ is within the normal range of 60% to 80% and the patient is not clinically compromised, the nurse can assume that oxygen supply and demand are balanced for that individual.

Assessment of Svo_2 or $Scvo_2$. If Svo_2 or $Scvo_2$ falls below 60% and is sustained, the clinician must assume that oxygen supply is not equal to demand (Table 11-6). It is helpful to assess the cause of decreased Svo_2 or $Scvo_2$ in a logical sequence that reflects knowledge of the meaning of the venous saturation value. The following is one such assessment sequence:

1. Clinically assess the patient.
2. Assess whether the decreased Svo_2 or $Scvo_2$ is caused by low oxygen supply. Verify the effectiveness of the ventilator or oxygen mask, or check arterial oxygen saturation (Sao_2) from arterial blood gas values.
3. Assess cardiac function by performing a CO measurement.
4. Assess the hemoglobin value by checking recent laboratory results or by withdrawing a blood sample for laboratory analysis.
5. Assess whether the decreased Svo_2 or $Scvo_2$ is the result of a recent patient movement or nursing action that may have temporarily increased tissue oxygen consumption.

Incorporating Svo_2 or $Scvo_2$ Values into the Hemodynamic Assessment.

Therapeutic Goals for Svo_2 or $Scvo_2$. The concept of therapeutic goals or targets is helpful when developing protocols for hemodynamic assessment. Accepted therapeutic values for venous oximetry are: an Svo_2 of 70% or above and an $Scvo_2$ of 65% or above. The concept is that patients with values below these values are at greater risk for organ hypoperfusion and increased mortality. This was seen in a study of intraoperative and postoperative surgical patients, in whom an $Scvo_2$ below 65% was associated with increased mortality.[86] However, cardiac surgery patients who were below the $Scvo_2$ 65% target did not have lower mortality rates.[87] Based on studies of patients with sepsis, the Surviving Sepsis Campaign guidelines recommend that $Scvo_2$ be maintained above 70% for septic patients.[83,84] This represents a clinically useful target to aim for even as research is ongoing to find the $Scvo_2$ value for optimal survival.

Low Svo_2 or $Scvo_2$. If Svo_2 or $Scvo_2$ falls below 40%, and is maintained at this low value, the imbalance of oxygen supply and demand will not be adequate to meet tissue needs

TABLE 11-6	ALTERATIONS IN OXYGEN CONSUMPTION, IDENTIFIED FROM MIXED VENOUS OXYGEN SATURATION MONITORING	
CONDITION OR ACTIVITY	% INCREASE OVER RESTING $\dot{V}o_2$	% DECREASE UNDER RESTING $\dot{V}o_2$
Clinical Conditions That Increase $\dot{V}o_2$		
Fever	10% (for each 1° C above normal)	
Skeletal injuries	10%-30%	
Work of breathing	40%	
Severe infection	60%	
Shivering	50%-100%	
Burns	100%	
Routine postoperative procedures	7%	
Nasal intubation	25%-40%	
Endotracheal tube suctioning	27%	
Chest trauma	60%	
Multiple organ dysfunction syndrome	20%-80%	
Sepsis	50%-100%	
Head injury, with patient sedated	89%	
Head injury, with patient not sedated	138%	
Critical illness in emergency department	60%	
Nursing Activities That Increase $\dot{V}o_2$		
Dressing change	10%	
Electrocardiogram	16%	
Agitation	18%	
Physical examination	20%	
Visitor	22%	
Bath	23%	
Chest x-ray examination	25%	
Weighing on sling scale	36%	
Conditions That Decrease $\dot{V}o_2$		
Anesthesia		25%
Anesthesia in burned patients		50%

the low $S\mathrm{vo}_2$ or $Scvo_2$ and to correct the oxygen supply-demand imbalance. To avoid the risk of lactic acidosis, it is helpful to watch the trend of the $S\mathrm{vo}_2$ or $Scvo_2$ and to intervene early with a goal of returning the venous oxygen saturation to 70%.[84]

High $S\mathrm{vo}_2$ or $Scvo_2$. In certain clinical conditions, $S\mathrm{vo}_2$ or $Scvo_2$ may increase to an above-normal level (>80%). This occurs during times of low oxygen demand, such as during anesthesia or hypothermia. In some cases of septic shock, the tissue cells cannot use the oxygen supplied to them, and the oxygen is not extracted from the blood at the tissue level. In this situation, the venous oxygen reserve remains elevated, and the $S\mathrm{vo}_2$ or $Scvo_2$ value is higher than normal (Table 11-7). If the $S\mathrm{vo}_2$ PA catheter drifts into a wedged position, the $S\mathrm{vo}_2$ increases because the fiberoptic tip of the catheter comes into contact with newly oxygenated blood.

ELECTROCARDIOGRAPHY

Nursing Management

Nursing priorities for the patient with bedside ECG monitoring focus on accurate: (1) selection of the ECG lead, (2) interpretation of the ECG, and (3) initiation of emergency measures to treat dysrhythmias when required.

Selecting ECG Leads

ECG Leads. The basic 3-lead ECG system consists of three bipolar electrodes that are applied to the chest wall and labeled right arm (RA), left arm (LA), and left leg (LL) (Figure 11-19). Three leads are created from this configuration, called simply Lead I, Lead II, and Lead III, (Figure 11-20). A 5-lead ECG system is typically used in critical care. This system incorporates Leads I-III, plus three augmented vector leads: aVR, aVL, and aVF, (see Figure 11-20) and at least one chest lead (precordial lead), also known as a "V" lead. Leads are color-coded to decrease the risk of misplacement. A multiselect function on the bedside monitor allows clinicians to switch between views and quickly obtain multiple images of the patient's ECG rhythm.[88]

A bipolar lead system means that each displayed ECG lead has a positive and a negative pole. One lead also acts as a ground. The function of the ground electrode is to prevent the appearance of background electrical interference on the ECG tracing. Leads do not transmit any electricity to the patient; they sense and record it.

ECG Paper. ECG paper records the speed and magnitude of electrical impulses on a grid composed of small and large boxes (Figure 11-21). Every large box has five small boxes in it. At a standard paper speed of 25 mm/sec, on the horizontal axis, one small box (1 mm) is equivalent to 0.04 second, and one large box (5 mm) represents 0.20 second. Distances along the horizontal axis represent speed and are stated in seconds rather than in millimeters or number of boxes. The vertical axis represents the magnitude, or force, of the electrical signal. One small vertical box equals 0.1 mm. The vertical scale is also standardized to a specific calibration, usually a rise of

at the cellular level. At some point, the cells change from an aerobic to anaerobic mode of metabolism, which results in the production of lactic acid and is representative of a shock state in which cellular injury or cell death may result. At this point, every attempt must be made to determine the cause of

TABLE 11-7	MEASUREMENTS OF MIXED VENOUS OXYGEN SATURATION	
S$\bar{v}o_2$ MEASUREMENT	PHYSIOLOGICAL BASIS FOR CHANGES IN S$\bar{v}o_2$/Sc$\bar{v}o_2$	CLINICAL DIAGNOSIS AND RATIONALE
High S$\bar{v}o_2$ (80%-95%)	Increased oxygen supply Decreased oxygen demand	Patient receiving more oxygen than required by clinical condition Anesthesia, which causes sedation and decreased muscle movement Hypothermia, which lowers metabolic demand (e.g., during cardiopulmonary bypass) Sepsis caused by decreased ability of tissues to use oxygen at a cellular level False high-positive result because the pulmonary artery catheter is wedged in a pulmonary arteriole S$\bar{v}o_2$ only)
Normal S$\bar{v}o_2$/Sc$\bar{v}o_2$ (60%-80%)	**Normal oxygen supply and metabolic demand**	Balanced oxygen supply and demand Anemia or bleeding with compromised cardiopulmonary system
Low S$\bar{v}o_2$/Sc$\bar{v}o_2$ (<60%)	Decreased oxygen supply caused by: Low hemoglobin (Hgb) Low arterial saturation (Sao$_2$) Low cardiac output (CO) Increased oxygen consumption ($\bar{v}o_2$)	Hypoxemia resulting from decreased oxygen supply or lung disease Cardiogenic shock caused by left ventricular pump failure Metabolic demand exceeds oxygen supply in conditions that increase muscle movement and increase metabolic rate, including physiological states such as shivering, seizures, and hyperthermia and nursing interventions such as being weighed on a bed scale and turning

Modified from White KM, et al: The physiologic basis for continuous mixed venous oxygen saturation monitoring, *Heart Lung* 19(5 Pt 2): 548, 1990.

10 mm (2 large boxes) in response to a 1 mV electrical signal, evident at the beginning of the ECG tracing.

Interpreting the ECG

The analysis of waveforms and intervals provide the basis for ECG interpretation (Figure 11-22).

P Wave. The P wave represents atrial depolarization.

QRS Complex. The QRS complex represents ventricular depolarization, corresponding to phase 0 of the ventricular action potential. It is referred to as a complex because it consists of several different waves. The letter Q is used to describe an initial negative deflection; only if the first deflection from the baseline is negative will it be labeled a Q wave. The letter R applies to any positive deflection. If there are two positive deflections in one QRS complex, the second is labeled R' ("R prime") and is commonly seen in lead V_1 in patients with right bundle branch block. The letter S refers to any subsequent negative deflections. Any combination of these deflections can occur and is collectively called the QRS complex (Figure 11-23). The QRS duration is normally less than 0.10 second (2.5 small horizontal boxes).

T Wave. The T wave represents ventricular repolarization. The onset of the QRS to approximately the midpoint or peak of the T wave represents an absolute refractory period, during which the heart muscle cannot respond to another stimulus no matter how strong that stimulus may be (Figure 11-24). From the midpoint to the end of the T wave, the heart muscle is in the relative refractory period. The heart muscle has not yet fully recovered, but it can be depolarized again if a strong enough stimulus is received. This can be a particularly dangerous time for ventricular ectopy to occur, especially if any portion of the myocardium is ischemic, because the ischemic

muscle takes even longer to fully repolarize. This sets the stage for the disorganized, self-perpetuating depolarization of various sections of the myocardium known as ventricular fibrillation (VF).

Intervals between Waveforms. The intervals between waveforms are evaluated (see Figure 11-22).

PR Interval. The PR interval is measured from the beginning of the P wave to the beginning of the QRS complex. Normally, the PR interval is 0.12 to 0.20 second long and represents the time between sinus node discharge and the beginning of ventricular depolarization (see Figure 11-22). Because most of this period results from delay of the impulse in the AV node, the PR interval is an indicator of AV nodal function.

In the electrophysiology laboratory and in some critical care units, these time values are described in milliseconds. There are 1000 milliseconds (msec) in 1 second. The normal PR interval value can also be written as 120 to 200 msec.

ST Segment. The ST segment is the portion of the wave that extends from the end of the QRS to the beginning of the T wave. Its duration is not measured. Instead, its shape and location are evaluated.[89,90] The ST segment is normally flat and at the same level as the isoelectric baseline. The baseline measurement is taken 60 to 80 msec after the J point (Figure 11-25). Any vertical change in the ST segment from baseline is expressed in millimeters and may indicate myocardial ischemia (one small box equals 1 mm). ST-segment elevation (vertical increase above baseline greater than 1 mm) is associated with acute myocardial injury[91] and pericarditis. ST-segment depression (decrease from baseline more than 1 mm) is associated with myocardial ischemia.[92] The ST segment must be monitored carefully in high-risk patients.[92]

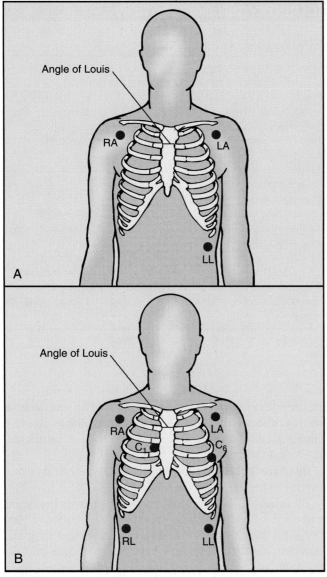

FIGURE 11-19 *A,* Three electrodes and lead-wire cables allow monitoring of three of the limb leads: I, II, and III. *B,* Five electrodes and lead-wire cables allow monitoring of any of the six standard limb leads (I, II, III, aVR, aVL, or aVF), and any one precordial or chest (C) lead from position V₁ to V₆. The label C₁ indicates the correct position of the chest electrode for monitoring lead V₁, and C₆ indicates the proper position of the chest electrode for monitoring V₆.

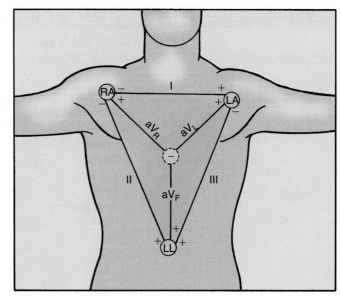

FIGURE 11-20 Standard limb leads. Leads are located on the extremities: right arm (RA), left arm (LA), and left leg (LL). The right leg electrode serves as a ground. Leads I, II, and III are bipolar, with each using a positive electrode and a negative electrode. Leads aVR, aVL, and aVF are augmented unipolar leads that use the calculated center of the heart as their negative electrode.

QT Interval. The QT interval is measured from the beginning of the QRS complex to the end of the T wave and indicates the total time interval from the onset of depolarization to the completion of repolarization (see Figure 11-22). There is no established bedside monitoring lead recommended for measuring the QT interval.[89] On the 12-lead ECG, the QT interval is usually the longest in precordial (chest) leads V₃ and V₄.[89] The important point is that each clinician measures the QT interval using the same ECG lead.[89] At normal heart rates, the QT interval is less than one half of the R-R interval when measured from one QRS complex to the next. However,

the length of a QT interval depends on heart rate and must be adjusted according to the heart rate to be evaluated accurately.

Because the QT interval shortens with faster heart rates and lengthens with slower heart rates, it is often written as a "corrected" value (QTc), meaning the QT value was mathematically corrected as if the heart rate were 60 beats/min.[93] This allows comparison of QTc across a range of heart rates. The normal QTc is less than 0.46 second (460 msec) in women and less than 0.45 second (450 msec) in men.[89] A prolonged QT interval is significant because it can predispose the patient to the development of polymorphic VT, also known as torsades de pointes. A long QT interval can be the result of a congenital chromosomal abnormality, or it can be acquired as a result of electrolyte imbalance or antidysrhythmic drug therapy.[94,95]

Heart Rate Determination. The first thing to assess when evaluating a rhythm strip is the ventricular rate. Regardless of the dysrhythmia involved, the ventricular rate holds the key to whether the patient can tolerate the dysrhythmia (i.e., maintain adequate blood pressure, CO, and mentation). If the ventricular rate is consistently greater than 200 or less than 30, emergency measures must be started to correct the rate. A detailed analysis of the underlying rhythm disturbance can proceed later, when the immediate crisis is over. The three methods for calculating rate when the rhythm is <u>regular</u> (Figure 11-26, *A*) follow:

1. Number of R-R intervals in 6 seconds times 10 (ECG paper is usually marked at the top in 3-second increments, making a 6-second interval easy to identify.)

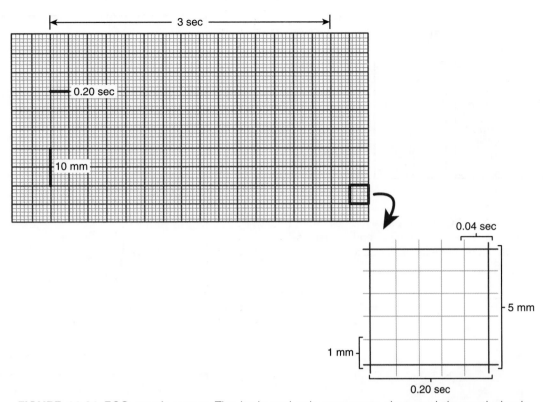

FIGURE 11-21 ECG graph paper. The horizontal axis represents time, and the vertical axis represents the magnitude of voltage. Horizontally, each small box is 0.04 second, and each large box is 0.20 second. Vertically, each large box is 5 mm. Markings are present every 3 seconds at the top of the paper for ease in calculating heart rate.

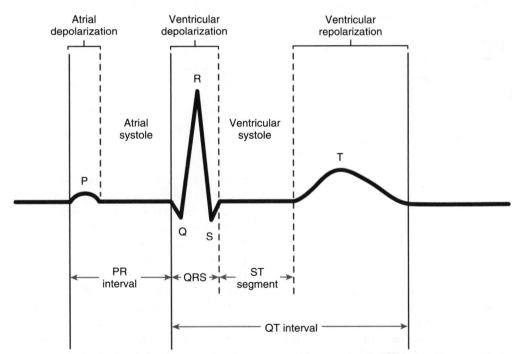

FIGURE 11-22 Normal ECG waveforms, intervals, and correlation with events of the cardiac cycle. The *P wave* represents atrial depolarization, followed immediately by atrial systole. The *QRS* represents ventricular depolarization, followed immediately by ventricular systole. The *ST segment* corresponds to phase 2 of the action potential, during which time the heart muscle is completely depolarized and contraction normally occurs. The *T wave* represents ventricular repolarization. The *PR interval,* measured from the beginning of the P wave to the beginning of the QRS, corresponds to atrial depolarization and impulse delay in the atrioventricular (AV) node. The *QT interval,* measured from the beginning of the QRS complex to the end of the T wave, represents the time from initial depolarization of the ventricles to the end of ventricular repolarization.

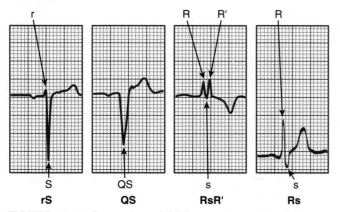

FIGURE 11-23 Examples of QRS complexes. Small deflections are labeled with lowercase letters, and uppercase letters are used for larger deflections. A second upward deflection is labeled R'.

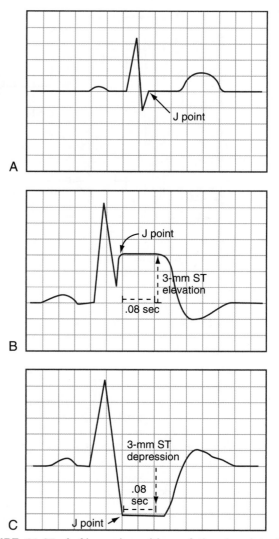

FIGURE 11-25 *A,* Normal position of the J point. *B,* A 3-mm ST-segment elevation. *C,* A 3-mm ST-segment depression. ST-segment changes are measured 60 to 80 msec (0.06 to 0.08 sec) after the J point.

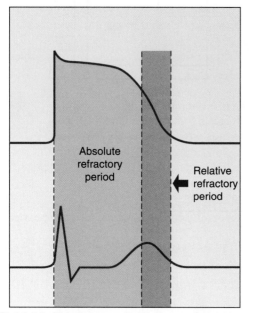

FIGURE 11-24 Absolute and relative refractory periods are correlated with the myocardial cell action potential and with an ECG.

2. Number of large boxes between QRS complexes divided into 300
3. Number of small boxes between QRS complexes divided into 1500

In the healthy heart, the atrial rate and the ventricular rate are the same. However, in many dysrhythmias, the atrial and ventricular rates are different, and both must be calculated. To find the atrial rate, the PP interval, instead of the R-R interval, is used in one of the three methods listed for determining rate.

When the rhythm is *irregular*, the first method (R-R intervals in 6 seconds × 10) is the only method that can be used (see Figure 11-26, *B*).

Rhythm Determination. The term rhythm refers to the regularity with which the P waves or R waves occur. Calipers assist in determining rhythm. One point of the calipers is placed on the beginning of one R wave, and the other point is placed on the next R wave. Leaving the calipers "set" at this interval, each succeeding R-R interval is checked to be sure it is the same width as the first one measured.

P-Wave Evaluation. The P wave is analyzed by answering the following questions. First, is the P wave present or absent? Second, is it related to the QRS? It is hoped that one P wave will be in front of every QRS. Sometimes, two, three, or four P waves may be in front of every QRS. If this pattern is consistent, the P wave and QRS are still related, although not on a 1:1 basis.

PR-Interval Evaluation. The duration of the PR interval, which normally is 0.12 to 0.20 second (120 to 200 msec), is measured first. This is measured from the start of a visible P wave to the beginning of the next QRS (see Figure 11-22). All PR intervals on the strip are verified to be sure they have the same duration as the original interval.

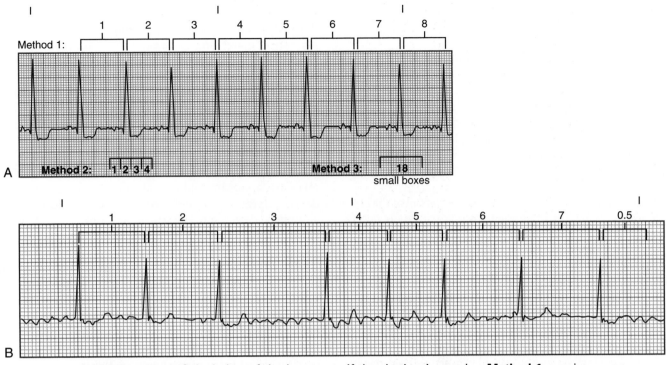

FIGURE 11-26 *A,* Calculation of the heart rate if the rhythm is regular. **Method 1:** number of R-R intervals in 6 seconds multiplied by 10 (e.g., 8 × 10 = 80/min). **Method 2:** number of large boxes between QRS complexes divided into 300 (e.g., 300 ÷ 4 = 75/min). **Method 3:** number of small boxes between QRS complexes divided into 1500 (e.g., 1500 ÷ 18 = 84/min). *B,* Rate calculation if the rhythm is irregular, as in this example of atrial fibrillation. Only method 1 can be used (e.g., 7.5 intervals × 10 = 75/min).

TABLE 11-8	SINUS RHYTHMS			
PARAMETERS	**NORMAL SINUS RHYTHM**	**SINUS BRADYCARDIA**	**SINUS TACHYCARDIA**	**SINUS DYSRHYTHMIA**
Rate	60-100/min	<60/min	>100/min	Variable
Rhythm	Regular	Regular	Regular	Irregular; respiratory variation
P wave	Present, with one per QRS	Present, with one per QRS	Present, with one per QRS	Present, with one per QRS
PR interval	0.12-0.20 sec and constant	0.12-0.20 sec and constant	0.12-0.20 sec and constant	0.12-0.20 sec and constant
QRS	0.06-0.10 sec	0.06-0.10 sec	0.06-0.10 sec	0.06-0.10 sec

QRS Complex Evaluation. The entire ECG strip must be evaluated to ascertain that the QRS complexes are consistently the same shape and width. The normal QRS duration is 0.06 to 0.10 second (60 to 100 msec). If more than one QRS shape is on the strip, each QRS must be measured. The QRS is measured from where it leaves the baseline to where it returns to the baseline (see Figure 11-22).

QT Evaluation. The length of the QT varies with the heart rate. The QT interval is shorter when the heart rate is faster. A QT interval corrected for heart rate (QTc) that is longer than 0.50 second (500 msec) is of concern, as discussed earlier under "QT Interval."

Dysrhythmia Interpretation

In clinical practice the terms "dysrhythmia" and "arrhythmia" often are used interchangeably. Both are correct, and either may be used in clinical practice; this text favors "dysrhythmia." A dysrhythmia is any disturbance in the normal cardiac conduction pathway. Patients in critical care units always have continuous ECG monitoring. ECG rhythm strips are recorded routinely, and any time a significant rhythm change occurs.

Sinus Rhythms. There are four rhythms that begin with the word sinus, indicating that the rhythm originates from within the sinus node. Table 11-8 provides a summary of the major features of this category of rhythms.

Normal Sinus Rhythm. (Figure 11-27.)
RATE: 60 to 100 beats/min.
RHYTHM: Regular (±10%).
P WAVE: Present, all the same shape, with only one preceding each QRS complex.
PR INTERVAL: 0.12 to 0.20 second.
QRS DURATION: 0.06 to 0.10 second.
QRS COMPLEX: Shape and whether deflection is positive or negative vary depending on lead placement and do not provide key diagnostic information.
ETIOLOGY: Normal conduction.
TREATMENT: None required.

Sinus Bradycardia. Sinus bradycardia meets all of the criteria for normal sinus rhythm except that the rate is fewer than 60 beats/min (see Table 11-8). Sinus bradycardia usually is not treated unless the patient displays symptoms of hypoperfusion, such as hypotension, dizziness, chest pain, or changes in level of consciousness.

Sinus Tachycardia. Sinus tachycardia meets all the criteria for normal sinus rhythm except that the rate is greater than 100 beats/min (see Table 11-8). Rates may be as high as 180 to 200 beats/min in healthy, young adults during strenuous exercise. However, in the critical care setting, bed rest is prescribed for most patients. It is wise to be skeptical of any "sinus tachycardia" with a rate greater than 150 and to search for a triggering focus other than the sinus node. Many drugs used in critical care can cause sinus tachycardia; common culprits are dopamine, hydralazine, atropine, and epinephrine. Tachycardia is detrimental to anyone with ischemic heart disease because it decreases the time for ventricular filling, decreases stroke volume, and compromises CO.

Tachycardia increases heart work and myocardial oxygen demand while decreasing oxygen supply by decreasing coronary artery filling time. If the cause of the tachycardia can be determined, such as fever or pain, that symptom is treated rather than trying to treat the heart rate directly.

Sinus Dysrhythmia. Sinus dysrhythmia, commonly called sinus arrhythmia in clinical practice, meets all of the criteria for normal sinus rhythm except that the rhythm is irregular (see Table 11-8). This irregularity coincides with the respiratory pattern; heart rate increases with inhalation and decreases with exhalation[96] (Figure 11-28). Sinus dysrhythmia often occurs in children and young adults, and the incidence decreases with age. No treatment is required. To accurately detect sinus dysrhythmia, look at all P waves closely to verify that they are all the same shape and that the PR intervals are all constant.

Atrial Dysrhythmias. Atrial dysrhythmias originate from an ectopic focus in the atria, somewhere other than the sinus node (Table 11-9). The ectopic impulse occurs prematurely, before the normal sinus impulse occurs. The premature atrial depolarization may initiate a normal QRS complex, an abnormal or aberrant complex, or an SVT. Huge advances have been made in the understanding of the pathogenesis and management of atrial dysrhythmias.

Premature Atrial Contractions. Premature atrial contractions (PACs) are isolated, early beats from an ectopic focus in the atria. The underlying rhythm is usually sinus. The regular sinus rhythm is interrupted by an early, abnormally shaped atrial P wave. The early atrial wave usually looks different from the sinus P wave and may be inverted. The PR interval may be longer, shorter, or the same as the PR interval of a sinus impulse. The QRS that follows the ectopic atrial P wave can vary in shape depending on the degree of refractoriness of the AV node.

- *PAC with Narrow QRS.* If the atrial impulse arrives in the AV node after the AV node is fully repolarized, the impulse is conducted to the ventricles as a normal QRS. If the ventricles are also fully repolarized, conduction through the bundle branches is expected and a normal QRS is recorded on the ECG (Figure 11-29, *A*).
- *PAC with Wide QRS.* Occasionally, the early ectopic P wave can be conducted through the AV node, but part of the conduction pathway through the ventricular bundle branches is blocked. Because the right bundle branch normally has the longest refractory period, it is usually

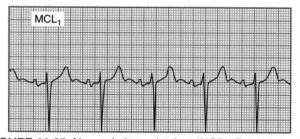

FIGURE 11-27 Normal sinus rhythm (NSR). The rate is 70, and the rhythm is regular. One P wave is present before each QRS complex. The PR interval is 0.18 second and does not vary throughout the strip. The QRS duration is 0.08 second. All evaluation criteria are within normal limits.

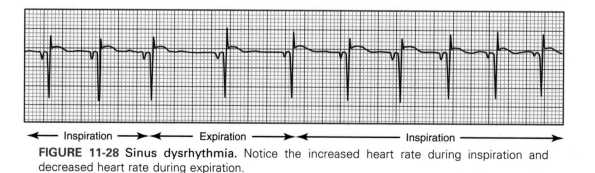

←—— Inspiration ——→←—— Expiration ——→←———— Inspiration ————→

FIGURE 11-28 Sinus dysrhythmia. Notice the increased heart rate during inspiration and decreased heart rate during expiration.

TABLE 11-9	ATRIAL DYSRHYTHMIAS			
PARAMETER	PAROXYSMAL SUPRAVENTRICULAR TACHYCARDIA	MULTIFOCAL ATRIAL TACHYCARDIA	ATRIAL FLUTTER	ATRIAL FIBRILLATION
Rate				
Atrial	150-250/min	100-160/min	250-350/min	>350/min (unable to count it)
Ventricular	Same or less	Same	250-350/min, one half or less	100-180/min (uncontrolled); <100/min (controlled)
Rhythm	Regular	Irregular	Atrial; regular; ventricular; may or may not be regular	Irregularly irregular
P Wave	Present; abnormally shaped	Present; three or more different shapes	F waves	Fibrillatory baseline
PR Interval	May be normal or prolonged	Variable	Conduction ratio: flutter waves per QRS	Absent
QRS	0.06-0.10 sec	0.06-0.10 sec	0.06-0.10 sec	0.06-0.10 sec

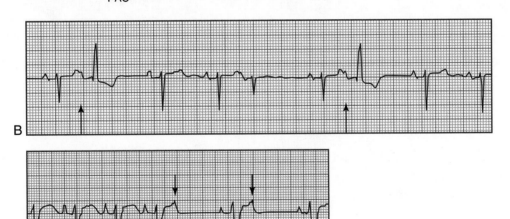

FIGURE 11-29 Premature atrial contractions (PACs). *A,* Normally conducted PAC. The early P wave is indicated by the *arrow,* and the QRS that follows has a normal shape and duration. *B,* Nonconducted (blocked) PACs. The early P waves are indicated by *arrows.* Notice how they distort the T waves, making them appear peaked compared with the normal T waves seen after the third and fourth QRS complexes. *C,* Right bundle branch block aberration after a PAC.

the right bundle branch that is still blocked when the early impulse arrives. This produces a QRS that is wider than 0.12 second (120 msec) or wider than three small horizontal boxes on the ECG paper (see Figure 11-29, *B*). Conduction through the ventricles that is different from normal is referred to as aberrant. Consequently, these early, abnormally conducted PACs are described as aberrantly conducted PACs.

- *Nonconducted PAC with Pause without QRS.* Sometimes, the ectopic P wave arrives so early that the AV node is still in its absolute refractory period. In this case, the wave of depolarization does not move past the AV node, and no QRS follows. All that is seen on the ECG is an early, abnormal P wave followed by a pause until the next sinus P wave occurs (see Figure 11-29, *C*). This is called a nonconducted PAC.

PACs are not restricted to individuals with heart disease, and are accentuated by emotional upheaval, nicotine, and caffeine. Heart failure is associated with PACs. As atrial pressure rises, the atrial walls are stretched, causing irritability of atrial cells and the occurrence of PACs.

Supraventricular Tachycardia. The term supraventricular tachycardia (SVT) is used clinically to describe a varied group of dysrhythmias that originate above the AV node. SVT is not a specific term; it includes sinus tachycardia, atrial tachycardia, multifocal atrial tachycardia, atrial flutter, atrial fibrillation, and junctional tachycardia. Each of these entities has a distinct pathophysiology, specific therapy, and expected outcome. SVT may also be described as a narrow-complex tachycardia, defined as a QRS that is less than 0.12 second (120 milliseconds).[97] After the specific dysrhythmia is identified, it usually is described by its specific name, such as 'atrial fibrillation with a rapid ventricular response'.[98] The term SVT is used to describe a rapid, sustained atrial or junctional tachycardia when the exact mechanism is unknown. Women are affected by episodic SVT at about twice the rate of men.[97]

SVT is not always benign. About 15% of people with SVT experience syncope (lose consciousness). Medications are used to limit the SVT rate and prevent "blackouts" or syncope.[97] SVT that is persistent for weeks or months may lead to a tachycardia-mediated cardiomyopathy.[85] A baseline 12-lead ECG is helpful, and when possible, a 12-lead ECG should be obtained during the palpitations.[85] SVT that is persistent for weeks or months may lead to a tachycardia-mediated cardiomyopathy. Paroxysmal means starting and stopping abruptly. Paroxysmal supraventricular tachycardia (PSVT) is a form of SVT that starts abruptly and stops as suddenly as it began (Figure 11-30).

Atrial Flutter. Atrial flutter is recognized on the ECG by the sawtooth atrial pattern. These sawtooth-shaped atrial wavelets are not P waves; they are more appropriately called F waves (atrial flutter waves), as shown in Figure 11-31. Fortunately, the AV node does not allow conduction of all these impulses to the ventricles.

RATE: Atrial rate 250 to 350 beats/min.

RHYTHM: Regular flutter waves. Ventricular response (QRS complexes) may be regular or irregular.

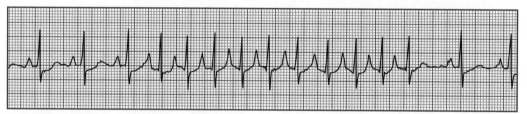

FIGURE 11-30 Paroxysmal supraventricular tachycardia (PSVT). Notice that the atrial rate during tachycardia is 158 beats/min. The run starts and stops abruptly.

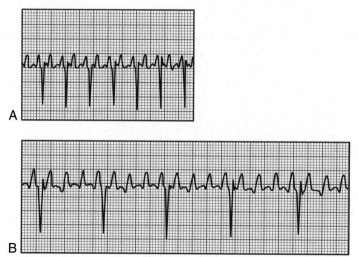

FIGURE 11-31 *A,* Initial strip shows atrial flutter with 2:1 conduction through the atrioventricular (AV) node. *B,* During carotid sinus massage, (a vagal maneuver) the AV conduction rate is decreased, more clearly revealing the flutter waves.

P WAVE: Replaced by Flutter (F) waves.

PR INTERVAL: No longer applies; instead a conduction ratio of flutter waves to QRS complexes (e.g., 2:1, 3:1, 4:1) is used. When evaluating the rate of atrial flutter, both atrial and ventricular rates must be calculated. The atrial rate is always faster.

QRS COMPLEX: Shape is usually narrow and normal.

PHYSIOLOGY: Atrial flutter can be started by any isolated atrial impulse, but in order to be maintained, the atrial flutter requires a reentry circular pathway around macroscopic structures in the atria. Typically, these structures are in the right atrium and involve the vena cava and the tricuspid valve in an area known as the cavotricuspid isthmus. The reentry loop typically circles counterclockwise around the tricuspid valve[97] and can circle the inferior vena cava (IVC) or the IVC and the tricuspid valve. To maintain a viable, self-perpetuating reentry pathway, the loop must avoid the sinoatrial node and be large enough to always meet tissue that is ready to be depolarized (accept a new electrical stimulus). The atrial reentry rate in atrial flutter is typically between 250 to 350 beats/min, producing the classic sawtooth or flutter wave pattern.[97] The atrial flutter wavelet always appears regular, because the circuit is always the same length and requires exactly the same amount of time to complete the reentry loop (see Table 11-9).

The ventricular response rate is the major factor that impacts how symptomatic a patient becomes following onset of atrial flutter. If the atrial rate is 300 beats/min and the AV conduction ratio is 4:1, the ventricular response rate is 75 beats/min and should be well tolerated. However, if the atrial rate is 300 beats/min and the AV conduction ratio is 2:1, the corresponding ventricular rate of 150 beats/min may cause symptoms of dizziness, or chest pain and palpitations. An atrial rate of 250 beats/min with a 1:1 AV conduction ratio yields a ventricular response rate of 250 beats/min; the patient will be extremely symptomatic, and emergency measures are needed to decrease the ventricular rate.

MANAGEMENT: Sometimes, it is difficult to identify the flutter waves on an ECG rhythm strip, especially if the conduction ratio is 2:1. Vagal maneuvers may permit visualization of the atrial waveform and thereby facilitate accurate diagnosis, as seen in Figure 11-31. Electrical cardioversion and atrial overdrive pacing are the most effective interventions to convert atrial flutter to sinus rhythm. The conversation rate with DC cardioversion is between 95% and 100%.[97] If atrial flutter has been present for more than 48 hours, up to one third of patients will have thrombi in the atria, and anticoagulation is mandated before pharmacological or electrical cardioversion. The risk of systemic emboli after cardioversion ranges from 2% to 7%.[97] Overdrive atrial pacing is often favored to convert atrial flutter after cardiac surgery. Epicardial wires that are placed at the time of surgery are connected to an external pacemaker. The overall success rate of atrial overdrive pacing is 83% (range, 55% to 100%).[97]

Pharmacological cardioversion using ibutilide (Corvert) is effective at converting hemodynamically stable atrial flutter to sinus rhythm in 38% to 76% of patients.[97] The reasons for the variance in conversion in clinical studies is unknown, but it was not related to the length of time the patients had been in atrial flutter. For patients who responded to the ibutilide, the average conversion time after infusion was 30 minutes.[97] One of the complications of ibutilide is polymorphic tachycardia—also known as torsades de pointes—but in studies of patients with atrial flutter, the rate of torsades de pointes was less than 3%.[97]

Antidysrhythmic drugs are administered for two reasons in atrial flutter: (1) to slow conduction through the AV node; and (2) to convert the atrial rhythm back to normal sinus rhythm (NSR). Amiodarone IV achieves both aims and is frequently administered in critical care. Further information about pharmacological management of atrial dysrhythmias is listed in Chapter 13 in Table 13-14. For patients with chronic atrial flutter unrelated to an acute disease process, permanent termination of the atrial flutter circuit can be achieved by radiofrequency ablation (RFA). RFA is a catheter procedure that creates a scar-line conduction block across one of more sections of the reentry pathway.

Atrial Fibrillation. Atrial fibrillation is the most frequently encountered dysrhythmia in the developed world (Figure 11-32). It affects an estimated 2.3 million individuals in the United States and 4.5 million people in the European Union. In the United States the estimated annual cost to treat atrial fibrillation is about $3,000 per patient per year.[99] When first detected, atrial fibrillation may be described as paroxysmal (self-terminating) or persistent (not self-terminating); when all attempts at conversion to sinus rhythm have failed, it is described as permanent (Figure 11-33). Atrial fibrillation is present in 0.4% to 1% of the general population, but the incidence rises to more than 8% among those older than 80 years.[99] The median age of patients with atrial fibrillation is 75 years.[99] Atrial fibrillation is the most common cardiac dysrhythmia in the United States and responsible for about one third of dysrhythmia-related hospital admissions.[99] The risk of developing atrial fibrillation is higher for people with a history of hypertension, heart failure, obesity, or MI.[99]

RATE: Atrial rate 350 to 600 fibrillatory waves per minute.

Ventricular rate 60 to 100 (when controlled by medication), greater than 100 (when uncontrolled by medication).

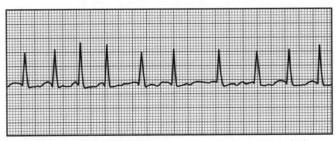

FIGURE 11-32 Atrial fibrillation. Notice the irregularly irregular ventricular rhythm.

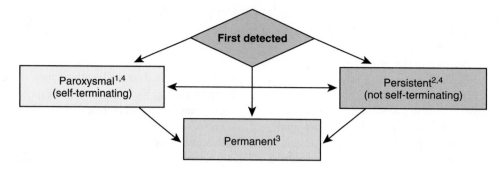

[1]Episodes that generally last less than or equal to 7 days (most less than 24 h);
[2]usually more than 6 days;
[3]cardioversion failed or not attempted; and
[4]both paroxysmal and persistent AF may be recurrent.

FIGURE 11-33 **Patterns of new-onset atrial fibrillation.** (From Fuster V, et al: ACC/AHA/ESC 2006 Guidelines for the Management of Patients with Atrial Fibrillation: a report of the American College of Cardiology/American Heart Association Task Force on Practice Guidelines and the European Society of Cardiology Committee for Practice Guidelines [Writing Committee to Revise the 2001 Guidelines for the Management of Patients With Atrial Fibrillation]: developed in collaboration with the European Heart Rhythm Association and the Heart Rhythm Society, *Circulation* 114[7]:e257, 2006.)

RHYTHM: Irregularly irregular ventricular rhythm.
P WAVE: Replaced by fibrillating baseline or waves.
PR INTERVAL: Absent. Replaced by fibrillating baseline.
QRS DURATION: 0.06 to 0.10 second.
QRS COMPLEX: Usually normal because pathway through ventricles is unchanged once impulse leaves AV node.

Atrial fibrillation may be classified under the broad category of SVT, because the heart rate is rapid and many patients have symptoms of hypotension and breathlessness during paroxysmal atrial fibrillation when uncontrolled by medication. Uncoordinated atrial electrical activation leads to a rapid deterioration in atrial mechanical function. The ECG tracing in atrial fibrillation is notable for an uneven atrial baseline that lacks clearly defined P waves and instead shows rapid oscillations or fibrillatory wavelets that vary in size, shape, and frequency.[99] The atrial fibrillatory waves are particularly easy to identify in the inferior ECG leads II, III, and aVF.

ETIOLOGY: The pathogenesis of atrial fibrillation has traditionally been ascribed to random electrical foci firing in the atria. Research using high-density atrial mapping, high-speed video recordings, and ECG analysis has uncovered distinct spatial organization within the atria.[99] Atrial fibrillation involves several reentry circuits within the atria, and in some cases, they originate at specific anatomic sites. The four pulmonary veins that drain into the left atrium are a trigger site for early foci to initiate and maintain atrial reentry circuits.[99] The earliest atrial ectopic foci have been electrically mapped 2 to 4 cm within the pulmonary veins.[100] The affected pulmonary veins contain thin myocardial sleeves of tissue that project into the pulmonary veins from the left atrium. The tissue ultimately becomes part of the venous wall. The spread of atrial fibrillation to the rest of the atria is thought to occur through multiple reentry wavelets that

are maintained in perpetual motion by a "mother rotor," or dominant reentry circuit, which functions at a higher frequency, drives the atrial fibrillation, and originates from the ectopic pulmonary vein tissue.[100]

MANAGEMENT: There continues to be debate about the most effective pharmacological treatment approach for atrial fibrillation, as shown in the algorithm to treat new-onset atrial fibrillation (Figure 11-34). In the past, the gold standard was to convert the patient out of the atrial fibrillation back to sinus rhythm. However, for many older patients, staying out of atrial fibrillation is an unattainable goal. Today, the major focus is on rhythm control versus rate control for atrial fibrillation. All patients with atrial fibrillation require anticoagulation to prevent thrombotic embolism and stroke.

Rhythm Control. For the hospitalized patient with new-onset atrial fibrillation with unstable hemodynamics, the focus is generally on rhythm control (conversion to sinus rhythm) using antidysrhythmic drugs or electrical cardioversion. Emergency drugs used to convert atrial fibrillation to sinus rhythm, also known as a chemical cardioversion, include amiodarone and ibutilide. Antidysrhythmic drugs used long-term to maintain the patient in sinus rhythm include amiodarone, disopyramide, flecainide, moricizine, procainamide, propafenone, quinidine, sotalol, and dofetilide or a combination of these medications as needed.[101] Even with drug therapy, recurrence of atrial fibrillation is likely.[101] Electrical cardioversion may be successful in converting the atria to sinus rhythm if attempted within a few days or weeks of the onset of atrial fibrillation. Its success is less likely if the atrial fibrillation has existed for a long time.[99] Without antidysrhythmic drug therapy, about 75% of cardioverted patients would be in atrial fibrillation at one year.[102]

Rate Control. The most frequently prescribed drugs used to control the ventricular rate in atrial fibrillation include

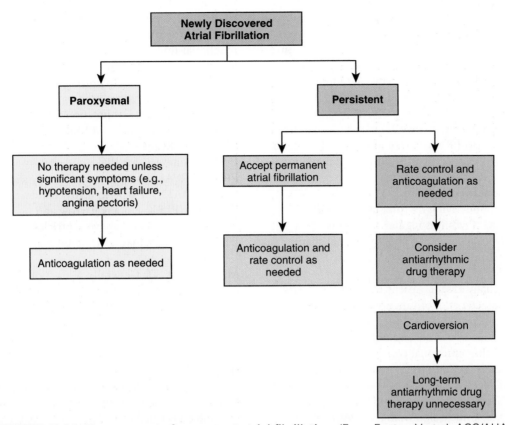

FIGURE 11-34 Management of new-onset atrial fibrillation. (From Fuster, V et al: ACC/AHA/ ESC 2006 Guidelines for the Management of Patients with Atrial Fibrillation: a report of the American College of Cardiology/American Heart Association Task Force on Practice Guidelines and the European Society of Cardiology Committee for Practice Guidelines [Writing Committee to Revise the 2001 Guidelines for the Management of Patients With Atrial Fibrillation]: developed in collaboration with the European Heart Rhythm Association and the Heart Rhythm Society, *Circulation* 114[7]:e257, 2006.)

calcium channel blockers, beta-blockers, and digoxin. These drugs work to slow conduction through the AV node. They have no impact on the fibrillating atria. In the past, it was assumed that rate control was an inferior strategy, because patients who remained in atrial fibrillation lost "atrial kick," and were presumed to have an increased risk of embolic stroke. The results of two multicenter trials have altered that perception: the *Atrial Fibrillation Follow-up: Investigation of Rhythm Management* (AFFIRM) and the *RAte Control vs. Electrical Cardioversion for Persistent Atrial Fibrillation* (RACE).[101] These two trials found similar morbidity, mortality, and quality of life in patients treated long-term with rhythm conversion, or rate control.[101] For long-term management of atrial fibrillation, rate control is the recommended approach, and therapeutic anticoagulation to prevent embolic stroke is mandatory.[103] Antidysrhythmic medications used to manage atrial fibrillation are listed in Chapter 13 (Table 13-15).

Anticoagulation. To prevent embolic stroke, it is important to pay attention to the 48-hour rule. Patients who have been in atrial fibrillation for 48 hours or longer (how long may not be known) must be adequately anticoagulated with an oral vitamin K antagonist (warfarin) to achieve a target

international normalized ration (INR) of 2.5 (range, 2.0 to 3.0) for at least 3 weeks before elective cardioversion.[103] A diagnostic echocardiogram may be used to verify that the atria are free from thrombi. After successful cardioversion, patients should continue to be anticoagulated for 4 weeks.[103] These antithrombotic recommendations apply equally to patients with atrial flutter.[103]

Catheter Ablation. Percutaneous catheter interventions to treat atrial fibrillation are available for younger patients who have atrial fibrillation without structural heart disease. Radiofrequency ablation (RFA) is employed to isolate foci that originate in the four pulmonary veins. Several different RFA options are available, encircling all four veins together, isolating pulmonary veins individually, or in pairs.[104] This catheter procedure is successfully used in many cardiac electrophysiology centers.[105,106]

Junctional Dysrhythmias. Only certain areas of the AV node have the property of automaticity. The entire area around the AV node is collectively called the AV junction; impulses generated there are called junctional. After an ectopic impulse arises in the junction, it spreads in two directions at once. One wave of depolarization spreads upward into the atria and depolarizes them, causing the recording of a P wave on the ECG. This is called retrograde (backward) conduction, and the P wave is inverted when viewed in lead II. At the same time, another wave of depolarization spreads downward into the ventricles through the normal conduction pathway, producing a normal QRS complex. This is called antegrade (forward) conduction.

Depending on timing, the P wave (1) may be seen in front of the QRS, with a short PR interval of less than 0.12 second, (2) may be obscured entirely by the QRS, or (3) may immediately follow the QRS.

Premature Junctional Contraction.
RATE: Depends on underlying rhythm, usually NSR.
RHYTHM: On ECG, rhythm is regular from sinus node except for early QRS complex (PJC) of normal shape.
P WAVE: May be entirely absent, may be seen in T wave, or may be inverted.
PR INTERVAL: Usually absent. Absent or short PR interval are defining characteristics of junctional rhythms.
QRS DURATION: 0.06 to 0.10 second.
QRS COMPLEX: Usually narrow and normal.
ETIOLOGY: Premature junctional contraction (PJC) is a single ectopic impulse that originates in AV junctional area.
MANAGEMENT: Usually none required. PJCs have virtually the same clinical significance as PACs. If the patient is receiving digoxin, however, digitalis toxicity should be considered. Although digoxin slows conduction through the AV node, it also increases automaticity in the junction.

Junctional Escape Rhythm. Sometimes, the junction becomes the dominant pacemaker of the heart (Table 11-10). Normally, the intrinsic rate of the junction is 40 to 60 beats/min. The intrinsic rate of the sinus node is 60 to 100 beats/min. Under normal conditions, the junction never has a chance to escape and depolarize the heart because it is overridden by the sinus node. However, if the sinus node fails, the junctional impulses can depolarize completely and pace the heart. This is called a junctional escape rhythm, and it is a protective mechanism to prevent asystole in the event of sinus node failure.
RATE: Intrinsic rate of junction is 40 to 60 beats/min if dominant pacemaker of heart.
RHYTHM: Regular.
P WAVE: Same as for PJC.
PR INTERVAL: Usually absent or very short.
QRS DURATION: 0.06 to 0.10 second.
QRS COMPLEX: Usually narrow and normal because impulse originates above ventricles.
ETIOLOGY: Originates in AV junction after failure of sinus node.
MANAGEMENT: Generally, a junctional escape rhythm (Figure 11-35) is well tolerated hemodynamically. Sometimes a pacemaker is inserted as a protective measure when there is evidence that the AV junction may fail completely.

A junctional tachycardia also shares the same junctional characteristics but has a rate faster than 100 beats/min.

Junctional Tachycardia and Accelerated Junctional Rhythm. A junctional rhythm can also occur at a faster rate (see Table 11-10). As with sinus rhythm, the term tachycardia is reserved for rates greater than 100 beats/min; junctional tachycardia is a junctional rhythm, usually regular, at a rate greater than 100 beats/min.

When the junctional rate is greater than 60 beats/min and less than 100 beats/min (faster than the intrinsic rate of the junction but not fast enough to be considered a tachycardia), the phrase accelerated junctional rhythm applies.[107] Accelerated junctional rhythm does not usually cause symptoms, mainly because the heart rate is within the normal range.

TABLE 11-10	JUNCTIONAL RHYTHMS		
PARAMETER	**JUNCTIONAL ESCAPE RHYTHM**	**ACCELERATED JUNCTIONAL RHYTHM**	**JUNCTIONAL TACHYCARDIA**
Rate	40-60/min	60-100/min	>100/min
Rhythm	Regular	Regular	Regular
P waves	May be present or absent; inverted in lead II	May be present or absent; inverted in lead II	May be present or absent; inverted in lead II
PR interval	<0.12 sec	<0.12 sec	<0.12 sec
QRS	0.06-0.10 sec	0.06-0.10 sec	0.06-0.10 sec

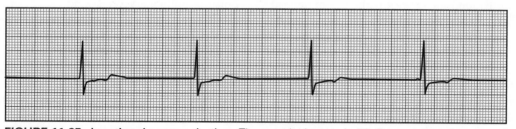

FIGURE 11-35 Junctional escape rhythm. The ventricular rate is 38. P waves are absent, and the QRS has a normal width.

Junctional tachycardia may not be tolerated as well, depending on the rate and the patient's underlying cardiac reserve.

Ventricular Dysrhythmias. Ventricular dysrhythmias result from an ectopic focus in any portion of the ventricular myocardium. The usual conduction pathway through the ventricles is not used, and the wave of depolarization must spread from cell to cell. As a result, the QRS complex is prolonged and is always greater than 0.12 second (wider than three small horizontal boxes on an ECG rhythm strip). It is the width of the QRS, not the height, that is important in the diagnosis of ventricular ectopy.

Premature Ventricular Contractions.

RATE: Depends on underlying HR, usually NSR.

RHYTHM: Early QRS complexes interrupt underlying rhythm.

PR INTERVAL: Absent or retrograde after PVC.

QRS DURATION: Greater than 0.12 second.

QRS COMPLEX: Wide, with bizarre shape.

- *Unifocal PVCs:* Probably all result from the same irritable focus (Figure 11-36, *A*).
- *Multifocal PVCs:* Ventricular ectopic beats have various shapes in the same lead. More serious than unifocal PVCs, multifocal PVCs indicate that a greater area of irritable myocardium is involved. Multifocal PVCs are more likely to deteriorate into ventricular tachycardia/fibrillation (Figure 11-36, *B*).
- *Ventricular Bigeminy:* One PVC follows each normal beat (Figure 11-36, *C*).
- *Compensatory Pause:* There is an apparently long "pause" following a PVC. However, the time-interval from the last normal QRS preceding the PVC to the QRS following the PVC is equal to two complete cardiac cycles. The compensatory pause allows the sinus node to resume the normal pattern (Figure 11-36, *D*).
- *Interpolated PVC:* PVC falls between two normal QRS complexes without disturbing the rhythm. RR interval between sinus beats remains the same (Figure 11-36, *E*).
- *Couplet:* Two consecutive PVCs.
- *Triplet:* Three consecutive PVCs.
- *R on T:* When a PVC occurs on the T wave during the *relative refractory period* (latter half of T wave) individual segments of myocardium can depolarize independently, increasing the risk of ventricular fibrillation (Figure 11-36, *F*).
- *Fusion Beat:* If the sinus impulse and the ventricular ectopic impulse meet in the middle of the ventricles, a fusion beat results.[108] Fusion beats are narrower than ventricular beats and look like a cross between the patient's sinus QRS and the ventricular ectopic QRS (Figure 11-36, *G*).

ETIOLOGY: Myocardial ischemia, electrolyte imbalances, hypoxia, acidosis, heart disease, myocardial scar tissue, and prodysrhythmic medications.[109]

PHYSIOLOGY: Ventricular dysrhythmias can arise from any ectopic focus in any portion of the ventricular myocardium. The usual conduction pathway through ventricles is not used, and the wave of depolarization spreads from cell to cell.

Idioventricular Rhythms. Sometimes an ectopic focus in the ventricle can become the dominant pacemaker of the heart (Table 11-11). If the sinus node and the AV junction fail, the ventricles depolarize at their own intrinsic rate of 20 to 40 times per minute. This is called an idioventricular escape rhythm and is protective in nature.

RATE: 20 to 40 beats/min (escape rhythm). When the rate is between 40 and 100 beats/min it is called an accelerated idioventricular rhythm (AIVR), (Figure 11-37).

RHYTHM: Regular.

PR INTERVAL: Absent.

QRS DURATION: Greater than 0.12 second.

P WAVE: Present, but not associated with QRS complex.

QRS COMPLEX: Wide and bizarre because complexes originate in ventricles.

ETIOLOGY: SA and AV nodes may be ischemic, infarcted, or depressed by drug toxicity.

MANAGEMENT: Rather than trying to abolish the ventricular beats, the aim of treatment is to increase the effective heart rate and reestablish a higher pacing site, such as the sinus node or the AV junction. Usually, a temporary pacemaker is used to increase heart rate until the underlying problems that caused failure of higher pacing sites can be resolved.

Antidysrhythmic drugs are not indicated. Lidocaine IV is *never* administered to a patient with an idioventricular rhythm; the lidocaine will suppress the ventricular ectopic pacing site, resulting in asystole.

Ventricular Tachycardia. Ventricular tachycardia (VT) is caused by a ventricular pacing site firing 100 times or more per minute, usually maintained by a reentry mechanism within the ventricular tissue (Figure 11-38). The complexes are wide, and the rhythm may be slightly irregular, often accelerating as the tachycardia continues (see Table 11-11). In most cases, the sinus node is not affected and it continues to depolarize the atria at a normal rate. P waves can sometimes be seen on the ECG tracing. They are not related to the QRS and may even appear to conduct a normal impulse to the ventricles if their timing is just right.

RATE: Greater than 100 beats/min.

RHYTHM: Mostly regular. May have some irregularities.

P WAVE: Not related to QRS. Sinus node is unaffected and will continue to depolarize atria, unrelated to the ventricular rate.

PR INTERVAL: Absent.

QRS DURATION: Greater than 0.12 second.

QRS COMPLEX: Wide, with bizarre shape compared with sinus QRS (see Figure 11-38).

- *Nonsustained Ventricular Tachycardia (VT):* Three or more consecutive PVCs, rate greater than 100 beats/min, lasts less than 30 seconds without hemodynamic collapse, and self-terminates.
- *Torsades de Pointes ("Twisting of the Points"):* A specific form of polymorphic VT that refers to the twisting appearance of VT on the ECG (Figure 11-39). Torsades may be precipitated by antidysrhythmic drugs that prolong the QT interval. The intent is to lengthen the ventricular

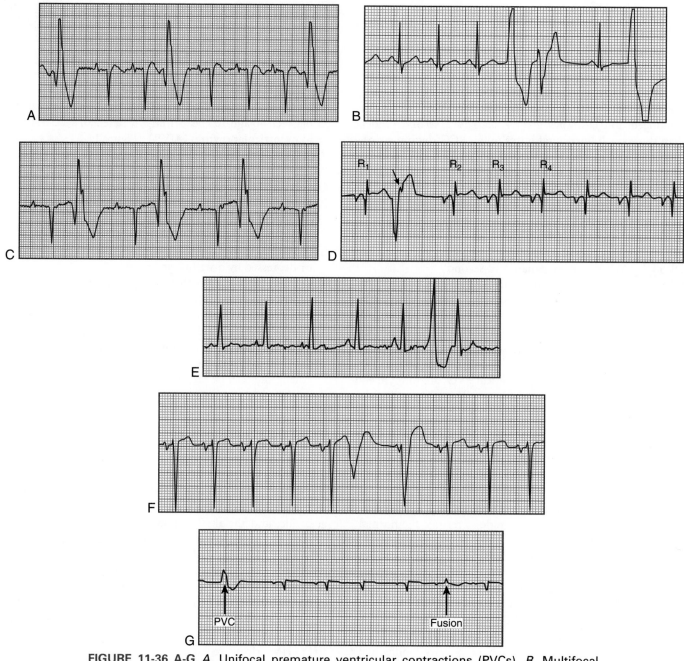

FIGURE 11-36 A-G *A,* Unifocal premature ventricular contractions (PVCs). *B,* Multifocal PVCs. *C,* Ventricular bigeminy. *D,* **Premature ventricular contraction (PVC) with a fully compensatory pause.** The interval between the two sinus beats that surround the PVC (R_1 and R_2) is exactly two times the normal interval between sinus beats (R_3 and R_4). The fully compensatory pause occurs because the sinus node continues to pace despite the PVC. Notice the sinus P wave *(arrow)* hidden in the ST segment of the PVC. This P wave did not conduct through to the ventricles because they had just been depolarized and were still in the absolute refractory period. *E,* **Interpolated PVC.** The PVC falls between two normal QRS complexes without disturbing the rhythm. Notice that the R-R interval between sinus beats remains the same. *F,* **R-on-T phenomenon.** *G,* **Ventricular fusion beat** *(arrows).* The QRS duration is only 0.08 second, and the shape represents the normal QRS and the previous PVC.

TABLE 11-11	VENTRICULAR RHYTHMS			
PARAMETER	IDIOVENTRICULAR RHYTHM	ACCELERATED IDIOVENTRICULAR RHYTHM	VENTRICULAR TACHYCARDIA	VENTRICULAR FIBRILLATION
Rate	20-40/min	40-100/min	>100/min	None
Rhythm	Usually regular	Usually regular	Usually regular	Irregular
P waves	Absent or retrograde	Absent or retrograde	Absent or retrograde	None
PR interval	None	None	None	None
QRS	>0.12 sec	>0.12 sec	>0.12 sec	Fibrillatory waves

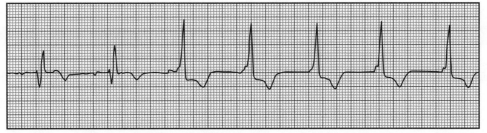

FIGURE 11-37 Accelerated idioventricular rhythm (AIVR). The QRS duration is 0.14 second, and the ventricular rate is 65.

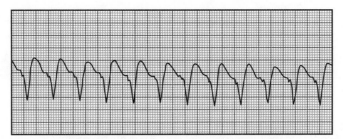

FIGURE 11-38 Ventricular tachycardia.

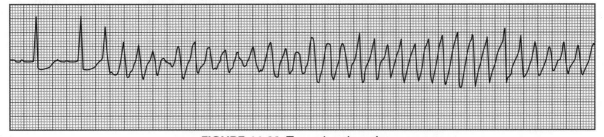

FIGURE 11-39 Torsades de pointes.

refractory period, but it can cause a *prodysrhythmic effect* (also described as a *proarrhythmic effect*), which can sometimes be fatal.[109]

More than 90% of VT occurs in the presence of structural cardiac disease, such as myocardial ischemia, congenital heart disease, valvular dysfunction, and cardiomyopathy. Other triggers include drug toxicity, electrolyte disturbances, and as an adverse reaction to certain antidysrhythmic drugs (prodysrhythmia).[109]

MANAGEMENT: VT is a potentially life-threatening dysrhythmia and must be treated quickly, especially when symptoms occur. How VT is clinically managed depends on the rate, whether the patient is stable or unstable, and whether a pulse and adequate blood pressure are present. Pulseless VT is a life-threatening

condition. The patient will lose consciousness and will need immediate cardiopulmonary resuscitation and defibrillation as described in the American Heart Association (AHA) protocols for advanced cardiac life support (ACLS).

Patients with stable or wide-complex "slow VT" who have a heart rate below 150 beats/min, palpable pulse, and stable blood pressure may be treated pharmacologically with amiodarone, beta-blockers, lidocaine, procainamide, or overdrive pacing as described in the ACLS protocols.

After the acute episode is resolved, patients who have already experienced sustained VT or cardiac arrest continue to be at risk for sudden cardiac death (SCD). An extensive clinical evaluation of these patients is warranted, including cardiac catheterization and electrophysiological testing with

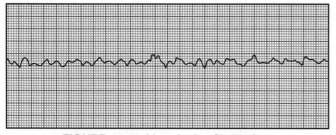

FIGURE 11-40 Ventricular fibrillation.

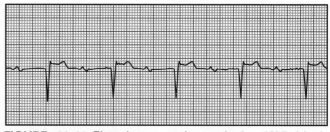

FIGURE 11-41 First-degree atrioventricular (AV) block. The PR interval is prolonged to 0.44 second.

TABLE 11-12 ATRIOVENTRICULAR BLOCK

PARAMETER	FIRST DEGREE	SECOND-DEGREE MOBITZ I (WENCKEBACH)	SECOND-DEGREE MOBITZ II	THIRD DEGREE (COMPLETE)
PR interval	>0.20 sec and constant	Increases with each consecutively conducted P wave	Constant	Varies randomly
P waves	1 P wave for each QRS	Intermittently not conducted, yielding more P waves than QRS complexes	Intermittently not conducted, yielding more P waves than QRS complexes	P waves independent and not related to QRS complexes
QRS	0.06-0.10 sec	0.06-0.10 sec	May be normal, but usually coexists with bundle branch block (>0.12 sec)	0.06-0.10 sec if junctional escape pacemaker activates the ventricles >0.12 sec if ventricular escape pacemaker activates the ventricles

programmed ventricular stimulation. Therapy is aimed at preventing a recurrence of sustained VT or VF. It may include treating the underlying cause, administering antidysrhythmic drugs, performing ablation of the reentrant pathway within the ventricle, or inserting an implantable cardioverter defibrillator (ICD). Chapter 13 provides more information on implantable cardioverter defibrillators; see Figure 13-6.

Ventricular Fibrillation. VF is the result of chaotic electrical activity. The ventricles merely quiver, and no forward flow of blood occurs. On the ECG, VF appears as a continuous, undulating pattern without clear P, QRS, or T waves (Figure 11-40), often with erratic undulations of the baseline (coarse VF) or as a mild tremor (fine VF).
RATE: Indeterminable.
RHYTHM: Irregular, wavy baseline without recognizable QRS complexes.
P WAVE: Absent. Cannot be distinguished from fibrillating ventricular baseline.
PR INTERVAL: Absent.
QRS DURATION: Absent. No QRS complexes present.
QRS COMPLEX: Normal P wave and QRS are replaced by a wavy baseline.
MANAGEMENT: In VF, the patient has no pulse, no blood pressure, and is unconscious. No blood is being pumped from the heart. Emergency electrical defibrillation is the only definitive therapy. Resuscitative measures such as cardiopulmonary resuscitation (CPR), intubation, and correction of metabolic abnormalities are performed concurrently per ACLS guidelines.

Atrioventricular Blocks. On the ECG, the ability of the AV node to conduct is evaluated by measuring the PR interval and the relationship of P waves to QRS complexes (Table 11-12). The normal PR interval, measured from the beginning of the P wave to the beginning of the QRS complex, ranges from 0.12 to 0.20 second.

First-Degree Atrioventricular Block. When all atrial impulses are conducted to the ventricles but the PR interval is greater than 0.20 second, this is known as first-degree AV block or as first-degree heart block (Figure 11-41).
RATE: Depends on underlying rhythm, usually NSR.
RHYTHM: Regular if NSR.
P WAVE: Present, normal shape.
PR INTERVAL: Greater than 0.20 second.
QRS DURATION: 0.06 to 0.10 second.
QRS COMPLEX: Unaffected.
MANAGEMENT: None required. Many older patients have first-degree AV block as a chronic condition associated with aging of AV junction. Acute myocardial infarction: Patients with acute MI should be monitored for degeneration into more serious forms of AV block. Drug side effect: If development of first-degree AV block is new and related to recent antidysrhythmic administration, the medication regimen must be evaluated.[110,111] If the associated QRS is narrow, it is likely that the only conduction abnormality is in the AV node. However, if the associated QRS complex is widened, it is likely that there is also damage to the bundle branches as a result of sclerosis, ischemia, or infarction.[111]

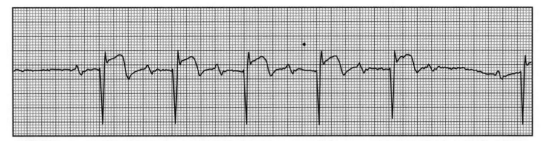

FIGURE 11-42 Mobitz type I (Wenckebach) second-degree atrioventricular (AV) block. Notice that the PR intervals gradually increase from 0.36 to 0.46 second until a P wave is not conducted to the ventricles.

Second-Degree Atrioventricular Block. Second-degree AV block can be broadly defined as a condition in which some atrial impulses are conducted to the ventricles, but others are "blocked" at the AV node. This description of intermittent AV conduction covers two patterns with markedly different clinical significance: second-degree AV block is divided into Mobitz type I (also known as Wenckebach block), and Mobitz type II.

- **Mobitz Type I.** This is a rhythm known by several different names, including Mobitz I and Wenckebach. The AV conduction times progressively lengthen until a P wave is not conducted. This typically occurs in a pattern of grouped beats and is observed on the ECG by a gradually lengthening PR interval, until ultimately the final P wave in the group fails to conduct (Figure 11-42). In Mobitz type I, the QRS complex is generally of normal width and appearance.[111]

RATE: Atrial rate depends on underlying sinus rate. Ventricular rate depends on P wave/QRS ratio.

RHYTHM: Regular, irregular pattern. P waves regular. As part of Mobitz I pattern, R-to-R intervals become progressively shorter until sinus P wave is not conducted, resulting in a pause. After the pause, the cycle repeats. The PR interval typically lengthens the most with the second beat of the cycle.

P WAVE: Normal shape.

PR INTERVALS: Progressively lengthen until a P wave is not conducted to ventricles and therefore is not followed by QRS complex.

QRS DURATION: 0.06 to 0.10 second.

QRS COMPLEX: Conducted complexes are normal.

TREATMENT: No treatment required if the ventricular rate is sufficient to sustain hemodynamic stability. In certain clinical conditions, such as acute MI, consider the risk of progression to a more severe form of heart block and if hemodynamic compromise is present or deemed likely, a temporary transvenous pacemaker may be inserted.

- **Mobitz Type II.** Mobitz type II block is always anatomically located below the AV node in the bundle of His in the bundle branches or even in the Purkinje fibers.[111] This results in an all-or-nothing situation with respect to AV conduction. Sinus P waves are or are not conducted. When conduction does occur, all PR intervals are the same. Because of the anatomic location of the block, on the

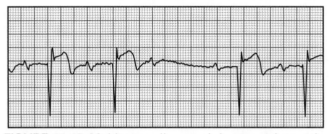

FIGURE 11-43 Mobitz type II second-degree atrioventricular (AV) block. Notice that the PR intervals remain constant.

surface ECG the PR interval is constant and the QRS complexes may be slightly wider than normal (Figure 11-43).

RATE: Atrial rate usually 60 to 100 beats/min. Ventricular rate slower and depends on number of conducted P waves.

RHYTHM: Regular if AV node consistently conducts every second or third P wave. Irregular if P waves conducted inconsistently.

P WAVE: Normal in shape. More P waves than QRS complexes.

PR INTERVAL: 0.12 to 0.20 second. Constant interval for P waves that conduct to ventricles.

QRS DURATION: 0.06 to 0.10 second. Wider if bundle branch block (BBB) is present.

QRS COMPLEX: May be narrow and normal or widened due to coexisting BBB.

MANAGEMENT: Mobitz II block is more ominous clinically than Mobitz I and often progresses to complete AV block. If the block involves the bundle branches, an escape rhythm may not develop.[112] For this reason, it is important to prepare for transcutaneous cardiac pacing (TCP) by bringing an external pacemaker (usually combined with a defibrillator) to the bedside. TCP refers to external pacing from outside the chest wall. When pacing is required, two large pacing electrodes are placed on the chest. There is always a diagram on the machine showing where to place the pads on the chest. Consider the possibility that the patient will need a temporary transvenous pacemaker inserted and possibly require a permanent pacemaker before hospital discharge.

Third-Degree Atrioventricular Block. Third-degree, or complete, AV block is a condition in which no atrial impulses

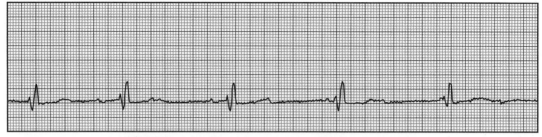

FIGURE 11-44 Third-degree (complete) heart block.

can conduct from the atria to the ventricles (Figure 11-44). This is also described by the terms complete heart block or AV dissociation to indicate that the atria and the ventricles are controlled by different pacemakers.[108] The block can be located at the level of the AV node, within the bundle of His, or on the bundle branches. It can be caused by infarction, digitalis toxicity, or age-related degeneration of the conduction system in older patients.[113]

RATE: Depends on underlying rhythm.

RHYTHM: Usually regular.

P WAVE: Normal shape.

PR INTERVAL: P waves are not related to QRS complexes, so PR interval varies widely.

QRS DURATION: Greater than 0.10 second.

QRS COMPLEX: If junctional focus is pacing heart, complex is narrow but is not related to P waves. If ventricular focus is pacing heart, QRS is wide and unrelated to P waves.

MANAGEMENT: Emergency ventricular pacemaker support is required. A ventricular focus may depolarize spontaneously at the idioventricular intrinsic rate of 20 to 40 beats/min. If not, asystole occurs and death will result if pacemaker support is not immediate.

LABORATORY ASSESSMENT

Nursing Management

The priorities for laboratory assessment for the patient with cardiovascular dysfunction focus on: (1) interpreting serum electrolytes and safely replacing electrolyte deficiencies, (2) monitoring cardiac biomarkers, (3) trending hematological studies, (4) assessing coagulation values, and (5) evaluating the serum lipid profile.

Interpreting Serum Electrolyte Levels

Potassium. During depolarization and repolarization of nerve and muscle fiber, potassium and sodium exchange occurs intracellularly and extracellularly. The potassium gradient across the cell membrane determines conduction velocity and helps confine pacing activity to the sinus node. An excess or deficiency of potassium can alter myocardial muscle function. Normal serum potassium levels are 3.5 to 4.5 mEq/L.

Hyperkalemia. Elevated serum potassium, called hyperkalemia, can be caused by a variety of conditions that include excess potassium administration, extensive skeletal muscle destruction (rhabdomyolysis), tumor lysis syndrome, kidney failure, and some drugs. Hyperkalemia elicits significant changes in the ECG because it decreases AV conduction velocity, slows ventricular depolarization, and accelerates repolarization.[114] As the serum levels of potassium rise above normal (>4.5 mEq/L), evidence is clearly visible on the ECG (Figure 11-45, *A*). Tall, narrow peaked T waves are usually, although not uniquely, associated with early hyperkalemia and are followed by prolongation of the PR interval, loss of the P wave, widening of the QRS complex, heart block, and asystole.[114] Severely elevated serum potassium (>8 mEq/L) causes a wide QRS tachycardia, as shown in the 12-lead ECG in Figure 11-45, *B*. If not corrected, severe hyperkalemia can lead to VF or cardiac standstill.

This life-threatening condition can be acutely managed with an intravenous insulin or glucose infusion that drives the potassium inside the cell and temporarily out of the serum. Potassium is permanently removed from the serum by cation-exchange resin products, such as Kayexalate, placed into the gastrointestinal tract or removed directly from the blood by hemodialysis. Coexisting low serum sodium, calcium, or pH levels potentiate the cardiac effects of hyperkalemia.

Hypokalemia. A low serum potassium (K^+) level, called hypokalemia (<3.5 mEq/L), is commonly caused by gastrointestinal losses, diuretic therapy with insufficient replacement, or chronic steroid therapy. Hypokalemia is also reflected by changes on the ECG (Figure 11-46, *A-E*). The earliest ECG change is often PVCs, which can deteriorate into VT or VF without appropriate potassium replacement.

Hypokalemia impairs myocardial conduction and prolongs ventricular repolarization. This can be seen by a prominent U wave (a positive deflection after the T wave on the ECG). The U wave is not totally unique to hypokalemia, but its presence is a signal for the clinician to check the serum potassium level. In the critical care unit, where patients are receiving diuretics or have nasogastric tubes to suction, the serum potassium level is checked frequently by the critical care nurse and replaced intravenously to normal levels to prevent dysrhythmias. Great care must be taken when replacing potassium intravenously to ensure it is diluted sufficiently and administered slowly to prevent accidental overdose.[115] Potassium is a high-alert medication, and additional safety procedures are recommended for this drug (see Patient Safety Priorities box on Medication Administration). If concomitant hypomagnesemia exists, successful replenishment of potassium deficit cannot be accomplished until the hypomagnesemia is reversed.

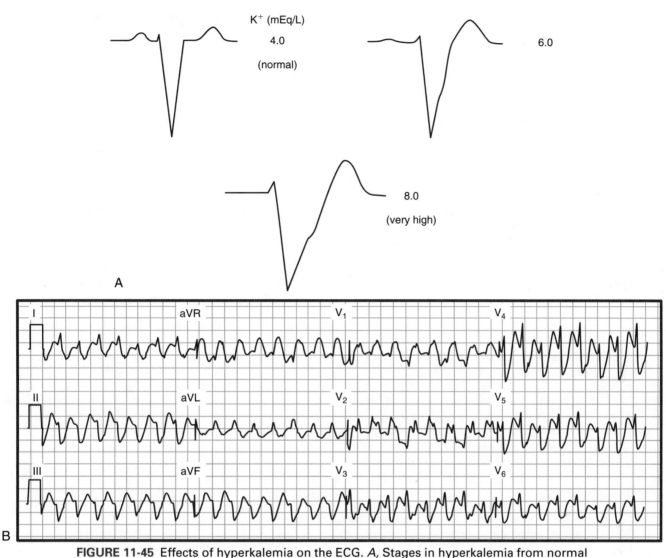

FIGURE 11-45 Effects of hyperkalemia on the ECG. *A,* Stages in hyperkalemia from normal potassium levels to plasma levels of 8 mEq/L. At approximately 6 mEq/L, the P wave flattens, the QRS broadens, and the ST segment disappears, with the S wave flowing into the tall, tented T wave. *B,* A 12-lead ECG of a patient with a serum potassium level of 9.1 mEq/L.

⚡ PATIENT SAFETY PRIORITIES

Medication Administration

1. Accurate patient identification
   - Use at least two patient identifiers (not the patient's room number) when taking blood samples or administering medications or blood products. Examples include patient name, date of birth, or hospital record number.
2. Effective communication among caregivers
   - Hospitals should have (or implement) a process for taking verbal or telephone orders that requires verification "read back" of the complete order by the person receiving the order.
   - An organizational method to decrease the number of medication errors is the use of computerized physician

order entry (CPOE), as advocated by the Leapfrog group (*www.leapfroggroup.org*).
   - Guidelines for development of safe medication order sets (paper or electronic) are available at www.ismp.org/Tools/guidelines/StandardOrderSets.pdf.
   - Standardize the abbreviations, acronyms, and symbols used throughout the organization, including a list of abbreviations, acronyms, and symbols to avoid. Examples of problematic abbreviations include "U" for units and "μg" for micrograms. When handwritten, a capital U can be mistaken for a zero (0); in numerous case reports, an insulin dosage written in U was interpreted as 0. Using the abbreviation "μg" instead of "mcg" for micrograms is

---

⚡ **PATIENT SAFETY PRIORITIES—cont'd**

Medication Administration

also problematic; when handwritten, the Greek letter μ can look like an "m."

- Use of trailing zeros (e.g., 2.0 versus 2) and use of a leading decimal point without a leading zero (e.g., .2 instead of 0.2) are dangerous prescription-writing practices. Misinterpretation has caused 10-fold dosing errors. Information on similar medication issues is available on the Joint Commission website (www.jointcommission.org).

3. High-alert medication safety
   - The Institute for Safe Medication Practices (ISMP) publishes a list of high-alert medications, available at www.ismp.org/Tools/highalertmedications.pdf; plus a list of commonly confused drug names, available at www.ismp.org/Tools/confuseddrugnames.pdf.
   - Remove concentrated electrolytes (including but not limited to potassium chloride, potassium phosphate, and hypertonic sodium chloride) from patient care units.
   - Standardize and limit the number of drug concentrations available in the hospital.
   - In the first 2 years after the Joint Commission enacted a sentinel event reporting mechanism, the most common category was medication errors, and the most frequently implicated drug was potassium chloride (KCl). The Joint Commission reviewed ten incidents of patient death resulting from misadministration of KCl. Eight were the result of direct infusion of concentrated KCl. In six of the eight cases, the KCl was mistaken for another medication, primarily because of similarities in packaging and labeling. Most often, KCl was mistaken for sodium chloride, heparin, or furosemide (Lasix).
   - The Joint Commission suggests that health care organizations not make concentrated KCl available outside the pharmacy unless appropriate, specific safeguards are in place.

4. Reporting errors
   - Because thousands of brand name and generic drugs are available, there is always the potential for error. Similar drug names, written or spoken, accounted for approximately 15% of all medication error reports to the U.S. Pharmacopeia (USP). The USP Drug Error Finder Tool

is available online at www.usp.org/hqi/similarProducts/drugErrorFinderTool.html.
   - Medication Errors can be reported to the National Coordinating Council for Medication Error Reporting and Prevention. (www.nccmerp.org/reportMedError.html); or to the Institute for Safe Medication Practices at https://www.ismp.org/orderforms/reporterrortoISMP.asp.
   - See ISMP list of high-alert medications and commonly confused drug names above.

5. Infusion pump safety
   - Ensure free-flow protection on all general-use and patient-controlled analgesia (PCA) intravenous (IV) infusion pumps used in the organization.
   - Infusion pumps that do not provide protection from the free flow of IV fluid or medication administration are hazardous, and should not be used. Free flow occurs when IV solution flows freely under the force of gravity without being controlled by the infusion pump. Free flow typically occurs after the administration set is temporarily removed from the pump to transfer a patient to another area, change a patient's gown, or place a patient on a radiography table. Clinicians can greatly reduce this risk by using administration sets with set-based anti-free-flow mechanisms that prevent gravity free flow by closing off the IV tubing to stop flow when the administration set is removed from the pump.

References and Resources

Additional medication safety information can be accessed on the web pages of the following patient safety organizations:

Institute for Safe Medication Practices, www.ismp.org (accessed January 2011)

The Joint Commission, www.jointcommission.org (accessed January 2011)

U.S. Pharmacopeia, www.usp.org (accessed January 2011)

The Leapfrog Group, www.leapfroggroup.org (Accessed January 2011)

National Coordinating Council for Medication Error Reporting and Prevention, www.nccmerp.org (Accessed January 2011)

Calcium. Calcium (Ca^{2+}) is an important cation in the body. Calcium metabolism is controlled by many factors, including normal parathyroid hormone (PTH) function, calcitonin, and vitamin D acting on target organs such as the kidney, bone, and gastrointestinal tract.[116] Calcium is an important mediator of many cardiovascular functions because of its effect on vascular tone, myocardial contractility, and cardiac excitability.[116]

Serum calcium values are recorded in three possible ways, depending on the hospital laboratory: milliequivalents per liter (mEq/L), milligrams per deciliter (mg/dL), or millimoles per liter (mmol/L).

Ionized Calcium. In the bloodstream, 55% of calcium is bound to protein (primarily albumin) and found in complexes with anions such as chloride and phosphate. As such, it is not physiologically available to the body.[116] The remaining 45% of calcium is biologically active and is called the ionized calcium.[116] The normal serum concentration of ionized calcium is maintained within very narrow limits; changes in ionized calcium levels are responsible for the clinical effects of hypercalcemia and hypocalcemia. If a patient has an extremely low total serum calcium (<7.0 mg/dL), it is highly likely that the ionized calcium will also be low.[117] However, the only accurate way to determine the level

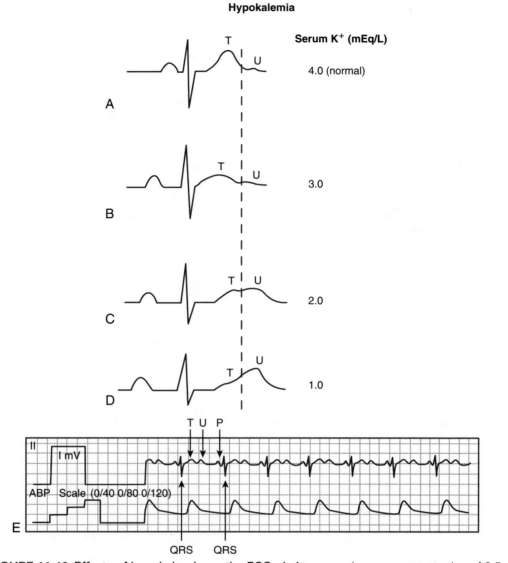

FIGURE 11-46 Effects of hypokalemia on the ECG. *A,* At a normal serum concentration of 3.5 to 4.5 mEq/L, the amplitude of the T wave is appreciably greater than that of the U wave. *B,* By the time the serum potassium level has dropped to 3 mEq/L, the amplitudes of the T and U waves are approaching each other. *C* and *D,* With a further drop in the level of potassium, the U wave begins to tower over and fuse with the T wave. *E,* ECG tracing from a patient with serum potassium of 2.6 mEq/L shows a prominent U wave.

of ionized calcium—described as physiologically active, unbound, or free—is to measure the ionized serum value with a laboratory assay. The mathematically calculated values that are extrapolates from total calcium and serum albumin levels have been shown to be inaccurate.[118]

Hypercalcemia. Hypercalcemia is defined as increased amounts of ionized calcium (>4.8 mg/dL or 1.30 mmol/L) or increased amounts of total serum calcium (>10.5 mg/dL or 2.60 mmol/L). Serum calcium levels are increased by bone tumors; primary hyperparathyroidism caused by elevated PTH levels; excessive intake of supplemental calcium and vitamin D, usually in oral antacids; hypomagnesemia; and

as a complication of kidney failure from decreased renal excretion of calcium.[120] Hypercalcemia affects many organs, causes smooth muscle relaxation, and can lead to neurological changes such as lethargy, confusion, and even coma.[118] Elevated serum calcium has the cardiovascular effect of strengthening contractility and shortening ventricular repolarization, demonstrated on the ECG by a shortened QTc interval.[118] Rhythm disturbances may include bradycardia; first-, second-, and third-degree heart block; and bundle branch block. Hypercalcemia can potentiate the effects of digitalis, precipitate digitalis toxicity, and cause hypertension.[116]

Management of hypercalcemia involves promotion of renal excretion of calcium by diuretics and high-volume intravenous normal saline at 200 to 300 mL/hr if tolerated by the cardiac, pulmonary, and renal systems. Patients who cannot tolerate this clinical regimen should be hemodialyzed using a low-calcium dialysate.[119]

Hypocalcemia. Hypocalcemia is defined as an ionized calcium level below normal (<4 mg/dL or <1.05 mmol/L) or a low total serum calcium level. Hypocalcemia (measured by ionized calcium) is a common finding and is reported to occur in 26% to 88% of critically ill patients, depending on the admitting diagnosis.[120] The more severe the patient's illness, the greater the risk of developing hypocalcemia.[120] Transfusions of blood from the blood bank lower serum calcium levels because the citrate used as an anticoagulant in banked blood binds to the calcium. This is called citrate chelation. If citrate is used during hemodialysis or plasmapheresis, it will have the same calcium-binding (chelating) effect.[120] Phosphate also binds to calcium and can lower the serum calcium level.[120] Metabolic alkalosis often coexists with hypocalcemia.[120] The cardiovascular effects of hypocalcemia include decreased myocardial contractility, decreased CO, and hypotension. Rhythm disturbances with severe hypocalcemia are variable, ranging from bradycardia to VT and asystole. When the ionized calcium is low, the ECG may show a prolonged QTc interval (Figure 11-47). A long QT interval predisposes a patient to the life-threatening ventricular dysrhythmia called torsades de pointes.

MANAGEMENT: Management of hypocalcemia, especially when the ionized calcium is low, involves infusion of intravenous calcium chloride or IV calcium gluconate.[120,121]

• Calcium chloride provides 27 mg of elemental calcium/mL.

• Calcium gluconate provides 9 mg of elemental calcium/mL.

Magnesium. Magnesium (Mg^{2+}) is essential for many enzyme, protein, lipid, and carbohydrate functions in the body and is critical for the production and use of energy. The body stores most magnesium in bone (53%), muscle (27%), and soft tissues (19%); only a tiny proportion resides within the bloodstream—red blood cells contain 0.5%, and serum contains 0.3%.[122] As with other electrolytes, the ionized portion of the serum magnesium is the biologically active component that is available for biochemical processes. Serum magnesium is 67% ionized, 19% protein bound, and 14% complexed.[122] The serum magnesium is what is normally measured in a routine blood test. Serum magnesium can be reported in units of mEq/L, mg/dL, or mmol/L, depending on the laboratory running the analysis. The normal serum range is from 1.5 to 2 mEq/L, 1.8 to 2.4 mg/dL, or 0.7 to 1.1 mmol/L. These represent the same serum level of magnesium despite different measurement guidelines used in the report. It is important to anticipate that normal reference values will vary between hospital laboratories.

Hypermagnesemia. The incidence of hypermagnesemia is rare in comparison with hypomagnesemia. It results from kidney failure, tumor lysis syndrome, or iatrogenic overtreatment.

Hypomagnesemia. A total serum magnesium concentration below 1.5 mEq/L defines hypomagnesemia. It is commonly associated with other electrolyte imbalances, most notably alterations in potassium, calcium, and phosphorus. Low serum magnesium levels can result from many causes. Hypomagnesemia is caused by insufficient intake in the diet or in total parenteral nutrition (TPN) and is associated with chronic alcohol abuse. In the critical care unit, aggressive diuresis with loop diuretics will lower serum potassium and

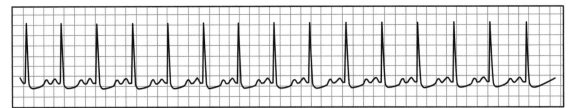

FIGURE 11-47 Abnormal QT prolongation in a hypocalcemic patient. The patient is a 50-year-old woman admitted to the critical care unit with a diagnosis of alcoholic liver disease and malnourishment. Total calcium concentration is 5.1 mg/dL, and the albumin level is 1.3 mg/dL. The QT interval (0.55 second) is markedly prolonged for the heart rate (100 beats/min). The QT interval varies with the heart rate and can be corrected (QTc) as if the heart rate were 60 beats/min using Bazett's formula:

$$QTc = \frac{QT}{\sqrt{RR}},$$

The QTc should be 0.44 second or less. The QTc in the ECG tracing shown is 0.55 second. Hypocalcemia lengthens ventricular repolarization. A quick method for assessing the QT interval is to remember that it is usually less than half of the R-R interval. If it is more than one half of the R-R interval, it is prolonged. (From Yucha CB, Toto KH: Calcium and phosphorus derangements, _Crit Care Nurs Clin North Am_ 6[4]:747, 1994.)

magnesium levels.[122] Diarrhea can be a significant cause of magnesium loss because lower gastrointestinal fluids contain up to 15 mEq/L magnesium; vomiting or gastric suction causes less depletion because the upper gastrointestinal fluids contain about 1 mEq/L.[122] Another cause of magnesium depletion is rapid administration of citrated blood products, which causes the citrate to bind to the magnesium, a condition known as citrate chelation. In patients with chronic hypomagnesemia, the serum levels are replenished from the bone stores.[122]

Hypokalemia and hypocalcemia are likely to be unresponsive to replacement therapy until the hypomagnesemia is corrected.[116, 122] Expected cardiac-related changes with hypomagnesemia include hypertension and vasospasm, including coronary artery spasm. Some studies have linked magnesium depletion to sudden cardiac death, to an increased incidence of acute MI, and to the occurrence of ventricular dysrhythmias.[122]

In hypomagnesemia, the ECG changes are similar to those seen with hypokalemia[122] and hypocalcemia: prolonged PR and QTc intervals, presence of U waves, T-wave flattening, and a widened QRS complex. Cardiac dysrhythmias may be supraventricular or ventricular and include torsades de pointes. Dysrhythmias associated with hypomagnesemia and long QT interval may not respond to the usual antidysrhythmic drugs, but they often respond well to magnesium infusions. The treatment of choice for torsades de pointes is intravenous magnesium sulfate. The dose of magnesium is adjusted based on the severity of the clinical situation as described in the American Heart Association (AHA) guidelines.[123] When VF or pulseless VT cardiac arrest is associated with long QT interval, hypomagnesemia, or torsades de pointes, 1 to 2 g magnesium in 10 mL D_5W is administered IV for 5 to 20 minutes.[123] In torsades de pointes without cardiac arrest (the patient has a pulse), magnesium is administered more slowly: 1 to 2 g magnesium in 50 to 100 mL D_5W IV over 5 to 60 minutes.[123] It is important to evaluate kidney function when administering magnesium to avoid precipitating a hypermagnesemia state.

Monitoring Cardiac Biomarkers

Cardiac biomarkers, previously described by the term cardiac enzymes, are proteins that are released from severely damaged myocardial tissue cells.[91,124] When myocardial cells are damaged, they release detectable proteins into the bloodstream so that a rise in biomarkers can be correlated with myocardial cellular damage. The biomarkers that are routinely measured include cardiac troponin I (cTnI), cardiac troponin T (cTnT), and CK-MB. Table 11-13 summarizes the cardiac biomarkers related to myocardial injury and infarction.[125] Unfortunately, in many hospitals, the laboratory turnaround time for results of cardiac biomarkers is between 60 and 90 minutes, which limits the usefulness of the biomarkers in the emergency room when the patient is first admitted with symptoms of acute coronary syndrome.[125] If point-of-care testing at the bedside is used, the results are available more quickly and may be more helpful in the clinical decision-making process.[125]

TABLE 11-13	SERUM BIOMARKERS AFTER ACUTE MYOCARDIAL INFARCTION		
SERUM BIOMARKER	**TIME TO INITIAL ELEVATION (HOURS)***	**PEAK ELEVATION[†] (HOURS)***	**RETURN TO BASELINE (DAYS)***
Cardiac troponin I (cTnI)	3-12	24	5-10
Cardiac troponin T (cTnT)	3-12	12-48	5-14
CK-MB[‡]	3-12	24	2-3

*Time periods represent average reported values.
[†]Does not include patients who have had reperfusion therapy.
[‡]The creatine kinase (CK) enzyme consists of two subunits, the brain type (B) and the muscle type (M).

Creatine Kinase-MB. The creatine kinase (CK) muscle/brain (MB) biomarker (CK-MB) is released as a result of myocardial damage, and serum levels rise 4 to 8 hours after MI, peak at 15 to 24 hours, and remain elevated for 2 to 3 days (see Table 11-13). Serial samples are drawn routinely at 6- or 8-hour intervals, and three samples are usually sufficient to support or rule out the diagnosis of MI. CK-MB is never an isolated test; it is always performed in conjunction with cardiac troponin levels.

Troponin T and Troponin I. The troponins are biomarkers for myocardial damage found in cardiac muscle. cTnI and cTnT are more sensitive markers of myocardial damage than CK-MB, and as a result, more patients with myocardial damage are now being dectected.[91] Several different methods of laboratory assay are available, which means that normal serum levels will vary between different clinical settings, although cardiac serum cTnI and cTnT levels are low in the absence of myocardial muscle damage.[125]

The initial elevation of cTnI, cTnT, and CK-MB occurs 3 to 6 hours after the acute myocardial damage. This means that if an individual comes to the emergency department as soon as chest pain is experienced, the biomarkers will not have risen. For this reason, it is clinical practice to diagnose an acute MI by 12-lead ECG and clinical symptoms without waiting for elevation of cardiac biomarkers.

Because cTnI is found only in cardiac muscle, it is a highly specific biomarker for myocardial damage, considerably more specific than CK-MB. As a consequence, patients with a positive cTnI result and a negative CK-MB result usually rule in an acute MI.[126] A negative cTnI result that remains negative many hours after an episode of chest pain is a strong indicator that the patient is not experiencing an acute MI. Even with a negative cTnI result, symptoms of chest pain still indicate that the patient should have a comprehensive cardiac evaluation to determine if there is underlying CAD present that may later lead to complications.

Cardiac Biomarkers and Reperfusion. Management of STEMI includes opening the coronary artery obstructed by a thrombus and reperfusing the injured area as rapidly as possible.[124] Individuals who have recent onset of chest pain (within 12 hours) are candidates for reperfusion therapies, including fibrinolytic agents ("clot busters"), and cardiac catheterization with PCIs such as balloon angioplasty, atherectomy, or stent placement. If successful, these interventions may totally abort the MI or limit the amount of cardiac muscle damage, resulting in an early rise and fall of the cardiac biomarkers as illustrated in Figure 13-9 of Chapter 13.[124] After reperfusion, the serum troponin levels rise dramatically and peak early. Cardiac biomarker samples are drawn at admission, before administration of fibrinolytic therapy or PCI, and then at 6- or 8-hour intervals for 18 to 24 hours to detect any biomarker rise and assess the return of effective myocardial reperfusion.

Natriuretic Peptide Biomarkers in Heart Failure. Natriuretic peptides are biomarkers that provide additional information with which to accurately evaluate the breathless patient. It can be difficult to identify whether a dyspneic patient has a primary pulmonary problem or is exhibiting symptoms of acute heart failure with pulmonary edema. Cardiac natriuretic peptides are used to help make the correct diagnosis. In decompensated heart failure, the myocytes in the volume-distended heart release atrial natriuretic peptide (ANP) from the atria and brain natriuretic peptide (BNP) from the ventricles.

BNP Tests. Three laboratory assays are commercially available to measure BNP: a point-of-care test, a laboratory test for BNP, and a different laboratory test to measure the amino-terminal fragment of pro-BNP (NT-pro-BNP).[127] BNP has a half-life of about 20 minutes, whereas pro-BNP has a longer half-life of 1 to 2 hours.[128] The choice of test is generally dependent on what is available in the hospital.[128]

The greater the ventricular wall stress, the higher the BNP level will rise. The BNP value is combined with the physical examination, the 12-lead ECG, and a chest radiograph to increase the accuracy of heart failure diagnosis (Figure 11-48).[128] A patient with a BNP level below 100 pg/mL is unlikely to be in heart failure, and a patient with a BNP level above 400 pg/dL is almost definitely in heart failure; the higher the BNP the greater the certitude. BNP is an excellent test to rule out acute heart failure.[127] The challenge lies in interpreting the results of patients with a BNP level between 100 and 400 pg/mL, sometimes described as an indeterminate zone, or gray zone.[128] This highlights the importance of using a spectrum of clinical and diagnostic tests. As the symptoms of heart failure are successfully treated, the BNP level usually decreases toward the normal range.

Natriuretic peptides are also released from the endothelium and from the kidney, and they can alter the measured BNP levels. Kidney filtration is one of the mechanisms by which BNP is cleared from the bloodstream. BNP levels are higher in patients with kidney failure, especially if the glomerular filtration rate (GFR) is below 60 mL/min/1.7 m².[127,128] BNP levels can also be elevated in high-CO septic shock, possibly because of endothelial natriuretic peptide release or myocardial damage.[127]

BNP levels are lower than expected in obese patients with heart failure, possibly because natriuretic peptide receptors in adipose tissue degrade BNP more rapidly.[128] Conditions such as mitral stenosis that cause pulmonary edema but protect the left ventricle are associated with lower BNP levels than expected from the clinical picture. Even with these caveats, the BNP remains an extremely useful addition in the diagnosis of heart failure.

Trending Hematological Studies

Hematological laboratory studies that are routinely ordered for the management of patients with altered cardiovascular status are red blood cell (RBC) or erythrocyte level, hemoglobin level, hematocrit level, and white blood cell (WBC) or leukocyte level.

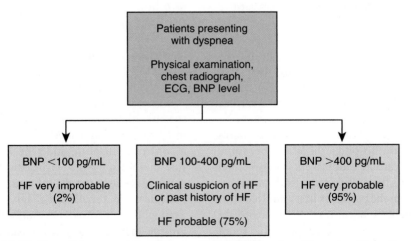

FIGURE 11-48 The B-type natriuretic peptide (BNP) algorithm in the diagnosis of heart failure.

Red Blood Cells. The normal amount of RBCs in a person varies with age, gender, environmental temperature, altitude, and exercise. Men produce 4.5 to 6 million RBCs/mm³, whereas the normal level for women is 4 to 5.5 million/mm³. Anemia is the clinical condition that occurs when not enough red blood cells are available to carry oxygen to the tissues. Polycythemia is the condition that occurs when excess RBCs are produced.

Hemoglobin. Hemoglobin levels normally range from 14 to 18 g/dL in men and from 12 to 16 g/dL in women.

Hematocrit. The hematocrit is the volume percentage of RBCs in whole blood. The value is 40% to 54% for men and 38% to 48% for women.

White Blood Cells. Most inflammatory processes that produce necrotic tissue within the heart muscle, such as rheumatic fever, endocarditis, and MI, increase the WBC level. WBCs are also known as leukocytes, and a WBC test may be called a serum leukocyte count. The normal WBC level for both genders is 5000 to 10,000 cells/mm³. The WBC level also increases in response to infection.

Platelets. The normal platelet count is 150,000 to 400,000 cells/mm³. Less commonly, the normal platelet count range will be written as 150 to 400 × 10⁹/L. Normally, the platelet count is the only laboratory value that is reported. Unfortunately, there is no routine test available for critical care patients that can evaluate platelet functionality. Platelets are important because they are the first cells to be activated when the coagulation system is stimulated. Many drugs inhibit platelet function and make the platelets "slippery" so that they do not clump together to activate the clotting process. Sometimes, the antiplatelet action of a drug is its intended role, such as with aspirin used to prevent acute coronary syndrome, and it can be an unintended side effect. A low platelet count is called thrombocytopenia.

Assessing Blood Coagulation Studies

Coagulation studies are ordered to determine blood-clotting effectiveness. Anticoagulants—most notably heparin, direct thrombin inhibitors, warfarin, and platelet inhibitory agents—are administered daily in critical care units for many clinical reasons. It is essential to understand the laboratory tests that are used to monitor the effectiveness of therapeutic anticoagulation.

Prothrombin Time. Most coagulation study results are reported as the length of time in seconds it takes for blood to form a clot in the laboratory test tube. The prothrombin time (PT) is no longer directly used to determine the therapeutic dosage of warfarin (Coumadin) necessary to achieve anticoagulation. The PT is not standardized between laboratories so the result of this test is always reported as a standardized international normalized ratio (INR).[129]

International Normalized Ratio. The INR was developed by the World Health Organization (WHO) in 1982 to standardize PT results among clinical laboratories worldwide. Table 11-14 shows target INR ranges for different cardiovascular conditions that require anticoagulation. It is recommended that the INR be used to guide anticoagulation therapy with warfarin rather than the PT, especially if the PT results are analyzed at more than one laboratory.

When a patient is first started on warfarin, it is important to know that it can take 72 hours or more to achieve a therapeutic level of anticoagulation. This is because the half-life of prothrombin is between 60 and 72 hours.[129] This delay in anticoagulation effectiveness also occurs if a patient is being converted from heparin anticoagulation—monitored by activated partial thromboplastin time (aPTT)—to warfarin anticoagulation (monitored by INR). To ensure a safe transition, a delay of 4 to 5 days must be anticipated in order to obtain two therapeutic INR values 24 hours apart before the heparin is discontinued.[129]

Activated Partial Thromboplastin Time. The aPTT is used to measure the effectiveness of intravenous or subcutaneous ultrafractionated heparin (UFH) administration. Coagulation monitoring is required with UFH, although not with subcutaneous low-molecular-weight heparin, because of lower levels of plasma protein binding. In cases of overanticoagulation with heparin, the antidote is protamine sulfate.

Activated Coagulation Time. An additional test of heparin effect is the activated coagulation time (ACT). The ACT can be performed outside of the laboratory setting in areas such as the cardiac catheterization laboratory, the operating room,

TABLE 11-14	NORMAL AND THERAPEUTIC COAGULATION VALUES		
TEST	**CLINICAL CONDITION**	**NORMAL VALUE**	**THERAPEUTIC ANTICOAGULANT TARGET VALUE**
INR	Normal coagulation	<1.0	
INR	Atrial fibrillation		2.0-3.0
INR	Treatment of DVT/PE		2.0-3.0
INR	Mechanical heart valves		2.5-3.5
aPTT	Normal coagulation	28-38 sec	1.5-2.5 × normal
PTT	Normal coagulation	60-90 sec	1.5-2.0 × normal
ACT*	Normal coagulation	0-120 sec	150-300 sec

ACT, activated coagulation time; *aPTT,* activated partial thromboplastin time; *DVT,* deep vein thrombosis; *INR,* international normalized ratio; *PE,* pulmonary embolism; *PTT,* partial thromboplastin time.
*ACT is normal, but therapeutic values may vary with type of activator used.

or specialized critical care units. Normal and therapeutic values for all of these coagulation studies are shown in Table 11-14.

Evaluating Serum Lipid Studies

Four primary blood lipid levels are important in evaluating an individual's risk of developing or having progression of CAD: total cholesterol; low-density lipoprotein cholesterol (LDL-C); triglycerides; and high-density lipoprotein cholesterol (HDL-C). When levels of cholesterol low-density lipoproteins (LDLs) and triglycerides are elevated or the level of high-density lipoproteins (HDLs) is low, the patient is considered at risk for developing or having progression of CAD and is offered intensive interventions in diet therapy, exercise prescription, and drug therapy.[130]

Total Cholesterol. Cholesterol is a fatlike substance (lipid) that is present in cell membranes, is produced by the liver, and is a precursor of bile acids and steroid hormones. The cholesterol level in the blood is determined partly by genetics and partly by acquired factors such as diet, calorie balance, and level of physical activity. Cholesterol in excess amounts (>200 mg/dL) in the serum forces the progression of atherosclerosis (atherogenesis). Table 11-15 lists the desirable lipid levels to lower the risk of CAD and to reduce morbidity and mortality in patients with established CAD.

Low-Density Lipoproteins. About 60% to 70% of the total serum cholesterol is carried in the bloodstream, complexed as LDL-C. The LDL-C and total serum cholesterol levels are directly correlated with risk for CAD, and high levels of each are significant predictors of future acute MI in persons with established coronary artery atherosclerosis. LDL-C is the major atherogenic lipoprotein and is the primary target for cholesterol-lowering efforts.[130,131] Guidelines recommend maintaining an LDL-C level below 130 mg/dL for the patient with no history of atherosclerotic disease. A patient with known CAD but who is not high risk should aim for an LDL-C level below 100 mg/dL. The recommended target LDL-C level for high-risk patients with CAD has been lowered to 70 mg/dL.[131]

Very-Low-Density Lipoproteins and Triglycerides. The very-low-density lipoproteins (VLDLs) contain 10% to 15% of the total serum cholesterol along with most of the triglycerides in fasting serum. Elevated triglyceride levels are often associated with reduced HDL-C levels.[130]

High-Density Lipoproteins. HDLs are particles that carry 20% to 30% of the total serum cholesterol. A low HDL-C level (below 35 mg/dL) is another independent, significant risk factor for CAD. Several studies also support the finding that HDL-C helps protect against atherogenesis, and a level greater than 50 mg/dL may act as a shield against the risk of CAD.[130,131]

DIAGNOSTIC PROCEDURES

An overview of the many diagnostic procedures used to evaluate cardiovascular dysfunction in critical care is provided in Table 11-16.

TABLE 11-15	DESIRABLE LIPID LEVELS
LIPID	**DESIRABLE LEVEL**
Total cholesterol	<200 mg/dL
LDL-C	<130 mg/dL without CAD
	<100 mg/dL with CAD but not considered high risk
	<70 mg/dL with CAD and considered at high risk for future coronary events
Triglycerides	<150 mg/dL
HDL-C	>40 mg/dL (male)
	>50 mg/dL (female)

Data from the Executive Summary of the Third Report of the National Cholesterol Education Program (NCEP) Expert Panel on Detection, Evaluation, and Treatment of High Blood Cholesterol in Adults (Adult Treatment Panel III), *JAMA* 285(19):2486, 2001; Grundy SM, et al: Implications of recent clinical trials for the National Cholesterol Education Program (NCEP) Adult Treatment Panel III (ATP III) Guidelines, *Circulation* 110(2):227, 2004. *CAD,* coronary artery disease; *HDL-C,* high-density lipoprotein cholesterol; *LDL-C,* low-density lipoprotein cholesterol.

TABLE 11-16	CARDIOVASCULAR DIAGNOSTIC STUDIES	
STUDY	**EVALUATES**	**COMMENTS**
Aortography	Aortic valve insufficiency Aneurysms or dissection of ascending aorta Coarctation of the aorta Injuries to the aorta and major branches	Contrast medium used: Check for allergy to iodine, shellfish, dye; ensure hydration following procedure. Monitor for clinical indications of anaphylaxis (e.g., flushing, urticaria, and stridor). Monitor puncture site.
Cardiac biopsy	Effect of cardiotoxic drugs Evidence of cardiac transplant rejection Inflammatory heart disease Tumors Cardiomyopathy	Observe closely for signs of cardiac perforation and/or cardiac tamponade.

TABLE 11-16   CARDIOVASCULAR DIAGNOSTIC STUDIES—cont'd

STUDY	EVALUATES	COMMENTS

Cardiac catheterization and coronary angiography	Severity of coronary artery stenosis
	Cardiac muscle function
	Pressures within the heart
	Cardiac output and ejection fraction
	Blood gas analysis within chambers
	Allows angioplasty, atherectomy, intracoronary stents, or lasers to reduce coronary artery obstruction
		Before test:
		  Check for allergy to iodine, shellfish, dye (contrast medium used).
		After the test:
		  Ensure hydration following procedure (contrast medium used).
		  Keep extremity in which catheter was placed immobilized in a straight position for 6-12 hours.
		  Monitor arterial puncture point for hemorrhage or hematoma.
		  Monitor neurovascular status of affected limb.
		  Note complaints of back pain and vital sign changes (may indicate retroperitoneal hemorrhage).

Chest radiography	Cardiac size and shape Presence of pulmonary congestion or pleural effusions Presence of thoracic aneurysm or calcification of the aorta Position of pulmonary artery and cardiac catheter, pacemaker, or wires	Inquire about possibility of pregnancy.
Computed tomography	Left ventricular wall motion Cardiac tumors Myocardial infarction Pericardial effusion Aortic aneurysm Aortic dissection	Examination may be done with or without contrast medium. If contrast medium used, check for allergy to iodine, shellfish, dye, and ensure hydration following procedure.
Digital subtraction angiography	Vascular disease and degree of occlusion	Contrast medium used: Check for allergy to iodine, shellfish, dye; ensure hydration following procedure. Monitor for clinical indications of anaphylaxis (e.g., flushing, urticaria, and stridor). Monitor puncture site.
Doppler ultrasonography Duplex ultrasonography	Vascular disease and degree of occlusion	

Echocardiography
• M-mode: single ultrasound beam
• Two-dimensional: planar ultrasound beam; wider view of heart and structures
• Doppler: addition of Doppler to demonstrate flow of blood through the heart
• Color flow: Doppler blood flow superimposed on two-dimensional echocardiogram
• Stress echocardiography: images before, during, and after exercise or pharmacological stress
• Transesophageal echocardiography: transducer placed in esophagus
	Chamber size and wall thickness
	Valve functioning
	  • Papillary muscle functioning
	  • Prosthetic valve functioning
	Ventricular wall motion abnormalities
	Intracardiac masses
	Presence of pericardial fluid
	Intracardiac pressures (Doppler)
	Ejection fraction and cardiac output (Doppler)
	Valve gradients (Doppler)
	Intracardiac shunts (Doppler)
	Thoracic aneurysm (transesophageal)
		Transesophageal echocardiography is better choice if patient is obese, has chronic obstructive pulmonary disease, chest wall deformity, chest trauma, or thick chest dressings.
		Monitor for methemoglobinemia if local anesthetic (e.g., Cetacaine) is used.

TABLE 11-16 **CARDIOVASCULAR DIAGNOSTIC STUDIES—cont'd**

STUDY	EVALUATES	COMMENTS
Electrocardiography	Dysrhythmias Conduction defects including intraventricular blocks Electrolyte imbalance Drug toxicity Myocardial ischemia, injury, infarction Chamber hypertrophy	List what drugs the patient is receiving on electrocardiogram request. Be alert to electrical safety hazards.
Electrophysiological studies	Dysrhythmias under controlled circumstances Best therapy for control of dysrhythmia: drug, required dosage of therapy; pacemaker; catheter ablation	Patients may have near-death experience during electrophysiological studies; encourage expression of fears, concerns, anxieties. Monitor puncture site.
Holter monitor	Suspected dysrhythmias over 24-hour period Pacemaker function Silent ischemia	Instruct patient regarding importance of diary-keeping.
Intravascular ultrasound	Coronary artery size and patency Structure of vessel wall Coronary artery stent position and patency Aorta and presence of aneurysm, aneurysm dissections	As for cardiac catheterization
Magnetic resonance imaging	Three-dimensional view of the heart Anatomy and structure of the heart and great vessels including cardiomyopathy; congenital defect; masses; aneurysm Changes in chemistry of tissues before structural changes occur	Test does not involve radiation or dyes. Test cannot be used in patients with any implanted metallic device, including pacemakers, implantable defibrillators, metallic heart valves, or intracranial aneurysm clips.
Multiple-gated acquisition scan (radionuclide angiography)	Ventricular size and ventricular wall motion Cardiac output, cardiac index, end-systolic volume, end-diastolic volume, and ejection fraction Intracardiac shunts	Assure patient that amount of radioactive material is minimal.
Pericardiocentesis and pericardial fluid analysis	Presence of blood, pus, pathogens, or malignancy Also used for emergency relief of cardiac tamponade	Observe closely for signs of cardiac tamponade.
Peripheral angiography	Atherosclerotic plaques, occlusion, aneurysms, or traumatic injury	Before test: Contrast medium is used—check for allergy to iodine, shellfish, or dye. After the test: Contrast medium is used—ensure hydration after procedure. Keep extremity in which catheter was placed immobilized in a straight position for 6-12 hours. Monitor arterial puncture point for hemorrhage or hematoma. Monitor neurovascular status of affected limb. Monitor for indications of systemic emboli.
Phonocardiography	Extra heart sounds and murmurs in relation to the cardiac cycle and electrocardiogram	Rarely used today.
Plethysmography: arterial or venous	Arterial Patency of peripheral arteries and presence of occlusive vascular disease Venous Patency of peripheral venous system and presence of deep vein thrombosis	Test requires one normal extremity because one extremity is compared to the other.
Positron emission tomography (cardiac PET scan)	Severity of coronary artery stenosis Collateral circulation Patency of bypass grafts Size and location of infarcted tissue	Assure patient that amount of radioactive material is minimal.

TABLE 11-16	CARDIOVASCULAR DIAGNOSTIC STUDIES—cont'd	
STUDY	**EVALUATES**	**COMMENTS**
Signal-averaged electrocardiogram	Presence of late electrical potentials that may be responsible for malignant ventricular dysrhythmias; may be performed before and after ablation	Patient must lie still for 10 minutes.
Stress electrocardiography	Persons with high risk for coronary artery disease, patients with known coronary artery disease, or postsurgical patients for ischemia with exercise or pharmacological agents (e.g., adenosine, dipyridamole, or dobutamine) Exercise-induced dysrhythmias	One millimeter or greater transient ST-segment depression 80 msec after the J point is suggestive of coronary artery disease. Monitor closely for exercise-induced hypotension or ventricular dysrhythmias.
Technetium-99 pyrophosphate scan	Size, location of acute myocardial infarction (infarcted areas show increased uptake of radioactivity [hot spots] 1-7 days after myocardial infarction)	Assure patient that amount of radioactive material is minimal. Peak accuracy is obtained at 12-48 hours after initial symptoms.
Thallium stress electrocardiography	Myocardial ischemia during exercise (ischemic areas show decreased uptake of radioactivity [cold spots])	Assure patient that amount of radioactive material is minimal.
Thallium-201 scan	Myocardial ischemia (ischemic areas show decreased uptake of radioactivity [cold spots])	Assure patient that amount of radioactive material is minimal.
Vectorcardiography	Chamber hypertrophy Bundle branch blocks and hemiblocks Myocardial ischemia or infarction	As for electrocardiography.
Venography (ascending contrast phlebography)	Deep leg veins Presence of deep vein thrombosis Competence of deep vein valves May be used to locate suitable vein for arterial bypass graft	Contrast medium used: Check for allergy to iodine, shellfish, dye; ensure hydration after procedure. Monitor for clinical indications of anaphylaxis (e.g., flushing, urticaria, and stridor). Monitor puncture site.
Ventriculography	Ventricular wall motion Wall thickness Ventricular aneurysm Mitral valve motion Left ventricular end-diastolic volume, end-systolic volume, stroke volume, ejection fraction Intracardiac shunt	Contrast medium used: Check for allergy to iodine, shellfish, dye; ensure hydration after procedure. Monitor for clinical indications of anaphylaxis (e.g., flushing, urticaria, and stridor). Monitor puncture site.

From Dennison RD: *Pass CCRN!*, ed 3, St Louis, 2007, Mosby.

MI, Myocardial infarction; *2D*, two-dimensional; *TEE*, transesophageal echocardiography; *COPD*, chronic obstructive pulmonary disease; *CAD*, coronary artery disease; *DVT*, deep vein thrombosis.

REFERENCES

1. Ang D, et al: Mechanisms of heartburn, *Nat Clin Pract Gastroenterol Hepatol* 5(7):383, 2008.
2. Faybush EM, Fass R: Gastroesophageal reflux disease in noncardiac chest pain, *Gastroenterol Clin North Am* 33(1):41, 2004.
3. Chun AA, McGee SR: Bedside diagnosis of coronary artery disease: a systematic review, *Am J Med* 117(5):334, 2004.
4. Marrie TJ, Brown N: Clubbing of the digits, *Am J Med* 120(11):940, 2007.
5. Spicknall KE, et al: Clubbing: an update on diagnosis, differential diagnosis, pathophysiology, and clinical relevance, *J Am Acad Dermatol* 52(6):1020, 2005.
6. Martinez-Lavin M: Exploring the cause of the most ancient clinical sign of medicine: finger clubbing, *Semin Arthritis Rheum* 36(6):380, 2007.
7. Vinayak AG, et al: Usefulness of the external jugular vein examination in detecting abnormal central venous pressure in critically ill patients, *Arch Intern Med* 166(19):2132, 2006.
8. Brennan JM, et al: A comparison by medicine residents of physical examination versus hand-carried ultrasound for estimation of right atrial pressure, *Am J Cardiol* 99(11):1614, 2007.
9. Drazner MH, et al: Prognostic importance of elevated jugular venous pressure and a third heart sound in patients with heart failure, *N Engl J Med* 345(8):574, 2001.
10. Drazner MH, et al: Third heart sound and elevated jugular venous pressure as markers of the subsequent development of heart failure in patients with asymptomatic left ventricular dysfunction, *Am J Med* 114(6):431, 2003.
11. Sinisalo J, et al: Simplifying the estimation of jugular venous pressure, *Am J Cardiol* 100(12):1779, 2007.

12. Wiese J: The abdominojugular reflux sign, *Am J Med* 109(1):59, 2000.

13. Khan NA, et al: Does the clinical examination predict lower extremity peripheral arterial disease? *JAMA* 295(5):536, 2006.

14. Lewin J, Maconochie I: Capillary refill time in adults, *Emerg Med J* 25(6):325, 2008.

15. Chobanian AV, et al: Seventh report of the Joint National Committee on Prevention, Detection, Evaluation, and Treatment of High Blood Pressure, *Hypertension* 42(6):1206, 2003.

16. Chobanian AV: Prehypertension revisited, *Hypertension* 48(5):812, 2006.

17. Fields LE, et al: The burden of adult hypertension in the United States 1999 to 2000: a rising tide, *Hypertension* 44(4):398, 2004.

18. Perloff D, et al: *Human blood pressure determination by sphygmomanometry*, ed 6, Dallas, 2001, American Heart Association.

19. Shadman R, et al: Subclavian artery stenosis: prevalence, risk factors, and association with cardiovascular diseases, *J Am Coll Cardiol* 44(3):618, 2004.

20. Naschitz JE, Rosner I: Orthostatic hypotension: framework of the syndrome, *Postgrad Med J* 83(983):568, 2007.

21. Marcus GM, et al: Relationship between accurate auscultation of a clinically useful third heart sound and level of experience, *Arch Intern Med* 166(6):617, 2006.

22. Swami A, Spodick DH: Pulsus paradoxus in cardiac tamponade: a pathophysiologic continuum, *Clin Cardiol* 26(5):215, 2003.

23. Stone MK, et al: Respiratory changes in the pulse-oximetry waveform associated with pericardial tamponade, *Clin Cardiol* 29(9):411, 2006.

24. Wu LA, Nishimura RA: Images in clinical medicine: pulsus paradoxus, *N Engl J Med* 349(7):666, 2003.

25. Treadway K: Heart sounds, *N Engl J Med* 354(11):1112, 2006.

26. Chizner MA: Cardiac auscultation: rediscovering the lost art, *Curr Probl Cardiol* 33(7):326, 2008.

27. Barrett MJ, et al: Mastering cardiac murmurs: the power of repetition, *Chest* 126(2):470, 2004.

28. Mehta NJ, Khan IA: Third heart sound: genesis and clinical importance, *Int J Cardiol* 97(2):183, 2004.

29. Shah SJ, et al: Physiology of the third heart sound: novel insights from tissue Doppler imaging, *J Am Soc Echocardiogr* 21(4):394, 2008.

30. Marcus GM, et al: Usefulness of the third heart sound in predicting an elevated level of B-type natriuretic peptide, *Am J Cardiol* 93(10):1312, 2004.

31. Halm MA: Flushing hemodynamic catheters: what does the science tell us? *Am J Crit Care* 17(1):73, 2008.

32. Del Cotillo M, et al: Heparinized solution vs. saline solution in the maintenance of arterial catheters: a double blind randomized clinical trial, *Intensive Care Med* 34(2):339, 2008.

33. Hall KF, et al: Effect of heparin in arterial line flushing solutions on platelet count: a randomised double-blind study, *Crit Care Resusc* 8(4):294, 2006.

34. Warkentin TE, et al: Treatment and prevention of heparin-induced thrombocytopenia: American College of Chest Physicians Evidence-Based Clinical Practice Guidelines (8th edition), *Chest* 133(suppl 6):340S, 2008.

35. Bridges E: AACN Practice Alert: Pulmonary artery pressure/central venous pressure measurement; revised 12/2009 (website). www.aacn.org/WD/Practice/Docs/PracticeAlerts/PAP_Measurement_05-2004.pdf. Accessed January 2011.

36. Figg KK, Nemergut EC: Error in central venous pressure measurement, *Anesth Analg* 108(4):1209, 2009.

37. American Association of Critical-Care Nurses (AACN): Audit of pulmonary artery/central venous pressure measurement (website). www.aacn.org/WD/Practice/Docs/PracticeAlerts/pap%20measurement%20audit%20tool%2009-2010%20final.pdf. Accessed January 2011.

38. Graham KC, Cvach M: Monitor alarm fatigue: standardizing use of physiological monitors and decreasing nuisance alarms, *Am J Crit Care* 19(1):28, 2010.

39. Kohonen M, et al: Is the Allen test reliable enough? *Eur J Cardiothorac Surg* 32(6):902, 2007.

40. Barone JE, Madlinger RV: Should an Allen test be performed before radial artery cannulation? *J Trauma* 61(2):468, 2006.

41. Agrifoglio M, et al: The Allen test is not adequate enough for the screening of hand circulation, *Eur J Cardiothorac Surg* 33(4):754, 2008.

42. Shiloh AL, et al: Ultrasound-guided catheterization of the radial artery: a systematic review and meta-analysis of randomized controlled trials, *Chest* 2010 Epub in press.

43. Hadian M, Pinsky MR: Functional hemodynamic monitoring, *Curr Opin Crit Care* 13(3):318, 2007.

44. Pickering TG, et al: Recommendations for blood pressure measurement in humans and experimental animals: Part 1: blood pressure measurement in humans: a statement for professionals from the Subcommittee of Professional and Public Education of the American Heart Association Council on High Blood Pressure Research, *Hypertension* 45(1):142, 2005.

45. Wang H, et al: Effectiveness of different central venous catheters for catheter-related infections: a network meta-analysis, *J Hosp Infect* 76(1):1, 2010.

46. Polderman KH, Girbes AR: Central venous catheter use. Part 1: Mechanical complications, *Intensive Care Med* 28(1):1, 2002.

47. Polderman KH, Girbes AR: Central venous catheter use. Part 2: Infectious complications, *Intensive Care Med* 28(1):18, 2002.

48. Maddukuri P, et al: Echocardiographic diagnosis of air embolism associated with central venous catheter placement: case report and review of the literature, *Echocardiography* 23(4):315, 2006.

49. Collyer TC, et al: Severe air embolism resulting from a perforated cap on a high-flow three-way stopcock connected to a central venous catheter, *Eur J Anaesthesiol* 24(5):474, 2007.

50. Deceuninck O, et al: Images in cardiovascular medicine. Massive air embolism after central venous catheter removal, *Circulation* 116(19):e516, 2007.

51. Wang AZ, et al: The differences between venous air embolism and fat embolism in routine intraoperative monitoring methods, transesophageal echocardiography, and fatal volume in pigs, *J Trauma* 65(2):416, 2008.

52. Garnacho-Montero J, et al: Risk factors and prognosis of catheter-related bloodstream infection in critically ill patients: a multicenter study, *Intensive Care Med* 34(12):2185, 2008.

53. O'Grady P, et al. Guidelines for the prevention of intravascular catheter-related infections, *Am J Infect Control* 39(4):S1-S34, 2011.

54. Boyce JM, Pittet D: Guideline for hand hygiene in health-care settings. Recommendations of the Healthcare Infection Control Practices Advisory Committee and the HIPAC/SHEA/APIC/IDSA Hand Hygiene Task Force, *Am J Infect Control* 30(8):S1, 2002.

55. Ruschulte H, et al: Prevention of central venous catheter related infections with chlorhexidine gluconate impregnated wound dressings: a randomized controlled trial, *Ann Hematol* 88(3):267, 2009.

56. Marx G, Reinhart K: Venous oximetry, *Curr Opin Crit Care* 12(3):263, 2006.

57. Shepherd SJ, Pearse RM: Role of central and mixed venous oxygen saturation measurement in perioperative care, *Anesthesiology* 111(3):649, 2009.

58. Richard C, et al: Early use of the pulmonary artery catheter and outcomes in patients with shock and acute respiratory distress syndrome: a randomized controlled trial, *JAMA* 290(20):2713, 2003.

59. Wheeler AP, et al: Pulmonary-artery versus central venous catheter to guide treatment of acute lung injury, *N Engl J Med* 354(21):2213, 2006.

60. Binanay C, et al: Evaluation study of congestive heart failure and pulmonary artery catheterization effectiveness: the ESCAPE trial, *JAMA* 294(13):1625, 2005.

61. Harvey S, Singer M: Managing critically ill patients with a pulmonary artery catheter, *Br J Hosp Med (Lond)* 67(8): 421, 2006.

62. Harvey S, et al: Post hoc insights from PAC-Man—the U.K. pulmonary artery catheter trial, *Crit Care Med* 36(6):1714, 2008.

63. Sandham JD, et al: A randomized, controlled trial of the use of pulmonary-artery catheters in high-risk surgical patients, *N Engl J Med* 348(1):5, 2003.

64. Harvey S, et al: Pulmonary artery catheters for adult patients in intensive care, *Cochrane Database Syst Rev* (3):CD003408, 2006.

65. Shah MR, et al: Impact of the pulmonary artery catheter in critically ill patients: meta-analysis of randomized clinical trials, *JAMA* 294(13):1664, 2005.

66. Bernard GR, et al: Pulmonary artery catheterization and clinical outcomes: National Heart, Lung, and Blood Institute and Food and Drug Administration Workshop Report. Consensus statement, *JAMA* 283(19):2568, 2000.

67. Wiener RS, Welch HG: Trends in the use of the pulmonary artery catheter in the United States, 1993-2004, *JAMA* 298(4):423, 2007.

68. Cotter G, et al: Hemodynamic monitoring in acute heart failure, *Crit Care Med* 36(suppl 1):S40, 2008.

69. Pulmonary Artery Catheter Education Project (PACEP) (website). www.learnicu.net/Clinical_Practice/Fundamentals/PACEP/Pages/default.aspx. Accessed January 2011.

70. American Thoracic Society: *Pulmonary Artery Catheter Primer* (website). www.thoracic.org/clinical/critical-care/clinical-education/hemodynamic-monitoring/pulmonary-artery-catheter-primer/index.php. Accessed January 2011.

71. Summerhill EM, Baram M: Principles of pulmonary artery catheterization in the critically ill, *Lung* 183(3):209, 2005.

72. Bridges EJ: Pulmonary artery pressure monitoring: when, how, and what else to use, *AACN Adv Crit Care* 17(3):286, 2006.

73. Wong FW: Where is end expiration? Measuring PAWP when the patient is on pressure support ventilation, *Dynamics* 21(1):11, 2010.

74. Pinsky MR: Hemodynamic evaluation and monitoring in the ICU, *Chest* 132(6):2020, 2007.

75. Frazier SK, Skinner GJ: Pulmonary artery catheters: state of the controversy, *J Cardiovasc Nurs* 23(2):113, 2008.

76. Antle DE: Ensuring competency in nurse repositioning of the pulmonary artery catheter, *Dimens Crit Care Nurs* 19(2):44, 2000.

77. Oztekin DS, et al: Comparison of complications and procedural activities of pulmonary artery catheter removal by critical care nurses versus medical doctors, *Nurs Crit Care* 13(2):105, 2008.

78. Baldwin IC, Heland M: Incidence of cardiac dysrhythmias in patients during pulmonary artery catheter removal after cardiac surgery, *Heart Lung* 29(3):155, 2000.

79. Gawlinski A: Measuring cardiac output: intermittent bolus thermodilution method, *Crit Care Nurse* 20(2):118, 2000.

80. Walsh E, et al: Iced vs room-temperature injectates for cardiac index measurement during hypothermia and normothermia, *Am J Crit Care* 19(4):365, 2010.

81. Wavra T, Bader MK: Bolus cardiac output and accuracy in therapeutic hypothermia, *Crit Care Nurse* 29(6):71, 2009.

82. Giuliano KK, et al: Backrest angle and cardiac output measurement in critically ill patients, *Nurs Res* 52(4):242, 2003.

83. Rivers E, et al: Early goal-directed therapy in the treatment of severe sepsis and septic shock, *N Engl J Med* 345(19):1368, 2001.

84. Dellinger RP, et al: Surviving Sepsis Campaign: international guidelines for management of severe sepsis and septic shock: 2008, *Crit Care Med* 36(1):296, 2008.

85. Jesurum J: Protocols for practice—Svo_2 monitoring, *Crit Care Nurse* 24(4):73, 2004.

86. Collaborative Study Group on Perioperative $Scvo_2$ Monitoring: Multicentre study on peri- and postoperative central venous oxygen saturation in high-risk surgical patients, *Crit Care* 10(6):R158, 2006.

87. Ospina-Tascón GA, et al: What type of monitoring has been shown to improve outcomes in acutely ill patients? *Intensive Care Med* 34(5):800, 2008.

88. Kligfield P, et al: Recommendations for the standardization and interpretation of the electrocardiogram: part I: The electrocardiogram and its technology: a scientific statement from the American Heart Association Electrocardiography and Arrhythmias Committee, Council on Clinical Cardiology; the American College of Cardiology Foundation; and the Heart Rhythm Society: endorsed by the International Society for Computerized Electrocardiology, *Circulation* 115(10):1306, 2007.

89. Drew BJ, et al: Practice standards for electrocardiographic monitoring in hospital settings: an American Heart Association scientific statement from the Councils on Cardiovascular Nursing, Clinical Cardiology, and Cardiovascular Disease in the Young: endorsed by the International Society of Computerized Electrocardiology and the American Association of Critical-Care Nurses, *Circulation* 110(17):2721, 2004.

90. Drew BJ, Funk M: Practice standards for ECG monitoring in hospital settings: executive summary and guide for implementation, *Crit Care Nurs Clin North Am* 18(2):157, 2006.

91. Anderson JL, et al: ACC/AHA 2007 guidelines for the management of patients with unstable angina/non ST-elevation myocardial infarction: a report of the American College of Cardiology/American Heart Association Task Force on Practice Guidelines (Writing Committee to Revise the 2002 Guidelines for the Management of Patients with Unstable Angina/Non ST-Elevation Myocardial Infarction): developed in collaboration with the American College of Emergency Physicians, the Society for Cardiovascular Angiography and Interventions, and the Society of Thoracic Surgeons: endorsed by the American Association of Cardiovascular and Pulmonary Rehabilitation and the Society for Academic Emergency Medicine, *Circulation* 116(7):e148, 2007.

92. AACN Practice Alert: ST-Segment Monitoring, *Crit Care Nurse* 28(4):70, 2008.

93. Sommargren CE, Drew BJ: Preventing torsades de pointes by careful cardiac monitoring in hospital settings, *AACN Adv Crit Care* 18(3):285, 2007.

94. Roden DM: Drug-induced prolongation of the QT interval, *N Engl J Med* 350(10):1013, 2004.

95. Drew BJ, et al: Prevention of torsade de pointes in hospital settings: a scientific statement from the American Heart Association and the American College of Cardiology Foundation, *Circulation* 121(8):1047, 2010.

96. Yasuma F, Hayano J: Respiratory sinus arrhythmia: why does the heartbeat synchronize with respiratory rhythm? *Chest* 125(2):683, 2004.

97. Blomström-Lundqvist C, et al: ACC/AHA/ESC guidelines for the management of patients with supraventricular arrhythmias—executive summary. a report of the American College of Cardiology/American Heart Association Task Force on Practice Guidelines and the European Society of Cardiology Committee for Practice Guidelines (Writing Committee to Develop Guidelines for the Management of Patients with Supraventricular Arrhythmias) developed in collaboration with NASPE-Heart Rhythm Society, *J Am Coll Cardiol* 42(8):1493, 2003.

98. Carey MG, Pelter MM: Rapid ventricular response, *Am J Crit Care* 17(1):83, 2008.

99. Fuster V, et al: ACC/AHA/ESC 2006 Guidelines for the Management of Patients with Atrial Fibrillation: a report of the American College of Cardiology/American Heart Association Task Force on Practice Guidelines and the European Society of Cardiology Committee for Practice Guidelines (Writing Committee to Revise the 2001 Guidelines for the Management of Patients With Atrial Fibrillation): developed in collaboration with the European Heart Rhythm Association and the Heart Rhythm Society, *Circulation* 114(7):e257, 2006.

100. Everett TH, Olgin JE: Basic mechanisms of atrial fibrillation, *Cardiol Clin* 22(1):9, 2004.

101. Kellen JC: Implications for nursing care of patients with atrial fibrillation: lessons learned from the AFFIRM and RACE studies, *J Cardiovasc Nurs* 19(2):128, 2004.

102. Weiss EM, Buescher T: Atrial fibrillation: treatment options and caveats, *AACN Clinical Issues* 15(3):362, 2004.

103. Singer DE, et al: Antithrombotic therapy in atrial fibrillation: American College of Chest Physicians Evidence-Based Clinical Practice Guidelines (8th edition), *Chest* 133(suppl 6):546S, 2008.

104. Calkins H, et al: HRS/EHRA/ECAS expert consensus statement on catheter and surgical ablation of atrial fibrillation: recommendations for personnel, policy, procedures and follow-up. A report of the Heart Rhythm Society (HRS) Task Force on Catheter and Surgical Ablation of Atrial Fibrillation developed in partnership with the European Heart Rhythm Association (EHRA) and the European Cardiac Arrhythmia Society (ECAS); in collaboration with the American College of Cardiology (ACC), American Heart Association (AHA), and the Society of Thoracic Surgeons (STS). Endorsed and approved by the governing bodies of the American College of Cardiology, the American Heart Association, the European Cardiac Arrhythmia Society, the European Heart Rhythm Association, the Society of Thoracic Surgeons, and the Heart Rhythm Society, *Europace* 9(6):335, 2007.

105. Calkins H, et al: Treatment of atrial fibrillation with antiarrhythmic drugs or radiofrequency ablation: two systematic literature reviews and meta-analyses, *Circ Arrhythm Electrophysiol* 2(4): 349, 2009.

106. Nair GM, et al: A systematic review of randomized trials comparing radiofrequency ablation with antiarrhythmic medications in patients with atrial fibrillation, *J Cardiovasc Electrophysiol* 20(2): 138, 2009.

107. Pelter MM, Carey MG: P wave alterations, *Am J Crit Care* 16(2):187, 2007.

108. Jacobson C: Tools for teaching arrhythmias: wide QRS beats and rhythms. Part I. P waves, fusion, and capture beats, *AACN Adv Crit Care* 17(4):462, 2006.

109. Roden DM: Proarrhythmia as a pharmacogenomic entity: a critical review and formulation of a unifying hypothesis, *Cardiovasc Res* 67(3):419, 2005.

110. Berdajs D, et al: Incidence and pathophysiology of atrioventricular block following mitral valve replacement and ring annuloplasty, *Eur J Cardiothorac Surg* 34(1):55, 2008.

111. Paul S: Understanding advanced concepts in atrioventricular block, *Crit Care Nurse* 21(1):56, 2001.

112. Adams-Hamoda MG, Pelter MM: Heart blocks, *Am J Crit Care* 12(1):77, 2003.

113. Pelter MM, Carey MG: Slow escape rhythms, *Am J Crit Care* 16(4):405, 2007.

114. Freeman K, et al: Effects of presentation and electrocardiogram on time to treatment of hyperkalemia, *Acad Emerg Med* 15(3):239, 2008.

115. Sladdin C, Lee G: Safely treating hypokalaemia in high dependency cardiac surgical patients, *Nurs Crit Care* 11(6):267, 2006.

116. Ariyan CE, Sosa JA: Assessment and management of patients with abnormal calcium, *Crit Care Med* 32(suppl 4):S146, 2004.

117. Dickerson RN, et al: Low serum total calcium concentration as a marker of low serum ionized calcium concentration in critically ill patients receiving specialized nutrition support, *Nutr Clin Pract* 22(3):323, 2007.

118. Dickerson RN, et al: Accuracy of methods to estimate ionized and "corrected" serum calcium concentrations in critically ill multiple trauma patients receiving specialized

nutrition support, *JPEN J Parenter Enteral Nutr* 28(3):133, 2004.

119. Ma G, et al: Electrocardiographic manifestations: digitalis toxicity, *J Emerg Med* 20(2):145, 2001.

120. Zivin JR, et al: Hypocalcemia: a pervasive metabolic abnormality in the critically ill, *Am J Kidney Dis* 37(4):689, 2001.

121. Dickerson RN, et al: Dose-dependent characteristics of intravenous calcium therapy for hypocalcemic critically ill trauma patients receiving specialized nutritional support, *Nutrition* 23(1):9, 2007.

122. Noronha JL, Matuschak GM: Magnesium in critical illness: metabolism, assessment, and treatment, *Intensive Care Med* 28(6):667, 2002.

123. ECC Committee, Subcommittees and Task Forces of the American Heart Association: 2005 American Heart Association guidelines for cardiopulmonary resuscitation and emergency cardiovascular care: Part 7.2 management of cardiac arrest, *Circulation* 112(suppl 24): IV-58, 2005.

124. Antman EM, et al: ACC/AHA guidelines for the management of patients with ST-elevation myocardial infarction–executive summary: a report of the American College of Cardiology/American Heart Association Task Force on Practice Guidelines (Writing Committee to Revise the 1999 Guidelines for the Management of Patients with Acute Myocardial Infarction), *Can J Cardiol* 20(10):977, 2004.

125. Novis DA, et al: Biochemical markers of myocardial injury test turnaround time: a College of American Pathologists Q-Probes study of 7020 troponin and 4368 creatine kinase-MB determinations in 159 institutions, *Arch Pathol Lab Med* 128(2):158, 2004.

126. Lin JC, et al: Rates of positive cardiac troponin I and creatine kinase MB mass among patients hospitalized for suspected acute coronary syndromes, *Clin Chem* 50(2):333, 2004.

127. Correa de Sa DD, Chen HH: The role of natriuretic peptides in heart failure, *Curr Cardiol Rep* 10(3):182, 2008.

128. Maisel A: Circulating natriuretic peptide levels in acute heart failure, *Rev Cardiovasc Med* 8(suppl 5):S13, 2007.

129. Ansell J, et al: Pharmacology and management of the vitamin K antagonists: American College of Chest Physicians Evidence-Based Clinical Practice Guidelines (8th edition), *Chest* 133(suppl 6):160S, 2008.

130. Grundy SM, et al: Implications of recent clinical trials for the National Cholesterol Education Program Adult Treatment Panel III guidelines, *Circulation* 110(2):227, 2004.

131. Grundy SM, et al: Diagnosis and management of the metabolic syndrome: an American Heart Association/National Heart, Lung, and Blood Institute Scientific Statement, *Circulation* 112(17):2735, 2005.

12

Cardiovascular Disorders

Elizabeth Scruth, Annette Haynes

⊖volve WEBSITE

Be sure to check out the bonus material, including free self-assessment exercises, on the Evolve web site at *http://evolve.elsevier.com/Urden/priorities/*.

OBJECTIVES

- Describe the etiology and pathophysiology of atherosclerotic coronary artery disease.
- Identify the pathophysiology and clinical manifestations of acute heart failure.

- Explain the treatment of selected cardiovascular disorders: coronary artery disease, cardiomyopathy, and valvular disease.
- Discuss the nursing priorities for managing a patient with an acute cardiovascular disorder.

Cardiovascular disease remains the leading cause of mortality in the United States. The estimated direct and indirect national cost of cardiovascular disease in 2010 was $503.2 billion.[1] Cardiovascular diseases are the leading cause of death for women and men. There are almost 80 million adults in the United States living with cardiovascular disease. Cardiovascular disease accounts for 1 of every 2.9 deaths in the United States.[1] In terms of disability, the number of disability-adjusted life-years (DALYs) attributable to cardiovascular disease on a global basis is projected to double by the year 2020. An understanding of the pathology of cardiovascular disease processes and clinical management allows the critical care nurse to accurately anticipate and plan interventions. This chapter focuses on cardiac disorders commonly seen in the critical care environment.

CORONARY ARTERY DISEASE

Description and Etiology

The biggest contributor to cardiovascular-related morbidity and mortality is coronary artery disease (CAD). Atherosclerosis is a progressive disease that affects arteries throughout the body. In the heart, atherosclerotic changes are clinically known as CAD. This disease process is also known by the term coronary heart disease (CHD) because other heart structures ultimately become involved in the disease process. The atherosclerotic vascular changes that lead to CAD may begin in childhood.[2] Research and epidemiological data collected during the past 50 years have demonstrated a strong association between specific risk factors and the development of CAD.[1] These risk factors are further delineated as nonmodifiable and modifiable coronary risk factors (Box 12-1).

Risk Factors for Coronary Artery Disease
Age, Gender, and Race

The severe effects of CAD occur as a person ages. In general, CAD symptoms are seen in middle and old age.[1] Traditionally, CAD has been regarded as a male disease, but it is increasingly obvious that in modern society it affects both genders.[1] The average age for a person having a first heart attack is 64.5 years for men and 70.3 years for women.[1] Starting at age 75 years, the prevalence of cardiovascular disease is higher among women than men.[2,3] CAD rates for postmenopausal women are two to three times higher than those for premenopausal women of the same age.[1] People of color and multiracial populations of both genders have higher CAD mortality rates than do white populations of similar socioeconomic status.[1]

Family History

A positive family history is one in which a close blood relative has had a myocardial infarction (MI) or stroke before the age of 60. This family history suggests a genetic or lifestyle predisposition to the development of CAD. Individuals with a

BOX 12-1   CORONARY ARTERY DISEASE RISK FACTORS

Nonmodifiable Risk Factors
- Age
- Gender
- Family history
- Race

Modifiable Risk Factors
- Elevated serum lipids
- Hypertension
- Cigarette smoking
- Prediabetes or diabetes mellitus
- Diet high in saturated fat, cholesterol, and calories
- Elevated homocysteine level
- Metabolic syndrome
- Obesity
- Physical inactivity
- Postmenopause (modification remains controversial)

TABLE 12-1   LIPID GUIDELINES AND RISK FOR CORONARY ARTERY DISEASE

LIPID	TARGET VALUE* (mg/dl)
Total cholesterol	<200
HDL cholesterol	
Men	>40
Women	>50
LDL cholesterol	
Very high risk	<70
High risk	<100
Low risk	<130
VLDL cholesterol	<30
Triglycerides	<150

HDL, high-density lipoprotein; *LDL,* low-density lipoprotein; *VLDL,* very-low-density lipoprotein.
*Values outside the target range increase the risk for coronary artery disease.

family history had a 50% greater risk of having an acute MI in the INTERHEART study.[4] This was a large, international, standardized case-control study of similar cohorts in 52 countries that was designed to examine the importance of risk factors for CAD on a worldwide basis.[4]

Hyperlipidemia

Hyperlipidemia is a leading factor responsible for severe atherosclerosis and the development of CAD. Determining total serum cholesterol and triglyceride levels is a helpful start in the evaluation process.[3,5] A lipid panel blood test can measure the following values:
- High-density lipoprotein (HDL) cholesterol
- Low-density lipoprotein (LDL) cholesterol
- Very-low-density lipoprotein (VLDL) cholesterol
- Triglycerides

Treatment of hyperlipidemia has advanced beyond the concept of lowering total cholesterol to treatment of specific lipoprotein abnormalities.[3,6-8] The target levels for specific serum lipids are listed in Table 12-1.

Total Cholesterol. The total cholesterol is the sum of the HDL, LDL, and VLDL cholesterol in the bloodstream. It is used as a starting point for lipid testing. A total cholesterol level higher than 200 mg/dL is an indication to investigate the lipid profile and other risk factors for CAD. More than 102 million American adults (46.8% of the adult population) have a total blood cholesterol level at or above 200 mg/dL.[1]

High-Density Lipoprotein Cholesterol. HDL cholesterol is frequently described as the "good cholesterol" because higher serum levels exert a protective effect against acute atherosclerotic events. All the reasons are not completely understood, but one recognized physiological effect is the ability of HDL to promote the efflux of cholesterol from cells. This process may minimize the accumulation of foam cells in the artery wall and decrease the risk of developing atherosclerosis.[9] High HDL cholesterol levels confer antiinflammatory and antioxidant benefits on the arterial wall.[9] In contrast, a low HDL cholesterol level is an independent risk factor for the development of CAD and other atherosclerotic conditions. HDL cholesterol is generally higher in women, and levels can be raised by physical exercise and by smoking cessation. In patients with low HDL cholesterol levels, when lifestyle changes are ineffective, the HDL level can be raised by drugs such as extended-release nicotinic acid (niacin) and fibrates. In 2006 16.2% of the adult U.S. population had HDL cholesterol levels below 40 mg/dL.[1]

Low-Density Lipoprotein Cholesterol. LDL cholesterol is usually described as the "bad cholesterol" because high levels are associated with an increased risk of acute coronary syndrome, stroke, and peripheral arterial disease (PAD). High LDL levels initiate the atherosclerotic process by infiltrating the vessel wall and binding to the matrix of cells beneath the endothelium.[9] LDL cholesterol also exerts an inflammatory effect on the arterial vessel wall.[9] A high LDL cholesterol level is initially managed by nonpharmacological lifestyle changes such as weight loss, smoking cessation, low-fat diet, physical exercise, and attainment of a normal body size as measured by the body mass index (BMI). If lifestyle changes are insufficient to reduce the LDL cholesterol level in the bloodstream, the drug category of choice is a statin. Numerous research studies have conclusively demonstrated that lowering the LDL cholesterol with statins for primary or secondary prevention is highly effective in lowering mortality due to CAD.[1,3] Therapy should be tailored to treat the individual cardiovascular risk profile. The target LDL cholesterol is determined according to the individual's risk profile as described in Table 12-1. Patients at highest risk are advised to maintain LDL cholesterol below 70 mg/dL; those at high risk, a level below 100 mg/dL; and those at low risk, LDL below 130 mg/dL. Controversy exists about whether the tiered LDL goals in the current guidelines are sufficiently low to prevent coronary atherosclerosis developing in persons without CAD. Some cardiologists advocate a reduction of the LDL goal to a 50 to 70 mg/dL range for everyone, not just those with a known cardiovascular disease.[10] In 2006 32.6% of the adult U.S. population had LDL cholesterol levels of 130 mg/dL or higher.[1]

Very-Low-Density Lipoprotein Cholesterol. VLDL cholesterol is not usually measured, although a normal value is about 30 mg/dL.[6] The value can be estimated by subtracting the sum of the HDL and LDL from the total cholesterol. When triglyceride levels are elevated, the VLDL cholesterol level also is high.

Triglycerides. Triglycerides are serum lipids that constitute an additional atherogenic risk factor. Triglycerides are carried by VLDL cholesterol in the bloodstream.[7] An optimal triglyceride level is below 150 mg/dL, and the more elevated the triglyceride serum level, the higher the risk of developing CAD. A value between 150 and 199 mg/dL is borderline high; a value between 200 and 500 mg/dL is high; and a value above 500 mg/dL signals a high risk of atherogenic complications and a strong risk for the presence or development of type 2 diabetes.

Lipoprotein(a). LDL cholesterol can be further analyzed by the category of lipid particles that make up the total LDL value. Researchers have investigated the function of several lipid particles to determine their role in the development of premature atherosclerotic CAD. One particle that has been extensively studied is lipoprotein(a), which is abbreviated Lp(a) and described verbally as "LP little a." Lp(a) is manufactured in the liver and circulates in the bloodstream bound to a large glycoprotein called apolipoprotein(a), abbreviated as apo(a).[11] The Lp(a)-apo(a) lipid particle concentration is elevated in the presence of inflammation, and it stimulates atheroma and clot formation in inflamed arteries.[11] This effect is thought to occur because the apo(a) is structurally similar to plasminogen, a protein essential for clot formation.

Lp(a) levels are 90% genetically determined. Elevated Lp(a) plasma levels constitute the most frequently encountered genetic lipid disorder in families with premature CAD.[11] Testing for Lp(a) is reserved for high-risk patient populations such as those with a strong family history of premature atherosclerotic disease and for patients with premature CAD who do not exhibit the expected cardiac risk factors. Reduction of Lp(a) levels to below 30 mg/dL is the therapeutic goal. This is usually achieved by ingesting high doses (1 to 2 grams/day) of extended-release nicotinic acid (niacin). The Lp(a) level is not reduced by statins, drugs that traditionally lower LDL levels, or by physical exercise, a low-fat diet, weight loss, or tight control of blood glucose levels.[11] Lifestyle changes are recommended, and research is ongoing, but a cure is not yet discernible.

High-Fat Diet

A diet rich in saturated fats leads to elevated cholesterol levels in the blood. The first line of treatment to lower elevated serum cholesterol is a low-fat, high-fiber diet and increased physical exercise.[7,8] If these measures are not effective, lipid-lowering drugs are indicated.[1] This approach sounds simple, but less than one half of the people who qualify for lipid reduction therapy are taking their medications; only one third of treated patients reach their LDL target; and fewer than 20% of patients with CAD are at their LDL goal.[1] Although lipid-lowering drugs are very helpful for some, they are not a panacea for everyone.

Obesity

Obesity is a disease of modern times. Global estimates are more than 1 billion overweight adults, and at least 300 million of these people are obese. Obesity is often associated with a sedentary lifestyle. A high risk of coronary heart disease is among the well-established adverse health effects associated with excess weight. Hypertension, hypercholesterolemia, and diabetes are among the clinical conditions that are important mediators of this association.[12] In the United States in 2001, 122 million adults were overweight or obese.[13] In 2006 144 million adults, or 66% of the U.S. adult population, were overweight or obese.[1] Obesity is defined using the body mass index (BMI).

The BMI is calculated as the weight in kilograms divided by the square of the height in meters (kg/m^2); it assesses body weight relative to height. BMI is used to evaluate the threat of excess pounds as a risk factor for CAD and permits comparisons of people of different gender, age, height, and body type.[1] BMI is calculated as the weight in kilograms divided by the square of the height in meters (kg/m^2). The BMI calculation in metric units is shown in Box 12-2. A normal BMI is between 18.5 and 25 kg/m^2. A BMI between 25 and 30 kg/m^2 indicates the person is overweight. A BMI greater than 30 kg/m^2 is the definition of obesity.[1]

The distribution pattern of fat on the body is a CAD risk factor. The more weight carried in the abdominal area, producing a large waist, the greater the risk of CAD. Excess

---

BOX 12-2 **HOW TO CALCULATE AND INTERPRET BODY MASS INDEX**

Use a Calculator to Determine the Body Mass Index (BMI)
Metric Units
Divide body weight in kilograms by height in meters; divide the result by height in meters:

$$BMI = (Weight_{kg}/Height_m) \div Height_m$$

Example: A person weighs 100 kg and is 1.90 m tall:

$$BMI = 100/1.90 \div 1.90 = 27.7$$

How to Interpret the BMI Result

BMI (kg/m^2)	Weight Status
<18.5	Underweight
18.5-24.9	Normal weight
25-29.5	Overweight
>30	Obese
>40	Extreme obesity

abdominal adiposity (apple body shape) indicates additional fat around the abdominal organs compared with individuals who have a smaller waist and larger hips (pear body shape). A waist size greater than 40 inches in men and 35 inches in women increases their risk for CAD. Physical exercise assists with weight reduction, lowers the risk for CAD, and decreases the risk of developing type 2 diabetes.

Physical Inactivity

Regular vigorous physical activity using large muscle groups promotes physiological adaptation to aerobic exercise that can prevent the development of CAD and reduce symptoms in patients with established cardiovascular disease.[14] Exercise also reduces the incidence of many other diseases, including type 2 diabetes, osteoporosis, obesity, depression, and cancers of the colon and breast.[14] Many research trials have demonstrated the positive effects of physical activity on the other major cardiac risk factors.[14] Exercise alters the lipid profile by decreasing LDL cholesterol and triglyceride levels and increasing HDL cholesterol levels.[14] Exercise reduces insulin resistance at the cellular level, lowering the risk for developing type 2 diabetes, especially if combined with a weight-loss program.[14] Epidemiological studies indicate that physical athletics as a young person do not confer protection in later years. A sedentary lifestyle has negative effects, regardless of age, gender, BMI, smoking status, presence or absence of hypertension, or abnormal lipoprotein profile. Lifelong physical activity is necessary to prevent atherosclerotic CAD and stroke.[14] In 2005 the prevalence of adults not engaging in any physical activity during leisure or work time was 10.3% in the United States.[1] In affluent countries, only one third of the population exercises moderately for the recommended 30 minutes, five times per week.

Hypertension

Normal blood pressure is described as a systolic blood pressure (SBP) below 120 mm Hg and a diastolic blood pressure (DBP) below 80 mm Hg. Hypertension is defined as an SBP greater than 140 mm Hg or DBP higher than 90 mm Hg. Controlled hypertension describes a situation in which administration of antihypertensive medications maintains the patient's blood pressure within the normal range.

Hypertension is a cardiac risk factor because the high SBP damages the arterial endothelium, leading to vascular inflammation that encourages formation of plaque. Hypertension is a complex, multifactorial disease process. Hypertension is divided into stages for the purposes of treatment, as shown in Table 12-2.

Prehypertension is an SBP of 120 to 139 mm Hg or DBP above 85 mm Hg.[1,13] In the United States, one in five adults is prehypertensive. Hypertension is diagnosed when the blood pressure is above 140/90 mm Hg. Hypertension affects another one in four adults in the United States. After the blood pressure is above 140/80 mm Hg, hypertension is described as stage 1 or stage 2 depending on the severity (see Table 12-2).

TABLE 12-2	BLOOD PRESSURE GUIDELINES AND RISK FOR CORONARY ARTERY DISEASE	
CATEGORY	SYSTOLIC BP* (mm Hg)	DIASTOLIC BP* (mm Hg)
Normal (optimal)*	<120	<80
Prehypertension	120-139	80-89
Stage 1 hypertension	140-159	90-99
Stage 2 hypertension	≥160	≥100

BP, blood pressure; CAD, coronary artery disease.
*Values greater than normal increase the risk for CAD and heart failure.

Hypertension is often described as the "silent killer," because 30% of those affected are unaware they have seriously elevated blood pressure.[1] A higher percentage of men than women have hypertension until age 45, but from the ages of 45 to 54 years, the percentage of men and women with hypertension is similar.[1] It is essential that patients understand that sustained elevation of blood pressure leads inexorably toward atherosclerosis, heart failure, kidney failure, stroke, and heart attack.[13] So widespread is hypertension in industrialized societies that even a normotensive person at age 55 has a 90% lifetime risk of developing hypertension. This implies that even normotensive persons should adopt interventions to maintain a normal blood pressure.[13] The estimated direct and indirect cost of hypertension in the United States for 2010 is $76.6 billion.[1]

According to recent guidelines, the goal of treatment for the hypertensive person without other risk factors is to achieve a blood pressure below 140/80 mm Hg. For the hypertensive person who already has diabetes or kidney disease, the target blood pressure is below 130/80 mm Hg. A normal blood pressure is below 120/80 mm Hg.[13]

Lifestyle interventions that can normalize blood pressure include physical exercise, a low-salt diet, limiting alcohol intake, and achieving normal body weight. Most patients are started on a diuretic, and if this is insufficient, they may be placed on an angiotensin-converting enzyme inhibitor (ACEI), angiotensin receptor blocker (ARB), beta-blocker, or calcium channel blocker. Most patients require at least two medications, each from different drug classifications, to normalize their blood pressure.[13] Hypertensive emergencies with acute organ damage are discussed in the last section of this chapter.

Cigarette Smoking

The greater the number of cigarettes smoked per day, the greater the risk of developing CAD, acute MI, and stroke.[14,16] In the United States, the prevalence of smoking has always been lower among women than men.[1] Cigarette smoking unfavorably alters serum lipid levels, decreases the HDL cholesterol level, and increases LDL cholesterol and triglyceride levels. In the United States, smoking remains common, with an overall prevalence of 20.6% of the adult population. Smoking increases the risk of coronary heart disease at all levels.[1] Smokers are two to four times more likely to develop CAD than nonsmokers.[1] Passive, secondhand smoke exposure also increases cardiovascular risk; 34.7% of nonsmoking adults are exposed to environmental tobacco smoke at home or at work.[15-17] Nicotine is addictive, and smoking cessation is difficult. People need tremendous support to be able to "kick the habit." Chapter 25 provides patient education guidelines on how to stop smoking.

Diabetes Mellitus

Individuals with diabetes mellitus (types 1 and 2) have a higher incidence of coronary heart disease compared with the general population. Data from the Framingham Heart Study indicates a doubling in the incidence of diabetes over the past 30 years and most dramatically during the 1990s.[1] Elevated blood glucose level is a known risk factor for development of vascular inflammation associated with atherosclerosis. The normoglycemia range is 70 to 100 mg/dL. It is recommended that patients in critical care have blood glucose levels maintained close to the normal range[18] while avoiding hypoglycemic episodes.

A fasting blood glucose concentration between 100 and 125 mg/dL represents a prediabetic state and is a risk factor for the development of diabetes and CAD (Table 12-3). A fasting blood glucose above 126 mg/dL is indicative of diabetes. Patients with diabetes have an increased risk of developing CAD and have worse clinical outcomes after acute coronary syndrome events.[19] In a multinational study of patients who were seen at hospitals with symptoms of acute coronary syndrome, almost one in four had a known history of diabetes.[20]

Chronic Kidney Disease

Chronic kidney disease is considered a risk equivalent for CAD.[2,3,21] This means patients with chronic kidney disease have as much risk of experiencing a coronary event as if they already had CAD.[2,3,22] The risk of death for the patient with acute MI rises as the serum creatinine level increases.[22] In one study, the in-hospital mortality rates for patients with an acute MI were 2% for patients with normal kidney function, 6% for those with mild kidney failure, 14% for those with moderate kidney failure, 21% for those with severe kidney failure, and 30% for patients with end-stage kidney disease.[22] Mortality following cardiac surgery is also higher for individuals with chronic kidney disease.[23]

Metabolic Syndrome

Metabolic syndrome refers to the clustering of risk factors associated with cardiovascular disease and type 2 diabetes.[1] The prevalence of metabolic syndrome in 2006 for adults in the United States was 34%.[1] Metabolic syndrome is diagnosed when three or more of the following risk factors are present:[24,25]

1. Waist circumference is greater than 40 inches (102 cm) in men and greater than 35 inches (88 cm) in women.
2. Serum triglyceride is level greater than 150 mg/dL (≥1.7 mmol/L).
3. High-density lipoprotein (HDL) cholesterol level is less than 40 mg/dL (≤1.04 mmol/L) in men; less than 50 mg/dL (≤1.29 mmol/L) in women.
4. Blood pressure is 130/85 mm Hg or higher, which is diagnostic for prehypertension or hypertension.
5. Fasting glucose level is 100 mg/dL or higher, which is diagnostic for prediabetes. A fasting blood glucose level greater than 126 mg/dL is diagnostic for diabetes.

It is perhaps obvious that individuals with the signs of metabolic syndrome are at increased risk for CAD; even so, it is surprising to what degree this holds true. In the Framingham epidemiological study, presence of the factors associated with metabolic syndrome predicted 25% of all new-onset CAD and almost 50% of new-onset diabetes.[23]

Women and Heart Disease: Premenopause and Postmenopause

Serious CAD symptoms occur approximately 5 years later in women than in men.[25] The average age for the first acute MI in men is 65.8 years and in women is 70.4 years.[1] Incidence of CAD is two to three times higher among postmenopausal women than women who are premenopausal.[1] In the past, it seemed logical to prescribe hormone replacement therapy (HRT) to treat the symptoms of menopause. However, well-designed research trials discovered an increase in cardiovascular events in the first year of HRT (estrogen plus progestin), although cardiac events declined after the first year.[25,26] Subsequent studies have confirmed this result.[24] In 2004 the estrogen-only HRT trial was stopped by the National Institutes of Health (NIH) because of an increased risk of stroke among the women taking estrogen. For these reasons, HRT is no longer recommended for prevention of atherosclerotic cardiovascular disease.[27] Data from the Framingham Heart Study indicate the lifetime risk for cardiovascular disease is more than one in two for women at age 40.[1]

Cardiovascular disease kills more than one-half million women annually in the United States. To emphasize the magnitude of the problem, this represents more deaths than the next seven fatal diseases for women combined.[28] Mortality rates for women after an acute MI are higher than for men: 38% and 25%, respectively. Risk factors more strongly associated with acute MI in women compared to men include

TABLE 12-3	FASTING BLOOD GLUCOSE AND RISK FOR CORONARY ARTERY DISEASE	
BLOOD GLUCOSE LEVEL	**FASTING PLASMA GLUCOSE LEVEL* (mg/dL)**
Normal	70-100
Prediabetic	100-125
Diabetic	126 or higher

CAD, coronary artery disease.
*Values greater than normal increase the risk for CAD and kidney failure.

hypertension, diabetes mellitus, alcohol intake, and physical inactivity.[26] Many reasons contribute to women having higher mortality from acute MI, including waiting longer to seek medical care, having smaller coronary arteries, being older when symptoms occur, and experiencing very different symptoms from those of men of the same age.[29] The 2007 evidence-based guidelines for cardiovascular disease prevention in women recommended a plan for a general approach to the female patient that classifies her as high risk, at risk, or at optimal risk.[28] In 2007 50% of women surveyed by the American Heart Association (AHA) recognized that heart disease was the leading cause of death among women.

Vascular Inflammation

The link between vascular inflammation and atherosclerotic disease is well established.[31] Measurement of this link has been more controversial, however.[30] Many researchers think the development of atherosclerotic plaque occurs in response to inflammation. Noxious inflammatory agents circulate in the bloodstream and stimulate chemical mediators that directly modify the arterial wall. The initial inflammatory stimuli include increased blood glucose, elevated blood lipids, nicotine, and hypertension. However, other clinical conditions, such as connective tissue disorders and systemic infection, also produce an inflammatory state, and it is not clear what the impact of inflammation produced by these stimuli is on the vessels.[30] Research to identify prognostic inflammatory markers is ongoing.

C-Reactive Protein

The inflammatory marker most frequently cited is C-reactive protein (CRP). It is measured as high-sensitivity C-reactive protein (hs-CRP).[30] The higher the hs-CRP value, the greater the risk of a coronary event, especially if all other potential causes of systemic inflammation such as infection can be ruled out. If other systemic inflammatory conditions such as bronchitis or a urinary tract infection are present, the hs-CRP test loses all predictive value.[31] CRP and other inflammatory markers are used to estimate the probability of future acute coronary events.[30,31] During acute coronary syndrome events, there is widespread activation of neutrophils in the cardiac circulation (measured from the coronary sinus), which suggests that inflammation is not limited to one unstable plaque.[32] Debate continues about whether CRP is simply a marker of vascular inflammation or also contributes to the proinflammatory state.[9]

Multifactorial Risk and Risk Equivalents

CAD has multifactorial causation; the greater the number of risk factors, the greater the risk of developing CAD.[1,3,24,33] The best time for an individual to make lifestyle changes is before symptoms of CAD occur. Patients with two or more risk factors or with one or more of the CAD risk-equivalent diseases have the greatest potential to benefit from risk-factor reduction and lifestyle change.[3]

Certain medical conditions are considered risk equivalents of CAD. A risk equivalent means the person has the same risk of having an acute MI as if they had coronary heart disease already. Two noncardiac medical conditions are considered risk equivalents for CAD: diabetes mellitus and chronic kidney disease. Peripheral arterial disease and cerebral vascular disease are atherosclerotic conditions that are also considered CAD risk equivalents.

Primary Versus Secondary Prevention of Coronary Artery Disease

If a person has symptoms of CAD or has previously had an acute coronary syndrome event, the goal of any lifestyle change or medication is called secondary prevention, or preventing another heart attack. If an individual matches the risk profile described previously but does not have symptoms of CAD or has not had an acute MI, the treatment plan is described as primary prevention. The constellation of cardiac risk factors is well established and can predict development of CAD for most populations in the developed industrial world.

Pathophysiology of Coronary Artery Disease

Coronary heart disease is a progressive atherosclerotic disorder of the coronary arteries that results in narrowing or complete occlusion. Atherosclerosis affects the medium-size arteries that perfuse the heart and other major organs. Normal arterial walls are composed of three layers: the intima (inner lining), the media (middle muscular layer), and the adventitia (outer coat).

Development of Atherosclerosis

Atherosclerosis is a chronic inflammatory disorder that is characterized by an accumulation of macrophages and T lymphocytes in the arterial intimal wall. A high LDL cholesterol concentration is one of the triggers of vascular inflammation. The inflammation injures the wall, allowing the LDL cholesterol to move into the vessel wall below the endothelial surface.[9] Blood monocytes adhere to endothelial cells and migrate into the vessel wall. Within the artery wall, some monocytes differentiate into macrophages that unite with and then internalize LDL cholesterol. The foam cells that result are the marker cells of atherosclerosis.[9]

Elevated LDL cholesterol levels promote low-level endothelial inflammation that allows lipoproteins to infiltrate the intimal vessel wall. After it has infiltrated under the endothelium, LDL cholesterol tends to stay within the vessel wall rather than return to the circulation.[9] This contrasts with the actions of HDL cholesterol, which enters the vessel wall, helps efflux cholesterol from cells, and then returns to the circulation.[9] The actions of HDL cholesterol may help minimize the number of foam cells in the artery wall.[9]

Atherosclerotic Plaque Rupture

When a mature atherosclerotic plaque develops, it is not uniform in composition. It has a lipid liquid center filled with procoagulant factors. A connective tissue fibrous cap covers the top of the fluid lipid center.[30-32] The abrupt rupture of this cap allows procoagulant lipids to flood into the vessel lumen and rapidly form a coronary thrombosis, as shown in Table 12-4. As the enlarging clot blocks blood flow through the coronary artery, a "heart attack" will occur unless there is adequate collateral circulation from other coronary vessels. Symptoms and suggested cardiac interventions at appropriate stages in development of CAD are listed in Table 12-4.

Plaques that are likely to rupture are saturated with macrophages and other inflammatory cells. These vulnerable plaques are usually not obstructive and are situated at bends or branch points in the arterial tree.[3] It is not known what factors cause the fibrous cap to rupture or erode. As deep fissures in the cap expose the procoagulant factors to the blood plasma, an unstoppable cycle is put into motion. When platelets in the bloodstream are exposed to collagen, necrotic debris, von Willebrand factor, and thromboxane, a clot is formed that can occlude the coronary artery. Highly fibrotic plaques do not rupture. The type of atherosclerotic

---

TABLE 12-4 TIMELINE OF ATHEROGENESIS DEVELOPMENT DEPICTED BY LONGITUDINAL SECTION OF AN ARTERY

ATHEROGENESIS/THROMBOGENESIS	ASSOCIATED SYMPTOMS	CARDIAC INTERVENTION
A. Normal artery, normal vessel wall.	No symptoms	Primary prevention of CAD recommended: consume a low-fat diet, take regular physical exercise, avoid smoking, and achieve normal BMI
B. Lipids in bloodstream.	No symptoms	
C. Extracellular lipid accumulates in the intima of the artery (atheroma).	No symptoms	
D. Lipid accumulation evolves to become a fatty-fibrous (atherosclerotic) lesion. Some lesions contain a lipid interior covered by a fibrous cap.	Chest pain with exercise that is relieved by rest or NTG (stable angina) or possibly no symptoms until the lesion fills more than 75% of the vessel lumen	PCI if stable angina is present and CAD is diagnosed by cardiac catheterization
E. Rupture of the cap allows lipid in the center to be released into the bloodstream, stimulating clot formation (thrombogenesis).	Chest pain not relieved by rest or NTG (ACS – unstable angina)	Call 911 for immediate transport to a hospital, preferably one with experience treating ACS
F. Fresh clot blocks the vessel; spasm of the artery may occur near the thrombus.	Chest pain unrelieved by rest or NTG – severity, location of angina, and associated symptoms vary greatly among individuals (ACS – acute MI)	Emergency intervention to open the artery: fibrinolytic or catheter-based procedure (PCI)
G. Vessel is open, but the atherosclerotic lesion remains.	No symptoms	Secondary prevention of CAD to prevent repeat MI; beta-blockers to prevent arrhythmias; ACE-1 drugs to prevent ventricular remodeling and heart failure; elective PCI

ACE-1, angiotensin-converting enzyme 1; *ACS*, acute coronary syndrome; *BMI*, body mass index; *CAD*, coronary artery disease; *MI*, myocardial infarction; *NTG*, nitroglycerin; *PCI*, percutaneous coronary intervention.
(Modified from Antman EM, et al: ACC/AHA guidelines for the management of patients with ST-elevation myocardial infarction – executive summary, *Circulation* 110(5):588, 2004.)

plaque that is prone to rupture has a weak fibrous cap and a large amount of liquid cholesterol within the core (see Table 12-4).[32]

Plaque Regression

A reduction in blood cholesterol decreases atherosclerotic plaque size by decreasing the amount of liquid cholesterol within the plaque core.[7] Lowering cholesterol levels does not change the dimensions of the fibrous or calcified portions of the plaque. However, lower cholesterol levels reduce vascular inflammation and make vulnerable plaque less likely to rupture.

If diet is not effective in lowering blood cholesterol, lipid-lowering drugs are prescribed to lower the LDL cholesterol level below 100 mg/dL for patients at risk for CAD and to aim for an LDL level below 70 mg/dL for individuals with the highest-risk profile.[7] Drugs, diet, and exercise are used to lower the triglyceride levels to less than 150 mg/dL, and to raise HDL cholesterol levels above 40 mg/dL for men and above 50 mg/dL for women (see Table 12-1).[3,7,8,33]

Acute Coronary Syndromes

The term acute coronary syndrome (ACS) is used to describe the array of clinical presentations of CAD that range from unstable angina to acute MI (see Table 12-4).[1,3,5] The general public and media describe an acute MI as a "heart attack."

The following section discusses stable manifestations of CAD (stable angina) and acute manifestations described as an acute coronary syndrome (unstable angina and acute MI).

Angina

Angina pectoris, or chest pain, caused by myocardial ischemia is not a separate disease, but rather a symptom of CAD. It is caused by a blockage or spasm of a coronary artery, leading to diminished myocardial blood supply. The lack of oxygen causes myocardial ischemia, which is felt as chest discomfort, pressure, or pain. Angina may occur anywhere in the chest, neck, arms, or back, but the most commonly described location is pain or pressure behind the sternum. The pain often radiates to the left arm but can also radiate down both arms and to the back, the shoulder, the jaw, or the neck (Figure 12-1). Angina symptoms are not the same for all individuals, many patients may describe pressure or discomfort rather than pain and presenting symptoms can be highly individualized, as described in Box 12-3. Patients and families must be taught that angina does not always present in the dramatic heart attack scenario seen on television and in movies, in which the person clutches the throat or chest and exhibits extreme distress.[3]

Women and Angina. Many women experience a variety of different symptoms before an acute MI and during the acute event, as shown in Box 12-4.[34] The recognition and publicity

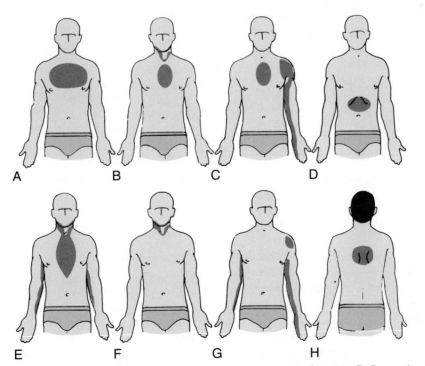

FIGURE 12-1 Common Sites for Anginal Pain. *A,* Upper part of chest. *B,* Beneath sternum, radiating to neck and jaw. *C,* Beneath sternum, radiating down left arm. *D,* Epigastric. *E,* Epigastric, radiating to neck, jaw, and arms. *F,* Neck and jaw. *G,* Left shoulder. *H,* Intrascapular.

BOX 12-3   CHARACTERISTICS OF ANGINA PECTORIS

Location
- Beneath sternum, radiating to neck and jaw
- Upper chest
- Beneath sternum, radiating down left arm
- Epigastric
- Epigastric, radiating to neck, jaw, and arms
- Neck and jaw
- Left shoulder, inner aspect of both arms
- Intrascapular

Duration
- Less than 5 minutes
- Less than 5 minutes (stable)
- Longer than 5 minutes or worsening symptoms without relief from rest or sublingual nitroglycerin indicates preinfarction symptoms (unstable)

Quality
- Sensation of pressure or heavy weight on the chest
- Feeling of tightness, like a vise
- Visceral quality (deep, heavy, squeezing, aching)

- Burning sensation
- Shortness of breath, with feeling of suffocation
- Most severe pain ever experienced

Radiation
- Medial aspect of left arm
- Jaw
- Left shoulder
- Right arm

Precipitating Factors
- Exertion/exercise
- Cold weather
- Exercising after a large, heavy meal
- Walking against the wind
- Emotional upset
- Fright, anger
- Coitus

Medication Relief
- Usually within 45 seconds to 5 minutes after sublingual nitroglycerin administration

BOX 12-4   CARDIOVASCULAR SYMPTOMS EXPERIENCED BY WOMEN BEFORE ACUTE MYOCARDIAL INFARCTION

SYMPTOMS 1 MONTH BEFORE ACUTE MI	SYMPTOMS DURING ACUTE MI
• Unusual fatigue (71%)	• Shortness of breath (58%)
• Sleep disturbance (48%)	• Weakness (55%)
• Shortness of breath (42%)	• Unusual fatigue (43%)
• Indigestion (39%)	• Cold sweat (39%)
• Anxiety (36%)	• Dizziness (39%)
• Heart racing (27%)	• Nausea (36%)
• Arms weak/heavy (25%)	• Arm heaviness or weakness (35%)
• Changes in thinking or memory (24%)	• Ache in arms (32%)
• Vision change (23%)	• Heat or flushing (32%)
• Loss of appetite (22%)	• Indigestion (31%)
• Hands or arms tingling (22%)	• Pain centered high in chest (31%)
• Difficulty breathing at night (19%)	• Heart racing (23%)

MI, myocardial infarction.
From McSweeney JC, et al: Women's early warning symptoms of acute myocardial infarction, *Circulation* 108(21):2619, 2003.

about the fact that many women do not experience "crushing chest pain" is important if women's symptoms are not to be trivialized by clinicians.[35] It is important that all patients are made aware of angina symptom equivalents, such as unexpected shortness of breath, breaking out in a cold sweat, or sudden fatigue, nausea, or lightheadedness.[3] More women die every year in the United States of cardiovascular disease than men, a fact that is largely unknown.[28]

Stable Angina. Stable angina is predictable and caused by similar precipitating factors each time; typically, it is exercise induced. Patients become used to the pattern of this type of angina and may describe it as "my usual chest pain." Pain control should be achieved within 5 minutes by rest and by taking sublingual nitroglycerin. Stable angina is the result of fixed lesions (blockages) of more than 75% of the coronary artery lumen. Ischemia and chest pain occur when myocardial demand from exertion exceeds the fixed blood oxygen supply.[6] Additional information on CAD and stable angina is provided in the box Evidence-Based Collaborative Practice: Coronary Artery Disease and Stable Angina.

EVIDENCE-BASED COLLABORATIVE PRACTICE
Coronary Artery Disease and Stable Angina

Summary of Evidence-Based Recommendations for Management of Coronary Artery Disease and Stable Angina

Strong evidence exists that the following lifestyle interventions help to prevent CAD:

- Diet
  - Diet low in salt and high in fiber, fruit, vegetables, and grains.
  - All dietary fat less than 30% of total calories; saturated fat less than 7%.
  - Multivitamin if homocysteine level is elevated.
  - Limit sugary foods.
  - Limit calories if overweight.
  - Omega-3 fatty acids included in diet.
- Exercise
  - Start by walking more often and increase physical exercise from there.
  - Refer to cardiac rehabilitation program.
- Obesity
  - Achieve healthy body weight.
- Addiction
  - Stop cigarette smoking.
  - Avoid exposure to environmental (second-hand) tobacco smoke at home and at work.
  - Limit alcohol intake.

Strong evidence exists that the following diagnostic procedures help the patient with angina:

- When a patient presents with chest pain, quickly obtaining a detailed history of symptoms, focused physical examination, and risk factor assessment can help determine whether the probability of CAD is low, intermediate, or high.
- Initial laboratory tests include hemoglobin, fasting blood glucose, lipid panel.
- Obtain a baseline 12-lead ECG at rest, even if chest pain is not present.
- Obtain a 12-lead ECG during an episode of chest pain.
- Obtain a chest radiograph if symptoms of heart failure are present.
- Obtain an exercise 12-lead ECG if the condition is stable and symptoms suggest CAD or if the condition is stable with complete LBBB or RBBB that makes the ECG difficult to interpret for ischemia.
- Obtain cardiac echocardiography for patients with a systolic murmur suggestive of aortic stenosis.
- Use cardiac echocardiography to determine extent of LV hypertrophy or dysfunction.
- Stress cardiac echocardiography is recommended for patients with greater than 1 mm of ST-segment depression at rest (stress may be by physical exercise or by pharmacological stimulation).
- Coronary angiography (typically as part of a cardiac catheterization procedure) is recommended for patients at high risk for adverse coronary events.

Initial Pharmacological and Lifestyle Treatment Recommendations

- The goal of treatment is to eliminate chest pain.
- The 10 most important elements of CAD and stable angina management can be remembered using the A to E mnemonic:

  A – Aspirin and antianginal drugs: Prescribe daily, low-dose (75 to 325 mg) aspirin; oral nitrates; and sublingual nitroglycerin for episodes of angina.

  B – Beta-blockers and blood pressure: Use ACEI and beta-blockers to decrease blood pressure to less than 140/90 mm Hg if no other CAD risk factors are present and to less than 130/80 mm Hg if diabetes or kidney disease are present.

  C – Cholesterol and cigarettes: Obtain a fasting lipid profile. Recommend diet or lipid-reduction drug therapy (statin) to lower LDL-C to less than 100 mg/dL (<70 mg/dL if achievable), increase HDL-C to more than 40 mg/dL for men or more than 50 mg/dL for women, and reduce triglycerides to less than 150 mg/dL. Recommend adding plant stanols or sterols (2 g/day) or viscous fiber (>10 g/day), or both, to the diet to further lower LDL-C; add dietary omega-3 fatty acids in the form of fish or capsule (1 g/day). Always ask about tobacco use; strongly recommend smoking cessation; encourage nicotine replacement therapy (nicotine patches or gum) as needed.

  D – Diet and diabetes: Prescribe a low-fat, calorie-appropriate diet and provide nutritional consultation as needed to achieve a fasting blood glucose level of 70 to 100 mg/dL and HbA_{1c} of less than 7%.

  E – Education and exercise: Provide education about risk factor modification and the CAD disease process; recommend daily exercise for 30 to 60 minutes (ideal) or at least seven times each week (minimum of 5 days per week). Achieve a BMI between 18.5 and 24.9 kg/m^2 and waist less than 40 inches for men or less than 35 inches for women. Treat depression if present. HRT is not recommended as a treatment for symptoms of coronary heart disease. Influenza vaccination is recommended.

Interventional and Surgical Recommendations for Stable High-Risk Patients

Patients are risk stratified according to their symptoms and the results of cardiac diagnostic tests.

- Percutaneous catheter interventions (PCI)
  - Angioplasty, atherectomy, stent
  - PCI is more frequently performed than open heart surgery for relief of anginal symptoms.
- Coronary artery bypass surgery (CABG)
  - For patients with left main occlusion or multivessel disease
  - For patients with two-vessel disease who have significant proximal LAD stenosis and an LV ejection fraction less than 50%

Data from Gibbons RJ, et al: ACC/AHA 2002 guideline update for the management of patients with chronic stable angina – summary article, *Circulation* 107(1):149, 2003; Fraker TD, et al: 2007 Chronic angina focused update of the ACC/AHA 2002 guidelines for the management of patients with chronic stable angina, *J Am Coll Cardio* 50(23):2264, 2007; Mosca L, et al. Evidence-based guidelines for cardiovascular disease prevention in women: 2007 update, *Circulation* 115(11):1481, 2007.
ACEI, angiotensin-converting enzyme inhibitors; *BMI,* body mass index; *CAD,* coronary artery disease; *ECG,* electrocardiogram; *HbA₁c,* glycosylated hemoglobin; *HDL-C,* high-density lipoprotein cholesterol; *HRT,* hormone replacement therapy; *LAD,* left anterior descending coronary artery; *LBBB,* left bundle branch block; *LDL-C,* low-density lipoprotein cholesterol; *LV,* left ventricle; *RBBB,* right bundle branch block.

Unstable Angina. Unstable angina is defined as a change in a previously established stable pattern of angina. It is part of the continuum of ACS. Unstable angina usually is more intense than stable angina, may awaken the person from sleep, or may necessitate more than nitrates for pain relief. A change in the level or frequency of symptoms requires immediate medical evaluation. Severe angina that persists for more than 5 minutes, is worsening in intensity, and is not relieved by one nitroglycerin tablet is a medical emergency, and the patient or a family member must call 911 immediately.[3] The 911 (Emergency Medical Services [EMS]) system is available to 90% of the population of the United States.[3] In one study, patients with an acute MI who used 911 and were transported to the hospital by ambulance had significantly faster receipt of initial reperfusion therapies.[36,37] Family and friends are discouraged from driving a person experiencing unstable angina to the hospital and instead are encouraged to call 911. Patients should be instructed never to drive themselves but to contact the EMS by calling 911.

Unstable angina is an indication of atherosclerotic plaque instability. It can signal atherosclerotic plaque rupture and thrombus formation that can lead to MI. The patient who comes to the emergency department with recent onset of unstable angina but who has nonspecific or nonelevated ST-segment changes on the 12-lead electrocardiogram (ECG) may be admitted to the critical care unit to rule out MI. If the symptoms are typical of MI, it is important to treat the patient according to the latest published guidelines, because not all patients who experience an MI have ST-segment elevation on the 12-lead ECG.[5]

Medical Management

Accurate assessment of chest pain symptoms is essential if unstable angina is to be recognized and treated effectively. An important reason to ask questions about the chest pain is to differentiate between stable and unstable angina. The change from stable to unstable angina is potentially life threatening for the patient. If the ST segments are elevated or there is a newly documented left bundle branch block on the 12-lead ECG, the patient will be treated for acute MI.[3] However, if these classic ECG signs are missing and the chest pain continues, the current pharmacological treatments of choice are aspirin, vasodilation by nitroglycerin, intravenous antiplatelet agents such as the glycoprotein (GP) IIb/IIIa inhibitors, and intravenous unfractionated heparin (UFH).[5] Low-molecular-weight heparin (LMWH) combined with fibrinolysis is an alternative to heparin fibrinolysis for patients younger than 75 years with a serum creatinine level below 2.5 mg/dL for men and below 2 mg/dL for women.[3]

Another option is to transport the patient directly to the cardiac catheterization laboratory for direct visualization of the coronary arteries by the cardiologist. Recanalization of the coronary arteries is recommended, provided the institution performs more than 200 procedures annually or the individual physician performs more than 75 interventional procedures annually.[3,5]

Nursing Management

Nursing management of the patient with CAD and angina incorporates a variety of nursing diagnoses (Nursing Diagnosis Priorities box on Coronary Artery Disease and Angina). **Nursing priorities focus on (1) recognizing myocardial ischemia, (2) controlling chest pain, (3) maintaining a calm environment, and (4) providing patient education.**

NURSING DIAGNOSIS PRIORITIES
Coronary Artery Disease and Angina

- Acute Pain related to transmission and perception of cutaneous, visceral, muscular, or ischemic impulses, p. A-5
- Ineffective Cardiopulmonary Tissue Perfusion related to decreased myocardial oxygen supply or increased myocardial oxygen demand, or both, p. A-28
- Activity Intolerance related to cardiopulmonary dysfunction, p. A-1
- Powerlessness related to lack of control over current situation, p. A-33
- Anxiety related to threat to biological, psychological, or social integrity, p. A-7
- Deficient Knowledge: Discharge Regimen related to lack of previous exposure to information, p. A-15

Recognizing Myocardial Ischemia

Complaints of chest discomfort (angina) must be evaluated quickly, because angina is an indicator of myocardial ischemia. The patient is asked to rate the intensity of the chest discomfort on a scale of 0 to 10. Pain levels must be assessed with sensitivity to differences in cultural manifestations of pain. The words "chest pain" are not to be used exclusively, because some patients describe their angina as "pressure" or "heaviness." It is important to document the characteristics of the pain and the patient's heart rate and rhythm, blood pressure, respirations, temperature, skin color, peripheral pulses, urine output, mentation, and overall tissue perfusion. A 12-lead ECG is used to identify the area of ischemic myocardium. The major concern is that the chest pain may represent preinfarction angina, and early identification is essential so that the patient can be immediately treated. A range of treatments are available that include fibrinolytic infusion immediately, or transfer to the cardiac catheterization laboratory for a coronary arteriogram and opening of a blocked artery. If the hospital does not have a cardiac catheterization laboratory, GP IIb/IIIa receptor blockers may be infused to prevent the evolution of the acute MI before transfer.[3,5] Figure 12-2 presents additional information about transfer between hospitals in this circumstance.

Relieving Chest Pain

In the critical care unit, control of angina is achieved by a combination of supplemental oxygen, nitrates, analgesia, and surveillance of the angina and of the effects of pharmacological therapy.

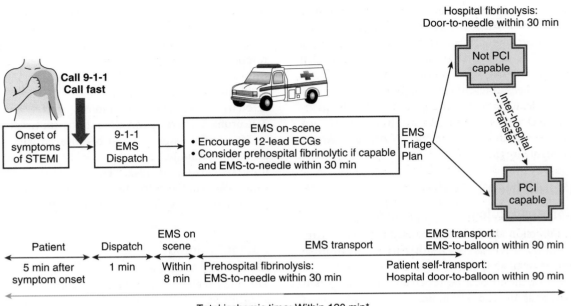

FIGURE 12-2 Evaluation of Prehospital Chest Pain, ACS and Treatment Options. *STEMI,* ST elevation myocardial infarction; *EMS,* emergency medical services; *PCI,* percutaneous catheter intervention. (Illustration modified from Antman EM, et al: ACC/AHA guidelines for the management of patients with ST-elevation myocardial infarction – executive summary: a report of the American College of Cardiology/American Heart Association Task Force on Practice Guidelines (Writing Committee to Revise the 1999 Guidelines for the Management of Patients with Acute Myocardial Infarction), *Circulation* 110(9):e82).

- *Oxygen:* All patients with acute ischemic pain are administered supplemental oxygen to increase myocardial oxygenation. Use of pulse oximetry is recommended to guide therapy and maintain oxygen saturation above 90%.[3] Patients who develop symptoms of acute heart failure may require emergency intubation and mechanical ventilation to correct significant hypoxemia.[3,5]

- *Nitrates:* A combination of intravenous and sublingual nitroglycerin is used to vasodilate the coronary arteries and decrease pain. After nitrate administration, the critical care nurse closely observes the patient for relief of chest pain, for return of the ST segment to baseline, and for the potential development of unwanted side effects such as hypotension and headache. Administration of a nitrate is avoided if the SBP is below 90 mm Hg. Drug interactions with nitrates are another potential cause for concern. The phosphodiesterase inhibitor medication sidenafil (Viagra) is prescribed for several conditions including pulmonary hypertension and erectile dysfunction. Sidenafil and nitrates in combination may contribute to a precipitous fall in blood pressure.[3,5]

- *Analgesia:* Morphine (2 to 4 mg given intravenously) is the analgesic opiate of choice for preinfarction angina. It relieves pain and decreases fear and anxiety. After administration, the critical care nurse assesses the patient for pain relief and the development of unwanted side effects such as hypotension and respiratory depression.[3,5]

- *Aspirin:* Chewing an oral nonenteric-coated aspirin (162 to 325 mg) at the beginning of chest pain has been shown to reduce mortality. The nonenteric formulation is preferred because it increases absorption in the mouth when chewed, not swallowed.[3,5]

Maintaining a Calm Environment

Patients admitted to a critical care unit with unstable angina experience extreme anxiety and fear of death. The critical care nurse is faced with the challenge of ensuring that the elements of a calm environment that can alleviate the patient's fear and anxiety are maintained, while being ready at all times to respond to an acute emergency, such as a cardiac arrest, or to assist with emergency intubation or insertion of hemodynamic monitoring catheters.

Providing Patient Education

In the critical care unit, the patient's ability to retain educational information is severely affected by stress and pain. Initial patient education stresses the importance of alerting the nurse to any symptoms of chest pain or discomfort, and avoiding the Valsalva maneuver, which is defined as forced expiration against a closed glottis. This can be explained to the patient as "bearing down" when going to the bathroom or breath-holding when repositioning in bed. The Valsalva maneuver causes an increase in intrathoracic pressure that decreases venous return to the right side of the heart and is associated with low blood pressure and symptomatic bradycardia.

After the anginal pain is controlled, longer-term patient and family education can begin. Points to cover include risk factor modification, signs and symptoms of angina, when to call the physician, medications, and dealing with emotions and stress. However, because the acute hospital length of stay for uncomplicated angina is usually less than three days, referral to a cardiac rehabilitation program for a controlled exercise program and risk-factor modification after discharge may be the most helpful teaching intervention a critical care nurse can provide. Clinical practice guidelines for the management of CAD and stable angina are listed in the box Evidence-Based Collaborative Practice: Coronary Artery Disease and Stable Angina.

MYOCARDIAL INFARCTION

Description and Etiology

Myocardial infarction (MI) is the term used to describe irreversible myocardial necrosis (cell death) that results from an abrupt decrease or total cessation of coronary blood flow to a specific area of the myocardium.[1] In the hospital, this is often referred to as an acute MI, indicating the sudden onset and the life-threatening nature of the event. Increasingly, an acute MI is described in relation to whether there was ST-segment elevation on the diagnostic 12-lead ECG. It may be labeled an acute non-ST-segment elevation MI (NSTEMI)[5] or an acute ST-segment elevation MI (STEMI).[3]

Three mechanisms can block the coronary artery and are responsible for the acute reduction in oxygen delivery to the myocardium:

1. Plaque rupture
2. New coronary artery thrombosis
3. Coronary artery spasm close to the ruptured plaque

Myocardial tissue can best be salvaged within the first 2 hours (120 minutes) after the onset of anginal symptoms, as illustrated in Figure 12-2.[3] The earlier the myocardium is revascularized, the better the survival.[5] Unfortunately, many persons do not seek treatment until the acute phase has passed.[3]

Pathophysiology

Myocardial Ischemia

The outer region of the infarcted myocardial area is the *zone of ischemia*, as illustrated in Figure 12-3. It is composed of viable cells. Priority interventions are targeted to save this viable muscle. Repolarization in this zone is temporarily impaired but eventually will be restored to normal. Electrical

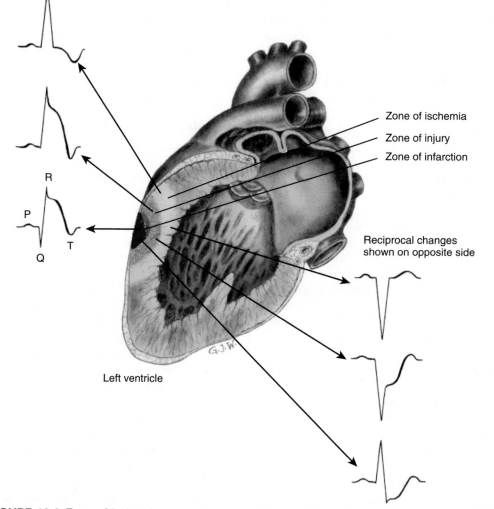

FIGURE 12-3 Zone of ischemia, zone of injury, and zone of infarction are shown through ECG waveforms and reciprocal waveforms corresponding to each zone.

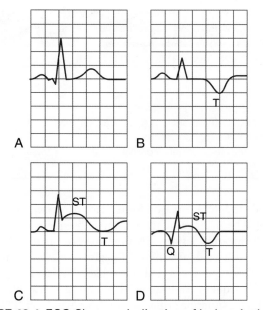

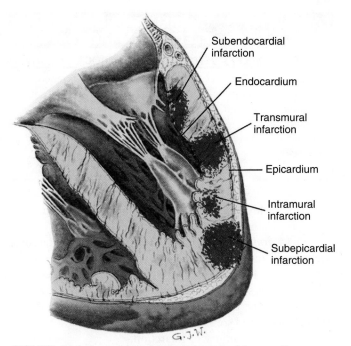

FIGURE 12-4 ECG Changes Indicative of Ischemia, Injury, and Infarction (Necrosis) of the Myocardium. *A,* Normal ECG. *B,* Ischemia indicated by inversion of the T wave. *C,* Ischemia and current of injury indicated by T-wave inversion and ST-segment elevation. The ST segment may be elevated above or depressed below the baseline, depending on whether the tracing is from a lead facing toward or away from the infarcted area and depending on whether epicardial or endocardial injury occurs. Epicardial injury causes ST-segment elevation in leads facing the epicardium. *D,* Ischemia, injury, and myocardial necrosis. The Q wave indicates necrosis of the myocardium.

FIGURE 12-5 Location of Infarctions in Myocardium.

conduction from areas of viable myocardium produces a normal QRS configuration as shown in Figure 12-4, *A.* Repolarization of ischemic myocardial cells manifests as T-wave inversion (see Figure 12-4, *B*).

Myocardial Injury

The infarcted zone is surrounded by injured but still potentially viable tissue in an area known as the zone of injury (see Figure 12-3). Cells in this area do not fully repolarize because of the deficient blood supply. This is recorded on the ECG as elevation of the ST segment (see Figure 12-4, *C*).

Myocardial Infarction

The area of dead muscle (necrosis) in the myocardium is known as the zone of infarction (see Figure 12-3). On the ECG, evidence of this zone is seen by new pathological Q waves, which reflect a lack of depolarization from the cardiac surface involved in the MI (see Figure 12-4, *D*). As healing takes place, the cells in this area are replaced by scar tissue.

MIs are classified according to the location on the myocardial surface and the muscle layers affected. Not all infarctions cause necrosis in all layers, as shown in Figure 12-5. A transmural MI involves all three cardiac layers—the endocardium, the myocardium, and the epicardium. A transmural (full-thickness) MI usually provokes significant ECG changes (see Figure 12-4). This is also described as a Q-wave MI. Not every

acute MI produces a recognizable series of Q waves on the 12-lead ECG. Some patients who had a demonstrated Q wave on a 12-lead ECG as a result of an acute MI lose the Q wave months or years later. The reasons for this are unknown, but it may represent the development of collateral circulation.

12-Lead Electrocardiographic Changes. The ECG changes produced by a transmural infarction demonstrate alteration in myocardial depolarization (QRS complex) and repolarization (ST segment). The changes in repolarization are seen by the presence of new Q waves. These new, pathological Q waves are deeper and wider than tiny Q waves found on the normal 12-lead ECG.[3]

Myocardial Infarction Location

The location of infarction is determined by correlating the ECG leads with Q waves and the ST-segment T-wave abnormalities (Table 12-5). Infarction most commonly affects the left ventricle and the interventricular septum; however, the right ventricle can be infarcted, and many patients who sustain an inferior MI have some right ventricular damage. The ECG manifestations that are used to diagnose an MI and pinpoint the area of damaged ventricle include inverted T waves, ST-segment elevation, and pathological Q waves in specific lead groupings as described subsequently.

Anterior Wall Infarction. Anterior wall infarction results from occlusion of the proximal left anterior descending artery (see Table 12-5). ST-segment elevation is expected in leads V_1 through V_4 on the 12-lead ECG, as shown in Figure 12-6. If the left main coronary artery is occluded, the ECG manifestations will involve almost all of the precordial leads V_1 through V_6 and leads I and aVL (augmented voltage left) as listed in Table 12-5. The specific groups of ECG changes that help to locate the part of the heart that is infarcting are called indicative changes. A large anterior wall MI may be

TABLE 12-5	CORRELATIONS AMONG VENTRICULAR SURFACES, ELECTROCARDIOGRAPHIC LEADS, AND CORONARY ARTERIES	
SURFACE OF LEFT VENTRICLE	**ELECTROCARDIOGRAPHIC LEADS**	**CORONARY ARTERY USUALLY INVOLVED**
Inferior	II, III, aVF	Right coronary artery
Lateral	V_5-V_6, I, aVL	Circumflex
Anterior	V_2-V_4	Left anterior descending
Anterior lateral	V_1-V_6, I, aVL	Left main coronary artery
Septal	V_1-V_2	Left anterior descending
Posterior	V_1-V_2	Circumflex or right coronary artery (reciprocal changes)
	V_7-V_9 (direct)	

associated with left ventricular pump failure, cardiogenic shock, or death.[3]

Left Lateral Wall Infarction. Left lateral wall infarction occurs as a result of occlusion of the circumflex coronary artery. On a 12-lead ECG, new Q waves and ST-segment T-wave changes are seen in leads I, aVL, V_5, and V_6 (Figure 12-7). In reality, few patients present with only lateral wall ECG changes, and some anterior wall leads (V_3 and V_4) may show evidence of injury or infarction.

Inferior Wall Infarction. Inferior wall infarction occurs with occlusion of the right coronary artery. This infarction manifests by ECG changes in leads II, III, and aVF (Figure 12-8). Conduction disturbances are expected with an inferior wall MI and are related to the anatomy of the coronary arterial supply. Because the right coronary artery perfuses the sinoatrial (SA) node in slightly more than half of the population and supplies the proximal bundle of His and atrioventricular (AV) node in more than 90% of individuals, heart block and other conduction disturbances should be anticipated. Inferior wall MI carries a mortality rate of about 6%. If the right ventricle is involved, the mortality rate increases to 25% to 30%.[3]

Right Ventricular Infarction. Right ventricular infarction occurs when there is a blockage in a proximal section of the right coronary artery. This places all of the right ventricle and the inferior wall at risk. Right ventricular ischemia can be demonstrated in up to one half of inferior wall STEMIs, although only 10% to 15% show the hemodynamic abnormalities associated with classic infarction of the right ventricle.[3] If massive infarction occurs, the patient can suffer cardiogenic shock, which carries a mortality rate of more than 50% in this population.[37,38]

Posterior Wall Infarction. Posterior wall infarction can occur because of a blockage in the right coronary artery or in the circumflex artery. This occurs because both arteries supply this section of the heart, although the right coronary artery is generally the dominant vessel. A posterior wall MI is difficult to detect but may be identified by specific leads placed in the left scapular area or by very tall R waves in leads V_1 and V_2.

Non-ST-Segment Elevation Myocardial Infarction

The 12-lead ECG is a highly useful diagnostic tool. For many years, it was considered the gold standard when diagnosing an acute MI. However, the ST segment is not elevated in every acute MI. One reason for the lack of ST-segment elevation may be that the infarction and subsequent necrosis are not full-thickness lesions. Because some of the muscle in the area can still be depolarized, ST-segment elevation may not occur. This type of MI is also less likely to develop Q waves on a subsequent 12-lead ECG after the acute phase has passed. This situation is diagnostically known as an NSTEMI.[5] This condition has previously been described by several names, including nontransmural MI, non-Q-wave MI, and subendocardial MI. Because patients who sustain an NSTEMI do have CAD, it is important that they be treated aggressively to minimize the size of the infarcted area. Without the visual clue of the ST-segment elevation on the 12-lead ECG, the patients cannot receive immediate intravenous fibrinolytic agents, but they can be appropriately managed in an interventional catheterization laboratory and receive GP IIb/IIIa inhibitor therapy, as illustrated in the timeline in Figure 12-2. The 12-lead ECG plays a vital role in identifying the treatment plan for an ACS. ST-segment elevation is helpful when present, but it would be a mistake to believe the patient is not in danger of MI if the ST segment is not elevated. In this case, the definitive diagnosis may be made in the cardiac catheterization laboratory or by elevation of specific cardiac biomarkers.

Cardiac Biomarkers During Myocardial Infarction

In the presence of damaged or necrotic myocardial muscle cells, cardiac biomarkers are released. These biomarkers are also called cardiac enzymes. To confirm the diagnosis of acute MI, the serum biomarkers creatine kinase-muscle/brain (CK-MB) and troponin I or troponin T are measured. If the coronary artery is opened by fibrinolytic therapy or a percutaneous catheter intervention (PCI), the biomarkers exhibit a more rapid rise and dramatic fall (Figure 12-9). Information on biomarkers is also shown in Table 11-14 in Chapter 11.

Complications of Acute Myocardial Infarction

Many patients experience complications occurring early or late in the postinfarction course. These complications may result from electrical dysfunction or from a cardiac contractility problem. The presence of a new murmur in a patient with an acute MI warrants special attention because it may indicate rupture of the papillary muscle. Electrical dysfunctions include bradycardia, bundle branch blocks, and various

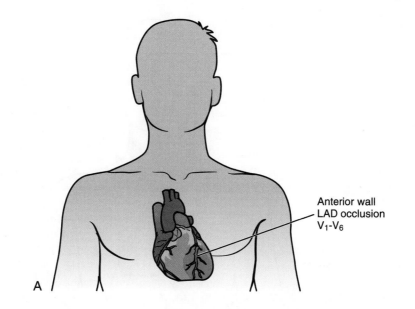

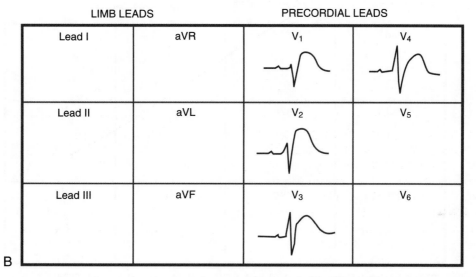

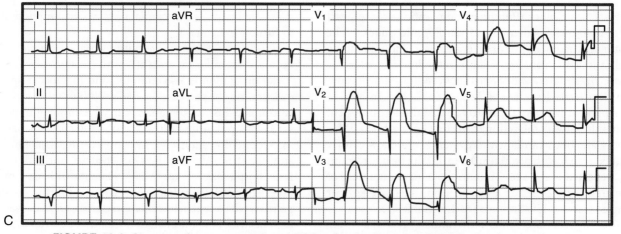

FIGURE 12-6 Changes Seen on a 12-Lead ECG with An Anterior Wall MI. *A,* Infarction location on the cardiac wall. *B,* ECG leads with expected ST-segment elevation. *C,* A 12-lead ECG from a patient experiencing left anterior wall MI. *LAD,* left anterior descending artery.

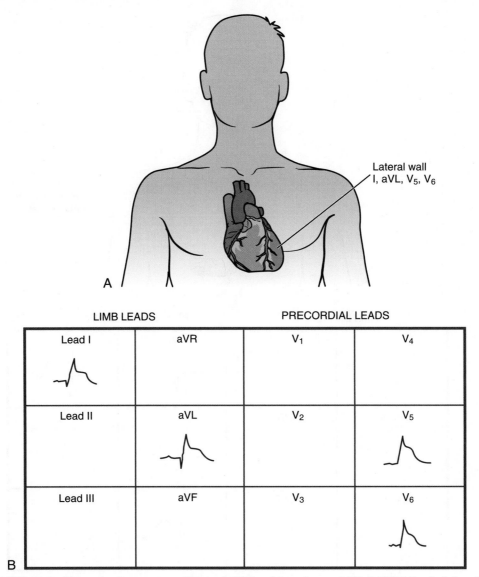

FIGURE 12-7 Changes Seen on a 12-Lead ECG with a Lateral Wall STEMI. *A,* Infarction location on the cardiac wall. *B,* ECG leads with expected ST-segment elevation.

degrees of heart block. Pumping complications cause heart failure, pulmonary edema, and cardiogenic shock.[3] The murmur can be indicative of severe damage and impending complications such as heart failure and pulmonary edema.

Sinus Bradycardia and Sinus Tachycardia. Sinus brady-cardia (heart rate less than 60 beats/min) occurs in 30% to 40% of patients who sustain an acute MI.[2] It is more prevalent with an inferior wall infarction in the first hour after STEMI.[2] Symptomatic bradycardia with hypotension and low cardiac output is treated with atropine (0.5 to 1.0 mg by intravenous push), repeated every 3 to 5 minutes to a maximum dose of 0.03 mg/kg (e.g., 2 mg for a person who weighs 70 kg) per Advanced Cardiac Life Support (ACLS) Guidelines.

Sinus Tachycardia. Sinus tachycardia (heart rate more than 100 beats/min) most often occurs with an anterior wall MI. Anterior infarctions impair left ventricular pumping ability, thereby reducing the ejection fraction and the stroke volume. In an attempt to maintain cardiac output, the heart rate increases. Sinus tachycardia must be corrected, because it greatly increases myocardial oxygen consumption, leading to further ischemia.

Atrial Dysrhythmias. Premature atrial contractions (PACs) occur frequently in patients who sustain an acute MI. Atrial fibrillation is also common and may occur spontane-ously or may be preceded by PACs. With onset of atrial fibril-lation, the loss of organized atrial contraction decreases cardiac output by up to 20%. A global registry of patients with ACS found that almost 8% have preexisting atrial fibrillation, and about 6% develop new-onset atrial fibrillation during their hospitalization for ACS.[39] Patients with new-onset or preexisting atrial fibrillation have a higher morbidity rate than patients without atrial fibrillation during an ACS event. ACS patients with new-onset atrial fibrillation experience a greater number of in-hospital adverse events such as reinfarction, shock, pulmonary edema, bleeding, and stroke.[39] Atrial fibril-lation during the hospitalization significantly affects risk of death in the setting of an acute MI; it increases in-hospital mortality by 20% and long-term mortality by 34%.[2]

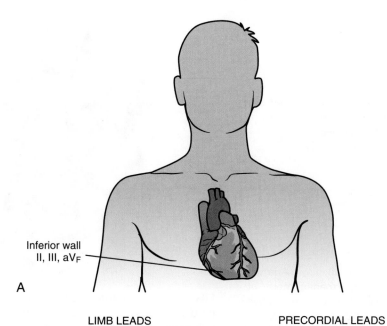

Inferior wall
II, III, aVF

A

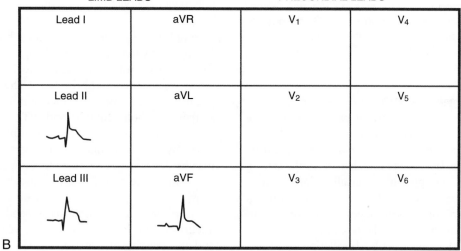

LIMB LEADS   PRECORDIAL LEADS

Lead I	aVR	V₁	V₄
Lead II	aVL	V₂	V₅
Lead III	aVF	V₃	V₆

B

Example of an Acute Inferior Wall MI

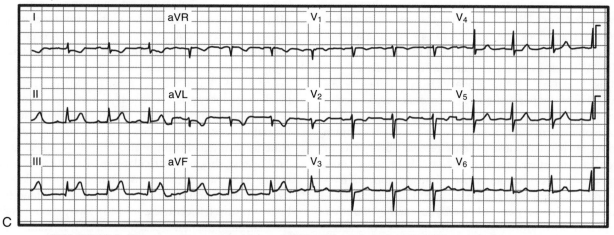

C

FIGURE 12-8 Changes Seen on a 12-Lead ECG with an Inferior Wall MI. *A,* Infarction location on cardiac wall. *B,* ECG leads with expected ST-segment elevation. *C,* A 12-lead ECG from a patient experiencing inferior wall MI.

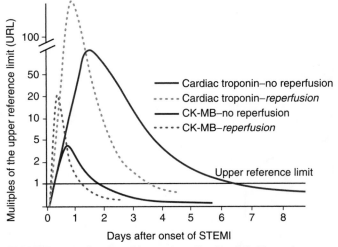

FIGURE 12-9 Cardiac Biomarkers During MI. (From Antman EM, et al: ACC/AHA guidelines for the management of patients with ST-elevation myocardial infarction – executive summary: a report of the American College of Cardiology/American Heart Association Task Force on Practice Guidelines (Writing Committee to Revise the 1999 Guidelines for the Management of Patients with Acute Myocardial Infarction), *Circulation* 110(9):e82, 2004.)

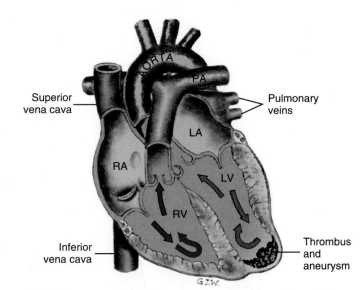

FIGURE 12-10 Ventricular Aneurysm After Acute Myocardial Infarction. *LA,* left atrium; *LV,* left ventricle; *PA,* pulmonary artery; *RA,* right atrium; *RV,* right ventricle.

Ventricular Dysrhythmias. Premature ventricular contractions (PVCs) are seen in almost all patients within the first few hours after an MI. They are initially controlled by administering oxygen to reduce myocardial hypoxia and by correcting acid-base or electrolyte imbalances. In the setting of an acute MI, PVCs are pharmacologically treated if they have the following characteristics: frequent, closely coupled (R-on-T phenomenon), multiform shapes, and occurrence in bursts of three or more, increasing the risk of sustained ventricular tachycardia (VT). Ventricular fibrillation (VF) is a life-threatening dysrhythmia associated with high mortality in acute MI. Beta-blockers are often prescribed after an acute MI to decrease mortality from ventricular dysrhythmias.[3]

Atrioventricular Heart Block During Myocardial Infarction. Heart block occurs in 6% to 14% of patients with STEMI, and those patients have increased mortality rates.[2] In STEMI, AV block most often occurs after an inferior wall infarction. Because the right coronary artery supplies the AV node in 90% of the population, right coronary artery occlusion leads to ischemia and infarction of the AV node cells. The development of sudden heart block has become much less common because most patients receive fibrinolysis or undergo PCI to open the occluded vessel. In most cases, transcutaneous pacing is the primary intervention; transvenous pacemakers are used less frequently.[2]

Ventricular Aneurysm After Myocardial Infarction. A ventricular aneurysm (Figure 12-10) is a noncontractile, thinned left ventricular wall that results from an acute transmural infarction. It most often occurs in the setting of an acute left anterior descending artery occlusion with a wide area of infarcted myocardium.[2] The most effective prevention is early reperfusion of the myocardium, accomplished by opening the thrombosed coronary artery. In one study, the rate of ventricular aneurysm was reduced from 19% in untreated patients to 7% when the coronary artery was opened by fibrinolysis.[2] The most common complications of a ventricular aneurysm are acute heart failure, systemic emboli, angina, and VT. Treatment is directed toward management of these complications and surgical repair by left ventricular aneurysmectomy. The affected area may be described as hypokinetic (contracts poorly), akinetic (noncontractile scar tissue), or dyskinetic (scar tissue that moves in the opposite direction of the normal contractile myocardium). The prognosis depends on the size of the aneurysm, the level of overall left ventricular dysfunction, and the severity of coexisting CAD.

Ventricular Septal Rupture After Myocardial Infarction. Postinfarction rupture of the ventricular septal wall is a rare but potentially lethal complication of an acute anterior wall MI (Figure 12-11). Ventricular septal rupture, also known as an acquired ventricular septal defect (VSD), is an abnormal communication between the right and left ventricle. This complication occurs in less than 1% of all MIs, and the incidence has declined because most STEMI patients have the blocked coronary artery opened.[2] Nevertheless, rupture of the ventricular septum carries an extremely high mortality rate.[40] Mortality rates between 35% and 73% are typical.[41,42] Most patients with septal rupture also have signs and symptoms of cardiogenic shock. Ventricular septal rupture manifests as severe chest pain, syncope, hypotension, and sudden hemodynamic deterioration caused by shunting of blood from the high-pressure left ventricle into the low-pressure right ventricle through the new septal opening. A holosystolic murmur (often accompanied by a thrill) can be auscultated and is best heard along the left sternal border. A diagnosis of postinfarction ventricular septal rupture can be made at the bedside with use of oxygen saturation assessment by means of a pulmonary artery catheter or by transesophageal

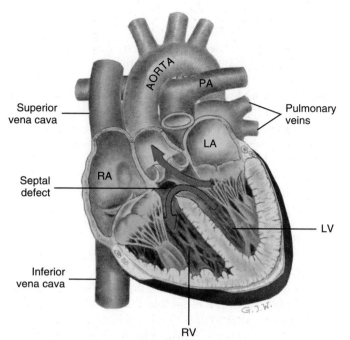

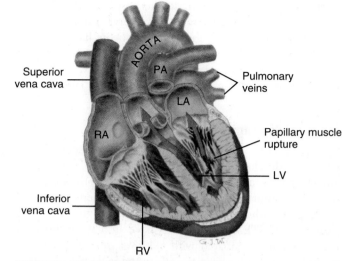

FIGURE 12-11 Ventricular Septal Rupture After Acute Myocardial Infarction. *LA,* left atrium; *LV,* left ventricle; *PA,* pulmonary artery; *RA,* right atrium; *RV,* right ventricle.

FIGURE 12-12 Papillary Muscle Rupture After Acute Myocardial Infarction. *LA,* left atrium; *LV,* left ventricle; *PA,* pulmonary artery; *RA,* right atrium; *RV,* right ventricle.

echocardiography (TEE). Rupture of the septum is a medical and surgical emergency. The patient's condition is stabilized with vasodilators and an intraaortic balloon pump (IABP) to decrease afterload.[42] The goal of afterload reduction in this patient population is to decrease the amount of blood being shunted to the right side of the heart and consequently to increase the flow of blood to the systemic circulation. If the septal rupture is very small, and the patient's condition is sufficiently stable to wait for scar tissue to form before surgical repair, survival improves. Unfortunately, when the septal opening is large, the massive left-to-right shunt across the septum makes the chances of survival dismal with or without surgery.[41,42]

Papillary Muscle Rupture After Myocardial Infarction. Papillary muscle rupture can occur when the infarct involves the area around one of the papillary muscles that support the mitral valve. Infarction of the papillary muscles results in ineffective mitral valve closure, and blood is forced back into the low-pressure left atrium during ventricular systole. The rupture may be partial or complete. Complete rupture is catastrophic and precipitates severe acute mitral regurgitation, cardiogenic shock, and high risk of death.

Partial rupture of the valve structures (Figure 12-12) also results in mitral regurgitation, but the condition can be stabilized with aggressive medical management using the IABP and vasodilators. Urgent surgical intervention is required to replace the mitral valve.[43] As with other structural complications during acute MI, the incidence is decreased in patients who have their myocardium reperfused early.[2] Of the patients with acute MI who are admitted to the critical care unit in cardiogenic shock, 10% have papillary muscle rupture with acute mitral regurgitation. The mortality rate is 71% with

medical treatment and 40% with surgical intervention to replace or repair the mitral valve.[2]

Cardiac Wall Rupture After Myocardial Infarction. Of the deaths that occur after MI, 1% to 6% can be attributed to cardiac rupture.[2] The incidence of cardiac wall rupture has two peak times. The first occurs within the first 24 hours and the second between the third and fifth postinfarction days when leukocyte scavenger cells are removing necrotic debris, thinning the myocardial wall.[2] The onset is sudden and usually catastrophic. Bleeding into the pericardial sac results in cardiac tamponade, cardiogenic shock, pulseless electrical activity (PEA), and death. Survival is rare. If rupture occurs in the hospital, emergency pericardiocentesis is required to relieve the tamponade until a surgical repair can be attempted. The best prevention is early reperfusion of the myocardium.[2]

Pericarditis After Myocardial Infarction. Pericarditis is inflammation of the pericardial sac. It can occur during a transmural MI or after an acute MI. Pericarditis may occur in 5% to 20% of transmural infarctions, but it is treated only if it is clinically significant.[44] The damaged epicardium becomes rough and inflamed and irritates the pericardium lying adjacent to it, precipitating pericarditis. Pain is the most common symptom of pericarditis, and a pericardial friction rub is the most common initial sign. The friction rub is best auscultated with a stethoscope at the sternal border and is described as a grating, scraping, or leathery scratching. Pericarditis frequently produces a pericardial effusion (fluid).[44] After the effusion occurs, the friction rub may disappear. On the 12-lead ECG, pericarditis may manifest as elevation of the ST segment in all of the typically upright leads.[45] Pericarditis is treated with nonsteroidal antiinflammatory drugs. Pericarditis that occurs as a late complication of acute MI is also known as Dressler's syndrome.[44,46]

Heart Failure and Acute Myocardial Infarction. Almost 20% of patients with acute STEMI also have acute heart failure on admission to the hospital. These patients have often waited longer to come to the hospital and are older and more likely to be female. Compared with acute MI patients without heart failure, these patients have a higher risk of adverse in-hospital events and have longer lengths of stay and higher in-hospital mortality rates.[47] More detailed information about heart failure is presented later in this chapter.

Medical Management

Quality-outcomes research shows that compliance with the guidelines developed by the American College of Cardiology and the American Heart Association (ACC/AHA) decreases in-hospital mortality after acute MI.[48,49] Patients admitted to hospitals who adhere to the AHA/ACC guidelines for treatment of STEMI or NSTEMI have an 8.3% in-hospital mortality rate, compared with a 15.3% mortality rate for patients managed at hospitals where the most recent guidelines are not fully used.[48,49] The guidelines are research-based and are designed to improve the outcome of patients admitted to the hospital with an acute MI. Clinical guidelines address the issues of interventions to open the coronary artery, anticoagulation, prevention of dysrhythmias, tight glucose control, and prevention of ventricular remodeling after STEMI.[3]

Recanalization of the Coronary Artery

The essential immediate interventions are fibrinolytic therapy or PCI to open the occluded artery for the patient with an acute STEMI.[2] All clinical guidelines emphasize the need for patients with symptoms of ACS to be rapidly triaged and treated.[2]

Anticoagulation

In the acute phase after STEMI, heparin is administered in combination with fibrinolytic therapy to recanalize (open) the coronary artery.[2] For patients who will receive fibrinolytic therapy, an initial heparin bolus of 60 units/kg (maximum 4000 units) is given intravenously, followed by a continuous heparin drip at 12 units/kg/hr (maximum 1000 units/hr) to maintain an activated partial thromboplastin time (aPTT) between 50 and 70 seconds (1.5 to 2.0 times control). Alternatively, LMWH may be used at doses that provide full anticoagulation.[2]

It is also prudent to administer intravenous UFH or subcutaneous LMWH if the person is at risk for thrombus development.[2] For patients with known heparin-induced thrombocytopenia (HIT),[50] a third class of antithrombotic drugs is available as an alternative to LMWH or UFH. These are direct antithrombotic agents (e.g., hirudin, bivalirudin, argatroban, fondaparinux). Use of newer antithrombotic drugs remains low in clinical practice, however.[52] Patients at risk for thrombotic emboli include those with an anterior wall infarction, atrial fibrillation, previous embolus, cardiomyopathy, or cardiogenic shock.

When the risk of systemic embolic complications remains high, especially in atrial fibrillation, the patient should be anticoagulated with warfarin (Coumadin).[2]

Dysrhythmia Prevention

The antidysrhythmic with the best safety record after STEMI is amiodarone. The reduction in death related to decreased dysrhythmias after MI is 13%.[2] Beta-blockers are another class of antidysrhythmics that are recommended for all patients after STEMI. Beta-blockers prevent ventricular dysrhythmias, lower blood pressure, and prevent reinfarction, especially in patients with left ventricular dysfunction.[2]

Tight Glucose Control

Achievement of normal blood glucose levels during the acute phase and after MI improves survival.[2]

Prevention of Ventricular Remodeling

Many patients are at risk of developing heart failure after STEMI. Vasodilating drugs known as ACEIs or ARBs can stop or limit the ventricular remodeling that leads to heart failure. An ACEI is used, or if it is not tolerated, an ARB is indicated for all patients after STEMI.[2] Information about the clinical effects of heart failure is provided later in this chapter.

Nursing Management

Nursing management of the patient with an acute MI incorporates a variety of nursing diagnoses (Nursing Diagnoses Priorities box on Myocardial Infarction). **Nursing priorities focus on (1) balancing myocardial oxygen supply and demand, (2) preventing complications, and (3) providing patient education.**

NURSING DIAGNOSIS PRIORITIES
Myocardial Infarction

- Acute Pain related to transmission and perception of cutaneous, visceral, muscular, or ischemic impulses, p. A-5
- Decreased Cardiac Output related to alterations in preload, p. A-10
- Decreased Cardiac Output related to alterations in afterload, p. A-10
- Decreased Cardiac Output related to alterations in contractility, p. A-11
- Decreased Cardiac Output related to alterations in heart rate or rhythm, p. A-11
- Activity Intolerance related to cardiopulmonary dysfunction, p. A-1
- Ineffective Cardiopulmonary Tissue Perfusion related to decreased myocardial oxygen supply or increased myocardial oxygen demand, or both, p. A-28
- Disturbed Sleep Pattern related to fragmented sleep, p. A-17
- Anxiety related to threat to biological, psychological, or social integrity, p. A-7
- Ineffective Coping related to situational crisis and personal vulnerability, p. A-30
- Powerlessness related to lack of control over current situation or disease progression, p. A-33
- Deficient Knowledge: Discharge Regimen related to lack of previous exposure to information, p. A-15

Balancing Myocardial Oxygen Supply and Demand

In the acute period, if severe heart muscle damage has occurred, myocardial oxygen supply is increased by the administration of supplemental oxygen to prevent tissue hypoxia. Drugs play an increasingly important role in balancing tissue oxygen supply and demand, and it is the critical care nurse who administers and monitors the effectiveness of these agents. For the patient with a low cardiac output, positive inotropic drugs such as dobutamine, dopamine, and milrinone are prescribed. These inotropic agents are used to increase cardiac contractility in the healthy areas of the heart (increasing oxygen supply), while avoiding damage to the recently infarcted areas. Myocardial oxygen supply can be further enhanced by the use of coronary artery vasodilators. Nitroglycerin is recommended for the first 48 hours to increase vasodilation and prevent myocardial ischemia.[2] Research evidence supports the administration of early beta-blockade therapy to decrease myocardial workload and to prevent dysrhythmias. Administration of beta-blockers reduces mortality by 14% in the first 7 days after an MI and by 23% in the long-term.[2] However, if the patient is in cardiogenic shock, beta-blockers are withheld until the cardiac output has improved.[2] Other interventions to decrease cardiac work and myocardial oxygen consumption include bed rest with bedside commode privileges when the patient is clinically stable.

Preventing Complications

A thorough grasp of the range of potential complications that can occur after STEMI is essential. Cardiac monitoring for early detection of ventricular dysrhythmias is ongoing. Assessment for signs of continued ischemic pain is important,

because angina is a warning sign of myocardium at risk. In response to angina, a 12-lead ECG is obtained to determine if there is an extension of the infarct, nitroglycerin is administered, and the physician is notified immediately so that interventions may be initiated to limit the size of the MI. Heart failure is a serious complication after STEMI. When the patient's blood pressure is stable, treatment with ACEI is initiated. These vasodilators are used to prevent the left ventricular remodeling and dilation that occurs in many patients after an acute MI. Hypotension is a potential complication of ACEI, especially with the first dose. It is an important nursing responsibility to monitor blood pressure and patient symptoms after taking this medication. Surveillance to detect obvious and subtle signs of bleeding is also a priority because so many acute MI patients receive antiplatelet, anticoagulant, and fibrinolytic medications.[2]

In the first 24 hours, stable patients with acute MI may be given only a light diet, because their appetite is often poor. It is no longer considered necessary to restrict iced fluids or caffeine. While the patient is in bed, an upright position is preferred to foster better lung expansion. Deep breathing decreases the risk of atelectasis. An upright position also decreases venous return, lowers preload, and decreases cardiac work. The patient is taught to avoid increasing intraabdominal pressure (Valsalva maneuver). Stool softeners are given to the patient to lessen the risk of constipation from analgesics and bed rest and to decrease the risk of straining. The nurse controls the critical care unit environment by decreasing noise, diminishing sensory overload, and allowing adequate rest periods. (Evidence-Based Collaborative Practice box on Acute Coronary Syndrome and Acute Myocardial Infarction (Non-STEMI and STEMI).)

EVIDENCE-BASED COLLABORATIVE PRACTICE
Acute Coronary Syndrome and Acute Myocardial Infarction (Non-STEMI and STEMI)

Prevention of Acute Coronary Syndrome
The term *ACS* is used to define the life-threatening consequences of CAD, notably unstable angina, non-STEMI, and STEMI:
- Unstable angina is a term that denotes chest pain that is not relieved by SL nitroglycerin or rest within 5 minutes.
- Non-STEMI is an acute MI without ST-segment elevation on the 12-lead ECG.
- STEMI is an acute MI with ST-segment elevation on the 12-lead ECG.

All of the recommendations are "class I," meaning that there is strong research evidence to support these recommendations.

Recommendations That Decrease the Risk of Developing Non-STEMI and STEMI
- Primary care providers should evaluate CAD risk factors for all patients every 3 to 5 years.
- The 10-year risk of ACS and acute MI should be assessed for all patients who have more than two major risk factors.

- An intensive risk factor modification program is recommended for patients with established CAD or high-risk equivalents such as diabetes or chronic kidney disease.

Recommendations That Patients Be Educated about Emergency ACS Symptoms
- A patient who has previously diagnosed CAD should take one SL nitroglycerin dose, and the patient (if alone) or a friend or relative should call 911 if chest pain or discomfort is unrelieved or worsening in 5 minutes.
- The same recommendation applies to a patient without known CAD. If pain is unrelieved with rest or worsening at 5 minutes, the patient (if alone) or a friend or relative should call 911.
- Patients with chest discomfort should be transported to the hospital by ambulance rather than be driven by a friend or relative.
- Family members should be advised to take a CPR course before an ACS emergency occurs. This will teach CPR skills, demonstrate use of an AED, and educate participants about the "chain of survival" concept.

Continued

EVIDENCE-BASED COLLABORATIVE PRACTICE—cont'd
Acute Coronary Syndrome and Acute Myocardial Infarction (Non-STEMI and STEMI)

Recommendations for Prehospital EMS-Paramedic First Responders

- First responders such as EMS-paramedics can provide early defibrillation and ACLS for patients in cardiac arrest.
- EMS personnel should administer 162 to 325 mg of nonenteric aspirin (chewed, not swallowed) to patients with chest pain and suspected STEMI.
- A prehospital fibrinolysis protocol is reasonable for patients with STEMI if there are physicians in the ambulance or if there is a well-organized EMS service with full-time paramedics plus 12-lead ECG transmission capability and online medical direction.
- Patients older than 75 years and those with cardiogenic shock should be transported to a hospital with the ability to provide fibrinolytics, emergency PCI, or emergency CABG. PCI or CABG, if needed, should be provided *within 18 hours* after the onset of cardiogenic shock.
- Patients with STEMI who have a contraindication to fibrinolytic therapy should be brought to a hospital capable of emergency PCI or CABG. At the scene, the door-to-departure time should be less than 30 minutes. PCI should be initiated within 90 minutes after initial medical contact.

Recommendations for Initial Emergency Clinical Management

- Hospitals should establish multidisciplinary teams to facilitate rapid triage of patients who present to the ED with chest pain.
- Use of written protocols is recommended to standardize care. An immediate cardiology consultation is advised if the patient's symptoms fall outside the written protocol.

STEMI

- Fibrinolytics for STEMI: Time from coming into contact with the health care system (paramedics or ED) to receiving fibrinolytics should be *less than 30 minutes.* A brief, focused neurological examination to determine prior stroke or presence of cognitive defects is necessary before administration of fibrinolytics.
- PCI for STEMI: Time from coming into contact with the health care system (paramedics or ED) to balloon inflation PCI should be *less than 90 minutes.*

Non-STEMI

- If the level of risk for the patient with non-STEMI is not immediately apparent, a "chest pain unit" within the ED permits close surveillance by competent clinicians without immediate hospital admission.
- Glycoprotein IIb/IIIa inhibitors for non-STEMI, in addition to aspirin and heparin, are indicated if cardiac catheterization or PCI is planned.
- PCI may be indicated for non-STEMI.

Recommendations for Initial Emergency Physical Assessment
Vital Signs

- HR, BP, RR, temperature Spo_2, ECG monitor to detect presence of dysrhythmias.

Physical Assessment

- Assess for warm or cool skin, color, capillary refill, peripheral pulses.
- Auscultate heart for cardiac murmur or new S_3 or S_4.
- Auscultate lungs for air entry plus crackles, wheezes.
- Observe for breathlessness, frothy pink sputum (pulmonary edema).
- Ask patient, family, significant others for relevant history.

Recommendations for Emergency Diagnostics
12-Lead ECG

- The 12-lead ECG should be shown to the ED physician within 10 minutes after the patient's arrival in the ED for all patients with chest discomfort or angina-equivalent symptoms.
- If the first ECG is normal but the patient continues to have symptoms of chest pain/discomfort, the 12-lead ECG should be repeated at 5- to 10-minute intervals, *or* continuous 12-lead ECG monitoring can be used.
- In patients with inferior wall infarction, RV infarction must be suspected and right-sided ECG leads recorded. V_4R is the diagnostic lead of choice to diagnose ST-segment elevation in the RV.

Laboratory Studies

- Laboratory tests should be performed as part of the general management of STEMI but should not delay the administration of reperfusion therapy.

Cardiac Biomarkers

- Measurement of cardiac-specific troponins is recommended for patients with coexistent skeletal muscle injury. Clinicians are advised not to wait for results of the biomarker assay before initiating reperfusion therapy. Point-of-care (handheld) biomarker assay results are permissible, but subsequent biomarker assays should be done by quantitative laboratory analysis.

Imaging Studies

- Portable chest radiograph: Obtaining the chest radiograph must not delay reperfusion therapy unless a major complication such as aortic dissection is suspected.
- Portable echocardiography (TTE or TEE) or MRI scan to distinguish aortic dissection from STEMI, for patients in whom the symptoms are not clear.

Recommendations for Care
Prevent Hypoxia

- Supplemental oxygen administered to maintain Sao_2 greater than 90%.

Coronary Vasodilation

- Nitroglycerin (0.04 mg SL every 5 minutes for three doses) is administered. If chest pain or discomfort is ongoing, start peripheral IV. Administer IV nitroglycerin for relief of chest pain, control of hypertension, or relief of pulmonary congestion.
- Proactively instruct patients with CAD prescribed NTG, who experience chest discomfort/pain to take one NTG

0.04 mg SL, and to call Emergency Medical Services (EMS-911) immediately if chest discomfort is unimproved or is worsening after one SL dose.

Pain Control
- Morphine sulfate (2 to 4 mg IV) is administered; can increase to 2- to 8-mg IV increments at 5- to 15-minute intervals for STEMI pain control.

NSAIDs
- Discontinue NSAIDs (except for aspirin), both nonselective and COX-2 selective agents, at time of presentation with STEMI because of increased risk of mortality, reinfarction, hypertension, heart failure, and myocardial rupture associated with NSAID use.

Aspirin
- Aspirin 162-325 mg to be chewed for rapid buccal absorption.

Beta-Blockers
- Oral beta-blocker therapy is administered to STEMI patients without contraindications to beta-blockade, irrespective of fibrinolytic or primary PCI reperfusion.
- Contraindications for beta-blockade with STEMI include signs of heart failure, low cardiac output, cardiogenic shock risk, heart block or prolonged PR interval (>0.24 second), and active asthma or reactive airway disease.
- While considering the options for reperfusion, beta-blockers are given if the patient has tachycardia or hypertension; otherwise, they are started as soon as possible after STEMI.

Angiotensin-Converting Enzymes Inhibitors
- Oral ACE inhibitors are indicated within the first 24 hours after STEMI.

Recommendations for Emergency Interventions for STEMI
Fibrinolytic Drugs
- Fibrinolytic drugs are administered to STEMI patients with ST-segment elevation greater than 0.1 mV (1 mm or one small box) in two contiguous precordial (chest) leads or two adjacent limb leads, new LBBB or presumed new LBBB, and onset of symptoms less than 12 hours earlier.
- Before administration of fibrinolytic therapy, rule out neurological contraindications.
- Rule out facial trauma, uncontrolled hypertension, or ischemic stroke within the last 3 months.
- If contraindications to fibrinolysis are present, PCI is the preferred method of reperfusion.

PCI
- Emergency diagnostic coronary angiography to identify blocked coronary artery before PCI.
- Emergency PCI is recommended over fibrinolytic therapy if symptom onset was longer than 3 hours ago.
- Emergency PCI can be performed within 12 hours after symptom onset for patients with new LBBB or presumed new LBBB.

- Emergency PCI balloon inflation within 90 minutes after arrival at the hospital
- If cardiogenic shock develops within 36 hours after MI, in patients younger than 75 years with ST-segment elevation, or in patients with new LBBB, "rescue PCI" is recommended within 18 hours after shock onset.

Cardiac Surgery
- Emergency CABG surgery is undertaken for specific indications in STEMI:
  - Failed PCI with persistent pain or hemodynamic instability
  - Recurrent ischemia refractory to medical therapy in patients with suitable anatomy who are not candidates for PCI
  - Post-MI VSR or papillary muscle rupture, both of which frequently lead to cardiogenic shock
  - Cardiogenic shock within 36 hours after MI, in patients younger than 75 years with ST-segment elevation, or in patients with new LBBB who have multivessel or left main disease
  - Recurrent ventricular dysrhythmias in patients with 50% or greater left main coronary artery lesion or triple-vessel disease or both

Recommendations for Secondary Prevention of Complications
Medications
- ACE inhibitors to prevent ventricular remodeling
- Beta-blockers to prevent ventricular dysrhythmias
- Diuretics if heart failure has developed
- Antihyperlipidemics if total cholesterol, LDL-C, or triglycerides are elevated

Recommendations for Management of Complications after STEMI
Cardiogenic Shock
- IABP for patients with hypotension (BP of 90 mm Hg or SBP of 30 mm Hg below baseline)

Ventricular Arrhythmias
- VF or pulseless VT is managed by standard ACLS criteria: unsynchronized biphasic shock of 200 joules, followed by 2 minutes (five cycles) of CPR; then another shock of 200 joules if patient has not converted, followed by 2 minutes of CPR. Vasopressors are given during CPR if intravenous or intraosseous access is available.
- Patients with hemodynamically significant VT more than 2 days after STEMI who have ongoing ventricular dysrhythmias are considered for implantation of an ICD.
- Patients with an EF between 30% and 40% at 1 month after STEMI should undergo an EPS; if they are inducible to VT/VF, an ICD is recommended to reduce risk of SCD.
- Patients with an EF of less than 30% at 1 month after STEMI are at high risk for SCD.

AV Block
- Transvenous pacemaker (emergency) or permanent pacemaker (later elective) is inserted for symptomatic second- or third-degree AV block.

Continued

- All patients after STEMI who require permanent pacing should also be evaluated for ICD indications.

Provide Relevant Education
Medications
- Written and verbal instructions about medication dosages, administration, and side effects.

Emergency Information
- Give patient and family information about calling 911 if pain/angina-equivalent symptoms persist or are worse after 5 minutes.

- Family members of high-risk patients are advised to take a CPR class and learn about AED.

Risk Factors
- Smoking cessation, hypertension control, weight control, normal blood glucose; low-fat diet; normal lipid panel.
- Increase physical activity, no new HRT for women.

Cardiac Rehabilitation
- Participation in a cardiac rehabilitation program will help the patient continue the process of risk factor and lifestyle modification.

Data from Antman EM, et al: ACC/AHA guidelines for the management of patients with ST-elevation myocardial infarction, *Circulation* 110(5):588, 2004; Antman EM, et al: 2007 focused update of the ACC/AHA 2004 guidelines for the management of patients with ST-elevation myocardial infarction, *Circulation* 117(2):296, 2008; Braunwald E, et al: ACC/AHA 2002 guideline update for the management of patients with unstable angina and non-ST-segment elevation myocardial infarction, *J Am Coll Cardiol* 40(7):1366, 2002; Anderson LJ, et al: ACC/AHA 2007 guidelines for the management of patients with unstable angina and non-ST-elevation myocardial infarction, *J Am Coll Cardiol* 50(7):e1, 2007; Kushner FG, et al: 2009 Focused Updates: ACC/AHA Guidelines for the Management of Patients With ST-Elevation Myocardial Infarction (updating the 2004 Guideline and 2007 Focused Update) and ACC/AHA/SCAI Guidelines on Percutaneous Coronary Intervention (updating the 2005 Guideline and 2007 Focused Update): a report of the American College of Cardiology Foundation/American Heart Association Task Force on Practice Guidelines *Circulation* 120(22):2271, 2009.
ACE, angiotensin-converting enzyme; *ACLS*, advanced cardiac life support; *ACS*, acute coronary syndrome; *AED*, automated external defibrillator; *AV*, atrioventricular; *BP*, blood pressure, *CABG*, coronary artery bypass graft surgery; *CAD*, coronary artery disease; *COX-2*, cyclooxygenase 2; *CPR*, cardiopulmonary resuscitation; *ECG*, electrocardiogram; *ED*, emergency department; *EF*, ejection fraction; *EMS*, emergency medical services; *EPS*, electrophysiology study; *HR*, heart rate; *HRT*, hormone replacement therapy; *IABP*, intraaortic balloon pump; *ICD*, implantable cardioverter defibrillator; *IV*, intravenous; *LBBB*, left bundle branch block; *LDL*, low-density lipoprotein cholesterol; *MI*, myocardial infarction; *MRI*, magnetic resonance imaging; *non-STEMI*, non-ST-segment elevation myocardial infarction; *NSAIDs*, nonsteroidal antiinflammatory drugs; *PCI*, percutaneous coronary intervention; *RR*, respiratory rate; *RV*, right ventricle; *Sao₂*, arterial oxygen saturation; *SCD*, sudden cardiac death; *SL*, sublingual; *Spo₂*, oxygen saturation from external pulse oximeter; *STEMI*, ST-segment elevation myocardial infarction; *TEE*, transesophageal echocardiogram; *TTE*, transthoracic echocardiogram; *VF*, ventricular fibrillation; *VSR*, ventricular septal rupture; *VT*, ventricular tachycardia.

Providing Patient Education

It is important to discuss the risk of depression following acute MI. The incidence of depression after an MI ranges from 17% to 27%. Key symptoms of depression mentioned frequently by cardiac patients are fatigue, change in appetite, and sleep disturbance. Depression is an independent risk factor for increased morbidity and mortality in those with coronary heart disease, and it is a treatable condition.

After the acute phase has passed, education for the patient and family focuses on risk-factor reduction, manifestations of angina, when to call a physician or emergency services, medications, and resumption of physical and sexual activity. If possible, a referral is made to a cardiac rehabilitation program so that this education can be reinforced outside the acute care hospital environment.[51]

CARDIAC ARREST AND SUDDEN CARDIAC DEATH

Description

Between 400,000 and 460,000 people die suddenly of cardiac causes each year.[1] This number represents 60% of all cardiac deaths.[1] These statistics represent deaths that occur outside the hospital with symptoms that last less than 1 hour or occur in a hospital emergency department.[52] Sudden cardiac death

represents about 5% of the total annual mortality rate for all causes.[53]

When the onset of symptoms is rapid, the most likely mechanism of death is VT, which degenerates into VF. This syndrome is called sudden cardiac death (SCD). Despite aggressive cardiopulmonary resuscitation (CPR) initiated outside the hospital, few who sustain an out-of-hospital cardiac arrest survive to hospital discharge. Strategies that have been shown to improve the resuscitation chain of survival involve huge community-wide programs to teach laypersons CPR and how to use an automated external defibrillator (AED). With such programs in place and with accessible AED units and rapid EMS support, survival to hospital discharge has been shown to improve.[54]

Etiology

Most SCD incidents occur in patients with preexisting ventricular dysfunction resulting from underlying heart disease that is either acquired or has a genetic component as listed in Box 12-5. Specific SCD risk factors include extensive coronary atherosclerosis with or without a history of an acute MI; dilated or hypertrophic cardiomyopathy; valvular heart disease; autonomic nervous system abnormalities; electrical system abnormalities, such as AV block, Wolff-Parkinson-White (WPW) syndrome, prolonged QT syndrome; and taking medications that prolong the QT interval.[55-57]

BOX 12-5 CAUSES OF SUDDEN CARDIAC DEATH

Acquired SCD Risk

Acquired SCD patients are older adults with a history of CAD, MI, and subsequent heart failure.

- Heart failure
  - Ejection fraction <30%.
  - Heart structure is abnormal (systolic or diastolic ventricular dysfunction).
  - CAD and a history of MI that has produced scar tissue is the most common cause of VT/VF leading to SCD.
- Cardiomyopathy (dilated or ischemic)
  - Patients who are inducible for VT/VF in EPS are at highest risk.
  - Risk is decreased by implantation of an ICD and antidysrhythmic drug therapy.

Genetic SCD Risk

Genetic cardiovascular disease accounts for 40% of SCD in young adults.

- Brugada syndrome ECG signs: coved-type ST-segment elevation (>2 mm) in right precordial leads, although ECG variations also occur.
  - Heart structure appears normal.
  - High risk of VT or VF in otherwise healthy young adult.
  - VT/VF often occurs at night, at rest.
  - Represents 4% of all SCD; average age, 41 years.
  - Represents up to 20% of genetic SCD patients.
  - Hereditary: autosomal-dominant genetic transmission.
  - Five times more common in males.

- Patients who are inducible in EPS are at increased risk.
  - Risk reduced by implantation of an ICD.
- Wolff-Parkinson-White syndrome
  - Congenital accessory conduction pathway connects the atria and ventricles.
  - Accessory pathway is in addition to the normal conduction system.
  - Accessory pathway allows very rapid transmission of impulses leading to "preexcitation" of the ventricle that can degenerate into VT/VF, especially if atrial dysrhythmias are present.
  - WPW syndrome is usually identified when patient is a teenager or young adult.
  - WPW syndrome is often recognized during exercise by palpitations or breathlessness.
  - It can be cured in many cases by radiofrequency ablation of the accessory pathway.
- Hypertrophic cardiomyopathy
  - There is a risk of VT/VF with exercise.
  - The HOCM form can be cured in many cases by alcohol ablation of the enlarged ventricular septum.
  - For other HCM patients, the risk is reduced by implantation of an ICD.
- Long QT syndrome
  - There is a risk of VT/VF with exercise with some long QT syndromes.
  - The risk is reduced by implantation of an ICD.

CAD, coronary artery disease; *CV*, cardiovascular; *ECG*, electrocardiogram; *EPS*, electrophysiology study; *HCM*, hypertrophic cardiomyopathy; *HOCM*, hypertrophic subaortic obstructive cardiomyopathy; *ICD*, implantable cardioverter defibrillator; *MI*, myocardial infarction; *SCD*, sudden cardiac death; *VF*, ventricular fibrillation; *VT*, ventricular tachycardia; *WPW*, Wolff-Parkinson-White.

An ejection fraction of less than 30% and a history of ventricular dysrhythmias are powerful predictors of SCD. Unfortunately, many individuals are unaware of their risk. In one longitudinal analysis, 48% of the SCD victims had not previously been diagnosed with cardiac disease.[52] Fifty percent of men and 64% of women who die suddenly of cardiovascular disease have no previous symptoms of the disease. Men account for 70% to 89% of SCD, an annual incidence that is three to four times higher for men than women.[1]

Therapeutic Hypothermia

Depending on the length of time the patient was unconscious following the cardiac arrest, cognitive defects can occur, caused by lack of cerebral blood flow and resultant hypoxia to the brain. For comatose patients at high risk for hypoxic brain injury after cardiac arrest, therapeutic hypothermia to about 33° centigrade is initiated for several hours to preserve brain function.[58,59] Only one tenth to one third of people who are resuscitated after cardiac arrest are discharged from the hospital and able to lead an independent life.[59] Post-arrest hypothermia treatment increases the likelihood that survivors of cardiac arrest will leave the hospital without major brain damage.[59]

Survivors receive antidysrhythmic agents and may also have an implantable cardioverter defibrillator (ICD) unit

inserted.[59-62] Prevention focuses on identification and treatment of high-risk cardiac patients (see "Implantable Cardioverter Defibrillator" and "Antidysrhythmic Drugs" in Chapter 13).

HEART FAILURE

Description and Etiology

The number of patients with heart failure is increasing in the United States. More than five million Americans have a diagnosis of heart failure, and about 550,000 new cases are diagnosed each year.[63] This represents about 2.5% of the adult population. More than 282,000 people die of heart failure each year.[1] Heart failure is primarily a disease of older persons; approximately 80% of patients hospitalized with heart failure are older than 65 years.[63] Total inpatient and outpatient costs for heart failure treatment exceed $27.9 billion each year,[63] with $2.9 billion required for heart failure drugs alone.[63]

Pathophysiology

Heart failure is a response to cardiac dysfunction, a condition in which the heart cannot pump blood at a volume required to meet the body's needs. Any condition that impairs the ability of the ventricles to fill or eject blood can cause heart failure.

CAD with resultant necrotic damage to the left ventricle is the underlying cause of heart failure in most patients. Other major conditions that lead to heart failure include valvular dysfunction, infection (myocarditis or endocarditis), cardiomyopathy, and uncontrolled hypertension.[63] Hypertension is a precursor of heart failure in 75% of heart failure cases.[1]

Assessment and Diagnosis

Heart failure is typically classified using the New York Heart Association (NYHA) criteria. Patients are assigned into four groups, I through IV, depending on the degree of symptoms and the amount of patient effort required to elicit symptoms (Table 12-6). Research-based clinical guidelines suggest adding a second level of classification that emphasizes the progressive nature of heart failure through stages identified by increasing symptom distress and intensified clinical interventions (Figure 12-13).[63] Heart failure can manifest in many different ways, depending on how far ventricular remodeling and dysfunction have advanced. Heart failure may be discovered because of a known clinical syndrome such as acute MI, or because of decreased exercise tolerance, fluid retention, or admission to the critical care unit for an unrelated condition.[63] The clinical assessment signs diagnostic of fluid volume overload are jugular venous distention (JVD) and a third heart sound.[63] The assessment procedures used to estimate JVD and auscultate a third heart sound are described in Chapter 11 (Box 11-1, Box 11-2; Figure 11-2, Figure 11-3). These clinical diagnostic skills, are also used to make the diagnosis of heart failure.[63]

The first step in the diagnosis is to determine the underlying structural abnormality creating the ventricular dysfunction and symptoms. Various imaging tests are available to visualize cardiac anatomy, and laboratory tests are used to evaluate the impact of hormonal or electrolyte imbalance. The results of these tests permit the cardiology team to design a treatment plan to control symptoms and possibly correct the underlying cause. All patients do not have the same type of heart failure.

Left Ventricular Failure

Failure of the left ventricle is defined as a disturbance of the contractile function of the left ventricle, resulting in a low

TABLE 12-6	NEW YORK HEART ASSOCIATION FUNCTIONAL CLASSIFICATION OF HEART FAILURE	
CLASS	**DEFINITION**	
I	Normal daily activity does not initiate symptoms.	
II	Normal daily activities initiate onset of symptoms, but symptoms subside with rest.	
III	Minimal activity initiates symptoms; patients are usually symptom-free at rest.	
IV	Any type of activity initiates symptoms, and symptoms are present at rest.	

cardiac output state. This leads to vasoconstriction of the arterial bed that raises systemic vascular resistance (SVR), a condition also described as "high afterload," and creates congestion and edema in the pulmonary circulation and alveoli. Clinical manifestations include decreased peripheral perfusion with weak or diminished pulses; cool, pale extremities; and in later stages, peripheral cyanosis (Table 12-7). Over time, with progression of the disease state the fluid accumulation behind the dysfunctional left ventricle elevates pulmonary pressures, contributes to pulmonary congestion and edema, and produces dysfunction of the right ventricle, resulting in failure of the right side of the heart.

Right Ventricular Failure

Failure of the right side of the heart is defined as ineffective right ventricular contractile function. Pure failure of the right ventricle may result from an acute condition such as a pulmonary embolus or a right ventricular infarction, but it is most commonly caused by failure of the left side of the heart. The common manifestations of right ventricular failure are jugular venous distention, elevated central venous pressure (CVP), weakness, peripheral or sacral edema, hepatomegaly (enlarged liver), jaundice, and liver tenderness. Gastrointestinal symptoms include poor appetite, anorexia, nausea, and an uncomfortable feeling of fullness (see Table 12-7).

Heart Failure with Systolic Dysfunction

Systolic dysfunction describes an abnormality of the heart muscle that markedly decreases contractility during systole (ejection) and lessens the quantity of blood that can be pumped out of the heart. Patients with a diagnosis of systolic heart failure have signs and symptoms of heart failure combined with a below-normal ejection fraction. Left ventricular systolic dysfunction is the classic picture that most clinicians consider when thinking about heart failure. In addition to the signs and symptoms of left heart failure (described earlier), the patient has a low ejection fraction. There is some debate about how low the ejection fraction has to be to qualify as systolic heart failure, but the value is usually below 50%;[64] some clinicians cite numbers below 45% or 40%.[65,66] Symptoms of heart failure with systolic dysfunction include dyspnea, exercise intolerance, and fluid volume overload.

Heart Failure with Diastolic Dysfunction

Diastolic dysfunction describes an abnormality of the heart muscle that makes it unable to relax, stretch, or fill during diastole. The ejection fraction can be normal or abnormal (low), and the patient may be symptomatic or symptom-free.[64,67,68] Half of patients with heart failure have diastolic muscle dysfunction.[69] The principal causes are similar to systolic heart failure: CAD, myocardial ischemia, uncontrolled hypertension, and left ventricular hypertrophy.[67] Some conditions that are known to markedly alter diastolic function include hypertrophic cardiomyopathy, restrictive cardiomyopathy, and infiltrative diseases such as amyloidosis and neoplastic infiltrate.

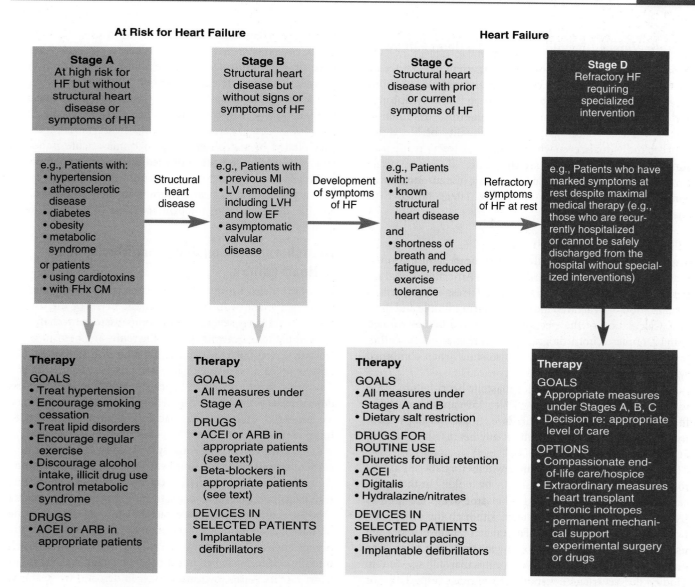

At Risk for Heart Failure

Heart Failure

Stage A
At high risk for HF but without structural heart disease or symptoms of HR

Stage B
Structural heart disease but without signs or symptoms of HF

Stage C
Structural heart disease with prior or current symptoms of HF

Stage D
Refractory HF requiring specialized intervention

e.g., Patients with:
• hypertension
• atherosclerotic disease
• diabetes
• obesity
• metabolic syndrome

or patients
• using cardiotoxins
• with FHx CM

→ Structural heart disease →

e.g., Patients with
• previous MI
• LV remodeling including LVH and low EF
• asymptomatic valvular disease

→ Development of symptoms of HF →

e.g., Patients with:
• known structural heart disease
and
• shortness of breath and fatigue, reduced exercise tolerance

→ Refractory symptoms of HF at rest →

e.g., Patients who have marked symptoms at rest despite maximal medical therapy (e.g., those who are recurrently hospitalized or cannot be safely discharged from the hospital without specialized interventions)

Therapy

GOALS
• Treat hypertension
• Encourage smoking cessation
• Treat lipid disorders
• Encourage regular exercise
• Discourage alcohol intake, illicit drug use
• Control metabolic syndrome

DRUGS
• ACEI or ARB in appropriate patients

Therapy

GOALS
• All measures under Stage A

DRUGS
• ACEI or ARB in appropriate patients (see text)
• Beta-blockers in appropriate patients (see text)

DEVICES IN SELECTED PATIENTS
• Implantable defibrillators

Therapy

GOALS
• All measures under Stages A and B
• Dietary salt restriction

DRUGS FOR ROUTINE USE
• Diuretics for fluid retention
• ACEI
• Digitalis
• Hydralazine/nitrates

DEVICES IN SELECTED PATIENTS
• Biventricular pacing
• Implantable defibrillators

Therapy

GOALS
• Appropriate measures under Stages A, B, C
• Decision re: appropriate level of care

OPTIONS
• Compassionate end-of-life care/hospice
• Extraordinary measures
  - heart transplant
  - chronic inotropes
  - permanent mechanical support
  - experimental surgery or drugs

FIGURE 12-13 Stages in the Development of Heart Failure, with Recommended Therapy by Stage. (Adapted from Hunt SA, et al: 2009 focused update incorporated into the ACC/AHA 2005 guidelines for the diagnosis and management of heart failure in adults, *Circulation* 119(14):e391, 2009.)

TABLE 12-7	CLINICAL MANIFESTATIONS OF RIGHT- AND LEFT-SIDED HEART FAILURE		
LEFT VENTRICULAR FAILURE		**RIGHT VENTRICULAR FAILURE**	
SIGNS	**SYMPTOMS**	**SIGNS**	**SYMPTOMS**
Tachypnea	Fatigue	Peripheral edema	Weakness
Tachycardia	Dyspnea	Hepatomegaly	Anorexia
Cough	Orthopnea	Splenomegaly	Indigestion
Bibasilar crackles	Paroxysmal nocturnal dyspnea	Hepatojugular reflux	Weight gain
Gallop rhythms (S_3 and S_4)	Nocturia	Ascites	Mental changes
Increased pulmonary artery pressures		Jugular venous distention	
Hemoptysis		Increased central venous pressure	
Cyanosis		Pulmonary hypertension	
Pulmonary edema			

Systolic Versus Diastolic Dysfunction Heart Failure

It is impossible to determine whether a patient has systolic or diastolic heart failure from clinical assessment alone.[64] Both types of heart failure produce similar signs and symptoms, and in most patients systolic and diastolic dysfunction coexist.[63] The level of symptoms and quality of life varies between individuals, even when the ejection fraction and presumed cardiac dysfunction are the same.[70] This may occur because most symptoms occur as a result of neurohormonal compensatory mechanisms (described later) rather than changes in cardiac output.

Doppler Echocardiography

The definitive diagnosis of the type of heart failure is often made using Doppler echocardiography. An echocardiogram performed at rest and during exercise (stress echo) permits visualization of heart wall movement during systole and diastole. Calculation of the ejection fraction can be determined using Doppler echocardiography or during a cardiac catheterization. These diagnostic tests also show when combined systolic and diastolic dysfunction coexist.[64]

The annual mortality rate for diastolic heart failure is 5% to 8%, markedly less than the 10% to 15% annual mortality for patients with systolic heart failure. To put this in perspective, age-matched controls without any heart failure have an annual mortality rate of just 1%.[64,67]

It is not possible to distinguish whether a patient has systolic or diastolic heart failure simply by looking at the medications he or she is prescribed. The same drugs are used to treat the two types of heart failure, although the underlying rationales may be different.[65] For example, beta-blockers are used in diastolic heart failure to slow the heart rate, to prolong diastole to give more time for ventricular filling, and to modify the ventricular response to exercise, especially for patients who have a preserved ejection fraction.[65] When beta-blockers are prescribed for treatment of systolic heart failure, the intent is to preserve long-term inotropic (contractile) function and prevent ventricular remodeling.[65] Diuretics are used to treat both types of heart failure, although a smaller dosage is generally needed in diastolic heart failure.[65] ACEIs and ARBs are also used to treat both types of heart failure. The medications used to treat heart failure are further discussed in Chapter 13 (see Table 13-19).

Acute Versus Chronic Heart Failure

Acute or chronic heart failure is determined by the rapidity with which the syndrome develops, the presence and activation of compensatory mechanisms, and the presence or absence of fluid accumulation in the interstitial space (see Figure 12-13). In clinical practice guidelines, the terms *acute* and *chronic* have replaced the older name of congestive heart failure (CHF), because not all heart failure involves pulmonary congestion.[63] However, the descriptor CHF remains in common parlance in clinical practice.

Acute heart failure has a sudden onset, with no compensatory mechanisms. The patient may experience acute pulmonary edema, low cardiac output, or even cardiogenic shock. Patients with chronic heart failure are hypervolemic, have sodium and water retention, and have structural heart chamber changes such as dilation or hypertrophy.[63]

Chronic heart failure is ongoing, with symptoms that may be made tolerable by medication, diet, and a reduced activity level. The deterioration into acute heart failure can be precipitated by the onset of dysrhythmias, acute ischemia, sudden illness, or cessation of medications. This may necessitate admission to a critical care unit. Hypertension is the primary precursor of heart failure in women, whereas CAD, specifically acute MI, is the primary cause of heart failure in men.[63]

Neurohormonal Compensatory Mechanisms in Heart Failure

When the heart begins to fail and the cardiac output is no longer sufficient to meet the metabolic needs of the tissues, the body activates several major compensatory mechanisms: the sympathetic nervous system, the renin-angiotensin-aldosterone system (RAAS), and if hypertension is present, the development of ventricular hypertrophy (see Figure 12-13). This process ultimately reshapes the ventricle in a process described as ventricular remodeling. These pathophysiological processes and the pharmacological measures taken to limit ventricular remodeling are described in this section.

The sympathetic nervous system compensates for low cardiac output by increasing heart rate and blood pressure. As a result, levels of circulating catecholamines are increased, resulting in peripheral vasoconstriction. In addition to raising blood pressure and heart rate, catecholamines cause shunting of blood from nonvital organs, such as the skin, to vital organs, such as the heart and brain. This mechanism, although initially helpful, may become a negative factor if elevation of heart rate increases myocardial oxygen demand while shortening the amount of time for diastolic filling and coronary artery perfusion.

Activation of RAAS in heart failure promotes fluid retention.[63,71] The RAAS is activated by low cardiac output that causes the hormone renin to be secreted by the kidneys. A physiological chain of events is then set in motion that leads to volume overload. The renin acts on angiotensinogen in the bloodstream and converts it to angiotensin I; when angiotensin passes through the lung tissues, it is activated by ACE, an enzyme that converts the angiotensin I to angiotensin II, a powerful vasoconstrictor that increases SVR, raises blood pressure, and increases the workload of the left ventricle; the increased SVR further lowers cardiac output. The mineralocorticoid hormone aldosterone is released from the adrenal glands and stimulates sodium retention by means of the distal tubules of the kidney. In response to the low cardiac output, the renal arterioles constrict, decrease glomerular filtration, and increase reabsorption of sodium from the proximal and distal tubules. To break the RAAS cycle of fluid retention in heart failure, two types of drugs are prescribed to interrupt the steps. To inhibit the conversion of angiotensin I to angiotensin II, an ACEI is prescribed (see Table 13-19 in Chapter

13). These agents prevent arterial vasoconstriction, decrease blood pressure and SVR, and decrease the amount of ventricular remodeling that often occurs with heart failure. A drug that inhibits angiotensin II directly may be prescribed instead. The drugs in this category are ARBs.[74] Aldactone (spironolactone) is a drug from a different category that is also prescribed to break the RAAS cycle. Aldactone is a mineralocorticoid receptor antagonist that inhibits (blocks) the retention of sodium from the distal tubules of the kidney.[71-73] Figure 12-14 shows the mechanism of action by which these drugs act on the RAAS.

Ventricular hypertrophy is the final compensatory mechanism. It is also strongly associated with preexisting hypertension. Because myocardial hypertrophy increases

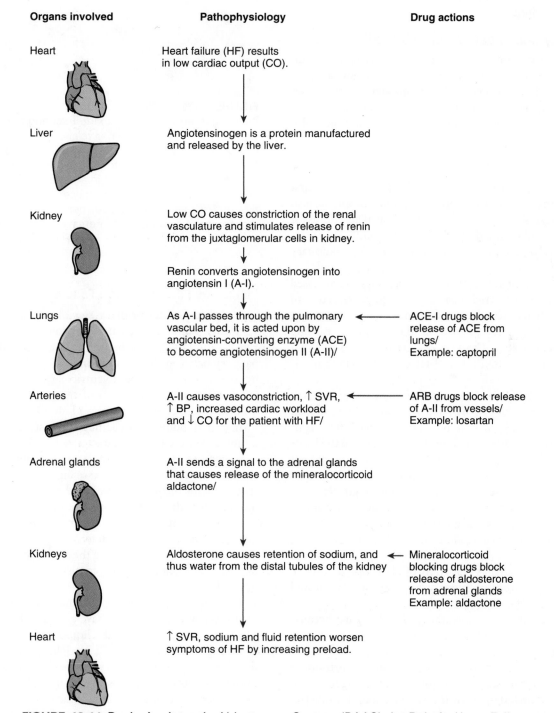

FIGURE 12-14 Renin-Angiotensin-Aldosterone System (RAAS), its Role in Heart Failure, and Drug Actions.

the force of contraction, hypertrophy helps the ventricle overcome an increase in afterload. When this mechanism is no longer efficient for the ventricle, it will remodel by dilation.

Ventricular remodeling occurs as a result of the previously described mechanisms. The shape of the ventricle is changed, or is remodeled, to resemble a round bowl. A dilated ventricle has poor contractility and is enlarged without hypertrophy. Research trial evidence indicates that synergistic use of drugs from different categories—ACEI or ARB, Aldactone, plus beta-blockade—can halt or reduce the progression of heart failure remodeling.[72,74,75]

Pulmonary Complications of Heart Failure

The respiratory manifestations of acute heart failure result from tissue hypoperfusion and organ congestion and are progressive. The severity of respiratory manifestations progresses as heart failure worsens. Initially, symptoms of breathlessness appear only with exertion, but eventually symptoms also occur at rest.[63]

Shortness of Breath in Heart Failure

The patient experiences the feeling of shortness of breath first with exertion, but as heart failure worsens, symptoms are also present at rest. A diagnostic blood test is available to assist clinicians in differentiating whether a patient's shortness of breath is caused by cardiac failure or by pulmonary complications.

BNP and NT-proBNP: Natriuretic peptides are released from the cardiac ventricles in response to increased wall tension. Heart failure increases left ventricular wall tension because of the excess preload in the ventricles causing increased wall stretch. The peptides are measured as brain natriuretic peptide (BNP) and N-terminal proB type natriuretic peptide (NT-proBNP).[63]

When the BNP blood level is greater than 100 pg/mL, the dyspnea is more likely to be related to cardiac rather than pulmonary failure.[76-78] A BNP result greater than 400 is considered indicative of heart failure. The more severe the heart failure, the higher the BNP test result.[79] If the patient has concomitant kidney failure, the BNP clinical diagnostic cut-point to diagnose heart failure rises to greater than 200 pg/mL.[80] See Chapter 11, Figure 11-48 for more information on using BNP to diagnose heart failure.

Breathlessness in heart failure is described by the following terms:

- *Dyspnea:* the patient's sensation of shortness of breath, which results from pulmonary vascular congestion and decreased lung compliance
- *Orthopnea:* difficulty in breathing when lying flat because of an increase in venous return that occurs in the supine position
- *Paroxysmal nocturnal dyspnea:* a severe form of orthopnea in which the patient awakens from sleep gasping for air
- *Cardiac asthma:* dyspnea with wheezing, a nonproductive cough, and pulmonary crackles that progress to the gurgling sounds of pulmonary edema

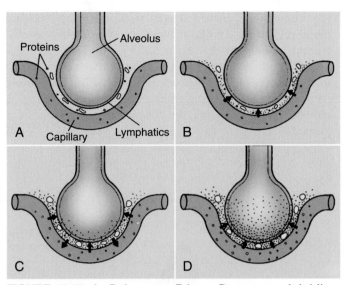

FIGURE 12-15 As Pulmonary Edema Progresses, it Inhibits Oxygen and Carbon Dioxide Exchange at the Alveolar Capillary Interface. *A,* Normal relationship. *B,* Increased pulmonary capillary hydrostatic pressure causes fluid to move from the vascular space into the pulmonary interstitial space. *C,* Lymphatic flow increases in an attempt to pull fluid back into the vascular or lymphatic space. *D,* Failure of lymphatic flow and worsening of left-sided heart failure results in further movement of fluid into the interstitial space and the alveoli.

Pulmonary Edema in Heart Failure

The alveolus is the primary site of gas exchange (Figure 12-15, *A*). Pulmonary edema, or protein-laden fluid in the alveoli, inhibits gas exchange by impairing the diffusion pathway between the alveolus and the capillary. It is caused by increased left atrial and ventricular pressures and results in an excessive accumulation of serous or serosanguineous fluid in the interstitial spaces and alveoli of the lungs. The formation of pulmonary edema has two stages. The first stage is not as severe and is characterized by interstitial edema, engorgement of the perivascular and peribronchial spaces, and increased lymphatic flow (see Figure 12-15, *B*). The later stage is characterized by alveolar edema resulting from fluid moving into the alveoli from the interstitium (see Figure 12-15, *C*). Eventually, blood plasma moves into the alveoli faster than the lymphatic system can clear it, interfering with diffusion of oxygen, depressing the arterial partial pressure of oxygen (PaO_2), and leading to tissue hypoxia (see Figure 12-15, *D*).

Heart failure patients in pulmonary edema are extremely breathless and anxious and have a sensation of suffocation. They expectorate pink, frothy liquid and feel as if they are drowning. They may sit bolt upright, gasp for breath, or thrash about. The respiratory rate is elevated, and accessory muscles of ventilation are used, with nasal flaring and bulging neck muscles. Respirations are characterized by loud inspiratory and expiratory gurgling sounds. Diaphoresis is profuse, and the skin is cold, ashen, and sometimes cyanotic, reflecting low cardiac output, increased sympathetic stimulation, peripheral vasoconstriction, and desaturation of arterial blood.

Arterial Blood Gases in Pulmonary Edema. Arterial blood gas values are variable. In the early stage of pulmonary edema, respiratory alkalosis may be present because of hyperventilation, which eliminates carbon dioxide. As the pulmonary edema progresses and gas exchange becomes impaired, acidosis (pH <7.35) and hypoxemia ensue. A chest radiograph usually confirms an enlarged cardiac silhouette, pulmonary venous congestion, and interstitial edema.

Dysrhythmias and Heart Failure

A ventricular ejection fraction below 30% and the presence of NYHA class III or IV heart failure are strongly associated with ventricular dysrhythmias and an increased risk of death.[63,81-84] Because sustained VT or VF initiates sudden cardiac death, high-risk patients with severe heart failure are prescribed antidysrhythmic drugs and have an ICD inserted.[82-84]

Many patients with heart failure also have atrial fibrillation. Digoxin is frequently prescribed in atrial fibrillation to control ventricular heart rate. Digoxin does not prolong life but decreases symptoms and hospitalizations associated with heart failure. Digoxin may also work synergistically with specific beta-blockers (e.g., carvedilol) and make the symptoms more tolerable for patients with severe heart failure.[83,85]

Medical Management

The goals of the medical management of heart failure are to relieve heart failure symptoms, enhance cardiac performance, and correct known precipitating causes of acute heart failure.

Relief of Symptoms and Enhancement of Cardiac Performance

In the acute phase of advanced heart failure, the patient may have a pulmonary artery catheter in place so that left ventricular function can be followed closely. Control of symptoms involves management of fluid overload and improvement of cardiac output by decreasing SVR and increasing contractility. Diuretics are administered to decrease preload and to eliminate excess fluid from the body.[73] If pulmonary edema develops, additional diuretics are used. Morphine is given to facilitate peripheral dilation and decrease anxiety. Afterload is decreased by vasodilators, such as sodium nitroprusside (Nipride) and nitroglycerin. Nitrates are used to decrease preload and vasodilate the coronary arteries if CAD is an underlying cause of the acute heart failure. For some patients, an intraaortic balloon pump (IABP) is temporarily required.[86] Contractility is initially increased by continuous infusion of positive inotropic drugs (dopamine) or by combination inodilators such as dobutamine or milrinone. Nesiritide (Natrecor) or intravenous BNP is indicated for the relief of patients with acutely decompensated heart failure who have dyspnea at rest. Nesiritide lowers pulmonary artery pressures and wedge pressure, which decreases symptoms of dyspnea.[87,88]

After the acute heart failure is controlled, the patient is weaned off intravenous medications, which are gradually replaced by oral agents. Before the transition out of the critical care unit, the heart failure patient will receive ACEIs to inhibit left ventricular chamber remodeling and to slow left ventricular dilation.[63,71,74] If the patient does not tolerate ACEIs, ARBs may be substituted.[74] Low dosage beta-blockers such as carvedilol may also be prescribed, although strict surveillance is required to anticipate and avoid untoward negative inotropic effects.[83,89] Digoxin may be added to the regimen, especially if the person has concomitant atrial fibrillation.[85]

Nonpharmacological interventions that are increasingly used include cardiac resynchronization therapy (CRT).[90] CRT is biventricular pacing where the right and left ventricles each have a pacing lead in contact with the myocardium. The right ventricular lead is inside the right ventricle, and the left ventricular lead is positioned into a left wall tributary of the coronary sinus vein.[90,91] In newer permanent pacemaker models, the right and left ventricular leads are paced to synchronize the ventricles and improve heart failure symptoms.

Correction of Precipitating Causes

After symptoms of heart failure are controlled, diagnostic studies such as cardiac catheterization, echocardiography, and thallium scanning are undertaken to uncover the cause of the heart failure and tailor long-term management to treat the cause. Some structural problems such as valvular disease may be amenable to surgical correction.

Palliative Care for End-Stage Heart Failure

In 2004 a consensus statement on palliative and supportive care in advanced heart failure was published.[92] Because heart failure is a progressive disease, some patients will not recover.[63] At some point, many NYHA class-IV heart failure patients will become candidates for palliative care.[92] The primary aim of palliative care is symptom management. Symptom-management strategies are deployed to emphasize relief from suffering. Fundamental to all symptom-management strategies for heart failure is the optimization of medications according to current guidelines. The most common symptoms of advanced heart failure are dyspnea, pain, and fatigue.[92]

Nursing Management

Nursing management of the patient with heart failure incorporates a variety of nursing diagnoses (see Nursing Diagnosis Priorities box on Acute Heart Failure). **Nursing priorities focus on (1) optimizing cardiopulmonary function, (2) promoting comfort and emotional support, (3) monitoring the effectiveness of pharmacological therapy, (4) providing adequate nutritional intake, and (5) providing patient education.**

Optimizing Cardiopulmonary Function

The patient's ECG is evaluated for any dysrhythmias that may be present or may develop as a result of drug toxicity or electrolyte imbalance. Patients with heart failure are prone to digoxin toxicity because of decreased renal perfusion; they are also prone to electrolyte imbalances. Breath sounds are auscultated frequently to determine the adequacy of respiratory effort and to assess for onset or worsening of pulmonary congestion. Oxygen through a nasal cannula is administered to relieve dyspnea. Diuretics or vasodilators are used to decrease excessive preload and afterload.[75,88] If the patient is not hypotensive, morphine may be administered to decrease hyperventilation and anxiety. If the patient's ventilatory status worsens, the nurse must be prepared for endotracheal intubation and mechanical ventilation. Obtaining daily weights is important until the weight stabilizes at a "dry" weight. Generally, the daily weight is used in fluid management and a weekly weight is optimally used for tracking body weight (e.g., muscle, fat).

Promoting Comfort and Emotional Support

During periods of breathlessness, activity must be restricted. Bed rest is usually prescribed for the patient, who is positioned with the head of the bed elevated to allow for maximal lung expansion. The arms can be supported on pillows so that no undue stress is placed on the shoulder muscles. The legs may be placed in a dependent position to encourage venous pooling, thereby decreasing venous return. Rest periods must be carefully planned and adhered to while independence within the patient's activity prescription is fostered. Vital signs are recorded before an activity is begun and after it is completed. Signs of activity intolerance, such as dyspnea, fatigue, sustained increase in pulse, and onset of dysrhythmias, are documented and reported to the physician. Activity is gradually increased according to the patient's tolerance. Skin breakdown is a risk because of the combination of bed rest, inadequate nutrition, peripheral edema, and decreased perfusion to the skin and subcutaneous tissue. Frequent position changes and mobilization can help to provide comfort and prevent this complication.

Monitoring the Effects of Pharmacological Therapy

Patients experiencing acute heart failure require aggressive pharmacological therapy.[82,88,93,94] The nurse must know the action, side effects, therapeutic levels, and toxic effects of the diuretics and vasodilators used to decrease preload, the positive inotropic agents used to increase ventricular contractility, the vasodilators used to decrease afterload, and any antidysrhythmics used to control heart rate and prevent dysrhythmias. The patient's hemodynamic response to these agents is closely monitored. Fluid intake and output balances are tabulated daily or even hourly in the critical care unit.

Providing Adequate Nutritional Intake

Patients experiencing heart failure often have decreased appetite and nausea, and small, frequent meals may be more appropriate than the standard three large meals. Food must be as tasty as possible; favorite foods and food from home may be incorporated into the diet as long as the foods are compatible with nutritional restrictions such as low levels of sodium to decrease the risk of fluid retention. Each patient must be assessed for nutritional imbalance individually. Some people with heart failure are well nourished, some are obese, and some are malnourished before they enter the hospital.

Providing Patient Education

The nurse assesses the patient's and family's understanding of the pathophysiology and individual risk-factor profile for heart failure.[95] Primary topics of education include the importance of a low-salt diet, daily weight, fluid restrictions, and written information about the multiple medications used to control the symptoms of heart failure.[63,96] Many patients with a diagnosis of heart failure also require education about lifestyle changes such as smoking cessation, weight loss, energy conservation, and how to incorporate exercise and sodium restriction into their daily lives.[74,97,98] Achieving the optimal outcomes for the patient with heart failure requires contributions from a team of educated health care clinicians.[63,74,97,98] Collaborative multidisciplinary goals, developed from clinical practice guidelines for management of the patient with symptoms of heart failure, are listed in the Evidence-Based Collaborative Practice box on Heart Failure.

CARDIOMYOPATHY

Description and Etiology

Cardiomyopathy is a disease of the heart muscle: *cardio* (heart), *myo* (muscle), and *pathy* (pathology). Cardiomyopathies are classified on the basis of structural abnormalities and, if known, genotype. The cardiomyopathic categories are hypertrophic, restrictive, and dilated, as illustrated in Figure 12-16.

Hypertrophic Obstructive Cardiomyopathy

Hypertrophic cardiomyopathy (HCM) is a genetically inherited disease that affects the myocardial sarcomere.[99-102] As HCM progresses, the left ventricle becomes stiff, noncompliant, and hypertrophied, sometimes in an asymmetric fashion.[99] HCM occurs in two forms. A well-known, but less frequent, manifestation is a stiff, noncompliant myocardial muscle with left ventricular hypertrophy and bizarre cellular hypertrophy of the upper ventricular septum. This left ventricular septal hypertrophy obstructs outflow through the aortic valve, especially during exercise (see Figure 12-16, *A*). It also pulls the papillary muscle out of alignment, causing mitral regurgitation. This form of HCM was previously known as idiopathic hypertrophic subaortic stenosis (IHSS); however, because IHSS does not describe all patients with hypertrophied hearts, the more general term of HCM is now used.[99] Other patients with HCM have generalized left ventricular hypertrophy, but the septum is not more enlarged than the rest of the myocardium.[99] HCM causes significant diastolic dysfunction because the muscle-bound, stiff, noncompliant heart muscle cannot fill adequately during diastole.

Two advances in diagnostic medicine have propelled understanding of the differences between these two forms of HCM. Two-dimensional transthoracic echocardiography (TTE) is often useful as the first diagnostic test to identify HCM.[99] TTE enables visualization of the septal anatomy, septal movement, and ventricular wall thickness and motion. The second advance is diagnostic genetics. Genetic testing for HCM usually is performed at a center with expertise in this area.[99] HCM is inherited as an autosomal dominant trait, and the clinical expression is caused by mutations in any of one of 10 genes. Each different gene encodes different protein components of the myocardial sarcomere.[99] Genetic analysis is an expanding research area that will help clarify diagnosis and treatment options for this cardiomyopathy.[101]

Symptoms are similar to those seen with heart failure plus the symptoms of myocardial ischemia, supraventricular tachycardia (SVT), VT syncope, and stroke. Symptoms usually are more intense with physical exercise, especially in the obstructive form of HCM, in which the aortic outflow tract is obstructed by the enlarged left ventricular septum. Because there is a known association between HCM and SCD, limitation of physical activity may be recommended. Causes of SCD are thought to stem from ventricular dysrhythmias and atrial fibrillation.[99] Episodes of paroxysmal atrial fibrillation occur in 20% to 25% of HCM patients.[99] The atrial dysrhythmias are related to increased age and atrial enlargement.[99] Pharmacological management includes beta-blockers to decrease left ventricular workload, medications to control and prevent atrial and ventricular dysrhythmias, anticoagulation if atrial fibrillation or left ventricular thrombi are present, and drugs to manage heart failure. Interventional procedures include insertion of an ICD to decrease the risk of SCD, and percutaneous alcohol ablation of the intraventricular septum

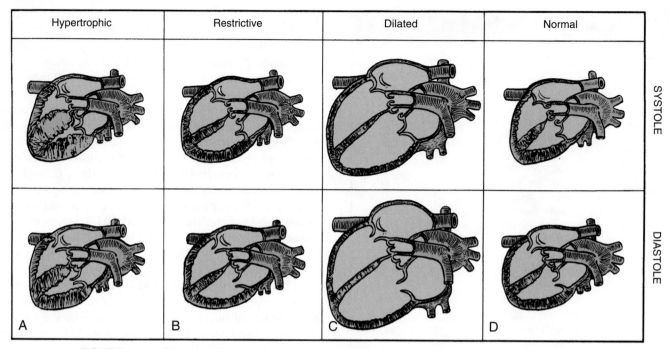

Hypertrophic	Restrictive	Dilated	Normal	
				SYSTOLE
A	B	C	D	DIASTOLE

FIGURE 12-16 Types of Cardiomyopathies and Differences in Ventricular Diameter during Systole and Diastole Compared with a Normal Heart. *A,* Hypertrophic. *B,* Restrictive. *C,* Dilated. *D,* Normal.

to decrease the size of the septal wall.[99,102] Surgical procedures such as septal myectomy and mitral valve replacement are options used less frequently than in the past.[99]

Dilated Cardiomyopathy

Dilated cardiomyopathy is characterized by gross dilation of both ventricles without muscle hypertrophy (see Figure 12-16, *C*). There are several distinct causes of dilated cardiomyopathy. It is estimated that 30% of patients with dilated cardiomyopathy may have a genetic cause.[63]

Ischemic Dilated Cardiomyopathy. Ischemic dilated cardiomyopathy results from repeated myocardial injury or infarction caused by the sequelae of CAD. It is the most common cause of dilated cardiomyopathy in the United States. Signs and symptoms of systolic heart failure and a low ejection fraction are present.

Familial Dilated Cardiomyopathy. When the cause of the dilated cardiomyopathy is unknown, it is called idiopathic. In some cases, the occurrence is linked to genetic inheritance. Scientific advances in molecular genetics permit detailed studies of families with a high incidence of dilated cardiomyopathy. It is estimated that 10% to 50% of familial idiopathic dilated cardiomyopathy cases reflect genetic transmission.[103-105] In affected families, various genetic mutations occur in the gene that codes for the sarcomere contractile protein in the heart. The heritable trait can be expressed as an autosomal dominant or recessive inheritance pattern.[103-105] Preliminary research indicates that the genetic picture is highly individual for different family groups, even if the clinical picture appears similar.[103-105]

Other Causes of Dilated Cardiomyopathy. There are many other nonischemic, nongenetic known causes of dilated cardiomyopathy. Injury can be caused by valvular heart dysfunction that has placed extreme pressure or volume on the chambers, and viral or bacterial infections such as myocarditis can lead to inflammatory changes that permanently remodel the heart.[106] Other noncardiac causes include infiltration by systemic collagens as in amyloidosis or sarcoidosis.[107]

In dilated cardiomyopathy, the myocardial muscle fibers contract poorly, resulting in global left ventricular dysfunction, low cardiac output, atrial and ventricular dysrhythmias, blood pooling that leads to ventricular thrombi and embolic episodes, refractory heart failure, and premature death. The goals of the medical management of dilated cardiomyopathy are similar to those for systolic heart failure: improvement of pump function, removal of excess fluid, control of heart failure symptoms, anticipation and management of complications, and prevention of SCD.

Restrictive Cardiomyopathy

Restrictive cardiomyopathy is the least commonly encountered cardiomyopathy in industrialized societies (see Figure 12-16, *B*). As with the other cardiomyopathies, this form can be idiopathic or can have a known cause.[108,109] Restrictive cardiomyopathy results in ventricular wall rigidity as a consequence of myocardial fibrosis. The overall effect is the diastolic inhibition of ventricular filling. Diastolic heart failure, low cardiac output, dyspnea, orthopnea, and liver engorgement are the most common clinical manifestations of restrictive cardiomyopathy. Medical management includes beta-blockers to slow the heart rate and allow more time for ventricular filling, diuretics to remove excess fluid, and a low-sodium diet.

Nursing Management

Nursing management of the patient with cardiomyopathy incorporates a variety of nursing diagnoses related to the symptoms of heart failure. These nursing diagnoses are reviewed in the Nursing Diagnosis Priorities box on Cardiomyopathy. **Nursing priorities are individualized according to the type of cardiomyopathy and heart failure and focus on (1) achieving a stable fluid balance, (2) monitoring the effects of pharmacological therapy, (3) safely increasing mobility, and (4) providing patient and family education.** As with heart failure, a collaborative team of compassionate, knowledgeable professionals is required to provide effective care and education for these challenging patients.[96]

NURSING DIAGNOSIS PRIORITIES

Cardiomyopathy

- Decreased Cardiac Output related to alterations in preload, p. A-10
- Decreased Cardiac Output related to alterations in afterload, p. A-10
- Decreased Cardiac Output related to alterations in contractility, p. A-11
- Decreased Cardiac Output related to alterations in heart rate or rhythm, p. A-11
- Impaired Gas Exchange related to ventilation/perfusion mismatch or intrapulmonary shunting, p. A-23
- Activity Intolerance related to cardiopulmonary dysfunction, p. A-1
- Anxiety related to threat to biological, psychological, or social integrity, p. A-7
- Powerlessness related to lack of control over current situation or disease progression, p. A-33
- Deficient Knowledge: Discharge Regimen related to lack of previous exposure to information, p. A-15

VALVULAR HEART DISEASE

Description and Etiology

Valvular heart disease describes structural and functional abnormalities of single or multiple cardiac valves. The result is an alteration in blood flow across the valve. The two types of valvular lesions are stenotic and regurgitant. These are described with reference to the specific cardiac valves involved.

Usually, if a person is admitted to the critical care unit with valve disease, he or she is experiencing acute heart failure or is being admitted for cardiac surgical valvular replacement. In the past in the United States, most valvular lesions were rheumatic in origin, and damage was a direct result of group A β-hemolytic streptococcal pharyngitis. As a result of aggressive treatment of "strep throat," this has become a rare problem, and older patients now are more likely to be seen with symptoms of heart failure and degenerative valve changes. These changes may be described as myxomatous leaflet degeneration or annular calcification.[110,111]

Pathophysiology

Mitral Valve Stenosis

Mitral valve stenosis describes a progressive narrowing of the mitral valve orifice. Primary cause is rheumatic endocarditis with rare occurrences related to congenital malformations. Mitral stenosis occurs in twice as many women as men.[111] Symptoms occur when the normal valve size is reduced to 2 cm^2 or less. Symptoms occur at rest when the valve area is reduced below 1 cm^2.[111] Narrowing is caused by aging valve tissue or by acute rheumatic valvulitis (Table 12-8, *A*). The diffuse valve leaflets fibrose and fuse, reducing mobility and thickening the chordae tendineae. As a result, the mitral valve can no longer open or close passively in response to left atrial and ventricular pressure changes. Blood flow across the valve is impeded. Mitral stenosis increases the risk of developing atrial fibrillation because of the high pressures in the left atrium that will stimulate left atrial remodeling and enlargement. Development of atrial fibrillation will significantly increase symptoms and may increase the need for surgical replacement of the valve.

Mitral Valve Regurgitation

Mitral valve regurgitation may result from rheumatic disease, aging of the valve, endocarditis, collagen vascular disease, or papillary muscle dysfunction[111] (see Table 12-8, *B*). In mitral regurgitation, the valve annulus, leaflets, chordae tendineae, and papillary muscles may all be dysfunctional, or the dysfunction may be isolated to just one component of the valve. Mitral valve regurgitation results in retrograde flow of blood into the left atrium with each ventricular contraction. It is always described as chronic or acute because of the very different impact on the left-sided chambers.

With chronic mitral valve regurgitation, the left atrium has dilated to accommodate the additional regurgitant volume, whereas the left ventricle has hypertrophied (increased muscle) to maintain an adequate stroke volume and cardiac output. In contrast, acute mitral valve regurgitation is precipitated by chordae tendineae or papillary muscle rupture resulting from an acute MI or infectious endocarditis.[111] This is a medical emergency. The left atrium cannot accommodate the sudden increase in volume and pressure, and use of an IABP and inotropic drug support is often required to increase forward output and reduce pulmonary congestion. After the patient's condition has stabilized, surgical replacement or repair of the incompetent valve is performed.[111]

Aortic Valve Stenosis

Aortic valve stenosis describes a narrowing of the aortic valve area. It can result from aging, rheumatic valvulitis, or deterioration of a congenital bicuspid valve[111] (see Table 12-8, *C*). The pathological hallmarks are inflammation, fibrous valvular thickening, and tissue calcification. When the aortic valvular opening is reduced to less than 1.5 cm^2, the condition is classified as mild. Cardiac catheterization or Doppler

TABLE 12-8 VALVULAR DYSFUNCTION

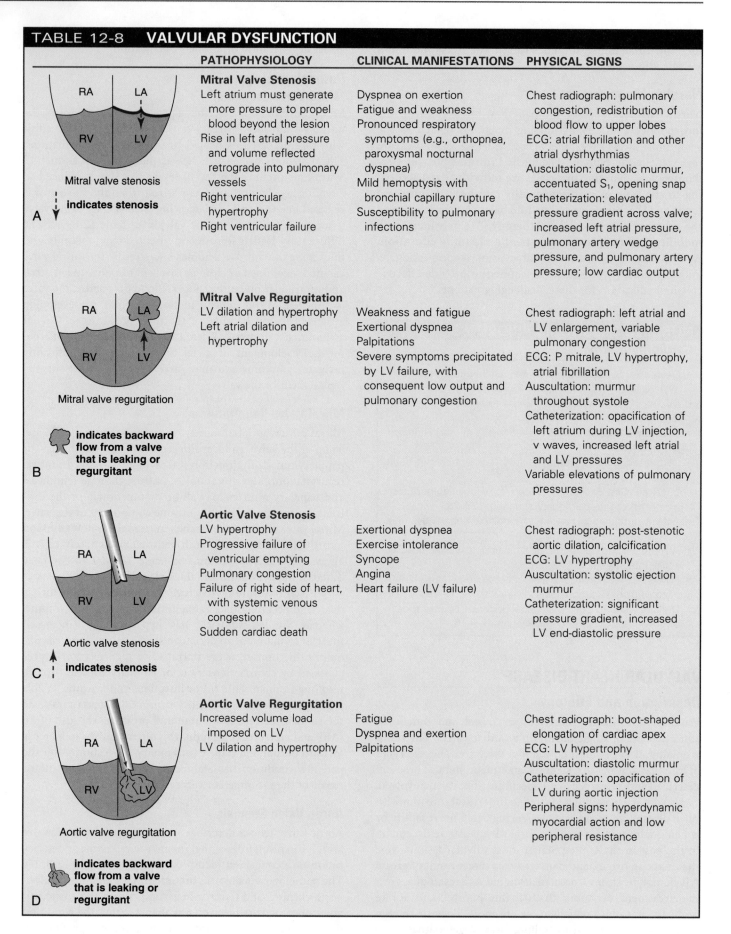

	PATHOPHYSIOLOGY	CLINICAL MANIFESTATIONS	PHYSICAL SIGNS
Mitral Valve Stenosis	Left atrium must generate more pressure to propel blood beyond the lesion Rise in left atrial pressure and volume reflected retrograde into pulmonary vessels Right ventricular hypertrophy Right ventricular failure	Dyspnea on exertion Fatigue and weakness Pronounced respiratory symptoms (e.g., orthopnea, paroxysmal nocturnal dyspnea) Mild hemoptysis with bronchial capillary rupture Susceptibility to pulmonary infections	Chest radiograph: pulmonary congestion, redistribution of blood flow to upper lobes ECG: atrial fibrillation and other atrial dysrhythmias Auscultation: diastolic murmur, accentuated S_1, opening snap Catheterization: elevated pressure gradient across valve; increased left atrial pressure, pulmonary artery wedge pressure, and pulmonary artery pressure; low cardiac output
Mitral Valve Regurgitation	LV dilation and hypertrophy Left atrial dilation and hypertrophy	Weakness and fatigue Exertional dyspnea Palpitations Severe symptoms precipitated by LV failure, with consequent low output and pulmonary congestion	Chest radiograph: left atrial and LV enlargement, variable pulmonary congestion ECG: P mitrale, LV hypertrophy, atrial fibrillation Auscultation: murmur throughout systole Catheterization: opacification of left atrium during LV injection, v waves, increased left atrial and LV pressures Variable elevations of pulmonary pressures
Aortic Valve Stenosis	LV hypertrophy Progressive failure of ventricular emptying Pulmonary congestion Failure of right side of heart, with systemic venous congestion Sudden cardiac death	Exertional dyspnea Exercise intolerance Syncope Angina Heart failure (LV failure)	Chest radiograph: post-stenotic aortic dilation, calcification ECG: LV hypertrophy Auscultation: systolic ejection murmur Catheterization: significant pressure gradient, increased LV end-diastolic pressure
Aortic Valve Regurgitation	Increased volume load imposed on LV LV dilation and hypertrophy	Fatigue Dyspnea and exertion Palpitations	Chest radiograph: boot-shaped elongation of cardiac apex ECG: LV hypertrophy Auscultation: diastolic murmur Catheterization: opacification of LV during aortic injection Peripheral signs: hyperdynamic myocardial action and low peripheral resistance

A Mitral valve stenosis — ↓ indicates stenosis

B Mitral valve regurgitation — indicates backward flow from a valve that is leaking or regurgitant

C Aortic valve stenosis — ↑ indicates stenosis

D Aortic valve regurgitation — indicates backward flow from a valve that is leaking or regurgitant

TABLE 12-8 VALVULAR DYSFUNCTION—cont'd

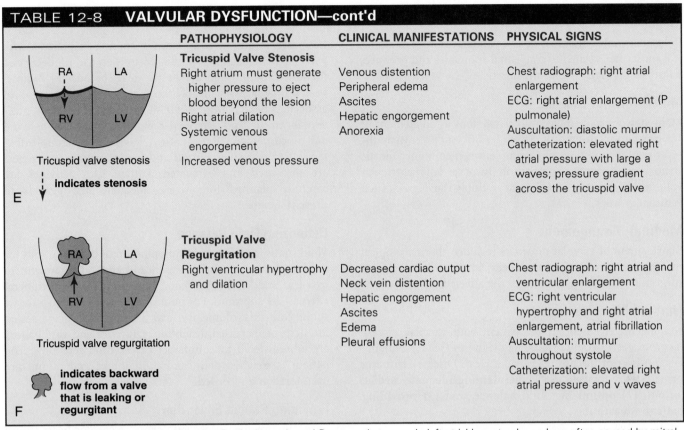

	PATHOPHYSIOLOGY	CLINICAL MANIFESTATIONS	PHYSICAL SIGNS
E	**Tricuspid Valve Stenosis** Right atrium must generate higher pressure to eject blood beyond the lesion Right atrial dilation Systemic venous engorgement Increased venous pressure	Venous distention Peripheral edema Ascites Hepatic engorgement Anorexia	Chest radiograph: right atrial enlargement ECG: right atrial enlargement (P pulmonale) Auscultation: diastolic murmur Catheterization: elevated right atrial pressure with large a waves; pressure gradient across the tricuspid valve
F	**Tricuspid Valve Regurgitation** Right ventricular hypertrophy and dilation	Decreased cardiac output Neck vein distention Hepatic engorgement Ascites Edema Pleural effusions	Chest radiograph: right atrial and ventricular enlargement ECG: right ventricular hypertrophy and right atrial enlargement, atrial fibrillation Auscultation: murmur throughout systole Catheterization: elevated right atrial pressure and v waves

ECG, electrocardiogram; *LV,* left ventricular; *P mitrale,* m-shaped P waves that occur in left atrial hypertrophy and are often caused by mitral stenosis; *P pulmonale,* tall, peaked P waves that occur in right atrial hypertrophy and are often caused by chronic pulmonary disease.

echocardiography can identify a gradient of less than 25 mm Hg across the valve.[112] The gradient represents the difference in systolic pressure between the left ventricle and the aorta. A significant pressure difference is a diagnostic hallmark of valvular stenosis. If the valve orifice has narrowed to 1 cm² or less, the gradient will be greater than 40 mm Hg, and the diagnosis will be upgraded to severe aortic valve stenosis.[111] The impedance of left ventricular ejection into the aorta results in increased left ventricular systolic pressure, left ventricular hypertrophy, and eventually left ventricular dilation. When symptoms such as angina, dyspnea, syncope, and other indicators of heart failure develop, it is critical to intervene to prevent further damage to the left ventricle. Aortic valve replacement is usually indicated. Balloon valvotomy (dilation) may be an option for carefully selected patients with aortic stenosis without calcification, or for patients whose mortality risk during surgical aortic valve replacement is unacceptably high.[111,112]

Aortic Valve Regurgitation

Aortic regurgitation, also known as aortic insufficiency, can occur as a result of rheumatic fever, systemic hypertension, Marfan syndrome, syphilis, rheumatoid arthritis, aging valve tissue, or discrete subaortic stenosis (see Table 12-8, D). Aortic valve incompetence results in a reflux of blood back into the left ventricle during ventricular diastole. To accommodate this extra volume, the left ventricle initially dilates and then hypertrophies in an attempt to empty more completely and to meet the needs of the peripheral circulation. Aortic valve replacement is recommended for symptomatic patients with well-preserved or moderate left ventricular dysfunction.[111]

Tricuspid Valve Stenosis

Tricuspid valve stenosis is rarely an isolated lesion (see Table 12-8, E). It often occurs in conjunction with mitral or aortic disease. Its origin most often is rheumatic fever or a complication of intravenous drug abuse and resultant endocarditis.[111] Tricuspid valve stenosis increases the pressure work of the usually low-pressure right atrium, resulting in right atrial hypertrophy. The right atrium dilates in an attempt to accommodate the residual right atrial volume and the incoming venous return. As a result, systemic venous congestion occurs—the consequences of which include jugular venous congestion, liver failure, hepatomegaly, ascites, and peripheral edema.

Tricuspid Valve Regurgitation

Tricuspid valve regurgitation usually results from advanced failure of the left side of the heart that eventually affects the right side of the heart, severe pulmonary hypertension, or as a complication of infectious endocarditis[111] (see Table 12-8, F).

Pulmonic Valve Disease

Pulmonary valve disease is not a common disorder in adults. It is most often related to congenital anomalies and produces failure of the right side of the heart.

Mixed Valvular Lesions

Many persons have mixed valvular lesions as an element of stenosis and regurgitation. Mixed lesions can accentuate the severity of a condition. For example, when combined, aortic stenosis and aortic regurgitation increase left ventricular volume and pressure and thereby multiply the degree of left ventricular work.

Medical Management

Management of valvular disorders includes pharmacological therapy to control symptoms of heart failure and then cardiac surgical repair or replacement of the affected valve.[111]

Nursing Management

Nursing management of the patient with valvular disease incorporates a variety of nursing diagnoses (see the Nursing Diagnosis Priorities box on Valvular Heart Disease). **Nursing priorities are focused on (1) maintaining adequate cardiac output, (2) optimizing fluid balance, and (3) providing patient education.**

NURSING DIAGNOSIS PRIORITIES

Valvular Heart Disease

- Decreased Cardiac Output related to alterations in preload, p. A-10
- Decreased Cardiac Output related to alterations in afterload, p. A-10
- Decreased Cardiac Output related to alterations in contractility, p. A-11
- Decreased Cardiac Output related to alterations in heart rate or rhythm, p. A-11
- Activity Intolerance related to cardiopulmonary dysfunction, p. A-1
- Deficient Knowledge: Discharge Regimen related to lack of previous exposure to information, p. A-15

Maintaining Cardiac Output

Low cardiac output is a common finding in patients with valvular heart disease. It can occur because of decreased forward flow through a stenotic valve, because of bidirectional flow across an incompetent valve, or because of associated heart failure. Vital signs and the effect of positive inotropic and afterload-reducing agents are assessed and documented. If the patient has hemodynamic catheters inserted, cardiac output and hemodynamic parameters are measured and evaluated. Patient care activities are carefully planned to provide adequate rest periods to prevent fatigue.

Optimizing Fluid Balance

Fluid status is evaluated by auscultation of breath sounds for crackles, heart sounds for presence of an S_3, daily weights to trend a "sudden weight gain," and presence of peripheral edema. The appearance of pulmonary crackles or an S_3 heart sound confirms volume overload. The jugular vein is assessed for signs of increased distention. Diuretics and vasodilators are administered to counteract excess fluid retention. The patient is weighed daily, and fluid intake and output are monitored and recorded.

Providing Patient Education

Education for the patient with acute or chronic heart failure caused by valvular dysfunction includes: (1) information related to diet, (2) fluid restrictions, (3) the actions and side effects of heart failure medications, (4) the need for prophylactic antibiotics before undergoing any invasive procedures such as dental work, and (5) when to call the health care provider to report a negative change in cardiac symptoms. Many patients also require information about valvular heart surgery. Achieving the optimal outcomes for the patient with valve disease requires contributions from a team of educated health care clinicians. Collaborative multidisciplinary priorities are listed in the box Evidence-Based Collaborative Practice: Valvular Heart Disease. The heart valve replacement section in Chapter 13 provides more information on surgical management.

EVIDENCE-BASED COLLABORATIVE PRACTICE

Valvular Heart Disease

Class I recommendations with strong evidence are provided.

Recommendations for Detection and Surveillance of Valvular Disease by Echocardiography
- Echocardiography is noninvasive and is used for all initial diagnosis and serial follow-up evaluations.

Recommendations for Aortic Stenosis
- Echocardiography is the primary diagnostic tool.
- Coronary arteriography is used before AVR if CAD is suspected.

- AVR recommended for symptomatic patients with severe AS; AVR can be combined with CABG surgery when CAD is present.

Recommendations for Aortic Regurgitation
- Echocardiography is the primary diagnostic tool.
- Cardiac catheterization is used if noninvasive tests are inconclusive.
- AVR is indicated for symptomatic patients with severe AR irrespective of LV systolic function.

EVIDENCE-BASED COLLABORATIVE PRACTICE—cont'd

Valvular Heart Disease

- AVR is indicated for nonsymptomatic patients with severe AR with LV systolic dysfunction (ejection fraction < 0.5 [50%]); AVR can be combined with CABG surgery if CAD is present.

Recommendations for Mitral Stenosis
- Echocardiography is the primary diagnostic tool.
- Anticoagulation is indicated in MS patients with atrial fibrillation (paroxysmal, persistent, or permanent) and for MS patients in sinus rhythm with a prior embolic event or left atrial thrombus.
- Cardiac catheterization if noninvasive tests are inconclusive

- Mitral valve repair (preferable), or mitral valve replacement is indicated for symptomatic (NYHA functional class III or IV) moderate or severe MS if percutaneous mitral balloon valvotomy is contraindicated.

Recommendations for Mitral Regurgitation
- Echocardiography is the primary diagnostic tool.
- Cardiac catheterization if noninvasive tests are inconclusive or if additional hemodynamic measurements are required.
- Mitral valve repair is the operation of choice over valve replacement in most patients with chronic MR.

Data from Bonow RO, et al: 2008 focused update incorporated into the ACC/AHA 2006 guidelines for the management of patients with valvular heart disease, *Circulation* 118(15):e523, 2008; Nishimura RA, et al: ACC/AHA guideline update on valvular heart disease: focused update on infective endocarditis, *Circulation* 118(8):887, 2008; *AR*, aortic regurgitation; *AS*, aortic stenosis; *AVR*, aortic valve replacement; *CABG*, coronary bypass graft; *CAD*, coronary valve disease; *IE*, infective endocarditis; *LV*, left ventricular; *MR*, mitral regurgitation; *MS*, mitral stenosis; *NYHA*, New York Heart Association.

REFERENCES

1. American Heart Association: *Heart disease & stroke statistics – 2010 update-at-a-glance (website)*, Dallas, 2010, American Heart Association. www.americanheart.org/downloadable/heart/1265665152970DS-3241%20HeartStrokeUpdate_2010.pdf. Accessed January 2011.
2. Antman EM, et al: 2007 Focused update of the ACC/AHA 2004 guidelines for the management of patients with ST-Elevation Myocardial Infarction: a report of the American College of Cardiology/American Heart Association Task Force on Practice Guidelines; developed in collaboration with the Canadian Cardiovascular Society endorsed by the American Academy of Family Physicians: 2007 Writing Group to Review New Evidence and Update the ACC/AHA 2004 Guidelines for the Management of Patients with ST-Elevation Myocardial Infarction, writing on behalf of the 2004 Writing Committee, *Circulation* 117(2):296, 2008.
3. Fraker TD, et al: 2007 Chronic angina focused update of the ACC/AHA 2002 guidelines for the management of patients with chronic stable angina: a report of the American College of Cardiology/American Heart Association Task Force on Practice Guidelines Writing Group to develop the focused update of the 2002 guidelines for the management of patients with chronic stable angina, *J Am Coll Cardiol* 50(23):2264, 2007.
4. Yusuf S, et al, INTERHEART Study Investigators: Effect of potentially modifiable risk factors associated with myocardial infarction in 52 countries (The INTERHEART Study): case-control study, *Lancet* 364(9438):937, 2004.
5. Anderson JL, et al: ACC/AHA 2007 guidelines for the management of patients with unstable angina/non-ST-elevation myocardial infarction: a report of the American College of Cardiology/American Heart Association Task Force on Practice Guidelines (Writing Committee to Revise the 2002 Guidelines for the Management of Patients with Unstable Angina/Non-ST-Elevation Myocardial Infarction), *J Am Coll Cardiol* 50(7):e1, 2007.
6. Gibbons RJ, et al: ACC/AHA 2002 guideline update for the management of patients with chronic stable angina – summary article: a report of the American College of Cardiology/American Heart Association Task Force on Practice Guidelines (Committee on the Management of Patients with Chronic Stable Angina), *Circulation* 107(1):149, 2003.
7. Expert Panel on Detection, Evaluation, and Treatment of High Blood Cholesterol in Adults: Executive summary of the third report of the National Cholesterol Education Program (NCEP) Expert Panel on Detection, Evaluation, and Treatment of High Blood Cholesterol in Adults (Adult Treatment Panel III), *JAMA* 285(19):2486, 2001.
8. Grundy SM, et al: Implications of recent clinical trials for the National Cholesterol Education Program Adult Treatment Panel III guidelines, *Circulation* 110(2):227, 2004.
9. Barter PJ, et al: Antiinflammatory properties of HDL, *Circ Res* 95(8):764, 2004.
10. O'Keefe JH Jr, et al: Optimal low-density lipoprotein is 50 to 70 mg/dL: lower is better and physiologically normal, *J Am Coll Cardiol* 43(11):2142, 2004.
11. Futterman LG, Lemberg L: Lp(a) lipoprotein: an independent risk factor for coronary heart disease after menopause, *Am J Crit Care* 10(1):63, 2001.
12. Jensen MK, et al: Obesity, behavioral lifestyle factors, and risk of acute coronary events, *Circulation* 117(24):3062, 2008.
13. Chobanian AV, et al: Seventh report of the Joint National Committee on Prevention, Detection, Evaluation, and Treatment of High Blood Pressure, *Hypertension* 42(6):1206, 2003.
14. Thompson PD, et al: Exercise and physical activity in the prevention and treatment of atherosclerotic cardiovascular disease: a statement from the Council on Clinical Cardiology (Subcommittee on Exercise, Rehabilitation, and Prevention) and the Council on Nutrition, Physical Activity, and Metabolism (Subcommittee on Physical Activity), *Circulation* 107(24):3109, 2003.
15. Brook RD, et al: Air pollution and cardiovascular disease: a statement for healthcare professionals from the Expert Panel on Population and Prevention Science of the American Heart Association, *Circulation* 109(21):2655, 2004.

16. Sargent RP, et al: Reduced incidence of admissions for myocardial infarction associated with public smoking ban: before and after study, *BMJ* 328(7446):977, 2004.

17. Houterman S, et al: Smoking, blood pressure and serum cholesterol-effects on 20-year mortality, *Epidemiology* 14(1):24, 2003.

18. Garber AJ, et al: American College of Endocrinology position statement on inpatient diabetes and metabolic control, *Endocr Pract* 10(1):77, 2004.

19. McGuire DK, et al: Association of diabetes mellitus and glycemic control strategies with clinical outcomes after acute coronary syndromes, *Am Heart J* 147(2):246, 2004.

20. Franklin K, et al: Implications of diabetes in patients with acute coronary syndromes. The Global Registry of Acute Coronary Events, *Arch Intern Med* 164(13):1457, 2004.

21. Sarnak MJ, et al: Kidney disease as a risk factor for development of cardiovascular disease: a statement from the American Heart Association Councils on Kidney in Cardiovascular Disease, High Blood Pressure Research, Clinical Cardiology, and Epidemiology and Prevention, *Hypertension* 42(5):1050, 2003.

22. Wright RS, et al: Acute myocardial infarction and renal dysfunction: a high-risk combination, *Ann Intern Med* 137(7):563, 2002.

23. Hedley AJ, et al: Impact of chronic kidney disease on patient outcome following cardiac surgery, *Heart Lung Circ* 19(8):453, 2010.

24. Grundy SM, et al: Clinical management of metabolic syndrome: report of the American Heart Association/ National Heart, Lung, and Blood Institute/American Diabetes Association conference on scientific issues related to management, *Circulation* 109(4):551, 2004.

25. Grady D, et al: Cardiovascular disease outcomes during 6.8 years of hormone therapy: Heart and Estrogen/progestin Replacement Study follow-up (HERS II), *JAMA* 288(1):49, 2002.

26. Hulley S, et al: Randomized trial of estrogen plus progestin for secondary prevention of coronary heart disease in postmenopausal women. Heart and Estrogen/progestin Replacement Study (HERS) Research Group, *JAMA* 280(7):605, 1998.

27. Anderson GL, et al: Effects of conjugated equine estrogen in postmenopausal women with hysterectomy: the Women's Health Initiative randomized controlled trial, *JAMA* 291(14):1701, 2004.

28. Mosca L, et al: Evidence-based guidelines for cardiovascular disease prevention in women: 2007 update, *Circulation* 115(11):1481, 2007.

29. Lefler LL, Bondy KN: Women's delay in seeking treatment with myocardial infarction: a meta synthesis, *J Cardiovasc Nurs* 19(4):251, 2004.

30. Pearson TA, et al: Markers of inflammation and cardiovascular disease: application to clinical and public health practice: a statement for healthcare professionals from the Centers for Disease Control and Prevention and the American Heart Association, *Circulation* 107(3):499, 2003.

31. Speidl WS, et al: High-sensitivity C-reactive protein in the prediction of coronary events in patients with premature coronary artery disease, *Am Heart J* 144(3):449, 2002.

32. Buffon A, et al: Widespread coronary inflammation in unstable angina, *N Engl J Med* 347(1):5, 2002.

33. King SB 3rd, et al: 2007 Focused update of the ACC/AHA/ SCAI 2005 guideline update for percutaneous coronary intervention: a report of the American College of Cardiology/American Heart Association Task Force on Practice Guidelines, 2007 Writing Group to Review New Evidence and Update the ACC/AHA/SCAI 2005 Guideline Update for Percutaneous Coronary Intervention, writing on behalf of the 2005 Writing Committee, *J Am Coll Cardiol* 51(2):172, 2008.

34. McSweeney JC, et al: Women's early warning symptoms of acute myocardial infarction, *Circulation* 108(21):2619, 2003.

35. Bairey Merz N, et al: Women's ischemic syndrome evaluation: current status and future research directions. Report of the National Heart, Lung and Blood Institute workshop, October 2-4, 2002: executive summary, *Circulation* 109(6):805, 2004.

36. Canto JG, et al: Use of emergency medical services in acute myocardial infarction and subsequent quality of care: observations from the National Registry of Myocardial Infarction 2, *Circulation* 106(24):3018, 2002.

37. Jacobs AK, et al: Cardiogenic shock caused by right ventricular infarction: a report from the SHOCK registry, *J Am Coll Cardiol* 41(8):1273, 2003.

38. Lanza M: Right ventricular myocardial infarction: when the power fails, *Dimens Crit Care Nurs* 21(4):122, 2002.

39. Mehta RH, et al: Comparison of outcomes of patients with acute coronary syndromes with and without atrial fibrillation, *Am J Cardiol* 92(9):1031, 2003.

40. Birnbaum Y, et al: Ventricular septal rupture after acute myocardial infarction, *N Engl J Med* 347(18):1426, 2002.

41. Crenshaw BS, et al: Risk factors, angiographic patterns, and outcomes in patients with ventricular septal defect complicating acute myocardial infarction. GUSTO-I (Global Utilization of Streptokinase and TPA for Occluded Coronary Arteries) Trial Investigators, *Circulation* 101(1):27, 2000.

42. Deja MA, et al: Post infarction ventricular septal defect – can we do better? *Eur J Cardiothorac Surg* 18(2):194, 2000.

43. Birnbaum Y, et al: Mitral regurgitation following acute myocardial infarction, *Coron Artery Dis* 13(6):337, 2002.

44. Maisch B, et al: Guidelines on the diagnosis and management of pericardial diseases executive summary: the Task Force on the Diagnosis and Management of Pericardial Diseases of the European Society of Cardiology, *Eur Heart J* 25(7):587, 2004.

45. Wang K, et al: ST-segment elevation in conditions other than acute myocardial infarction, *N Engl J Med* 349(22):2128, 2003.

46. Paelinck B, Dendale PA: Images in clinical medicine: cardiac tamponade in Dressler's syndrome, *N Engl J Med* 348(23):e8, 2003.

47. Wu AH, et al: Hospital outcomes in patients presenting with congestive heart failure complicating acute myocardial infarction: a report from the Second National Registry of Myocardial Infarction (NRMI-2), *J Am Coll Cardiol* 40(8):1389, 2002.

48. Szekendi MK: Compliance with acute MI guidelines lowers inpatient mortality, *J Cardiovasc Nurs* 18(5):356, 2003.

49. Eagle KA, et al: Adherence to evidence-based therapies after discharge for acute coronary syndromes: an ongoing prospective, observational study, *Am J Med* 117(2):73, 2004.

50. Crespo EM, et al: Evaluation and management of thrombocytopenia and suspected heparin-induced

thrombocytopenia in hospitalized patients: The Complications after Thrombocytopenia Caused by Heparin (CATCH) registry, *Am Heart J* 157(4):651, 2009.

51. Balady GJ, et al: Core components of cardiac rehabilitation/secondary prevention programs: a statement for healthcare professionals from the American Heart Association and the American Association of Cardiovascular and Pulmonary Rehabilitation Writing Group, *Circulation* 102(9):1069, 2000.

52. Fox CS, et al: Temporal trends in coronary heart disease mortality and sudden cardiac death from 1950 to 1999: the Framingham Heart Study, *Circulation* 110(5):522, 2004.

53. Chugh SS, et al: Current burden of sudden cardiac death: multiple source surveillance versus retrospective death-certificate based review in a large U.S. community, *J Am Coll Cardiol* 44(6):1268, 2004.

54. Hallstrom AP, et al: Public-access defibrillation and survival after out-of-hospital cardiac arrest, *N Engl J Med* 351(7):637, 2004.

55. Priori SG, et al: Task Force on Sudden Cardiac Death of the European Society of Cardiology, *Eur Heart J* 22(16):1374, 2001.

56. Antzelevitch C, et al: Brugada syndrome: report of the second consensus conference: endorsed by the Heart Rhythm Society and the European Heart Rhythm Association, *Circulation* 111(5):659, 2005.

57. Goldberger JJ, et al: American Heart Association/American College of Cardiology Foundation/Heart Rhythm Society scientific statement on noninvasive risk stratification techniques for identifying patients at risk for sudden cardiac death: a scientific statement from the American Heart Association Council on Clinical Cardiology Committee on Electrocardiography and Arrhythmias and Council on Epidemiology and Prevention, *J Am Coll Cardiol* 52(14):1179, 2008.

58. Neumar RW, et al: Post-Cardiac Arrest Syndrome: Epidemiology, Pathophysiology, Treatment, and Prognostication A consensus statement from the International liaison Committee on Resuscitation, *Circulation* 118(23):2452, 2008.

59. Arrich J, et al: Hypothermia for neuroprotection in adults after cardiopulmonary resuscitation, *Cochrane Database Syst Rev* (4):CD004128, 2009.

60. Epstein AE, et al: ACC/AHA/HRS 2008 guideline for device-based therapy of cardiac rhythm abnormalities: a report of the American College of Cardiology/American Heart Association Task Force on Practice Guidelines (Writing Committee to Revise the ACC/AHA/NASPE 2002 Guideline Update for Implantation of Cardiac Pacemakers and Antiarrhythmic Devices) developed in collaboration with American Association for Thoracic Surgery and the Society of Thoracic Surgeons, *J Am Coll Cardiol* 51(21):e1, 2008.

61. Steinbeck G: Evolution of implantable cardioverter defibrillator indications: comparison of guidelines in the United States and Europe, *J Cardiovasc Electrophysiol* 13(suppl 1):S96, 2002.

62. Epstein AE: An update on implantable cardioverter-defibrillator guidelines, *Curr Opin Cardiol* 19(1):23, 2004.

63. Hunt SA, et al: 2009 focused update incorporated into the ACC/AHA 2005 guidelines for the diagnosis and management of heart failure in adults: a report of the American College of Cardiology/American Heart Association

Task Force on Practice Guidelines, *Circulation* 119(14):e391, 2009.

64. Zile MR, Brutsaert DL: New concepts in diastolic dysfunction and diastolic heart failure: Part I. Diagnosis, prognosis, and measurements of diastolic function, *Circulation* 105(11):1387, 2002.

65. Zile MR, Brutsaert DL: New concepts in diastolic dysfunction and diastolic heart failure: Part II. Causal mechanisms and treatment, *Circulation* 105(12):1503, 2002.

66. Henry LB: Left ventricular systolic dysfunction and ischemic cardiomyopathy, *Crit Care Nurs Q* 26(1):16, 2003.

67. Aurigemma GP, Gaasch WH: Clinical practice. Diastolic heart failure, *N Engl J Med* 351(11):1097, 2004.

68. Bolliger K, Sadar AM: Care and management of the patient with right heart failure secondary to diastolic dysfunction: an advanced practice perspective and case review, *Crit Care Nurs Q* 26(1):22, 2003.

69. Gradman AH, Wilson JT: Hypertension and diastolic heart failure, *Curr Cardiol Rep* 11(6):422, 2009.

70. Riedinger MS, et al: Quality of life in patients with heart failure: do gender differences exist? *Heart Lung* 30(2):105, 2001.

71. Thohan V, et al: Aldosterone antagonism and congestive heart failure: a new look at an old therapy, *Curr Opin Cardiol* 19(4):301, 2004.

72. Patten RD, Soman P: Prevention and reversal of LV remodeling with neurohormonal inhibitors, *Curr Treat Options Cardiovasc Med* 6(4):313, 2004.

73. Paul S: Balancing diuretic therapy in heart failure: loop diuretics, thiazides, and aldosterone antagonists, *Congest Heart Fail* 8(6):307, 2002.

74. Paul S: Ventricular remodeling, *Crit Care Nurs Clin North Am* 15(4):407, 2003.

75. Dimopoulos K, et al: Meta-analyses of mortality and morbidity effects of an angiotensin receptor blocker in patients with chronic heart failure already receiving an ACE inhibitor (alone or with a beta-blocker), *Int J Cardiol* 93(2-3):105, 2004.

76. McCullough PA, Sandberg KR: B-type natriuretic peptide and renal disease, *Heart Fail Rev* 8(4):355, 2003.

77. Maisel AS, et al: Bedside B-type natriuretic peptide in the emergency diagnosis of heart failure with reduced or preserved ejection fraction. Results from the Breathing Not Properly (BNP) multinational study, *J Am Coll Cardiol* 41(11):2010, 2003.

78. Maisel AS, et al: Impact of age, race, and sex on the ability of B-type natriuretic peptide to aid in the emergency diagnosis of heart failure: results from the Breathing Not Properly (BNP) multinational study, *Am Heart J* 147(6):1078, 2004.

79. Maisel AS, et al: Rapid measurement of B-type natriuretic peptide in the emergency diagnosis of heart failure, *N Engl J Med* 347(3):161, 2002.

80. McCullough PA, et al: Uncovering heart failure in patients with a history of pulmonary disease: rationale for the early use of B-type natriuretic peptide in the emergency department, *Acad Emerg Med* 10(3):198, 2003.

81. Buxton AE, et al: Relation of ejection fraction and inducible ventricular tachycardia to mode of death in patients with coronary artery disease: an analysis of patients enrolled in the multicenter unsustained tachycardia trial, *Circulation* 106(19):2466, 2002.

82. Stroe AF, Gheorghiade M: Carvedilol: beta-blockade and beyond, *Rev Cardiovasc Med* 5(suppl 1):S18, 2004.

83. Zhang J: Sudden cardiac death: implantable cardioverter defibrillators and pharmacological treatments, *Crit Care Nurs Q* 26(1):45, 2003.

84. Whang W, et al: Heart failure and the risk of shocks in patients with implantable cardioverter defibrillators: results from the Triggers of Ventricular Arrhythmias (TOVA) study, *Circulation* 109(11):1386, 2004.

85. Khand AU, et al: Carvedilol alone or in combination with digoxin for the management of atrial fibrillation in patients with heart failure? *J Am Coll Cardiol* 42(11):1944, 2003.

86. Chen EW, et al: Relation between hospital intra-aortic balloon counterpulsation volume and mortality in acute myocardial infarction complicated by cardiogenic shock, *Circulation* 108(8):951, 2003.

87. Burger AJ, et al: Effect of nesiritide (B-type natriuretic peptide) and dobutamine on ventricular arrhythmias in the treatment of patients with acutely decompensated congestive heart failure: the PRECEDENT study, *Am Heart J* 144(6):1102, 2002.

88. Colbert K, Greene MH: Nesiritide (Natrecor): a new treatment for acutely decompensated congestive heart failure, *Crit Care Nurs Q* 26(1):40, 2003.

89. Abraham WT, Iyengar S: Practical considerations for switching beta-blockers in heart failure patients, *Rev Cardiovasc Med* 5(suppl 1):S36, 2004.

90. Abraham WT, Hayes DL: Cardiac resynchronization therapy for heart failure, *Circulation* 108(21):2596, 2003.

91. Young JB, et al: Combined cardiac resynchronization and implantable cardioversion defibrillation in advanced chronic heart failure: the MIRACLE ICD Trial, *JAMA* 289(20):2685, 2003.

92. Goodlin SJ, et al: Consensus statement: palliative and supportive care in advanced heart failure, *J Card Fail* 10(3):200, 2004.

93. Rudisill PT, et al: The use of beta-blockers in the treatment of chronic heart failure, *Crit Care Nurs Clin North Am* 15(4):439, 2003.

94. Fonarow GC, et al: Organized Program to Initiate Lifesaving Treatment in Hospitalized Patients with Heart Failure (OPTIMIZE-HF): rationale and design, *Am Heart J* 148(1):43, 2004.

95. Callahan HE: Families dealing with advanced heart failure: a challenge and an opportunity, *Crit Care Nurs Q* 26(3):230, 2003.

96. Grady KL, et al: Team management of patients with heart failure: a statement for healthcare professionals from the Cardiovascular Nursing Council of the American Heart Association, *Circulation* 102(19):2443, 2000.

97. Coviello JS, Nyström KV: Obesity and heart failure, *J Cardiovasc Nurs* 18(5):360, 2003.

98. Sneed NV, Paul SC: Readiness for behavioral changes in patients with heart failure, *Am J Crit Care* 12(5):444, 2003.

99. Maron BJ, et al: American College of Cardiology/European Society of Cardiology clinical expert consensus document on hypertrophic cardiomyopathy. A report of the American College of Cardiology Foundation Task Force on Clinical Expert Consensus Documents and the European Society of Cardiology Committee for Practice Guidelines, *J Am Coll Cardiol* 42(9):1687, 2003.

100. Nishimura RA, Holmes DR Jr: Clinical practice. Hypertrophic obstructive cardiomyopathy, *N Engl J Med* 350(13):1320, 2004.

101. Marian AJ: Hypertrophic cardiomyopathy: from genetics to treatment, *Eur J Clin Invest* 40(4):360, 2010

102. Elliott P, McKenna WJ: Hypertrophic cardiomyopathy, *Lancet* 363(9424):1881, 2004.

103. Kamisago M, et al: Mutations in sarcomere protein genes as a cause of dilated cardiomyopathy, *N Engl J Med* 343(23):1688, 2000.

104. Li D, et al: Novel cardiac troponin T mutation as a cause of familial dilated cardiomyopathy, *Circulation* 104(18):2188, 2001.

105. Murphy RT, et al: Novel mutation in cardiac troponin I in recessive idiopathic dilated cardiomyopathy, *Lancet* 363(9406):371, 2004.

106. Noutsias M, et al: Current insights into the pathogenesis, diagnosis and therapy of inflammatory cardiomyopathy, *Heart Fail Monit* 3(4):127, 2003.

107. Syed J, Myers R: Sarcoid heart disease, *Can J Cardiol* 20(1):89, 2004.

108. Ammash NM, et al: Clinical profile and outcome of idiopathic restrictive cardiomyopathy, *Circulation* 101(21):2490, 2000.

109. Felker GM, et al: Underlying causes and long-term survival in patients with initially unexplained cardiomyopathy, *N Engl J Med* 342(15):1077, 2000.

110. Nishimura RA, et al: ACC/AHA 2008 guideline update on valvular heart disease: focused update on infective endocarditis: a report of the American College of Cardiology/American Heart Association Task Force on Practice Guidelines, *Circulation* 118(8):887, 2008.

111. Bonow RO, et al: ACC/AHA 2006 guidelines for the management of patients with valvular heart disease: a report of the American College of Cardiology/American Heart Association Task Force on Practice Guidelines (Writing Committee to Revise the 1988 Guidelines for the Management of Patients with Valvular Heart Disease) developed in collaboration with the Society of Cardiovascular Anesthesiologists; endorsed by the Society for Cardiovascular Angiography and Interventions and the Society of Thoracic Surgeons, *Circulation* 114(5):e84, 2006.

112. Rosengart TK, et al: Percutaneous and minimally invasive valve procedures: a scientific statement from the American Heart Association Council on Cardiovascular Surgery and Anesthesia, Council on Clinical Cardiology, Function Genomics and Translation Biology Interdisciplinary Working Group, and Quality of Care and Outcomes Research Interdisciplinary Working Group, *Circulation* 117(13):1750, 2008.

Cardiovascular Therapeutic Management

Joni L. Dirks

OBJECTIVES

- Describe the functions of a temporary pacemaker and an implantable cardioverter-defibrillator.
- Identify the signs of reperfusion in a patient undergoing fibrinolytic therapy.
- Outline the nursing management for a patient undergoing cardiac surgery and cardiac interventional procedures.
- List the most important categories of cardiovascular drugs, their intended actions, and major significance.

A wide variety of therapeutic interventions is employed in the management of the patient with cardiovascular dysfunction. This chapter focuses on the priority interventions used to manage acute cardiovascular disorders in the critical care setting.

TEMPORARY PACEMAKERS

Pacemakers are electronic devices that can be used to initiate the heartbeat when the heart's intrinsic electrical system cannot effectively generate a rate adequate to support cardiac output. Pacemakers may be used temporarily, either supportively or prophylactically, until the condition responsible for the rate or conduction disturbance resolves.[1]

Indications

The clinical indications for instituting temporary pacemaker therapy are similar regardless of the cause of the rhythm disturbance that necessitates the placement of a pacemaker. The causes range from drug toxicities and electrolyte imbalances to sequelae related to acute myocardial infarction (MI) or cardiac surgery.

The Pacemaker System

A pacemaker system is a simple electrical circuit consisting of a pulse generator and a pacing lead (an insulated electrical wire) with one, two, or three electrodes.

Pacing Pulse Generator

The pulse generator is designed to generate an electrical current that travels through the pacing lead and exits through an electrode (exposed portion of the wire) that is in direct contact with the heart. This electrical current initiates a myocardial depolarization. The current then seeks to return by one of several pathways to the pulse generator to complete the circuit. The power source for a temporary external pulse generator is a standard 9-volt alkaline battery inserted into the generator.

Pacing Lead Systems

The pacing lead used for temporary pacing may be bipolar or unipolar. In a bipolar system, two electrodes (positive and negative) are located within the heart, whereas in a unipolar system, only one electrode (negative) is in direct contact with the myocardium. In both systems, the current flows from the negative terminal of the pulse generator, down the pacing lead to the negative electrode, and into the heart. The current is then picked up by the positive electrode (ground) and flows back up the lead to the positive terminal of the pulse generator.

The bipolar lead used in transvenous pacing has two electrodes on one catheter (Figure 13-1). The distal, or negative, electrode is at the tip of the pacing lead and is in direct contact with the heart, usually inside the right atrium or ventricle. Approximately 1 cm from the negative electrode is

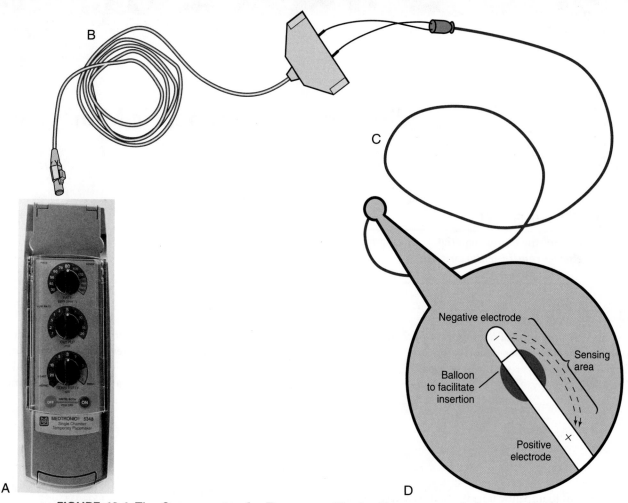

FIGURE 13-1 The Components of a Temporary Bipolar Transvenous Catheter. *A,* Single-chamber temporary (external) pulse generator. *B,* Bridging cable. *C,* Pacing lead. *D,* Enlarged view of the pacing lead tip. (*A,* Courtesy Medtronic Inc., Minneapolis, Minn.)

a positive electrode. The negative electrode is attached to the negative terminal, and the positive electrode is attached to the positive terminal of the pulse generator, either directly or by means of a bridging cable (see Figure 13-1, *B*).

Pacing Routes

Several routes are available for temporary cardiac pacing. Permanent pacing usually is accomplished transvenously, although when a thoracotomy is otherwise indicated, as in cardiac surgery, the physician may elect to insert permanent epicardial pacing wires.

Transcutaneous Pacing

Transcutaneous cardiac pacing involves the use of two large skin electrodes, one placed anteriorly and the other posteriorly on the chest, connected to an external pulse generator. It is a rapid, noninvasive procedure that nurses can perform in the emergency setting and is recommended as a primary intervention in the advanced cardiac life support (ACLS) algorithm for the treatment of symptomatic bradycardia.[2] Improved technology related to stimulus delivery

and the development of large electrode pads that help disperse the energy have helped reduce the pain associated with cutaneous nerve and muscle stimulation. Discomfort may still be an issue for some patients, particularly when higher energy levels are required to achieve capture. This route is typically used as a short-term therapy until the situation resolves or another route of pacing can be established.

Epicardial Pacing

The insertion of temporary epicardial pacing wires has become a routine procedure during most cardiac surgical cases. Ventricular and, in many cases, atrial pacing wires are loosely sewn to the epicardium. The terminal pins of these wires are pulled through the skin before the chest is closed. If both chambers have pacing wires attached, the atrial wires exit subcostally to the right of the sternum and the ventricular wires exit in the same region but to the left of the sternum. These wires can be removed several days after surgery by gentle traction at the skin surface with minimal risk of bleeding.[3]

TABLE 13-1	**NASPE/BPEG GENERIC CODE**			
POSITION I: CHAMBERS PACED	**POSITION II: CHAMBERS SENSED**	**POSITION III: RESPONSE TO SENSING**	**POSITION IV: RATE MODULATION**	**POSITION V: MULTISITE PACING**
0 = None	0 = None	0 = None	0 = None	0 = None
A = Atrium	A = Atrium	T = Triggered	R = Rate Modulation	A = Atrium
V = Ventricle	V = Ventricle	I = Inhibited		V = Ventricle
D = Dual (A + V)	D = Dual (A + V)	D = Dual (T + I)		D = Dual (A + V)

Modified from Bernstein AD, et al: The Revised NASPE/BPEG generic code for antibradycardia, adaptive-rate and multisite pacing, *Pacing Clin Electrophysiol* 25(2):260, 2002.
BPEG, British Pacing and Electrophysiology Group; *NASPE*, North American Society of Pacing and Electrophysiology.

Transvenous Pacing

Temporary transvenous endocardial pacing is accomplished by advancing a pacing electrode wire through a vein, often the subclavian or internal jugular vein, and into the right atrium or right ventricle (RV). Insertion can be facilitated through direct visualization with fluoroscopy or by the use of the standard electrocardiogram (ECG). In some cases, the pacing wire is inserted through a special pulmonary artery catheter by means of a port that exits in the right atrium or right ventricle.

Codes and Modes

Three-Letter Pacemaker Code

The Inter-Society Commission for Heart Disease (ICHD) has a standardized code for describing the various pacing modes. A three-letter code is used to describe temporary pacing modes. The first letter refers to the cardiac chamber that is paced. The second letter designates which chamber is sensed, and the third letter indicates the pacemaker's response to the sensed event.[4]

Five-Letter Pacemaker Code

The five-letter pacemaker code contains the three-letter code categories plus two sections that list additional programming functions (Table 13-1).[4]

Synchronous Pacing Modes

Synchrony implies that the pacemaker only delivers a stimulus when the heart's intrinsic pacemaker fails to function at a predetermined rate. The most physiological of the synchronous modes are those in which the normal sequential relationship between atrial and ventricular depolarization and contraction is maintained. Atrioventricular (AV) synchrony increases the volume in the ventricle before contraction and thus improves cardiac output. When atrial-to-ventricular conduction is impaired, as during heart block, AV synchrony can be maintained through a dual-chamber (both atrial and ventricular) pacing mode.

DDD Pacing. The most physiological of the AV pacing modes is the DDD mode. In DDD pacing, atrial and ventricular leads are used for both pacing and sensing (Table 13-2). In response to sensed activity, the pacemaker inhibits the pacing stimulus. Therefore a sensed P wave in the atrium will

TABLE 13-2	**EXAMPLES OF TEMPORARY PACING MODES**
PACING MODE	**DESCRIPTION**
Asynchronous	
AOO	Atrial pacing, no sensing
VOO	Ventricular pacing, no sensing
DOO	Atrial and ventricular pacing, no sensing
Synchronous	
AAI	Atrial pacing, atrial sensing, inhibited response to sensed P waves
VVI	Ventricular pacing, ventricular sensing, inhibited response to sensed QRS complexes
DVI	Atrial and ventricular pacing, ventricular sensing; both atrial and ventricular pacing are inhibited if a spontaneous ventricular depolarization is sensed
Universal	
DDD	Both chambers are paced and sensed; inhibited response of the pacing stimuli to sensed events in their respective chambers; triggered response to sensed atrial activity to allow for rate-responsive ventricular pacing

inhibit the atrial pacing stimulus, whereas a sensed R wave in the ventricle will inhibit the ventricular pacing stimulus. DDD pacing is also described as "universal pacing" or "physiological pacing" because it most closely resembles the heart's intrinsic conduction system.

VVI Pacing. The VVI mode is designed to pace the ventricle when the pacemaker does not sense an intrinsic (patient initiated) ventricular depolarization. Other names that are popularly used for this mode include "backup pacing" or "demand pacing" (see Table 13-2). VVI pacing is necessary in specific circumstances; the classic example is symptomatic bradycardia with atrial fibrillation. Because a fibrillating atrium is impossible to pace, one effective intervention is to use VVI pacing to maintain ventricular function.

Asynchronous Pacing Modes

Fixed-rate or asynchronous pacing modes ignore the patient's intrinsic heartbeat. These modes are uncommon with the exception of two situations. Emergency DOO or VOO pacing may be used in asystole as a lifesaving measure. These modes are sometimes used in the operating room, where electromagnetic interference (EMI) from electrocautery and other electrical equipment can interfere with normal pacemaker function.

Pacemaker Settings

The controls on all external temporary pulse generators are similar. Their functions must be thoroughly understood so that pacing can be initiated quickly in an emergency situation and troubleshooting can be facilitated if problems with the pacemaker arise.

The rate control regulates the number of impulses that can be delivered to the heart per minute. The rate setting depends on the physiological needs of the patient, but it usually is maintained between 60 and 80 beats/min.

The output dial regulates the amount of electrical current, measured in milliamperes (mA), that is delivered to the heart to initiate depolarization. The point at which depolarization occurs, called threshold, is indicated by a myocardial response to the pacing stimulus (i.e., capture). Threshold can be determined by gradually decreasing the output setting until 1:1 capture is lost. The output setting is then slowly increased until 1:1 capture is reestablished; this threshold to pace is less than 1 mA with a properly positioned pacing electrode. The output is set two to three times higher than threshold, because thresholds tend to fluctuate over time. Box 13-1 details the procedure for measuring pacing thresholds. Separate output controls for atrium and ventricle are used with a dual-chamber pulse generator.

The sensitivity control regulates the ability of the pacemaker to detect the heart's intrinsic electrical activity. Sensitivity is measured in millivolts (mV) and determines the size of the intracardiac signal that the generator will recognize. If the sensitivity is adjusted to its most sensitive setting —a setting of 0.5 to 1.0 mV—the pacemaker can respond even to low-amplitude electrical signals coming from the heart. Turning the sensitivity to its least sensitive setting (i.e., adjusting the dial to a setting of 20 mV or to the area labeled *async*) results in inability of the pacemaker to sense any intrinsic electrical activity and causes the pacemaker to function at a fixed rate. A sense indicator (often a light) on the pulse generator signals each time intrinsic cardiac electrical activity is sensed. A pulse generator may be designed to sense atrial activity, ventricular activity, or both. Box 13-2 describes the procedure for measuring sensitivity.

The AV interval control (available only on dual-chamber generators) regulates the time interval between the atrial and ventricular pacing stimuli. This interval is analogous to the PR interval that occurs in the intrinsic ECG. Proper adjustment of this interval to between 150 and 250 milliseconds (msec) preserves AV synchrony and permits maximal ventricular stroke volume and enhanced cardiac output.

Temporary DDD pacemakers have several other digital controls that are unique to this type of temporary pulse generator. The lower rate, or base rate, determines the rate at which the generator will pace when intrinsic activity falls below the set rate of the pacemaker. The upper rate determines the fastest ventricular rate the pacemaker will deliver in response to sensed atrial activity. This setting is needed to protect the patient's heart from being paced in response to rapid atrial dysrhythmias. The pulse width, which can be adjusted from 0.05 to 2 msec, controls the length of time that the pacing stimulus is delivered to the heart. There is also an atrial refractory period, programmable from 150 to 500 msec, which regulates the length of time, after a sensed or paced ventricular event, during which the pacemaker cannot respond to another atrial stimulus. An emergency button is

---

BOX 13-1 DETERMINING THE TEMPORARY PACEMAKER PACING THRESHOLD

1. Adjust the pacemaker rate setting so that patient is 100% paced. It may be necessary to increase the pacing rate to achieve this setting.
2. Gradually decrease the output (milliampere, mA) setting until 1:1 capture is lost. The pacing threshold is the point at which capture is lost.
3. Slowly increase the output setting until 1:1 capture is reestablished. With a properly positioned pacing electrode, the pacing threshold should be less than 1.0 mA.
4. Set the output setting two to three times higher than measured threshold, because thresholds tend to fluctuate over time.
5. If a dual-chamber pulse generator is being used, evaluate pacing thresholds for the atrial and ventricular leads separately.

BOX 13-2 DETERMINING THE TEMPORARY PACEMAKER SENSITIVITY THRESHOLD

- Set the sensitivity control to its most sensitive setting.
- Adjust the pulse generator rate to 10 beats/min less than the patient's intrinsic rate (the flash indicator should flash regularly).
- Reduce the generator output to the minimal value to eliminate the risk of competing with the intrinsic rhythm.
- Gradually increase the sensitivity value until the sense indicator stops flashing and the pace indicator starts flashing.
- Decrease sensitivity until the sense indicator begins to flash again; this is the sensitivity threshold.
- Adjust the sensitivity setting on the generator to half of the threshold value; restore the generator output and rate to their original values.

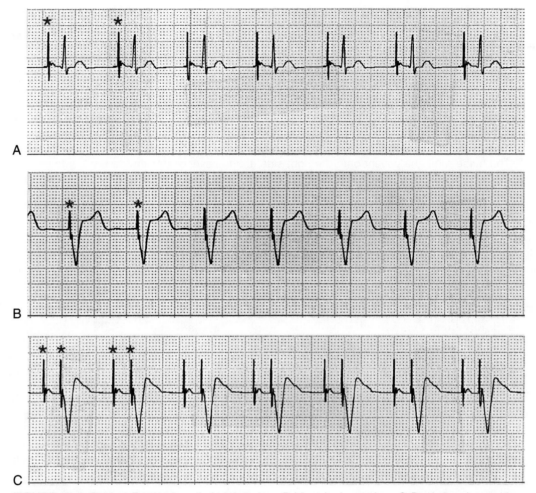

FIGURE 13-2 Pacing Examples. *A,* Atrial pacing. *B,* Ventricular pacing. *C,* Dual-chamber pacing. Each *asterisk* represents a pacemaker impulse.

also available on most models to allow for rapid initiation of asynchronous (DOO) pacing during an emergency.

On all temporary pacemakers, an on/off switch is provided with a safety feature that prevents the accidental termination of pacing. Also a "lock" feature is used to prevent unintended changes to the prescribed settings.

Pacing Artifacts

All patients with temporary pacemakers require continuous ECG monitoring. The pacing artifact is the spike that is seen on the ECG tracing as the pacing stimulus is delivered to the heart. A *P wave* is visible after the pacing artifact if the atrium is being paced (Figure 13-2, *A*). Similarly, a *QRS complex* follows a ventricular pacing artifact (see Figure 13-2, *B*). With dual-chamber pacing, a pacing artifact precedes both the P wave and the QRS complex (see Figure 13-2, *C*).

Pacemaker Malfunctions
Pacing Abnormalities

Most pacemaker malfunctions can be categorized as abnormalities of either pacing or sensing. Immediate and accurate recognition of these malfunctions is critically important in a pacemaker-dependent individual.

Failure to Pace. Failure of the pacemaker to deliver the pacing stimulus results in the disappearance of the pacing artifact on the bedside ECG monitor, even though the patient's intrinsic rate is less than the set rate on the pacemaker (Figure 13-3). This can occur either intermittently or continuously and can be attributed to failure of the pulse generator or its battery, a loose connection between the various components of the pacemaker system, broken lead wires, or stimulus inhibition as a result of EMI. Tightening connections, replacing the batteries or the pulse generator itself, or removing the source of EMI may restore pacemaker function.

Failure to Capture. If the pacing stimulus fires but fails to initiate a myocardial depolarization, a pacing artifact will be present but will not be followed by the expected P wave or QRS complex, depending on the chamber being paced (Figure 13-4). This "loss of capture" most often can be attributed either to displacement of the pacing electrode or to an increase in the threshold (electrical stimulus necessary to elicit a myocardial depolarization) as a result of medications, metabolic disorders, electrolyte imbalances, or fibrosis or myocardial ischemia at the site of electrode placement. In many cases, increasing the output (mA) may elicit capture.

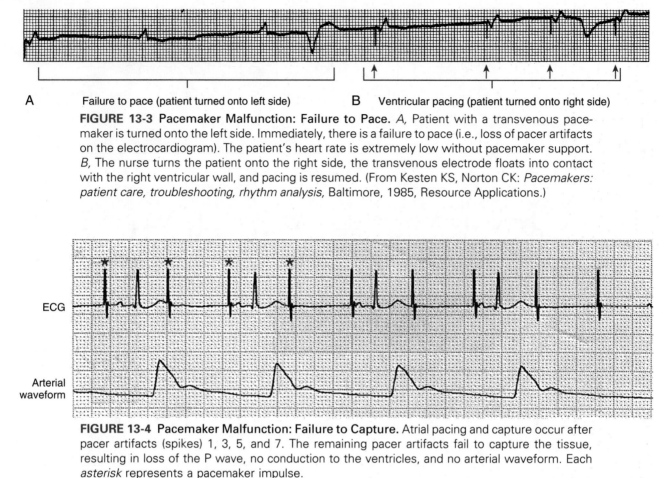

A Failure to pace (patient turned onto left side)   **B** Ventricular pacing (patient turned onto right side)

FIGURE 13-3 Pacemaker Malfunction: Failure to Pace. *A,* Patient with a transvenous pacemaker is turned onto the left side. Immediately, there is a failure to pace (i.e., loss of pacer artifacts on the electrocardiogram). The patient's heart rate is extremely low without pacemaker support. *B,* The nurse turns the patient onto the right side, the transvenous electrode floats into contact with the right ventricular wall, and pacing is resumed. (From Kesten KS, Norton CK: *Pacemakers: patient care, troubleshooting, rhythm analysis,* Baltimore, 1985, Resource Applications.)

FIGURE 13-4 Pacemaker Malfunction: Failure to Capture. Atrial pacing and capture occur after pacer artifacts (spikes) 1, 3, 5, and 7. The remaining pacer artifacts fail to capture the tissue, resulting in loss of the P wave, no conduction to the ventricles, and no arterial waveform. Each *asterisk* represents a pacemaker impulse.

For transvenous leads, repositioning the patient to the left side may improve lead contact and restore capture.[1]

Pacing can occur at inappropriate rates. For example, impending battery failure in a permanent pacemaker can result in a gradual decrease in the paced rate, also referred to as rate drift. Inappropriate stimuli from a pacemaker may result in a pacemaker-mediated tachycardia. This usually is caused by sensing of inappropriate signals in a dual-chamber pacemaker that is in a trigger mode, such as DDD. Placing a magnet over the generator to transiently suspend sensing can terminate the tachycardia.[1]

Sensing Abnormalities

Sensing abnormalities include both undersensing and oversensing.

Undersensing. Undersensing is the inability of the pacemaker to sense spontaneous myocardial depolarizations. Undersensing results in competition between paced complexes and the heart's intrinsic rhythm. This malfunction is manifested on the ECG by pacing artifacts that occur after or are unrelated to spontaneous complexes (Figure 13-5). Undersensing can result in the delivery of pacing stimuli into a relative refractory period of the cardiac depolarization cycle. A ventricular pacing stimulus delivered into the downslope of the T wave (R-on-T phenomenon) is a

real danger with this type of pacer aberration, because it may precipitate a lethal dysrhythmia. The nurse must act quickly to determine the cause and initiate appropriate interventions. Frequently the cause can be attributed to inadequate wave amplitude (height of the P or R wave). If this is the case, the situation can be promptly remedied by increasing the sensitivity by moving the sensitivity dial toward its lowest setting. Other possible causes include inappropriate (asynchronous) mode selection, lead displacement or fracture, loose cable connections, and pulse generator failure.

Oversensing. Oversensing occurs as a result of inappropriate sensing of extraneous electrical signals that leads to unnecessary triggering or inhibition of stimulus output, depending on the pacer mode. The source of these electrical signals can range from tall peaked T waves to EMI in the critical care environment. Because most temporary pulse generators are programmed in demand modes, oversensing results in unexplained pauses in the ECG tracing as the extraneous signals are sensed and inhibit pacing. Often, moving the sensitivity dial toward 20 mV (less sensitive) stops the pauses. With permanent pacemakers, a magnet may be placed over the generator to restore pacing in an asynchronous mode until appropriate changes in the generator settings can be programmed.

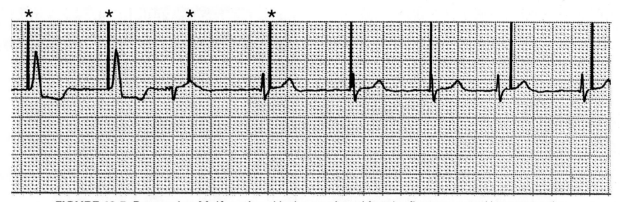

FIGURE 13-5 Pacemaker Malfunction: Undersensing. After the first two paced beats, a series of intrinsic beats occur; the pacemaker unit fails to sense these intrinsic QRS complexes. These pacer artifacts do not capture the ventricle because they occur during the refractory period of the cardiac cycle. Each *asterisk* represents a pacemaker impulse.

Medical Management

The physician determines the pacing route based on the patient's clinical situation. Transcutaneous pacing typically is used in emergent situations until a transvenous lead can be secured. If the patient is undergoing heart surgery, epicardial leads may be electively placed at the end of the operation. The physician places the transvenous or epicardial pacing lead or leads, repositioning them as needed to obtain adequate pacing and sensing thresholds. Decisions regarding lead placement may later limit the pacing modes available to the clinician. For example, to perform dual-chamber pacing, both atrial and ventricular leads must be placed. In an emergency, however, interventions are focused on establishing ventricular pacing, and atrial lead placement may not be feasible. After lead placement, the initial settings for output and sensitivity are determined, the pacing rate and mode are selected, and the patient's response to pacing is evaluated.

Nursing Management

Nursing priorities in the care of a patient with a temporary pacemaker can be combined into four primary areas: (1) preventing pacemaker malfunction, (2) protecting against microshock, (3) monitoring for complications, and (4) providing patient education.

Preventing Pacemaker Malfunction

Continuous ECG monitoring is essential to facilitate prompt recognition of and appropriate intervention for pacemaker malfunction. Proper care of the pacing system can prevent pacing abnormalities.

The temporary pacing lead and bridging cable must be properly secured to the body with tape to prevent accidental displacement of the electrode, which can result in failure to pace or sense. The external pulse generator can be secured to the patient's waist with a strap or placed in a telemetry bag for the mobile patient. If the patient is on a regimen of bed rest, the pulse generator can be suspended with twill tape from an IV pole mounted overhead on the ceiling. This prevents tension on the lead while the patient is moved (given adequate length of bridging cable) and alleviates the possibility of accidental disconnection or dropping of the pulse generator.

The nurse inspects for loose connections between the leads and pulse generator on a regular basis.[5] Replacement batteries and pulse generators must always be available on the unit. Although the battery has an anticipated life span of 1 month, it probably is sound practice to change the battery if the pacemaker has been operating continually for several days. Newer generators provide a low-battery signal 24 hours before complete loss of battery function occurs to prevent inadvertent interruptions in pacing. The pulse generator must always be labeled with the date on which the battery was replaced.

Protecting against Microshock

It is important to be aware of all sources of EMI within the critical care environment that may interfere with the pacemaker's function. Sources of EMI in the clinical area include electrocautery, defibrillation current, radiation therapy, magnetic resonance imaging devices, and transcutaneous electrical nerve stimulation (TENS) units.[3] In most cases, if EMI is suspected of precipitating pacemaker malfunction, conversion to the asynchronous mode (fixed rate) can maintain pacing until the cause of the EMI is removed.

Because the pacing electrode provides a direct, low-resistance path to the heart, the nurse takes special care while handling the external components of the pacing system to avoid conducting stray electrical current from other equipment. Even a small amount of stray current transmitted through the pacing lead could precipitate a lethal dysrhythmia. The possibility of *microshock* can be minimized by wearing rubber gloves when handling the pacing wires and by proper insulation of terminal pins of pacing wires when they are not in use. The latter precaution can be accomplished by the use of caps provided by the manufacturer or by improvising with a plastic syringe or section of disposable rubber glove. The wires are taped securely to the patient's chest to prevent accidental electrode displacement. Additional safety measures include using a nonelectric or a properly grounded electric bed, keeping all electrical equipment away from the bed, and permitting the use of only rechargeable electric razors.

Monitoring for Complications

Infection at the lead insertion site is a rare but serious complication associated with temporary pacemakers. The site is carefully inspected for purulent drainage, erythema, and edema, and the patient is observed for signs of systemic infection. Site care is performed according to the institution's policies and procedures. Although most infections remain localized, endocarditis can occur in patients with endocardial pacing leads.

During transvenous pacing insertion, a balloon at the tip of the catheter is inflated with air to facilitate transvenous insertion. Once the tip of the pacing catheter is correctly positioned within the heart chamber, the balloon is deflated. It is important that the external balloon port is labeled to avoid inadvertent access.[5] A rare complication associated with transvenous pacing is myocardial perforation, which can result in rhythmic hiccoughs or cardiac tamponade.

Providing Patient Education

Patient teaching for the person with a temporary pacemaker emphasizes the prevention of complications. The patient is instructed not to handle any exposed portion of the lead wire and to notify the nurse if the dressing over the insertion site becomes soiled, wet, or dislodged. When epicardial pacemaker wires are removed following cardiac surgery, explain that a pulling sensation may be experienced.[6] The patient is advised not to use any electrical devices brought in from home that could interfere with pacemaker functioning.

Patients with temporary transvenous pacemakers need to be taught to restrict movement of the affected extremity to prevent lead displacement.

PERMANENT PACEMAKERS

More than 195,000 permanent pacemakers are implanted annually in the United States, and critical care nurses are likely to encounter these devices in their clinical practice.[7] These pacemakers were originally designed to provide an adequate ventricular rate in patients with symptomatic bradycardia. Today, the goal of pacemaker therapy is to simulate, as much as possible, normal physiological cardiac depolarization and conduction. Sophisticated generators permit rate-responsive pacing, affecting responses to sensed atrial activity (DDD) or to a variety of physiological sensors (body motion, QT interval, minute ventilation). For patients who do not have a functional sinus node that can increase their heart rate, rate-responsive pacemakers have been shown to improve exercise capacity and quality of life.[8] Table 13-3 describes the types of rate-responsive pacing modes in clinical use.

TABLE 13-3	PERMANENT PACEMAKER RATE-RESPONSE PACING MODES
PULSE GENERATOR	**DESCRIPTION**
AAIR	AAI features plus rate-responsive pacing; used for patients with a symptomatic bradycardia who have a paceable atrium and intact AV conduction
VVIR	VVI features plus rate-responsive pacing; used for patients with an atrium that is unpaceable as a result of chronic atrial fibrillation or other atrial dysrhythmia
DDDR	DDD features plus rate-responsive pacing; used for patients with symptomatic bradycardia in which the atrium is paceable but AV conduction is, or may become, unreliable

The concept of physiological pacing continues to evolve, because studies have indicated that pacing initiated from the RV apex—even in a dual-chamber mode—may promote heart failure in patients with permanent pacemakers.[1] This has prompted further research to identify alternative sites for pacing and modes that can maximize intrinsic AV conduction and minimize ventricular pacing.[8]

Technological advances in the computer industry have had a major impact on today's permanent pacemakers. Microprocessors have allowed for the development of increasingly smaller generators despite the incorporation of more complex features. Today's pacemaker generators are smaller, more energy-efficient, and more reliable than previous models. A new trend in permanent pacemakers is to use these devices as nonpharmacological therapy in treatment of heart failure.

Cardiac Resynchronization Therapy

About one third of patients with severe heart failure have ventricular conduction delays (prolonged QRS duration or bundle branch block). These conduction delays have been shown to create a lack of synchrony between the contractions of the LV and RV. The hemodynamic consequences of this dyssynchrony include impaired ventricular filling with decreased ejection fraction, cardiac output, and mean arterial pressure.[9] Cardiac resynchronization therapy (CRT) uses atrial pacing plus stimulation of both the LV and RV (biventricular pacing), in an attempt to optimize atrial and ventricular mechanical activity. The CRT device uses three pacing leads, one each in the right atrium and the RV and a specially designed transvenous lead that is inserted through the coronary sinus to pace the LV.[9] Because many patients with heart failure are also at risk for sudden cardiac death, biventricular pacing is available on some implantable cardioverter defibrillators (ICDs). A number of clinical trials have shown symptomatic and structural cardiac improvement with this new therapy.[10]

Atrial Arrhythmia Suppression

There is a growing incidence of atrial fibrillation, and atrial pacing has been proposed as a possible preventative therapy for this dysrhythmia in selected patients. Atrial pacing in patients with bradycardia has been shown to lower the recurrence of atrial fibrillation, especially compared with ventricular pacing.[11] Most pacemakers can be programmed to mode switch to a non-P wave tracking mode if rapid atrial rates are sensed.[1] Strategies for patients with paroxysmal atrial fibrillation, which include pacing both atriums (bi-atrial pacing) and transiently pacing the atrium at a rate higher than the patient's intrinsic sinus rate, require further study.[12]

Medical Management

Permanent pacemakers may be implanted with the patient under local anesthesia in the operating room or in the cardiac catheterization laboratory. Transvenous leads usually are inserted through the cephalic or subclavian vein and positioned in the right atrium or RV, or both, with fluoroscopic guidance. Satisfactory lead placement is determined by testing the stimulation and sensitivity thresholds with a pacing system analyzer. The leads are then attached to the generator, which is inserted into a surgically created pocket in the subcutaneous tissue below the clavicle.

Nursing Management

Nursing management for patients after permanent pacemaker implantation includes monitoring for complications related to insertion and for pacemaker malfunction. Postoperative complications are rare but include cardiac perforation and tamponade, pneumothorax, hematoma, lead displacement, and infection.[13,14]

Identification of permanent pacemaker malfunction is the same as that described previously for temporary pacemakers. To evaluate pacemaker function, the nurse must know at least the pacemaker's programmed mode of pacing and the lower rate setting. With permanent pacemakers, settings are adjusted noninvasively through a specialized programmer that uses pulsed magnetic fields or an RF signal. If a pacemaker problem is suspected, ECG strips are obtained, and the physician is notified so that the pacemaker settings can be reprogrammed as needed. If the patient experiences symptoms of decreased cardiac output, he or she may require support with temporary transcutaneous pacing until the problem is corrected.

Critical care nurses also may be involved in monitoring patients with permanent pacemakers after discharge. Some units are equipped with transtelephonic monitoring equipment that allows patients to transmit information over the telephone from a monitoring device in their home. Transmission of the patient's ECG can provide information to confirm proper pacemaker function (capture and sensing) and to determine battery status (rate). Newer technology that uses an Internet-based remote monitoring system for pacemaker follow-up may soon replace standard transtelephonic ECG evaluation.[15]

The foregoing discussion provides an introduction to the basic concepts of pacemaker therapy. However, the nurse who cares for patients with permanent or temporary pacemakers must be familiar with even the most sophisticated modes of pacemaker function. Only by keeping pace with current technology can the nurse accurately interpret pacer function and thereby safely and effectively care for patients with pacemakers.

IMPLANTABLE CARDIOVERTER DEFIBRILLATORS

An implantable cardioverter defibrillator (ICD) is an electronic device that is used in the treatment of tachydysrhythmias. The ICD is capable of identifying and terminating life-threatening ventricular dysrhythmias; 114,000 are implanted annually in the U.S.[7] Initially, an ICD was recommended only for patients who had survived an episode of cardiac arrest caused by ventricular fibrillation (VF) or ventricular tachycardia (VT). Later, a number of clinical trials compared ICD therapy for such secondary prevention of sudden cardiac death with antidysrhythmic drug therapy and found improved survival with the ICD.[1] As a result, ICD use was expanded to include primary prevention of sudden cardiac death in patients with coronary artery disease (CAD), previous MI, or LV dysfunction in whom VT or VF was inducible during EPS. Trials have shown improved survival with ICD implantation in high-risk patients (i.e., those with previous MI and an ejection fraction <35%) even without evidence of VT or VF on an EPS.[10] These results have further increased the number of patients who receive an ICD.

The ICD System

The ICD system contains (1) sensing electrodes to recognize the dysrhythmia and (2) defibrillation electrodes or patches that are in contact with the heart and can deliver a shock. These electrodes are connected to a generator that is surgically placed in the subcutaneous tissue of the pectoral region in the upper chest (Figure 13-6). The early-model generators could defibrillate or cardiovert only lethal dysrhythmias. The current generation of devices delivers a tiered therapy, with options for programmable antitachycardia pacing, bradycardia backup pacing, low-energy cardioversion, and high-energy defibrillation. With tiered therapy, antitachycardia pacing is used as the first line of treatment in some cases of VT. If the VT can be pace-terminated successfully, the patient will not receive a shock from the generator and may not even realize that the ICD terminated the dysrhythmia. If programmed bursts of pacing do not terminate the VT, the ICD will cardiovert the rhythm. If the dysrhythmia deteriorates into VF, the ICD is programmed to defibrillate at a higher energy. If the dysrhythmia terminates spontaneously, the

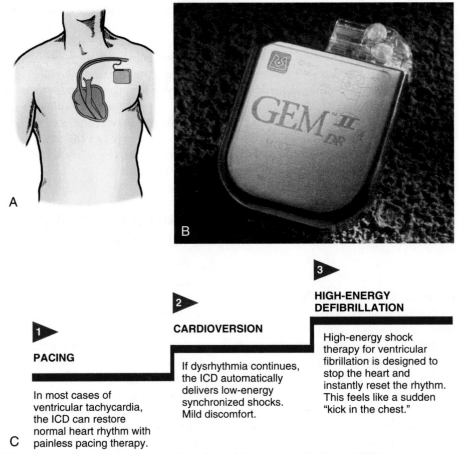

FIGURE 13-6 *A,* Placement of an implantable cardioverter defibrillator (ICD) with a transvenous lead system in the pectoral region of the upper chest. Pacing, cardioversion, and defibrillation functions are all contained in a lead (or leads) inserted into the right atrium and ventricle. *B,* An example of a dual-chamber ICD (Medtronic Gem II DR) with tiered therapy and pacing capabilities. *C,* Tiered therapy is designed to use increasing levels of intensity to terminate ventricular dysrhythmias. (Courtesy Medtronic Inc., Minneapolis, Minn.)

device will not discharge. Occasionally, the electrical rhythm may deteriorate to asystole or a slow idioventricular rhythm; in such cases, the bradycardia backup pacing function is activated.

ICDs are dual-chamber devices with leads in both atria and ventricles. The atrial leads allows for dual-chamber pacing to optimize hemodynamic performance and atrial sensing to more accurately discriminate between atrial and ventricular tachycardias and to decrease the incidence of inappropriate shocks. Implantable defibrillators with atrial capabilities may also be used to deliver therapies such as cardioversion or antitachycardia pacing to patients with atrial tachydysrhythmias, but their use may be limited because of the painful nature of the shocks.[12] ICDs may also incorporate triple-lead systems (leads in one atrium and both ventricles) to allow for CRT and defibrillation in one device. Other developments in ICD technology include improved diagnostic and telemetry functions, such as the ability to provide real-time electrograms obtained from the ICD electrodes or the ability to perform remote device interrogation by telephone or Internet.[16]

ICD Insertion

The ICD has progressed in both programmable functions and insertion design. Transvenous electrode leads are inserted into the subclavian vein and advanced into the right side of the heart, where contact with the endocardium is achieved. The endocardial leads are used for sensing, pacing, cardioversion, and defibrillation, and are connected to the generator by tunneling through the subcutaneous tissue. Technical advances and the development of smaller ICDs have made it feasible to implant these devices in the pectoral position, similar to permanent pacemakers.

Medical Management

Medical management in the ICD patient begins before implantation with a thorough evaluation of the patient's dysrhythmia and underlying cardiac function. Patients at risk for sudden cardiac death (SCD) undergo an electrophysiology study to determine the origin of the dysrhythmia and the effect of antidysrhythmic agents in suppressing or altering the rate of the dysrhythmia. Further assessment of cardiac status is made to determine whether additional interventions (e.g., cardiac surgery, angioplasty or stent) are indicated to improve cardiac function and decrease SCD risk.

ICD Programming

An electrophysiologist performs the initial programming of the device at the time of implantation. During implantation, defibrillation threshold measurements are obtained. This involves inducing the dysrhythmia and then evaluating the device's ability to terminate it. After it has been determined that the ICD functions appropriately, further follow-up is conducted on an outpatient basis to monitor the number of discharges and the battery life of the device.

Nursing Management

It is important to know the type of ICD implanted, how the device functions, and whether it is activated (i.e., on). If the patient experiences a shockable rhythm, the nurse should be prepared to defibrillate in the rare event that the device fails. During external defibrillation, the paddles or patches should not be placed directly over the ICD generator. Standard paddle placement may need to be altered in patients with ICDs to achieve successful defibrillation.[2] Most patients continue to take antidysrhythmic medications to decrease the number of shocks required and to slow the rate of the tachycardia. Complications associated with the permanent ICD include infection from the implanted system,[14] broken leads, and sensing of supraventricular tachydysrhythmias resulting in unneeded discharges.

Providing Patient Education

To facilitate a positive psychological adjustment to the ICD, patient education about the device is vital.[17,18] Preoperative teaching for the ICD patient includes information about how the device works and what to expect during the implantation procedure. After implantation, education is focused on aspects of living with an ICD. Patients need information pertaining to scheduled device follow-up and instructions about what to do if they experience a shock. Many institutions have successfully used family support groups for this patient population.

FIBRINOLYTIC THERAPY

Fibrinolytic therapy is an important clinical intervention for the patient experiencing acute ST-elevation myocardial infarction (STEMI). Before the introduction of fibrinolytic agents, medical management of acute MI was focused on decreasing myocardial oxygen demands to minimize myocardial necrosis and preserve ventricular function. Today, efforts to limit the size of the infarction are directed toward timely reperfusion of the jeopardized myocardium through restoration of blood flow in the culprit vessel (the open artery theory). Two options are available for opening the artery—fibrinolytics and mechanical intervention. Although mechanical catheter-based intervention has been proven to yield better outcomes when performed in a timely fashion, only

25% of U.S. hospitals are estimated to have this capability.[19] For this reason, fibrinolytic therapy continues to play a major role in the treatment of acute MI.

The use of fibrinolytic therapy is predicated on the theory that the significant event in acute coronary syndromes (e.g., unstable angina, acute MI) is the rupture of an atherosclerotic plaque with thrombus formation (Figure 13-7). The thrombus, which is composed of aggregated platelets bound together with fibrin strands, occludes the coronary artery, depriving the myocardium of oxygen previously supplied by that artery. The administration of a fibrinolytic agent results in lysis of the acute thrombus, resulting in recanalization, or opening, of the obstructed coronary artery and restoration of blood flow to the affected tissue. After perfusion is restored, adjunctive measures are taken to prevent further clot formation and repeat occlusion.

Eligibility Criteria
Inclusion Criteria

Certain criteria have been developed, based on research findings, to determine the patient population that would most likely benefit from the administration of fibrinolytic therapy. Patients with recent onset of chest pain (<12 hours' duration) and persistent ST elevation (>0.1 mV in two or more contiguous leads) are considered candidates for fibrinolytic therapy.[20] Patients who present with bundle branch blocks that may obscure ST-segment analysis and a history suggesting an acute MI are also considered candidates for therapy. The goal of therapy is to administer fibrinolytic therapy within 30 minutes after presentation at the hospital, described as "door-to-needle" time. Time is crucial because early reperfusion yields the greatest benefit.[21]

Exclusion criteria are usually based on the increased risk of bleeding incurred from the use of fibrinolytics. Patients who have stable clots that might be disrupted by fibrinolytic therapy (recent surgery, trauma, or stroke) usually are not considered candidates for fibrinolytic therapy. Other selection criteria for the use of fibrinolytic therapy are presented in Box 13-3.

Exclusion Criteria

Currently, fibrinolytic therapy is not indicated for patients with unstable angina or non-ST-elevation myocardial infarction (NSTEMIs). It is believed that these conditions result from plaque rupture with the formation of an only partially occlusive thrombus. Fibrinolysis breaks up the clot and releases thrombin, and this can paradoxically increase the material necessary for further thrombosis.[22] Instead, these patients are treated with antiplatelet agents (e.g., aspirin, clopidogrel, glycoprotein IIb/IIIa inhibitors) and antithrombin drugs (e.g., heparin).

Fibrinolytic Agents

Four fibrinolytic agents are currently available for intravenous treatment of acute STEMI. All of these agents stimulate lysis of the clot by converting inactive plasminogen to plasmin, an enzyme responsible for degradation of fibrin.

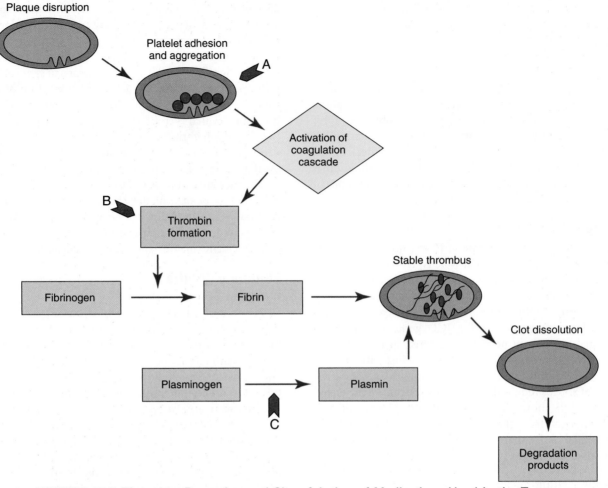

FIGURE 13-7 Thrombus Formation and Site of Action of Medications Used in the Treatment of Acute Myocardial Infarction. *A,* Site of action of antiplatelet agents such as aspirin and glycoprotein IIb/IIIa inhibitors. *B,* Heparin bonds with antithrombin III and thrombin to create an inactive complex. *C,* Fibrinolytic agents convert plasminogen to plasmin, an enzyme responsible for degradation of fibrin clots.

BOX 13-3   FIBRINOLYTIC THERAPY SELECTION CRITERIA

- No more than 12 hours from onset of chest pain (less if possible)
- ST-segment elevation on electrocardiogram or new-onset left bundle branch block
- Ischemic chest pain unresponsive to sublingual nitroglycerin
- No conditions that might cause a predisposition to hemorrhage

---

Streptokinase (SK) and urokinase were the first generation of fibrinolytic agents and had their primary effect on circulating plasminogen. Urokinase availability has been limited because of manufacturing problems. Newer fibrinolytic agents (e.g., alteplase, reteplase, tenecteplase) have a greater effect on clot plasminogen than on circulating plasminogen and are described as clot selective. A comparison of currently approved fibrinolytic agents is provided in Table 13-4.

Because patients with an area of plaque disruption are still at risk for clot formation and reocclusion, fibrinolytic therapy is used in conjunction with anticoagulants and antiplatelet agents. Current guidelines recommend that heparin be administered for a minimum of 48 hours after fibrinolytic therapy. Low-molecular-weight heparin (LMWH) is considered an acceptable alternative in patients younger than 75 years who have adequate kidney function. Antiplatelet therapy with clopidogrel is recommended for 14 days, and aspirin should be continued indefinitely[20] (Table 13-5).

Outcomes of Fibrinolytic Therapy

The benefit of fibrinolytic therapy correlates with the degree of restoration of normal blood flow in the infarct-related artery. Coronary artery patency is defined by angiographic perfusion grades developed by the Thrombolysis in Myocardial Infarction (TIMI) study group in 1985 (Box 13-4).[23] Achievement of TIMI grade 3 flow is associated with the best long-term survival. Studies also indicate that rapid restoration of normal blood flow, within 90 minutes after treatment,

TABLE 13-4	PHARMACOLOGICAL MANAGEMENT: FIBRINOLYTIC AGENTS FOR USE IN ACUTE MYOCARDIAL INFARCTION		
DRUG	**DOSAGE**	**MECHANISM OF ACTION**	**SPECIAL CONSIDERATIONS**
Clot-Specific			
tPA (alteplase)	IV: 100 mg over 90 min with the first 15 mg given as a bolus	Binds to fibrin at the clot and promotes activation of plasminogen to plasmin	Short half-life, so heparin is usually given with the drug as a bolus and afterward as an infusion. Aspirin is begun with administration of the drug and continued daily.
rPA (reteplase)	IV: 10 units given as a bolus over 2 min, repeated in 30 min	Binds to fibrin at the clot and promotes activation of plasminogen to plasmin	Heparin is started with administration of the drug and continued for 24 hours. Aspirin is begun with administration of the drug and continued daily.
TNKase (tenecteplase)	IV: 30-50 mg based on body weight, given as a single bolus	Binds to fibrin at the clot and promotes activation of plasminogen to plasmin	Heparin is started with administration of the drug. Aspirin is begun with administration of the drug and continued daily.
Non-Clot-Specific			
SK (streptokinase)	IV: 1.5 million units given over 60 min	Catalyzes the conversion of plasminogen to plasmin, which causes lysis of fibrin; has systemic lytic effects	May cause allergic reactions and hypotension. Heparin may be administered IV or SQ. Aspirin is begun with administration of the drug and continued daily.

IV, intravenous; *rPA,* recombinant plasminogen activator; *SQ,* subcutaneous; *tPA,* tissue plasminogen activator.

TABLE 13-5	PHARMACOLOGICAL MANAGEMENT: ANTICOAGULANTS		
CLASSIFICATION AND DRUG	**MECHANISM OF ACTION**	**INDICATIONS**	**SPECIAL CONSIDERATIONS**
Heparin			
Heparin sodium	Enhances activity of antithrombin III, a natural anticoagulant	Prevention of clotting in patients with MI and those undergoing PCI or cardiac surgery	Effectiveness of treatment may be monitored by aPTT or ACT. Response is variable because of binding with plasma proteins. Effects may be reversed with protamine sulfate. Risk of developing HIT exists.
Low-Molecular-Weight Heparin			
Dalteparin (Fragmin) Enoxaparin (Lovenox)	Enhances activity of antithrombin III	Prophylaxis and treatment of thromboembolic complications after surgery Prevention of clots in patients with unstable angina and MI	More predictable response than heparin, because the drug is not largely bound to protein. aPTT not particularly useful in monitoring treatment.
Direct Thrombin Inhibitor			
Lepirudin (Refludan) Bivalirudin (Angiomax) Argatroban (Argatroban)	Directly inhibits thrombin	Prophylaxis and treatment of thrombosis in patients with HIT Prevention of clots in patients with unstable angina or PCI	aPTT may be monitored daily. Dose should be adjusted for patients with renal insufficiency. No reversal agent is available.

ACT, activated clotting time; *aPTT,* activated partial thromboplastin time; *HIT,* heparin-induced thrombocytopenia; *MI,* myocardial infarction; *PCI,* percutaneous coronary intervention.

results in improved LV function and reduced mortality. The three fibrin-specific fibrinolytics have been shown to achieve TIMI 3 flow in 54% to 63% of patients at 90 minutes.[24]

The area of fibrinolytic therapy continues to evolve, and drug dose ranges and regimens are subject to change when research findings are updated. Whereas fibrinolytic agents target the fibrin portion of the clot, other treatment strategies are focusing on the platelet portion of the clot (see Figure 13-7). Clinical trials evaluating the combination of glycoprotein IIb/IIIa receptor antagonists with fibrinolytic agents (at half-dose) found outcomes equivalent to those of fibrinolytics alone, but with an increased risk for bleeding.[25] There was

BOX 13-4	**FLOW IN THE INFARCT-RELATED ARTERY AS DESCRIBED IN THE THROMBOLYSIS IN MYOCARDIAL INFARCTION TRIAL**
Perfusion Grades	Flow in the Infarct-Related Artery
TIMI 3	Normal or brisk flow through the coronary artery
TIMI 2	Partial flow, slower than in normal vessels
TIMI 1	Sluggish flow with incomplete distal filling
TIMI 0	No flow beyond the point of occlusion

Modified from TIMI Study Group: The thrombolysis in myocardial infarction (TIMI) trial. Phase I findings, *N Engl J Med* 312(14):932, 1985.
TIMI, Thrombolysis in Myocardial Infarction Trial.

also speculation that a planned strategy for administering fibrinolytics or glycoprotein IIb/IIIa receptor antagonists, or both, to patients who must be transported to another facility for percutaneous intervention would improve outcomes. Although promising in theory, this facilitated approach to revascularization has not been shown to be beneficial and may increase the risk for bleeding complications in some patients.[26]

Evidence of Reperfusion

In the cardiac catheterization laboratory, the blood flow of a vessel that has been occluded by a thrombus and then opened by fibrinolytic therapy can be observed directly under fluoroscopy. The adequacy of the flow of blood through the coronary artery is described using the standardized thrombolysis in myocardial infarction (TIMI) scale (Box 13-4).

Nursing Management

Nursing priorities for the patient receiving fibrinolytic therapy are directed toward (1) identifying candidates for reperfusion therapy, (2) observing for signs of reperfusion, (3) monitoring for signs of bleeding, and (4) providing patient education.

Identifying Candidates for Reperfusion Therapy

Nursing management of the patient undergoing fibrinolytic therapy begins with identifying potential candidates. In many institutions, checklists are used to facilitate the rapid identification of patients who are candidates for fibrinolytics. The nurse prepares the patient for fibrinolytic therapy by starting intravenous lines and obtaining baseline laboratory values and vital signs.

Observing for Signs of Reperfusion

Reperfusion of the ischemic myocardium may be observed noninvasively by several means, as follows:

- Ischemic chest pain ceases abruptly as blood flow is restored.
- Reperfusion ventricular dysrhythmias may occur; generally these are self-limiting or nonsustained, and aggressive antidysrhythmic therapy is not required.
- Normalization of the previously elevated ST segments. To monitor the ST segment changes, a monitoring lead should be chosen that clearly demonstrates the ST elevation before initiation of therapy.[27]
- The serum concentration of myocardial biomarkers released by damaged myocardial cells, such as myocardial creatine kinase (CK-MB) or troponin, are monitored. These biomarkers rise rapidly and markedly after reperfusion of the ischemic heart muscle.

Monitoring for Signs of Bleeding

The most common complication related to thrombolysis is bleeding, from the fibrinolytic therapy itself and also because patients routinely receive anticoagulation therapy for several days to minimize the possibility of rethrombosis. The nurse must continually monitor for clinical manifestations of bleeding. Mild gingival bleeding and oozing around venipuncture sites is common and not a cause of concern. Should serious bleeding occur, such as intracranial or internal bleeding, all fibrinolytic and heparin therapies are discontinued and volume expanders or coagulation factors, or both, are administered.

In addition to accurate assessment of the patient for evidence of bleeding, nursing management includes preventive measures to minimize the potential for bleeding. For example, patient handling is limited, injections are avoided if at all possible, and additional pressure is provided to ensure hemostasis at venipuncture and arterial puncture sites. Intravenous lines are placed before lytic therapy is administered. A heparin lock may be used for obtaining laboratory specimens during treatment.

Providing Patient Education

Education for the patient receiving fibrinolytic therapy includes information regarding the actions of fibrinolytic agents, with emphasis on precautions to minimize bleeding. For example, the patient is cautioned against vigorous tooth brushing and told to refrain from using straight-edge razors. Information is provided regarding ongoing risk-factor management in the prevention of atherosclerotic CAD.

CATHETER INTERVENTIONS FOR CORONARY ARTERY DISEASE

During the past three decades, the use of catheter procedures to open coronary arteries blocked or narrowed by CAD has expanded dramatically. These procedures are grouped by the term percutaneous coronary intervention (PCI). Today, PCI includes percutaneous transluminal coronary angioplasty (PTCA), atherectomy, and stent implantation. Advances in device technology, along with more effective anticoagulant and antiplatelet regimens, have reduced complication rates and improved procedural outcomes.[28]

Indications for Catheter-Based Interventions

Indications for catheter-based interventions have been considerably broadened since the initial application of balloon angioplasty. Whereas only patients with single-vessel CAD were once considered for PTCA, patients with multivessel disease, even those who have previously undergone saphenous vein grafting, internal mammary artery (IMA) grafting, or fibrinolytic therapy for acute MI, may now be candidates for catheter intervention. Previously seen as a rescue procedure to reduce a severe stenosis that persisted after fibrinolytic therapy, PCI is now preferred as the initial method of treatment for acute MI (primary PCI) when this therapy is available in the hospital.[29] See "Coronary Artery Disease" in Chapter 12.

Surgical Backup

Initially, most institutions required that patients preparing to undergo angioplasty be candidates for coronary artery bypass graft (CABG) surgery. Complications such as intimal dissection with abrupt closure of the vessel could arise during the procedure, requiring the patient to undergo emergency CABG. Today, most dissections are effectively treated with stent placement, with less than 1% of patients requiring emergency bypass surgery. As a result, most institutions use an informal surgical backup plan, such as the first available operating room. Nevertheless, the availability of cardiac surgical services on site is still recommended. The one exception is in institutions that offer PCI only for treatment of acute STEMI. In this setting, an organized plan for emergent transfer to a surgical center may be used in lieu of on-site surgical access.[30]

Angioplasty

PTCA involves the use of a balloon-tipped catheter that, when advanced through an atherosclerotic lesion (atheroma), can be inflated intermittently for the purpose of dilating the stenotic area and improving blood flow through it (Figure 13-8). The high inflation pressure of the balloon stretches the vessel wall, fractures the plaque, and enlarges the vessel lumen. After balloon deflation, the vessel exhibits some degree of elastic recoil, resulting in a residual stenosis of approximately 30%.[31] A successful angioplasty procedure is one in which the stenosis is reduced to less than 50% of the vessel lumen diameter.[30]

Restenosis occurred in more than one third of patients who underwent PTCA as a solo procedure. Restenosis within the first 6 months was diagnosed when patients experienced a recurrence of anginal symptoms.[32] Studies showed that restenosis was influenced by the final lumen diameter after PTCA, the severity of elastic recoil of the vessel walls in response to the balloon inflation, and the amount of intimal hyperplasia that occurred as the vessel healed over the treated area. Patient characteristics such as a history of diabetes or unstable angina were also found to increase the risk of restenosis.[33] Today, PTCA is rarely used alone as an intervention, except to treat lesions in very small coronary arteries.[31] Nevertheless, balloon angioplasty remains an essential technique in PCI for dilating vessels and for deploying intracoronary stents.

Atherectomy

Atherectomy is the excision and removal of the atherosclerotic plaque by cutting, shaving, or grinding. Specialized coronary catheters are used. Initially, atherectomy devices were used alone in an attempt to avoid the trauma to the vessel that was known to occur with balloon angioplasty and to more efficiently remove the atherosclerotic plaque, thereby decreasing the rate of restenosis. Later, as restenosis was also found to occur with these devices, balloon angioplasty was added as an adjunctive therapy to optimize the diameter of the vessel lumen and offset the intimal hyperplasia that occurred as a result of the procedure. Despite significant improvements in initial procedural success, atherectomy failed to significantly reduce the rate of restenosis.[34] In the current era of stenting, atherectomy devices are used in less than 5% of procedures.[31]

Two atherectomy devices are used in PCI: directional coronary atherectomy (DCA) (Figure 13-9, A) and rotational ablation (Rotablator) (Figure 13-9, B). A randomized clinical trial showed no clinical benefit for the use of DCA in combination with stent, compared with stenting alone.[35] As a result, DCA is currently used only for noncalcified lesions that involve a bifurcation of a major side branch or in the ostium of the left anterior descending (LAD) artery.[28] Rotational atherectomy is used for chronic total occlusion and for calcified bifurcation lesions.[28]

Coronary Stents

A major development in the field of interventional cardiology has been the coronary stent prosthesis. A stent is a metal structure that is introduced into the coronary artery over a guidewire and expanded into the vessel wall at the site of the lesion (Figure 13-10). Bare metal stents were first used to treat acute or threatened vessel closure after failed PTCA.[32] The stent acted as a scaffold to tack dissection flaps against the vessel wall and provided mechanical support to minimize elastic recoil. Multiple stents may be implanted sequentially

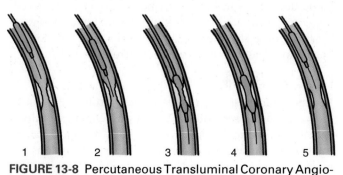

FIGURE 13-8 Percutaneous Transluminal Coronary Angioplasty (PTCA) is used to open a stenotic vessel occluded by atherosclerosis.

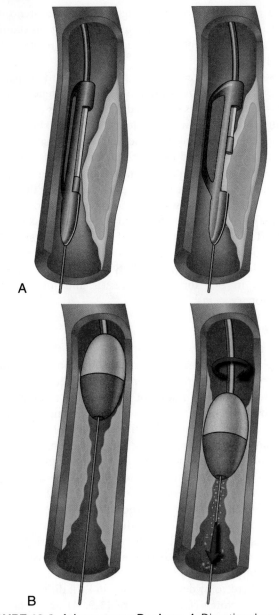

FIGURE 13-9 Atherectomy Devices. *A,* Directional coronary atherectomy catheter. *B,* Rotational atherectomy catheter.

within a vessel to fully cover the area of the lesion. Stents are currently the predominant form of PCI and are used in more than 90% of all interventional procedures.[7] Numerous stent models are available. They are composed of various types of metal (stainless steel, titanium, cobalt chromium) and come in a variety of configurations (e.g., mesh, coil). Most stents are balloon expandable (see Figure 13-10).

Stent Thrombosis

Specific interventions are used to prevent subacute stent thrombosis. High-pressure balloon inflations within the stent are employed to fully open the stent within the vessel, so reduced anticoagulation is sufficient to maintain stent patency. Dual antiplatelet therapy (aspirin and thienopyridine) has been shown to be more important than anticoagulation in preventing stent thrombosis.[36] These agents are administered before the procedure and continued at discharge.[37] Two potent antiplatelet glycoprotein IIb/IIIa inhibitors, eptifibatide (Integrilin) and tirofiban (Aggrastat), also reduce the formation of intracoronary thrombosis and are used across the spectrum of interventional procedures, from PTCA to atherectomy to stenting.[37] Indications and dosing of glycoprotein IIb/IIIa inhibitors are provided in Table 13-6.

Drug-Eluting Stents

In an effort to minimize restenosis, drug-eluting stents (DES) were developed. These stents have polymer coatings impregnated with drugs that are released slowly into the endothelium at the site of stent placement to inhibit cellular proliferation. DES coated with sirolimus (an immunosuppressive drug used to prevent organ transplant rejection) and paclitaxel (an anticancer agent) have been approved by the FDA.[38] In initial trials, DES were found to decrease the 6-month restenosis rate to less than 10%, and they soon became the predominant stent, implanted in 90% of patients. Some trials demonstrated similar efficacy between bare metal stents and DES in long-term outcomes (stent thrombosis, MI, or death) and raised concerns regarding the possibility of late stent thrombosis (>1 year) in DES.[39,40] As a result, DES usage has decreased somewhat to between 60% and 70% of patients.[30] Because a DES delays endothelialization, dual antiplatelet therapy must be continued for a longer period to prevent stent thrombosis. A DES is also considerably more expensive than a bare metal stent. A comparison of bare metal stents and DES is provided in Table 13-7.

PCI Complications
Acute Complications

The incidence of serious cardiac complications after PCI, including coronary spasm, coronary artery dissection, and acute coronary thrombosis, has decreased significantly with improvements in technology. Stents have proved efficacious in the repair of coronary dissections, decreasing the need for emergency bypass surgery. Acute thrombosis has decreased with the use of glycoprotein IIb/IIIa inhibitors (see Table 13-6). Other complications that can occur in the period immediately after PCI include bleeding and hematoma formation at the site of vascular cannulation, compromised blood flow to the involved extremity, retroperitoneal bleeding, contrast-induced kidney failure, dysrhythmias, and vasovagal response (hypotension, bradycardia, and diaphoresis) during manipulation or removal of introducer sheaths.

Late Complications

Restenosis after PCI continues to be a problem, although rates are much lower with DES than with angioplasty alone. Patients at greatest risk are those with complex lesions, multivessel disease, or diabetes.[41] Treatment options for in-stent restenosis include balloon dilation, debulking with an atherectomy device, implantation of another DES or brachytherapy—the localized delivery of intracoronary

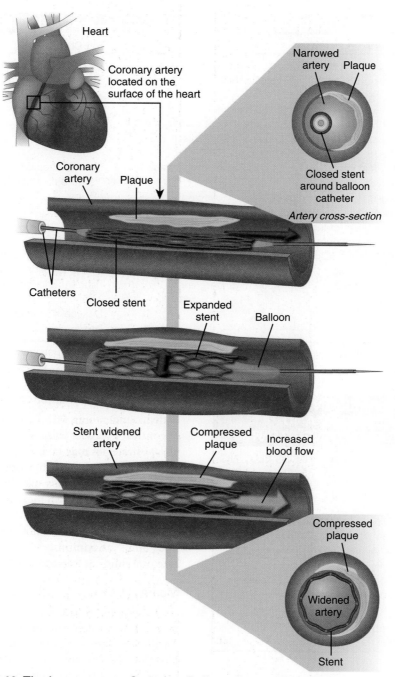

FIGURE 13-10 The Intracoronary Stent is a Balloon-Expandable Stent.

radiation through specialized catheters. Because healing within the stent is delayed, late thrombosis may occur in patients with DES. Late thrombosis, although rare, is associated with a 45% mortality rate. Premature discontinuation of antiplatelet therapy is the strongest predictor of late stent thrombosis, especially with DES.[32]

Nursing Management

Nursing management after PCI is focused on accurate assessment of the patient's condition and prompt intervention. **Nursing priorities are directed toward (1) monitoring for recurrent angina, (2) protecting kidney function,** **(3) monitoring the femoral access site, (4) monitoring peripheral pulses, promoting mobility, and (5) providing patient education.**

Monitoring for Recurrent Angina

It is essential that the nurse observe the patient for recurrent angina or ST elevation, which are clinical indicators of myocardial ischemia. Monitoring leads should be selected that will reflect ischemia in the vessels that were treated during the intervention.[29] Angina during interventional cardiology procedures is an expected occurrence at the time of balloon inflation or manipulation within the coronary

TABLE 13-6 PHARMACOLOGICAL MANAGEMENT: GLYCOPROTEIN IIB/IIIA INHIBITORS

DRUG	INDICATIONS AND DOSAGE	SPECIAL CONSIDERATIONS
Abciximab (ReoPro)	ACS: 0.25 mg/kg IVP, then 10 mcg/min until PCI PCI: 0.25 mg/kg IVP, then 0.125 mcg/kg/min × 12 hr	Used concomitantly with heparin and aspirin May affect platelet function for up to 48 hours after infusion
Eptifibatide (Integrilin)	ACS: IV bolus of 180 mcg/kg followed by an infusion of 2 mcg/kg/min for up to 72 hours; if the patient undergoes PCI, the infusion should be continued up to hospital discharge, or for up to 18 to 24 hours after the procedure, whichever comes first, and continued for 24 hours after the procedure, for a total of 96 hours PCI: 180 mcg/kg IVP immediately before PCI followed by a continuous infusion of 2.0 mcg/kg/min and a second 180-mcg/kg bolus 10 minutes after the first bolus. Infusion should be continued for a minimum of 12 hours	Concomitant heparin and aspirin may be administered Platelet function returns to baseline within 6-8 hours Dosage should be reduced in patients with severe renal dysfunction
Tirofiban (Aggrastat)	ACS (with or without PCI): 0.4 mcg/kg/min for 30 min, then continued at 0.1 mcg/kg/min for 48-108 hours after ACS or 12-24 hours post-procedure for patients undergoing PCI	Administered in combination with heparin for patients undergoing PCI Platelet function returns to baseline within 4-8 hours Dosage should be reduced in patients with severe kidney dysfunction

ACS, acute coronary syndrome; *IV*, intravenous; *IVP*, intravenous push; *PCI*, percutaneous coronary intervention.

TABLE 13-7 COMPARISON OF BARE METAL AND DRUG-ELUTING STENTS

CHARACTERISTICS	BARE METAL STENT	DRUG-ELUTING STENT
Restenosis rate (at 6 months)	15-20%	5-10%
Cost	$800-1000 per stent	$2400-3000 per stent
Duration of dual antiplatelet therapy	2-4 weeks	12 months
Recommended lesion features	Short lesions <20 mm Large vessel diameter >3.0 mm	Longer lesions >20 mm Small vessel diameter <3.5 mm

Protecting Kidney Function

Patients undergoing PCI are exposed to significant amounts of contrast dye, with its associated nephrotoxicity. Renal protective strategies may be implemented before the procedure, especially for patients with evidence of baseline impairment of kidney function. This may include preprocedural hydration, infusion of sodium bicarbonate, and administration of *N*-acetylcysteine (Mucomyst).[42] After PCI, hydration is essential to maintain adequate flow through the kidneys. Intravenous fluids are administered, and patients are encouraged to take oral fluids as tolerated.[43]

Monitoring the Femoral Access Site

Assessing for Bleeding. While the femoral sheath is in place or after its removal, bleeding or hematoma at the sheath insertion site may occur due to the effects of anticoagulation. The nurse observes the patient for bleeding or swelling at the puncture site and frequently assesses adequacy of circulation to the involved extremity. The nurse also assesses the patient for back pain, which can indicate retroperitoneal bleeding from the internal arterial puncture site. The patient is instructed to keep the involved leg straight and not to elevate the head of the bed any more than 30 degrees while the sheath is in place (to prevent dislodgment) and for several hours after its removal (to prevent bleeding), unless a vascular closure device is used. After sheath removal, direct pressure is applied to the puncture site for 15 to 30 minutes; a sandbag may be ordered if direct pressure is inadequate for hemostasis. For stent placement or atherectomy, which require a larger sheath size, a C-clamp or femoral compression device may be used to apply continuous pressure for 1 to 2 hours to ensure adequate hemostasis.

artery. Intraprocedural angina is caused by the temporary interruption of blood flow through the involved artery, which should subside with deflation or removal of the balloon or nitroglycerin administration, or both. Angina after a coronary interventional procedure may be caused by transient coronary vasospasm, or it may signal a more serious complication—acute thrombosis. In any case, the nurse must act quickly to assess for manifestations of myocardial ischemia and initiate clinical interventions as indicated. The physician usually orders intravenous nitroglycerin to be titrated to alleviate chest pain. Continued angina despite maximal vasodilator therapy usually rules out transient coronary vasospasm as the source of ischemic pain, and a return to the cardiac catheterization laboratory must be considered.

Hemostatic Devices. In the last decade, percutaneous vascular hemostatic devices have been introduced to address the problem of achieving adequate hemostasis at the femoral access site after sheath removal. Active closure devices utilize mechanical sutures, collagen plugs, or metal clips to close the vessel when the sheath is removed. Advantages of these devices include a reduced time to hemostasis of less than 5 minutes regardless of the patient's level of anticoagulation, earlier ambulation, and increased patient comfort.[44] Perclose has marketed a percutaneous vascular surgical device that is inserted into the femoral artery in the same position as a conventional introducer sheath. The device contains needles and sutures that are used to suture the artery closed after the interventional procedure. Angio-Seal is a vascular hemostatic device that uses a collagen plug to seal the arterial puncture site. Gentle pressure is maintained over the puncture site for approximately 5 minutes, until hemostasis is achieved. The StarClose vascular closure device consists of a tiny circumferential nitinol (nickel and titanium) clip that is applied to the surface of the vessel to close the femoral artery at the end of the procedure.

Reports of complications and increased cost have limited the use of active closure devices by some clinicians.[44,45] To avoid these complications, a number of products have been developed to enhance manual compression and shorten the time required to achieve hemostasis. Some of these devices rely on the delivery of prothrombotic materials by a patch, whereas others increase local pressure over the puncture site. These devices do not offer immediate closure, but may decrease the time to ambulation.[44] A comparison of vascular closure systems is provided in Table 13-8.

Monitoring Peripheral Pulses

Excessive bleeding or hematoma formation can become a serious problem if it results in hypotension or compromised blood flow to the involved extremity. Pulses are usually monitored every 15 minutes for the first 2 hours after the procedure and then every 1 to 2 hours until the sheaths are removed. After sheath removal, pulses are again monitored at 15-minute intervals for a brief period.

Promoting Mobility

Patients usually are allowed to resume ambulation 6 to 8 hours after the procedure, depending on institutional protocol, and effectiveness of hemostatic closure of the vascular access site.

Providing Patient Education

In most cases, patients undergoing elective angioplasty, atherectomy, or stent procedures are hospitalized for approximately 24 hours. All patients require education about their medication regimen and about risk-factor modification. Because of the abbreviated hospital stay, the nurse often has time to do little more than identify the offending risk factors and initiate basic instruction. Patients are referred to local cardiac rehabilitation centers for more extensive teaching and follow-up to facilitate understanding and compliance with risk-factor modification.

TABLE 13-8	**VASCULAR CLOSURE DEVICES**		
TECHNOLOGY AND EXAMPLES	**DESCRIPTION**		**COMMENTS**
Patch Chito-Seal Clo-Sur P.A.D. D-Stat SyvekPatch	Patches that contain materials to promote clotting are applied directly to the puncture site, along with manual compression.		Less expensive than active closure devices. No foreign material is left in the patient.
Suture Perclose A-TProGlide	Sutures deployed through the sheath are used to close the arteriotomy site.		Allows for immediate reaccess through the site if needed. Device failure may require surgical repair.
Plug or Sealant Angio-Seal Duett Mynx	Placement of a procoagulant sealant such as collagen or thrombin is used to close the artery. Angio-Seal also includes an intravascular suture to anchor the collagen plug in place. The Mynx system uses a balloon catheter to inject sealant into the puncture site tract.		Reaccess must be done 1 cm above the previous arterial access site to avoid dislodging the sealant. Extrusion of the sealant into the vessel may compromise the arterial lumen. Components are absorbed within 30-90 days, depending on the sealant used.
Clip or Staple EVS-Angiolink StarClose	Circumferential staples or clips are deployed at the site of the arteriotomy to close the vessel.		Extravascular clip does not compromise the artery lumen.

Another point of instruction that must be addressed is the patient's knowledge deficit related to discharge medications. Patients are sent home on a regimen of antiplatelet drugs and drugs for secondary prevention, such as lipid-lowering agents and blood pressure medications. A nitrate such as isosorbide may be prescribed to promote vasodilation, or, if the patient has demonstrated evidence of a vasospastic component to the disease, calcium channel blockers may be used. It is essential that the patient clearly understand the rationale for therapy and the potential side effects of each drug. Patients also need to understand the importance of not discontinuing their antiplatelet therapy; deaths have been reported when patients discontinued this therapy before elective procedures.[46] It is important that patients be provided with written information and a number to call if problems occur.

PERCUTANEOUS VALVE REPAIR

Percutaneous catheter technology has also been adapted to allow for nonsurgical interventions for stenotic cardiac valves. Percutaneous balloon valvuloplasty, also known as balloon valvotomy, has become an accepted alternative to surgical approaches in patients with mitral or pulmonic valve stenosis. Aortic valvotomy has a limited role in adults, because restenosis and clinical deterioration occur within 6 to 12 months in most patients, and the procedure is associated with significant morbidity and mortality.[47] Eligibility criteria for balloon valvuloplasty are listed in Box 13-5.

Balloon valvotomy is performed in the cardiac catheterization laboratory. The procedure is similar to a routine cardiac catheterization, including cannulation of the femoral artery and vein with percutaneous introducer sheaths. The balloon dilation catheter is then threaded over a guidewire across the stenotic valvular orifice. The valves may be approached retrograde through the aorta, or antegrade across the interatrial septum. In the antegrade transseptal approach, the balloon catheter is passed across the interatrial septum, which results in the creation of a small atrial septal defect.[48] Subsequent inflations of the balloon increase the valve opening by

separating fused valve leaflets, cracking calcified leaflets, and stretching valve structures. Inflations are continued until the balloon "waist" disappears, which indicates full inflation. Regurgitant flow can result, particularly after mitral valvotomy, and may result in the need for emergent valve replacement if severe. The risks of balloon valvotomy are similar to those inherent in most catheterization procedures and include cardiac perforation, thromboembolic events, dysrhythmias, and vascular complications caused by the sheath. Postprocedural nursing management is similar to that for other percutaneous cardiac catheter procedures.

A number of additional percutaneous procedures for valve repair are being evaluated in clinical trials. Percutaneous aortic valve replacement has shown promising results as a possible treatment for aortic stenosis. This procedure involves the use of a valvuloplasty balloon catheter to deliver a stainless steel stent with an attached bovine valve within the native aortic valve. After the stent is in position, the balloon is inflated to deploy the stent valve.[49] Investigational percutaneous treatments for mitral valve repair include correction of mitral regurgitation with a leaflet clip or an annular ring.[50]

CARDIAC SURGERY

Nursing management of the patient undergoing cardiac surgery is demanding but exciting work that requires the talents of an experienced team of critical care nurses. The following discussion introduces basic cardiac surgical techniques and principles of cardiopulmonary bypass and highlights the key points about postoperative care of the adult patient who requires valve replacement or coronary artery revascularization.

Coronary Artery Bypass Surgery

Since its introduction more than 2 decades ago, CABG has proved to be safe and effective in relieving uncontrolled angina pectoris in most patients. Information on coronary artery disease is presented in Chapter 12 and catheter interventions for coronary artery disease are discussed earlier in this chapter.

The combined results of three major randomized trials support the view that CABG affords dramatic improvement of symptoms and quality of life. CABG is more effective than medical therapy (i.e., pharmacological therapy and PCI) for improving survival in patients with left main coronary artery disease, triple-vessel disease, or double-vessel disease involving the LAD artery, and for relief of exercise-induced ischemia or chronic ischemia leading to LV dysfunction. Medical therapy is recommended if the ischemia is prevented by antianginal drugs that are well tolerated by the patient.[51] Surgical revascularization has been shown to be more efficacious than stenting in patients with multivessel disease.[52] If arterial grafts are used, CABG has superior long-term patency rates, surpassing those of angioplasty or stents.[53] Bypass surgery may allow for more complete revascularization, because it can be used on vessels that are not amenable to treatment with a

---

BOX 13-5 **INDICATIONS FOR BALLOON VALVULOPLASTY**

Aortic
- Nonsurgical candidate with incapacitating symptoms
- Patient with aortic stenosis who requires urgent noncardiac surgery
- Patient with severe heart failure or cardiogenic shock because of aortic stenosis whose condition needs to be stabilized until valve replacement is deemed safer
- Patient with poor left ventricular function, low cardiac output, and a small gradient across a stenotic aortic valve whose need for aortic valve replacement requires assessment

Mitral
- As an alternative to open mitral commissurotomy

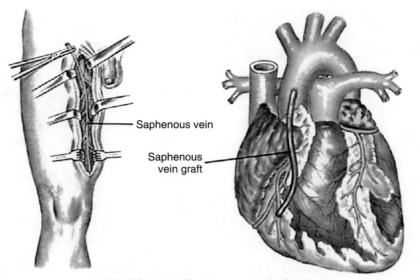

FIGURE 13-11 Saphenous Vein Graft.

percutaneous approach, such as those with total occlusions or excessive tortuosity.

Myocardial revascularization involves the use of a conduit, or channel, designed to bypass an occluded coronary artery. The two most common conduits are the saphenous vein graft and the internal mammary artery (IMA) graft.

Saphenous Vein Graft

Saphenous vein grafting involves the anastomosis of an excised portion of the saphenous vein proximal to the aorta and distal to the coronary artery below the obstruction (Figure 13-11). Traditionally, the saphenous vein graft was obtained through an open incision, but endoscopic harvesting of this vessel is now possible. This minimally invasive technique of graft procurement decreases postoperative pain and reduces leg wound infection.[54]

Internal Mammary Artery Graft

The IMA, which usually remains attached to its origin at the subclavian artery, is swung down and anastomosed distal to the coronary artery (Figure 13-12). Either the right IMA or the left IMA may be used as a conduit. Of note, emergency CABG may preclude the use of the IMA because of the extra time required to mobilize the artery and the inability to effect cardioplegia through this conduit. However, the current trend is to use arterial conduits such as the IMA whenever possible, because their long-term patency rates are superior to those of the saphenous vein graft.[55]

Right Gastroepiploic Artery Graft

The right gastroepiploic artery (GEA) has also been introduced as an alternative conduit for CABG. The artery, which is a branch of the gastroduodenal artery, is pulled up through the diaphragm to the pericardial cavity, and anastomosed to a distal portion of the coronary artery. Although it is a little smaller in diameter than the IMA, studies indicate that patency rates are excellent.[56] Because of its size and anatomic

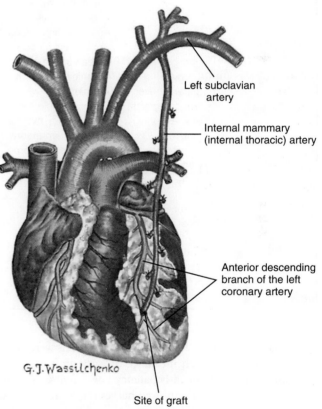

G.J. Wassilchenko

FIGURE 13-12 Internal Mammary Artery Graft.

location, the gastroepiploic artery is well suited for bypassing the right coronary artery, the circumflex artery, or the posterior descending artery. However, the technical aspects of obtaining this conduit may limit its widespread use.

Radial Artery Grafts

The potential benefit of long-term patency associated with arterial conduits has revived interest in the use of radial artery grafts. First introduced as a potential conduit for myocardial

TABLE 13-9	CONDUITS USED FOR CORONARY ARTERY BYPASS GRAFTS	
TYPE OF GRAFT	**ADVANTAGES**	**DISADVANTAGES**
Saphenous vein	Easily harvested Length allows for multiple grafts No anatomic limitations to graft sites	Long-term patency is not as good as that of arterial grafts Requires at least two anastomosis sites Associated with leg edema postoperatively
Internal mammary artery	Improved patency over venous grafts Requires only one anastomosis	Requires extensive dissection Not accessible for emergency bypass Associated with increased chest wall discomfort postoperatively Anatomic limitations to bypassing some areas of the heart
Gastroepiploic artery	Improved patency over venous grafts Requires only one anastomosis Associated with increased gastrointestinal complications postoperatively	Technically difficult to harvest Not accessible for emergency bypass Anatomic limitations to bypassing some areas of the heart Requires adequate collateral flow to the hand through the ulnar artery May be associated with higher rates of vasospasm Requires two anastomosis sites

revascularization in the 1970s, radial artery grafts were abandoned because of a high incidence of early graft occlusion and vasospasm. Current early patency rates of 90% or better have been attributed to improved harvesting techniques and the use of postoperative calcium channel blockers to minimize vasospasm.[57] A comparison of conduits used for myocardial revascularization is provided in Table 13-9.

Valvular Surgery

Valvular disease results in various hemodynamic dysfunctions that usually can be managed medically as long as the patient remains symptom-free. There is reluctance to intervene surgically early in the course of this disease because of the surgical risks and long-term complications associated with prosthetic valve replacement. These consequences, however, must be weighed against the possibility of irreversible deterioration in LV function that may develop during the compensated asymptomatic phase (see "Valvular Heart Disease" in Chapter 12).

Surgical therapy for aortic valve disease consists primarily of aortic valve replacement, although repairs may be done for selected regurgitant valves.[48] Three surgical procedures are available to treat mitral valve disease: commissurotomy, valve repair, and valve replacement. Commissurotomy is performed for mitral stenosis; the fused leaflets are incised, and calcium deposits are débrided to increase valve mobility. Repair of damaged leaflets may be accomplished with pericardial patches. In the setting of mitral regurgitation, valve repair may include reshaping of the leaflets and the use of a ring to reduce the size of the dilated mitral annulus, enhancing leaflet coaptation (annuloplasty). Although it is technically more demanding, valve repair is preferred over replacement to avoid the complications inherent with a prosthetic valve: the risk of thromboembolic events and the need for long-term anticoagulation.[58] If reconstruction of the mitral valve is not possible, it is replaced.

The patient undergoing valvular surgery has an anticipated length of hospital stay from 5 to 9 days. The longer length of stay is for patients who undergo cardiac catheterization in addition to valvular surgery. Prosthetic heart valves are designed with an orifice, through which blood flows, and an occluding structure that opens and closes. The two categories of prosthetic heart valves are mechanical valves and biological valves, also described as tissue valves. Mechanical valves are made from combinations of metal alloys, Pyrolite carbon, Dacron, and Teflon, and have rigid occluding devices (Figure 13-13). Their construction renders them highly durable, but all patients with mechanical valves require anticoagulation to reduce the incidence of thromboembolism.[59] Biological valves are constructed from animal or human cardiac tissue and have flexible occluding mechanisms. Because of their low thrombogenicity, tissue valves offer the patient freedom from therapeutic anticoagulation. Their durability, however, is limited by their tendency toward early calcification. Box 13-6 provides a description of various valvular prostheses.

Heart Transplant

Heart transplant is performed for end-stage heart failure with a life expectancy of only 6 to 12 months.[60] A median incision and sternotomy is for visualization of the thorax. All of the diseased heart is removed except the posterior walls of the atria that contain the openings of the pulmonary veins and the vena cava. There are four major anastomoses to connect the donor heart to the remaining atrial wall. The right atria, left atria, aorta, and pulmonary artery are connected in that order (Figure 13-14). Immediate postoperative management is similar to other cardiac surgical procedures. For the rest of their lives, recipients must take immunosuppressive drugs to prevent rejection of the new heart.[61] Surveillance for rejection, prevention of infection, and comprehensive education about transplant self-care are essential to ensure a long-term success.

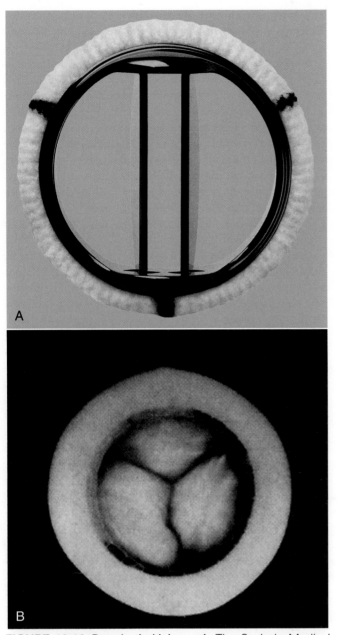

FIGURE 13-13 Prosthetic Valves. *A,* The St Jude Medical mechanical heart valve is a mechanical central-flow disk. *B,* In the Hancock II porcine aortic valve, the flexible Delrin stent and sewing ring are covered in Dacron cloth. (*A,* Courtesy St Jude Medical, Inc., copyright 1993, St Paul, Minn; *B,* from Eagle K, et al, editors: *The practice of cardiology,* ed 2, Boston, 1989, Little, Brown.)

BOX 13-6 CLASSIFICATION OF PROSTHETIC CARDIAC VALVES

Mechanical Valves
- Medtronic Hall
- Omniscience
- Monostrut
  Bi-leaflet: two semicircular leaflets, mounted on a circular sewing ring that opens centrally
- St Jude Medical
- Duromedics
- CarboMedics
- On-X
- ATS

Biological Or Tissue Valves (Bioprostheses)
Porcine heterograft: a porcine aortic valve mounted on a semiflexible stent and preserved in glutaraldehyde
- Hancock
- Carpentier-Edwards
- Toronto Stentless (St Jude)
- Freestyle Stentless (Medtronic)
  Homograft: a human heart valve (aortic or pulmonic) harvested from a donated heart and cryopreserved; may or may not be mounted on a support ring

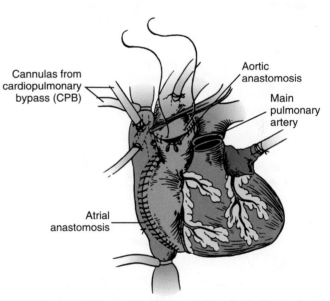

FIGURE 13-14 Heart Transplant Surgical Procedure. (Modified from Hurst JW, et al: *Hurst's The Heart,* ed 7, New York, 1990, McGraw-Hill.)

Cardiopulmonary Bypass

Cardiopulmonary bypass (CPB) is a mechanical means of circulating and oxygenating a patient's blood while diverting most of the circulation from the heart and lungs during cardiac surgical procedures. Numerous clinical sequelae can result from CPB (Table 13-10). Knowledge of these effects allows the nurse to anticipate problems and intervene effectively.

Nursing Management

Nursing priorities are directed toward (1) optimizing cardiac output, (2) temperature regulation, (3) controlling bleeding, (4) maintaining chest tube patency, (5) recognizing cardiac tamponade, (6) promoting early extubation, (7) assessing for neurological complications, (8) preventing infection, (9) preserving kidney function, and (10) providing patient education.

TABLE 13-10	PHYSIOLOGICAL EFFECTS OF CARDIOPULMONARY BYPASS
EFFECTS	**CAUSES**
Intravascular fluid deficit (hypotension)	Third-spacing
	Postoperative diuresis
	Sudden vasodilation (drugs, rewarming)
Third-spacing (weight gain, edema)	Decreased plasma protein concentration
	Increased capillary permeability
Myocardial depression (decreased cardiac output)	Hypothermia
	Increased systemic vascular resistance
	Prolonged cardiopulmonary bypass pump run
	Preexisting heart disease
	Inadequate myocardial protection
Coagulopathy (bleeding)	Systemic heparinization
	Mechanical trauma to platelets
	Depressed release of clotting factors from liver as a result of hypothermia
Pulmonary dysfunction (decreased lung mechanics and impaired gas exchange)	Decreased surfactant production
	Pulmonary microemboli
	Interstitial fluid accumulation in lungs
Hemolysis (hemoglobinuria)	Red blood cells damaged in pump circuit
Hyperglycemia (rise in serum glucose concentration)	Decreased insulin release
	Stimulation of glycogenolysis
Hypokalemia (low serum potassium concentration)	Intracellular shifts during bypass and postoperative diuresis
Hypomagnesemia (low serum magnesium concentration)	Postoperative diuresis resulting from hemodilution
Neurological dysfunction (decreased level of consciousness, motor/sensory deficits)	Inadequate cerebral perfusion
	Microemboli to brain (air, plaque fragments, fat globules)
Hypertension (transient rise in blood pressure)	Catecholamine release and systemic hypothermia causing vasoconstriction

Optimizing Cardiac Output

Postoperative cardiovascular support often is indicated because of a low-output state resulting from preexisting heart disease, a prolonged cardiopulmonary bypass pump run, inadequate myocardial protection, or some combination of these factors. Cardiac output can be maximized by adjustments in heart rate, preload, afterload, and contractility.

Heart Rate. In the presence of low cardiac output, the heart rate can be appropriately regulated by means of temporary pacing or drug therapy. Temporary epicardial pacing usually is instituted when the heart rate of the adult patient who has had cardiac surgery drops to less than 80 beats/min. In the case of tachycardia, intravenous beta-blockers (esmolol) or calcium channel blockers (diltiazem) may be used in the acute postoperative period to slow supraventricular rhythms with a ventricular response that exceeds 110 beats/min. Because ventricular ectopy can result from hypokalemia, serum potassium levels are maintained in the high-normal range (4.5 to 5 mEq/L) to provide some margin for error. Maintaining serum magnesium in a therapeutic range (2 mEq/L) has also been shown to reduce the incidence of dysrhythmias in the postoperative period.[62]

Atrial fibrillation occurs in one third of patients after cardiac surgery, with a peak occurrence in the first 2 to 3 days after surgery. This rhythm may induce hemodynamic compromise, prolong hospitalization, and increase the patient's risk of stroke. Prophylactic administration of antidysrhythmic agents such as beta-blockers has been shown to decrease the incidence of atrial fibrillation and its clinical sequelae.[63]

Preload. In most patients, reduced preload is the cause of low postoperative cardiac output. If a pulmonary artery catheter has been inserted during surgery, monitoring of the pulmonary artery occlusion pressure (PAOP), also known as the wedge pressure, can provide a more convenient and accurate guide to LV preload than monitoring of central venous pressure (CVP) alone. To enhance preload, volume may be administered in the form of crystalloid, colloid, or packed red cells. It is not uncommon to achieve the greatest hemodynamic stability in cardiac surgery patients when filling pressures (PAOP or pulmonary artery diastolic pressure [PADP]) are in the range of 18 to 20 mm Hg (normally 5 to 12 mm Hg).

Afterload. Partly as a result of the peripheral vasoconstrictive effects of hypothermia, many patients who have had cardiac surgery demonstrate postoperative hypertension. Although it is transient, postoperative hypertension can precipitate or exacerbate bleeding from the mediastinal chest tubes. The high SVR (afterload) resulting from the intense vasoconstriction can increase LV workload. Vasodilator therapy with intravenous sodium nitroprusside or nitroglycerin often is used to reduce afterload, control hypertension, and improve cardiac output.

A significant percentage of patients experience hypotension after cardiopulmonary bypass, associated with peripheral vasodilation and a low SVR. This is believed to occur, in part, because of the systemic inflammatory response to cardiopulmonary bypass. Therapy for hypotension after cardiac surgery usually includes volume loading and vasopressors such as phenylephrine or vasopressin to tighten the peripheral vasculature and maintain an adequate mean arterial pressure.[64]

Contractility. If the adjustments in heart rate, preload, and afterload fail to produce significant improvement in cardiac output, contractility can be enhanced with positive inotropic support or intraaortic balloon pumping (IABP) to augment circulation (discussed later).

Temperature Regulation

Hypothermia can contribute to depressed myocardial contractility in the patient who has had cardiac surgery. Hypothermia may contribute to postoperative bleeding, because the functioning of clotting factors is depressed during hypothermia. After surgery, patients may be rewarmed with the use of warmed air or water blankets. To prevent subsequent excessive temperature elevations, care must be taken to remove the blankets promptly when the body temperature reaches 98.6° F (37° C).

Controlling Bleeding

Postoperative bleeding from the mediastinal chest tubes can be caused by inadequate hemostasis, disruption of suture lines, or coagulopathy associated with cardiopulmonary bypass or hypothermia. Bleeding is more likely to occur with IMA grafts as a result of the extensive chest wall dissection required to free the IMA. If bleeding in excess of 150 mL/hr occurs early in the postoperative period, clotting factors (fresh-frozen plasma, fibrinogen, and platelets) and additional protamine (used to reverse the effects of heparin) may be administered, along with prompt blood replacement. Other medications used in the treatment of postoperative bleeding are described in Table 13-11.

TABLE 13-11	PHARMACOLOGICAL MANAGEMENT: POSTOPERATIVE BLEEDING	
DRUG	**DOSAGE**	**ACTION AND SIDE EFFECTS**
Aminocaproic acid (Amicar)	Loading dose: 5 g over 1 hour, followed by continuous infusion of 1 g/hr for 8 hr or until bleeding is controlled	Inhibits conversion of plasminogen to plasmin to prevent fibrinolysis, helping to stabilize clots
Desmopressin acetate (DDAVP)	0.3 mg/kg IV over 20-30 minutes	Improves platelet function by increasing levels of factor VIII side effects include facial flushing, tachycardia, headache, and hypotension
Protamine sulfate	25-50 mg IV slowly over 10 minutes	Neutralizes the anticoagulant effect of heparin Can cause hypotension, bradycardia, and allergic reactions

Autotransfusion devices, which facilitate the collection and reinfusion of shed mediastinal blood, were used in some institutions in the past. Routine autotransfusion of shed mediastinal blood is no longer recommended, because it may further exacerbate bleeding by activating the extrinsic clotting pathway and increase the risk of infection.[65] The use of positive end-expiratory pressure (PEEP) in conjunction with mechanical ventilation may be helpful in controlling excessive bleeding in some cases by increasing the intrathoracic pressure enough to effect tamponade of oozing mediastinal blood vessels.[65] Rewarming the patient reverses the depressed manufacture and release of clotting factors that results from hypothermia. However, persistent mediastinal bleeding—usually in excess of 500 mL in 1 hour or 300 mL/hr for 2 consecutive hours despite normalization of clotting studies—is an indication for reexploration of the surgical site.

Maintaining Chest Tube Patency

Chest tube stripping to maintain patency of the tubes is controversial because of the high negative pressure generated by routine methods of stripping. It is believed to result in tissue damage that can contribute to bleeding. This risk must be carefully weighed against the real danger of cardiac tamponade if blood is not effectively drained from around the heart. Chest tube stripping often is advocated in instances of excessive postoperative bleeding. However, the technique of "milking" the chest tubes is advisable for routine postoperative care, because this technique generates less negative pressure and decreases the risk of bleeding.

Recognizing Cardiac Tamponade

Cardiac tamponade may occur after surgery if blood accumulates in the mediastinal space, impairing the heart's ability to pump. Signs of tamponade include elevated and equalized filling pressures (e.g., CVP, PADP, PAOP), decreased cardiac output, decreased blood pressure, jugular venous distention, pulsus paradoxus, muffled heart sounds, sudden cessation of chest tube drainage, and a widened cardiac silhouette on chest x-ray films. Interventions for tamponade may include emergency sternotomy in the intensive care unit or a return to the operating room for surgical evacuation of the clot.

Promoting Early Extubation

Until recently, overnight intubation to facilitate lung expansion and optimize gas exchange was common for patients who had undergone cardiac surgery. Newer protocols that facilitate early extubation (within the first 4 to 8 hours) have been implemented in most institutions.[66] Early extubation requires a multidisciplinary approach that incorporates anesthesiologists, surgeons, nurses, and respiratory therapists. Potential candidates must be identified before surgery so that the anesthetic regimen can be modified to support early extubation. One approach is to use short-acting anesthetic agents such as propofol (Diprivan) at the end of the surgery and to minimize the use of opioids. Another option is to administer neostigmine and glycopyrrolate at the end of the surgery to reverse the neuromuscular blockade used during the procedure.

After surgery, patients are evaluated for hemodynamic stability, adequate control of bleeding, and normothermia. After these criteria have been met, the patient is weaned off propofol or given neuromuscular reversal agents, and ventilator weaning can begin. If needed, opioids are given in small increments to manage pain and anxiety. Patients who exhibit hemodynamic instability or intraoperative complications or who have underlying pulmonary disease related to long-term valvular dysfunction may require longer periods of mechanical ventilation. After extubation, supplemental oxygen is administered, and patients are medicated for incisional pain to facilitate adequate coughing and deep breathing.

Assessing for Neurological Complications

The transient neurological dysfunction often seen in patients who have had cardiac surgery has been attributed to decreased cerebral perfusion, cerebral microemboli, and the systemic inflammatory response. It was once thought to be primarily caused by cardiopulmonary bypass, but newer evidence indicates that cognitive decline may be influenced more by patient-related factors such as the degree of preexisting cerebral vascular disease or diabetes.[67] Compounding these are environmental factors such as sensory deprivation and sensory overload associated with being in a critical care unit. The term postcardiotomy delirium has been used to describe this postoperative syndrome that initially may manifest as only a mild impairment of orientation but that may progress to agitation, hallucinations, and paranoid delusions. One study indicated that mild preoperative cognitive impairment might be a useful predictor of who is likely to develop postcardiotomy delirium.[68]

Treatment of delirium may require the use of medications such as benzodiazepines or haloperidol (Haldol).

Environmental modifications such as noise reduction, restoring normal day/night lighting patterns, and placing familiar objects at the bedside may help to calm and reorient the patient. Liberalization of visitation policies to allow family members a prolonged presence at the bedside is also highly desirable. Nursing management is organized to maximize optimal sleep patterns whenever possible.

Preventing Infection

Postoperative fever is fairly common after cardiopulmonary bypass. However, persistent temperature elevation to greater than 101° F (38.3° C) must be investigated. Sternal wound infections and infective endocarditis are the most devastating infectious complications, but leg wound infection, pneumonia, and urinary tract infection also can occur. Infection rates are greater in diabetic patients. Studies have shown that maintaining the blood glucose concentration between 80 and 110 mg/dL in the perioperative period by means of a continuous insulin infusion may decrease the risk of infection in this population.[69]

Preserving Kidney Function

Hemolysis caused by trauma to the red blood cells in the extracorporeal circuit results in hemoglobinuria, which can damage kidney tubules. Small amounts of furosemide (Lasix) usually are given to promote urine flow if the urine output is low (<25 to 30 mL/hr) and tinged pink.

Guidelines for Coronary Artery Bypass Grafting

The American College of Cardiology and the American Heart Association have developed a set of clinical practice guidelines for care of the patient undergoing CABG.[51] These guidelines are designed to support clinical decision making with research evidence (Evidence-Based Collaborative Practice box on Coronary Artery Bypass Graft Surgery).

EVIDENCE-BASED COLLABORATIVE PRACTICE
Coronary Artery Bypass Graft Surgery

A summary is provided of evidence and evidence-based review recommendations for management of the coronary artery bypass graft (CABG) surgery patient.

Strong Evidence to Support CABG in the Following Circumstances:
CABG for Stable and Unstable Angina
- Significant left main coronary artery stenosis.
- Left main equivalent stenosis: significant (≥70%) stenosis of the proximal left anterior descending (LAD) artery and proximal left circumflex artery.
- Three-vessel disease. Survival benefit is greater in patients with abnormal left ventricular function; such as left ventricular ejection fraction (LVEF) less than 0.50 (50%), or large areas of demonstrable myocardial ischemia.
- One- or two-vessel disease plus extensive ischemia and LVEF less than 0.50 (50%).

- Disabling or unstable angina despite maximal noninvasive therapy if surgery can be performed with acceptable risk. If the angina is not typical, objective evidence of ischemia should be obtained.
- Unstable angina or non-ST-elevation myocardial infarction (NSTEMI) if emergency percutaneous coronary intervention (PCI) revascularization is not optimal or possible, or ongoing ischemia is not responsive to maximal nonsurgical therapy.

CABG during ST-Elevation Myocardial Infarction
- Emergent or urgent CABG in patients with ST-elevation myocardial infarction (STEMI) should be undertaken in the following circumstances:
  1. Failed angioplasty with persistent pain or hemodynamic instability in patients with coronary anatomy suitable for surgery

Coronary Artery Bypass Graft Surgery

2. Persistent or recurrent ischemia refractory to medical therapy in patients with coronary anatomy suitable for surgery who have a significant area of myocardium at risk and who are not candidates for PCI
3. At the time of surgical repair of postinfarction ventricular septal rupture or mitral valve insufficiency
4. Cardiogenic shock in patients younger than 75 years old with STEMI or left bundle branch block or posterior myocardial infarction (MI) who develop shock within 36 hours after MI and are suitable candidates for revascularization that can be performed within 18 hours after shock, unless further support is futile because of the patient's wishes or because of contraindications or unsuitability for further invasive care

CABG Criteria for Life-Threatening Ventricular Dysrhythmias
- Life-threatening ventricular dysrhythmias in the presence of left main coronary artery stenosis greater than or equal to 50% or three-vessel coronary disease.

CABG Plus Valve Surgery Criteria
- Patients undergoing CABG who also have severe aortic stenosis should undergo aortic valve replacement (AVR). Severe aortic stenosis is measured by a mean gradient greater than or equal to 50 mm Hg or a Doppler velocity greater than or equal to 4 m/sec.

Reduction in Intraoperative Complications
- Significant atherosclerosis of the ascending aorta mandates a surgical approach that minimizes the possibility of arteriosclerotic emboli and stroke.
- Blood cardioplegia should be considered in patients undergoing cardiopulmonary bypass accompanying CABG surgery for acute MI or unstable angina.
- In every patient undergoing CABG, the left internal mammary artery should be given primary consideration for revascularization of the LAD artery.

Transmyocardial Revascularization
- Transmyocardial surgical laser revascularization, alone or in combination with CABG surgery, is reasonable in patients with angina refractory to medical therapy who are not candidates for PCI or surgical revascularization.

Reduction in Risk of Infection
- Preoperative antibiotic administration should be used in all patients to reduce the risk of postoperative infection.
- A deep sternal wound infection should be treated with aggressive surgical débridement and early revascularized muscle flap coverage, unless there are complicating circumstances.

Prevention of Postoperative Dysrhythmias
- Preoperative or early postoperative administration of beta-blockers in patients without contraindications should be used as the standard therapy to reduce the incidence and clinical sequelae of atrial fibrillation after CABG surgery.

Antiplatelet Therapy
- Aspirin is the drug of choice for prophylaxis against early saphenous vein graft closure.
- If clinical circumstances permit, clopidogrel should be withheld for 5 days before the performance of CABG surgery.

Pharmacological Management of Hyperlipidemia
- All CABG surgery patients should receive statin therapy unless otherwise contraindicated.

Smoking Cessation is Important
- All smokers should receive educational counseling and be offered smoking cessation therapy after CABG surgery.
- Pharmacological therapy including nicotine replacement and bupropion (in selected patients) should be offered to patients indicating a willingness to quit.

Cardiac Rehabilitation is Beneficial
- Cardiac rehabilitation should be offered to all eligible patients after CABG.

Moderate Evidence Exists to Support the Following:
Assessment of Preoperative Risk
- Preoperative statistical risk models may be used to obtain objective estimates of cardiac surgical operative mortality.
- After MI that leads to clinically significant right ventricular dysfunction, it is reasonable to delay surgery for 4 weeks to allow recovery.

CABG Risk-Benefit Analysis for Stable and Unstable Angina
- CABG can be beneficial for patients who have proximal or nonproximal LAD stenosis with one- or two-vessel disease. The decision depends on extent of ischemia and LVEF (see section on *Strong Evidence*).

CABG during ST-Elevation Myocardial Infarction
- CABG may be performed as primary reperfusion in patients who have suitable anatomy, who are not candidates for or have had previous failed fibrinolysis or PCI, and who are not in the early hours (6 to 12 hours) of evolving STEMI. In patients who have had a STEMI or an NSTEMI, CABG mortality is elevated for the first 3 to 7 days after infarction, and the benefit of revascularization must be balanced against this increased risk. Beyond 7 days after infarction, the revascularization criteria described in the section on *Strong Evidence* are applicable.

CABG Plus Valve Surgery Criteria
- For patients with a preoperative diagnosis of clinically significant mitral regurgitation, concomitant mitral valve repair or replacement at the time of CABG is probably indicated.
- For patients undergoing CABG who have moderate aortic stenosis, concomitant AVR is probably indicated. Moderate aortic stenosis is measured by a mean transvalve gradient of 30 to 50 mm Hg or a Doppler velocity of 3 to 4 m/sec.

Continued

- Patients undergoing CABG who have mild aortic stenosis may be considered candidates for AVR if the risk of the combined procedure is acceptable. Mild aortic stenosis is measured by a mean gradient less than 30 mm Hg or a Doppler velocity less than 3 m/sec.

Reduction in Risk of Thrombus Formation
- After cardiac surgery, patients with atrial fibrillation that is recurrent or that persists longer than 24 hours should receive warfarin anticoagulation for 4 weeks.
- Long-term anticoagulation (3 to 6 months) is indicated for the patient with recent anteroapical infarct and persistent wall-motion abnormality after CABG surgery.
- Preoperative screening with echocardiography is considered for patients who have had a recent anterior MI to detect left ventricular thrombus; if thrombus is present, the timing or surgical approach may be altered.

Reduction in Risk of Carotid Disease and Stroke
- Carotid endarterectomy is probably indicated before CABG surgery or concomitant with CABG in patients who have a symptomatic carotid stenosis and in asymptomatic patients who have a unilateral or bilateral internal carotid stenosis of 80% or greater.
- Carotid screening is probably indicated in the following subsets of patients: age greater than 65 years, left main coronary artery stenosis, peripheral arterial disease, history of smoking, history of transient ischemic attack or stroke, carotid bruit on examination.

Cardiac Biomarker Elevation and Outcome
- Assessment of cardiac biomarkers in the first 24 hours after CABG may be considered. Patients with the highest elevations of creatine kinase-MB (>5 times the upper limit of normal) are at increased risk for subsequent adverse events.

Adjuncts to Myocardial Protection
- Use of prophylactic intraaortic balloon pump (IABP) support as an adjunct to myocardial protection is probably indicated in patients with evidence of ongoing myocardial ischemia or a subnormal cardiac index.

Reduction in Risk of Infection
- The risk for deep sternal wound infection is reduced by aggressive control of perioperative hyperglycemia with a continuous intravenous insulin infusion.

Prevention of Postoperative Dysrhythmias
- Preoperative administration of amiodarone reduces the incidence of postcardiotomy atrial fibrillation and is an appropriate prophylactic therapy for patients at high risk for postoperative atrial fibrillation who have contraindications to therapy with beta-blockers (see section on *Strong Evidence*).
- Digoxin and nondihydropyridine calcium channel blockers are useful for control of ventricular rate but at present have no indication for prophylactic use.
- Low-dose sotalol can be considered to reduce the incidence of atrial fibrillation after CABG in patients who are not candidates for traditional beta-blockers.

Data from Eagle KA, et al: ACC/AHA 2004 guideline update for coronary artery bypass graft surgery: a report of the American College of Cardiology/American Heart Association Task Force on Practice Guidelines (Committee to Update the 1999 Guidelines for Coronary Artery Bypass Graft Surgery), *Circulation* 110(14):e340, 2004.

Providing Patient Education

Patient education includes information related to the surgical procedure, risk-factor management, and postoperative self-care. Patients who have undergone valve surgery may also require information regarding the need for antibiotic prophylaxis before invasive procedures and specific instructions pertaining to their anticoagulation regimen.

Minimally Invasive Cardiac Surgery

Over the past decade, new techniques have been developed to address some of the problems associated with traditional cardiac surgery procedures. Many of these procedures can be accomplished without a median sternotomy, by means of a series of holes, or ports, in the chest and small thoracotomy incisions. CABG or valve surgery is then performed using a thoracoscope for visualization and specially designed instruments.[70] As technology has improved, minimally invasive procedures have become an option for an expanding number of patients.[74] These procedures may be performed without cardiopulmonary bypass and are described as "off-pump" or "beating heart." Other options

are to use a less invasive, catheter-based system of cardiopulmonary bypass with access through the femoral artery and vein.[70]

OPCAB and MIDCABG

In an effort to avoid the adverse effects of cardiopulmonary bypass, off-pump coronary artery bypass (OPCAB) is performed in approximately 20% to 30% of cases.[70] A variety of incisional approaches can be used. In minimally invasive direct coronary artery bypass graft (MIDCABG) surgery, a small left anterior thoracotomy incision is used to directly harvest the left IMA, which is then anastomosed to the LAD artery. Alternative approaches may use a segment of saphenous vein or radial artery, one end of which is attached to the left IMA and the other to accessible coronary arteries.[70] Some surgeons may opt for a standard median sternotomy approach to allow for bypassing of distal vessels. Several techniques are used to stabilize the operative area during an OPCAB procedure. Immobilization devices that use compression or suction to create an immobile area have been developed to stabilize cardiac wall motion at the site of the anastomosis. Drugs that temporarily decrease the heart rate (e.g., esmolol, diltiazem) or cause transient cardiac asystole (e.g., adenosine) may also be used to further limit cardiac motion.[71]

Results from OPCAB surgery have been mixed. Some studies have demonstrated improvements in morbidity, including decreased transfusion requirements, shortened time on the ventilator, decreased length of stay, and a lower incidence of stroke and renal complications.[72] Others have shown no advantage over conventional surgery.[73,74] OPCAB may be most beneficial in patients with significant comorbid conditions and in those with contraindications to cardiopulmonary bypass.[75]

Minimally invasive procedures will continue to be refined with the use of robotic equipment in cardiac surgery, currently under clinical investigation at a small number of centers. Robotic-assisted surgery allows the surgeon to view a computer-enhanced image while manipulating instruments through small portholes using robotic arms. This provides increased surgical precision and the ability to perform conventional procedures with smaller incisions.[70]

INTRAAORTIC BALLOON PUMP

IABP is the most widely used temporary mechanical circulatory assist device for supporting failing circulation (Box 13-7). Its therapeutic effects are based on the hemodynamic principles of diastolic augmentation and afterload reduction.

The most commonly used intraaortic balloon (IAB) catheter consists of a single, sausage-shaped polyurethane balloon that is wrapped around the distal end of a vascular catheter and positioned in the descending thoracic aorta just distal to the takeoff of the left subclavian artery. The second generation of IAB catheters is more flexible; they can be wrapped to a smaller diameter than their predecessors and therefore can be inserted into the femoral artery percutaneously rather than surgically. When attached to a bedside pumping console and properly synchronized to the patient's cardiac cycle, the IAB inflates during diastole and deflates just before systole.

Initially, as the balloon is inflated in diastole concurrent with aortic valve closure, the blood in the aortic arch above the level of the balloon is displaced retrograde (backward) toward the aortic root, augmenting diastolic coronary arterial blood flow and increasing myocardial oxygen supply (Figure 13-15, A). The blood volume in the aorta below the level of the balloon is propelled forward toward the peripheral vascular system, which may enhance renal perfusion. Subsequently, the deflation of the balloon just before the opening of the aortic valve creates a potential space or vacuum in the

BOX 13-7	**INDICATIONS FOR USE OF THE INTRAAORTIC BALLOON PUMP**

- Left ventricular failure after cardiac surgery
- Unstable angina refractory to medications
- Recurrent angina after acute myocardial infarction
- Complications of acute myocardial infarction
  - Cardiogenic shock
  - Papillary muscle dysfunction or rupture with mitral regurgitation
  - Ventricular septal rupture
- Refractory ventricular dysrhythmias

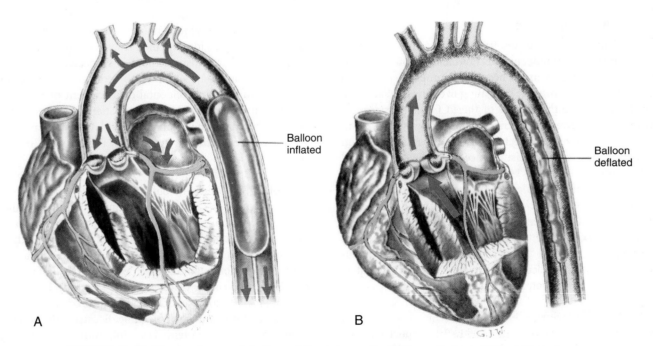

Balloon inflated

Balloon deflated

A   B

FIGURE 13-15 Mechanisms of Action of the Intraaortic Balloon Pump. *A,* Diastolic balloon inflation augments coronary blood flow. *B,* Systolic balloon deflation decreases afterload.

aorta, toward which blood flows unimpeded during ventricular ejection (see Figure 13-15, *B*). This decreased resistance to LV ejection, or decreased afterload, facilitates ventricular emptying and reduces myocardial oxygen demands. The overall physiological effect of IABP therapy is an improvement in the balance between myocardial oxygen supply and demand. Contraindications to IABP include aortic aneurysm, aortic valve insufficiency, and severe peripheral vascular disease.[76]

Medical Management

The IAB may be inserted in the operating room, the cardiac catheterization laboratory, or the critical care unit. The IAB catheter is usually inserted percutaneously through the femoral artery and advanced to the correct position in the descending thoracic aorta. The physician may insert the balloon through an introducer sheath, or perform a sheathless insertion. The sheathless insertion decreases the degree of vessel occlusion created by the catheter. In the rare situation where percutaneous catheter placement is not feasible, the catheter can be placed through surgical cutdown or by a direct thoracic approach. After insertion, the balloon is attached to the console and filled with the prescribed volume of helium, and pumping is initiated. If the balloon fails to unwrap completely during filling, the physician may rapidly inflate and deflate the balloon manually, using a syringe.

Nursing Management

The management of the IAB pumping console and its timing functions may be performed by the nurse caring for the patient or delegated to specially trained personnel on the unit. In either situation, several important nursing management responsibilities relate to care of the patient receiving IABP therapy.

Preventing Dysrhythmias

The ECG and arterial pressure tracings are constantly monitored to verify the timing and effect of balloon counterpulsation. For counterpulsation to occur, the pump must receive a trigger signal to identify the beginning of a new cardiac cycle. The trigger can be the R wave of the ECG, the upstroke of the arterial pressure waveform, or a pacemaker spike.[76] Dysrhythmias can adversely affect the timing of balloon inflation and deflation, so rhythm disturbances must be detected and treated promptly. Modern IABPs have automatic timing features that use internal algorithms to adjust inflation and deflation in response to changes in the patient's heart rate or rhythm. New catheters are available that incorporate a fiberoptic sensor to enhance the quality of the arterial waveform obtained from the IAB catheter and improve timing. Mean arterial pressure is ideally maintained at approximately 80 mm Hg with adequate pumping.

Preventing Peripheral Ischemia

The most common complication of IABP support is lower extremity ischemia resulting from occlusion of the femoral artery by the catheter itself or by emboli caused by thrombus

formation on the balloon.[77] Although ischemic complications have decreased with sheathless insertion techniques and the introduction of smaller balloon catheters (7.5 versus 9.5 Fr), evaluation of peripheral circulation remains an important nursing assessment.[78] The presence and quality of peripheral pulses distal to the catheter insertion site are assessed frequently, along with color, temperature, and capillary refill of the involved extremity. Doppler localization of peripheral pulses may be required if pulses are difficult to palpate on the cannulated extremity. Signs of diminished perfusion must be reported immediately. Anticoagulation (e.g., heparin infusion) may be prescribed to decrease the incidence of thrombosis. Other vascular complications associated with IABP include acute aortic dissection and the development of pseudoaneurysms at the catheter insertion site.

Monitoring for Balloon Complications

Another potential complication of IABP therapy is balloon perforation. Perforation occurs because of repeated contact of the balloon membrane with calcified plaque in the aorta as the balloon inflates and deflates. The patient is monitored for evidence of a balloon leak, such as a gas leak alarm from the pump console or the presence of blood in the IAB tubing. If a balloon leak is detected, pumping is stopped and the physician is immediately notified so that the balloon can be removed. If the balloon is not promptly removed or pumping is attempted after the perforation, the IAB may become entrapped as the blood hardens within the catheter, creating a mass. If this occurs, the balloon must be surgically removed.

Monitoring Balloon-Catheter Position

The balloon catheter must be maintained in proper position to optimize its effectiveness and minimize complications. The balloon may migrate proximally and occlude the left subclavian artery, which is detected clinically by a diminished left radial pulse; or the catheter may move distally, compromising circulation to the kidney, which is detected by a fall in urine output. If catheter displacement is suspected, x-rays of the chest or abdomen are obtained to verify balloon placement. Measures to prevent accidental displacement of the balloon catheter include ensuring that the patient observes complete bed rest, with the head of the bed elevated no more than 30 degrees, and avoids any flexion of the involved hip.

Preventing Complications

Log rolling, in which the patient is moved from side to side every 2 hours, is used to maintain skin integrity and to prevent pulmonary atelectasis. Some institutional protocols call for implementation of continuous lateral rotation therapy to help facilitate pulmonary toilet in the patient with an IABP. Because thrombocytopenia may occur as a result of mechanical destruction of the platelets by the pumping action of the balloon, platelet counts are closely monitored and the patient is observed for evidence of bleeding. Because infection of the insertion site is a potential complication, the dressing is changed in accordance with the hospital policy for other invasive lines.

Providing Psychological Support

The psychological needs of the patient must be considered while on IABP therapy. Sleep deprivation is common and is related in part to the continuous nursing management requirements for the patient and the noise level in the unit, including the sounds made by the balloon pumping device. Anxiety related to fear of non-recovery and loss of control because of forced immobility is a common occurrence.

Weaning from the IABP

Weaning from the IABP is considered after hemodynamic stability has been achieved with no, or only minimal, pharmacological support. One weaning procedure consists of slowly decreasing the pumping frequency from every beat to every eighth beat, as tolerated. Another weaning method involves a gradual decrease in balloon volume.[79] To prevent thrombus formation on the balloon surface, the IABP must remain at a minimal pumping ratio (or volume) until its removal.

PHARMACOLOGICAL MANAGEMENT

Antidysrhythmic Drugs

Antidysrhythmic drugs comprise a diverse category of pharmacological agents used to terminate or prevent an array of abnormal cardiac rhythms. These drugs commonly are classified according to their primary effect on the action potential of cardiac cells (Figure 13-16). The classification scheme shown in Table 13-12 is the most commonly used system. Classification of newer agents is more difficult, because some of these agents have characteristics of more than one class and others have no characteristics of the current system.

Class I Drugs

Class I agents are sodium channel blockers that decrease the influx of sodium ions through "fast" channels during phase 0 depolarization. This prolongs the absolute (effective) refractory period, thereby decreasing the risk of premature impulses from ectopic foci. These drugs also depress automaticity by slowing the rate of spontaneous depolarization of pacemaker cells during the resting phase (phase 4).

Class II Drugs

Class II drugs are β-adrenergic blockers (beta-blockers). They inhibit dysrhythmias mediated by the sympathetic nervous system by competing with endogenous catecholamines for available receptor sites. As a result, spontaneous depolarization during the resting phase (phase 4) is depressed, and AV conduction is slowed. Drugs in this class can be further subdivided into cardioselective agents (those that block only β_1-receptors) and noncardioselective agents (those that block both β_1- and β_2-receptors). Knowledge of the effects of adrenergic-receptor stimulation allows for anticipation of both the therapeutic responses brought about by beta-blockade and the potential adverse effects of these agents

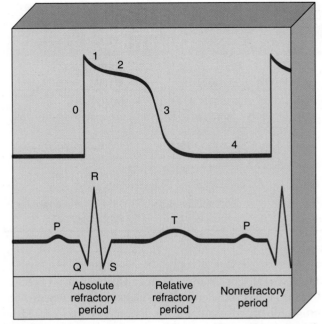

FIGURE 13-16 The phases of the cardiac action potential and their relationship to the heart's refractory periods. *Phase 0*, Depolarization with rapid influx of sodium. *Phase 1*, Rapid repolarization with rapid efflux of potassium ions and decreased sodium conductance. *Phase 2*, Plateau with slow influx of sodium and calcium ions. *Phase 3*, Repolarization with continued efflux of potassium ions. *Phase 4*, Resting phase with restoration of ionic balance by sodium and potassium pumps.

TABLE 13-12	CLASSIFICATION OF ANTIDYSRHYTHMIC AGENTS	
CLASS	**ACTION**	**DRUG**
I	Blocks sodium channels (stabilizes cell membrane)	
IA	Blocks sodium channels and delays repolarization, lengthening the duration of the action potential	Quinidine Procainamide Disopyramide
IB	Blocks sodium channels and accelerates repolarization, shortening the duration of the action potential	Lidocaine Mexiletine Tocainide
IC	Blocks sodium channels and slows conduction through the His-Purkinje system, prolonging the QRS duration	Flecainide Encainide Propafenone
II	Blocks beta-receptors	Esmolol Metoprolol Propranolol
III	Slows repolarization and prolongs the duration of the action potential	Amiodarone Ibutilide Sotalol Dofetilide
IV	Blocks calcium channels	Diltiazem Verapamil

TABLE 13-13	EFFECTS OF ADRENERGIC RECEPTORS	
RECEPTOR	LOCATION	RESPONSE TO STIMULATION
Alpha(α)	Vessels of skin, muscles, kidneys, and intestines	Vasoconstriction of peripheral arterioles
Beta₁ (β₁)	Cardiac tissue	Increased heart rate Increased conduction Increased contractility
Beta₂ (β₂)	Vascular and bronchial smooth muscle	Vasodilation of peripheral arterioles Bronchodilation

(Table 13-13). For example, bronchospasm can be precipitated by noncardioselective beta-blockers in a patient with chronic obstructive pulmonary disease (COPD) caused by blockade of the effects of β_2-receptors in the lungs. Beta-blockers also are negative inotropes and must be used cautiously in patients with LV dysfunction. Although numerous beta-blockers are marketed, only esmolol, metoprolol, and propranolol are available as intravenous agents for the treatment of acute dysrhythmias. Of these, esmolol (Brevibloc) offers significant advantages for the critically ill patient because of its short half-life (approximately 9 minutes). It is used in the treatment of supraventricular tachycardias, such as atrial fibrillation and atrial flutter.

Class III Drugs

Class III agents include amiodarone, dofetilide, ibutilide, and sotalol. These agents markedly slow the rate of phase 3 repolarization, increasing the effective refractory period and the action potential duration. Although their effects on the action potential are similar, these drugs differ greatly in their mechanism of action and their side effects. At this time, sotalol is approved only for oral use. Intravenous amiodarone was originally approved for the treatment of serious ventricular dysrhythmias refractory to other medications. Because of its effectiveness, it is now used for both atrial and ventricular dysrhythmias.[80] Dofetilide (Tikosyn) is a new class III antidysrhythmic agent used for the conversion to and maintenance of normal sinus rhythm in patients with highly symptomatic atrial fibrillation or atrial flutter. Because dofetilide prolongs the refractoriness of both atrial and ventricular tissue, prolongation of the QT interval can occur and is associated with an increased risk of torsades de pointes.[81] Therapy with dofetilide is initiated in a hospital setting under close monitoring. Ibutilide (Covert) is a short-term antidysrhythmic agent used for the rapid conversion of acute atrial fibrillation or atrial flutter to sinus rhythm. The drug is administered as a 10-minute infusion in a carefully monitored clinical setting. The most serious side effect of ibutilide is its potential for inducing life-threatening dysrhythmias, especially torsades de pointes.[82]

Class IV Drugs

Class IV agents are calcium channel blockers that inhibit the influx of calcium through slow calcium channels during the plateau phase (phase 2). This effect occurs primarily in tissue in which slow calcium channels predominate, primarily the sinus and AV nodes and the atrial tissue. Verapamil was the first drug in this category available as an intravenous antidysrhythmic. It depresses sinus and AV node conduction and is effective in terminating supraventricular tachycardias caused by AV nodal reentry. Diltiazem (Cardizem) has become available in intravenous form and is thought to be as effective as verapamil in treating supraventricular dysrhythmias, with fewer hypotensive side effects. Because accessory pathways are not affected by calcium channel blockade, both of these agents must be avoided when treating atrial fibrillation in patients with Wolff-Parkinson-White syndrome.[80]

Unclassified Antidysrhythmics

Adenosine (Adenocard) is an antidysrhythmic agent that remains unclassified under the current system. Adenosine occurs endogenously in the body as a building block of adenosine triphosphate (ATP). Given in intravenous boluses, adenosine slows conduction through the AV node, causing transient AV block. It is used clinically to convert supraventricular tachycardias and to facilitate differential diagnosis of rapid dysrhythmias. Because of its short half-life, the drug is administered intravenously as a rapid bolus, followed by a saline flush. The bolus is delivered as centrally as possible, so that the drug reaches the heart before it is metabolized.[80] Side effects are transient, because the drug is rapidly taken up by the cells and is cleared from the body within 10 seconds.

Magnesium is also unclassified under the present system. Although its action as an antidysrhythmic agent is not entirely understood, clinical studies suggest that it may reduce the incidence of both ventricular and supraventricular dysrhythmias in selected patient populations. It is considered the treatment of choice in patients with torsades de pointes. For acute treatment, 1 to 2 g of magnesium is administered over 1 to 2 minutes. In patients with confirmed hypomagnesemia, this bolus may be followed with a 24-hour infusion.[80]

Side Effects

Antidysrhythmic drugs carry the risk of serious side effects, some of which can be life threatening. The major side effects of the intravenous antidysrhythmic agents are listed in Table 13-14. The most severe complication is the potential for a prodysrhythmic effect. This may result in worsening of the underlying dysrhythmia, the occurrence of a new dysrhythmia, or the development of a bradydysrhythmia. For example, torsades de pointes is a prodysrhythmia caused by a number of drugs. Because the development of a prodysrhythmia is unpredictable, the nurse plays an important role in evaluating ECG changes, monitoring drug levels, and assessing patient symptoms. Antidysrhythmic agents may also alter the amount of energy required for defibrillation and pacing. For example, increases in the dose of an antidysrhythmic drug may increase

TABLE 13-14 PHARMACOLOGICAL MANAGEMENT: SELECTED ANTIDYSRHYTHMIC AGENTS

DRUG AND SITE OF ACTION	INDICATIONS	DOSAGE	MAJOR SIDE EFFECTS
Sinus Node, Atria, or AV Node			
Adenosine	SVT, PSVT	6 mg IV rapid push; if unsuccessful, repeat with 12 mg over 1-2 seconds; follow with IV fluid 10 mL flush (NS or D_5W)	Transient; flushing, dyspnea, hypotension
Digoxin	AFib, AF, PSVT	0.5-1 mg loading dose in divided doses; maintenance dose of 0.125-0.375 mg daily	Bradycardia, heart block Toxicity: CNS and GI symptoms
Diltiazem	SVT, AFib, AF	Bolus dose of 0.25 mg/kg IV over 2 minutes, followed by an infusion of 5-15 mg/hr	Bradycardia, hypotension, AV block
Esmolol	ST, SVT	Loading dose of 500 mcg/kg over 1 minute, followed by an infusion of 50 mcg/kg/min for 4 minutes; repeat procedure every 5 minutes, increasing infusion by 25-50 mcg/kg/min to maximum of 200 mcg/kg/min	Hypotension, bradycardia, heart failure
Ibutilide	AFib, AF	0.010-0.025 mg/kg infused over 10 minutes (may repeat once) or 1 mg diluted in 50 mL infused over 10 minutes (may repeat once)	Minimal side effects except for rare polymorphic VT (torsades de pointes)
Propranolol	SVT	1-3 mg IV every 5 minutes, not to exceed 0.1 mg/kg	Bradycardia, heart block, heart failure
Verapamil	AF, PSVT	5-10 mg IV over 2 minutes, may repeat in 15-30 minutes	Hypotension, bradycardia, heart failure
Ventricle			
Lidocaine	PVCs, VT, VF	1-1.5 mg/kg bolus, followed by continuous infusion of 1-4 mg/min	CNS toxicity, nausea, vomiting with repeated doses
Atria and Ventricle			
Amiodarone	VT/VT arrest	300 mg IV push; may repeat with 150 mg in 3-5 minutes (maximum dose, 2.2 g/24 hr)	Hypotension, abnormal liver function tests
	Stable VT, AFib, AF	150 mg IV over 10 minutes, followed by 360 mg over 6 hours (1 mg/min); maintenance infusion of 0.5 mg/min	
Procainamide	AF, SVT, PVCs, VT	Loading dose of 12-17 mg/kg at a rate of 20 mg/min, followed by infusion of 1-4 mg/min	Hypotension, GI effects Widening of QRS and QT lengthening

AF, atrial flutter; *AFib*, atrial fibrillation; *AV*, atrioventricular; *CNS*, central nervous system; *D_5W*, 5% dextrose in water; *GI*, gastrointestinal; *IV*, intravenous; *NS*, normal saline; *PSVT*, paroxysmal supraventricular tachycardia; *PVCs*, premature ventricular contractions; *ST*, sinus tachycardia; *SVT*, supraventricular tachycardia; *VT*, ventricular tachycardia; *VF*, ventricular fibrillation.

the amount of output (mA) required to depolarize the myocardium.

Treatment of Atrial Fibrillation

More than 2 million people in the United States have atrial fibrillation, and extensive research has been done on the treatment of this disorder. The goals of pharmacological therapy for atrial fibrillation include reestablishing and maintaining sinus rhythm, decreasing the rapid ventricular response during episodes of atrial fibrillation, and preventing the risk of thromboembolism. Table 13-15 reviews current drugs used in the treatment of atrial fibrillation. Results of

some clinical trials suggest that rate control is equivalent to restoration of sinus rhythm in terms of mortality.[82,83]

Inotropic Drugs

Critically ill patients with compromised cardiac function often require the use of medications to enhance myocardial contractility (positive inotropes). Clinically available inotropes include cardiac glycosides, sympathomimetics, and phosphodiesterase inhibitors. These agents increase myocardial contractility, resulting in improved cardiac output, more complete emptying of the ventricles, and decreased filling pressures.

TABLE 13-15	PHARMACOLOGICAL MANAGEMENT: ATRIAL FIBRILLATION	
TREATMENT GOAL	**CLASSIFICATION AND DRUG**	**SPECIAL CONSIDERATIONS**
Conversion or maintenance of sinus rhythm	**Class IA** Quinidine Procainamide (Pronestyl) Disopyramide (Norpace)	Class IA drugs prolong QT intervals and may cause torsades de pointes. Rate control should be achieved before initiation of therapy.
	Class IC Flecainide (Tambocor) Propafenone (Rythmol)	Class IC drugs are prodysrhythmic in patients with CAD or previous MI and should be avoided in these patients.
	Class III Amiodarone (Cordarone) Dofetilide (Tikosyn) Ibutilide (Corvert) Sotalol (Betapace)	Amiodarone and sotalol also have beta-blocking properties and may help with rate control. Treatment with dofetilide requires careful monitoring for prodysrhythmic effects. Ibutilide is an IV agent and is used for conversion only.
Control of ventricular rate	**Beta-blockers** Esmolol (Brevibloc) Metoprolol (Lopressor) Propranolol (Inderal)	IV esmolol may be used in acute settings to control ventricular rate. Oral agents are used for maintenance therapy. Beta-blockers provide good rate control during exercise.
	Calcium channel blockers Diltiazem (Cardizem) Verapamil (Isoptin)	Intravenous calcium channel blockers may be used in emergency situations, followed by oral agents for maintenance therapy.
	Digitalis compounds Digoxin (Lanoxin)	Digoxin does not effectively control rate with exercise, so it may be used in combination with other drugs.
Prevention of thromboembolism	**Anticoagulants** Heparin Warfarin (Coumadin)	Heparin may be used in emergency situations, before cardioversion. Warfarin is used long term, with monitoring to achieve an INR of 2.0-3.0.
	Antiplatelet agents Aspirin	Aspirin may be used in patients with contraindications to warfarin or in low-risk patients younger than 65 years.

CAD, coronary artery disease; *INR*, international normalized ratio; *IV*, intravenous; *MI*, myocardial infarction.

Cardiac Glycosides

Cardiac glycosides include digitalis and its derivatives. Although these drugs have been used for centuries, their slow onset of action and risk of toxicity make them more appropriate for management of chronic heart failure. Because digoxin also causes slowing of the sinus rate and a decrease in AV conduction, it may be administered intravenously in the acute care setting to control supraventricular dysrhythmias.

Sympathomimetic Agents

Sympathomimetic agents stimulate adrenergic receptors, thereby simulating the effects of sympathetic nerve stimulation. Included in this category are naturally occurring catecholamines (epinephrine, dopamine, and norepinephrine) and synthetic catecholamines (dobutamine and isoproterenol). The cardiovascular effects of these drugs, which vary according to their selectivity for specific receptor sites, are often dose dependent as well. Table 13-16 describes the cardiovascular effects of sympathomimetic drugs at various dosages.

Dopamine. Dopamine (Intropin) is one of the most widely used drugs in the critical care setting. It is a chemical precursor of norepinephrine, which, in addition to both α- and β-receptor stimulation, can activate dopaminergic receptors in the renal and mesenteric blood vessels. The actions of this drug are entirely dose related.[84] At low dosages of 1 to 2 mcg/kg/min, dopamine stimulates dopaminergic receptors, causing vasodilation of the renal and mesenteric vascular beds. The resultant increase in kidney perfusion increases urinary output. However, it is clear that this increase in urine output does not confer protection against the development of acute kidney injury. Moderate dosages result in stimulation of β_1-receptors to increase myocardial contractility and improve cardiac output. At dosages greater than 10 mcg/kg/min, dopamine predominantly stimulates α-receptors, resulting in vasoconstriction that often negates both the β-adrenergic and the dopaminergic effects. (Priority Medications box on Dopamine.)

TABLE 13-16 PHYSIOLOGICAL EFFECTS OF SYMPATHOMIMETIC AGENTS

RECEPTOR ACTIVATED*	CARDIOVASCULAR EFFECTS							
DRUG	DOSAGE	ALPHA	BETA$_1$	BETA$_2$	DOPA	CO	HR	SVR
Dobutamine	<5 mcg/kg/min	0	↑↑	↑	0	↑↑	↑	↓
	5-20 mcg/kg/min	0	↑↑↑	↑↑	0	↑↑↑	↑↑	↓↓
Dopamine	<3 mcg/kg/min	0	↑	↑	↑↑↑	0/↑	0/↑	0
	3-10 mcg/kg/min	↑↑	↑↑↑	↑	↑↑↑	↑↑↑	↑	↑
	11-20 mcg/kg/min	↑↑↑	↑↑↑	↑	↑↑	↑↑	↑↑	↑↑↑
Epinephrine	<2 mcg/min	0	↑	↑↑	0	0/↑	0/↑	↓
	2-8 mcg/min	↑↑	↑↑↑	↑↑	0	↑↑↑	↑↑	↑
	9-20 mcg/min	↑↑↑	↑↑↑	↑↑	0	↑↑	↑↑	↑↑↑
Isoproterenol	1-7 mcg/min	0	↑↑↑	↑↑↑	0	↑↑↑	↑↑↑	↓↓↓
Norepinephrine	<2 mcg/min	↑↑↑	↑↑	0	0	↑	0/↑	↑↑↑
	2-16 mcg/min	↑↑↑↑	↑↑	0	0	↓	↑	↑↑↑↑
Phenylephrine	10-100 mcg/min	↑↑↑↑	0	0	0	0	↓	↑↑↑

*See Table 13-13 for actions of receptors.
0, no effect; ↑, increased (number of arrows indicates degree of effect); ↓, decreased (number of arrows indicates degree of effect); *CO*, cardiac output; *HR*, heart rate; *SVR*, systemic vascular resistance.

PRIORITY MEDICATIONS

Dopamine

Drug Class: Catecholamine/Inotrope

DRUG ACTION	DRUG DOSAGE AND DRUG DELIVERY
Increase urine output	low dose: ≤ 3 mcg/kg/min, IV infusion
Increase cardiac output	moderate dose: 3-5 mcg/kg/min, IV infusion
Increase blood pressure	high dose: 10-20 mcg/kg/min, IV infusion

Priority Nursing Considerations
The actions of dopamine are strongly dose related (see above).

Side Effects and Clinical Assessment
Low-dose dopamine to increase urine output: Few systemic side effects expected, although sinus tachycardia. PACs and PVCs occur in some patients. Assess adequacy of urine output.

Moderate-dose dopamine to increase cardiac output: Few systemic side effects expected, although dysrhythmias may occur. Assess cardiac output, BP, peripheral pulses, and color of extremities to avoid any evidence of peripheral vasoconstriction.

High-dose dopamine to treat shock: High-dose dopamine activates peripheral vascular alpha-receptors to cause vasoconstriction with the intent of raising blood pressure in shock states. As with other vasopressors, dopamine should never be administered to a hypovolemic patient, because the resulting vasoconstriction may increase tissue and organ ischemia. The Surviving Sepsis campaign recommends either dopamine or norepinephrine through a central venous catheter (CVC) as a first-line vasopressor to treat shock states following appropriate volume resuscitation. In a study that compared dopamine with norepinephrine to treat shock, patient mortality was identical, but dysrhythmias occurred more frequently in the dopamine group including: sinus tachycardia, atrial fibrillation, PVCs, and ventricular tachycardia.[1,2]

Always palpate peripheral pulses and check peripheral capillary refill to verify that peripheral circulation is not compromised by the dopamine infusion.

Extravasation Risk & Antidote: Dopamine should not be administered via peripheral IV. The reason is that should the IV infiltrate and dopamine extravasate into the surrounding soft tissues, necrosis can occur.

If extravasation occurs, stop the dopamine infusion. The antidote is phentolamine (an alpha-receptor blocker). Phentolamine 5 to 10 mg is diluted in 10 mL normal saline and administered intradermally into the affected tissues as soon as possible.

Dopamine should be administered via a central venous catheter to avoid this complication.

Clinical Examples
Dopamine is a versatile drug that is used in a variety of clinical situations in critical care. In shock states, high-dose dopamine can be used to maintain blood pressure in combination with volume resuscitation. For the patient with heart failure or following cardiac surgery, dopamine at moderate dose is frequently used to support cardiac output. The aim is to increase cardiac contractility by stimulating the beta-adrenergic receptors in the myocardium. Dopamine is also infused at low dose to increase urine output.

The specificity of the dose-related effects requires the nurse to carefully monitor for both expected and untoward changes in cardiac output, blood pressure, dysrhythmias, urine output and peripheral perfusion.

References
1. De Backer D, et al: Comparison of dopamine and norepinephrine in the treatment of shock, *N Engl J Med* 362(9):779, 2010.
2. Patel GP, et al: Efficacy and safety of dopamine versus norepinephrine in the management of septic shock, *Shock* 33(4):375, 2010.

Dobutamine. Dobutamine (Dobutrex) is a synthetic catecholamine with predominantly β_1-adrenergic effects. It also produces some β_2 stimulation, resulting in a mild vasodilation. Dobutamine is as effective as dopamine in increasing myocardial contractility and is useful in the treatment of heart failure, especially in hypotensive patients who cannot tolerate vasodilator therapy. The usual dosage range is 2.5 to 20 mcg/kg/min, titrated on the basis of hemodynamic parameters.

Epinephrine. Epinephrine (Adrenalin) is produced by the adrenal gland as part of the body's response to stress. This agent has the ability to stimulate both α- and β-receptors, depending on the dose administered (see Table 13-14). At doses of 1 to 2 mg/min, epinephrine binds with β-receptors to increase heart rate, cardiac conduction, contractility, and vasodilation, thereby increasing cardiac output. As the dosage is increased, α-receptors are stimulated, resulting in increased vascular resistance and increased blood pressure. At these doses, epinephrine's impact on cardiac output depends on the heart's ability to pump against the increased afterload. Epinephrine accelerates the sinus rate and may precipitate ventricular dysrhythmias in the ischemic heart. Other side effects include restlessness, angina, and headache.

Norepinephrine. Norepinephrine (Levophed) is similar to epinephrine in its ability to stimulate β- and α-receptors, but it lacks the β_2 effects of epinephrine. At low infusion rates, β_1-receptors are activated to produce increased contractility, augmenting cardiac output. At higher doses, the inotropic effects are limited by marked vasoconstriction mediated by α-receptors. Clinically, norepinephrine is used most often as a vasopressor to elevate blood pressure in shock states.

Phosphodiesterase Inhibitors

Phosphodiesterase inhibitors are inotropic agents that also are potent vasodilators (inodilators). Drugs in this classification inhibit the enzyme phosphodiesterase, resulting in increased levels of cyclic adenosine monophosphate (AMP) and intracellular calcium. Amrinone (Inocor) and milrinone (Primacor) were the first of these agents approved for use in the United States. Increases in cardiac output occur as a result of increased contractility (inotropic effects) and decreased afterload (vasodilative effects). Filling pressures tend to decrease, while heart rate and blood pressure remain fairly constant. Amrinone may cause thrombocytopenia, so platelet counts are monitored and patients are observed for hemorrhagic complications. Milrinone is associated with a lower rate of thrombocytopenia but can induce ventricular dysrhythmias (PVCs, VT) in a significant number of patients.[85]

Vasodilator Drugs

Vasodilators are pharmacological agents that improve cardiac performance by various degrees of arterial or venous dilation, or both. The goal of vasodilator therapy may be reduction of preload or of afterload, or both. Afterload reduction is accomplished by vasodilation of arterial vessels. This results in decreased resistance to LV ejection and may improve cardiac

output without increasing myocardial oxygen demands. Reduction of preload is accomplished by dilation of venous vessels to increase capacitance. This results in decreased filling pressures for a failing heart. These drugs may be classified into four groups on the basis of mechanism of action (Table 13-17).

Direct Smooth Muscle Relaxants

Direct-acting vasodilators include sodium nitroprusside, nitroglycerin, and hydralazine. These drugs produce relaxation of vascular smooth muscle through the activation of nitric oxide, which results in decreased systemic vascular resistance (SVR). Hypotension may occur as a result of peripheral vasodilation, and headaches may be caused by cerebral vasodilation. Compensatory mechanisms can occur in response to the drop in blood pressure. These include baroreceptor activation that causes reflex tachycardia and activation of the renin-angiotensin-aldosterone system (RAAS) (see Figure 12-14 in Chapter 12), with resultant sodium and water retention.

Sodium Nitroprusside. Sodium nitroprusside (Nipride) is a potent, rapidly acting venous and arterial vasodilator that is particularly suitable for rapid reduction of blood pressure in hypertensive emergencies and perioperatively. It also is effective for afterload reduction in the setting of severe heart failure. The drug is administered by continuous intravenous infusion, with the dosage titrated to maintain the desired blood pressure and SVR. Prolonged administration can result in thiocyanate toxicity, manifested by nausea, confusion, and tinnitus.[86]

Nitroglycerin. Intravenous nitroglycerin (Tridil) causes both arterial and venous vasodilation, but its venous effect is more pronounced. It is used in the critical care setting for the treatment of acute heart failure because it reduces cardiac filling pressures, relieves pulmonary congestion, and decreases cardiac workload and oxygen consumption. Nitroglycerin dilates the coronary arteries and is a useful adjunct in the treatment of unstable angina and acute MI. The initial dosage is 10 mcg/min, and the infusion is titrated upward to achieve the desired clinical effect: a reduction or elimination of chest pain, decreased PAOP (wedge pressure), or a decrease in blood pressure. Nitroglycerin is administered prophylactically to prevent coronary vasospasm after coronary angioplasty, atherectomy, stent insertion, or fibrinolytic therapy. The most common side effects of this drug are hypotension, flushing, and headache.[85]

Calcium Channel Blockers

Calcium channel blockers are a chemically diverse group of drugs with differing pharmacological effects (Table 13-18).

Nifedipine (Procardia) and nicardipine (Cardene) are dihydropyridines. Drugs in this group of calcium channel blockers (with the suffix *pine*) are used primarily as arterial vasodilators. These agents reduce the influx of calcium in the arterial resistance vessels. Both coronary and peripheral arteries are affected. They are used in the critical care setting to treat hypertension. Nifedipine is available only in an oral

TABLE 13-17	PHARMACOLOGICAL MANAGEMENT: CHARACTERISTICS OF SELECTED VASODILATORS				
CLASSIFICATION AND DRUGS	**DOSAGE**	**PRELOAD**	**AFTERLOAD**	**SIDE EFFECTS**	
Direct Smooth Muscle Relaxants					
Sodium nitroprusside (Nipride)	0.25-6 mcg/kg/min IV infusion	Moderate	Strong	Hypotension, thiocyanate toxicity, reflex tachycardia	
Nitroglycerin (Tridil)	5-300 mcg/min IV infusion	Strong	Mild	Headache, reflex tachycardia, hypotension	
Calcium Channel Blockers					
Nicardipine (Cardene)	5 mg/hr IV, titrated to 15 mg/hr	None	Strong	Hypotension, headache, reflex tachycardia	
Nifedipine (Procardia)	10-30 mg PO	None	Strong	Hypotension, headache, reflex tachycardia	
Angiotensin-Converting Enzyme Inhibitors					
Captopril (Capoten)	6.25-100 mg PO every 8-12 hr	Moderate	Moderate	Hypotension, chronic cough, neutropenia	
Enalapril (Vasotec)	0.625 mg IV over 5 minutes, then every 6 hours	Moderate	Moderate	Hypotension, elevation of liver enzymes	
α-Adrenergic Blockers					
Labetalol (Normodyne)	20-80 mg IV bolus every 10 minutes, then 1-2 mg/min infusion	Moderate	Moderate	Orthostatic hypotension, bronchospasm, AV block	
Phentolamine (Regitine)	1-5 mg IV slowly every 6 hours	Moderate	Moderate	Hypotension, tachycardia	

AV, atrioventricular; *IV,* intravenous; *PO,* orally.

TABLE 13-18	PHARMACOLOGICAL MANAGEMENT: CHARACTERISTICS OF CALCIUM CHANNEL BLOCKERS			
DRUG	**ACTIONS**	**DOSAGE**	**SPECIAL CONSIDERATIONS**	
Dihydropyridines				
Nicardipine (Cardene)	Short-term control of hypertension	5 mg/hr IV, titrated to 15 mg/hr	Hypotension, headache, nausea	
Nifedipine (Procardia)	Hypertension	10-30 mg PO	Hypotension, headache, reflex tachycardia	
Benzothiazepines				
Diltiazem (Cardizem)	SVT, AFib, AF, angina	Bolus dose of 0.25 mg/kg IV over 2 minutes, followed by an infusion of 5-15 mg/hr	Bradycardia, hypotension, atrioventricular block	
Phenylalkylamines				
Verapamil (Calan, Isoptin)	AF, PSVT	5-10 mg IV, may repeat in 15-30 minutes	Hypotension, bradycardia, heart failure	

AF, atrial flutter; *AFib,* atrial fibrillation; *IV,* intravenous; *PO,* by mouth; *PSVT,* paroxysmal supraventricular tachycardia; *SVT,* supraventricular tachycardia.

form, but in the past it was prescribed sublingually during hypertensive emergencies. Reports of adverse events associated with sublingual nifedipine have prompted the FDA to strongly discourage sublingual use.[87] Nicardipine has become available as an intravenous calcium channel blocker, and it offers more accurate titration for effective control of hypertension. Side effects of nifedipine and nicardipine are related to vasodilation and include hypotension, reflex tachycardia, flushing, headache, and ankle edema.

Diltiazem (Cardizem) is from the benzothiazepine group of calcium channel blockers. *Verapamil* (Calan, Isoptin) is part of the phenylalkylamine group. The different classifications account for the differing actions of these calcium channel blockers. These drugs dilate coronary arteries but have little effect on the peripheral vasculature. They are used in the treatment of angina, especially that which has a vasospastic component, and as antidysrhythmics in the treatment of supraventricular tachycardias.

Angiotensin-Converting Enzyme Inhibitors

Angiotensin-converting enzyme (ACE) inhibitors produce vasodilation by blocking the conversion of angiotensin I to angiotensin II. Because angiotensin is a potent vasoconstrictor, limiting its production decreases SVR. In contrast to the direct vasodilators and nifedipine, ACE inhibitors do not cause reflex tachycardia or induce sodium and water retention. However, these drugs may cause a profound fall in blood pressure, especially in patients who are volume-depleted. Blood pressure must be monitored carefully, especially at the initiation of therapy.

Captopril (Capoten) and enalapril (Vasotec) are used in patients with heart failure to decrease SVR (afterload) and PAOP (preload). Captopril is available only in an oral form, but it has a relatively rapid onset of action (approximately 1 hour). Enalapril is available in an intravenous form and may be used to decrease afterload in more emergent situations.

Atrial Natriuretic Peptide

Nesiritide (Natrecor) is a new vasodilator used in the treatment of acute heart failure. This agent is a recombinant form of human brain natriuretic peptide (BNP), the hormone released by cardiac cells in response to ventricular distention. The primary effects of nesiritide include decreased filling pressures (PAOP, CVP), reduced SVR, and increased urine output. Compared with traditional vasodilator therapy for acute heart failure, nesiritide reportedly is as effective as the traditional agents and has fewer side effects (e.g., headache).[85] The recommended dose is an intravenous bolus of 2 mcg/kg, followed by a continuous infusion of 0.01 mcg/kg/min. The primary side effect is hypotension. If this occurs, nesiritide may need to be discontinued for a time and then restarted at a lower dose after the patient has stabilized.[85] Low-dose nesiritide may have a protective effect on kidney function.[88] High dose administration is associated with hypotension and dysrhythmias.[88]

Alpha-Adrenergic Blockers

Peripheral adrenergic blockers block α-receptors in arteries and veins, resulting in vasodilation. Orthostatic hypotension is a common side effect and may result in syncope. Long-term therapy also may be complicated by fluid and water retention.

Labetalol (Normodyne), a combined peripheral alpha-blocker and cardioselective beta-blocker, is used in the treatment of acute stroke and hypertensive emergencies.[89] Because the blockade of β₁-receptors permits the decrease of blood pressure without the risk of reflexive tachycardia and increased cardiac output, this drug is also useful in the treatment of acute aortic dissection.[90]

Phentolamine (Regitine) is a nonselective peripheral alpha-blocker that decreases blood pressure through arterial vasodilation. The half-life is 19 minutes when given intravenously. It is administered by slow IV push, 1 to 5 mg every 6 hours to reduce blood pressure.[86] This drug is used only in very specific circumstances. Phentolamine is the drug of choice to control blood pressure and sweating caused by pheochromocytoma, an epinephrine (adrenaline)-secreting tumor that can arise from the adrenal medulla.[86]

Phentolamine also is used to treat the extravasation of dopamine or other vasopressors into peripheral tissues. If this occurs, 5 to 10 mg is diluted in 10 mL normal saline and administered intradermally into the infiltrated area as soon as possible following the extravasation.

Dopamine Receptor Agonists

Fenoldopam (Corlopam) is the first of a new class of vasodilators called selective, specific dopamine (D₁) receptor agonists.[86] The drug is a potent vasodilator that affects peripheral, renal, and mesenteric arteries. It is administered by continuous intravenous infusion beginning at 0.1 mcg/kg/min and titrated up to the desired blood pressure effect, with a maximum recommended dose of 1.6 mcg/kg/min. It can be administered as an alternative to sodium nitroprusside or other antihypertensives in the treatment of hypertensive emergencies. Fenoldopam can be used safely in patients with kidney dysfunction.[86]

Vasopressors

Vasopressors are sympathomimetic agents that mediate peripheral vasoconstriction through stimulation of α-receptors (see Table 13-16). This results in increased SVR and elevates blood pressure. Some of these drugs (epinephrine and norepinephrine) also have the ability to stimulate β-receptors. Vasopressors are not widely used in the treatment of critically ill cardiac patients, because the dramatic increase in afterload is taxing to a damaged heart. Vasopressors are also used to maintain organ perfusion in shock states. For example, norepinephrine (Levophed) may be administered as a continuous intravenous infusion to maintain organ perfusion by increasing SVR in cases of severe sepsis or septic shock.

Vasopressin

Vasopressin, also known as antidiuretic hormone (ADH), has become popular in the critical care setting for its vasoconstrictive effects. At higher doses, vasopressin directly stimulates V1 receptors in vascular smooth muscle, resulting in vasoconstriction of capillaries and small arterioles. A one-time dose of 40 units intravenously is recommended in the ACLS guidelines as first-line drug therapy for VF, pulseless VT asystole, or pulseless electrical activity (PEA).[91] Continuous infusions of 0.02 unit/min up to 0.1 unit/min have been used in the treatment of vasodilatory shock in patients with refractory hypotension after cardiopulmonary bypass.[62]

TABLE 13-19	PHARMACOLOGICAL MANAGEMENT: HEART FAILURE		
CLASSIFICATION AND DRUGS	**MECHANISM OF ACTION**	**EFFECTS**	**SPECIAL CONSIDERATIONS**
ACE Inhibitors Captopril (Capoten) Enalapril (Vasotec) Lisinopril (Prinivil)	Interferes with the renin-angiotensin-aldosterone system by preventing conversion of angiotensin I to angiotensin II	Decreases afterload Decreases preload Reverses ventricular remodeling	Agents appear equivalent in treatment of heart failure Monitor closely for hypotension when initiating therapy May be contraindicated in patients with renal insufficiency
Angiotensin Receptor Blockers Losartan (Cozaar) Valsartan (Diovan)	Interferes with the renin-angiotensin-aldosterone system by blocking the effect of angiotensin II at the angiotensin II receptor site	Decreases afterload Decreases preload Reverses ventricular remodeling	Reserved for patients who cannot tolerate ACE inhibitors due to side effects such as severe cough or angioedema
Beta-Blockers Metoprolol (Lopressor) Carvedilol (Coreg)	Counteracts the SNS response activated in heart failure by blocking receptor sites	Slows heart rate Prevents dysrhythmias Decreases blood pressure Reverses ventricular remodeling	Not initiated during decompensated stage of heart failure Use cautiously in patients with reactive airway disease, poorly controlled diabetes, bradydysrhythmias, or heart block Carvedilol dose is increased slowly, while monitoring for symptoms caused by vasodilation, such as dizziness or hypotension
Aldosterone Antagonists Spironolactone (Aldactone)	Counteracts the effects of aldosterone, which include sodium and water retention	Decreases preload Decreases myocardial hypertrophy	May increase serum potassium
Inotropes Digoxin (Lanoxin)	Affects the Na^+,K^+-ATPase pump in myocardial cells to increase the strength of contraction	Increases contractility Increases cardiac output Prevents atrial dysrhythmias	Risk of toxicity is increased with hypokalemia

ACE, Angiotensin-converting enzyme; *Na^+/K^+-ATPase,* sodium-potassium adenosine triphosphatase; *SNS,* sympathetic nervous system.

In septic shock, vasopressin levels have been reported to be lower than anticipated for a shock state.[92] Vasopressin continuous infusion of 0.03 unit/min may be added to the norepinephrine infusion in refractory shock per the 2008 surviving sepsis guidelines.[92] Patients must be assessed for side effects such as heart failure caused by the antidiuretic effects, and monitored for increased risk of ischemia in the myocardium, spleen, and periphery.[92] Vasopressin should be infused through a central line to avoid the risk of peripheral extravasation and resultant tissue necrosis. Placement of an arterial line in shock states to monitor blood pressure and SVR is recommended.[92]

Drug Treatment of Heart Failure

Almost 5 million Americans have heart failure, making it a major chronic health issue.[93] The goals of treatment in heart failure include alleviating symptoms, slowing the progression of the disease, and improving survival. Findings from a number of randomly controlled clinical trials have resulted in guidelines for the pharmacological treatment of heart failure.[94,95] Please see the Concept Map on Heart Failure, which integrates pharmacological management of heart failure. Additional information about heart failure is available in Chapter 12. Table 13-19 reviews the drugs currently recommended for the treatment of heart failure.

Concept Map:
Heart Failure-Decreased Cardiac Output

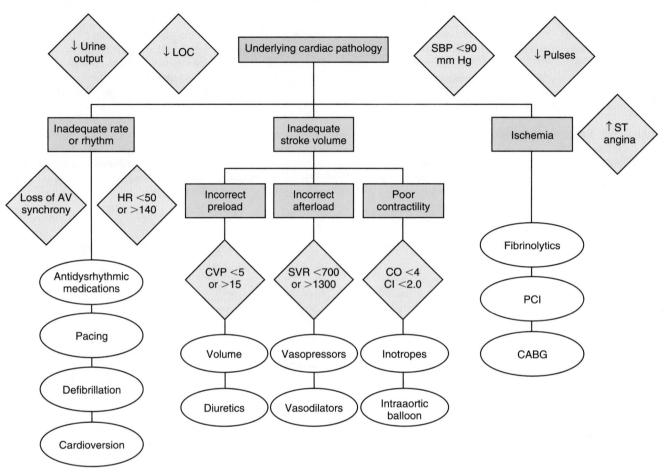

Concept Map: Heart Failure-Decreased Cardiac Output.

CASE STUDY   PATIENT WITH A CARDIAC PROBLEM

Answers to the Case Study Questions can be found on the Evolve web site at http://evolve.elsevier.com/Urden/priorities/.

Brief Patient History

Mrs. G is a 54-year-old African-American woman who has been having intermittent indigestion for the past month. She has a history of hypertension and hyperlipidemia. She was admitted as an inpatient on a medical floor for management of her blood pressure and is scheduled to undergo endoscopy tomorrow. Mrs. G suddenly becomes diaphoretic and complains of nausea and epigastric pain.

Clinical Assessment

The rapid response team is called to evaluate Mrs. G. When the team arrives at her bedside, she continues to complain of pain, which now radiates to her neck and back. She has some slight shortness of breath and is vomiting.

Diagnostic Procedures

The admission electrocardiogram (ECG) shows ST-segment elevation in II, III, and AVF. Baseline vital signs include

the following: blood pressure of 160/90 mm Hg, heart rate of 98 beats/min (sinus rhythm), respiratory rate of 18 breaths/min, temperature of 99° F, and O_2 saturation of 94%.

Medical Diagnosis

Mrs. G is diagnosed with an inferior myocardial infarction.

Questions

1. What major outcomes do you expect to achieve for this patient?
2. What problems or risks must be managed to achieve these outcomes?
3. What interventions must be initiated to monitor, prevent, manage, or eliminate the problems and risks identified?
4. What interventions should be initiated to promote optimal functioning, safety, and well-being of the patient?
5. What possible learning needs do you anticipate for this patient?
6. What cultural and age-related factors may have a bearing on the patient's plan of care?

REFERENCES

1. Schoenfeld MH: Contemporary pacemaker and defibrillator device therapy: challenges confronting the general cardiologist, *Circulation* 115(5):638, 2007.
2. American Heart Association: ECC Guidelines. Part 5. Electrical therapies: automated external defibrillators, defibrillation, cardioversion and pacing, *Circulation* 112(8):IV-35, 2005.
3. Reade MC: Temporary epicardial pacing after cardiac surgery: a practical review. Part I. General considerations in the management of epicardial pacing, *Anaesthesia* 62(3):264, 2007.
4. Bernstein AD, et al: The revised NASPE/BPEG generic pacemaker code for antibradycardia, adaptive-rate and multi-site pacing, *Pacing Clin Electrophysiol* 25(2):260, 2002.
5. Dwyer D, Bauer K: Take the lead on safety with temporary cardiac pacing, *Nursing* 40(3):63, 2010.
6. Mullin MH, et al: Sensations during removal of epicardial pacing wires after coronary artery bypass graft surgery, *Heart Lung* 38(5):377, 2009.
7. Lloyd-Jones D, et al: Heart disease and stroke statistics – 2010 update: a report from the American Heart Association Statistics Committee and Stroke Statistics Subcommittee, *Circulation* 121(7):e46, 2010.
8. Epstein AE, et al: ACC/AHA/HRS 2008 guidelines for device-based therapy of cardiac rhythm abnormalities: executive summary, *Circulation* 117(21):2820, 2008.
9. Saul L: Cardiac resynchronization therapy, *Crit Care Nurse Q* 30(1):58, 2007.
10. Jeevanantham V, et al: Cardiac resynchronization therapy in heart failure patients: an update, *Cardiol J* 16(3):197, 2009.
11. Palazzo MO: Atrial fibrillation and the postoperative cardiac surgery patient, *Crit Care Nurs Clin North Am* 19(4):395, 2007.
12. Kalahasty G, Ellenbogen K: The role of pacemakers in the management of patients with atrial fibrillation, *Cardiol Clin* 27(1):137, 2009.
13. McMullan J, et al: Care of the pacemaker/implantable cardioverter defibrillator patient in the ED, *Am J Emerg Med* 25(7):812, 2007.
14. Baddour LM, et al: Update on cardiovascular implantable electronic device infections and their management: A scientific statement from the American Heart Association, *Circulation* 121(3):458, 2010.
15. Crossley GH, et al: Clinical benefits of remote versus transtelephonic monitoring of implanted pacemakers, *J Am Coll Cardiol* 54(22):2012, 2009.
16. Angerstein RL, et al: Enhancing care for cardiac resynchronization therapy patients: device diagnostics and clinical application, *J Cardiovasc Nurs* 21(5):397, 2006.
17. Wheeler EC, et al: Psychological impact of implantable cardioverter defibrillator on their recipients, *Dimens Crit Care Nurs* 28(4):176, 2009.
18. Dunbar SB, et al: Effect of a psychoeducational intervention on depression, anxiety, and health resource use in implantable cardioverter defibrillator patients, *Pacing Clin Electrophysiol* 32(10):1259, 2009.
19. Faxon DP: Development of systems of care for ST-elevation myocardial infarction patients: current state of ST-elevation myocardial infarction care, *Circulation* 116(2):e29, 2007.
20. Antman EM, et al: 2007 Focused update of the ACC/AHA 2004 guidelines for the management of patients with ST-elevation myocardial infarction, *Circulation* 117(2):296, 2008.
21. Peacock WF, et al: Reperfusion strategies in the emergency treatment of ST-segment elevation myocardial infarction, *Am J Emerg Med* 25(3):353, 2007.
22. Anderson JL, et al: ACC/AHA 2007 guidelines for the management of patients with unstable angina/non-ST-elevation myocardial infarction, *Circulation* 116(7):e148, 2007.
23. TIMI Study Group: The Thrombolysis in Myocardial Infarction (TIMI) trial. Phase I findings, *N Engl J Med* 312(14):932, 1985.
24. Kiernan TJ, Gersh BJ: Thrombolysis in acute myocardial infarction: current status, *Med Clin North Am* 91(4):617, 2007.
25. Gelfand EV, Cannon CP: Myocardial infarction: contemporary management strategies, *J Intern Med* 262(1):59, 2007.
26. Zimarino M, et al: Facilitated PCI: rationale, current evidence, open questions, and future directions, *J Cardiovasc Pharmacol* 51(1):3, 2008.
27. Drew BJ, et al: Practice standards for electrocardiographic monitoring in hospital settings: an AHA scientific statement, *Circulation* 110(17):2721, 2004.
28. Sharma SK, Chen V: Coronary interventional devices: balloon, atherectomy, thrombectomy and distal protection devices, *Cardiol Clin* 24(2):201, 2006.
29. Singh KP, Harrington RA: Primary percutaneous coronary intervention in acute myocardial infarction, *Med Clin North Am* 91(4):639, 2007.
30. King SB, et al: ACCF/AHA/SCAI 2007 update of the clinical competence statement on cardiac interventional procedures, *Circulation* 116(1):98, 2007.
31. Pompa JJ, Baim DS, Resnic FS: Percutaneous coronary and valvular intervention. In Libby P, et al, editors: *Braunwald's heart disease*, ed 8, Philadelphia, 2007, Saunders.
32. Newsome LT, Kutcher MA, Royster RL: Coronary artery stents: Part I. Evolution of percutaneous intervention, *Anesth Analg* 107(2):552, 2008.
33. Rajagopal V, Rockson SG: Coronary restenosis: a review of mechanisms and management, *Am J Med* 115(7):547, 2003.
34. Bittl JA, et al: Meta-analysis of randomized trials of percutaneous transluminal coronary angioplasty versus atherectomy, cutting balloon atherotomy, or laser angioplasty, *J Am Coll Cardiol* 43(6):936, 2004.
35. Stankovic G, et al: Comparison of directional coronary atherectomy and stenting versus stenting alone for the treatment of de novo and restenotic coronary artery narrowing, *Am J Cardiol* 93(8):953, 2004.
36. King SB, et al: 2007 focused update of the ACC/AHA/SCAI 2005 guideline update for percutaneous coronary intervention, *Circulation* 117(2):261, 2008.
37. Levine GN, et al: Newer pharmacotherapy in patients undergoing percutaneous interventions: a guide for pharmacists and other health care professionals, *Pharmacotherapy* 26(11):1537, 2006.
38. Sims JM: Update on drug-eluting stents, *Dimens Crit Care Nurs* 26(6):237, 2007.
39. Kastrati A, et al: Analysis of 14 trials comparing sirolimus-eluting stents with bare-metal stents, *N Engl J Med* 356(10):1030, 2007.
40. Stone GW, et al: Safety and efficacy of sirolimus- and paclitaxel-eluting coronary stents, *N Engl J Med* 356(10):998, 2007.

41. Camenzind E: Treatment of in-stent restenosis: back to the future? *N Engl J Med* 355(20):2149, 2006.

42. Wong EM, et al: A review of the management of patients after percutaneous coronary intervention, *Int J Clin Pract* 60(5):582, 2006.

43. Shoulders-Odom B: Management of patients after percutaneous coronary interventions, *Crit Care Nurs* 28(5):26, 2008.

44. Dauerman HL, et al: Vascular closure devices: the second decade, *J Am Coll Cardiol* 50(17):1617, 2007.

45. Jozic J, et al: Timing and correlates of very early major adverse clinical events following percutaneous coronary intervention, *J Invasive Cardiol* 20(3):113, 2008.

46. Grines CL, et al: Prevention of premature discontinuation of dual antiplatelet therapy in patients with coronary artery stents, *Circulation* 115(6):813, 2007.

47. Rosengart TK, et al: Percutaneous and minimally invasive valve procedures: a scientific statement from the American Heart Association Council on Cardiovascular Surgery and Anesthesia, Council on Clinical Cardiology, Functional Genomics and Translational Biology Interdisciplinary Working Group, and Quality of Care and Outcomes Research Interdisciplinary Working Group, *Circulation* 117(13):1750, 2008.

48. Bonow RO, et al: 2008 focused update incorporated into the ACC/AHA 2006 guidelines for the management of patients with valvular heart disease, *Circulation* 118(15):e523, 2008.

49. Lauck S, et al: A new option for the treatment of aortic stenosis: percutaneous aortic valve replacement, *Crit Care Nurse* 28(3):40, 2008.

50. Mack MJ: Percutaneous treatment of mitral regurgitation: so near, yet so far! *J Thorac Cardiovasc Surg* 135(2):237, 2008.

51. Eagle KA, et al: ACC/AHA 2004 guideline update for coronary artery bypass graft surgery: a report of the American College of Cardiology/American Heart Association Task Force on Practice Guidelines (Committee to Update the 1999 Guidelines for Coronary Artery Bypass Graft Surgery), *Circulation* 110(14):e340, 2004.

52. Booth J, et al: Randomized, controlled trial of coronary artery bypass surgery versus percutaneous coronary intervention in patients with multivessel coronary artery disease: six-year follow-up from the Stent or Surgery Trial (SoS), *Circulation* 118(4):381, 2008.

53. Bravata DM, et al: Systematic review: The comparative effectiveness of percutaneous coronary interventions and coronary artery bypass graft surgery, *Ann Intern Med* 147(10):703, 2007.

54. Lai T, et al: The transition from open to endoscopic saphenous vein harvesting and its clinical impact, *Tex Heart Inst J* 33(3):316, 2006.

55. Desai ND, Fremes SE: Radial artery conduit for coronary revascularization: as good as the internal thoracic artery? *Curr Opin Cardiol* 22(6):534, 2007.

56. Barner HB: Operative treatment of coronary atherosclerosis, *Ann Thorac Surg* 85(3):1473, 2008.

57. Collins P, et al: Radial artery versus saphenous vein patency randomized trial: five-year angiographic follow-up, *Circulation* 117(22):2859, 2008.

58. Hill KM: Surgical repair of cardiac valves, *Crit Care Nurs Clin North Am* 19(4):353, 2007.

59. Rahimtoola SH: Choice of prosthetic heart valve in adults: an update, *J Am Coll Cardiol* 55(22):2413, 2010.

60. McCalmont V, Ohler L: Cardiac transplantation: candidate identification, evaluation, and management, *Crit Care Nurs Q* 31(3):216, 2008.

61. De Bleser L, et al: Interventions to improve medication-adherence after transplantation: a systematic review, *Transpl Int* 22(8):780, 2009.

62. Katz EA: Pharmacologic management of the postoperative cardiac surgery patient, *Crit Care Nurs Clin North Am* 19(4):487, 2007.

63. Mayson SE, et al: The changing face of postoperative atrial fibrillation prevention: a review of current medical therapy, *Cardiol Rev* 15(5):231, 2007.

64. St André AC, DelRossi A: Hemodynamic management of patients in the first 24 hours after cardiac surgery, *Crit Care Med* 33(9):2082, 2005.

65. Ferraris VA, et al: Perioperative blood transfusion and blood conservation in cardiac surgery: The Society of Thoracic Surgeons and The Society of Cardiovascular Anesthesiologists clinical practice guideline, *Ann Thorac Surg* 83(suppl 5):S27, 2007.

66. Martin CG, Turkelson SL: Nursing care of the patient undergoing coronary artery bypass grafting, *J Cardiovasc Nurs* 21(2):109, 2006.

67. Selnes OA: Etiology of cognitive change after CABG surgery: more than just the pump? *Nat Clin Pract Cardiovasc Med* 5(6):314, 2008.

68. Veliz-Reissmüller G, et al: Pre-operative mild cognitive dysfunction predicts the risk for post-operative delirium after elective cardiac surgery, *Aging Clin Exp Res* 19(3):172, 2007.

69. Streeter NB: Considerations in prevention of surgical site infections following cardiac surgery: when your patient is diabetic, *J Cardiovasc Nurs* 21(3):E14, 2006.

70. Miga KC: Trends in cardiac surgery: exploring the past and looking into the future, *Crit Care Nurs Clin North Am* 19(4):343, 2007.

71. Shatzer MB, et al: To pump or not to pump? *Crit Care Nurse Q* 30(1):67, 2007.

72. Puskas JD, et al: Off-pump vs conventional coronary artery bypass grafting: early and 1-year graft patency, cost, and quality-of-life outcomes: a randomized trial, *JAMA* 291(15):1841, 2004.

73. Légaré JF, et al: Coronary bypass surgery performed off pump does not result in lower in-hospital morbidity than coronary artery bypass grafting on pump, *Circulation* 109(7):887, 2004.

74. Hravnak M, et al: Short-term complications and resource utilization in matched subjects after on-pump or off-pump primary isolated coronary artery bypass, *Am J Crit Care* 13(6):499, 2004.

75. Sellke FW, et al: Comparing on-pump and off-pump coronary artery bypass grafting: numerous studies but few conclusions. A scientific statement from the American Heart Association council on Cardiovascular Surgery and Anesthesia in collaboration with the interdisciplinary working group on quality of care and outcomes research, *Circulation* 111(21):2858, 2005.

76. Trost JC, Hillis LD: Intra-aortic balloon counterpulsation, *Am J Cardiol* 97(9):1391, 2006.

77. Erdogan HB, et al: In which patients should sheathless IABP be used? An analysis of vascular complications in 1211 cases, *J Card Surg* 21(4):342, 2006.

78. Reid MB, Cottrell D: Nursing care of patients receiving intra-aortic balloon counterpulsation, *Crit Care Nurse* 25(5):40, 2005.

79. Lewis PA, Courtney M: Weaning intraaortic balloon counterpulsation: the evidence, *Br J Card Nurs* 1(8):385, 2006.

80. American Heart Association: ECC Guidelines. Part 7.4. Monitoring and medications, *Circulation* 112(suppl 1):IV, 2005.

81. Friedman L, Alexander E: Update on the clinical impact and issues surrounding dofetilide (Tikosyn) therapy, *AACN Adv Crit Care* 17(2):102, 2006.

82. Fuster V, et al: ACC/AHA/ESC 2006 guidelines for the management of patients with atrial fibrillation: a report of the American College of Cardiology/American Heart Association Task Force on Practice Guidelines and the European Society of Cardiology Committee for Practice Guidelines, *Circulation* 114(7):e257, 2006.

83. Steinberg JS, et al: Analysis of cause-specific mortality in the Atrial Fibrillation Follow-up Investigation of Rhythm Management (AFFIRM) study, *Circulation* 109(16):1973, 2004.

84. Cooper BE: Review and update on inotropes and vasopressors, *AACN Adv Crit Care* 19(1):5, 2008.

85. Coons JC, Seidl E: Cardiovascular pharmacotherapy update for the intensive care unit, *Crit Care Nurse Q* 30(1):44, 2007.

86. Schulenburg M: Management of hypertensive emergencies: implications for the critical care nurse, *Crit Care Nurse Q* 30(2):86, 2007.

87. Mansoor AF, von Hagel Keefer LA: The dangers of immediate-release nifedipine for hypertensive crises, *Pharm Ther* 27(7):362, 2002.

88. Nigwekar SU, et al: Atrial natriuretic peptide for preventing and treating acute kidney injury, *Cochrane Database Syst Rev* (4):CD006028, 2009.

89. Feldstein C: Management of hypertensive crisis, *Am J Ther* 14(2):135, 2007.

90. Jain AR, et al. Treatment of hypertension in acute ischemic stroke, *Curr Treat Options Neurol* 11(2):120, 2009.

91. Hays AJ, Corso Y: Pharmacotherapy for a pulseless cardiac arrest, *AACN Adv Crit Care* 18(4):337, 2007.

92. Dellinger RP, et al: Surviving Sepsis Campaign: International guidelines for management of severe sepsis and septic shock, *Crit Care Med* 36(1):296, 2008.

93. Schocken DD, et al: Prevention of heart failure. A scientific statement from the American Heart Association Councils on Epidemiology and Prevention, Clinical Cardiology, Cardiovascular Nursing, and High Blood Pressure Research; Quality of Care and Outcomes Research Interdisciplinary Working Group; and Functional Genomics and Translational Biology Interdisciplinary Working Group, *Circulation* 117(19):2544, 2008.

94. Hunt SH, et al: 2009 focused update incorporated into the ACC/AHA 2005 guidelines for the diagnosis and management of heart failure in adults, *Circulation* 119(14):e391, 2009.

95. Quinn B: Pharmacological treatment of heart failure, *Crit Care Nurs Q* 30(4):299, 2007.

CHAPTER

14

Pulmonary Clinical Assessment and Diagnostic Procedures

Kathleen M. Stacy, Jeanne M. Maiden

evolve WEBSITE

Be sure to check out the bonus material, including free self-assessment exercises, on the Evolve web site at *http://evolve.elsevier.com/Urden/priorities/*.

OBJECTIVES

- Identify the components of a pulmonary history.
- Describe inspection, palpation, percussion, and auscultation of the patient with pulmonary dysfunction.
- Outline the steps in analyzing an arterial blood gas.
- Identify key diagnostic procedures used in assessment of the patient with pulmonary dysfunction.
- Discuss the nursing management of a patient undergoing a pulmonary diagnostic procedure.
- Delineate the use of pulse oximetry for bedside monitoring.

Assessment of the patient with pulmonary dysfunction is a systematic process that incorporates both a history and a physical examination. The purpose of the assessment is twofold: (1) to recognize changes in the patient's pulmonary status that would necessitate nursing or medical intervention and (2) to determine the ways in which the patient's pulmonary dysfunction is interfering with self-care activities. To complete the assessment, the patient's laboratory studies and diagnostic tests must be reviewed. This chapter focuses on priority clinical assessments, laboratory studies, and diagnostic tests for the critically ill patient with pulmonary dysfunction.

HISTORY

The initial presentation of the patient determines the rapidity and direction of the interview. For a patient in acute distress, the history is curtailed to just a few questions about the patient's chief complaint and precipitating events. For a patient in no obvious distress, the history focuses on four different areas: (1) review of the patient's present illness, (2) overview of the patient's general respiratory status, (3) examination of the patient's general health status, and (4) survey of the patient's lifestyle.[1] Questions to be included in the interview are outlined in Box 14-1.

A description of the patient's current symptoms is also obtained. Symptoms that are common in the pulmonary patient include dyspnea, cough, wheezing, edema, palpitations, fatigue, chest pain, hemoptysis, and sputum. Information is elicited regarding the location, onset and duration, characteristics, setting, aggravating and alleviating factors, associated symptoms, and efforts to treat the symptoms. If the cough is productive, the patient is asked questions about the color, amount, odor, and consistency of the sputum.[2-5]

BOX 14-1   PULMONARY HISTORY QUESTIONS

Present Illness
What brought you to the hospital?
What were the precipitating events?
When did the problem start?

Respiratory Status
Do you currently have a chronic lung disease, such as asthma, bronchitis, or emphysema?
Do you have a history of any lung disease, such as chronic respiratory infections or tuberculosis?
Have you had any chest surgery?

General Health Status
Do you have any other chronic disease or illness?
Do you have a history of any other disease, illness, or surgery?
Are you currently taking any medications, prescription or nonprescription?

Lifestyle
Do you smoke, or have you smoked in the past?
Have you been exposed to secondhand smoke?
Have you ever been exposed to lung irritants or cancer-causing agents, such as asbestos, chemicals, fumes, beryllium, coal or stone quarry dust, or Agent Orange?

CLINICAL ASSESSMENT

Inspection

Inspection of the patient focuses on three priorities: (1) observation of the tongue and sublingual area, (2) assessment of chest-wall configuration, and (3) evaluation of respiratory effort. If possible, the patient is positioned upright, with the arms resting at the sides.[3]

Observation of the Tongue and Sublingual Area

The patient's tongue and sublingual area are observed for a blue, gray, or dark purple tint or discoloration, indicating the presence of central cyanosis. Central cyanosis is a sign of hypoxemia, or inadequate oxygenation of the blood, and is considered to be life threatening. The fingers and toes may also appear discolored, an indication of the presence of peripheral cyanosis.[6]

Assessment of Chest-Wall Configuration

The size and shape of the patient's chest wall are assessed for an increase in the anteroposterior (AP) diameter and for structural deviations. Normally the ratio of AP diameter to lateral diameter ranges from 1:2 to 5:7.[2,4,5] An increase in the AP diameter is suggestive of chronic obstructive pulmonary disease (COPD).[2,4,5] The shape of the chest is inspected for any structural deviations. Some of the more commonly seen abnormalities are pectus excavatum, pectus carinatum, barrel chest, and spinal deformities. In pectus excavatum (funnel chest), the sternum and lower ribs are displaced posteriorly, creating a funnel or pit-shaped depression in the chest. This causes a decrease in the AP diameter of the chest and may interfere with respiratory function. In pectus carinatum (pigeon breast), the sternum projects forward, causing an increase in the AP diameter of the chest. A barrel chest also results in an increase in AP diameter of the chest and is characterized by displacement of the sternum forward and the ribs outward. Spinal deformities such as kyphosis, lordosis, and scoliosis may also be present and can interfere with respiratory function.[7]

Evaluation of Respiratory Effort

The patient's respiratory effort is evaluated for rate, rhythm, symmetry, and quality of ventilatory movements.[2] Normal breathing at rest is effortless and regular and occurs at a rate of 12 to 20 breaths per minute.[3] Some of the more commonly seen patterns in patients with pulmonary dysfunction are tachypnea, hyperventilation, and air trapping. Tachypnea is manifested by an increase in the rate and decrease in the depth of ventilation. Hyperventilation is manifested by an increase in both the rate and depth of ventilation. Patients with COPD often experience obstructive breathing, or air trapping. As the patient breathes, air becomes trapped in the lungs and ventilations become progressively shallower until the patient actively and forcefully exhales.[8]

Additional Assessment Areas

Other areas assessed are patient position, use of accessory muscles, presence of intercostal retractions, unequal movement of the chest wall, flaring of nares, and pausing midsentence to take a breath.[2,4,5] The presence of other iatrogenic features, such as chest tubes, central venous lines, artificial airways, and nasogastric tubes, should be noted as they may affect assessment findings.

Palpation

Palpation of the patient focuses on three priorities: (1) confirmation of tracheal position, (2) assessment of respiratory excursion, and (3) evaluation of fremitus. In addition, the thorax is assessed for any areas of tenderness, lumps, or bony deformities. The anterior, posterior, and lateral areas of the chest are evaluated in a systematic fashion.[2]

Confirmation of Tracheal Position

The patient's tracheal position is confirmed at midline. It is assessed by placing the fingers in the suprasternal notch and moving upward.[8] Deviation of the trachea to either side can indicate pneumothorax, unilateral pneumonia, diffuse pulmonary fibrosis, a large pleural effusion, or severe atelectasis. With atelectasis, the trachea shifts to the same side as the problem, and with pneumothorax the trachea shifts to the opposite side of the problem.[7]

Assessment of Respiratory Excursion

The patient's respiratory excursion is assessed for the degree and symmetry of movement. It is evaluated by placing the hands on the anterolateral chest with the thumbs extended along the costal margin, pointing to the xiphoid process, or by placing the hands on the posterolateral chest with the thumbs on either side of the spine at the level of the tenth rib. The patient is instructed to take a few normal breaths, then a few deep breaths. Chest movement is assessed for equality, which signifies symmetry of thoracic expansion.[3,7,8] Asymmetry is an abnormal finding that can occur with pneumothorax, pneumonia, or other disorders that interfere with lung inflation. The degree of chest movement is felt to ascertain the extent of lung expansion. The thumbs should separate 3 to 5 cm during deep inspiration.[5,8] Lung expansion of a hyperinflated chest is less than that of a normal one.[5,8]

Evaluation of Tactile Fremitus

Assessment of tactile fremitus is performed to identify, describe, and localize any areas of increased or decreased fremitus. Fremitus refers to the palpable vibrations felt through the chest wall when the patient speaks. It is assessed by placing the palmar surface of the hands against opposite sides of the chest wall and having the patient repeat the word "ninety-nine." The hands are moved systematically around the thorax until the anterior, posterior, and both lateral areas have been assessed.[7,8] Fremitus varies from patient to patient and depends on the pitch and intensity of the voice. Fremitus is described as normal, decreased, or increased. With normal fremitus, vibrations can be felt over the trachea but are barely palpable over the periphery.[2] With decreased fremitus, there is interference with the transmission of vibrations. Examples of disorders that decrease fremitus include pleural effusion, pneumothorax, bronchial obstruction, pleural thickening, and emphysema. With increased fremitus, there is an increase in the transmission of vibrations. Examples of disorders that increase fremitus include pneumonia, lung cancer, and pulmonary fibrosis.[5]

Percussion

Percussion of the patient focuses on two priorities: (1) evaluation of the underlying lung structure and (2) assessment of diaphragmatic excursion. Although not often used,

percussion is a useful technique for confirming suspected abnormalities.

Evaluation of Underlying Lung Structure

The patient's underlying lung structure is evaluated to estimate the amounts of air, liquid, or solid material present. It is performed by placing the middle finger of the nondominant hand on the chest wall. The distal portion, between the last joint and the nailbed, is then struck with the middle finger of the dominant hand. The hands are moved side to side, systematically around the thorax, to compare similar areas, until the anterior, posterior, and both lateral areas have been assessed. Five different tones can be elicited: resonance, hyperresonance, tympany, dullness, and flatness. These tones are distinguished by differences in intensity, pitch, duration, and quality. Table 14-1 describes the different percussion tones and their associated conditions.[3,7]

Assessment of Diaphragmatic Excursion

Diaphragmatic excursion is assessed by measuring the difference in the level of the diaphragm on inspiration and expiration. It is performed by instructing the patient to inhale and hold the breath. The posterior chest is percussed downward, over the intercostal spaces, until the dull sound produced by the diaphragm is heard. The spot is marked. The patient is then instructed to take a few breaths in and out, exhale completely, and then hold his or her breath. The posterior chest is percussed again, and the new area of dullness over the diaphragm is then located and marked. The difference between the two spots is noted and measured. Normal diaphragmatic excursion is 3 to 5 cm.[8] It is decreased in disorders or conditions such as ascites, pregnancy, hepatomegaly, and emphysema. It is increased in pleural effusion or disorders that elevate the diaphragm, such as atelectasis or paralysis.[7]

Auscultation

Auscultation of the patient focuses on three priorities: (1) evaluation of normal breath sounds, (2) identification

TABLE 14-1	PERCUSSION TONES: DESCRIPTION AND ASSOCIATED CONDITIONS				
TONE	**INTENSITY**	**PITCH**	**DURATION**	**QUALITY**	**CONDITIONS**
Resonance	Loud	Low	Long	Hollow	Normal lung Bronchitis
Hyperresonance	Very loud	Very low	Long	Booming	Asthma Emphysema Pneumothorax
Tympany	Loud	Musical	Medium	Drumlike	Large pneumothorax Emphysematous blebs
Dullness	Medium	Medium to high	Medium	Thudlike	Atelectasis Pleural effusion Pulmonary edema Pneumonia Lung mass
Flatness	Soft	High	Short	Extremely dull	Massive atelectasis Pneumonectomy

of abnormal breath sounds, and (3) assessment of voice sounds. Auscultation requires a quiet environment, proper positioning of the patient, and a bare chest.[9] Breath sounds are best heard with the patient in the upright position.[5]

Evaluation of Normal Breath Sounds

The patient's breath sounds are auscultated to evaluate the quality of air movement through the pulmonary system and to identify the presence of abnormal sounds. It is performed by placing the diaphragm of the stethoscope against the chest wall and instructing the patient to breathe in and out slowly with his or her mouth open.[2] Both the inspiratory and expiratory phases are assessed. Auscultation is done in a systematic sequence—side to side, top to bottom, posteriorly, laterally, and anteriorly[5] (Figure 14-1).

Normal breath sounds are different, depending on their location. They are classified into three categories: bronchial, bronchovesicular, and vesicular. Table 14-2 describes the characteristics of normal breath sounds.[2,5,9]

Identification of Abnormal Breath Sounds

Abnormal breath sounds are identified once the normal breath sounds have been clearly delineated. There are three categories of abnormal breath sounds: absent or diminished breath sounds, displaced bronchial breath sounds, and adventitious breath sounds. Table 14-3 describes the various abnormal breath sounds and their associated conditions.[2,5,9]

An absent or diminished breath sound indicates that there is little or no airflow to a particular portion of the lung (either a small segment or an entire lung).[9] Displaced bronchial breath sounds are normal bronchial sounds heard in the peripheral lung fields instead of over the trachea. This condition is usually indicative of fluid or exudate present in the alveoli.[9]

Adventitious breath sounds are extra or added sounds heard in addition to the other sounds already discussed. They are classified as crackles, rhonchi, wheezes, and friction rubs. Crackles (also referred to as rales) are short, discrete, popping or crackling sounds produced by fluid in the small airways or alveoli or by the snapping open of collapsed airways during inspiration. They are mainly heard on inspiration and are not clear by coughing.[8] Crackles can be further classified as fine, medium, or coarse, depending on pitch.[9] Rhonchi are coarse, rumbling, low-pitched sounds produced by airflow over secretions in the larger airways or by narrowing of the large airways. They are mainly heard on

TABLE 14-2	CHARACTERISTICS OF NORMAL BREATH SOUNDS
SOUND	**CHARACTERISTICS**
Vesicular	Heard over most of lung field; low pitch; soft and short exhalation, and long inhalation
Bronchovesicular	Heard over main bronchus area and over upper right posterior lung field; medium pitch; exhalation equals inhalation
Bronchial	Heard only over trachea; high pitch; loud and long exhalation

Modified from Thompson JM, et al: *Mosby's clinical nursing*, ed 5, St Louis, 2002, Mosby.

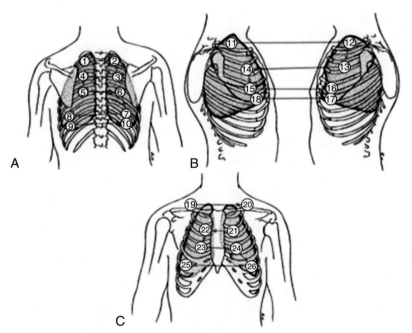

FIGURE 14-1 Auscultation Sequence. *A,* Posterior. *B,* Lateral. *C,* Anterior. (From Perry AG, Potter PA: *Clinical nursing skills and techniques,* ed 7, St Louis, 2010, Mosby.)

TABLE 14-3 ABNORMAL BREATH SOUNDS AND THEIR ASSOCIATED CONDITIONS

ABNORMAL SOUND	DESCRIPTION	CONDITION
Absent breath sounds	No airflow to particular portion of lung	Pneumothorax Pneumonectomy Emphysematous blebs Pleural effusion Lung mass Massive atelectasis Complete airway obstruction
Diminished breath sounds	Little airflow to particular portion of lung	Emphysema Pleural effusion Pleurisy Atelectasis Pulmonary fibrosis
Displaced bronchial sounds	Bronchial sounds heard in peripheral lung fields	Atelectasis with secretions Lung mass with exudates Pneumonia Pleural effusion Pulmonary edema
Crackles (rales)	Short, discrete popping or crackling sounds	Pulmonary edema Pneumonia Pulmonary fibrosis Atelectasis Bronchiectasis
Rhonchi	Coarse, rumbling, low-pitched sounds	Pneumonia Asthma Bronchitis Bronchospasm
Wheezes	High-pitched, squeaking, whistling sounds	Asthma Bronchospasm
Pleural friction rub	Creaking, leathery, loud, dry, coarse sounds	Pleural effusion Pleurisy

expiration and may be cleared with coughing.[8] Rhonchi can further be classified as bubbling, gurgling, or sonorous, depending on the characteristics of the sound.[9] Wheezes are high-pitched, squeaking, whistling sounds produced by airflow through narrowed small airways. They are mainly heard on expiration but may be heard throughout the ventilatory cycle.[8] Depending on their severity, wheezes can be further classified as mild, moderate, or severe.[9] Pleural friction rubs are creaking, leathery, loud, dry, coarse sounds produced by irritated pleural surfaces rubbing together. They are usually heard best in the lower anterolateral chest area during the latter portion of inspiration and the beginning of expiration. Pleural friction rubs are caused by inflammation of the pleura.[3,8,9]

Assessment of Voice Sounds

Assessment of the patient's voice sounds is particularly useful in detecting lung consolidation or lung compression. Three abnormal types of voice sounds are bronchophony, whispering pectoriloquy, and egophony. Bronchophony describes a condition in which the spoken voice is heard on auscultation with higher intensity and clarity than usual. Normally the spoken word is muffled when heard through the stethoscope. It is assessed by placing the diaphragm of the stethoscope against the posterior side of the patient's chest and instructing the patient to say "ninety-nine." Bronchophony is present when the sound heard is clear, distinct, and loud. Whispering pectoriloquy describes a condition of unusually clear transmission of the whispered voice on auscultation. Normally the whispered word is unintelligible when heard through the stethoscope. It is assessed by placing the stethoscope against the posterior side of the patient's chest and instructing the patient to whisper "one, two, three." Whispering pectoriloquy is present when the sound heard is clear and distinct. Egophony describes a condition in which the voice sounds increase in intensity and develop a nasal bleating quality on auscultation. It is assessed by placing the stethoscope against the posterior side of the patient's chest and instructing the patient to say "e-e-e." Egophony is present when the "e" sound changes to an "a" sound.[2,4,9]

LABORATORY STUDIES

Arterial Blood Gases

Interpretation of arterial blood gas (ABG) levels can be difficult, especially if one is under pressure to do it quickly and accurately. One method that can help ensure accuracy when analyzing arterial blood gas levels is to follow the same steps of interpretation each time. A specific method to be used each time that blood gas values must be interpreted is presented in brief in Box 14-2.

Step 1: Look at the PaO_2 level and answer the question, "Does the PaO_2 level show hypoxemia?" The PaO_2 is a measure of the partial pressure of oxygen dissolved in arterial blood plasma, with *P* standing for *partial pressure* and *a* standing for *arterial*. It is reported in millimeters of mercury (mm Hg). PaO_2 reflects 3% of total oxygen in the blood.[10]

The normal range in PaO_2 for persons breathing room air at sea level is 80 to 100 mm Hg. However, the normal range is age-dependent in two groups: infants and persons 60 years and older. The normal level for infants breathing room air is 50 to 70 mm Hg.[11] The normal level for persons 60 years and older decreases with age as changes occur in the ventilation/perfusion (V/Q) matching in the aging lung.[12] The correct PaO_2 for older persons can be ascertained as follows: 80 mm Hg (the lowest normal value) minus 1 mm Hg for every year that a person is over the age of 60. Using this formula, a 65-year-old individual can have a PaO_2 as low as 75 mm Hg and still be within the normal range (formula for 5 years over 60 years of age: 80 mm Hg − 5 mm Hg = 75 mm Hg). An acceptable range for an 80-year-old person

---

BOX 14-2 **STEPS FOR INTERPRETATION OF BLOOD GAS LEVELS**

Step 1

Look at the PaO_2 level, and answer this question:
- Does the Pao_2 level show hypoxemia?

Step 2

Look at the pH level, and answer this question:
- Is the pH level on the acid or alkaline side of 7.40?

Step 3

Look at the $Paco_2$ level, and answer this question:
- Does the $Paco_2$ level show respiratory acidosis, alkalosis, or normalcy?

Step 4

Look at the HCO_3^- level, and answer this question:
- Does the HCO_3^- level show metabolic acidosis, alkalosis, or normalcy?

Step 5

Look again at the pH level, and answer this question:
- Does the pH show a compensated or an uncompensated condition?

---

is 60 mm Hg (formula for 20 years over the age of 60: 80 mm Hg − 20 mm Hg = 60 mm Hg). At any age, a Pao_2 lower than 40 mm Hg represents a life-threatening situation that requires immediate action.[13] In addition, a Pao_2 less than the predicted lowest value indicates hypoxemia, which means that a lower-than-normal amount of oxygen is dissolved in plasma.[10]

Step 2: Look at the pH level and answer the question, "Is the pH on the acid or alkaline side of 7.40?" The pH is the hydrogen ion (H^+) concentration of plasma. Calculation of pH is accomplished by using the partial pressure of carbon dioxide ($Paco_2$) and the plasma bicarbonate level (Hco_3^-).[10]

The normal pH of arterial blood is 7.35 to 7.45, with the mean being 7.40. If the pH level is less than 7.40, it is on the acid side of the mean. A pH level less than 7.35 is known as *acidemia,* and the overall condition is called acidosis. If the pH level is greater than 7.40, it is on the alkaline side of the mean. A pH level greater than 7.45 is known as *alkalemia,* and the overall condition is called *alkalosis.*[10,14,15]

Step 3: Look at the $Paco_2$ level and answer the question, "Does the $Paco_2$ show respiratory acidosis, alkalosis, or normalcy?" The $Paco_2$ is a measure of the partial pressure of carbon dioxide dissolved in arterial blood plasma and is reported in mm Hg. It is the acid-base component that reflects the effectiveness of ventilation in relation to the metabolic rate.[10] In other words, the $Paco_2$ value indicates whether the patient can ventilate well enough to rid the body of the carbon dioxide produced as a consequence of metabolism.

The normal range for $Paco_2$ is 35 to 45 mm Hg. This range does not change as a person ages. A $Paco_2$ value of greater than 45 mm Hg defines respiratory acidosis, which is caused by alveolar hypoventilation. Hypoventilation can result from COPD, oversedation, head trauma, anesthesia, drug overdose, neuromuscular disease, or hypoventilation with mechanical ventilation.[14,15] A $Paco_2$ value that is less than 35 mm Hg defines respiratory alkalosis, which is caused by alveolar hyperventilation. Hyperventilation can result from hypoxia, anxiety, pulmonary embolism, pregnancy, and hyperventilation with mechanical ventilation or as a compensatory mechanism to metabolic acidosis.[14,15]

Step 4: Look at the HCO_3^- level and answer the question, "Does the HCO_3^- show metabolic acidosis, alkalosis, or normalcy?" The bicarbonate (HCO_3^-) is the acid-base component that reflects kidney function. The bicarbonate is reduced or increased in the plasma by renal mechanisms. The normal range is 22 to 26 mEq/L.[13,14] A bicarbonate level of less than 22 mEq/L defines metabolic acidosis, which can result from ketoacidosis, lactic acidosis, renal failure, or diarrhea. The cumulative effect is a gain of acids or a loss of base. A bicarbonate level that is greater than 26 mEq/L defines metabolic alkalosis, which can result from fluid loss from the upper gastrointestinal tract (vomiting or nasogastric suction), diuretic therapy, severe hypokalemia, alkali administration, or steroid therapy.[14,15]

Step 5: Look back at the pH level and answer the question, "Does the pH show a compensated or an uncompensated condition?" If the pH level is abnormal (less than 7.35 or greater than 7.45), the $Paco_2$ value or the Hco_3^- level, or both, will also be abnormal. This is an uncompensated condition because there has not been enough time for the body to return the pH to its normal range (Box 14-3).[14,15] If the pH level is within normal limits and both the $Paco_2$ value and the Hco_3^- level are abnormal, the condition is compensated because there has been enough time for the body to restore the pH to within its normal range.[14,15] Differentiating the primary disorder from the compensatory response can be difficult. The primary disorder is the abnormality that caused the pH level to shift initially; thus on whichever side of 7.40 the pH level occurs is considered the primary disorder (Box 14-4).[14,15] Partial compensation may also be present and is evidenced by abnormal pH, $Paco_2$, and Hco_3^- levels, indications that the body is attempting to return the pH to its normal range.[14,15]

Table 14-4 summarizes the changes in the acid-base components that accompany various acid-base disorders.[14,15] In addition to the parameters previously discussed, other factors must be considered when reviewing a patient's ABGs, including oxygen saturation, oxygen content, expected Pao_2, and base excess and deficit.

Oxygen Saturation

Oxygen saturation is a measure of the amount of oxygen bound to hemoglobin, compared with hemoglobin's maximal capability for binding oxygen. It can be assessed as a component of the ABG (Sao_2) or can be measured noninvasively using a pulse oximeter (Spo_2).[10] Oxygen saturation is reported as a percentage or as a decimal, with normal being greater than 95% on room air. Normally, the saturation level cannot reach 100% (on room air) because of the physiological shunting.[10,13] However, when supplemental oxygen is administered, oxygen saturation may approach 100% so closely that it is reported as 100%.

Proper evaluation of the oxygen saturation level is vital. For example, an Sao_2 of 97% means that 97% of the available hemoglobin is bound with oxygen. The word "available" is essential to evaluating the Sao_2 level, because the hemoglobin level is not always within normal limits and oxygen can bind only with what is available. A 97% saturation level associated with 10 g of hemoglobin does not deliver as much oxygen to the tissues as does a 97% saturation associated with 15 g of hemoglobin. Thus assessing only the Sao_2 level and finding it within normal limits must not lead one to believe that the patient's oxygenation status is normal. The hemoglobin level must also be evaluated before a decision on oxygenation status can be made.[10,16]

Oxygen Content

Oxygen content (Cao_2) is a measure of the total amount of oxygen carried in the blood, including the amount dissolved in plasma (measured by the Pao_2) and the amount bound to the hemoglobin molecule (measured by the Sao_2). Cao_2 is reported in milliliters (ml) of oxygen carried per 100 ml of

---

BOX 14-3   UNCOMPENSATED ARTERIAL BLOOD GAS VALUES

Example 1
Pao_2: 90 mm Hg
pH: 7.25
$Paco_2$: 50 mm Hg
Hco_3^-: 22 mEq/L
Interpretation: Uncompensated respiratory acidosis

Example 2
Pao_2: 90 mm Hg
pH: 7.25
$Paco_2$: 40 mm Hg
Hco_3^-: 17 mEq/L
Interpretation: Uncompensated metabolic acidosis

BOX 14-4   COMPENSATED ARTERIAL BLOOD GAS VALUES

Example 1
Pao_2: 90 mm Hg
pH: 7.37
$Paco_2$: 60 mm Hg
Hco_3^-: 38 mEq/L
Interpretation: Compensated respiratory acidosis with metabolic alkalosis. (The acidosis is considered the main disorder and the alkalosis the compensatory response, because the pH is on the acid side of 7.40.)

Example 2
Pao_2: 90 mm Hg
pH: 7.42
$Paco_2$: 48 mm Hg
Hco_3^-: 35 mEq/L
Interpretation: Compensated metabolic alkalosis with respiratory acidosis. (The alkalosis is considered the main disorder and the acidosis the compensatory response, because the pH is on the alkaline side of 7.40.)

TABLE 14-4   ARTERIAL BLOOD GAS ASSESSMENT

DISORDER	PH	$Paco_2$	Hco_3^-
Respiratory Acidosis			
Uncompensated	<7.35	>45 mm Hg	22-26 mEq/L
Partially compensated	<7.35	>45 mm Hg	>26 mEq/L
Compensated	7.35-7.39	>45 mm Hg	>26 mEq/L
Respiratory Alkalosis			
Uncompensated	>7.45	<35 mm Hg	22-26 mEq/L
Partially compensated	>7.45	<35 mm Hg	<22 mEq/L
Compensated	7.41-7.45	<35 mm Hg	<22 mEq/L
Metabolic Acidosis			
Uncompensated	<7.35	35-45 mm Hg	<22 mEq/L
Partially compensated	<7.35	<35 mm Hg	<22 mEq/L
Compensated	7.35-7.39	<35 mm Hg	<22 mEq/L
Metabolic Alkalosis			
Uncompensated	>7.45	35-45 mm Hg	>26 mEq/L
Partially compensated	>7.45	>45 mm Hg	>26 mEq/L
Compensated	7.41-7.45	>45 mm Hg	>26 mEq/L
Combined (or mixed) respiratory and metabolic acidosis	<7.35	>45 mm Hg	<22 mEq/L
Combined (or mixed) respiratory and metabolic alkalosis	>7.45	<35 mm Hg	>26 mEq/L

blood. The normal value is 20 ml of oxygen per 100 ml of blood. To calculate the oxygen content, the Pao_2, the Sao_2, and the hemoglobin level are used (see Appendix B). A change in any one of these parameters will affect the Cao_2.[10,16]

Classic Shunt Equation and Oxygen Tension Indices

The efficiency of oxygenation can be assessed by measuring the degree of intrapulmonary shunting that occurs in a patient at any one time, using the classic shunt equation and oxygen tension indices. Intrapulmonary shunting (QS/QT [the portion of cardiac output not exchanging with alveolar blood divided by the total cardiac output]) refers to venous blood that flows to the lungs without being oxygenated because of nonfunctioning alveoli.[17] Other names for this condition include shunt effect, low V/Q, wasted blood flow, and venous admixture.[10] Direct determination of intrapulmonary shunting requires the use of the classic shunt equation, which is both invasive and cumbersome. A shunt of 5% to 15% is considered mild, of 15% to 30% is considered major, and a shunt greater than 30% is a serious and potentially life-threatening condition.[10]

Often times, intrapulmonary shunting is estimated by using the oxygen tension indices. One advantage to these methods is the ease of performance, though they have been found to be unreliable in critically ill patients.[10] An estimate of intrapulmonary shunting can be determined by computing the difference between the alveolar and arterial oxygen concentrations. Normally, alveolar and arterial Po_2 values are approximately equal.[13] When they are not, it indicates that venous blood is passing malfunctioning alveoli and returning unoxygenated to the left side of the heart.[10,13] The most common oxygen tension indices used to estimate intrapulmonary shunting are the Pao_2/Fio_2 ratio, the Pao_2/PAo_2 ratio, and the A-a gradient (see Appendix B for formulas).[16]

Pao_2/Fio_2 Ratio

The Pao_2/Fio_2 ratio is clinically the easiest formula to calculate because it does not call for the computation of the alveolar Po_2. Normally, the Pao_2/Fio_2 ratio is greater than 300, with the lower the value the worse the lung function.[16]

Pao_2/PAo_2 Ratio

The Pao_2/PAo_2 ratio (arterial/alveolar O_2 ratio) is normally greater than 75%.[16] The disadvantage to using this formula is that it calls for the computation of the alveolar Po_2, but the advantage is that it is unaffected by changes in the Fio_2 as long as the underlying lung condition is stable.[10,16]

Alveolar-Arterial Gradient

The A-a gradient $(P[A-a]o_2)$ is normally less than 15 mm Hg on room air.[17] This estimate of intrapulmonary shunting is the least reliable clinically but is frequently used in clinical decision making. One of the major disadvantages to using this formula is that it is greatly influenced by the amount of oxygen the patient is receiving.[10,17]

Dead Space/Tidal Volume Ratio

The efficiency of ventilation can be measured using the dead space/tidal volume ratio (V_D/V_T) (see Appendix B). The formula measures the fraction of tidal volume not participating in gas exchange. Dead space greater than 0.4 indicates a dead-space-producing disorder and is considered abnormal.[18] The major limitations to using this formula are that it requires the measurement of exhaled carbon dioxide to complete and that the work of breathing by patients must remain stable during the collection.[10]

Sputum Studies

Careful analysis of sputum specimens is crucial for the rapid identification and treatment of pulmonary infections. The most difficult aspect of sputum examination is proper collection of the specimen. In general, collection of a good sputum sample requires a conscious, cooperative, sufficiently hydrated patient. When the patient has difficulty producing sputum, heated, nebulized saline may help to loosen secretions for expectoration. Chest physiotherapy combined with nebulization can improve the success rate. Collection of a sputum specimen is best done in the morning because there is a greater volume of secretions as a result of nighttime pooling. Brushing the teeth and rinsing the oropharyngeal area is recommended to reduce contamination before collecting a sample.[19]

Many critically ill patients cannot cough effectively, and thus sputum collection by other means is required. These methods include tracheobronchial aspiration, transtracheal aspiration, and the use of a fiberoptic bronchoscopy with a protected brush catheter. Because each method has its own benefits and risks, the patient's clinical condition determines the appropriate technique. Many critically ill patients have endotracheal or tracheostomy tubes already in place. Collecting sputum specimens from these patients requires special attention to technique (Box 14-5). Deep specimens are obtained to avoid collecting specimens that contain resident upper airway flora that may have migrated down the tube.[19]

Once a sputum specimen is obtained, it is examined for volume, physical properties, mucopurulence, and color. Next, a microscopic examination is done to identify the source of the specimen. If a bacterial infection is suspected, a Gram stain followed by a culture and sensitivity (C&S) is performed.[20]

DIAGNOSTIC PROCEDURES

Table 14-5 presents an overview of the various diagnostic procedures used to evaluate the patient with pulmonary dysfunction.

Nursing Management

The nursing management of a patient undergoing a diagnostic procedure involves a variety of interventions. **Priorities are directed toward (1) preparing the patient psychologically and physically for the procedure, (2) monitoring the patient's responses to the procedure, and (3) assessing the**

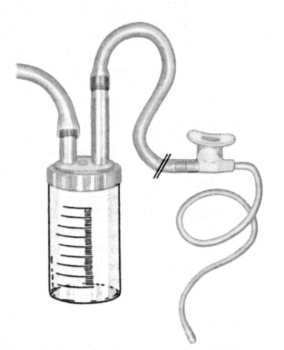

FIGURE 14-2 Specimen Container. (From Wilkins RL, et al, editors: *Egan's fundamentals of respiratory care*, ed 9, St Louis, 2008, Mosby.)

patient after the procedure. Preparing the patient includes teaching the patient about the procedure, answering any questions, and transporting and/or positioning the patient for the procedure. Monitoring the patient's responses to the procedure includes observing the patient for signs of pain, anxiety, or respiratory decompensation (Box 14-6) and monitoring vital signs. Assessing the patient after the procedure includes observing for complications of the procedure and medicating the patient for any postprocedure discomfort.

Any evidence of respiratory distress should be immediately reported to the physician and emergency measures to maintain breathing must be initiated.

BEDSIDE MONITORING

Pulse Oximetry

Pulse oximetry is a noninvasive method for monitoring oxygen saturation (SpO_2). It is indicated in any situation in which the patient's oxygenation status requires continuous observation. It consists of a microprocessor and a probe that attaches to the patient's forehead, finger, ear, toe, or nose. The probe consists of two light-emitting diodes and a photodetector. The diodes transmit red and infrared light wavelengths through the pulsating arterial vascular bed to the photodetector on the other side. The percentage of oxygen saturation is determined by the difference in absorbance of the red and infrared light caused by the difference in color between oxygen-bound (bright red) and oxygen-unbound (dark red) hemoglobin. The photodetector converts the light signals into an electric signal, which is then sent to the microprocessor, which converts it to a digital reading. The pulse oximeter is considered very accurate, within ±2% at saturation greater than 70%.[21,22] **Nursing priorities are directed toward minimizing the physiological and technical factors that can limit the monitoring system.**

Physiological Limitations

Physiological limitations include elevated levels of abnormal hemoglobins, presence of vascular dyes, and poor tissue perfusion. The pulse oximeter cannot differentiate between normal and abnormal hemoglobin. Elevated levels of abnormal hemoglobin falsely elevate the SpO_2. Vascular dyes, such as methylene blue, indigo carmine, indocyanine green, and fluorescein, also interfere with pulse oximetry and can lead to falsely low readings. Poor tissue perfusion to the area with the probe leads to loss of pulsatile flow and signal failure (Patient Safety Priorities box on Pulse Oximetry).[17,21]

⚡ PATIENT SAFETY PRIORITIES

Pulse Oximetry

In the critically ill patient, pulse oximetry is reliable only for monitoring the patient's oxygenation status. It is not a reliable method for monitoring the patient's ventilatory status. The ability of a pulse oximeter to detect hypoventilation is accurate only when the patient is breathing room air.* Because most critically ill patients require some form of oxygen therapy, pulse oximetry is not a reliable method of detecting hypercapnia and should *not* be used for this purpose.

*Witting MD, et al: The sensitivity of room-air pulse oximetry in the detection of hypercapnia, *Am J Emerg Med* 23(4):497, 2005.

Technical Limitations

Technical limitations include bright lights, excessive motion, and incorrect placement of the probe. Bright lights may interfere with the photodetector and cause inaccurate results. The

TABLE 14-5   PULMONARY DIAGNOSTIC STUDIES

STUDY	EVALUATION	COMMENTS
Bronchography	Detect obstruction or malformation of the tracheobronchial tree	Patient inspires radiopaque substance and then x-rays are taken. Inquire about possibility of pregnancy.
Chest x-ray	Detect pathological lung condition (e.g., pneumonia, pulmonary edema, atelectasis, or tuberculosis) Determine size and location of lung lesions and tumors Verify placement of endotracheal tube, central venous catheters, and chest tubes	Noninvasive test with minimal radiation exposure. Inquire about possibility of pregnancy. Posteroanterior and lateral films are done most commonly, but in critical care areas, anteroposterior portable films are frequently necessary because of inability to transport patient. Lateral decubitus films aid in identification of pleural effusion.
Exercise testing	Identify early disability Differentiate between cardiac and pulmonary disease	Monitor for changes in functional oxygen saturation during exercise. Monitor closely for exercise-induced hypotension or ventricular dysrhythmias.
Laryngoscopy, bronchoscopy, mediastinoscopy	Obtain cytological specimen or biopsy Identify tumors, obstructions, secretions, or foreign bodies in tracheobronchial tree Locate a bleeding site May be used therapeutically to remove secretions, foreign bodies, and other contaminants	Patient is sedated before the procedure, usually with a benzodiazepine (e.g., diazepam or midazolam). Monitor the patient for subcutaneous emphysema after study; indicates tracheal or bronchial tear. Monitor for hemoptysis; some blood in sputum is normal after biopsy but frank hemoptysis requires immediate attention.
Lung biopsy Transthoracic needle lung biopsy Open lung biopsy	Obtain specimen for cytological evaluation	Transthoracic needle biopsy performed under fluoroscopy; inquire about possibility of pregnancy. Open lung biopsy requires thoracotomy.
Magnetic resonance imaging	Distinguishes tumors from other structures (e.g., tumor, pleural thickening, or fibrosis)	Noninvasive test. Contraindicated for patients with pacemakers or implanted metallic devices.
Pulmonary angiography	Detects changes in lung tissue (e.g., masses) Diagnoses abnormalities in pulmonary vasculature, including thrombi and emboli Identifies congenital abnormalities of the circulation	Invasive test. Inquire about possibility of pregnancy. Contrast media injected into pulmonary artery: ensure adequate hydration after study. Monitor arterial puncture point for hematoma or hemorrhage.
Pulmonary function studies • Spirometry • Ventilator mechanics • Flow-volume loop • Diffusing capacity	Measures lung volumes, capacities, and flow rates Residual volume, functional residual capacity, and total lung capacity require nitrogen washout technique Identifies features of restrictive or obstructive lung disease Evaluates responsiveness to bronchodilator therapy Aids in evaluation of surgical risk Documents a disability or cause of dyspnea	Noninvasive studies. Frequently repeated after bronchodilator therapy.
Sleep studies	Diagnose and differentiate between obstructive, central, and cardiac sleep apnea	Restrict caffeine before testing. Usually done during normal sleep hours.
Thoracentesis (may include pleural biopsy)	Obtain pleural fluid and/or tissue specimen May be used therapeutically to remove pleural fluid	Monitor patient for indications of pneumothorax. Monitor for leakage from puncture point.
Thoracic computerized tomography	Defines lesions, masses, cavities, or shadows seen on normal chest x-rays Evaluates tracheal or bronchial narrowing Aids in planning radiation therapy	X-rays are taken at different angles.

Continued

TABLE 14-5	PULMONARY DIAGNOSTIC STUDIES—cont'd	
STUDY	**EVALUATION**	**COMMENTS**
Ultrasonography	Evaluates pleural disease Visualizes diaphragm and detects disease around diaphragm (e.g., subphrenic hematoma or abscess)	Noninvasive test
Ventilation scan Lung perfusion scan Ventilation/perfusion scan	Diagnoses ventilation and/or perfusion abnormalities including emphysema and pulmonary emboli	Invasive test: radioisotope inspired and injected intravascularly Inquire about possibility of pregnancy. Nuclear scan study: assure patient that amount of radioactive material is minimal.

From Dennison RD: *Pass CCRN!*, ed 3, St Louis, 2007, Mosby.

BOX 14-6 CLINICAL MANIFESTATIONS OF RESPIRATORY DECOMPENSATION

Inadequate Airway
Stridor
Noisy respirations
Supraclavicular and intercostal retractions
Flaring of nares
Labored breathing with use of accessory muscles

Inadequate Ventilation
Absence of air exchange at nose and mouth (breathlessness)
Minimal/absent chest wall motion
Manifestations of obstructed airway
Central cyanosis
Decreased or absent breath sounds (bilateral, unilateral)
Restlessness, anxiety, confusion
Paradoxical motion involving significant portion of chest wall
Decreased Pao_2, increased $Paco_2$, decreased pH

Inadequate Gas Exchange
Tachypnea
Decreased Pao_2
Increased dead space
Central cyanosis
Chest infiltrates on radiographic evaluation

---

probe must be covered to limit optical interference. Excessive motion can mimic arterial pulsations and can lead to false readings. Incorrect placement of the probe can lead to inaccurate results because part of the light can reach the photodetector without having passed through blood (optical shunting). Interventions to limit these problems include using the proper probe in the appropriate spot (e.g., not using a finger probe on the ear), applying the probe according to the directions, and ensuring that the area being monitored has adequate perfusion.[17,22]

Capnography

Capnography is the measurement of exhaled carbon dioxide (CO_2) gas and is also known as end-tidal CO_2 monitoring. Normally, alveolar and arterial CO_2 concentrations are equal in the presence of normal ventilation/perfusion relationships. In a patient who is hemodynamically stable, the end-tidal CO_2 ($Petco_2$) can be used to estimate the $Paco_2$, with the $Petco_2$ levels normally registering 1 to 5 mm Hg less than $Paco_2$ levels. The practitioner must determine first that a normal V/Q relationship exists before correlation of the $Petco_2$ and the $Paco_2$ can be assumed.[17,23] Causes of increased $Petco_2$ include situations in which CO_2 production is increased, such as hyperthermia, sepsis and seizures, or in which alveolar ventilation is decreased such as respiratory depression. Causes of decreased $Petco_2$ include situations in which CO_2 production is decreased, such as hypothermia, cardiac arrest, and pulmonary embolism, or in which alveolar ventilation is increased such as hyperventilation.[17]

In the critical care area, continuous capnography is used for assessment and monitoring of the patient's ventilatory status in a variety of situations including weaning from mechanical ventilation and undergoing procedural sedation. Assessment of changes in physiological dead space can be carried out with end-tidal CO_2 monitoring, based on the degree of difference between the $Paco_2$ and the $Petco_2$. As the severity of pulmonary impairment increases, so does the disparity between the $Paco_2$ and the $Petco_2$, as indicated by an increased gradient. A gradient of greater than 5 mm Hg can be seen with underperfused alveolar-capillary units (dead-space-producing situations) and nonperfused alveolar-capillary units (alveolar dead space). Increased dead-space ventilation is a result of decreased pulmonary blood flow/cardiac output and lung disease. This leads to an abnormality in the transfer of CO_2 from the blood to the lung. The result is a $Petco_2$ level that is lower than the $Paco_2$ because of the mixing of carbon dioxide between perfused and nonperfused units. The end result is an increased or widened $Paco_2$-to-$Petco_2$ gradient.[17,23]

The noninvasive measurement of $Petco_2$ enables assessment of the adequacy of cardiopulmonary resuscitation and endotracheal tube placement. Decreased pulmonary blood flow is associated with lower $Petco_2$ values, reflected clinically by decreased cardiac output, as in the case of cardiopulmonary resuscitation. During endotracheal intubation, a low $Petco_2$ reading indicates that the tube is positioned in the stomach, because the amount of carbon dioxide in the esophagus is expected to be low.[24]

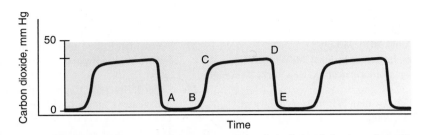

FIGURE 14-3 Normal Findings on a Capnogram. *A→B*, indicated the baseline; *B→C*, expiratory upstroke; *C→D*, alveolar plateau; *D*, partial pressure of end-tidal carbon dioxide (PetCO₂); *D→E*, inspiratory downstroke. (From Frakes M: Measuring end-tidal carbon dioxide: clinical applications and usefulness, *Crit Care Nurse* 21[5]:23, 2001.)

There are three forms of capnography: mainstream, sidestream, and microstream. All forms can be used in intubated patients but sidestream and microstream can also be used in non-intubated patients thus broadening the application of end-tidal CO_2 monitoring. Mainstream capnography measures the CO_2 level directed via a sensor in the exhalation port of the ventilator tubing. During exhalation, gas passes over the sensor and the information is transferred via an electrical cable to the display unit. The display unit produces a waveform, called a capnogram (Figure 14-3), and a numerical recording (PetCO₂). Disadvantages to this form of capnography include the weight of the sensor on the ventilator tubing and secretions and condensation can obstruct the sensor. In sidestream capnography, the CO_2 gas is continuously aspirated via a side port in the ventilator tubing or nasal cannula and is measured and analyzed by a side unit. Disadvantages to this form of capnography include obstruction of the sampling tube with secretions and slow response time. Microstream capnography is a newer and improved version of sidestream capnography that minimizes the disadvantages (Patient Safety Priorities box on Capnography).[23]

⚡ PATIENT SAFETY PRIORITIES
Capnography

Capnography and partial pressure of end-tidal carbon dioxide (PetCO₂) analysis have many diverse applications in the critical care area, but the practitioner must never assume the PetCO₂ values reflect arterial values of the partial pressure of carbon dioxide (PaCO₂) without waveform analysis. Any change in the waveform can indicate a change in the patient's pulmonary status and warrants further evaluation. Loss of the waveform may signal loss of effective respirations.

REFERENCES

1. Baid H: The process of conducting a physical assessment: a nursing perspective, *Br J Nurs* 15(13):710, 2006.
2. Simpson H: Respiratory assessment, *Br J Nurs* 15(9):484, 2006.
3. Reinke LF: Respiratory assessment. In Geiger-Bronksy M, Wilson DJ, editors: *Respiratory nursing: a core curriculum*, New York, 2008, Springer.
4. Finesilver C: Pulmonary assessment; what you need to know, *Prog Cardiovasc Nurs* 18(2):83, 2003.
5. Wilkins RL: Bedside assessment of the patient. In Wilkins RL, Stoller JK, Kacmarek RM, editors: *Egan's fundamentals of respiratory care*, ed 9, St Louis, 2008, Mosby.
6. DeWolfe CC: Apparent life-threatening event: a review, *Pediatr Clin North Am* 52(4):1127, 2005.
7. Barkauskas V, et al: *Health and physical assessment*, ed 3, St Louis, 2002, Mosby.
8. Seidel HM, et al: *Mosby's guide to physical examination*, ed 7, St Louis, 2010, Mosby.
9. Wilkins RL, et al: *Fundamentals of lung and heart sounds*, ed 3, St Louis, 2004, Mosby.
10. Levitzky M: *Pulmonary physiology*, ed 7, New York, 2007, McGraw-Hill.
11. Whitaker K: *Comprehensive perinatal and pediatric respiratory care*, Albany, N.Y., 2001, Delmar.
12. Ramadan F, El Solh AA: Overview of respiratory failure in older adults, *J Intensive Care Med* 21(6):345, 2006.
13. Wilkins RL: Gas exchange and transport. In Wilkins RL, Stoller JK, Kacmarek RM, editors: *Egan's fundamentals of respiratory care*, ed 9, St Louis, 2008, Mosby.
14. Ruholl L: Arterial blood gases: analysis and responses, *Medsurg Nurs* 15(6):343, 2006.
15. Beachey W: Acid-base balance. In Wilkins RL, Stoller JK, Kacmarek RM, editors: *Egan's fundamentals of respiratory care*, ed 9, St Louis, 2008, Mosby.
16. Wettstein R, Wilkins RL: Interpretation of blood gases. In Wilkins RL, Dexter JR, Heuer AJ, editors: *Clinical assessment in respiratory care*, ed 6, St Louis, 2010, Mosby.
17. Vines DL: Respiratory monitoring in the intensive care unit. In Wilkins RL, Dexter JR, Heuer AJ, editors: *Clinical assessment in respiratory care*, ed 6, St Louis, 2010, Mosby.
18. Adams AB: Monitoring and management of the patient in the intensive care unit. In Wilkins RL, Stoller JK, Kacmarek RM, editors: *Egan's fundamentals of respiratory care*, ed 8, St Louis, 2008, Mosby.

19. Wilkins RL, Dexter JR: Clinical laboratory studies. In Wilkins RL, Dexter JR, Heuer AJ, editors: *Clinical assessment in respiratory care*, ed 6, St Louis, 2010, Mosby.

20. Siela D: Diagnostic studies. In Geiger-Bronksy M, Wilson DJ, editors: *Respiratory nursing: a core curriculum*, New York, 2008, Springer.

21. Valdez-Lowe C, Ghareeb SA, Artinian NT: Pulse oximetry in adults, *Am J Nurs* 109(6):52, 2009.

22. Fernandez M, et al: Evaluation of a new pulse oximeter sensor, *Am J Crit Care* 16(2):146, 2007.

23. Zwerneman K: End-tidal carbon dioxide monitoring: a VITAL sign worth watching, *Crit Care Nurs Clin North Am* 18(2):217, 2006.

24. Nagler J, Krauss B: Capnography: a valuable tool for airway management, *Emerg Med Clin North Am* 26(4):881, 2008.

CHAPTER 15

Pulmonary Disorders

Kathleen M. Stacy

evolve WEBSITE

Be sure to check out the bonus material, including free self-assessment exercises, on the Evolve web site at *http://evolve.elsevier.com/Urden/priorities/.*

OBJECTIVES

- Describe the etiology and pathophysiology of selected pulmonary disorders.
- Identify the clinical manifestations of selected pulmonary disorders.
- Explain the treatment of selected pulmonary disorders.
- Discuss the nursing priorities for managing the patient with selected pulmonary disorders.

Understanding the pathology of the disease, the areas of assessment on which to focus, and the usual medical management allows the critical care nurse to more accurately anticipate and plan nursing interventions. This chapter focuses on pulmonary disorders commonly seen in the critical care environment.

ACUTE RESPIRATORY FAILURE

Acute respiratory failure (ARF) is a clinical condition in which the pulmonary system fails to maintain adequate gas exchange.[1] It is the most common organ failure seen in the intensive care unit today,[2,3] with a mortality rate of 22% to 75%.[2] Mortality varies directly with the number of additional organ failures.[2] Additional risk factors for mortality include history of liver, renal, or hematological dysfunction, presence of shock, and age greater than 55 years.[3]

ARF results from a deficiency in the performance of the pulmonary system (Concept Map: Acute Respiratory Failure).[1,4] It usually occurs secondary to another disorder that has altered the normal function of the pulmonary system in such a way as to decrease the ventilatory drive, decrease muscle strength, decrease chest wall elasticity, decrease the lung's capacity for gas exchange, increase airway resistance, or increase metabolic oxygen requirements.[5]

ARF can be classified as hypoxemic normocapnic respiratory failure (type I) or hypoxemic hypercapnic respiratory failure (type II), depending on analysis of the patient's arterial blood gases (ABGs). In type I respiratory failure, the patient presents with a low Pao_2 and a normal $Paco_2$, whereas in type II respiratory failure, Pao_2 is low and $Paco_2$ is high.[1,4]

Etiology

The etiologies of ARF may be classified as *extrapulmonary* or *intrapulmonary,* depending on the component of the respiratory system that is affected. Extrapulmonary causes include disorders that affect the brain, the spinal cord, the neuromuscular system, the thorax, the pleura, and the upper airways. Intrapulmonary causes include disorders that affect the lower airways and alveoli, the pulmonary circulation, and the alveolar-capillary membrane.[6] Table 15-1 lists the different etiologies of ARF and their associated disorders.

Pathophysiology

Hypoxemia is the result of impaired gas exchange and is the hallmark of acute respiratory failure. Hypercapnia may be present, depending on the underlying cause of the problem. The main causes of hypoxemia are alveolar hypoventilation, ventilation/perfusion (V/Q) mismatching, and intrapulmonary shunting.[1,7] Type I respiratory failure usually results from V/Q mismatching and intrapulmonary shunting, whereas type II respiratory failure usually results from alveolar hypoventilation, which may or may not be accompanied by V/Q mismatching and intrapulmonary shunting.[1]

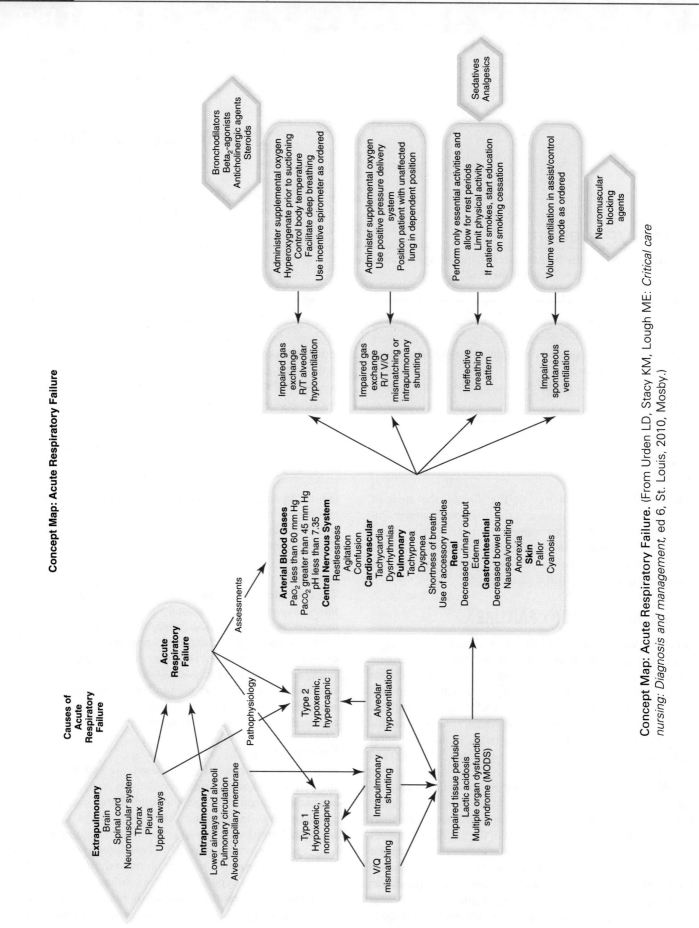

Concept Map: Acute Respiratory Failure. (From Urden LD, Stacy KM, Lough ME: *Critical care nursing: Diagnosis and management*, ed 6, St. Louis, 2010, Mosby.)

TABLE 15-1 ETIOLOGIES OF ACUTE RESPIRATORY FAILURE

AFFECTED AREA	DISORDERS*
Extrapulmonary	
Brain	Drug overdose
	Central alveolar hypoventilation syndrome
	Brain trauma or lesion
	Postoperative anesthesia depression
Spinal cord	Guillain-Barré syndrome
	Poliomyelitis
	Amyotrophic lateral sclerosis
	Spinal cord trauma or lesion
Neuromuscular system	Myasthenia gravis
	Multiple sclerosis
	Neuromuscular-blocking antibiotics
	Organophosphate poisoning
	Muscular dystrophy
Thorax	Massive obesity
	Chest trauma
Pleura	Pleural effusion
	Pneumothorax
Upper airways	Sleep apnea
	Tracheal obstruction
	Epiglottitis
Intrapulmonary	
Lower airways and alveoli	Chronic obstructive pulmonary disease (COPD)
	Asthma
	Bronchiolitis
	Cystic fibrosis
	Pneumonia
Pulmonary circulation	Pulmonary emboli
Alveolar-capillary membrane	Acute lung injury (ALI)
	Inhalation of toxic gases
	Near-drowning

*Not an inclusive list.

Alveolar Hypoventilation

Alveolar hypoventilation occurs when the amount of oxygen being brought into the alveoli is insufficient to meet the metabolic needs of the body.[6] This can be the result of increasing metabolic oxygen needs or decreasing ventilation.[5] Hypoxemia caused by alveolar hypoventilation is associated with hypercapnia and commonly results from extrapulmonary disorders.[1,7]

Ventilation/Perfusion Mismatching

Ventilation/perfusion (V/Q) mismatching occurs when ventilation and blood flow are mismatched in various regions of the lung in excess of what is normal. Blood passes through alveoli that are underventilated for the given amount of perfusion, leaving these areas with a lower-than-normal amount of oxygen. V/Q mismatching is the most common cause of hypoxemia and is usually the result of alveoli that are partially collapsed or partially filled with fluid.[1,7]

Intrapulmonary Shunting

The extreme form of V/Q mismatching, intrapulmonary shunting, occurs when blood reaches the arterial system without participating in gas exchange. The mixing of unoxygenated (shunted) blood and oxygenated blood lowers the average level of oxygen present in the blood. Intrapulmonary shunting occurs when blood passes through a portion of a lung that is not ventilated. This may be the result of (1) alveolar collapse secondary to atelectasis or (2) alveolar flooding with pus, blood, or fluid.[1,7]

If allowed to progress, hypoxemia can result in a deficit of oxygen at the cellular level. As the tissue demands for oxygen continue and the supply diminishes, an oxygen supply/demand imbalance occurs and tissue hypoxia develops. Decreased oxygen to the cells contributes to impaired tissue perfusion and the development of lactic acidosis and multiple organ dysfunction syndrome.[8]

Assessment and Diagnosis

The patient with ARF may experience a variety of clinical manifestations, depending on the underlying cause and the extent of tissue hypoxia. The clinical manifestations commonly seen in the patient with ARF are usually related to the development of hypoxemia, hypercapnia, and acidosis.[9] Because the clinical symptoms are so varied, they are not considered reliable in predicting the degree of hypoxemia or hypercapnia[1] or the severity of ARF.[3]

Diagnosing and following the course of respiratory failure is best accomplished by ABG analysis. ABG analysis confirms the level of $Paco_2$, Pao_2, and blood pH. ARF is generally accepted as being present when the Pao_2 is less than 60 mm Hg. If the patient is also experiencing hypercapnia, the $Paco_2$ will be greater than 45 mm Hg. In patients with chronically elevated $Paco_2$ levels, these criteria must be broadened to include a pH less than 7.35.[9]

A variety of additional tests are performed depending on the patient's underlying condition. These include bronchoscopy for airway surveillance or specimen retrieval, chest radiography, thoracic ultrasound, thoracic computed tomography, and selected lung function studies.[10]

Medical Management

Medical management of the patient with ARF is aimed at treating the underlying cause, promoting adequate gas exchange, correcting acidosis, initiating nutrition support, and preventing complications. Medical interventions to promote gas exchange are aimed at improving oxygenation and ventilation.

Oxygenation

Actions to improve oxygenation include supplemental oxygen administration and the use of positive airway pressure.[8] The purpose of oxygen therapy is to correct hypoxemia, and although the absolute level of hypoxemia varies in each patient, most treatment approaches aim to keep the arterial hemoglobin oxygen saturation greater than 90%.[9] The goal is to keep the tissues' needs satisfied but not produce hypercapnia or oxygen toxicity.[9] Supplemental oxygen administration is effective in treating hypoxemia related to alveolar hypoventilation and V/Q mismatching. When intrapulmonary shunting exists, supplemental oxygen alone is ineffective.[11] In this situation, positive pressure is necessary to open collapsed alveoli and facilitate their participation in gas exchange. Positive pressure is delivered via invasive and noninvasive mechanical ventilation. To avoid intubation, positive pressure is usually administered initially noninvasively via a mask.[12,13] For further information on noninvasive ventilation, see Chapter 16.

Ventilation

Interventions to improve ventilation include the use of noninvasive and invasive mechanical ventilation. Depending on the underlying cause and the severity of the ARF, the patient may be initially treated with noninvasive ventilation.[12] However, one study found that those patients with a pH of less than 7.25 at initial presentation had an increased likelihood of the need for invasive mechanical ventilation.[14] The selection of ventilatory mode and settings depends on the patient's underlying condition, severity of respiratory failure, and body size. Initially the patient is started on volume ventilation in the assist/control mode. In the patient with chronic hypercapnia, the settings should be adjusted to keep the arterial blood gas values within the parameters expected to be maintained by the patient after extubation.[15] For further information on mechanical ventilation see Chapter 16.

Pharmacology

Medications to facilitate dilation of the airways may also be of benefit in the treatment of the patient with ARF. Bronchodilators, such as beta$_2$-agonists and anticholinergic agents, aid in smooth muscle relaxation and are of particular benefit to patients with airflow limitations. Methylxanthines, such as aminophylline, are no longer recommended because of their negative side effects. Steroids also are often administered to decrease airway inflammation and enhance the effects of the beta$_2$-agonists. Mucolytics and expectorants are also no longer used since they have been found to be of no benefit in this patient population.[16]

Sedation is necessary in many patients to assist with maintaining adequate ventilation. It can be used to comfort the patient and decrease the work of breathing, particularly if the patient is fighting the ventilator. Analgesics should be administered for pain control.[17,18] In some patients, sedation does not decrease spontaneous respiratory efforts enough to allow adequate ventilation. Neuromuscular paralysis may be necessary to facilitate optimal ventilation. Paralysis also may be necessary to decrease oxygen consumption in the severely compromised patient.[18]

Acidosis

Acidosis may occur in the patient for a number of reasons. Hypoxemia causes impaired tissue perfusion, which leads to the production of lactic acid and the development of metabolic acidosis. Impaired ventilation leads to the accumulation of carbon dioxide and the development of respiratory acidosis. Once the patient is adequately oxygenated and ventilated, the acidosis should correct itself. The use of sodium bicarbonate to correct the acidosis has been shown to be of minimal benefit to the patient and thus is no longer recommended as first-line treatment. Bicarbonate therapy shifts the oxygen-hemoglobin dissociation curve to the left and can worsen tissue hypoxia. Sodium bicarbonate may be used if the acidosis is severe (pH <7.1), refractory to therapy, and causing dysrhythmias or hemodynamic instability.[19]

Nutrition Support

The initiation of nutrition support is of utmost importance in the management of the patient with ARF. The goals of nutrition support are to meet the overall nutritional needs of the patient while avoiding overfeeding, to prevent nutrition delivery-related complications, and to improve patient outcomes.[20] Failure to provide the patient with adequate nutrition support results in the development of malnutrition. Both malnutrition and overfeeding can interfere with the performance of the pulmonary system, further perpetuating ARF. Malnutrition decreases the patient's ventilatory drive and muscle strength, whereas overfeeding increases carbon dioxide production, which then increases the patient's ventilatory demand, resulting in respiratory muscle fatigue.[21]

The enteral route is the preferred method of nutrition administration. If the patient cannot tolerate enteral feedings or cannot receive enough nutrients enterally, he or she will be started on parenteral nutrition. Because the parenteral route is associated with a higher rate of complications, the goal is to switch to enteral feedings as soon as the patient can tolerate them.[20,21] Nutrition support should be initiated before the third day of mechanical ventilation for the well-nourished patient and within 24 hours for the malnourished patient.[20,21]

Complications

The patient with acute respiratory failure may experience a number of complications including ischemic-anoxic encephalopathy,[22] cardiac dysrhythmias,[23] venous thromboembolism,[24] and gastrointestinal bleeding.[25] Ischemic-anoxic encephalopathy results from hypoxemia, hypercapnia, and acidosis.[22] Dysrhythmias are precipitated by hypoxemia, acidosis, electrolyte imbalances, and the administration of beta$_2$-agonists.[23] Maintaining oxygenation, normalizing electrolytes, and monitoring drug levels will facilitate the prevention and treatment of encephalopathy and dysrhythmias.[22,23] Venous thromboembolism is precipitated by venous stasis resulting from immobility and can be prevented through the use of graduated compression stockings or pneumatic compression devices and low-dose unfractionated heparin or low-molecular-weight heparin.[24] Gastrointestinal bleeding can be prevented through the use of histamine$_2$-antagonists, cytoprotective agents, or proton pump inhibitors.[25] In addition, the patient is at risk for the complications associated with an artificial airway, mechanical ventilation, enteral and parenteral nutrition, and peripheral arterial cannulation.

Nursing Management

Nursing management of the patient with acute respiratory failure incorporates a variety of nursing diagnoses (Nursing Diagnosis Priorities box on Acute Respiratory Failure). Nursing care is directed by the specific etiology of the respiratory failure, although some common interventions are used. **Nursing priorities are directed toward (1) optimizing oxygenation and ventilation, (2) providing comfort and emotional support, (3) maintaining surveillance for complications, and (4) educating the patient and family.**

NURSING DIAGNOSIS PRIORITIES
Acute Respiratory Failure

- Impaired Gas Exchange related to alveolar hypoventilation, p. A-22
- Impaired Gas Exchange related to ventilation/perfusion mismatching or intrapulmonary shunting, p. A-23
- Ineffective Breathing Pattern related to musculoskeletal fatigue or neuromuscular impairment, p. A-27
- Risk for Aspiration, p. A-35
- Imbalanced Nutrition: Less Than Body Requirements related to lack of exogenous nutrients or increased metabolic demand, p. A-22
- Risk for Infection, p. A-36
- Impaired Spontaneous Ventilation related to respiratory muscle fatigue or metabolic factors, p. A-23
- Acute Confusion related to sensory overload, sensory deprivation, and sleep pattern disturbance, p. A-2
- Anxiety related to threat to biological, psychological, and/or social integrity, p. A-7
- Disturbed Body Image related to functional dependence on life-sustaining technology, p. A-16
- Compromised Family Coping related to critically ill family member, p. A-9
- Deficient Knowledge: Discharge Regimen related to lack of previous exposure to information (Patient Education special box on Acute Respiratory Failure), p. A-15

Optimizing Oxygenation and Ventilation

Nursing interventions to optimize oxygenation and ventilation include positioning, preventing desaturation, and promoting secretion clearance.

Positioning. Positioning of the patient with ARF depends on the type of lung injury and the underlying cause of hypoxemia. For those patients with V/Q mismatching, positioning is used to facilitate better matching of ventilation with perfusion to optimize gas exchange.[26] Because gravity normally facilitates preferential ventilation and perfusion to the dependent areas of the lungs, the best gas exchange would take place in the dependent areas of the lungs.[11] Thus the goal of positioning is to place the least affected area of the patient's lung in the most dependent position. Patients with unilateral lung disease should be positioned with the healthy lung in a dependent position.[26,27] Patients with diffuse lung disease may benefit from being positioned with the right lung down, because it is larger and more vascular than the left lung.[27,28] For those patients with alveolar hypoventilation, the goal of positioning is to facilitate ventilation. These patients benefit from nonrecumbent positions such as sitting or a semierect position.[29] In addition, semirecumbency has been shown to decrease the risk of aspiration and inhibit the development of hospital-acquired pneumonia.[30] Frequent repositioning (at least every 2 hours) is beneficial in optimizing the patient's ventilatory pattern and V/Q matching.[31]

Preventing Desaturation. A number of activities can prevent desaturation from occurring. These include performing procedures only as needed, hyperoxygenating the patient before suctioning, providing adequate rest and recovery time between various procedures, and minimizing oxygen consumption. Interventions to minimize oxygen consumption include limiting the patient's physical activity, administering sedation to control anxiety, and providing measures to control fever.[29] The patient should be continuously monitored with a pulse oximeter to warn of signs of desaturation.

Promoting Secretion Clearance. Interventions to promote secretion clearance include providing adequate systemic hydration, humidifying supplemental oxygen, coughing, and suctioning. Postural drainage and chest percussion and vibration have been found to be of little benefit in the critically ill patient[32,33] and thus are not discussed here.

To facilitate deep breathing, the patient's thorax should be maintained in alignment and the head of the bed elevated 30 to 45 degrees. This position best accommodates diaphragmatic descent and intercostal muscle action.

Once the patient is extubated, deep breathing and incentive spirometry should be started as soon as possible. Deep breathing involves having the patient take a deep breath and holding it for approximately 3 seconds or longer. Incentive spirometry involves having the patient take at least 10 deep, effective breaths per hour using an incentive spirometer. These actions help prevent atelectasis and reexpand any collapsed lung tissue. The chest should be auscultated during inflation to ensure that all dependent parts of the lung are well ventilated and to help the patient understand the depth of breath necessary for optimal effect. Coughing should be avoided unless secretions are present because it promotes collapse of the smaller airways.

Educating the Patient and Family

Early in the patient's hospital stay, the patient and family should be taught about acute respiratory failure, its etiologies, and its treatment. As the patient moves toward discharge, teaching should focus on the interventions necessary for preventing the reoccurrence of the precipitating disorder (Patient Education box on Acute Respiratory Failure). If the patient smokes, he or she should be encouraged to stop smoking and be referred to a smoking cessation program (Evidence-Based Collaborative Practice box on Smoking Cessation Guidelines). In addition, the importance of participating in a pulmonary rehabilitation program should be stressed. Additional information for the patient can be found at the American Lung Association website (www.lungusa.org).

PATIENT EDUCATION
Acute Respiratory Failure

- Pathophysiology of disease
- Specific etiology
- Precipitating factor modification
- Importance of taking medications
- Breathing techniques (e.g., pursed-lip breathing, diaphragmatic breathing)
- Energy conservation techniques
- Measures to prevent pulmonary infections (e.g., proper nutrition, hand washing, immunization against *Streptococcus pneumoniae* and influenza viruses)
- Signs and symptoms of pulmonary infections (e.g., sputum color change, shortness of breath, fever)
- Cough enhancement techniques (e.g., cascade cough, huff cough, end-expiratory cough, augmented cough)

EVIDENCE-BASED COLLABORATIVE PRACTICE
Smoking Cessation Guidelines

The following are the key recommendations of the updated guideline, *Treating Tobacco Use and Dependence*, based on the literature review and expert panel opinion:

1. Tobacco dependence is a chronic disease that often requires repeated intervention and multiple attempts to quit. Effective treatments exist, however, that can significantly increase rates of long-term abstinence.
2. It is essential that clinicians and health care delivery systems consistently identify and document tobacco use status and treat every tobacco user seen in a health care setting.
3. Tobacco dependence treatments are effective across a broad range of populations. Clinicians should encourage every patient willing to make a quit attempt to use the counseling treatments and medications recommended in this Guideline.
4. Brief tobacco dependence treatment is effective. Clinicians should offer every patient who uses tobacco at least the brief treatments shown to be effective in this Guideline.
5. Individual, group, and telephone counseling are effective, and their effectiveness increases with treatment intensity. Two components of counseling are especially effective, and clinicians should use these when counseling patients making a quit attempt:
   - Practical counseling (problem solving/skills training)
   - Social support delivered as part of treatment
6. Numerous effective medications are available for tobacco dependence, and clinicians should encourage their use by all patients attempting to quit smoking—except when medically contraindicated or with specific populations for which there is insufficient evidence of effectiveness (i.e., pregnant women, smokeless tobacco users, light smokers, and adolescents).

- Seven first-line medications (5 nicotine and 2 non-nicotine) reliably increase long-term smoking abstinence rates:
  - Bupropion SR
  - Nicotine gum
  - Nicotine inhaler
  - Nicotine lozenge
  - Nicotine nasal spray
  - Nicotine patch
  - Varenicline
- Clinicians also should consider the use of certain combinations of medications identified as effective in this Guideline.

7. Counseling and medication are effective when used by themselves for treating tobacco dependence. The combination of counseling and medication, however, is more effective than either alone. Thus, clinicians should encourage all individuals making a quit attempt to use both counseling and medication.
8. Telephone quitline counseling is effective with diverse populations and has broad reach. Therefore, clinicians and health care delivery systems should both ensure patient access to quitlines and promote quitline use.
9. If a tobacco user currently is unwilling to make a quit attempt, clinicians should use the motivational treatments shown in this Guideline to be effective in increasing future quit attempts.
10. Tobacco dependence treatments are both clinically effective and highly cost-effective relative to interventions for other clinical disorders. Providing coverage for these treatments increases quit rates. Insurers and purchasers should ensure that all insurance plans include the counseling and medication identified as effective in this Guideline as covered benefits.

From Fiore MC, et al: *Treating Tobacco Use and Dependence: 2008 Update* (Clinical Practice Guideline), Rockville, Md., 2008, U.S. Department of Health and Human Services, Public Health Service.

Collaborative management of the patient with acute respiratory failure is outlined in the Collaborative Management box on Acute Respiratory Failure.

COLLABORATIVE MANAGEMENT
Acute Respiratory Failure

- Identify and treat underlying cause.
- Administer oxygen therapy.
- Intubate patient.
- Initiate mechanical ventilation.
- Administer medications:
  - Bronchodilators
  - Steroids
  - Sedatives
  - Analgesics
- Position patient to optimize ventilation/perfusion matching.
- Suction as needed.
- Provide adequate rest and recovery time between various procedures.
- Correct acidosis.
- Initiate nutritional support.
- Maintain surveillance for complications:
  - Encephalopathy
  - Cardiac dysrhythmias
  - Venous thromboembolism
  - Gastrointestinal bleeding
- Provide comfort and emotional support.

ACUTE LUNG INJURY

Acute lung injury (ALI) is a systemic process that is considered to be the pulmonary manifestation of multiple organ dysfunction syndrome.[34] It is characterized by noncardiac pulmonary edema and disruption of the alveolar-capillary membrane as a result of injury to either the pulmonary vasculature or the airways.[35]

Many different diagnostic criteria have been used to identify ALI, which has led to confusion, particularly among researchers. In an attempt to standardize the identification of this disorder, the American-European Consensus Committee on ARDS recommended the following criteria be used to diagnose ALI:

- Acute in onset
- Ratio of partial pressure of oxygen (Pa_{O_2}) to fraction of inspired oxygen (Fi_{O_2}) less than or equal to 300 mm Hg (regardless of positive end-expiratory pressure [PEEP] level)
- Bilateral infiltrates on chest radiography
- Pulmonary artery occlusion pressure (PAOP) less than or equal to 18 mm Hg or no clinical evidence of left atrial hypertension[36,37]

The severest form of ALI is called acute (formerly called "adult") respiratory distress syndrome (ARDS).[36] ARDS is identified by the same diagnostic criteria as ALI except that the ratio of Pa_{O_2} to Fi_{O_2} is less than or equal to 200 mm Hg. As the etiology, pathophysiology, and treatment of ALI is the

BOX 15-1   RISK FACTORS FOR ACUTE LUNG INJURY

Direct Injury
Aspiration
Near-drowning
Toxic inhalation
Pulmonary contusion
Pneumonia
Oxygen toxicity
Transthoracic radiation

Indirect Injury
Sepsis
Nonthoracic trauma
Hypertransfusion
Cardiopulmonary bypass
Severe pancreatitis
Embolism—air, fat, amniotic fluid
Disseminated intravascular coagulation (DIC)
Shock states

same as for ARDS, the discussion will use the broader term of ALI.[37]

Etiology

A wide variety of clinical conditions is associated with the development of ALI. These are categorized as *direct* or *indirect*, depending on the primary site of injury (Box 15-1).[35,38] Direct injuries are those in which the lung epithelium sustains a direct insult. Indirect injuries are those in which the insult occurs elsewhere in the body and mediators are transmitted via the blood stream to the lungs. Sepsis, aspiration of gastric contents, diffuse pneumonia, and trauma were found to be major risk factors for the development of ALI.[37]

The mortality rate for ARDS is estimated to be 34% to 58%.[37]

Pathophysiology

The progression of ALI can be described in three phases: exudative, fibroproliferative, and resolution. ALI is initiated with stimulation of the inflammatory-immune system as a result of a direct or indirect injury (Figure 15-1). Inflammatory mediators are released from the site of injury, resulting in the activation and accumulation of the neutrophils, macrophages, and platelets in the pulmonary capillaries. These cellular mediators initiate the release of humoral mediators that cause damage to the alveolar-capillary membrane.[38]

Exudative Phase

Within the first 72 hours after the initial insult, the exudative phase or acute phase ensues. Once released, the mediators cause injury to the pulmonary capillaries, resulting in increased capillary membrane permeability leading to the leakage of fluid filled with protein, blood cells, fibrin, and activated cellular and humoral mediators into the pulmonary interstitium. Damage to the pulmonary capillaries also causes

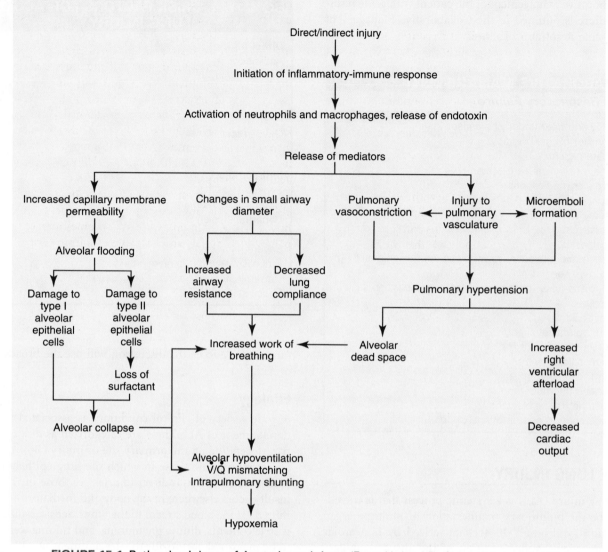

FIGURE 15-1 Pathophysiology of Acute Lung Injury. (From Urden LD, Stacy KM, Lough ME: *Critical care nursing: Diagnosis and management,* ed 6, St. Louis, 2010, Mosby.)

the development of microthrombi and elevation of pulmonary artery pressures. As fluid enters the pulmonary interstitium, the lymphatics are overwhelmed and unable to drain all the accumulating fluid, resulting in the development of interstitial edema. Fluid is then forced from the interstitial space into the alveoli, resulting in alveolar edema. Pulmonary interstitial edema also causes compression of the alveoli and small airways. Alveolar edema causes swelling of the type I alveolar epithelial cells and flooding of the alveoli. Protein and fibrin in the edema fluid precipitate the formation of hyaline membranes over the alveoli. Eventually, the type II alveolar epithelial cells are also damaged, leading to impaired surfactant production. Injury to the alveolar epithelial cells and the loss of surfactant lead to further alveolar collapse.[38,39]

Hypoxemia occurs as a result of intrapulmonary shunting and V/Q mismatching secondary to compression, collapse, and flooding of the alveoli and small airways. Increased work of breathing occurs as a result of increased airway resistance, decreased functional residual capacity (FRC), and decreased

lung compliance secondary to atelectasis and compression of the small airways. Hypoxemia and the increased work of breathing lead to patient fatigue and the development of alveolar hypoventilation. Pulmonary hypertension occurs as a result of damage to the pulmonary capillaries, microthrombi, and hypoxic vasoconstriction leading to the development of increased alveolar dead space and right ventricular afterload. Hypoxemia worsens as a result of alveolar hypoventilation and increased alveolar dead space. Right ventricular afterload increases and leads to right ventricular dysfunction and a decrease in cardiac output.[38]

Fibroproliferative Phase

This phase begins as disordered healing and starts in the lungs. Cellular granulation and collagen deposition occur within the alveolar-capillary membrane. The alveoli become enlarged and irregularly shaped (fibrotic) and the pulmonary capillaries become scarred and obliterated. This leads to further stiffening of the lungs, increasing pulmonary hypertension, and continued hypoxemia.[38,39]

Resolution Phase

Recovery occurs over several weeks as structural and vascular remodeling take place to reestablish the alveolar-capillary membrane. The hyaline membranes are cleared and intraalveolar fluid is transported out of the alveolus into the interstitium. The type II alveolar epithelial cells multiply, some of which differentiate to type I alveolar epithelial cells, facilitating the restoration of the alveolus. Alveolar macrophages remove cellular debris.[38,39]

Assessment and Diagnosis

Initially the patient with ALI may be seen with a variety of clinical manifestations, depending on the precipitating event. As the disorder progresses, the patient's signs and symptoms can be associated with the phase of ALI that he or she is experiencing (Table 15-2). During the exudative phase, the patient presents with tachypnea, restlessness, apprehension, and moderate increase in accessory muscle use. During the fibroproliferative phase, the patient's signs and symptoms progress to agitation, dyspnea, fatigue, excessive accessory muscle use, and fine crackles as respiratory failure develops.[40,41]

Arterial blood-gas analysis reveals a low Pao_2, despite increases in supplemental oxygen administration (refractory hypoxemia).[40] Initially the $Paco_2$ is low as a result of hyperventilation, but eventually the $Paco_2$ increases as the patient fatigues. The pH is high initially but decreases as respiratory acidosis develops.[40,41]

Initially the chest x-ray film may be normal, because changes in the lungs do not become evident for up to 24 hours. As the pulmonary edema becomes apparent, diffuse, patchy interstitial and alveolar infiltrates appear. This

TABLE 15-2	PHYSIOLOGY AND ASSOCIATED PHYSICAL EXAMINATION OF PATIENT WITH ALI	
PHASE	**PHYSIOLOGY**	**PHYSICAL EXAMINATION**
Exudative phase	Parenchymal surface hemorrhage	Restless, apprehensive, tachypneic
	Interstitial or alveolar edema	Respiratory alkalosis
	Compression of terminal bronchioles	Pao_2 normal
	Destruction of type 1 alveolar cells	CXR: normal
		Chest examination: moderate use of accessory muscles, lungs clear
		Pulmonary artery pressures: elevated
		Pulmonary artery occlusion pressure: normal or low
Fibroproliferative phase	Destruction of type 2 alveolar cells	Pulmonary artery pressures: elevated
	Gas exchange compromised	Increased workload on right ventricle
	Increased peak inspiratory pressure	Increased use of accessory muscles
	Decreased compliance (static and dynamic)	Fine crackles
		Increasing agitation related to hypoxia
	Refractory hypoxemia:	CXR: interstitial or alveolar infiltrates; elevated diaphragm
	• Intraalveolar atelectasis	Hyperventilation; hypercarbia
	• Increased shunt fraction	Decreased Svo_2
	• Decreased diffusion	Widening alveolar-arterial gradient
	Decreased functional residual capacity	Increased work of breathing
	Interstitial fibrosis	Worsening hypercarbia and hypoxemia
	Increased dead space ventilation	Lactic acidosis (related to aerobic metabolism)
		Alteration in perfusion:
		• Increased heart rate
		• Decreased blood pressure
		• Change in skin temperature and color
		• Decreased capillary filling
		End-organ dysfunction:
		• Brain: change in mentation, agitation, hallucinations
		• Heart: decreased cardiac output→angina, CHF, papillary muscle dysfunction, dysrhythmias, MI
		• Renal: decreased urinary or GFR
		• Skin: mottled, ischemic
		• Liver: elevated SGOT, bilirubin, alkaline phosphatase, PT/PTT; decreased albumin

Modified from Phillips JK: Management of patients with acute respiratory distress syndrome, *Crit Care Nurs Clin North Am* 11(2):233, 1999. *ALI*, Acute lung injury; *PaO₂*, arterial oxygen pressure; *CXR*, chest radiograph; *SvO₂*, venous oxygen saturation; *HF*, heart failure; *MI*, myocardial infarction; *GFR*, glomerular filtration rate; *SGOT*, serum glutamate oxaloacetate transaminase; *PT*, prothrombin time; *PTT*, partial thromboplastin time.

progresses to multifocal consolidation of the lungs, which appears as a "whiteout" on the chest x-ray film.[40]

Medical Management

Medical management of the patient with ALI involves a multifaceted approach. This strategy includes treating the underlying cause, promoting gas exchange, supporting tissue oxygenation, and preventing complications. Given the severity of hypoxemia, the patient is intubated and mechanically ventilated to facilitate adequate gas exchange.[42]

Ventilation

Traditionally the patient with ALI was ventilated with a mode of volume ventilation, such as assist/control ventilation (A/CV) or synchronized intermittent mandatory ventilation (SIMV), with tidal volumes adjusted to deliver 10 to 15 ml/kg. Current research now indicates that this approach may have actually led to further lung injury. It is now known that repeated opening and closing of the alveoli cause injury to the lung units (atelectrauma), resulting in inhibited surfactant production, and increased inflammation (biotrauma), resulting in the release of mediators and an increase in pulmonary capillary membrane permeability. In addition, excessive pressure in the alveoli (barotrauma) or excessive volume in the alveoli (volutrauma) leads to excessive alveolar wall stress and damage to the alveolar-capillary membrane, resulting in air escaping into the surrounding spaces.[42] Thus several different approaches have been developed to facilitate the mechanical ventilation of the patient with ALI.

Low Tidal Volume. Low tidal volume ventilation uses smaller tidal volumes (6 ml/kg) to ventilate the patient, in an attempt to limit the effects of barotrauma and volutrauma. The goal is to provide the maximum tidal volume possible while maintaining end-inspiratory plateau pressure less than 30 cm H_2O. To allow for adequate carbon dioxide elimination, the respiratory rate is increased to 20 to 30 breaths/min.[42,43]

Permissive Hypercapnia. Permissive hypercapnia uses low tidal volume ventilation in conjunction with normal respiratory rates, in an attempt to limit the effects of atelectrauma and biotrauma. Normally, to maintain normocapnia the patient's respiratory rate would have to be increased to compensate for the small tidal volume. In ALI though, increasing the respiratory rate can lead to worsening alveolar damage. Thus the patient's carbon dioxide level is allowed to rise, and the patient becomes hypercapnic. As a general rule, the patient's Pa_{CO_2} should not rise faster than 10 mm Hg per hour and overall should not exceed 80 to 100 mg Hg. Because of the negative cardiopulmonary effects of severe acidosis, the arterial pH is generally maintained at 7.20 or greater. To maintain the pH, the patient is given intravenous sodium bicarbonate or the respiratory rate and/or tidal volume are increased. Permissive hypercapnia is contraindicated in patients with increased intracranial pressure, pulmonary hypertension, seizures, and cardiac failure.[44]

Pressure Control Ventilation. In pressure control ventilation (PCV) mode, each breath is delivered or augmented with a preset amount of inspiratory pressure as opposed to tidal volume, which is used in volume ventilation. Thus the actual tidal volume the patient receives varies from breath to breath. PCV is used to limit and control the amount of pressure in the lungs and decrease the incidence of volutrauma. The goal is to keep the patient's plateau pressure (end-inspiratory static pressure) lower than 30 cm H_2O. A known problem with this mode of ventilation is that as the patient's lungs get stiffer, it becomes harder and harder to maintain an adequate tidal volume and severe hypercapnia can occur.[42,43]

Inverse Ratio Ventilation. Another alternative ventilatory mode that is used in managing the patient with ALI is inverse ratio ventilation (IRV), either pressure-controlled or volume-controlled. IRV prolongs the inspiratory (I) time and shortens the expiratory (E) time, thus reversing the normal I:E ratio. The goal of IRV is to maintain a more constant mean airway pressure throughout the ventilatory cycle, which helps keep alveoli open and participating in gas exchange. It also increases FRC and decreases the work of breathing. In addition, as the breath is delivered over a longer period of time, the peak inspiratory pressure in the lungs is decreased. A major disadvantage to IRV is the development of auto-positive end-expiratory pressure (PEEP). As the expiratory phase of ventilation is shortened, air can become trapped in the lower airways, creating unintentional PEEP (also known as auto-PEEP), which can cause hemodynamic compromise and worsening gas exchange. Patients on IRV usually require heavy sedation with neuromuscular blockade to prevent them from fighting the ventilator.[42,43]

High-Frequency Oscillatory Ventilation. Another alternative ventilatory mode that is used in patients who remain severely hypoxemic despite the treatments previous described is high-frequency oscillatory ventilation (HFOV). The goal of this method of ventilation is similar to that of IRV in that it uses a constant airway pressure to promote alveolar recruitment while avoiding overdistention of the alveoli. HFOV uses a piston pump to deliver very low tidal volumes at very high rates or oscillations (300 to 3000 breaths/min).[45]

Oxygen Therapy

Oxygen is administered at the lowest level possible to support tissue oxygenation. Continued exposure to high levels of oxygen can lead to oxygen toxicity, which perpetuates the entire process. The goal of oxygen therapy is to maintain an arterial hemoglobin oxygen saturation of 90% or greater using the lowest level of oxygen—preferably less than 0.50.[35]

Positive End-Expiratory Pressure (PEEP). Because the hypoxemia that develops with ALI is often refractory or unresponsive to oxygen therapy, it is necessary to facilitate oxygenation with PEEP. The purpose of using PEEP in the patient with ALI is to improve oxygenation while reducing Fio_2 to less toxic levels. PEEP has several positive effects on the lungs, including opening collapsed alveoli, stabilizing flooded alveoli, and increasing FRC. Thus PEEP decreases intrapulmonary shunting and increases compliance. PEEP also has several negative effects including (1) decreasing cardiac output (CO) as a result of decreasing venous return secondary to increased intrathoracic pressure and (2) barotrauma, as a result of gas escaping into the surrounding spaces secondary to alveolar rupture. The amount of PEEP a patient requires is determined by evaluating both arterial hemoglobin oxygen saturation and cardiac output. In most cases, a PEEP of 10 to 15 cm H_2O is adequate. If PEEP is too high, it can result in overdistention of the alveoli, which can impede pulmonary capillary blood flow, decrease surfactant production, and worsen intrapulmonary shunting. If PEEP is too low, it allows the alveoli to collapse during expiration, which can result in more damage to alveoli.[42]

Tissue Perfusion

Adequate tissue perfusion depends on an adequate supply of oxygen being transported to the tissues. An adequate CO and hemoglobin level is critical to oxygen transport. CO depends on heart rate, preload, afterload, and contractility. A variety of fluids and medications are used to manipulate this parameter. Newer approaches to fluid management include maintaining a very low intravascular volume (pulmonary artery occlusion pressure of 5 to 8 mm Hg) with fluid restriction and diuretics, while supporting the CO with vasoactive and inotropic medications. The goal is to decrease the amount of fluid leakage into the lungs.[46]

Nursing Management

Nursing management of the patient with ALI incorporates a variety of nursing diagnoses (Nursing Diagnosis Priorities box on Acute Lung Injury). **Nursing priorities are directed toward (1) optimizing oxygenation and ventilation, (2) providing comfort and emotional support, and (3) maintaining surveillance for complications.**

NURSING DIAGNOSIS PRIORITIES
Acute Lung Injury

- Impaired Gas Exchange related to ventilation/perfusion mismatching or intrapulmonary shunting, p. A-23
- Decreased Cardiac Output related to alterations in preload, p. A-10
- Imbalanced Nutrition: Less Than Body Requirements related to lack of exogenous nutrients or increased metabolic demand, p. A-22
- Risk for Aspiration, p. A-35
- Risk for Infection, p. A-36
- Anxiety related to threat to biological, psychological, and/or social integrity, p. A-7
- Disturbed Body Image related to functional dependence on life-sustaining technology, p. A-16
- Compromised Family Coping related to critically ill family member, p. A-9

Optimizing Oxygenation and Ventilation

Nursing interventions to optimize oxygenation and ventilation include positioning, preventing desaturation, and promoting secretion clearance. For further discussion on these interventions, see Nursing Management of Acute Respiratory Failure earlier in this chapter. One additional nursing intervention that can be used to improve the oxygenation and ventilation of the patient with ALI is prone positioning.

Prone Positioning. A number of studies have shown that prone positioning the patient with ALI results in an improvement in oxygenation. Although a number of theories propose how prone positioning improves oxygenation, the discovery that with ALI there is greater damage to the dependent areas of the lungs probably provides the best explanation. It was originally thought that ALI was a diffuse homogenous disease that affected all areas of the lungs equally. It is now known that the dependent lung areas are more heavily damaged than the nondependent lung areas. Turning the patient prone improves perfusion to less damaged parts of lungs and improves V/Q matching and decreases intrapulmonary shunting. Prone positioning appears to be more effective when initiated during the early phases of ALI.[47] For more information on prone positioning see Chapter 16.

Collaborative management of the patient with ALI is outlined in the Collaborative Management box on Acute Lung Injury.

COLLABORATIVE MANAGEMENT
Acute Lung Injury

- Administer oxygen therapy.
- Intubate patient.
- Initiate mechanical ventilation:
  - Permissive hypercapnia
  - Pressure control ventilation
  - Inverse ratio ventilation
- Use PEEP.
- Administer medications:
  - Bronchodilators
  - Sedatives
  - Analgesics
  - Neuromuscular blocking agents
- Maximize cardiac output:
  - Preload
  - Afterload
  - Contractility
- Prone patient.
- Suction as needed.
- Provide adequate rest and recovery time between various procedures.
- Initiate nutritional support.
- Maintain surveillance for complications:
  - Encephalopathy
  - Cardiac dysrhythmias
  - Venous thromboembolism
  - Gastrointestinal bleeding
  - Atelectrauma
  - Biotrauma
  - Volutrauma
  - Barotrauma
  - Oxygen toxicity
- Provide comfort and emotional support.

PNEUMONIA

Pneumonia is an acute inflammation of the lung parenchyma that is caused by an infectious agent that can lead to alveolar consolidation. Pneumonia can be classified as community-acquired (CAP) or hospital-acquired (HAP). Community-acquired pneumonia is acquired outside of the hospital.[48] Severe CAP requires admission to the intensive care unit and accounts for about 10% of all patients with pneumonia. The mortality for this patient group is in excess of 50%.[49] Hospital-acquired pneumonia is acquired while in the hospital for at least 48 hours.[54] Ventilator-associated pneumonia (VAP) is a subgrouping of HAP that refers to development of pneumonia after the insertion of an artificial airway. VAP represents 80% of all HAP cases.[50]

Etiology

The spectra of etiological pathogens of pneumonia vary with the type of pneumonia, as do the risk factors for the disease.

Severe Community-Acquired Pneumonia

Pathogens that can cause severe community-acquired pneumonia (CAP) include *Streptococcus pneumoniae*, *Legionella* species, *Haemophilus influenzae*, *Staphylococcus aureus*, *Mycoplasma pneumoniae*, respiratory viruses, *Chlamydia pneumoniae*, and *Pseudomonas aeruginosa*.[51] A number of factors increase the risk for developing CAP, including alcoholism; chronic obstructive pulmonary disease (COPD); and comorbid conditions such as diabetes, malignancy, and coronary artery disease.[48] Impaired swallowing and altered mental status also contribute to the development of CAP, because they result in an increased exposure to the various pathogens due to chronic aspiration of oropharyngeal secretions.[48]

Hospital-Acquired Pneumonia

Pathogens that can cause hospital-acquired pneumonia (HAP) include *S. aureus*, *S. pneumoniae*, *P. aeruginosa*, *Acinetobacter baumannii*, *Klebsiella spp.*, *Proteus spp.*, *Serratia spp.*, fungi, and respiratory viruses.[50] Two of the pathogens most frequently associated with VAP are *S. aureus* and *P. aeruginosa*.[30] Risk factors for HAP can be categorized as host-related, treatment-related, and infection-control-related (Box 15-2).[30]

Pathophysiology

Development of acute pneumonia implies a defect in host defenses, a particularly virulent organism, or an overwhelming inoculation event. Bacterial invasion of the lower respiratory tract can occur by inhalation of aerosolized infectious particles, aspiration of organisms colonizing the oropharynx, migration of organisms from adjacent sites of colonization, direct inoculation of organisms into the lower airway, spread of infection to the lungs from adjacent structures, spread of infection to the lung through the blood, and reactivation of latent infection (usually in the

---

BOX 15-2   RISK FACTORS FOR HOSPITAL-ACQUIRED PNEUMONIA

Host-Related
Advanced age
Altered level of consciousness
Chronic obstructive pulmonary disease
Severity of illness
Malnutrition
Shock
Trauma
Smoking
Dental plaque

Treatment-Related
Mechanical ventilation
Unintentional extubation
Reintubation
Bronchoscopy
Nasogastric tube
Previous antibiotic therapy
Elevated gastric pH secondary to histamine$_2$-blockers, antacid therapy, and enteral feedings
Upper abdominal surgery
Thoracic surgery
Supine position

Infection-Control-Related
Poor hand-washing practices

---

setting of immunosuppression). The most common mechanism appears to be aspiration of oropharyngeal organisms.[52] Table 15-3 lists the precipitating conditions that can facilitate the development of pneumonia.

Figure 15-2 depicts the pathophysiology of HAP. Colonization of the patient's oropharynx with infectious organisms is a major contributor to the development of HAP. Normally the oropharynx has a stable population of resident flora that may be anaerobic or aerobic. When stress occurs, such as with illness, surgery, or infection, pathogenic organisms replace normal resident flora. Previous antibiotic therapy also affects the resident flora population, making replacement by pathological organisms more likely. The pathogens are then able to invade the sterile lower respiratory tract.[30]

Disruption of the gag and cough reflexes, altered consciousness, abnormal swallowing, and artificial airways all predispose the patient to aspiration and colonization of the lungs and subsequent infection. Histamine$_2$ agonists, antacids, and enteral feedings also contribute to this problem because they raise the pH of the stomach and promote bacterial overgrowth. The nasogastric tube then acts as a wick, facilitating the movement of bacteria from the stomach to the pharynx, where the bacteria can be aspirated.[48]

Infection results in pulmonary inflammation with or without significant exudates. Increased capillary permeability occurs, leading to increased interstitial and alveolar fluid. V/Q mismatching and intrapulmonary shunting occurs,

TABLE 15-3 PRECIPITATING CONDITIONS OF PNEUMONIA

CONDITION	ETIOLOGIES
Depressed epiglottal and cough reflexes	Unconsciousness, neurological disease, endotracheal or tracheal tubes, anesthesia, aging
Decreased cilia activity	Smoke inhalation, smoking history, oxygen toxicity, hypoventilation, intubation, viral infections, aging, COPD
Increased secretion	COPD, viral infections, bronchiectasis, general anesthesia, endotracheal intubation, smoking
Atelectasis	Trauma, foreign body obstruction, tumor, splinting, shallow ventilations, general anesthesia
Decreased lymphatic flow	Heart failure, tumor
Fluid in alveoli	Heart failure, aspiration, trauma
Abnormal phagocytosis and humoral activity	Neutropenia, immunocompetent disorders, patients receiving chemotherapy
Impaired alveolar macrophages	Hypoxemia, metabolic acidosis, cigarette smoking history, hypoxia, alcohol use, viral infections, aging

COPD, Chronic obstructive pulmonary disease.

resulting in hypoxemia as lung consolidation progresses. Untreated pneumonia can result in ARF and initiation of the inflammatory-immune response. In addition, the patient may develop a pleural effusion. This is the result of the vascular response to inflammation, whereby capillary permeability is increased and fluid from the pulmonary capillaries diffuses into the pleural space.[48,53]

Prevention of VAP is discussed under the mechanical ventilation section of Chapter 16.

Assessment and Diagnosis

The clinical manifestations of pneumonia will vary with the offending pathogen. The patient may first be seen with a variety of signs and symptoms including dyspnea, fever, and cough (productive or nonproductive). Coarse crackles on auscultation and dullness to percussion may also be present.[53] Patients with severe CAP may manifest confusion and disorientation, tachypnea, hypoxemia, uremia, leukopenia, thrombocytopenia, hypothermia, and hypotension.[52]

Chest radiography is used to evaluate the patient with suspected pneumonia. The diagnosis is established by the presence of a new pulmonary infiltrate. The radiographic pattern of the infiltrates will vary with the organism.[54] A sputum Gram stain and culture are done to facilitate the identification of the infectious pathogen. In 50% of cases, though, a causative agent is not identified.[48] A diagnostic bronchoscopy may be needed, particularly if the diagnosis is unclear or current therapy is not working.[49] In addition, a complete blood count with differential, chemistry panel, blood cultures, and arterial blood gases is obtained.[51]

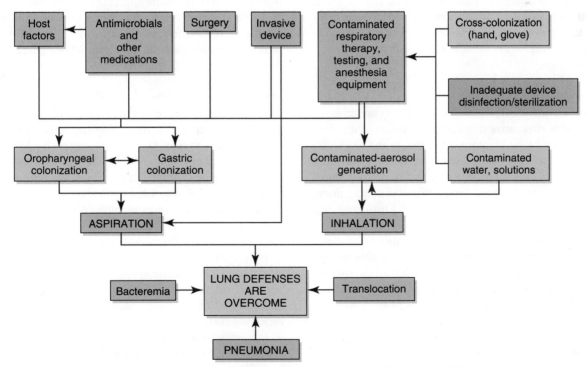

FIGURE 15-2 Pathophysiology of Pneumonia. (From Tablan OC, et al: Guideline for prevention of nosocomial pneumonia. The Hospital Infection Control Practices Advisory Committee, Centers for Disease Control and Prevention, *Am J Infect Control* 22(4):247, 1994.)

Medical Management

Medical management of the patient with pneumonia should include antibiotic therapy, oxygen therapy for hypoxemia, mechanical ventilation if acute respiratory failure develops, fluid management for hydration, nutritional support, and treatment of associated medical problems and complications. For patients having difficulty mobilizing secretions, a therapeutic bronchoscopy may be necessary.[53,54]

Antibiotic Therapy

Although bacteria-specific antibiotic therapy is the goal, this may not always be possible because of difficulties in identifying the organism and the seriousness of the patient's condition. The time involved obtaining cultures should be balanced against the need to begin some treatment based on the patient's condition. Empiric therapy has become a generally acceptable approach. In this approach, choice of antibiotic treatment is based on the most likely etiological organism while avoiding toxicity, superinfection, and unnecessary cost. If available, Gram stain results should be used to guide choices of antibiotics. Antibiotics should be chosen that offer broad coverage of the usual pathogens in the hospital or community. Failure to respond to such therapy may indicate that the chosen antibiotic regimen does not appropriately cover all of the etiological pathogens or that a new source of infection has developed.[50,51]

Currently the Centers for Medicare and Medicaid Services (CMS) and The Joint Commission (TJC) standards for managing patients with CAP require that the first dose of antibiotics be administered within 6 hours of arrival to the hospital. This timeframe is very controversial and has been the subject of much debate. Those in favor of the standard believe that early antibiotic administration leads to improved outcomes while those not in favor of the standard believe it leads to the overuse of antibiotics. More research is needed to clarify the issue.[55]

Independent Lung Ventilation

In patients with unilateral pneumonia or severely asymmetric pneumonia, this alternative mode of mechanical ventilation may be necessary to facilitate oxygenation. As the alveoli in the affected lung become flooded with pus, the lung becomes less compliant and difficult to ventilate. This results in a shifting of ventilation to the good lung without a concomitant shift in perfusion and thus an increase in V/Q mismatching. Independent lung ventilation (ILV) allows each lung to be ventilated separately, thus controlling the amount of flow, volume, and pressure each lung receives. A double-lumen endotracheal tube is inserted, and each lumen is usually attached to a separate mechanical ventilator. The ventilator settings are then customized to the needs of each lung to facilitate optimal oxygenation and ventilation.[56]

Nursing Management

Nursing management of the patient with pneumonia incorporates a variety of nursing diagnoses (Nursing Diagnosis Priorities box on Pneumonia). **Nursing priorities are directed toward (1) optimizing oxygenation and ventilation, (2) preventing the spread of infection, (3) providing comfort and emotional support, and (4) maintaining surveillance for complications.** In addition, the patient's response to the antibiotic therapy should be monitored for adverse effects.

NURSING DIAGNOSIS PRIORITIES
Pneumonia

- Ineffective Airway Clearance related to excessive secretions or abnormal viscosity of mucus, p. A-26
- Impaired Gas Exchange related to ventilation/perfusion mismatching or intrapulmonary shunting, p. A-23
- Imbalanced Nutrition: Less Than Body Requirements related to lack of exogenous nutrients or increased metabolic demand, p. A-22
- Risk for Aspiration, p. A-35
- Risk for Infection, p. A-36
- Anxiety related to threat to biological, psychological, and/or social integrity, p. A-7
- Powerlessness related to lack of control over current situation or disease progression, p. A-33
- Compromised Family Coping related to critically ill family member, p. A-9

Optimizing Oxygenation and Ventilation

Nursing interventions to optimize oxygenation and ventilation include positioning, preventing desaturation, and promoting secretion clearance. For further discussion on these interventions, see Nursing Management of Acute Respiratory Failure earlier in this chapter.

Preventing the Spread of Infection

Prevention should be directed at eradicating pathogens from the environment and interrupting the spread of organisms from person to person. Significant progress has been made in removing contaminants from the patient environment through proper disinfection of respiratory equipment and increased use of disposable supplies. Other possible environmental sources of pathogens include suctioning equipment and indwelling lines. These invasive tools must be given proper aseptic care.[30]

Proper hand hygiene is the single most important measure available to prevent the spread of bacteria from person to person (Evidence-Based Collaborative Practice box on Hand Hygiene Guidelines). In addition, meticulous oral care, including suctioning of the secretions pooling above the cuff of the artificial airway, is critical to decreasing the bacterial colonization of the oropharynx.[30]

Collaborative management of the patient with pneumonia is outlined in the Collaborative Management box on Pneumonia.

EVIDENCE-BASED COLLABORATIVE PRACTICE

Hand Hygiene Guidelines

- Wash hands with soap and water when visibly dirty or contaminated with blood and other body fluids.
- When washing hands with soap and water, wet hands first with water, apply an amount of product recommended by the manufacturer to hands, and rub hands together vigorously for at least 15 seconds, covering all surfaces of the hands and fingers. Rinse hands with water and dry thoroughly with a disposable towel. Use towel to turn off the faucet. Avoid using hot water, because repeated exposure to hot water may increase the risk of dermatitis.
- If hands are not visibly soiled, use an alcohol-based hand rub for routinely decontaminating hands.
- When decontaminating hands with an alcohol-based hand rub, apply product to palm of one hand and rub hands together, covering all surfaces of hands and fingers, until hands are dry (follow the manufacturer's recommendations regarding the volume of product to use).
- Decontaminate hands before and after having direct contact with patients.
- Decontaminate hands before and after donning gloves.
- Wear gloves when contact with blood or other potentially infectious materials, mucous membranes, or nonintact skin could occur.
- Change gloves during patient care if moving from a contaminated body site to a clean body site.
- Remove gloves after caring for a patient. Do not wear the same pair of gloves for the care of more than one patient, and do not wash gloves between uses with different patients.
- Decontaminate hands after contact with inanimate objects (including medical equipment).
- Do not wear artificial fingernails or extenders when having direct contact with patients at high risk (e.g., those in critical care units or operating rooms).
- Keep natural nails tips less than 1/4-inch long.

From Boyce, JM, et al, Advisory Committee and the HICPAC/SHEA/APIC/IDSA Hand Hygiene Task Force: Recommendations of the Healthcare Infection Control Practices Advisory Committee, *MMWR Recomm Rep* 51(RR16):1, 2002.

COLLABORATIVE MANAGEMENT

Pneumonia

- Administer oxygen therapy.
- Initiate mechanical ventilation as required.
- Administer medications:
  - Antibiotics
  - Bronchodilators
- Position patient to optimize ventilation/perfusion matching.
- Suction as needed.
- Provide adequate rest and recovery time between various procedures.
- Maintain surveillance for complications:
  - Acute respiratory failure
- Provide comfort and emotional support.

ASPIRATION PNEUMONITIS

The presence of abnormal substances in the airways and alveoli as a result of aspiration is misleadingly called *aspiration pneumonia*. This term is misleading because the aspiration of toxic substances into the lung may or may not involve an infection. *Aspiration pneumonitis* is a more accurate title, because injury to the lung can result from the chemical, mechanical, and/or bacterial characteristics of the aspirate.

Etiology

A number of factors have been identified that place the patient at risk for aspiration (Table 15-4). Gastric contents and oropharyngeal bacteria (see Pneumonia earlier in this chapter) are the most common aspirates of the critically ill patient.[57,58] The effects of gastric contents on the lungs will vary based on the pH of the liquid. If the pH is less than 2.5, the patient will develop a severe chemical pneumonitis resulting in hypoxemia. If the pH is greater than 2.5, the immediate damage to the lungs will be lessened but the elevated pH may have promoted bacterial overgrowth of the stomach.[57,58] Once the bacteria-laden gastric contents are aspirated into the lungs, overwhelming bacterial pneumonia can develop.[58]

Pathophysiology

The type of lung injury that develops after aspiration is determined by a number of factors, including the quality of the aspirate and the status of the patient's respiratory defense mechanisms.

Acid Liquid

The aspiration of acid (pH <2.5) liquid gastric contents results in the development of bronchospasm and atelectasis almost immediately. Over the next 4 hours, tracheal damage, bronchitis, bronchiolitis, alveolar-capillary breakdown, interstitial edema, and alveolar congestion and hemorrhage occur.[59] Severe hypoxemia develops as a result of intrapulmonary shunting and V/Q mismatching. As the disorder progresses, necrotic debris and fibrin fill the alveoli, hyaline membranes form, and hypoxic vasoconstriction occurs, resulting in elevated pulmonary artery pressures.[58,59] The clinical course will follow one of three patterns: (1) rapid improvement in 1 week, (2) initial improvement followed by deterioration and development of ARDS or pneumonia, or (3) rapid death from progressive ARF.[59]

Acid Food Particles

The aspiration of acid (pH <2.5) nonobstructing food particles can produce the most severe pulmonary reaction because of extensive pulmonary damage.[63] Severe hypoxemia, hypercapnia, and acidosis occur.[58,59]

Nonacid Liquid

The aspiration of nonacid (pH >2.5) liquid gastric contents is similar to acid liquid aspiration initially, but minimal structural damage occurs.[63] Intrapulmonary shunting and V/Q

TABLE 15-4   RISK FACTORS FOR ASPIRATION/ASPIRATION-RELATED PNEUMONIA

RISK FACTOR	RATIONALE
Decreased LOC, either because of CNS problems or use of sedatives	Decreased ability to protect airway from oropharyngeal secretions and regurgitated gastric contents Cough and gag reflexes diminish as LOC diminishes, whether from CNS disorder or sedation Slowed gastric emptying Decreased tone of lower esophageal sphincter
Supine position	Increases probability of gastroesophageal reflux
Presence of a nasogastric tube	Interferes with closure of lower esophageal sphincter Biofilm on tube predisposes to aspiration of pathogenic organisms
Vomiting	Sudden and forceful entry of gastric contents into oropharynx predisposes to aspiration Predisposes to displacement of feeding tube ports into esophagus
Feeding tube ports positioned in esophagus	Infused feedings reflux into oropharynx
Tracheal intubation	Reduction in upper airway defense related to ineffective cough, desensitization of the oropharynx and larynx, disuse atrophy of laryngeal muscles, and esophageal compression by an inflated cuff
Mechanical ventilation	Positive abdominal pressure predisposes to aspiration of gastric contents, probably by increasing gastroesophageal reflux
Accumulation of subglottic secretions above endotracheal cuff	Subglottic secretions can leak around cuff into the lower respiratory tract, especially when cuff is deflated
Inadequate cuff inflation of tracheal devices	Persistent low cuff pressure (e.g., 20 cm H_2O) predisposes to aspiration of oropharyngeal secretions and refluxed gastric contents
Gastric feeding site when gastric emptying significantly impaired	Accumulation of formula and gastrointestinal secretions predisposes to gastroesophageal reflux and aspiration
High GRVs	High GRVs predispose to gastroesophageal reflux and aspiration
Bolus feedings	Volume of infused formula may exceed the tolerance of patients who have poor cough and gag reflexes
Poor oral health	Colonized oropharyngeal secretions may be aspirated into respiratory tract
Advanced age	Older patients tend to have a reduced swallowing ability and are more likely to have neurological disorders that increase aspiration risks Strong association between advanced age and probability of developing pneumonia once aspiration has occurred
Hyperglycemia	Even mild hyperglycemia can cause delayed gastric emptying by disrupting postprandial antral contractions

From Metheny NA: Strategies to prevent aspiration-related pneumonia in tube-fed patients, *Respir Care Clin N Am* 12(4):603, 2006.
CNS, central nervous system; *GRVs*, gastric residual volumes; *LOC*, level of consciousness.

mismatching usually start to reverse within 4 hours, and hypoxemia clears within 24 hours.[58,59]

Nonacid Food Particles

The aspiration of nonacid (pH >2.5) nonobstructing food particles is similar to acid aspiration initially, with significant edema and hemorrhage occurring within 6 hours. After the initial reaction, the response changes to a foreign-body-type reaction with granuloma formation occurring around the food particles within 1 to 5 days.[59] In addition to hypoxemia, hypercapnia and acidosis occur as a result of hypoventilation.[57,58]

Assessment and Diagnosis

Clinically, the patient presents with signs of acute respiratory distress, and gastric contents may be present in the oropharynx. The patient will have shortness of breath, coughing, wheezing, cyanosis, and signs of hypoxemia. Tachypnea, tachycardia, hypotension, fever, and crackles also are present. Copious amounts of sputum are produced as alveolar edema develops.[57,58]

ABGs reflect severe hypoxemia. Chest x-ray film changes appear 12 to 24 hours after the initial aspiration, with no one pattern being diagnostic of the event. Infiltrates will appear in a variety of distribution patterns depending on the position of the patient during aspiration and the volume of the aspirate. If bacterial infection becomes established, leukocytosis and positive sputum cultures occur.[58]

Medical Management

Management of the patient with aspiration lung disorder includes both emergency and follow-up treatment. When aspiration is witnessed, emergency treatment should be instituted to secure the airway and minimize pulmonary damage. The upper airway should be suctioned immediately to remove the gastric contents.[57,58] Direct visualization by bronchoscopy is indicated to remove large particulate aspirate[61] or to confirm an unwitnessed aspiration event.[59] Bronchoalveolar lavage is not recommended because this practice disseminates the aspirate in lungs and increases damage. Prophylactic antibiotics are not recommended either.[59]

After airway clearance, attention should be given to supporting oxygenation and hemodynamics. Hypoxemia should be corrected with supplemental oxygen or mechanical ventilation with PEEP, if necessary.[57-59] Hemodynamic changes result from fluid shifts into the lungs that can occur after massive aspirations. Monitoring intravascular volume is essential, and judicious amounts of replacement fluids should be instituted to maintain adequate urinary output and vital signs.[59]

Initially antibiotic therapy is not indicated. If symptoms fail to resolve within 48 hours, empiric antibiotic therapy should be initiated. Corticosteroids have not demonstrated to be of any benefit in the treatment of aspiration pneumonitis and thus are not recommended either.[58]

Nursing Management

Nursing management of the patient with aspiration lung disorder incorporates a variety of nursing diagnoses (Nursing Diagnosis Priorities box on Aspiration). **Nursing priorities are directed toward (1) optimizing oxygenation and ventilation, (2) preventing further aspiration events, (3) providing comfort and emotional support, and (4) maintaining surveillance for complications.**

NURSING DIAGNOSIS PRIORITIES

Aspiration Pneumonitis

- Impaired Gas Exchange related to ventilation/perfusion mismatching or intrapulmonary shunting, p. A-23
- Ineffective Airway Clearance related to excessive secretions or abnormal viscosity of mucus, p. A-26
- Risk for Aspiration, p. A-35
- Risk for Infection, p. A-36
- Anxiety related to threat to biological, psychological, and/or social integrity, p. A-7
- Ineffective Coping related to situational crisis and personal vulnerability, p. A-30
- Compromised Family Coping related to critically ill family member, p. A-9

Optimizing Oxygenation and Ventilation

Nursing interventions to optimize oxygenation and ventilation include positioning, preventing desaturation, and promoting secretion clearance. For further discussion on these interventions, see Nursing Management of Acute Respiratory Failure earlier in this chapter.

Preventing Aspiration

One of the most important interventions for preventing aspiration is identifying the patient at risk for aspiration. Actions to prevent aspiration include confirming feeding tube placement, checking for signs and symptoms of feeding intolerance, elevating the head of the bed at least 30 degrees, feeding the patient via a small-bore feeding tube or gastrostomy tube, avoiding the use of a large-bore nasogastric tube, ensuring proper inflation of artificial airway cuffs, and frequent suctioning of the oropharynx of an intubated patient to prevent secretions from pooling above the cuff of the tube. For patients at risk for aspiration or intolerant of gastric feedings, the feeding tube should be placed in the small bowel.[60]

Collaborative management of the patient with aspiration pneumonitis is outlined in the Collaborative Management box on Aspiration Pneumonitis.

COLLABORATIVE MANAGEMENT

Aspiration Pneumonitis

- Administer oxygen therapy.
- Secure the patient's airway.
- Place patient in slight Trendelenburg position.
- Turn patient to right lateral decubitus position.
- Suction patient's oropharyngeal area.
- Initiate mechanical ventilation as required.
- Maintain surveillance for complications:
  - Pneumonia
  - Acute respiratory failure
  - Acute lung injury
- Provide comfort and emotional support.

PULMONARY EMBOLISM

Description

A pulmonary embolism (PE) occurs when a clot (thrombotic embolus) or other matter (nonthrombotic embolus) lodges in the pulmonary arterial system, disrupting the blood flow to a region of the lungs (Figure 15-3). The majority of thrombotic emboli arise from the deep leg veins, particularly the iliac, femoral, and popliteal veins.[61] Other sources include the right ventricle, the upper extremities, and the pelvic veins. Nonthrombotic emboli arise from fat, tumors, amniotic fluid, air, and foreign bodies. This section of the chapter focuses on thrombotic emboli.

Etiology

A number of predisposing factors and precipitating conditions put a patient at risk for developing a PE (Box 15-3). Of the three predisposing factors (i.e., hypercoagulability, injury to vascular endothelium, and venous stasis [Virchow's triad]), endothelial injury appears to be the most significant.[61]

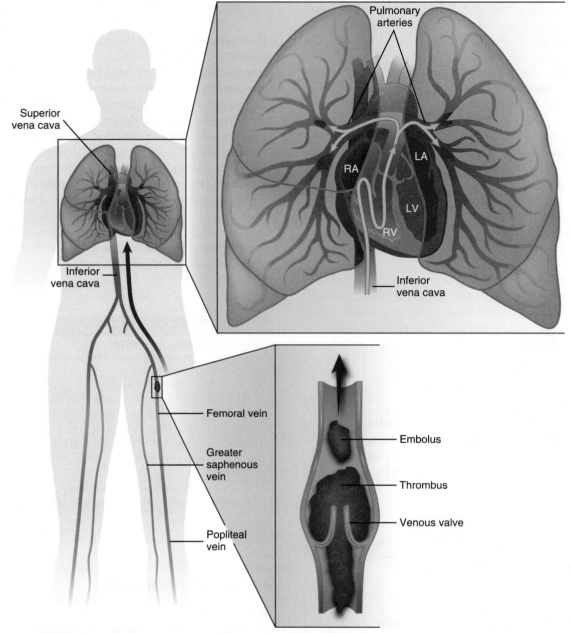

FIGURE 15-3 Pathophysiology of Pulmonary Embolism. Pulmonary embolism usually originates from the deep veins of the legs, most commonly the calf veins. These venous thrombi originate predominantly in venous valve pockets and at other sites of presumed venous stasis (inset, bottom). If a clot propagates to the knee vein or above, or if it originates above the knee, the risk of embolism increases. Thromboemboli travel through the right side of the heart to reach the lungs. *LA*, left atrium; *LV*, left ventricle; *RA*, right atrium; *RV*, right ventricle. (Modified from Tapson VF: Acute pulmonary embolism, *N Engl J Med* 358[10]:1037, 2008.)

Pathophysiology

A massive PE occurs with the blockage of a lobar or larger artery, resulting in occlusion of more than 40% of the pulmonary vascular bed. Blockage of the pulmonary arterial system has both pulmonary and hemodynamic consequences.[62] The effects on the pulmonary system are increased alveolar dead space, bronchoconstriction, and compensatory shunting.[67] The hemodynamic effects include an increase in pulmonary vascular resistance and right ventricular workload.[62,63]

Increased Dead Space

An increase in alveolar dead space occurs because an area of the lung is receiving ventilation without being perfused. The ventilation to this area is known as *wasted ventilation,* because it does not participate in gas exchange. This effect leads to alveolar dead space ventilation and an increase in the work of breathing. To limit the amount of dead space ventilation, localized bronchoconstriction occurs.[63]

BOX 15-3 RISK FACTORS FOR PULMONARY THROMBOEMBOLISM

Predisposing Factors
Venous stasis
   Atrial fibrillation
   Decreased cardiac output (CO)
   Immobility
Injury to vascular endothelium
   Local vessel injury
   Infection
   Incision
   Atherosclerosis
Hypercoagulability
   Polycythemia

Precipitating Conditions
Previous pulmonary embolus
Cardiovascular disease
   Heart failure
   Right ventricular infarction
   Cardiomyopathy
   Cor pulmonale
Surgery
   Orthopedic
   Vascular
   Abdominal
Cancer
   Ovarian
   Pancreatic
   Stomach
   Extrahepatic bile duct system
Trauma (injury or burns)
   Lower extremities
   Pelvis
   Hips
Gynecological status
   Pregnancy
   Postpartum
   Birth control pills
   Estrogen replacement therapy

Bronchoconstriction

Bronchoconstriction develops as a result of alveolar hypocarbia, hypoxia, and the release of mediators. Alveolar hypocarbia occurs as a consequence of decreased carbon dioxide in the affected area and leads to constriction of the local airways, increased airway resistance, and redistribution of ventilation to perfused areas of the lungs. A variety of mediators are released from the site of the injury, either from the clot or the surrounding lung tissue, which further causes constriction of the airways. Bronchoconstriction promotes the development of atelectasis.[63]

Compensatory Shunting

Compensatory shunting occurs as a result of the unaffected areas of the lungs having to accommodate the entire cardiac output. This creates a situation in which perfusion exceeds ventilation and blood is returned to the left side of the heart without participating in gas exchange. This leads to the development of hypoxemia.[63]

Hemodynamic Consequences

The major hemodynamic consequence of a PE is the development of pulmonary hypertension, which is part of the effect of a mechanical obstruction when more than 50% of the vascular bed is occluded. In addition, the mediators released at the injury site and the development of hypoxia cause pulmonary vasoconstriction, which further exacerbates pulmonary hypertension. As the pulmonary vascular resistance increases, so does the workload of the right ventricle as reflected by a rise in PA pressures. Consequently, right ventricular failure occurs, which can lead to decreases in left ventricular preload, CO, and blood pressure, and shock.[61-63]

Assessment and Diagnosis

The patient with a pulmonary embolism may have any number of presenting signs and symptoms, with the most common being tachycardia and tachypnea. Additional signs and symptoms that may be present include dyspnea, apprehension, increased pulmonic component of the second heart sound (P_1), fever, crackles, pleuritic chest pain, cough, evidence of a deep vein thrombosis, and hemoptysis.[61] Syncope and hemodynamic instability can occur as a result of right ventricular failure.[64]

Initial laboratory studies and diagnostic procedures that may be done are ABG analysis, D-dimer, electrocardiogram (ECG), chest radiography, and echocardiography (ECHO). ABGs may show a low Pao_2, indicating hypoxemia; a low $Paco_2$, indicating hypocarbia; and a high pH, indicating a respiratory alkalosis. The hypocarbia with resulting respiratory alkalosis is caused by tachypnea.[63] An elevated D-dimer will occur with a PE and a number of other disorders. A normal D-dimer will not occur with a PE and thus can be used to rule out a PE as the diagnosis.[62] The most frequent ECG finding seen in the patient with a PE is sinus tachycardia.[61] The classic ECG pattern associated with a PE—S wave in lead I, and Q wave with inverted T wave in lead III—is seen in fewer than 20% of patients.[64] Other ECG findings associated with a PE include right bundle branch block, new-onset atrial fibrillation, T-wave inversion in the anterior or inferior leads[65], and ST-segment changes.[65] Chest x-ray findings vary from normal to abnormal and are of little value in confirming the presence of a PE. Abnormal findings include cardiomegaly, pleural effusion, elevated hemidiaphragm, enlargement of the right descending pulmonary artery (Palla's sign), a wedge-shaped density above the diaphragm (Hampton's hump), and the presence of atelectasis.[63] An ECHO, either transthoracic or transesophageal, is also useful in the identification of a PE, because it can provide visualization of any emboli in the central pulmonary arteries. In addition, it can be used for assessing the hemodynamic consequences of the PE on the right side of the heart.[62]

Differentiating a PE from other illnesses can be difficult because many of its clinical manifestations are found in a variety of other disorders.[61] Thus a variety of other tests may be necessary, including a V/Q scintigraphy, pulmonary angiogram, and deep vein thrombosis (DVT) studies.[61-63] Given the advent of more sophisticated computed tomography (CT) scanners, the spiral CT is also being used to diagnose a PE.[63,64] A definitive diagnosis of a PE requires confirmation by a high-probability V/Q scan, an abnormal pulmonary angiogram or CT, or strong clinical suspicion coupled with abnormal findings on lower extremity DVT studies.[63]

Medical Management

Medical management of the patient with a pulmonary embolism involves both prevention and treatment strategies. Prevention strategies include the use of prophylactic anticoagulation with low-dose or adjusted-dose heparin, low-molecular-weight heparin, or oral anticoagulants (Table 15-5). The use of graduated compression stockings and pneumatic compression have also been demonstrated as effective methods of prophylaxis in low-risk patients.[65]

Treatment strategies include preventing the recurrence of a PE, facilitating clot dissolution, reversing the effects of pulmonary hypertension, promoting gas exchange, and preventing complications. Medical interventions to promote gas exchange include supplemental oxygen administration, intubation, and mechanical ventilation.[62]

Prevention of Recurrence

Interventions to prevent the recurrence of a PE include the administration of unfractionated or low-molecular-weight heparin and warfarin (Coumadin).[64] Heparin is administered to prevent further clots from forming and has no effect on the existing clot. The heparin should be adjusted to maintain the activated partial thromboplastin time (aPTT) in the range of 2 to 3 times of upper normal.[64] Warfarin should be started at the same time, and when the international normalized ratio (INR) reaches 3.0, the heparin should be discontinued. The INR should be maintained between 2.0 and 3.0. The patient should remain on warfarin for 3 to 12 months depending on his or her risk for thromboembolic disease.[64]

Interruption of the inferior vena cava is reserved for patients in whom anticoagulation is contraindicated. The procedure involves placement of a percutaneous venous filter (e.g., Greenfield filter) into the vena cava, usually below the renal arteries. The filter prevents further thrombotic emboli from migrating into the lungs.[64]

Clot Dissolution

The administration of fibrinolytic agents in the treatment of PE has had limited success. Currently, fibrinolytic therapy is reserved for the patient with a massive PE and concomitant hemodynamic instability. Either recombinant tissue-type plasminogen activator (rt-PA) or streptokinase may be used. The therapeutic window for using thrombolytic therapy is up to 14 days though the most benefit is usually obtained when given within 48 hours.[66]

Although often considered as a last resort, a surgical embolectomy may be performed to remove the clot.

TABLE 15-5	REGIMENS FOR VENOUS THROMBOEMBOLISM PROPHYLAXIS
CONDITION	**PROPHYLAXIS**
General surgery	Unfractionated heparin 5000 units SC TID or Enoxaparin 40 mg SC QD or Dalteparin 2500 or 5000 units SC QD
Orthopedic surgery	Warfarin (target INR 2.0 to 3.0) or Enoxaparin 30 mg SC BID or Enoxaparin 40 mg SC QD or Dalteparin 2500 or 5000 units SC QD or Fondaparinux 2.5 mg SC QD
Neurosurgery	Unfractionated heparin 5000 units SC BID or Enoxaparin 40 mg SC QD and Graduated compression stockings/ intermittent pneumatic compression Consider surveillance lower extremity ultrasonography
Oncological surgery	Enoxaparin 40 mg SC QD
Thoracic surgery	Unfractionated heparin 5000 units SC TID and Graduated compression stockings/ intermittent pneumatic compression
Medical patients	Unfractionated heparin 5000 units SC TID or Enoxaparin 40 mg SC QD or Dalteparin 5000 units SC QD or Fondaparinux 2.5 mg SC QD or Graduated compression stockings/ intermittent pneumatic compression for patients with contraindications to anticoagulation Consider combination pharmacological and mechanical prophylaxis for very high-risk patients Consider surveillance lower extremity ultrasonography for intensive care unit patients

SC, subcutaneous; *TID*, 3 times daily; *QD*, daily; *BID*, twice daily.
From Piazza G, Goldhaber SZ: Acute pulmonary embolism: part II: treatment and prophylaxis, *Circulation* 114(3):e42, 2006.

Generally it is performed as an open procedure while the patient is on cardiopulmonary bypass.[69] An emerging alternative to surgical embolectomy is catheter embolectomy. It appears to be particularly useful if surgical embolectomy is not available or is contraindicated. It appears to be most successful when performed within 5 days of the occurrence of the PE.[67]

Reversal of Pulmonary Hypertension

To reverse the hemodynamic effects of pulmonary hypertension, additional measures may be taken. These include the administration of inotropic agents and fluid. Fluids should be administered to increase right ventricular preload, which would stretch the right ventricle and increase contractility, thus overcoming the elevated pulmonary arterial pressures. Inotropic agents also can be used to increase contractility to facilitate an increase in CO.[64]

Nursing Management

Prevention of pulmonary embolism should be a major nursing focus, because the majority of critically ill patients are at risk for this disorder. Nursing actions are aimed at preventing the development of DVT, which is a major complication of immobility and a leading cause of PE. These measures include the use of graduated compression stockings or pneumatic compression devices, active/passive range-of-motion exercises involving foot extension, adequate hydration, and progressive ambulation.[24]

Nursing management of the patient with a PE incorporates a variety of nursing diagnoses (Nursing Diagnosis Priorities box on Pulmonary Embolus). **Nursing priorities are directed toward (1) optimizing oxygenation and ventilation, (2) monitoring for bleeding, (3) providing comfort and emotional support, (4) maintaining surveillance for complications, and (5) educating the patient and family.**

NURSING DIAGNOSIS PRIORITIES
Pulmonary Embolus

- Impaired Gas Exchange related to ventilation/perfusion mismatching or intrapulmonary shunting, p. A-23
- Acute Pain related to transmission and perception of cutaneous, visceral, muscular, or ischemic impulses, p. A-5
- Risk for Aspiration, p. A-35
- Anxiety related to threat to biological, psychological, and/or social integrity, p. A-7
- Powerlessness related to lack of control over current situation or disease progression, p. A-33
- Compromised Family Coping related to critically ill family member, p. A-9
- Deficient Knowledge: Discharge Regimen related to lack of previous exposure to information (see Patient Education box on Pulmonary Embolus), p. A-15

Optimizing Oxygenation and Ventilation

Nursing interventions to optimize oxygenation and ventilation include positioning, preventing desaturation, and promoting secretion clearance. For further discussion on these interventions, see Nursing Management of Acute Respiratory Failure earlier in this chapter.

Monitoring for Bleeding

The patient receiving anticoagulant or thrombolytic therapy should be observed for signs of bleeding. The patient's gums, skin, urine, stool, and emesis should be screened for signs of overt or covert bleeding. In addition, monitoring the patient's

INR or aPTT is critical to managing the anticoagulation therapy.

Educating the Patient and Family

Early in the patient's hospital stay, the patient and family should be taught about pulmonary embolus, its etiologies, and its treatment (Patient Education box on Pulmonary Embolus). As the patient moves toward discharge, teaching should focus on the interventions necessary for preventing the reoccurrence of deep vein thrombosis and subsequent emboli, signs and symptoms of deep vein thrombosis and anticoagulant complications, and measures to prevent bleeding. If the patient smokes, he or she should be encouraged to stop smoking and be referred to a smoking cessation program.

PATIENT EDUCATION
Pulmonary Embolus

- Pathophysiology of disease
- Specific etiology
- Precipitating factor modification
- Measures to prevent deep vein thrombosis (e.g., avoid tight-fitting clothes, crossing legs, and prolonged sitting or standing; elevate legs when sitting; exercise)
- Signs and symptoms of deep vein thrombosis (e.g., redness, swelling, sharp or deep leg pain)
- Importance of taking medications
- Signs and symptoms of anticoagulant complications (e.g., excessive bruising, discoloration of the skin, changes in color of urine or stools)
- Measures to prevent bleeding (e.g., use soft-bristle toothbrush, caution when shaving)

Collaborative management of the patient with a pulmonary embolus is outlined in the Collaborative Management box on Pulmonary Embolus.

COLLABORATIVE MANAGEMENT
Pulmonary Embolus

- Administer oxygen therapy.
- Intubate patient.
- Initiate mechanical ventilation.
- Administer medications:
  - Thrombolytic therapy
  - Anticoagulants
  - Bronchodilators
  - Inotropic agents
  - Sedatives
  - Analgesics
- Administer fluids.
- Position patient to optimize ventilation/perfusion matching.
- Maintain surveillance for complications:
  - Bleeding
  - Acute lung injury
- Provide comfort and emotional support.

STATUS ASTHMATICUS

Asthma is a chronic obstructive pulmonary disease that is characterized by partially reversible airflow obstruction, airway inflammation, and hyperresponsiveness to a variety of stimuli.[68] Status asthmaticus is a severe asthma attack that fails to respond to conventional therapy with bronchodilators, which may result in acute respiratory failure.[69]

Etiology

The precipitating cause of the attack is usually an upper respiratory infection, allergen exposure, or a decrease in antiinflammatory medications. Other factors that have been implicated include overreliance on bronchodilators, environmental pollutants, lack of access to health care, failure to identify worsening airflow obstruction, and noncompliance with the health care regimen.[69]

Pathophysiology

An asthma attack is initiated when exposure to an irritant or trigger occurs, resulting in the initiation of the inflammatory-immune response in the airways. Bronchospasm occurs along with increased vascular permeability and increased mucus production. Mucosal edema and thick, tenacious mucus further increase airway responsiveness. The combination of bronchospasm, airway inflammation, and hyperresponsiveness results in narrowing of the airways and airflow obstruction. These changes have significant effects on the pulmonary and cardiovascular systems.[69]

Pulmonary Effects

As the diameter of the airways decreases, airway resistance increases, resulting in increased residual volume, hyperinflation of the lungs, increased work of breathing, and abnormal distribution of ventilation. V/Q mismatching occurs, which results in hypoxemia. Alveolar dead space also increases as hypoxic vasoconstriction occurs, resulting in hypercapnia.[69]

Cardiovascular Effects

Inspiratory muscle force also increases in an attempt to ventilate the hyperinflated lungs. This results in a significant increase in negative intrapleural pressure, leading to an increase in venous return and pooling of blood in the right ventricle. The stretched right ventricle causes the intraventricular septum to shift, thereby impinging on the left ventricle. In addition, the left ventricle has to work harder to pump blood from the markedly negative pressure in the thorax to elevated pressure in systemic circulation. This leads to a decrease in cardiac output and a fall in systolic blood pressure on inspiration (pulsus paradoxus).[69]

Assessment and Diagnosis

Initially the patient may present with a cough, wheezing, and dyspnea. As the attack continues, the patient develops tachypnea, tachycardia, diaphoresis, increased accessory muscle use, and pulsus paradoxus greater than 25 mm Hg. Decreased level of consciousness, inability to speak, significantly diminished or absent breath sounds, and inability to lie supine herald the onset of acute respiratory failure.[70-73]

Initial ABGs indicate hypocapnia and respiratory alkalosis caused by hyperventilation. As the attack continues and the patient starts to fatigue, hypoxemia and hypercapnia develop.[70] Lactic acidosis also may occur as a result of lactate overproduction by the respiratory muscles. The end result is the development of respiratory and metabolic acidosis.[71]

Deterioration of pulmonary function tests despite aggressive bronchodilator therapy is diagnostic of status asthmaticus and indicates the potential need for intubation. A peak expiratory flow rate (PEFR) less than 40% of predicted or an FEV_1 (maximum volume of gas that the patient can exhale in 1 second [forced expiratory volume in 1 second]) less than 20% of predicted indicates severe airflow obstruction, and the need for intubation with mechanical ventilation may be imminent.[72]

Medical Management

Medical management of the patient with status asthmaticus is directed toward supporting oxygenation and ventilation. Bronchodilators, corticosteroids, oxygen therapy, and intubation and mechanical ventilation are the mainstays of therapy.[70]

Bronchodilators

Inhaled beta$_2$-agonists and anticholinergics are the bronchodilators of choice for status asthmaticus. Beta$_2$-agonists promote bronchodilation and can be administered by nebulizer or metered-dose inhaler (MDI). Usually larger and more frequent doses are given, and the drug is titrated to the patient's response. Anticholinergics that inhibit bronchoconstriction are not very effective by themselves, but in conjunction with beta$_2$-agonists, they have a synergistic effect and produce a greater improvement in airflow. The routine use of xanthines is not recommended in the treatment of status asthmaticus because they have been shown to have no therapeutic benefit.[69-72]

A number of studies have focused on the bronchodilator abilities of magnesium. Although it has been demonstrated that magnesium is inferior to beta$_2$-agonists as a bronchodilator, in patients who are refractory to conventional treatment, magnesium may be beneficial. A bolus of 1 to 4 g of intravenous magnesium given over 10 to 40 minutes has been reported to produce desirable effects.[69,70,72]

A number of other studies are evaluating the effects of leukotriene inhibitors such as zafirlukast, montelukast, and zileuton in the treatment of status asthmaticus. Leukotrienes are inflammatory mediators known to cause bronchoconstriction and airway inflammation. Research suggests that these agents may be beneficial as bronchodilators in those patients who are refractory to beta$_2$-agonists.[72]

Systemic Corticosteroids

Intravenous or oral corticosteroids also are used in the treatment of status asthmaticus. Their antiinflammatory effects limit mucosal edema, decrease mucus production, and potentiate beta$_2$-agonists. It usually takes 6 to 8 hours for the effects of the corticosteroids to become evident.[70] The use of inhaled corticosteroids for the treatment of status asthmaticus remains undecided at this time.[69,73] Initial studies indicate they may be beneficial in certain patient populations.[73]

Oxygen Therapy

Initial treatment of hypoxemia is with supplemental oxygen. High-flow oxygen therapy is administered to keep the patient's Sao$_2$ greater than 92%.[69] Another therapy currently under investigation is the use of heliox. A mixture of helium and oxygen, heliox has a lower density and higher viscosity than an oxygen and air mixture. Heliox is believed to reduce the work of breathing and improve gas exchange because it flows more easily through constricted areas. Studies have shown that it reduces air trapping and carbon dioxide and helps relieve respiratory acidosis.[69]

Intubation and Mechanical Ventilation

Indications for mechanical ventilation include cardiac or respiratory arrest, disorientation, failure to respond to bronchodilator therapy, and exhaustion.[69,71,72] A large endotracheal tube (8 mm) should be used to decrease airway resistance and to facilitate suctioning of secretions. Ventilating the patient with status asthmaticus can be very difficult. High inflation pressures should be avoided because they can result in barotrauma. The use of PEEP should be monitored closely because the patient is prone to developing air trapping. Patient-ventilator asynchrony also can be a major problem. Sedation and neuromuscular paralysis may be necessary to allow for adequate ventilation of the patient.[69,71]

Nursing Management

Nursing management of the patient with status asthmaticus incorporates a variety of nursing diagnoses (Nursing Diagnosis Priorities box on Status Asthmaticus). **Nursing priorities are directed toward (1) optimizing oxygenation and ventilation, (2) providing comfort and emotional support, (3) maintaining surveillance for complications, and (4) educating the patient and family.**

NURSING DIAGNOSIS PRIORITIES

Status Asthmaticus

- Impaired Gas Exchange related to alveolar hypoventilation, p. A-22
- Impaired Gas Exchange related to ventilation/perfusion mismatching or intrapulmonary shunting, p. A-23
- Ineffective Breathing Pattern related to musculoskeletal fatigue or neuromuscular impairment, p. A-27
- Ineffective Airway Clearance related to excessive secretions or abnormal viscosity of mucus, p. A-26
- Risk for Infection, p. A-36
- Anxiety related to threat to biological, psychological, and/or social integrity, p. A-7

- Disturbed Body Image related to actual change in body structures, function, or appearance, p. A-16
- Compromised Family Coping related to critically ill family member, p. A-9
- Deficient Knowledge: Discharge Regimen related to lack of previous exposure to information (see Patient Education special box on Status Asthmaticus), p. A-15

Optimizing Oxygenation and Ventilation

Nursing interventions to optimize oxygenation and ventilation include positioning, preventing desaturation, and promoting secretion clearance. For further discussion on these interventions, see Nursing Management of Acute Respiratory Failure earlier in this chapter.

Educating the Patient and Family

Early in the patient's hospital stay, the patient and family should be taught about asthma, its triggers, and its treatment (Patient Education box on Status Asthmaticus). As the patient moves toward discharge, teaching should focus on the interventions necessary for preventing the recurrence of status asthmaticus, early warning signs of worsening airflow obstruction, correct use of an inhaler and a peak flowmeter, measures to prevent pulmonary infections, and signs and symptoms of a pulmonary infection. If the patient smokes, he or she should be encouraged to stop smoking and be referred to a smoking cessation program. In addition, the importance of participating in a pulmonary rehabilitation program should be stressed.

PATIENT EDUCATION

Status Asthmaticus

- Pathophysiology of disease
- Specific etiology
- Early warning signs of worsening airflow obstruction (20% drop in peak expiratory flow rate [PEFR] below predicted or personal best, increase in cough, shortness of breath, chest tightness, wheezing)
- Treatment of attacks
- Importance of taking prescribed medications and avoidance of over-the-counter asthma medications
- Correct use of an inhaler (with and without spacer device)
- Correct use of a peak flow meter
- Removal or avoidance of environmental triggers (e.g., pollen; dust; mold spores; cat and dog dander; cold, dry air; strong odors; household aerosols; tobacco smoke; air pollution)
- Measures to prevent pulmonary infections (e.g., proper nutrition and hand washing, immunization against *Streptococcus pneumoniae* and influenza viruses)
- Signs and symptoms of pulmonary infection (e.g., sputum color change, shortness of breath, fever)
- Importance of participating in pulmonary rehabilitation program

Collaborative management of the patient with status asthmaticus is outlined in the Collaborative Management box on Status Asthmaticus.

COLLABORATIVE MANAGEMENT

Status Asthmaticus

- Administer oxygen therapy.
- Intubate patient.
- Initiate mechanical ventilation.
- Administer medications:
  - Bronchodilators
  - Corticosteroids
  - Sedatives
- Maintain surveillance for complications:
  - Acute respiratory failure
- Provide comfort and emotional support.

LONG-TERM MECHANICAL VENTILATOR DEPENDENCE

Long-term mechanical ventilator dependence (LTMVD) is a secondary disorder that occurs when a patient requires assisted ventilation longer than expected given the patient's underlying condition.[73] It is the result of complex medical problems that do not allow the weaning process to take place in a normal and timely manner. A review of the literature reveals a great deal of confusion regarding an exact definition of LTMVD, particularly with regards to an actual time frame. In 2005, the National Association for Medical Direction of Respiratory Care (NAMDRC) Consensus Panel recommended that LTMVD (which they referred to as prolonged mechanical ventilation) be defined as "the need for ≥21 consecutive days of mechanical ventilation for ≥6 hours per day."[74]

Etiology and Pathophysiology

A wide variety of physiological and psychological factors contribute to the development of LTMVD. Physiological factors include those conditions that result in decreased gas exchange, increased ventilatory workload, increased ventilatory demand, decreased ventilatory drive, and increased respiratory muscle fatigue (Box 15-4).[75] Psychological factors include those conditions that result in loss of breathing pattern control, lack of motivation and confidence, and delirium (Box 15-5).[76] The development of LTMVD also is affected by the severity and duration of the patient's current illness and any underlying chronic health problems.[77]

Medical and Nursing Management

The goal of medical and nursing management of the patient with LTMVD is successful weaning. The Third National Study Group on Weaning from Mechanical Ventilation, sponsored by the American Association of Critical-Care Nurses, proposed the Weaning Continuum Model that divides weaning into three stages: preweaning, weaning process, and weaning outcome.[78] It is within this framework that the management of the long-term ventilator-dependent patient is described. In addition, the common nursing diagnoses for this patient population are listed in the Nursing Diagnosis Priorities box on Long-Term Mechanical Ventilation.

BOX 15-4   PHYSIOLOGICAL FACTORS CONTRIBUTING TO LONG-TERM MECHANICAL VENTILATION DEPENDENCE

Decreased gas exchange
  Ventilation/perfusion mismatching
  Intrapulmonary shunting
  Alveolar hypoventilation
  Anemia
  Acute heart failure
Increased ventilatory workload
  Decreased lung compliance
  Increased airway resistance
  Small endotracheal tube
  Decreased ventilatory sensitivity
  Improper positioning
  Abdominal distention
  Dyspnea
Increased ventilatory demand
  Increased pulmonary dead space
  Increased metabolic demands
  Improper ventilator mode/settings

Metabolic acidosis
  Overfeeding
Decreased ventilatory drive
  Respiratory alkalosis
  Metabolic alkalosis
  Hypothyroidism
  Sedatives
  Malnutrition
Increased respiratory muscle fatigue
  Increased ventilatory workload
  Increased ventilatory demand
  Malnutrition
  Hypokalemia
  Hypomagnesemia
  Hypophosphatemia
  Hypothyroidism
  Critical illness polyneuropathy
  Inadequate muscle rest

BOX 15-5   PSYCHOLOGICAL FACTORS CONTRIBUTING TO LONG-TERM MECHANICAL VENTILATION DEPENDENCE

Loss of breathing pattern control
  Anxiety
  Fear
  Dyspnea
  Pain
  Ventilator asynchrony
  Lack of confidence in ability to breathe
Lack of motivation and confidence
  Inadequate trust in staff
  Depersonalization
  Hopelessness
  Powerlessness
  Depression
  Inadequate communication
Delirium
  Sensory overload
  Sensory deprivation
  Sleep deprivation
  Pain
  Medications

NURSING DIAGNOSIS PRIORITIES
Long-Term Mechanical Ventilation Dependence

- Impaired Spontaneous Ventilation related to respiratory muscle fatigue or neuromuscular impairment, p. A-23
- Dysfunctional Ventilatory Weaning Response related to physical, psychosocial, or situational factors, p. A-18
- Risk for Aspiration, p. A-35
- Imbalanced Nutrition: Less Than Body Requirements related to lack of exogenous nutrients or increased metabolic demand, p. A-22
- Risk for Infection, p. A-36
- Acute Confusion related to sensory overload, sensory deprivation, and sleep pattern disturbance, p. A-2
- Disturbed Body Image related to functional dependence on life-sustaining technology, p. A-16
- Relocation Stress Syndrome related to transfer out of the intensive care unit, p. A-34
- Powerlessness related to lack of control over current situation or disease progression, p. A-33
- Compromised Family Coping related to critically ill family member, p. A-9

Preweaning Stage

For the long-term ventilator-dependent patient, the preweaning phase consists of resolving the precipitating event that necessitated ventilatory assistance and preventing the physiological and psychological factors that can interfere with weaning. Before any attempts at weaning, the patient should be assessed for weaning readiness, an approach should be determined, and a method should be selected.[76,77]

Weaning Preparedness. The patient should be physiologically and psychologically prepared to initiate the weaning process by addressing those factors that can interfere with weaning. Aggressive medical management to prevent and treat ventilation/perfusion mismatching, intrapulmonary shunting, anemia, cardiac failure, decreased lung compliance, increased airway resistance, acid-base disturbances, hypothyroidism, abdominal distention, and electrolyte imbalances should be initiated. In addition, interventions to decrease the work of breathing should be implemented, such as replacing a small endotracheal tube with a larger tube or a tracheostomy, suctioning airway secretions, administering bronchodilators, optimizing the ventilator settings and trigger sensitivity, and positioning the patient in straight alignment with the head of the bed elevated at least 30 degrees. Enteral or parenteral nutrition should be started and the patient's nutritional state optimized. Physical therapy should be initiated for the patient with critical illness polyneuropathy because increased mobility facilitates weaning. A means of communication should be established with the patient. Sedatives can be administered to provide anxiety control, but the avoidance of respiratory depression is critical.[79]

Weaning Readiness. Although a variety of different methods for assessing weaning readiness have been developed, none has proven to be very accurate in predicting weaning success in the patient with LTMVD. One study did indicate that the presence of left ventricular dysfunction, fluid imbalance, and nutritional deficiency increased the duration of mechanical ventilation. Another study suggested that the upward trending of the albumin level may be predictive of weaning success. Because so many variables can affect the patient's ability to wean, any assessment of weaning readiness should incorporate these variables. Cardiac function, gas exchange, pulmonary mechanics, nutritional status, electrolyte and fluid balance, and motivation should all be considered when making the decision to wean. This assessment should be ongoing to reflect the dynamic nature of the process.[80]

Weaning Approach. Although weaning the patient requiring short-term mechanical ventilation is a relatively simple process that can usually be accomplished with a nurse and respiratory therapist, weaning the patient with LTMVD is a much more complex process that usually requires a multidisciplinary team approach. Multidisciplinary weaning teams that use a coordinated and collaborative approach to weaning have demonstrated improved patient outcomes and decreased weaning times. The team should consist of a physician; a nurse; a respiratory therapist; a dietitian; a physical therapist; and a case manager, a clinical outcomes manager, or a clinical nurse specialist. Additional members, if possible, should include an occupational therapist, a speech therapist, a discharge planner, and a social worker. Working together, the team members should develop a comprehensive plan of care for the patient that is efficient, consistent, progressive, and cost-effective.[81] Several studies have demonstrated successful weaning through the use of nurse and respiratory therapist managed protocols.[82]

Weaning Method. A variety of weaning methods are available, but no one method has consistently proven to be superior to the others. These methods include T-tube (T-piece), constant positive airway pressure (CPAP), pressure support ventilation (PSV), and synchronized intermittent mandatory ventilation (SIMV). One recent multicenter study lends evidence to support the use of PSV for weaning over T-tube or SIMV weaning. Often these weaning methods are used in combination with each other, such as SIMV with PSV, CPAP with PSV, or SIMV with CPAP.[75,77]

Weaning Process Stage

For the long-term ventilator patient, the weaning process phase consists of initiating the weaning method selected and minimizing the physiological and psychological factors that can interfere with weaning.[77] It is imperative that the patient not become exhausted during this phase, because this can result in a setback in the weaning process.[79] During this phase, the patient is assessed for weaning progress and signs of weaning intolerance.[76]

Weaning Initiation. Weaning should be initiated in the morning while the patient is rested. Before starting the weaning process, the patient is provided with an explanation of how the process works, a description of the sensations to expect, and reassurances that he or she will be closely monitored and returned to the original ventilator mode and settings if any difficulty occurs.[77] This information should be reinforced with each weaning attempt. One study showed that family presence during the weaning trial was beneficial and that the trials were longer when the family was present.[83]

T-tube and CPAP weaning are accomplished by removing the patient from the ventilator and then placing the patient on a T-tube or by placing the patient on CPAP mode for a specified duration of time, known as a weaning trial, for a specified number of times per day. When the weaning trial is over, the patient is placed on the assist-control mode or similar mode and allowed to rest to prevent respiratory muscle fatigue. Gradually the duration of time spent weaning is increased, as is the frequency, until the patient is able to breathe spontaneously for 24 hours. If PSV is used in conjunction with CPAP, the PSV is initially set to provide the patient with an assisted tidal volume of 10 to 12 mL/kg, and this is gradually weaned until a level of 6 to 8 cm H_2O of pressure support is achieved. SIMV and PSV weaning are accomplished by gradually decreasing the number of breaths or the amount of pressure support the patient receives by a specified amount until the patient is able to breathe spontaneously for 24 hours.[77]

Weaning Progress. Weaning progress can be evaluated using various methods. Evaluation of weaning progress when using a weaning method that gradually withdraws ventilatory support, such as SIMV or PSV, can be accomplished by measuring the percentage of the minute ventilation requirement that is provided by the ventilator. If the percentage steadily decreases, weaning is progressing. Evaluation of weaning progress when using a weaning method that removes ventilatory support, such as T-tube or CPAP, can be accomplished by measuring the amount of time the patient remains free from support. If the time steadily increases, weaning is progressing.[77]

Weaning Intolerance. Once the weaning process has begun, the patient should be continuously assessed for signs of intolerance. When present, these signs indicate when to place the patient back on the ventilator or to return the patient to the previous ventilator settings. Commonly used indicators include dyspnea; accessory muscle use; restlessness; anxiety; change in facial expression; changes in heart rate and blood pressure; rapid, shallow breathing; and discomfort.[80] Table 15-6 lists the different weaning intolerance indicators and actions that can be taken to control or prevent them.

Facilitative Therapies. Additional therapies may be needed to facilitate weaning in the patient who is having difficulty making weaning progress. These therapies include ventilatory muscle training and biofeedback. Inspiratory muscle training is used to enhance the strength and endurance of the respiratory muscles. Biofeedback can be used to promote relaxation and assist in the management of dyspnea and anxiety.[77]

Weaning Outcome Stage

Two outcomes are possible for a patient with LTMVD: weaning completed and incomplete weaning.[77]

Weaning Completed. Weaning is deemed successful when a patient is able to breathe spontaneously for 24 hours without ventilatory support. Once this occurs, the patient may be extubated or decannulated at any time, though this is not necessary for weaning to be considered successful.[78]

Incomplete Weaning. Weaning is deemed incomplete when a patient has reached a plateau (5 days at the same ventilatory support level without any changes) in the weaning process despite managing the physiological and psychological factors that impede weaning. Thus the patient is unable to breathe spontaneously for 24 hours without full or partial ventilatory support. Once this occurs, the patient should be placed in a subacute ventilator facility or discharged home on a ventilator with home care nursing follow-up.[78]

TABLE 15-6 WEANING INTOLERANCE INDICATIONS AND INTERVENTIONS

INDICATOR	ETIOLOGY	INTERVENTION
Pulmonary Signs (Emotional)		
Altered breathing pattern	Inadequate understanding of weaning process	Build trust in staff; consistent care providers
Dyspnea intensity		Encouragement; concrete goals for extubation
Change in facial expression	Inability to control breathing pattern	Involve patient in process and planning daily activities
		Efficient communication established
	Environmental factors	Organize care; avoid interruptions during weaning
		Adequate sleep
		Calm, caring presence of nurse; nonsedating anxiolytics
		Measure dyspnea
		Fan; music
		Biofeedback; relaxation; breathing control
		Family involvement; normalizing daily activities
Pulmonary Signs (Physiological)		
Accessory muscle use	Airway obstruction	Suction/air-mask bag unit ventilation; manually ventilate patient
Prolonged expiration	Secretions/atelectasis	
Asynchronous movements of chest and abdomen	Bronchospasm	Bronchodilators
	Patient position/kinked	Sitting upright in bed or chair or per patient preference
Retractions	ET tube	
Facial expression changes	Increased workload or muscle	
Dyspnea	Fatigue	
Shortened inspiratory time	Caloric intake	Dietary assessment
Increased breathing frequency, decreased V_T	Electrolyte imbalances	Assess electrolytes; give replacements as necessary
	Inadequate rest	Rest between weaning trials (i.e., SIMV frequency rate >5)
	Patient/ventilator interactions	Assess ventilator settings (i.e., flow rate, trigger sensitivity)
	Increased V_E requirement	Muscle training if appropriate
	Infection	Check for infection (treat if indicated)
	Overfeeding	Appropriate caloric intake
	Respiratory alkalosis	Baseline ABGs achieved (ventilate according to pH)
	Anxiety	Coaching to regularize breathing pattern; give nonsedating anxiolytics
	Pain	Judicious use of analgesics
CNS Changes		
Restless/irritable	Hypoxemia/hypercarbia	Increase FiO_2
Decreased responsiveness		Return to mechanical ventilation
		Discern etiology and treat
CV Deterioration		
Excessive change in BP or HR	Heart failure	Diuretics as ordered
	Increase venous return	Beta-blockers
Dysrhythmias	Ischemia	Increase FiO_2
Angina		Return to mechanical ventilation
Dyspnea		Discern etiology and treat

Modified from Knebel AR: When weaning from mechanical ventilation fails, *Am J Crit Care* 1(3):19, 1992.
ET, endotracheal; *SIMV,* synchronized intermittent mandatory ventilation; V_E, respiratory minute volume; V_T, tidal volume; *ABGs,* arterial blood gases; *FiO_2,* fraction of inspired oxygen; *CNS,* central nervous system; *CV,* cardiovascular; *BP,* blood pressure; *HR,* heart rate.

REFERENCES

1. Aboussouan LS: Respiratory failure and the need for ventilatory support. In Wilkins RL, Stoller JK, Kacmarek RM, editors: *Egan's fundamentals of respiratory care*, ed 9, St Louis, 2009, Mosby.
2. Flaatten H, et al: Outcome after acute respiratory failure is more dependent on dysfunction in other vital organs than on severity of the respiratory failure, *Crit Care* 7(4):R72, 2003.
3. Vincent JL, et al: The epidemiology of acute respiratory failure in critically ill patients, *Chest* 121(5):1602, 2002.
4. Balk R, Bone RC: Classification of acute respiratory failure, *Med Clin North Am* 67(3):551, 1983.
5. Curtis JR, Hudson LD: Emergent assessment and management of acute respiratory failure in COPD, *Clin Chest Med* 15(3):481, 1994.
6. Raju P, Manthous CA: The pathogenesis of respiratory failure: an overview, *Respir Care Clin N Am* 6(2):195, 2000.
7. Del Sorbo L, et al: Hypoxemic respiratory failure. In Mason RJ, et al, editors: *Murray and Nadel's textbook of respiratory medicine*, ed 5, Philadelphia, 2010, Saunders.
8. Walshe TE, D'Amore PA: The role of hypoxia in vascular injury and repair, *Annu Rev Pathol* 3:615, 2008.
9. Sigillito RJ, DeBlieux PM: Evaluation and initial management of the patient in respiratory distress, *Emerg Med Clin North Am* 21(2):239, 2003.
10. Dakin J, Griffiths M: The pulmonary physician in critical care 1: pulmonary investigations for acute respiratory failure, *Thorax* 57(1):79, 2002.
11. Misasi RS, Keyes JL: Matching and mismatching ventilation and perfusion in the lung, *Crit Care Nurse* 16(3):23, 1996.
12. Barreiro TJ, Gemmel DJ: Noninvasive ventilation, *Crit Care Clin* 23(2):201, 2007.
13. Peñuelas O, Frutos-Vivar F, Esteban A: Noninvasive positive-pressure ventilation in acute respiratory failure, *CMAJ* 177(10):1211, 2007.
14. Soo Hoo GW, Hakimian N, Santiago SM: Hypercapnic respiratory failure in COPD patients: response to therapy, *Chest* 117(1):169, 2000.
15. Ward NS, Dushay KM: Clinical concise review: mechanical ventilation of patients with chronic obstructive pulmonary disease, *Crit Care Med* 36(5):1614, 2008.
16. Grimes GC, et al: Medications for COPD: a review of effectiveness, *Am Fam Physician* 76(8):1141, 2007.
17. Sessler CN, Varney K: Patient-focused sedation and analgesia in the ICU, *Chest* 133(2):552, 2008.
18. Luer J: Sedation and neuromuscular blockade in mechanically ventilated patients. In Burns SM, editor: *Care of mechanically ventilated patients*, ed 2, Sudbury, Md., 2007, Jones and Bartlett.
19. Kraut JA, Madias NE: Metabolic acidosis: pathophysiology, diagnosis and management, *Nat Rev Nephrol* 6(5):274, 2010.
20. Martindale RG, et al: Guidelines for the provision and assessment of nutrition support therapy in the adult critically ill patient: Society of Critical Care Medicine and American Society for Parenteral and Enteral Nutrition: Executive Summary, *Crit Care Med* 37(5):1757, 2009.
21. Parrish CR, Krenitsky J, Willcutts K: Nutritional support for mechanically ventilated patients. In Burns SM, editor: *Care of mechanically ventilated patients*, ed 2, Sudbury, Md., 2007, Jones and Bartlett.
22. Gunther ML, Morandi A, Ely EW: Pathophysiology of delirium in the intensive care unit, *Crit Care Clin* 24(1):45, 2008.
23. Frazier SK: Cardiovascular effects of mechanical ventilation and weaning, *Nur Clin North Am* 43(1):1, 2008.
24. Francis CW: Prophylaxis for thromboembolism in hospitalized medical patients, *N Engl J Med* 356(14):1438, 2007.
25. Martin B: Prevention of gastrointestinal complications in the critically ill patient, *AACN Adv Crit Care* 18(2):158, 2007.
26. Wong WP: Use of body positioning in the mechanically ventilated patient with acute respiratory failure: application of Sackett's rules of evidence, *Physiother Theory Pract* 15(1):25, 1999.
27. Force TR, et al: Acute respiratory distress syndrome. Patient position and motion strategies, *Respir Care Clin N Am* 4(4):665, 1998.
28. Lasater-Erhard M: The effect of patient position on arterial oxygen saturation, *Crit Care Nurse* 15(5):31, 1995.
29. Cosenza JJ, Norton LC: Secretion clearance: state-of-the-art from a nursing perspective, *Crit Care Nurse* 6(4):23, 1986.
30. Flanders SA, Collard HR, Saint S: Nosocomial pneumonia: state of the science, *Am J Infect Control* 34(2):84, 2006.
31. Krishnagopalan S, et al: Body positioning of intensive care patients: clinical practice versus standards, *Crit Care Med* 30(11):2588, 2002.
32. Stiller K: Physiotherapy in intensive care: towards an evidence-based practice, *Chest* 118(6):1801, 2000.
33. McCool FD, Rosen M: Nonpharmacologic airway clearance therapies: ACCP evidence-based clinical practice guidelines, *Chest* 129(suppl 1):250S, 2006.
34. Krau SD: Making sense of multiple organ dysfunction syndrome, *Crit Care Nurs Clin North Am* 19(1):87, 2007.
35. Crouser ED, Fahy RJ: Acute lung injury, pulmonary edema, and multiple system organ failure. In Wilkins RL, Stoller JK, Kacmarek RM, editors: *Egan's fundamentals of respiratory care*, ed 9, St Louis, 2009, Mosby.
36. Bernard GR, et al: The American-European consensus conference on ARDS: definitions, mechanisms, relevant outcomes, and clinical trial coordination, *Am J Respir Crit Care Med* 149(3 pt 1):818, 1994.
37. Fan E, et al: Recruitment maneuvers for acute lung injury: a systematic review, *Am J Respir Crit Care Med* 178(11):1156, 2008.
38. George KJ: A systematic approach to care: adult respiratory distress syndrome, *J Trauma Nurs* 15(1):19, 2008.
39. Tsushima K, et al: Acute lung injury review, *Intern Med* 48(9):621, 2009.
40. Taylor MM: ARDS diagnosis and management, *Dimens Crit Care Nurs* 24(5):197, 2005.
41. Perina DG: Noncardiogenic pulmonary edema, *Emerg Med Clin North Am* 21(2):385, 2003.
42. Putensen C, et al: Meta-analysis: ventilation strategies and outcomes of the acute respiratory distress syndrome and acute lung injury, *Ann Intern Med* 151(8):566, 2009.
43. Malhotra A: Low-tidal-volume ventilation in the acute respiratory distress syndrome, *N Engl J Med* 357(11):1113, 2007.
44. Yilmaz M, Gajic O: Optimal ventilator settings in acute lung injury and acute respiratory distress syndrome, *Eur J Anaesthesiol* 25(1):89, 2008.
45. Chan KP, Stewart TE, Mehta S: High-frequency oscillatory ventilation for adult patients with ARDS, *Chest* 131(6):1907, 2007.

46. Liu KD, Matthay MA: Advances in critical care for the nephrologist: acute lung injury/ARDS, *Clin J Am Soc Nephrol* 3(2):578, 2008.

47. Alsaghir AH, Martin CM: Effect of prone positioning in patients with acute respiratory distress syndrome: a meta-analysis, *Crit Care Med* 36(2):603, 2008.

48. Pimentel L, McPherson SJ: Community-acquired pneumonia in the emergency department: a practical approach to diagnosis and management, *Emerg Med Clin North Am* 21(2):395, 2003.

49. Baudouin SV: The pulmonary physician in critical care. 3: critical care management of community acquired pneumonia, *Thorax* 57(3):267, 2002.

50. Rello J, Díaz E, Rodríguez A: Etiology of ventilator-associated pneumonia, *Clin Chest Med* 26(1):87, 2005.

51. Apisarnthanarak A, Mundy LM: Etiology of community-acquired pneumonia, *Clin Chest Med* 26(1):47, 2005.

52. Mandell LA, et al: Infectious Diseases Society of America/American Thoracic Society consensus guidelines on the management of community-acquired pneumonia in adults, *Clin Infect Dis* 44(suppl 2):S27, 2007.

53. Miskovich-Riddle L, Keresztes PA: CAP management guidelines, *Nurse Pract* 31(1):43, 2006.

54. Tarver RD, et al: Radiology of community-acquired pneumonia, *Radiol Clin North Am* 43(3):497, 2005.

55. Pines JM: Timing of antibiotics for acute, severe infections, *Emerg Med Clin North Am* 26(2):245, 2008.

56. Anantham D, Jagadesan R, Tiew PE: Clinical review: independent lung ventilation in critical care, *Crit Care* 9(6):594, 2005.

57. Johnson JL, Hirsch CS: Aspiration pneumonia: recognizing and managing a potentially growing disorder, *Postgrad Med* 113(3):99, 2003.

58. Marik PE: Aspiration pneumonitis and aspiration pneumonia, *N Engl J Med* 344(9):665, 2001.

59. Tietjen PA, Kaner RJ, Quinn CE: Aspiration emergencies, *Clin Chest Med* 15(1):117, 1994.

60. Metheny NA: Strategies to prevent aspiration-related pneumonia in tube-fed patients, *Respir Care Clin N Am* 12(4):603, 2006.

61. Piazza G, Goldhaber SZ: Acute pulmonary embolism: part I: epidemiology and diagnosis, *Circulation* 114(2):e28, 2006.

62. Carlbom DJ, Davidson BL: Pulmonary embolism in the critically ill, *Chest* 132(1):313, 2007.

63. Dweik RA, Arroliga AC: Pulmonary vascular disease. In Wilkins RL, Stoller JK, Kacmarek R, editors: *Egan's fundamentals of respiratory care*, ed 9, St Louis, 2008, Mosby.

64. Tapson VF: Acute pulmonary embolism, *N Eng J Med* 358(10):1037, 2008.

65. Piazza G, Goldhaber SZ: Acute pulmonary embolism: part II: treatment and prophylaxis, *Circulation* 114(3):e42, 2006.

66. Kearon C, et al: Antithrombotic therapy for venous thromboembolic disease: American College of Chest Physicians Evidence-Based Clinical Practice Guidelines (8th Edition), *Chest* 133(suppl 6):454S, 2008.

67. Kucher N: Catheter embolectomy for acute pulmonary embolism, *Chest* 132(2):657, 2007.

68. Fanta CH: Asthma, *N Engl J Med* 360(10):1002, 2009.

69. Holgate ST: The mechanisms, diagnosis, and management of severe asthma in adults, *Lancet* 368(9537):780, 2006.

70. Sims JM: An overview of asthma, *Dimens Crit Care Nurs* 25(6):264, 2006.

71. Cairns CB: Acute asthma exacerbations: phenotypes and management, *Clin Chest Med* 27(1):99, 2006.

72. Restrepo RD, Peters J: Near-fatal asthma: recognition and management, *Curr Opin Pulm Med*, 14(1):13, 2008.

73. Knebel AR, et al: Weaning from mechanical ventilation: concept development, *Am J Crit Care* 3(6):416, 1994.

74. MacIntyre NR, et al: Management of patients requiring prolonged mechanical ventilation: report of a NAMDRC Consensus Conference, *Chest* 128(6):3937, 2005.

75. Caroleo S, et al: Weaning from mechanical ventilation: an open issue, *Minerva Anestesiol* 73(7-8):417, 2007.

76. MacIntyre NR: Psychological factors in weaning from mechanical ventilatory support, *Respir Care* 40(3):277, 1995.

77. Burns SM: Weaning from mechanical ventilation. In Burns SM, editor: *Care of mechanically ventilated patients*, ed 2, Sudbury, Md., 2007, Jones and Bartlett.

78. Knebel AR, et al: Weaning from mechanical ventilatory support: refinement of a model, *Am J Crit Care* 7(2):149, 1998.

79. El-Khatib MF, Bou-Khalil P: Clinical review: Liberation from mechanical ventilation, *Crit Care* 12(4):221, 2008.

80. Cox CE, Carson SS: Prolonged mechanical ventilation. In MacIntyre NR, Branson RD, editors: *Mechanical ventilation*, ed 2, St Louis, 2009, Saunders.

81. White V, et al: Multidisciplinary team developed and implemented protocols to assist mechanical ventilation weaning: a systematic review of literature, *Worldviews Evid Based Nurs* Aug 31, 2010. [Epub ahead of print].

82. Girard TD, Ely EW: Protocol-driven ventilator weaning: reviewing the evidence, *Clin Chest Med* 29(2):241, 2008.

83. Happ MB, et al: Family presence and surveillance during weaning from prolonged mechanical ventilation, *Heart Lung* 36(1):47, 2007.

16

Pulmonary Therapeutic Management

Kathleen M. Stacy

⊖volve WEBSITE

Be sure to check out the bonus material, including free self-assessment exercises, on the Evolve web site at *http://evolve.elsevier.com/Urden/priorities/.*

OBJECTIVES

- Describe nursing management of a patient receiving oxygen therapy.
- List the indications and complications of the different artificial airways.
- Outline the principles of airway management.
- Discuss the various modes of invasive and noninvasive mechanical ventilation.

- Describe the management of a patient on mechanical ventilation.
- Delineate the care of the postoperative thoracic surgery patient and the lung transplant patient.

OXYGEN THERAPY

Normal cellular function depends on the delivery of an adequate supply of oxygen to the cells to meet their metabolic needs. The goal of oxygen therapy is to provide a sufficient concentration of inspired oxygen to permit full use of the oxygen-carrying capacity of the arterial blood; this ensures adequate cellular oxygenation, provided the cardiac output and hemoglobin concentration are adequate.[1,2]

Principles of Therapy

Oxygen is an atmospheric gas that must also be considered a drug, because—like most other drugs—it has detrimental and beneficial effects. Oxygen is one of the most commonly used and misused drugs. As a drug, it must be administered for good reason and in a proper, safe manner. Oxygen is usually ordered in liters per minute (L/min), as a concentration of oxygen expressed as a percentage, such as 40%, or as a fraction of inspired oxygen (Fio_2), such as 0.4.

The primary indication for oxygen therapy is hypoxemia.[3] The amount of oxygen administered depends on the pathophysiological mechanisms affecting the patient's oxygenation status. In most cases, the amount required should provide an arterial partial pressure of oxygen (Pao_2) of greater than 60 mm Hg or an arterial hemoglobin saturation (Sao_2) of greater than 90% during rest and exercise.[2] The concentration

of oxygen given to an individual patient is a clinical judgment based on the many factors that influence oxygen transport, such as hemoglobin concentration, cardiac output, and arterial oxygen tension.[1,2]

After oxygen therapy has begun, the patient is continuously assessed for level of oxygenation and the factors affecting it. The patient's oxygenation status is evaluated several times daily until the desired oxygen level has been reached and has stabilized. If the desired response to the amount of oxygen delivered is not achieved, the oxygen supplementation is adjusted, and the patient's condition is re-evaluated. It is important to use this dose-response method so that the lowest possible level of oxygen is administered that will still achieve a satisfactory Pao_2 or Sao_2.[2,3]

Methods of Delivery

Oxygen therapy can be delivered by many different devices (Table 16-1). Common problems with these devices include system leaks and obstructions, device displacement, and skin irritation. These devices are classified as low-flow, reservoir, or high-flow systems.[3]

Low-Flow Systems

A low-flow oxygen delivery system provides supplemental oxygen directly into the patient's airway at a flow of 8 L/min or less. Because this flow is insufficient to meet the patient's

CATEGORY	DEVICE	FLOW	FiO$_2$ RANGE (%)	FiO$_2$ STABILITY	ADVANTAGES	DISADVANTAGES	BEST USE
Low-flow	Nasal cannula	0.25-8 L/min (adults) ≤2 L/min (infants)	22-45	Variable	Use on adults, children, infants; easy to apply; disposable, low cost; well tolerated	Unstable, easily dislodged; high flows uncomfortable; can cause dryness/bleeding; polyps, deviated septum may block flow	Stable patient needing low FiO$_2$; home care patient requiring long-term therapy
	Nasal catheter	0.25-8 L/min	22-45	Variable	Use on adults, children, infants; good stability; disposable, low cost	Difficult to insert; high flows increase back pressure; needs regular changing; polyps, deviated septum may block insertion; may provoke gagging; air swallowing, aspiration	Procedures where cannula is difficult to use (bronchoscopy); long-term care for infants
	Transtracheal catheter	0.25-4 L/min	22-35	Variable	Lower O$_2$ usage/cost; eliminates nasal/skin irritation; improved compliance; increased exercise tolerance; increased mobility; enhanced image	High cost; surgical complications; infection; mucus plugging; lost tract	Home care or ambulatory patients who need increased mobility or who do not accept nasal oxygen
Reservoir	Reservoir cannula	0.25-4 L/min	22-35	Variable	Lower O$_2$ usage/cost; increased mobility; less discomfort because of lower flows	Unattractive, cumbersome; poor compliance; must be regularly replaced; breathing pattern affects performance	Home care or ambulatory patients who need increased mobility
	Simple mask	5-12 L/min	35-50	Variable	Use on adults, children, infants; quick, easy to apply; disposable, inexpensive	Uncomfortable; must be removed for eating; prevents radiant heat loss; blocks vomitus in unconscious patients	Emergencies, short-term therapy requiring moderate FiO$_2$
	Partial rebreathing mask	6-10 L/min (prevent bag collapse on inspiration)	35-60	Variable	Same as simple mask; moderate to high FiO$_2$	Same as simple mask; potential suffocation hazard	Emergencies, short-term therapy requiring moderate to high FiO$_2$
	Nonrebreathing mask	6-10 L/min (prevent bag collapse on inspiration)	55-70	Variable	Same as simple mask; high FiO$_2$	Same as simple mask; potential suffocation hazard	Emergencies, short-term therapy requiring high FiO$_2$
High-flow	Nonrebreathing circuit (closed)	3 × V$_E$ (prevent bag collapse on inspiration)	21-100	Fixed	Full range of FiO$_2$	Potential suffocation hazard; requires 50 psi air/O$_2$; blender failure common	Patients requiring precise FiO$_2$ at any level (21%-100%)
	Air-entrainment mask (AEM)	Varies; should provide output flow >60 L/min	24-50	Fixed	Easy to apply; disposable, inexpensive; stable, precise FiO$_2$	Limited to adult use; uncomfortable, noisy; must be removed for eating; FiO$_2$ >0.40 not ensured; FiO$_2$ varies with back-pressure	Unstable patients requiring precise low FiO$_2$
	Air-entrainment nebulizer	10-15 L/min input; should provide output flow ≥60 L/min	28-100	Fixed	Provides temperature control and extra humidification	FiO$_2$ <28% or >0.40 not ensured; FiO$_2$ varies with back-pressure; high infection risk	Patients with artificial airways requiring low to moderate FiO$_2$

Modified from Wilkins RL, et al, editors: *Egan's fundamentals of respiratory care*, ed 8, St Louis, 2003, Mosby.

$\dot{V}E$, minute volume.

inspiratory volume requirements, it results in a variable Fio_2 as the supplemental oxygen is mixed with room air. The patient's ventilatory pattern affects the Fio_2 of a low-flow system: as the ventilatory pattern changes, differing amounts of room air gas are mixed with the constant flow of oxygen. A nasal cannula is an example of a low-flow device.[3]

Reservoir Systems

A reservoir system incorporates some type of device to collect and store oxygen between breaths. When the patient's inspiratory flow exceeds the oxygen flow of the oxygen delivery system, the patient is able to draw from the reservoir of oxygen to meet his or her inspiratory volume needs. There is less mixing of the inspired oxygen with room air than in a low-flow system. A reservoir oxygen delivery system can deliver a higher Fio_2 than a low-flow system. Examples of reservoir systems are simple face masks, partial rebreathing masks, and nonrebreathing masks.[3]

High-Flow Systems

With a high-flow system, the oxygen flows out of the device and into the patient's airways in an amount sufficient to meet all inspiratory volume requirements. This type of system is not affected by the patient's ventilatory pattern. An air-entrainment mask is an example of a high-flow system.[3]

Complications of Oxygen Therapy

Oxygen, like most drugs, has adverse effects and complications resulting from its use. The adage "if a little is good, a lot is better" does not apply to oxygen. The lung is designed to handle a concentration of 21% oxygen, with some adaptability to higher concentrations, but adverse effects and oxygen toxicity can result if a high concentration is administered for too long.[4]

Oxygen Toxicity

The most detrimental effect of breathing a high concentration of oxygen is the development of oxygen toxicity. It can occur in any patient who breathes oxygen concentrations of greater than 50% for longer than 24 hours. Patients most likely to develop oxygen toxicity are those who require intubation, mechanical ventilation, and high oxygen concentrations for extended periods.[3]

Hyperoxia, or the administration of higher-than-normal oxygen concentrations, produces an overabundance of oxygen free radicals. These radicals are responsible for the initial damage to the alveolar-capillary membrane. Oxygen free radicals are toxic metabolites of oxygen metabolism. Normally, enzymes neutralize the radicals, preventing any damage from occurring. During the administration of high levels of oxygen, the large number of oxygen free radicals produced exhausts the supply of neutralizing enzymes. Damage to the lung parenchyma and vasculature occurs, resulting in the initiation of acute lung injury (ALI).[2,4]

A number of clinical manifestations are associated with oxygen toxicity. The first symptom is substernal chest pain that is exacerbated by deep breathing. A dry cough and

tracheal irritation follow. Eventually, there is definite pleuritic pain on inhalation, followed by dyspnea. Upper airway changes may include a sensation of nasal stuffiness, sore throat, and eye and ear discomforts. Chest radiographs and pulmonary function tests show no abnormalities until symptoms are severe. Complete, rapid reversal of these symptoms occurs as soon as normal oxygen concentrations are restored.[4]

Carbon Dioxide Retention

In patients with severe chronic obstructive pulmonary disease (COPD), carbon dioxide (CO_2) retention may occur as a result of administration of oxygen in high concentrations. A number of theories have been proposed for this phenomenon. One states that the normal stimulus to breathe (i.e., increasing CO_2 levels) is muted in patients with COPD and that decreasing oxygen levels become the stimulus to breathe. If hypoxemia is corrected by the administration of oxygen, the stimulus to breathe is abolished; hypoventilation develops, resulting in a further increase in the arterial partial pressure of carbon dioxide ($Paco_2$).[2,3] Another theory is that the administration of oxygen abolishes the compensatory response of hypoxic pulmonary vasoconstriction. This results in an increase in perfusion of underventilated alveoli and the development of dead space, producing ventilation/perfusion mismatching. As alveolar dead space increases, so does the retention of CO_2.[2,3,5] One further theory states that the rise in CO_2 is related to the ratio of deoxygenated to oxygenated hemoglobin (Haldane effect). Deoxygenated hemoglobin carries more CO_2 than oxygenated hemoglobin. Administration of oxygen increases the proportion of oxygenated hemoglobin, which causes increased release of CO_2 at the lung level.[5] Because of the risk of CO_2 accumulation, all chronically hypercapnic patients require careful low-flow oxygen administration.[3]

Absorption Atelectasis

Another adverse effect of high concentrations of oxygen is absorption atelectasis. Breathing high concentrations of oxygen washes out the nitrogen that normally fills the alveoli and helps hold them open (residual volume). As oxygen replaces the nitrogen in the alveoli, the alveoli start to shrink and collapse. This occurs because oxygen is absorbed into the bloodstream faster than it can be replaced in the alveoli, particularly in areas of the lungs that are minimally ventilated.[2,3]

Nursing Management

Nursing priorities for the patient receiving oxygen focus on (1) ensuring the oxygen is being administered as ordered and (2) observing for complications of the therapy. Confirming that the O_2 therapy device is properly positioned and replacing it after removal is important. During meals, an oxygen mask should be changed to a nasal cannula if the patient can tolerate one. The patient receiving O_2 therapy should also be transported with the oxygen. In addition, Spo_2 should be periodically monitored using a pulse oximeter.

ARTIFICIAL AIRWAYS

Pharyngeal Airways

Pharyngeal airways are used to maintain airway patency by keeping the tongue from obstructing the upper airway. The two types of pharyngeal airways are *oropharyngeal* and *nasopharyngeal*. Complications of these airways include trauma to the oral or nasal cavity, obstruction of the airway, laryngospasm, gagging, and vomiting.[6,7]

Oropharyngeal Airway

An oropharyngeal airway is made of plastic and is available in various sizes. The proper size is selected by holding the airway against the side of the patient's face and ensuring that it extends from the corner of the mouth to the angle of the jaw. If the airway is improperly sized, it will occlude the airway.[6,7] An oral airway is placed by inserting a tongue depressor into the patient's mouth to displace the tongue downward and then passing the airway into the patient's mouth, slipping it over the patient's tongue.[7] When properly placed, the tip of the airway lies above the epiglottis at the base of the tongue. It should be used only in an unconscious patient who has an absent or diminished gag reflex.[6,7]

Nasopharyngeal Airway

A nasopharyngeal airway is usually made of plastic or rubber and is available in various sizes. The proper size is selected by holding the airway against the side of the patient's face and ensuring that it extends from the tip of the nose to the earlobe.[6,7] A nasal airway is placed by lubricating the tube and inserting it midline along the floor of the naris into the posterior pharynx.[7] When properly placed, the tip of the airway lies above the epiglottis at the base of the tongue.[6,7]

Endotracheal Tubes

An endotracheal tube (ETT) is the most commonly used artificial airway for providing short-term airway management. Indications for endotracheal intubation include maintenance of airway patency, protection of the airway from aspiration, application of positive-pressure ventilation, facilitation of pulmonary toilet, and use of high oxygen concentrations.[8] An ETT may be placed through the orotracheal or the nasotracheal route.[9,10] In most situations involving emergency placement, the orotracheal route is used, because it is simpler and allows the use of a larger-diameter ETT.[10,11] Nasotracheal intubation provides greater patient comfort over time and is preferred in patients with a jaw fracture.[9,11,12] The advantages of orotracheal and nasotracheal intubation are presented in Table 16-2.

ETTs are available in various sizes, based on the inner diameter of the tube, and have a radiopaque marker that runs the length of the tube. On one end of the tube is a cuff that is inflated with the use of the pilot balloon. Because of the high incidence of cuff-related problems, low-pressure, high-volume cuffs are preferred. On the other end of the tube is a 15-mm adaptor that facilitates connection of the tube to a manual resuscitation bag (MRB), T-tube, or ventilator (Figure 16-1).[13]

Intubation

Before intubation, the necessary equipment is gathered and organized to facilitate the procedure. Readily available equipment should include a suction system with catheters and tonsil suction, an MRB with a mask connected to 100% oxygen, a laryngoscope handle with assorted blades, a variety of sizes of ETTs, and a stylet. Before the procedure is initiated, all equipment is inspected to ensure that it is in working order. The patient should be prepared for the procedure, if possible, with an intravenous catheter in place, and should be monitored with a pulse oximeter. The patient is sedated before the procedure (as clinical condition allows), and a topical anesthetic is applied to facilitate placement of the tube. In some cases, a paralytic agent may be necessary if the patient is extremely agitated.[9,11,14]

The procedure is initiated by positioning the patient with the neck flexed and head slightly extended in the "sniff" position. The oral cavity and pharynx are suctioned, and any dental devices are removed. The patient is preoxygenated and ventilated using the MRB and mask with 100% oxygen. Each

TABLE 16-2	**ADVANTAGES OF OROTRACHEAL, NASOTRACHEAL, AND TRACHEOSTOMY TUBES**	
OROTRACHEAL TUBES	**NASOTRACHEAL TUBES**	**TRACHEOSTOMY TUBES**
Easier access	Easily secured and stabilized	Easily secured and stabilized
Avoids nasal and sinus complications	Reduces risk of unintentional extubation	Reduces risk of unintentional decannulation
Allows for larger-diameter tube, which facilitates:	Well tolerated by patient	Well tolerated by patient
• Work of breathing	Enables swallowing and oral hygiene	Enables swallowing, speech, and oral hygiene
• Suctioning	Facilitates communication	Avoids upper airway complications
• Fiberoptic bronchoscopy	Avoids need for bite block	Allows for larger-diameter tube, which facilitates:
		• Work of breathing
		• Suctioning
		• Fiberoptic bronchoscopy

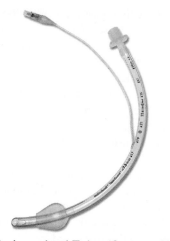

FIGURE 16-1 Endotracheal Tube. (Courtesy Nellcor Puritan Bennett, Pleasanton, Calif.)

intubation attempt is limited to 30 seconds. After the ETT is inserted, the patient is assessed for bilateral breath sounds and chest movement. Absence of breath sounds is indicative of an esophageal intubation, whereas breath sounds heard over only one side is indicative of a main stem intubation. A disposable end-tidal CO_2 detector is used to initially verify correct airway placement, after which the cuff of the tube is inflated and the tube is secured. Finally, a chest radiograph is obtained to confirm placement.[9-11] The tip of the ETT should be approximately 3 to 4 cm above the carina when the patient's head is in the neutral position.[10] After final adjustment of the position is complete, the level of insertion (marked in centimeters on the side of the tube) at the teeth is noted.[9,10,14]

A number of complications can occur during the intubation procedure, including nasal and oral trauma, pharyngeal and hypopharyngeal trauma, vomiting with aspiration, and cardiac arrest.[14] Hypoxemia and hypercapnia can also occur, resulting in bradycardia, tachycardia, dysrhythmias, hypertension, and hypotension.[8,12,14]

Complications

Several complications can occur while the ETT is in place, including nasal and oral inflammation and ulceration, sinusitis and otitis, laryngeal and tracheal injuries, and tube obstruction and displacement. Other complications can occur days to weeks after the ETT is removed, including laryngeal and tracheal stenosis and a cricoid abscess (Table 16-3). Delayed complications usually require some form of surgical intervention.[15]

Tracheostomy Tubes

A tracheostomy tube is the preferred method of airway maintenance in the patient who requires long-term intubation. Although no ideal time to perform the procedure has been identified, it is commonly accepted that if a patient has been intubated or is anticipated to be intubated for longer than 7

to 10 days, a tracheostomy should be performed.[16] A tracheostomy is also indicated in several other situations, such as the presence of an upper airway obstruction due to trauma, tumors, or swelling and the need to facilitate airway clearance due to spinal cord injury, neuromuscular disease, or severe debilitation.[17]

A tracheostomy tube provides the best route for long-term airway maintenance, because it avoids the oral, nasal, pharyngeal, and laryngeal complications associated with an ETT. The tube is shorter, of wider diameter, and less curved than an ETT; the resistance to air flow is less, and breathing is easier. Additional advantages of a tracheostomy tube include easier secretion removal, increased patient acceptance and comfort, capability of the patient to eat and talk if possible, and easier ventilator weaning.[11,17] Table 16-2 presents a list of the advantages of a tracheostomy tube.

Tracheostomy tubes are made of plastic or metal and may have one or two lumens. Single-lumen tubes consist of the tube; a built-in cuff, which is connected to a pilot balloon for inflation purposes; and an obturator, which is used during tube insertion. The double-lumen tubes consist of the tube with the attached cuff, the obturator, and an inner cannula that can be removed for cleaning and then reinserted or, if disposable, replaced by a new sterile inner cannula. The inner cannula can quickly be removed if it becomes obstructed, making the system safer for patients with significant secretion problems. Single-lumen tubes provide a larger internal diameter for airflow, so airflow resistance is reduced, and the patient can ventilate through the tube with greater ease. Plastic tracheostomy tubes also have a 15-mm adaptor on the end (Figure 16-2).[17,18]

Tracheostomy

A tracheostomy tube is inserted by an open procedure or a percutaneous procedure. An open procedure is usually performed in the operating room, whereas a percutaneous procedure can be done at the patient's bedside.[18]

A number of complications can occur during the tracheostomy procedure, including misplacement of the tracheal tube, hemorrhage, laryngeal nerve injury, pneumothorax, pneumomediastinum, and cardiac arrest.[15,18]

Complications

Several complications can occur while the tracheostomy tube is in place, including stomal infection, hemorrhage, tracheomalacia, tracheoesophageal fistula, tracheoinnominate artery fistula, and tube obstruction and displacement.[18] A number of complications can occur days to weeks after the tracheostomy tube is removed, including tracheal stenosis and tracheocutaneous fistula (Table 16-4). Delayed complications usually require some form of surgical intervention.[18]

Nursing Management

The patient with an endotracheal or tracheostomy tube requires some additional measures to address the effects associated with tube placement on the respiratory and other body

TABLE 16-3 COMPLICATIONS OF ENDOTRACHEAL TUBES

COMPLICATIONS	CAUSES	PREVENTION AND TREATMENT
Tube obstruction	Patient biting tube Tube kinking during repositioning Cuff herniation Dried secretions, blood, or lubricant Tissue from tumor Trauma Foreign body	*Prevention:* Place bite block. Sedate patient PRN. Suction PRN. Humidify inspired gases. *Treatment:* Replace tube.
Tube displacement	Movement of patient's head Movement of tube by patient's tongue Traction on tube from ventilator tubing Self-extubation	*Prevention:* Secure tube to upper lip. Restrain patient's hands as needed. Sedate patient PRN. Ensure that only 2 inches of tube extend beyond lip. Support ventilator tubing. *Treatment:* Replace tube.
Sinusitis and nasal injury	Obstruction of the paranasal sinus drainage Pressure necrosis of nares	*Prevention:* Avoid nasal intubations. Cushion nares from tube and tape or ties. *Treatment:* Remove all tubes from nasal passages. Administer antibiotics.
Tracheoesophageal fistula	Pressure necrosis of posterior tracheal wall, resulting from overinflated cuff and rigid nasogastric tube	*Prevention:* Inflate cuff with minimal amount of air necessary. Monitor cuff pressures every 8 hours. *Treatment:* Position cuff of tube distal to fistula. Place gastrostomy tube for enteral feedings. Place esophageal tube for secretion clearance proximal to fistula.
Mucosal lesions	Pressure at tube and mucosal interface	*Prevention:* Inflate cuff with minimal amount of air necessary. Monitor cuff pressures every 8 hours. Use appropriate size tube. *Treatment:* May resolve spontaneously. Perform surgical intervention.
Laryngeal or tracheal stenosis	Injury to area from end of tube or cuff, resulting in scar tissue formation and narrowing of airway	*Prevention:* Inflate cuff with minimal amount of air necessary. Monitor cuff pressures every 8 hours. Suction area above cuff frequently. *Treatment:* Perform tracheostomy. Place laryngeal stent. Perform surgical repair.
Cricoid abscess	Mucosal injury with bacterial invasion	*Prevention:* Inflate cuff with minimal amount of air necessary. Monitor cuff pressures every 8 hours. Suction area above cuff frequently. *Treatment:* Perform incision and drainage of area. Administer antibiotics.

PRN, as needed.

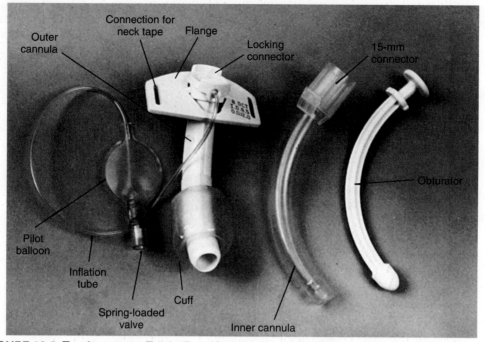

FIGURE 16-2 Tracheostomy Tube. (From Scanlan CL: Airway management. In Wilkins RL, et al, editors: *Egan's fundamentals of respiratory care,* ed 8, St Louis, 2003, Mosby.)

systems. **Nursing priorities for the patient with an artificial airway focus on (1) providing humidification, (2) maintaining the cuff management, (3) suctioning, (4) establishing a method of communication, and (5) providing oral hygiene.** Because the tube bypasses the upper airway system, warming and humidifying of air must be performed by external means. Because the cuff of the tube can cause damage to the walls of the trachea, proper cuff inflation and management is imperative. In addition, the normal defense mechanisms are impaired and secretions may accumulate; thus suctioning may be needed to promote secretion clearance. Because the tube does not allow air flow over the vocal cords, developing a method of communication is also very important. Last, observing the patient to ensure proper placement of the tube and patency of the airway is essential. Patient safety issues are addressed in the Patient Safety Priorities box on Artificial Airways.

⚡ **PATIENT SAFETY PRIORITIES**
Artificial Airways

In the event of unintentional extubation or decannulation, the patient's airway should be opened with the head tilt-chin lift maneuver and maintained with an oropharyngeal or nasopharyngeal airway. If the patient is not breathing, he or she should be manually ventilated with a manual resuscitation bag and face mask with 100% oxygen. In the case of a tracheostomy, the stoma should be covered to prevent air from escaping through it.

Humidification

Humidification of air normally is performed by the mucosal layer of the upper respiratory tract. When this area is bypassed, as occurs with ETT and tracheostomy tubes, or when supplemental oxygen is used, humidification by external means is necessary. Various humidification devices add water to inhaled gas to prevent drying and irritation of the respiratory tract, to prevent undue loss of body water, and to facilitate secretion removal.[19,20] The humidification device should provide inspired gas conditioned (heated) to body temperature and saturated with water vapor.[21]

Cuff Management

Because the cuff of the ETT or tracheostomy tube is a major source of the complications associated with artificial airways, proper cuff management is essential. To prevent the complications associated with cuff design, only low-pressure, high-volume cuffed tubes are used in clinical practice.[13,22] Even with these tubes, cuff pressures can be generated that are high enough to lead to tracheal ischemia and injury. Proper cuff inflation techniques and cuff pressure monitoring are critical components of the care of the patient with an artificial airway.[10,22]

Cuff Inflation Techniques. Two cuff inflation techniques are used: the minimal leak (ML) technique and the minimal occlusion volume (MOV) technique. The ML technique consists of injecting air into the cuff until no leak is heard and then withdrawing the air until a small leak is heard on inspiration. Problems with this technique include difficulty maintaining positive end-expiratory pressure (PEEP) and aspiration around the cuff. The MOV technique consists

TABLE 16-4	COMPLICATIONS OF TRACHEOSTOMY TUBES	
COMPLICATIONS	**CAUSES**	**PREVENTION AND TREATMENT**
Hemorrhage	Vessel opening after surgery Vessel erosion caused by tube	*Prevention:* Use appropriate size tube. Treat local infection. Suction gently. Humidify inspired gases. Position tracheal window not lower than third tracheal ring. *Treatment:* Pack lightly. Perform surgical intervention.
Wound infection	Colonization of stoma with hospital flora	*Prevention:* Perform routine stoma care. *Treatment:* Remove tube, if necessary. Perform aggressive wound care and debridement. Administer antibiotics.
Subcutaneous emphysema	Positive-pressure ventilation Coughing against a tight, occlusive dressing or sutured or packed wound	*Prevention:* Avoid suturing or packing wound closed around tube. *Treatment:* Remove any sutures or packing if present.
Tube obstruction	Dried blood or secretions False passage into soft tissues Opening of cannula positioned against tracheal wall Foreign body Tissue from tumor	*Prevention:* Suction PRN. Humidify inspired gases. Use a tube with a removable inner cannula. Position tube so that opening does not press against tracheal wall. *Treatment:* Remove/replace inner cannula. Replace tube.
Tube displacement	Patient movement Coughing Traction on ventilatory tubing	*Prevention:* Use commercial tube holder. Use tubes with adjustable neck plates for patients with short necks. Support ventilatory tubing. Sedate patient PRN. Restrain patient as needed. *Treatment:* Cover stoma and manually ventilate patient by mouth. Replace tube.
Tracheal stenosis	Injury to area from end of tube or cuff, resulting in scar tissue formation and narrowing of airway	*Prevention:* Inflate cuff with minimal amount of air necessary. Monitor cuff pressures every 8 hours. *Treatment:* Perform surgical repair.
Tracheoesophageal fistula	Pressure necrosis of posterior tracheal wall, resulting from overinflated cuff and rigid nasogastric tube	*Prevention:* Inflate cuff with minimal amount of air necessary. Monitor cuff pressures every 8 hours. *Treatment:* Perform surgical repair.
Tracheoinnominate artery fistula	Direct pressure from the elbow of the cannula against the innominate artery Placement of tracheal stoma below fourth tracheal ring Downward migration of the tracheal stoma, resulting from traction on tube High-lying innominate artery	*Prevention:* Position tracheal window not lower than third tracheal ring. *Treatment:* Hyperinflate cuff to control bleeding. Remove tube and replace with endotracheal tube and apply digital pressure through stoma against the sternum. Perform surgical repair.
Tracheocutaneous fistula	Failure of stoma to close after removal of tube	*Treatment:* Perform surgical repair.

PRN, as needed.

of injecting air into the cuff until no leak is heard at peak inspiration. This technique generates higher cuff pressures than does the ML technique. The selection of one technique over the other is determined by individual patient needs. If the patient needs a seal to provide adequate ventilation or is at high risk for aspiration, the MOV technique is used. If these are not concerns, usually the ML technique is used.[10,11,22]

Cuff Pressure Monitoring. Cuff pressures are monitored at least every shift with a cuff pressure manometer. Cuff pressures should be maintained at 20 to 25 mm Hg (24 to 30 cm H_2O), because greater pressures decrease blood flow to the capillaries in the tracheal wall and lesser pressures increase the risk of aspiration. Pressures in excess of 25 mm Hg (30 cm H_2O) should be reported to the physician. Cuffs are not routinely deflated, because this increases the risk of aspiration.[10,22]

Foam Cuff Tracheostomy Tubes. One tracheostomy tube on the market has a cuff made of foam that is self-inflating. It is deflated during insertion, after which the pilot port is opened to atmospheric pressure (room air), and the cuff self-inflates. After inflation, the foam cuff conforms to the size and shape of the patient's trachea, thereby reducing the pressure against the tracheal wall. The pilot port can be left open to atmospheric pressure or attached to the mechanical ventilator tubing, allowing the cuff to inflate and deflate with the cycling of the ventilator. Routine maintenance of a foam cuff tracheostomy tube includes aspirating the pilot port every 8 hours to measure cuff volume, to remove any condensation from the cuff area, and to assess the integrity of the cuff. Removal is accomplished by deflating the cuff; this can be complicated if the plastic sheath covering the foam is perforated. If perforation occurs, the foam may not be deflatable because the air cannot be totally aspirated.[23]

Suctioning

Suctioning is often required to maintain a patent airway in the patient with an ETT or tracheostomy tube. Suctioning is a sterile procedure that is performed only when the patient needs it and not on a routine schedule.[10,24] Indications for suctioning include coughing, secretions in the airway, respiratory distress, presence of rhonchi on auscultation, increased peak airway pressures on the ventilator, and decreasing oxygenation saturation.[11] Complications associated with suctioning include hypoxemia, atelectasis, bronchospasms, dysrhythmias, increased intracranial pressure, and airway trauma.[11,24]

Complications. Hypoxemia can result because the oxygen source is disconnected from the patient or the oxygen is removed from the patient's airways when the suction is applied. Atelectasis is thought to occur when the suction catheter is larger than one half of the diameter of the ETT. Excessive negative pressure occurs when suction is applied, promoting collapse of the distal airways. Bronchospasms are the result of stimulation of the airways with the suction catheter. Cardiac dysrhythmias, particularly bradycardias, are attributed to vagal stimulation. Airway trauma occurs with

impaction of the catheter in the airways and excessive negative pressure applied to the catheter.[10,11,24]

Suctioning Protocol. A number of protocols regarding suctioning have been developed. Several practices have been found helpful in limiting the complications of suctioning. Hypoxemia can be minimized by giving the patient three hyperoxygenation breaths (breaths at 100% Fio_2) with the ventilator before the procedure begins and again after each pass of the suction catheter.[10,25] If the patient exhibits signs of desaturation, hyperinflation (breaths at 150% tidal volume) should be added to the procedure.[10] Atelectasis can be avoided by using a suction catheter with an external diameter of less than one half of the internal diameter of the ETT.[24] Using no greater than 120 mm Hg of suction decreases the chances of hypoxemia, atelectasis, and airway trauma.[10] Limiting the duration of each suction pass to 10 to 15 seconds[10,24] and the number of passes to a maximum of three also helps minimize hypoxemia, airway trauma, and cardiac dysrhythmias.[26] The process of applying intermittent (instead of continuous) suction has been shown to be of no benefit.[27] The instillation of normal saline to help remove secretions has not proved to be of any benefit[24,28] and may actually contribute to the development of hypoxemia[10,29] and lower airway colonization, resulting in hospital-acquired pneumonia (HAP).[10,30]

Closed Tracheal Suction System. One device to facilitate the suctioning of a patient on a ventilator is the closed tracheal suction system (CTSS) (Figure 16-3). This device consists of a suction catheter in a plastic sleeve that attaches directly to the ventilator tubing. It allows the patient to be suctioned while remaining on the ventilator. Advantages of the CTSS include maintenance of oxygenation and PEEP during suctioning, reduction of hypoxemia-related complications, and protection of staff members from the patient's secretions. The CTSS is convenient to use, requiring only one person to perform the procedure.

Concerns related to the CTSS include autocontamination, inadequate removal of secretions, and increased risk of unintentional extubation resulting from the extra weight of the system on the ventilator tubing. Autocontamination has been shown not to be an issue if the catheter is cleaned properly after every use. Inadequate removal of secretions may or may not be a problem, and further investigation is required to settle this issue.[11] Although recommendations for changing the catheter vary, one study indicated that the catheter could be changed on an as-needed basis without increasing the incidence of HAP.[31]

Communication

One of the major stressors for the patient with an artificial airway is impaired communication. This is related to the inability to speak, insufficient explanations from staff members, inadequate understanding, fear of being unable to communicate, and difficulty with communication methods.[32] A number of interventions can facilitate communication in the patient with an ETT or tracheostomy tube. These include performing a complete assessment of the patient's ability to

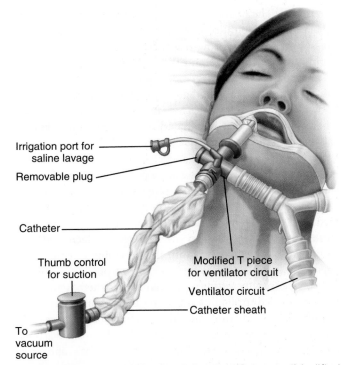

FIGURE 16-3 Closed Tracheal Suction System. (Modified from Sills JR: *Entry-level respiratory therapist exam guide,* St Louis, 2000, Mosby.)

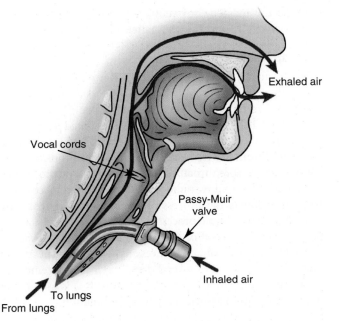

FIGURE 16-4 Passy-Muir Valve Mechanism of Action. (From Hodder RV: A 55-year-old patient with advanced COPD, tracheostomy tube, and sudden respiratory distress, *Chest* 121[1]:279, 2002.)

communicate, teaching the patient how to communicate, using a variety of methods to communicate, and facilitating the patient's ability to communicate by providing the patient with his or her eyeglasses or hearing aid.[33]

Methods to facilitate communication in this patient population include the use of verbal and nonverbal language and a variety of devices to assist the patient on short-term and long-term ventilator assistance. Nonverbal communication may include the use of sign language, gestures, lip-reading, pointing, facial expressions, or eye blinking. Simple devices available include pencil and paper; Magic Slates; magnetic boards with plastic letters; picture, alphabet, or symbol boards; and flash cards. More sophisticated devices include typewriters, computers, talking ETT and tracheostomy tubes, and external handheld vibrators. Regardless of the method selected, the patient must be taught how to use the device.[10,33]

Passy-Muir Valve. One device used to assist the mechanically ventilated patient with a tracheostomy to speak is the Passy-Muir valve. This one-way valve opens on inhalation, allowing air to enter the lungs through the tracheostomy tube, and closes on exhalation, forcing air over the vocal cords and out the mouth, permitting the patient to speak (Figure 16-4). Before the valve can be placed on a tracheostomy tube, the cuff must be deflated to allow air to pass around the tube, and the tidal volume of the ventilator must be increased to compensate for the air leak. In addition to aiding communication, the Passy-Muir valve can assist the ventilator-dependent patient with relearning normal breathing patterns. The valve is contraindicated in patients with laryngeal or pharyngeal dysfunction, excessive secretions, or poor lung compliance.[34]

Oral Hygiene

Patients with artificial airways are extremely susceptible to developing HAP due to microaspiration of subglottic secretions. Subglottic secretions are fluids from the oropharyngeal area that pool above the inflated cuff of the ETT or tracheostomy tube. These secretions are full of microorganisms from the patient's mouth. Because the cuff of the artificial airway does not create a tight seal in the patient's airway, these secretions seep around the cuff and into the patient's lungs, promoting the development of HAP.[35] Although bacteria are normally present in a patient's mouth, in the critically ill patient there are increased amounts of bacteria and more resistant bacteria. Decreased salivary flow, poor mucosal status, and dental plaque all contribute to this problem.[36]

Proper oral hygiene has the potential to decrease the incidence of HAP.[37] However, recent studies have shown that routine oral care is not a priority intervention for many nurses.[38] Currently there is no evidence-based protocol for oral care. Research studies are lacking, particularly with regard to frequency and effectiveness of different procedures.[39] Most experts agree, however, that oral care should consist of brushing the patient's teeth with a soft toothbrush to reduce plaque, brushing the patient's tongue and gums with a foam swab to stimulate the tissue, and performing deep oropharyngeal suctioning to remove any secretions that have pooled above the patient's cuff.[37-39] One intervention that has evidence supporting its use is rinsing the patient's mouth with chlorhexidine (15 mL of 0.12% oropharyngeal rinse applied twice daily for 30 seconds). This procedure has been shown to reduce oral colonization of bacteria and to decrease the incidence of ventilator-associated pneumonia, particularly in cardiac surgery patients.[40]

Extubation and Decannulation

After the airway is no longer needed, it is removed. Extubation is the process of removing an ETT. It is a simple procedure that can be accomplished at the bedside.[10,11] Before the cuff of an ETT or tracheostomy tube is deflated in preparation for removal, it is very important to ensure that secretions are cleared from above the tube cuff. Complications of extubation include sore throat, stridor, hoarseness, odynophagia, vocal cord immobility, pulmonary aspiration, and cough.[15] Decannulation is the process of removing a tracheostomy tube. It is also a simple process that can be performed at the bedside. After removal of the tracheostomy tube, the stoma is usually covered with a dry dressing, with the expectation that it will close within several days.[10,11] Difficulty removing the tracheostomy tube because of a tight stoma is usually the only complication associated with decannulation.[15]

INVASIVE MECHANICAL VENTILATION

Indications

Mechanical ventilation is the process of using an apparatus to facilitate the transport of oxygen and carbon dioxide between the atmosphere and the alveoli for the purpose of enhancing pulmonary gas exchange. It is indicated for physiological and clinical reasons. Physiological objectives include supporting cardiopulmonary gas exchange (alveolar ventilation and arterial oxygenation), increasing lung volume (end-expiratory lung inflation and functional residual capacity), and reducing the work of breathing. Clinical objectives include reversing hypoxemia and acute respiratory acidosis, relieving respiratory distress, preventing or reversing atelectasis and respiratory muscle fatigue, permitting sedation and neuromuscular blockade, decreasing oxygen consumption, reducing intracranial pressure, and stabilizing the chest wall.[41]

Use of Mechanical Ventilators

Types of Ventilators

The two main types of ventilators currently available are positive-pressure ventilators and negative-pressure ventilators. Negative-pressure ventilators are applied externally to the patient and decrease the atmospheric pressure surrounding the thorax to initiate inspiration. They generally are not used in the critical care environment. Positive-pressure ventilators use a mechanical drive mechanism to force air into the patient's lungs through an ETT or tracheostomy tube.[42]

Ventilator Mechanics

The ventilator must complete four phases of ventilation to properly ventilate the patient: (1) change from exhalation to inspiration; (2) inspiration; (3) change from inspiration to exhalation; and (4) exhalation. The ventilator uses four different variables to begin, sustain, and terminate each of these phases. These variables are described in terms of *volume, pressure, flow,* and *time*.[7,43,44]

Trigger. The phase variable that initiates the change from exhalation to inspiration is called the *trigger*. Breaths may be pressure-triggered or flow-triggered, based on the sensitivity setting of the ventilator and the patient's inspiratory effort; or they may be time-triggered, based on the rate setting of the ventilator. A breath that is initiated by the patient is known as a *patient-triggered* or *patient-assisted* breath, whereas a breath that is initiated by the ventilator is known as a *machine-triggered* or *machine-controlled* breath.

A *time-triggered breath* is a machine-controlled breath that is initiated by the ventilator after a preset length of time has elapsed. It is controlled by the rate setting on the ventilator (e.g., a rate of 10 breaths/minute yields 1 breath every 6 seconds). *Flow-triggered* and *pressure-triggered* breaths are patient-assisted breaths that are initiated by decreased flow or pressure, respectively, within the breathing circuit. Flow-triggering (also known as *flow-by*) is controlled by adjusting the flow-sensitivity setting of the ventilator, whereas pressure-triggering is controlled by adjusting the pressure-sensitivity setting. Many ventilators offer the various types of triggers in combination. For example, a breath may be time-triggered and flow-triggered, depending on the patient's ability to interact with the ventilator and initiate a breath.[7,42,43]

Limit. The variable that maintains inspiration is called the *limit* or *target*. Inspiration can be pressure-limited, flow-limited, or volume-limited. A *pressure-limited breath* is one in which a preset pressure is attained and maintained during inspiration. A *flow-limited breath* is one in which a preset flow is reached before the end of inspiration. A *volume-limited breath* is one in which a preset volume is delivered during the inspiration. However, the limit variable does not end inspiration; it only sustains it.[7,42,43]

Cycle. The variable that ends inspiration is called the *cycle*. The classification of positive-pressure ventilators is based on this variable: volume-cycled, pressure-cycled, flow-cycled, and time-cycled. *Volume-cycled ventilators* are designed to deliver a breath until a preset volume is delivered. *Pressure-cycled ventilators* deliver a breath until a preset pressure is reached within the patient's airways. *Flow-cycled ventilators* deliver a breath until a preset inspiratory flow rate is achieved. *Time-cycled ventilators* deliver a breath over a preset time interval.[7,42,43]

Baseline. The variable that is controlled during exhalation is called the *baseline*. Pressure is almost always used to adjust this variable. The patient exhales to a certain baseline pressure that is set on the ventilator. It may be set at zero (i.e., atmospheric pressure) or above atmospheric pressure (i.e., PEEP).[7,42,43]

Modes of Ventilation

The term *ventilator mode* refers to how the machine ventilates the patient. Selection of a particular mode of ventilation determines how much the patient will participate in his or her own ventilatory pattern. The choice depends on the patient's situation and the goals of treatment. The mode is determined by the combination of phase variables selected. Many modes are available (Table 16-5),[7,42-44] and some may be used in conjunction with others. Because brands of ventilators vary in their ability to perform certain functions, not all modes are available on all ventilators.[43]

Ventilator Settings

Settings on the ventilator allow the ventilator parameters to be individualized to the patient and also allow selection of the desired ventilation mode (Table 16-6). Each ventilator has a patient-monitoring system that allows all aspects of the patient's ventilatory pattern to be assessed, monitored, and displayed.[42-45]

Complications

Mechanical ventilation is often life-saving, but, like other interventions, it is not without complications. Some complications are preventable, whereas others can be

TABLE 16-5 MODES OF MECHANICAL VENTILATION		
MODE OF VENTILATION	**CLINICAL APPLICATION**	**NURSING IMPLICATIONS**
Continuous mandatory (volume or pressure) ventilation (CMV) also known as assist-control (AC) ventilation: delivers gas at preset tidal volume or pressure (depending on selected cycling variable) in response to patient's inspiratory efforts and initiates breath if patient fails to do so within preset time	Volume-controlled (VC) CMV is used as the primary mode of ventilation in spontaneously breathing patients with weak respiratory muscles. Pressure-controlled (PC) CMV is used in patients with decreased lung compliance or increased airway resistance, particularly when the patient is at risk for volutrauma.	Hyperventilation can occur in patients with increased respiratory rates. Sedation may be necessary to limit the number of spontaneous breaths. Patient on VC-CMV should be monitored for volutrauma. Patient on PC-CMV should be monitored for hypercapnia.
Pressure-regulated volume control ventilation (PRVCV): a variation of CMV that combines volume and pressure features; delivers a preset tidal volume using the lowest possible airway pressure; airway pressure will not exceed preset maximum pressure limit	PRVCV is used in patients with rapidly changing pulmonary mechanics (airway resistance and lung compliance), limiting potential complications.	
Pressure-controlled inverse ratio ventilation (PC-IRV): PC-CMV mode in which the inspiratory-to-expiratory (I:E) time ratio is greater than 1:1	PC-IRV is used in patients with hypoxemia refractory to positive end-expiratory pressure (PEEP); the longer inspiratory time increases functional residual capacity and improves oxygenation by opening collapsed alveoli, and the shorter expiratory time induces auto-PEEP that prevents alveoli from recollapsing.	Requires sedation or pharmacological paralysis, or both, because of discomfort. Increased intrathoracic pressure can result in excessive air trapping and decreased cardiac output.
Intermittent mandatory (volume or pressure) ventilation (IMV), also known as synchronous intermittent mandatory ventilation (SIMV): delivers gas at preset tidal volume or pressure (depending on selected cycling variable) and rate while allowing patient to breathe spontaneously; ventilator breaths are synchronized to patient's respiratory effort	VC-IMV is used as a primary mode of ventilation in many clinical situations and as a weaning mode. PC-IMV is used in patients with decreased lung compliance or increased airway resistance when the need to preserve the patient's spontaneous effects is important.	May increase the work of breathing and promote respiratory muscle fatigue. Patient should be monitored for hypercapnia, particularly with PC-IMV.
Adaptive support ventilation (ASV): ventilator automatically adjusts settings to maintain 100 mL/min/kg of minute ventilation; pressure support	ASV is a computerized mode of ventilation that increases or decreases ventilatory support based on patient needs; can be used with any patient requiring volume-controlled ventilation.	Not intended as a weaning mode. Adapts to changes in patient position.
Constant positive airway pressure (CPAP): positive pressure applied during spontaneous breaths; patient controls rate, inspiratory flow, and tidal volume	CPAP is a spontaneous breathing mode used in patients to increase functional residual capacity and improve oxygenation by opening collapsed alveoli at end expiration; it is also used for weaning.	Side effects include decreased cardiac output, volutrauma, and increased intracranial pressure. No ventilator breaths are delivered in PEEP or CPAP mode unless used with CMV or IMV.

Continued

TABLE 16-5 MODES OF MECHANICAL VENTILATION—cont'd

MODE OF VENTILATION	CLINICAL APPLICATION	NURSING IMPLICATIONS
Airway pressure release ventilation (APRV): two different levels of CPAP (inspiratory and expiratory) are applied for set periods of time, allowing spontaneous breathing to occur at both levels	APRV is a spontaneous breathing mode used to maintain alveolar recruitment without imposing additional peak inspiratory pressures that could lead to barotrauma.	Patient needs to be monitored for hypercapnia.
Pressure support ventilation (PSV): preset positive pressure used to augment patient's inspiratory efforts; patient controls rate, inspiratory flow, and tidal volume	PSV is a spontaneous breathing mode used as the primary mode of ventilation in patients with stable respiratory drive to overcome any imposed mechanical resistance (e.g., artificial airway). PSV can also be used with IMV to support spontaneous breaths.	Patient should be monitored for hypercapnia. Advantages include reduced patient work of breathing and improved patient-ventilator synchrony.
Volume-assured pressure support ventilation (VAPSV), also known as pressure augmentation (PA): a variation of PSV with a set tidal volume to ensure that patient receives minimum tidal volume with each pressure support breath	VAPSV is a spontaneous breathing mode used to treat acute respiratory illness and to facilitate weaning.	Advantages include increased patient comfort, decreased work of breathing, decreased respiratory muscle fatigue, and promotion of respiratory muscle conditioning.
Independent lung ventilation (ILV): each lung is ventilated separately	ILV is used in patients with unilateral lung disease, bronchopleural fistulas, or bilateral asymmetric lung disease.	Requires a double-lumen endotracheal tube, two ventilators, sedation, and/or pharmacological paralysis.
High-frequency ventilation (HFV): delivers a small volume of gas at a rapid rate High-frequency positive-pressure ventilation (HFPPV): delivers 60-100 breaths/min High-frequency jet ventilation (HFJV): delivers 100-600 cycles/min High-frequency oscillation (HFO): delivers 900-3000 cycles/min	HFV is used in situations in which conventional mechanical ventilation compromises hemodynamic stability, in patients with bronchopleural fistulas, during short-term procedures, and with diseases that create a risk of volutrauma.	Patients require sedation and/or pharmacological paralysis. Inadequate humidification can compromise airway patency. Assessment of breath sounds is difficult.

TABLE 16-6 VENTILATOR SETTINGS

PARAMETER	DESCRIPTION	TYPICAL SETTINGS
Respiratory rate (f)	Number of breaths the ventilator delivers per minute	6-20 breaths/min
Tidal volume (Vt)	Volume of gas delivered to patient during each ventilator breath	10-12 mL/kg 6-8 mL/kg in acute lung injury (ALI)
Oxygen concentration (FiO_2)	Fraction of inspired oxygen delivered to patient	May be set between 21% and 100%; adjusted to maintain PaO_2 level greater than 60 mm Hg or SpO_2 level greater than 90%
Positive end-expiratory pressure (PEEP)	Positive pressure applied at the end of expiration of ventilator breaths	3-5 cm H_2O
Pressure support (PS)	Positive pressure used to augment patient's inspiratory efforts	5-10 cm H_2O
Inspiratory flow rate and time	Speed with which the tidal volume is delivered	40-80 L/min Time: 0.8-1.2 sec
I:E ratio	Ratio of duration of inspiration to duration of expiration	1:2 to 1:1.5 unless inverse ratio ventilation is desired
Sensitivity	Determines the amount of effort the patient must generate to initiate a ventilator breath; it may be set for pressure-triggering or flow-triggering	Pressure trigger: 0.5-1.5 cm H_2O below baseline pressure Flow trigger: 1-3 L/min below baseline flow
High pressure limit	Regulates the maximal pressure the ventilator can generate to deliver the tidal volume; when the pressure limit is reached, the ventilator terminates the breath and spills the undelivered volume into the atmosphere	10-20 cm H_2O above peak inspiratory pressure

minimized but not eradicated. Physiological complications associated with mechanical ventilation include ventilator-induced lung injury, cardiovascular compromise, gastrointestinal disturbances, patient-ventilator dyssynchrony, and HAP.

Ventilator-Induced Lung Injury

Mechanical ventilation can cause two different types of injury to the lungs: air leaks and biotrauma.[44,46] Air leaks related to mechanical ventilation are the result of excessive pressure in the alveoli (barotrauma), excessive volume in the alveoli (volutrauma), or shearing due to repeated opening and closing of the alveoli (atelectrauma).[44,47] Barotrauma, volutrauma, and atelectrauma can lead to excessive alveolar wall stress and damage to the alveolar-capillary membrane, resulting in air leakage into the surrounding spaces. The air then travels out through the hilum and into the mediastinum (pneumomediastinum), pleural space (pneumothorax), subcutaneous tissues (subcutaneous emphysema), pericardium (pneumopericardium), peritoneum (pneumoperitoneum), and retroperitoneum (pneumoretroperitoneum). The resultant disorders vary from the fairly benign to the potentially lethal—the most lethal of which is a pneumothorax or pneumopericardium resulting in cardiac tamponade.[44,48]

Barotrauma, volutrauma, and atelectrauma can also cause the release of cellular mediators and initiation of the inflammatory-immune response. This type of ventilator-induced injury is known as biotrauma.[44,49] Biotrauma can result in the development of ALI.[50] To limit ventilator-induced lung injury, the plateau pressure (pressure needed to inflate the alveoli) should be kept at less than 32 cm H_2O, PEEP should be used to avoid end-expiratory collapse and reopening, and the tidal volume should be set at 6 to 10 mL/kg.[46,49]

Cardiovascular Compromise

Positive-pressure ventilation increases intrathoracic pressure, which decreases venous return to the right side of the heart. Impaired venous return decreases preload, which results in a decrease in cardiac output. As a secondary consequence, hepatic and renal dysfunction may occur. Positive-pressure ventilation impairs cerebral venous return. In patients with impaired autoregulation, positive-pressure ventilation can result in increased intracranial pressure.[44,51]

Gastrointestinal Disturbances

Gastrointestinal disturbances can occur as a result of positive-pressure ventilation. Gastric distention occurs when air leaks around the ETT or tracheostomy tube cuff and overcomes the resistance of the lower esophageal sphincter.[7] Vomiting can occur as a result of pharyngeal stimulation from the artificial airway.[15] These problems can be prevented by inserting a nasogastric tube and ensuring appropriate cuff inflation. Hypomotility and constipation may occur as a result of immobility and the administration of paralytic agents, analgesics, and sedatives.[7]

Patient-Ventilator Dyssynchrony

Because the ventilatory pattern is normally initiated by the establishment of negative pressure within the chest, the application of positive pressure can lead to patient difficulties in breathing while on the ventilator. To achieve optimal ventilatory assistance, the patient should breathe in synchrony with the machine. The selected mode of ventilation, the settings, and the type of ventilatory circuitry used can increase the work of breathing and lead to breathing out of synchrony with the ventilator. Patient-ventilatory dyssynchrony can result in decreased effectiveness of mechanical ventilation, the development of auto-PEEP, and psychological distress. Patients who are not breathing in synchrony with the ventilator appear to be fighting or "bucking" the ventilator. To minimize this problem, the ventilator is adjusted to accommodate the patient's spontaneous breathing pattern and to work with the patient. If this is not possible, the patient may need to be sedated or pharmacologically paralyzed.[43,52]

Ventilator-Associated Pneumonia

Ventilator-associated pneumonia (VAP) is a subgroup of HAP that refers to the development of pneumonia 48 to 72 hours after endotracheal intubation.[53] There is great potential for the development of pneumonia after placement of an artificial airway, because the tube bypasses or impairs many of the lung's normal defense mechanisms. After an artificial airway has been placed, contamination of the lower airways follows within 24 hours. This results from a number of factors that directly and indirectly promote airway colonization. The use of respiratory therapy devices (e.g., ventilators, nebulizers, intermittent positive-pressure breathing machines) also can increase the risk of pneumonia. The severity of the patient's illness and the presence of ALI or malnutrition significantly increase the likelihood that an infection will ensue. Therapeutic measures such as nasogastric tubes and gastric alkalinization with enteral feedings or medications facilitate the development of pneumonia. Nasogastric tubes promote aspiration by acting as a wick for stomach contents, whereas enteral feedings, antacids, histamine inhibitors, and proton-pump inhibitors increase the pH level of the stomach, promoting the growth of bacteria that can then be aspirated.[53] Additional information on managing the patient with pneumonia is provided in Chapter 15.

Prevention of VAP is critical. Several strategies may assist with prevention, including semirecumbent positioning, continuous aspiration of subglottic secretions (CASS), meticulous oral hygiene with antiseptics such as chlorhexidine (discussed earlier), and proper hand hygiene (Evidence-Based Practice box on Hand Hygiene Guidelines in Chapter 15).[53-55]

Semirecumbency. Positioning of the patient who requires mechanical ventilation is very important. Semirecumbent positioning (elevation of the head of the bed 30 to 45 degrees) reduces the incidence of gastroesophageal reflux and subsequent aspiration and decreases the incidence of VAP. The head of the patient's bed should be elevated to 30 to

45 degrees at all times unless contraindicated (e.g., hemodynamic instability, presence of intraaortic balloon pump, physician's order to the contrary).[53] However, this intervention does increase the risk of skin shear on the coccyx, and extra surveillance is mandatory for prevention of pressure ulcers.

Continuous Aspiration of Subglottic Secretions. Artificial airways are a significant risk factor for the development of VAP, because they allow for aspiration of bacteria-laden oropharyngeal and gastrointestinal secretions into the lungs. This occurs as a result of pooling of secretions from the mouth and stomach above the cuff of the artificial airway and leaking of the secretions around the cuff into the patient's airways.[35] Removal of the secretions from above the cuff by continuous aspiration has been shown to decrease the incidence of VAP.[56] CASS requires the use of a specialized ETT. A CASS tube has an additional lumen, with an opening above the cuff, which is connected to continuous (−20 mm Hg) or intermittent (−100 to −150 mm Hg) suction.[35,56] The tubes are recommended for patients who are expected to be intubated for longer than 48 hours. One problem with the CASS tube is that the aspiration lumen can become clogged with thick secretions, food particles, and clots.[35]

Other Measures to Reduce the Incidence of Ventilator-Associated Pneumonia. Recent studies have shown that use of an ETT with a polyurethane cuff may decrease the incidence of VAP. A traditional ETT has a polyvinyl low-pressure high-volume cuff. When the cuff is inflated, folds form in the cuff, allowing fluids and air to leak around the cuff and into the lungs. This is why subglottic secretion removal is so important. Polyurethane cuffs are much thinner than the traditional polyvinyl cuffs and do not form folds when they are inflated. There is no leakage of fluids into the lungs.[57]

Another recent study found that the use of silver-coated ETTs significantly reduced the incidence and delayed the onset of VAP, compared with a regular ETT. The tube decreased the incidence of VAP by preventing bacterial colonization and biofilm formation.[58] Biofilm is formed when bacteria cling to the inner lumen of the ETT and then secrete an exopolysaccharide substance. This substance forms a gelatinous matrix that allows bacteria to thrive on a non-biological surface.[59]

Weaning

Weaning is the gradual withdrawal of the mechanical ventilator and the reestablishment of spontaneous breathing. Weaning should begin only after the original process for which ventilator support was required has been corrected and patient stability has been achieved. Other factors to consider when weaning are length of time on ventilator, sleep deprivation, and nutritional status. Major factors that affect the patient's ability to wean include the ability of the lungs to participate in ventilation and respiration, cardiovascular performance, and psychological readiness.[60] This discussion focuses on weaning of the patient from short-term (≤3 days) mechanical ventilation. Management of weaning in the patient on long-term mechanical ventilation is discussed in Chapter 15.

Readiness to Wean

Patients should be screened every day for their readiness to wean. The screen should include an evaluation of the patient's level of consciousness, physiological and hemodynamic stability, adequacy of oxygenation and ventilation, spontaneous breathing capability, and respiratory rate and pattern. The rapid, shallow breathing index (RSBI) can predict weaning success. To calculate an RSBI, the patient's respiratory rate and minute ventilation are measured for 1 minute during spontaneous breathing. The measured respiratory rate is then divided by the tidal volume (expressed in liters). An RSBI of less than 105 is considered predictive of weaning success. If the patient is receiving sedation, the medication should be discontinued at least 1 hour before the RSBI is measured. If the patient meets criteria for weaning readiness and has an RSBI of less than 105, a spontaneous breathing trial can be performed.[61] One study showed that implementation of a weaning program that incorporated daily spontaneous-breathing trials had a positive impact on extubation rates and no effect on reintubation rates.[62]

After readiness to wean has been established, the patient is prepared for the weaning trial. The patient is positioned upright to facilitate breathing and suctioned to ensure airway patency. The process is explained to the patient, and the patient is offered reassurance and diversional activities. The patient is assessed immediately before the start of the trial and frequently during the weaning period for signs of weaning intolerance (Box 16-1).[60,61,63,64]

BOX 16-1 WEANING INTOLERANCE INDICATORS

- Decrease in level of consciousness
- Systolic blood pressure increased or decreased by 20 mm Hg
- Diastolic blood pressure greater than 100 mm Hg
- Heart rate increased by 20 beats/min
- Premature ventricular contractions greater than 6/min, couplets, or runs of ventricular tachycardia
- Changes in ST segment (usually elevation)
- Respiratory rate greater than 30 breaths/min or less than 10 breaths/min
- Respiratory rate increased by 10 breaths/min
- Spontaneous tidal volume less than 250 mL
- $Paco_2$ increased by 5 to 8 mm Hg and/or pH less than 7.30
- Spo_2 less than 90%
- Use of accessory muscles of ventilation
- Complaints of dyspnea, fatigue, or pain
- Paradoxical chest wall motion or chest abdominal asynchrony
- Diaphoresis
- Severe agitation or anxiety unrelieved by reassurance

Weaning Methods

A number of methods can be used to wean a patient from the ventilator. The method selected depends on the patient, his or her pulmonary status, and length of time on the ventilator. The three main methods for weaning are (1) T-tube (T-piece) trials, (2) synchronized intermittent mandatory ventilation (SIMV), and (3) pressure support ventilation (PSV).[60,63,65]

T-Piece Trials. T-piece weaning trials consist of alternating periods of ventilatory support (usually assist-control ventilation [ACV] or continuous mandatory ventilation [CMV]) with periods of spontaneous breathing. The trial is initiated by removing the patient from the ventilator and having the patient breathe spontaneously on a T-piece oxygen delivery system. After a set amount of time, the patient is placed back on the ventilator. The goal is to progressively increase the duration of time spent off the ventilator. During the weaning process, the patient is observed closely for respiratory muscle fatigue.[60-63,65] Constant positive airway pressure (CPAP) may be added to prevent atelectasis and improve oxygenation.[63,65]

Synchronized Intermittent Mandatory Ventilation Trials. The goal of SIMV weaning is the gradual transition from ventilatory support to spontaneous breathing. It is initiated by placing the ventilator in the SIMV mode and slowly decreasing the rate, usually one to three breaths at a time, until a rate of zero or near-zero is reached. An arterial blood gas (ABG) sample is usually obtained 30 minutes after the trial. This method of weaning can increase the work of breathing, and the patient must be closely monitored for signs of respiratory muscle fatigue.[60,63,65]

Pressure Support Ventilation Trials. PSV weaning consists of placing the patient on the pressure support mode and setting the pressure support at a level that facilitates the patient's achieving a spontaneous tidal volume of 10 to 12 mL/kg. PSV augments the patient's spontaneous breaths with a positive-pressure boost during inspiration. During the weaning process, the level of pressure support is gradually decreased in increments of 3 to 6 cm H_2O, while the tidal volume is maintained at 10 to 15 mL/kg, until a level of 5 cm H_2O is achieved. If the patient is able to maintain adequate spontaneous respirations at this level, extubation is considered. PSV also can be used with SIMV weaning to help overcome the resistance in the ventilator system.[60,63,65]

Nursing Management

Nursing priorities for the patient with invasive mechanical ventilation focus on (1) evaluating the patient for patient-related complications and (2) monitoring the patient for ventilator-related complications. Routine assessment of these patients includes monitoring for patient-related and ventilator-related complications. It includes a total patient assessment, with particular emphasis on the pulmonary system, placement of the ETT, and observation for subcutaneous emphysema and dyssynchrony with the ventilator. Assessment of the ventilator includes a review of all the ventilator settings and alarms. A clear understanding of the alarms and their related problems is important (Table 16-7).

TABLE 16-7	**TROUBLESHOOTING VENTILATOR ALARMS**	
PROBLEM	**CAUSES**	**INTERVENTIONS**
Low exhaled Vᴛ	Altered settings; any condition that triggers high- or low-pressure alarm; patient stops spontaneous respirations; leak in system preventing Vᴛ from being delivered; cuff insufficiently inflated; leak through chest tube; airway secretions; decreased lung compliance; spirometer disconnected or malfunctioning	Check settings; evaluate patient, check respiratory rate; check all connections for leaks; suction patient's airway; check cuff pressure; calibrate spirometer.
Low inspiratory pressure	Altered settings; unattached tubing or leak around ETT; ETT displaced into pharynx or esophagus; poor cuff inflation or leak; tracheoesophageal fistula; peak flows that are too low; low Vᴛ; decreased airway resistance resulting from decreased secretions or relief of bronchospasm; increased lung compliance resulting from decreased atelectasis; reduction in pulmonary edema; resolution of ALI; change in position	Reset alarm; reconnect tubing; modify cuff pressures; tighten humidifier; check chest tube; adjust peak flow to meet or exceed patient demand and correct for the patient's Vᴛ; reposition or change ETT.
Low exhaled minute volume	Altered settings; leak in system; airway secretions; decreased lung compliance; malfunctioning spirometer; decreased patient-triggered respiratory rate resulting from drugs, sleep, hypocapnia, alkalosis, fatigue, change in neurological status	Check settings; assess patient's respiratory rate, mental status, and work of breathing; evaluate system for leaks; suction airway; assess patient for changes in disease state; calibrate spirometer.
Low PEEP/CPAP pressure	Altered settings; increased patient inspiratory flows; leak; decreased expiratory flows from ventilator	Check settings and correct; observe for leaks in system; if unable to correct problem, increase PEEP settings.

TABLE 16-7   TROUBLESHOOTING VENTILATOR ALARMS—cont'd

PROBLEM	CAUSES	INTERVENTIONS
High respiratory rate	Increased metabolic demand; drug administration; hypoxia; hypercapnia; acidosis; shock; pain; fear; anxiety	Evaluate ABGs; assess patient; calm and reassure patient.
High-pressure limit	Improper alarm setting; airway obstruction resulting from patient fighting ventilator (holding breath as ventilator delivers VT); patient circuit collapse; tubing kinked; ETT in right main stem bronchus or against carina; cuff herniation; increased airway resistance resulting from bronchospasm, airway secretions, plugs, and coughing; water from humidifier in ventilator tubing; decreased lung compliance resulting from tension pneumothorax, change in patient position, ALI, pulmonary edema, atelectasis, pneumonia, or abdominal distention	Reset alarms; clear obstruction from tubing; unkink and reposition patient off of tubing; empty water from tubing; check breath sounds; reassure patient and sedate if necessary; check ABGs for hypoxemia; observe for abdominal distention that would put pressure on the diaphragm; check cuff pressures; obtain chest radiograph and evaluate for ETT position, pneumothorax, and pneumonia; reposition ETT; give bronchodilator therapy.
Low-pressure oxygen inlet	Improper oxygen alarm setting; oxygen not connected to ventilator; dirty oxygen intake filter	Correct alarm setting; reconnect or connect oxygen line to a 50-psi source; clean or replace oxygen filter.
I:E ratio	Inspiratory time longer than expiratory time; use of an inspiratory phase that is too long with a fast rate; peak flow setting too low while rate too high; machine too sensitive	Change inspiratory time or adjust peak flow; check inspiratory phase, or hold; check machine sensitivity.
Temperature	Sensor malfunction; overheating resulting from too low or no gas flow; sensor picking up outside airflow (from heater, open door or window, air conditioner); improper water levels	Test or replace sensor; check gas flow; protect sensor from outside source that would interfere with readings; check water levels.

Modified from Flynn JBM, Bruce NP: *Introduction to critical care nursing skills*, St. Louis, 1993, Mosby.
ABGs, arterial blood gases; *ALI*, acute lung injury; *CPAP*, constant positive airway pressure; *ETT*, endotracheal tube; *PEEP*, positive end-expiratory pressure; *Vt*, tidal volume.

The peak inspiratory pressure, exhaled tidal volume, and ABGs are also monitored. Issues regarding patient safety and patient transport are addressed, respectively, in the Patient Safety Priorities box on Invasive Mechanical Ventilation and the Evidence-Based Collaborative Practice box on Guidelines for Intrahospital Transport of Critically Ill Patients.

⚡ PATIENT SAFETY PRIORITIES

Invasive Mechanical Ventilation

Several measures are required to maintain a trouble-free ventilator system. These include maintaining a functional manual resuscitation bag connected to oxygen at the bedside, ensuring that the ventilator tubing is free of water, positioning the ventilator tubing to avoid kinking, maintaining the patency of ventilator tubing and connections, changing ventilator tubing per hospital policy, and monitoring the temperature of the inspired air. If the ventilator malfunctions, the patient is removed from the ventilator and ventilated manually with a manual resuscitation bag. Alarms should be sufficiently audible with respect to distance and competing noise within the unit.

EVIDENCE-BASED COLLABORATIVE PRACTICE

Summary of Guidelines for Intrahospital Transport of Critically Ill Patients

1. Pretransport Coordination and Communication
   * Confirm receiving unit readiness to receive patient.
   * Nurse to nurse handoff (if patient care responsibility is being transferred to a nurse in the receiving area)
   * Notify respiratory therapist and/or other members of the health care team of timing of transport and request equipment support as needed.
   * Mechanical ventilator in receiving unit (for mechanically ventilated patients)
2. Accompanying Personnel
   * A minimum of two people should accompany a critically ill patient (one of which should be a critical care nurse).
   * Unstable patients should be accompanied by a physician.
3. Accompanying Equipment
   * Blood pressure monitor or cuff
   * Pulse oximeter
   * Cardiac monitor with defibrillator

*Summary of Guidelines for Intrahospital
Transport of Critically Ill Patients*

- Basic resuscitation drugs (emergency cart should be readily available in receiving unit)
- Additional sedatives and narcotic analgesics
- Additional intravenous fluids and medications
- Oxygen delivery device attached to oxygen source with at least a 30-minute reserve or manual resuscitation bag and/or transport ventilator (for mechanically ventilated patients)
- Transport ventilator must have alarms and back up battery.

4. Monitoring During Transport
   - Continuous electrocardiographic monitoring
   - Continuous pulse oximetry
   - Periodic measurement of blood pressure, pulse rate, and respiratory rate

From Warren J, et al: Guidelines for the inter- and intrahospital transport of critically ill patients, *Crit Care Med* 32(1):256, 2004.

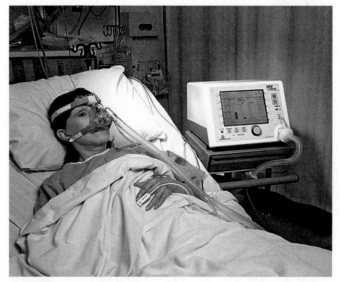

FIGURE 16-5 BiPAP Vision Face Mask in Use. (Courtesy Respironics Inc., Murrysville, Pa.)

Bedside evaluation of vital capacity, minute ventilation, ABG values, and other pulmonary function tests may be warranted, according to the patient's condition. The use of pulse oximetry can facilitate continuous, noninvasive assessment of oxygenation. Static and dynamic compliance should also be monitored to assess for changes in lung compliance (see Appendix B).[66]

NONINVASIVE POSITIVE-PRESSURE VENTILATION

Noninvasive positive-pressure ventilation (NPPV) is an alternative method of ventilation that uses a mask instead of an ETT to deliver the therapy. Advantages of this type of ventilation include decreased frequency of HAP, increased comfort, and the noninvasive nature of the procedure, which allows easy application and removal. It is indicated in type I and type II acute respiratory failure, cardiogenic pulmonary edema, and other situations in which intubation is not an option. Contraindications to NPPV include hemodynamic instability, dysrhythmias, apnea, uncooperativeness, intolerance of the mask, recent upper airway or esophageal surgery, and inability to maintain a patent airway, clear secretions, or properly fit the mask.[67]

NPPV can be applied with a nasal or facial mask and ventilator or with a BiPAP machine (Respironics Inc., Murrysville, Pa.) (Figure 16-5). One study found that a full-face mask is better tolerated than a nasal mask.[68] This type of ventilation uses a combination of PSV and PEEP supplied by a ventilator, or inspiratory and expiratory positive airway pressure (IPAP and EPAP, respectively) supplied by a BiPAP machine, to assist the spontaneously breathing patient with ventilation. On inspiration, the patient receives PSV or IPAP to increase tidal volume and minute ventilation, resulting in increased alveolar ventilation, a decreased $PaCO_2$ level, relief of dyspnea, and reduced accessory muscle use. On expiration, the patient receives PEEP or EPAP to increase functional residual capacity, resulting in an increased PaO_2 level. Humidified supplemental oxygen is administered to maintain a clinically acceptable PaO_2 level, and timed breaths may be added if necessary.[69]

Nursing Management

Nursing priorities for the patient with noninvasive mechanical ventilation focus on (1) evaluating the patient for patient-related complications and (2) monitoring the patient for ventilator-related complications. As with invasive mechanical ventilation, the patient must be closely monitored while receiving noninvasive mechanical ventilation. Respiratory rate, accessory muscle use, and oxygenation status are continually assessed to ensure that the patient is tolerating this method of ventilation. Continuous pulse oximetry with a set alarm parameter is also performed.[69,70]

The key to ensuring adequate ventilatory support is a properly fitted mask. A nasal mask or a full-face mask may be used, depending on the patient. A properly fitted mask minimizes air leakage and discomfort for the patient. Transparent dressings placed over the pressure points of the face help minimize air leakage and prevent facial skin necrosis caused by the mask. The BiPAP machine is able to compensate for air leaks.[70]

The patient is positioned with the head of the bed elevated at 45 degrees to minimize the risk of aspiration and to facilitate breathing. Insufflation of the stomach is a complication of this mode of therapy and places the patient at risk for aspiration. The patient is closely monitored for gastric distention, and a nasogastric tube is placed for decompression as necessary. Often patients are very anxious and have high levels of dyspnea before the initiation of noninvasive mechanical ventilation. After adequate ventilation has been established, anxiety and dyspnea are usually sufficiently relieved. Heavy sedation should be avoided, but if it is needed, it would constitute the need for intubation and invasive mechanical ventilation. It is important to spend 30 minutes with the patient after initiation of noninvasive ventilation, because the patient needs reassurance and must learn how to breathe on the machine.[68,70] Patient safety issues are addressed in the Patient Safety Priorities box on Noninvasive Mechanical Ventilation.

POSITIONING THERAPY

Positioning therapy can help match ventilation and perfusion through the redistribution of oxygen and blood flow in the lungs, which improves gas exchange. Based on the concept that there is preferential blood flow to the gravity-dependent areas of the lungs, positioning therapy is used to place the least damaged portion of the lungs into a dependent position. The least damaged portions of the lungs receive preferential blood flow, resulting in less ventilation/perfusion mismatching.[71] Currently, there are two approaches to position therapy: prone positioning and rotation therapy.

Prone Positioning

Prone positioning is a therapeutic modality that is used to improve oxygenation in patients with ALI.[72] It involves turning the patient completely over onto his or her stomach in the face-down position. Although a number of theories have been proposed to explain how prone positioning improves oxygenation, the discovery that ALI causes greater damage to the dependent areas of the lungs probably provides the best explanation. It was originally thought that ALI was a diffuse, homogenous disease that affected all areas of the lungs equally. It is now known that the dependent lung areas are more heavily damaged than the nondependent lung areas. Turning the patient prone improves perfusion to less damaged areas of the lungs, improves ventilation/perfusion matching, and decreases intrapulmonary shunting. Prone positioning can be used to facilitate the mobilization of secretions and provide pressure relief. Prone positioning is contraindicated in patients with increased intracranial pressure, hemodynamic instability, spinal cord injuries, or abdominal surgery.

Patients who are unable to tolerate a face-down position are also not appropriate candidates for this type of therapy.[73]

No standard has been established for the length of time a patient should remain in the prone position. A review of the research on this subject revealed a wide variation, anywhere from 30 minutes to 40 hours.[73] The therapy is considered successful if the patient has an improvement in Pao_2 of greater than 10 mm Hg within 30 minutes of being placed in the prone position.[73] The positioning schedule (length of time in prone position and frequency of turning) is usually based on the patient's tolerance of the procedure, the success of the procedure in improving the patient's Pao_2, and whether the patient is able to sustain improvements in Pao_2 when turned back to the supine position. Prone positioning is discontinued when the patient no longer demonstrates a response to the position change.[73]

The biggest limitation to prone positioning is the actual mechanics of turning the patient. A number of procedures have been discussed in the literature that advise using pillows to support the patient or using the Vollman Prone Positioner (Hill-Rom Inc., Batesville, Ind.) The latter is a steel frame with four cushions to support the patient's forehead, chin, chest, and pelvic area. The device is applied to the patient in the supine position and then used to turn the patient to the prone position (Figure 16-6). Regardless of the method used, the abdomen must be allowed to hang free to facilitate diaphragmatic descent.[73]

Before the patient is turned to the prone position, his or her eyes are lubricated and taped closed, tubes and drains are secured, and the procedure is explained to the patient and family. A team is organized to implement the turning procedure, and one member is positioned at the head of the bed to maintain the patient's airway. Complications of the procedure include dislodgment or obstruction of tubes and drains, hemodynamic instability, massive facial edema, pressure ulcers, aspiration, and corneal ulcerations.[73]

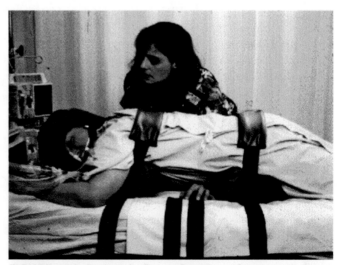

FIGURE 16-6 Patient in Prone Position. (Courtesy Kathleen Vollman.)

Rotation Therapy

Automated turning beds to provide rotation therapy are often used in the critical care setting. Kinetic therapy and continuous lateral rotation therapy (CLRT) are two forms of rotation therapy. The patient is continuously turned from side to side with a rotation of 40 degrees or greater (kinetic therapy) or with a rotation of less than 40 degrees (CLRT).[74] Two types of beds can perform this type of therapy: an oscillation bed, in which the mattress inflates and deflates to provide rotation; and a kinetic bed, in which the entire platform of the bed rotates.[75]

Rotation therapy is thought to improve oxygenation through better matching of ventilation to perfusion[76] and to prevent pulmonary complications associated with bed rest and mechanical ventilation.[77] However, to achieve such benefits, rotation must be aggressive, and the patient must be turned at least 40 degrees per side, with a total arc of at least 80 degrees,[78] for at least 18 hours a day.[77] CLRT has been shown to be of minimal pulmonary benefit to the critically ill patient.[74] Kinetic therapy decreases the incidence of VAP, particularly in neurological and postoperative patients.[78] In one study, kinetic therapy decreased the incidence of VAP and lobar atelectasis in medical, surgical, and trauma patients.[77]

Complications of the procedure include dislodgment or obstruction of tubes, drains, and lines; hemodynamic instability; and pressure ulcers. Lateral rotation does not replace manual repositioning to prevent pressure ulcers.[79] Repositioning changes the relationship of the patient's posterior surface to the mattress. This gives the skin a chance to reperfuse and to ventilate. Repositioning shifts weight-bearing points. To prevent pressure ulcers, the patient should be positioned 30 degrees from the surface of the mattress regardless of the degree of rotational turn. One study found that patients receiving rotational therapy still developed pressure ulcers of the sacrum, occiput, and heels.[80]

THORACIC SURGERY

Thoracic surgery refers to a number of surgical procedures that involve opening the thoracic cavity (thoracotomy) and/or the organs of respiration. Indications for thoracic surgery range from tumors and abscesses to repair of the esophagus and thoracic vessels.[81] Table 16-8 describes a variety

TABLE 16-8	THORACIC SURGERIES	
PROCEDURE	**DEFINITION**	**INDICATIONS**
Pneumonectomy	Removal of entire lung with or without resection of the mediastinal lymph nodes	Malignant lesions Unilateral tuberculosis Extensive unilateral bronchiectasis Multiple lung abscesses Massive hemoptysis Bronchopleural fistula
Lobectomy	Resection of one or more lobes of lung	Lesions confined to a single lobe Pulmonary tuberculosis Bronchiectasis Lung abscesses or cysts Trauma
Segmental resection	Resection of bronchovascular section of lung lobe	Small peripheral lesions Bronchiectasis Congenital cysts or blebs

Continued

TABLE 16-8   THORACIC SURGERIES—cont'd

PROCEDURE	DEFINITION	INDICATIONS
Wedge resection 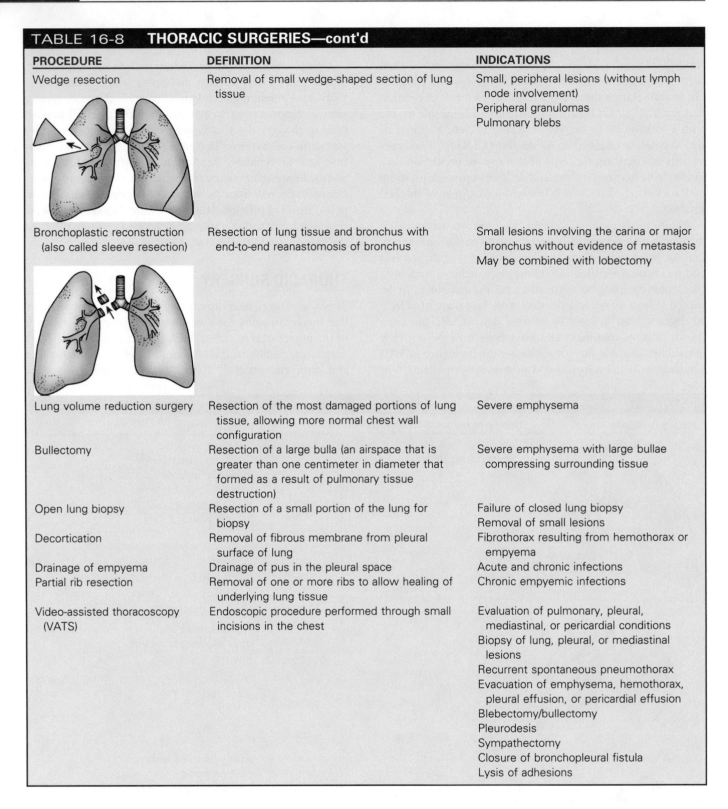	Removal of small wedge-shaped section of lung tissue	Small, peripheral lesions (without lymph node involvement) Peripheral granulomas Pulmonary blebs
Bronchoplastic reconstruction (also called sleeve resection)	Resection of lung tissue and bronchus with end-to-end reanastomosis of bronchus	Small lesions involving the carina or major bronchus without evidence of metastasis May be combined with lobectomy
Lung volume reduction surgery	Resection of the most damaged portions of lung tissue, allowing more normal chest wall configuration	Severe emphysema
Bullectomy	Resection of a large bulla (an airspace that is greater than one centimeter in diameter that formed as a result of pulmonary tissue destruction)	Severe emphysema with large bullae compressing surrounding tissue
Open lung biopsy	Resection of a small portion of the lung for biopsy	Failure of closed lung biopsy Removal of small lesions
Decortication	Removal of fibrous membrane from pleural surface of lung	Fibrothorax resulting from hemothorax or empyema
Drainage of empyema	Drainage of pus in the pleural space	Acute and chronic infections
Partial rib resection	Removal of one or more ribs to allow healing of underlying lung tissue	Chronic empyemic infections
Video-assisted thoracoscopy (VATS)	Endoscopic procedure performed through small incisions in the chest	Evaluation of pulmonary, pleural, mediastinal, or pericardial conditions Biopsy of lung, pleural, or mediastinal lesions Recurrent spontaneous pneumothorax Evacuation of emphysema, hemothorax, pleural effusion, or pericardial effusion Blebectomy/bullectomy Pleurodesis Sympathectomy Closure of bronchopleural fistula Lysis of adhesions

of thoracic surgical procedures and their indications. This discussion focuses only on the surgical procedures that involve the removal of lung tissue.

Preoperative Care

Before surgery, a complete evaluation of the patient is needed to determine the appropriateness of surgery as a treatment and to determine whether lung tissue can be removed without jeopardizing respiratory function. This is especially important when a lobectomy or pneumonectomy is being considered. When resection is being undertaken for tumor treatment, preoperative care includes evaluation of the type and extent of the tumor and the physical condition of the patient.[81]

The evaluation of the patient's physical status should focus on the adequacy of cardiopulmonary function. The preoperative evaluation should include pulmonary function tests to determine the patient's ability to manage with less lung tissue. Cardiac function also should be evaluated. Uncontrolled dysrhythmias, acute myocardial infarction, severe chronic heart failure, and unstable angina are all contraindications to surgery.[82]

Surgical Considerations

The type and location of surgery will dictate the type of surgical approach that is used. The most common approach is the posterolateral thoracotomy, which allows for exposure of both the lung and mediastinum. Other approaches that are used include anterolateral thoracotomy and median sternotomy.[81]

Special care is taken to avoid drainage of blood or secretions into the unaffected lung during surgery, because such an occurrence could cause hypoxemia and cardiac dysfunction. A double-lumen endotracheal tube is used during the surgery to protect the unaffected lung from secretions and necrotic tumor fragments. To decrease the incidence of hypoxemia during the procedure, 5 to 10 cm H_2O of PEEP is maintained to the deflated lung. In addition, the deflated lung is intermittently ventilated during the procedure.[83]

Complications and Medical Management

A number of complications are associated with a lung resection. These include acute respiratory failure, bronchopleural fistula, hemorrhage, cardiovascular disturbances, and mediastinal shift.

Acute Respiratory Failure

In the postoperative period, acute respiratory failure may result from atelectasis or pneumonia. Atelectasis can occur as a result of anesthesia, the surgical procedure, immobilization, and pain. Treatment should be aimed at correcting the underlying problems and supporting gas exchange. Supplemental oxygen and mechanical ventilation with PEEP may be necessary.[83]

Bronchopleural Fistula

Development of a postoperative bronchopleural fistula is a major cause of mortality after a lung resection. A bronchopleural fistula develops when the suture line fails to secure occlusion of the bronchial stump and an opening develops into the pleural space. This can result from an imperfect stump closure, perforation of the stump (e.g., with a suction catheter), high pressure within the airways (e.g., caused by mechanical ventilation),[84] or infection.[85] During surgery, careful attention is given to isolating and closing the bronchus in an attempt to secure a lasting seal with subsequent stump healing.[81] In addition, early extubation is encouraged to eliminate the possibility of perforation of the stump and high airway pressures.[84] Clinical manifestations of a bronchopleural fistula include shortness of breath and coughing up serosanguineous sputum. Immediate surgery is usually necessary to close the stump and prevent flooding of the remaining lung with fluid from the residual space.[85] If this occurs, the patient should be placed with the operative side down (remaining lung up) and a chest tube should be inserted to drain the residual space.[81]

Hemorrhage

Hemorrhage is an early, life-threatening complication that can occur after a lung resection. It can result from bronchial or intercostal artery bleeding or disruption of a suture or clip around a pulmonary vessel.[84] Excessive chest tube drainage can signal excessive bleeding. During the immediate postoperative period, chest tube drainage should be measured every 15 minutes; this frequency should be decreased as the patient stabilizes. If chest tube loss is greater than 100 ml/hour, fresh blood is noted, or a sudden increase in drainage occurs, hemorrhage should be suspected.

Cardiovascular Disturbances

Cardiovascular complications after thoracic surgery include dysrhythmias and pulmonary edema. Resections of a large lung area or a pneumonectomy may be followed by a rise in central venous pressure. With the loss of one lung, the right ventricle must empty its stroke volume into a vascular bed that has been reduced by 50%. This means a higher pressure system is created, which increases right ventricular workload and precipitates right ventricular failure. Depending on previous heart function, acute decompensation of both ventricles can result. Measures are aimed at supporting cardiac function and avoiding intravascular volume excess. These measures include optimizing preload, afterload, and contractility with vasoactive agents.[84]

Postoperative Nursing Management

Nursing care of the patient who has had thoracic surgery incorporates a number of nursing diagnoses (Nursing Diagnosis box on Thoracic Surgery). **Nursing priorities focus on (1) optimizing oxygenation and ventilation, (2) preventing atelectasis, (3) monitoring chest tubes, (4) assisting the patient to return to an adequate activity level, (5) providing comfort and emotional support, and (6) maintaining surveillance for complications.**

NURSING DIAGNOSIS PRIORITIES
Thoracic Surgery

- Ineffective Breathing Pattern related to decreased lung expansion, p. A-27
- Impaired Gas Exchange related to ventilation/perfusion mismatching or intrapulmonary shunting, p. A-23
- Impaired Gas Exchange related to alveolar hypoventilation, p. A-22
- Acute Pain related to transmission and perception of cutaneous, visceral, muscular, or ischemic impulses, p. A-5
- Anxiety related to threat to biological, psychological, or social integrity, p. A-7
- Disturbed Body Image related to actual change in body structures, function, or appearance, p. A-16
- Compromised Family Coping related to critically ill family member, p. A-9

Optimizing Oxygenation and Ventilation

Nursing interventions to optimize oxygenation and ventilation include positioning, preventing desaturation during procedures, and promoting secretion clearance.

Preventing Atelectasis

Nursing interventions to prevent atelectasis include proper patient positioning and early ambulation, deep-breathing exercises, incentive spirometry (IS), and pain management. The goal is to promote maximal lung ventilation and prevent hypoventilation.

Patient Positioning and Early Ambulation. The nurse should consider the surgical incision site and the type of surgery when positioning the patient. After a lobectomy, the patient should be turned onto the nonoperative side to promote V/Q matching. When the good lung is dependent and blood flow is greater to the area with better ventilation, V/Q matching is better. V/Q mismatching results when the affected lung is positioned down because of the increase in blood flow to an area with less ventilation. The patient should be turned frequently to promote secretion removal but should have the affected lung dependent as little as possible. The patient who has had a pneumonectomy should be positioned supine or on the operative side during the initial period. Turning onto the operative side promotes splinting of the incision and facilitates deep-breathing exercises. Tilting the patient slightly toward the unaffected side is possible, but the surgeon should indicate when free side-to-side positioning is safe.[85]

When sitting at the bedside or ambulating, patients must be encouraged to keep the thorax in straight alignment while they breathe deeply. This position best accommodates diaphragmatic descent and intercostal muscle action. The sitting or standing position provides enhanced ventilation to areas of the lung that are dependent in the supine position, thus accommodating maximal inflation and promoting gas exchange. Ambulation is essential in restoring lung function and should be initiated as soon as possible.[86]

Deep Breathing and Incentive Spirometry. Deep breathing and incentive spirometry should be performed regularly by patients who have undergone a thoracotomy. Deep breathing involves having the patient take a deep breath and holding it for approximately 3 seconds or longer. Incentive spirometry involves having the patient take at least 10 deep, effective breaths per hour using an incentive spirometer. These activities help reexpand collapsed lung tissue, thus promoting early resolution of the pneumothorax in patients with partial lung resections. The chest should be auscultated during inflation to ensure that all dependent parts of the lung are well ventilated and to help the patient understand the depth of breath necessary for optimal effect. Coughing, which should be encouraged only when secretions are present, assists in mobilizing secretions for removal.[86]

Pain Management. Pain can be a major problem after thoracic surgery. Pain can increase the workload of the heart, precipitate hypoventilation, and inhibit mobilization of secretions. Clinical manifestations of pain include tachypnea, tachycardia, elevated blood pressure, facial grimacing, splinting of the incision, hypoventilation, moaning, and restlessness. Several alternatives for pain management after thoracic surgery can be used. The two most common methods are systemic narcotic administration and epidural narcotic administration. Opioids can be administered intravenously or via patient-controlled analgesia (PCA) method. In addition, the patient should be assisted with splinting the incision with a pillow or blanket when deep breathing and coughing. Splinting stabilizes the area and reduces pain when moving, deep breathing, or coughing.[87]

Maintaining the Chest Tube System

Chest tubes are placed after most thoracic surgery procedures to remove air and fluid. The drainage will initially appear bloody, becoming serosanguineous and then serous over the first 2 to 3 days postoperatively. Approximately 100 to 300 mL of drainage will occur during the first 2 hours postoperatively, which will decrease to less than 50 mL/hour over the next several hours. Routine stripping of chest tubes is not recommended because excessive negative pressure can be generated in the chest. If blood clots are present in the drainage tubing or an obstruction is present, the chest tubes may be carefully milked. The chest tube may be placed to suction or water seal.[88]

During auscultation of the lungs, air leaks should be evaluated. In the early phase, an air leak is commonly heard over the affected area, because the pleura have not yet tightly sealed. As healing occurs, this leak should disappear. An increase in an air leak or the appearance of a new air leak should prompt investigation of the chest drainage system to discover whether air is leaking into the system from outside or whether the leak is originating from the incision. Increased air leaks not related to the thoracic drainage system may indicate disruption of sutures.[84]

Assisting Patient to Return to Adequate Activity Level

Within a few days after surgery, range-of-motion exercises for the shoulder on the operative side should be performed. The patient frequently splints the operative side and avoids shoulder movement because of pain. If immobility is allowed, stiffening of the shoulder joint can result. This is referred to as *frozen shoulder* and may require physical therapy and rehabilitation to regain satisfactory range of motion of the shoulder joint.[85]

Usually on the day after surgery, the patient is able to sit in a chair. Activity should be systematically increased, with attention to the patient's activity tolerance. With adequate pulmonary function before surgery and a surgical approach designed to preserve respiratory function, full return to previous activity levels is possible. This may take as long as 6 months to 1 year, depending on the tissue resected and the patient's general condition.[81]

SINGLE-LUNG AND DOUBLE-LUNG TRANSPLANTATIONS

Lung transplantation includes the transplantation of one or two lungs depending on the patient's underlying condition. Generally speaking, single-lung transplantation (SLT) is most appropriate for patients with restrictive lung diseases such as idiopathic pulmonary fibrosis and sarcoidosis or noninfectious obstructive lung diseases such as emphysema in the absence of significant cardiac dysfunction.[81] Pulmonary diseases that typically are associated with chronic lung infections, such as cystic fibrosis and bronchiectasis, require transplantation of both lungs because of the risk of cross-infection from the native lung into the transplanted lung.[89]

Single-Lung Transplant Surgical Procedure

Transplantation contralateral (opposite side) to a previous thoracotomy is preferable in order to avoid adhesions that require further surgical dissection. The left lung is sometimes preferred because it is easier to expose and has a longer left main bronchus. The longer bronchus gives the surgeon more flexibility in trimming the suture site as needed for anastomosis (Figure 16-7).[81] If there is a significant disproportion of ventilation and perfusion to one side, transplantation of the worse side may be the preferred option. With SLT, the remaining native lung, which has either restrictive or obstructive pathophysiology, will have a higher vascular resistance than the transplanted lung. The blood flow is then automatically directed toward the new lung.[90]

Use of cardiopulmonary bypass (CPB) is becoming less and less common during lung transplantation. However, patients with moderate to severe pulmonary hypertension generally require CPB because the clamping of the pulmonary artery necessary for removal of the diseased lung may cause sudden right heart failure. Inability to maintain adequate oxygenation and ventilation with a single lung, sudden increases in pulmonary artery pressure, poor right ventricular function, and hemodynamic compromise indicate the need for CPB.[89]

Double-Lung Transplant Surgical Procedure

The surgical procedure for both single- and double-lung transplantation (DLT) is similar, with a few exceptions. In fact, a DLT is performed as a bilateral, sequential SLT. The surgical incision for an SLT can be through either an anterolateral or posterolateral thoracotomy at the level of the fourth or fifth intercostal space. A DLT is performed through bilateral anterior thoracosternotomies extending from the midaxillary line and across the sternum at the fourth intercostal space. This approach is also known as a *clamshell incision*. The clamshell incision is exquisitely painful for the majority of patients, necessitating frequent pain assessment and intervention by the nurse. A median sternotomy or bilateral anterior thoracotomies are alternative surgical approaches.[81,91]

The anastomotic sites for DLT include the back wall of the atria (containing the four pulmonary vein orifices), the bronchus, and the main pulmonary artery as illustrated in Figure 16-8. Donor and recipient arteries are trimmed to suitable lengths, and an end-to-end anastomosis is performed. Bronchial anastomosis is performed with a running suture. After the atrial clamp is slowly removed, the patient is assessed for bleeding. In some transplant centers, the omentum is brought through the diaphragm from the abdomen and is wrapped around the bronchus for added stability of the anastomosis and increased vascular supply. Disadvantages of this maneuver include a larger incision and involvement of the abdominal cavity.[81]

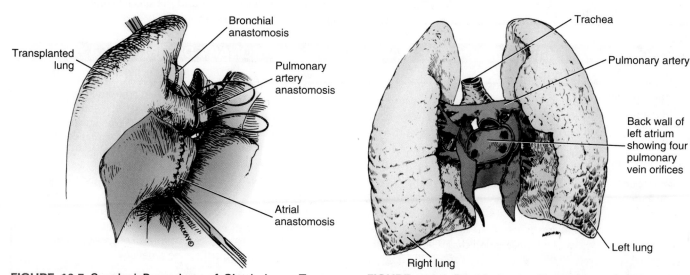

FIGURE 16-7 Surgical Procedure of Single-Lung Transplantation. (Modified from Baumgartner WA, et al: *Heart and heart-lung transplantation*, ed 2, Philadelphia, 2002, WB Saunders.)

FIGURE 16-8 Double-Lung Transplant Graft before Implantation into a Recipient. (Modified from Baumgartner WA, et al: *Heart and heart-lung transplantation*, ed 2, Philadelphia, 2002, WB Saunders.)

Living-Donor Lung Transplantation

Another alternative to traditional lung transplantation is living-donor lung transplantation. In living-donor transplantation, the lungs are harvested, not from a brain-dead donor, but from two living donors who provide either a right or left lower lobe to the recipient. The two donated lobes essentially function as new lungs. Recipients of this type of transplant tend to be patients with cystic fibrosis or other patients who are smaller in size. Smaller recipients increase the likelihood that two lobes are able to provide adequate pulmonary function. Living-donor lung transplantation is still fairly specialized and is therefore not as commonly practiced as cadaveric lung transplantation.[92]

Postoperative Medical and Nursing Management

Several nursing diagnoses are associated with the care of single-lung and double-lung transplant patients (Nursing Diagnosis Priorities box on Single-Lung and Double-Lung Transplantation). **Nursing priorities focus on (1) optimizing oxygenation and ventilation, (2) providing comfort and emotional support, and (3) maintaining surveillance for complications.** SLT patients generally require mechanical ventilation for a shorter duration. Less bleeding can be anticipated because of the brevity of the surgical procedure. A single pleural chest tube usually is sufficient for drainage. A pulmonary artery catheter may be used to measure right ventricular response when significant ventilation/perfusion (V/Q) mismatch occurs. In the event of elevated pulmonary artery pressures, pharmacological vasodilation or afterload reduction can be instituted. Patients with pulmonary hypertension potentially may have a greater V/Q mismatch, resulting in larger alveolar-arterial (A-a)O$_2$ gradients.

Surveillance for rejection and infection is critical. Pulmonary function testing is not initiated until the second or third week postoperatively to allow for surgical recovery. Decreased lung function because of fluid shifts, microatelectasis, and splinting from incisional pain would interfere with accurate testing. In unilateral lung transplantation, the transplanted lung functions in parallel with the native lung, which can be expected to retain any pathology. The patient must be measured by a comparison with his or her own baseline and not with normal standards. This concept also can be applied to the immediate postoperative period of intubation during the evaluation of arterial blood gases. Oxygenation and ventilation occur in both the diseased and transplanted lungs, and parameters for evaluation need to be adjusted accordingly.[93]

It is important that patient education is provided to cover all aspects of the immunosuppressive medication regimen, signs and symptoms of infection, role of pulmonary function tests, transbronchial biopsy, and clinical signs of pulmonary failure. In addition, a discussion of lifestyle adjustments, long-term considerations, and follow-up visits is included.

PHARMACOLOGY

A number of pharmacological agents are used in the care of the critically ill patient with pulmonary dysfunction. Table 16-9 reviews these agents and the special considerations necessary for administering them.[94]

NURSING DIAGNOSIS PRIORITIES

Single-Lung and Double-Lung Transplantation

- Ineffective Airway Clearance related to excessive secretions or abnormal viscosity of mucus, p. A-26
- Impaired Gas Exchange related to ventilation/perfusion mismatching or intrapulmonary shunting, p. A-23
- Risk for Infection, p. A-36
- Disturbed Body Image related to actual change in body structure, function, or appearance, p. A-16
- Anxiety related to threat to biological, psychological, and social integrity, p. A-7

TABLE 16-9 PHARMACOLOGICAL MANAGEMENT: PULMONARY DISORDERS

DRUG	DOSAGE	ACTIONS	SPECIAL CONSIDERATIONS
Neuromuscular Blocking Agents			Boxed Warning from FDA: Risk of anaphylactic and anaphylactoid type adverse reactions, including fatalities reported in association with use of neuromuscular blockers.
Vecuronium (Norcuron)	Loading dose: 0.08-0.1 mg/kg IV IV infusion: 0.8-1.2 mcg/kg/min	Used to paralyze patient to decrease oxygen demand and avoid ventilator dyssynchrony	Administer sedative and analgesic agents concurrently, because NMBAs have no sedative or analgesic properties.
Pancuronium (Pavulon)	Loading dose: 0.06-0.1 mg/kg IV IV infusion: 0.02-0.04 mg/kg/hr		Evaluate level of paralysis q4h using a peripheral nerve stimulator.
Rocuronium (Zemuron)	Loading dose: 0.6 mg/kg IV IV infusion: 10-12 mcg/kg/min		Protect patients from the environment, because they are unable to respond.

TABLE 16-9	PHARMACOLOGICAL MANAGEMENT: PULMONARY DISORDERS—cont'd		
DRUG	**DOSAGE**	**ACTIONS**	**SPECIAL CONSIDERATIONS**
Atracurium (Tracrium)	Loading dose: 0.30-0.50 mg/kg IV IV infusion: 4-12 mcg/kg/min		Prolonged muscle paralysis may occur after discontinuation of the paralytic agent.
Cisatracurium (Nimbex)	Loading dose: 0.15 to 0.2 mg/kg IV IV infusion: 0.5 to 10.2 mcg/kg/min)		
Mucolytics			
Acetylcysteine (Mucomyst)	Nebulizer, 20% solution: 3-5 mL tid-qid Nebulizer, 10% solution: 6-10 mL tid-qid	Used to decrease viscosity and elasticity of mucus by breaking down disulfide bonds within the mucus	May be administered with a bronchodilator, because drug can cause bronchospasms and inhibit ciliary function. Treatment is considered effective when bronchorrhea develops and coughing occurs. Antidote for acetaminophen overdose.
B₂-Agonists			
Epinephrine (Adrenalin)	Nebulizer, 1% solution: 2.5-5 mg (0.25-0.5 mL) qid	Used to relax bronchial smooth muscle and dilate airways to prevent bronchospasms	May cause skeletal muscle tremors. Higher doses may cause tachycardia, palpitations, increased blood pressure, dysrhythmias, and angina.
Racemic epinephrine	Nebulizer, 2.25% solution: 5.625-11.25 mg (0.25-0.5 mL) qid		
Isoetharine 1% (Bronkosol)	Nebulizer, 1% solution: 2.5-5 mg (0.25-0.5 mL) qid		May increase serum glucose and decrease serum potassium levels.
Terbutaline	MDI, 340 mcg/puff: 1-2 puffs qid MDI, 200 mcg/puff: 2 puffs q4-6h		Treatment is considered effective when breath sounds improve and dyspnea is lessened.
Metaproterenol (Alupent, Metaprel)	Nebulizer, 5% solution: 15 mg (0.3 mL) tid-qid MDI, 650 mcg/puff: 2-3 puffs tid-qid		Only approximately 10% of the administered dose reaches the site of action within the lungs.
Albuterol (Proventil, Ventolin)	Nebulizer, 5% solution: 2.5 mg (0.5 mL) tid-qid MDI, 90 mcg/puff: 2 puffs tid-qid		
Levalbuterol (Xopenex)	Nebulizer: 0.63 mg q6-8h		
Anticholinergic Agents			
Ipratropium (Atrovent)	Nebulizer, 0.02% solution: 0.5 mg (2.5 mL) q6-8h	Used to block the constriction of bronchial smooth muscle and reduce mucus production	There are relatively few adverse effects, because systemic absorption is poor.
Xanthines			
Theophylline	Loading dose: 4.6 mg/kg IV IV infusion: 0.4-0.8 mg/kg/hr	Used to dilate bronchial smooth muscle and reverse diaphragmatic muscle fatigue	Administer loading dose over 30 minutes. Monitor serum blood levels; therapeutic level is 10-20 mg/dL.
Aminophylline	Loading dose: 5.7mg/kg IV IV infusion: 0.5-1 mg/kg/hr		Administer with caution to patients with cardiac, renal, or hepatic disease. Signs of toxicity include central nervous system excitation, seizures, confusion, irritability, hyperglycemia, headache, nausea, hypotension, and dysrhythmias.

Continued

TABLE 16-9	PHARMACOLOGICAL MANAGEMENT: PULMONARY DISORDERS—cont'd		
DRUG	DOSAGE	ACTIONS	SPECIAL CONSIDERATIONS
Inhaled Corticosteroids			
Beclomethasone (Vanceril, Beclovent)	MDI, 42 mcg/puff: 2 puffs tid-qid	Used to decrease airway inflammation and enhance effectiveness of beta-agonists	Suppresses inflammatory response and interferes with ability to fight infection.
Flunisolide (AeroBid)	MDI, 250 mcg/puff: 2 puffs bid		Oral candidiasis is a side effect that can be minimized by having patients rinse their mouths after treatment.
Triamcinolone (Azmacort)	MDI, 100 mcg/puff: 2 puffs tid-qid		

MDI, metered-dose inhaler, NMBAs, neuromuscular blocking agents.

CASE STUDY   PATIENT WITH ACUTE RESPIRATORY FAILURE

Answers to the Case Study Questions can be found on the Evolve web site at http://evolve.elsevier.com/Urden/priorities/.

Brief Patient History

Mr. B is a 63-year-old obese man. He has a long history of chronic obstructive pulmonary disease (COPD) associated with smoking two packs of cigarettes a day for 40 years. During the past week, Mr. B has experienced a flulike illness with fever, chills, malaise, anorexia, diarrhea, nausea, vomiting, and a productive cough with thick, brownish, purulent sputum.

Clinical Assessment

Mr. B is admitted to the intermediate care unit from the emergency department with acute respiratory insufficiency. He is sitting up in bed, leaning forward, with his elbows resting on the over-the-bed table. Mr. B is breathing through his mouth, taking rapid shallow breaths, using his accessory muscles to ventilate. On inhalation, his nostrils flare and his accessory muscles retract. During exhalation, Mr. B uses pursed-lip breathing and his intercostal muscles bulge. He appears anxious and irritable and is able to speak only one or two barely audible words between each breath. Auscultation reveals crackles posteriorly over the right and left lower lung fields.

Diagnostic Procedures

His admission chest radiograph reveals infiltrates in the right lower lobe and left lower lobe. Gram stain of Mr. B's sputum shows numerous gram-positive diplococci. His baseline vital signs are as follows: blood pressure of 110/60 mm Hg, heart rate of 108 beats/min (sinus tachycardia), respiratory rate of 30 breaths/min, and temperature of 101.3° F. His baseline arterial blood gas (ABG) values on a 28% Venturi face mask are as follows: PaO_2 of 58 mm Hg, $PaCO_2$ of 33 mm Hg, pH of 7.52, HCO_3^- level of 28, and O_2 saturation of 88%.

Medical Diagnosis

Mr. B is diagnosed with community-associated pneumococcal pneumonia.

Questions

1. What major outcomes do you expect to achieve for this patient?
2. What problems or risks must be managed to achieve these outcomes?
3. What interventions must be initiated to monitor, prevent, manage, or eliminate the problems and risks identified?
4. What interventions should be initiated to promote optimal functioning, safety, and well-being of the patient?
5. What possible learning needs do you anticipate for this patient?
6. What cultural and age-related factors may have a bearing on the patient's plan of care?

REFERENCES

1. Henderson Y: Delivering oxygen therapy to acutely breathless adults, *Nurs Stand* 22(35):46, 2008.
2. O'Driscoll BR, et al: BTS guideline for emergency oxygen use in adult patients, *Thorax* 63(suppl 6):vi1, 2008.
3. Heuer AJ, Scanlan CL: Medical gas therapy. In Wilkins RL, Stoller JK, Kacmarek RM, editors: *Egan's fundamentals of respiratory care*, ed 9, St Louis, 2009, Mosby.
4. White AC: The evaluation and management of hypoxemia in the chronic critically ill patient, *Clin Chest Med* 22(1):123, 2001.
5. Kim V, et al: Oxygen therapy in chronic obstructive pulmonary disease, *Proc Am Thorac Soc* 5(4):513, 2008.
6. Barnes TA: Emergency cardiovascular life support. In Wilkins RL, Stoller JK, Kacmarek RM, editors: *Egan's fundamentals of respiratory care*, ed 9, St Louis, 2009, Mosby.
7. Pierce LNB: *Management of the mechanically ventilated patient*, ed 2, St Louis, 2007, Saunders.
8. McCorstin P, et al: Management of the mechanically ventilated patient in the emergency department, *J Emerg Nurs* 34(2):121, 2008.
9. Walz JM, Zayaruzny M, Heard SO: Airway management in critical illness, *Chest* 131(2):608, 2007.
10. St John RE, Seckel MA: Airway management. In Burns SM, editor: *AACN protocols for practice: care of the mechanically ventilated patient*, ed 2, Sudbury, Mass., 2007, Jones and Bartlett.

11. Simmons KF, Scanlan CL: Airway management. In Wilkins RL, Stoller JK, Kacmarek RM, editors: *Egan's fundamentals of respiratory care*, ed 9, St Louis, 2009, Mosby.

12. Chethan DB, Hughes RC: Tracheal intubation, tracheal tubes and laryngeal mask airways, *J Perioper Pract* 18(3):88, 2008.

13. Colice GL: Technical standards for tracheal tubes, *Clin Chest Med* 12(3):433, 1991.

14. Kabrhel C, et al: Orotracheal intubation, *N Eng J Med* 356(17):e15, 2007.

15. Feller-Kopman D: Acute complications of artificial airways, *Clin Chest Med* 24(3):445, 2003.

16. Durbin CG: Tracheostomy: why, when, and how? *Respir Care* 55(8):1056, 2010.

17. St John RE, Malen JF: Contemporary issues in adult tracheostomy management, *Crit Care Nurs Clin North Am* 16A(3):413, 2004.

18. Morris LL, Afifi, MS: *Tracheostomies: the complete guide*, New York, 2010, Springer.

19. Züchner K: Humidification: measurement and requirements, *Respir Care Clin N Am* 12(2):149, 2006.

20. Fink J: Humidity and bland aerosol therapy. In Wilkins RL, Stoller JK, Kacmarek RM, editors: *Egan's fundamentals of respiratory care*, ed 9, St Louis, 2009, Mosby.

21. Schulze A: Respiratory gas conditioning and humidification, *Clin Perinatol* 34(1):19, 2007.

22. Wright SE, VanDahm K: Long-term care of the tracheostomy patient, *Clin Chest Med* 24(3):473, 2003.

23. Bivona: *Fome-Cuf users manual*, Gary, Ind., 1991, Bivona.

24. American Association for Respiratory Care: AARC Clinical Practice Guidelines. Endotracheal suctioning of mechanically ventilated patients with artificial airways 2010, *Respir Care* 55(6):758, 2010.

25. Grap MJ, et al: Endotracheal suctioning: ventilator vs. manual delivery of hyperoxygenation breaths, *Am J Crit Care* 5(3):192, 1996.

26. Stone KS: Ventilator versus manual resuscitation bag as the method of delivering hyperoxygenation before endotracheal suctioning, *AACN Clin Issues Crit Care Nurs* 1(2):289, 1990.

27. Czarnik RE, et al: Differential effects of continuous versus intermittent suction on tracheal tissue, *Heart Lung* 20(2):144, 1991.

28. Raymond SJ: Normal saline instillation before suctioning: helpful or harmful? A review of the literature, *Am J Crit Care* 4(4):267, 1995.

29. Kinloch D: Instillation of normal saline during endotracheal suctioning: effects on mixed venous oxygen saturation, *Am J Crit Care* 8(4):231, 1999.

30. Hagler DA, Traver GA: Endotracheal saline and suction catheters: sources of lower airway contamination, *Am J Crit Care* 3(6):444, 1994.

31. Jelic S, Cunningham JA, Factor P: Clinical review: airway hygiene in the intensive care unit, *Crit Care* 12(2):209, 2008.

32. Jablonski RS: The experience of being mechanically ventilated, *Qual Health Res* 4(2):186, 1994.

33. Williams ML: An algorithm for selecting a communication technique with intubated patients, *Dimens Crit Care Nurs* 11(4):222, 1992.

34. Hodder RV: A 55-year-old patient with advanced COPD, tracheostomy tube, and sudden respiratory distress, *Chest* 121(1):279, 2002.

35. Scherzer R: Subglottic secretion aspiration in the prevention of ventilator-associated pneumonia, *Dimens Crit Care Nurs* 29(6):276, 2010.

36. Yoon MN, Steele CM: The oral care imperative: the link between oral hygiene and aspiration pneumonia, *Top Geri Rehab* 23(3):280, 2007.

37. Munro CL, Grap MJ: Oral health and care in the intensive care unit: state of the science, *Am J Crit Care* 13(1):25, 2004.

38. Binkley C, et al: Survey of oral care practices in U.S. intensive care units, *Am J Infect Control* 32(3):161, 2004.

39. Garcia R: A review of the possible role of oral and dental colonization on the occurrence of health-care associated pneumonia: underappreciated risk and a call for interventions, *Am J Infect Control* 33(9):527, 2005.

40. Chlebicki MP, Safdar N: Topical chlorhexidine for prevention of ventilator-associated pneumonia: a meta-analysis, *Crit Care Med* 35(2):595, 2007.

41. Haitsma JJ: Physiology of mechanical ventilation, *Crit Care Clin* 23(2):117, 2007.

42. Chatburn RL, Volsko TA: Mechanical ventilators. In Wilkins RL, Stoller JK, Kacmarek RM, editors: *Egan's fundamentals of respiratory care*, ed 9, St Louis, 2009, Mosby.

43. Pilbeam SP, Cairo SP: *Mechanical ventilation: physiological and clinical applications*, ed 4, St Louis, 2006, Mosby.

44. MacIntyre NR, Branson RD: *Mechanical ventilation*, ed 2, St Louis, 2009, Saunders.

45. Shelledy DC: Initiating and adjusting ventilatory support. In Wilkins RL, Stoller JK, Kacmarek RM, editors: *Egan's fundamentals of respiratory care*, ed 9, St Louis, 2009, Mosby.

46. Adams AB, Simonson DA, Dries DJ: Ventilator-induced lung injury, *Respir Care Clin N Am* 9(3):343, 2003.

47. Sarge T, Talmor D: Targeting transpulmonary pressure to prevent ventilator induced lung injury, *Minerva Anestesiol* 75(5):293, 2009.

48. Hemmila MR, Napolitano LM: Severe respiratory failure: advanced treatment options, *Crit Care Med* 34(suppl 9):S278, 2006.

49. Sarge T, Talmor D: Transpulmonary pressure: its role in preventing ventilator-induced lung injury, *Minerva Anestesiol* 74(6):335, 2008.

50. Oeckler RA, Hubmayr RD: Cell wounding and repair in ventilator injured lungs, *Respir Physiol Neurobiol* 163(1-3):44, 2008.

51. Frazier SK: Cardiovascular effects of mechanical ventilation and weaning, *Nurs Clin North Am* 43(1):1, 2008.

52. Unroe M, MacIntyre N: Evolving approaches to assessing and monitoring patient-ventilator interactions, *Curr Opin Crit Care* 16(3):261, 2010.

53. Rebmann T, Green LR: Preventing ventilator-associated pneumonia: An executive summary of the Association for Professionals in Infection Control and Epidemiology, Inc, Elimination Guide, *Am J Infect Control* 38(8):647, 2010.

54. Flanders SA, Collard HR, Saint S: Nosocomial pneumonia: state of the science, *Am J Infect Control* 34(2):84, 2006.

55. Aragon D, Sole ML: Implementing best practice strategies to prevent infection in the ICU, *Crit Care Nurs Clin North Am* 18(4):441, 2006.

56. Dezfulian C, et al: Subglottic secretion drainage for preventing ventilator-associated pneumonia: a meta-analysis, *Am J Med* 118(1):11, 2005.

57. Lorente L, et al: Influence of an endotracheal tube with polyurethane cuff and subglottic secretion drainage on pneumonia, *Am J Respir Crit Care Med* 176(11):1079, 2007.

58. Kollef MH, et al: Silver-coated endotracheal tubes and incidence of ventilator-associated pneumonia: the NASCENT randomized trial, *JAMA* 300(7):805, 2008.

59. Ramirez P, Ferrer M, Torres A: Prevention measures for ventilator-associated pneumonia: a new focus on the endotracheal tube, *Curr Opin Infect Dis* 20(2):190, 2007.

60. Shelledy DC: Discontinuing ventilatory support. In Wilkins RL, Stoller JK, Kacmarek RM, editors: *Egan's fundamentals of respiratory care*, ed 9, St Louis, 2009, Mosby.

61. MacIntyre N: Discontinuing mechanical ventilatory support, *Chest* 132(3):1049, 2007.

62. Robertson TE, et al: Improved extubation rates and earlier liberation from mechanical ventilation with implementation of a daily spontaneous-breathing trial protocol, *J Am Coll Surg* 206(3):489, 2008.

63. Burns SM: Weaning from mechanical ventilation. In Burns SM, editor: *AACN protocols for practice: care of the mechanically ventilated patient*, ed 2, Sudbury, Mass., 2007, Jones and Bartlett.

64. Siner JM, Manthous CA: Liberation from mechanical ventilation: what monitoring matters? *Crit Care Clin* 23(3):613, 2007.

65. Caroleo S, et al: Weaning from mechanical ventilation: an open issue, *Minerva Anestesiol* 73(7-8):417, 2007.

66. Bekos V, Marini JJ: Monitoring the mechanically ventilated patient, *Crit Care Clin* 23(3):575, 2007.

67. Garpestad E, Brennan J, Hill NS: Noninvasive ventilation for critical care, *Chest* 132(2):711, 2007.

68. Kwok H, et al: Controlled trial of oronasal versus nasal mask ventilation in the treatment of acute respiratory failure, *Crit Care Med* 31(2):468, 2003.

69. Barreiro TJ, Gemmel DJ: Noninvasive ventilation, *Crit Care Clin* 23(2):201, 2007.

70. Pierce LNB: Invasive and noninvasive modes and methods of mechanical ventilation. In Burns SM, editor: *AACN protocols for practice: care of the mechanically ventilated patient*, ed 2, Sudbury, Mass., 2007, Jones and Bartlett.

71. Misasi RS, Keyes JL: Matching and mismatching ventilation and perfusion in the lung, *Crit Care Nurse* 16(3):23, 1996.

72. Alsaghir AH, Martin CM: Effect of prone positioning in patients with acute respiratory distress syndrome: a meta-analysis, *Crit Care Med* 36(2):603, 2008.

73. Vollman KM: Prone positioning in the patient who has acute respiratory distress syndrome: the art and science, *Crit Care Nurs Clin North Am* 16(3):319, 2004.

74. Goldhill DR, et al: Rotational bed therapy to prevent and treat respiratory complications: a review and meta-analysis, *Am J Crit Care* 16(1):50, 2007.

75. Stiller K: Physiotherapy in intensive care: towards an evidence-based practice, *Chest* 118(6):1801, 2000.

76. Rance M: Kinetic therapy positively influences oxygenation in patients with ALI/ARDS, *Nurs Crit Care* 10(1):35, 2005.

77. Ahrens T, et al: Effect of kinetic therapy on pulmonary complications, *Am J Crit Care* 13(5):376, 2004.

78. Collard HR: Prevention of ventilator-associated pneumonia: an evidence-based systematic review, *Ann Intern Med* 138(6):494, 2003.

79. Powers J, Daniels D: Turning points: implementing kinetic therapy in the ICU, *Nurs Manage* 35(5):1, 2004.

80. Russell T, Logsdon A: Pressure ulcers and lateral rotation beds: a case study, *J Wound Ostomy Continence Nurs* 30(3):143, 2003.

81. Gregory Crum BS: Thoracic surgery. In Rothrock JC, editor: *Alexander's care of the patient in surgery*, ed 13, St Louis, 2007, Mosby.

82. Wadlund DL: Prevention, recognition, and management of nursing complications in the intraoperative and postoperative surgical patient, *Nurs Clin North Am* 41(2):151, 2006.

83. Grichnik KP, Clark JA: Pathophysiology and management of one-lung ventilation, *Thorac Surg Clin* 15(1):85, 2005.

84. Kopec SE, et al: The postpneumonectomy state, *Chest* 114(4):1158, 1998.

85. Brenner Z, Addona C: Caring for the pneumonectomy patient: challenges and changes, *Crit Care Nurse* 15(5):65, 1995.

86. Brooks JA: Postoperative nosocomial pneumonia: nurse-sensitive interventions, *AACN Clin Issues* 12(2):305, 2001.

87. Hazelrigg SR, Cetindag IB, Fullerton J: Acute and chronic pain syndromes after thoracic surgery, *Surg Clin North Am* 82(4):849, 2002.

88. Cerfolio RJ: Advances in thoracostomy tube management, *Surg Clin North Am* 82(4):833, 2002.

89. Hartwig MG, Davis RD Surgical considerations in lung transplantation: transplant operation and early postoperative management, *Respir Care Clin N Am* 10(4):473, 2004.

90. Trindade AJ, Palmer SM: Current concepts and controversies in lung transplantation, *Respir Care Clin N Am* 10(4):427, 2004.

91. Roselli EE, Smedira NG: Surgical advances in heart and lung transplantation, *Anesthesiol Clin North America* 22(4):789, 2004.

92. Bowdish ME, Barr ML: Living lobar lung transplantation, *Respir Care Clin N Am* 10(4):563, 2004.

93. Arcasoy SM: Medical complications and management of lung transplant recipients, *Respir Care Clin N Am* 10(4):505, 2004.

94. MICROMEDEX.

Neurological Clinical Assessment and Diagnostic Procedures

Kathleen M. Stacy

evolve WEBSITE

Be sure to check out the bonus material, including free self-assessment exercises, on the Evolve web site at
http://evolve.elsevier.com/Urden/priorities/.

OBJECTIVES

- Identify the components of a neurological history.
- Describe the five components of the neurological assessment.
- Discuss the neurological changes associated with intracranial hypertension.
- Identify key diagnostic procedures used in assessment of the patient with neurological dysfunction.

- Discuss the nursing management of a patient undergoing a neurological diagnostic procedure.
- Identify the different types of intracranial pressure monitoring devices.

Assessment of the critically ill patient with neurological dysfunction includes a review of the patient's health history, a thorough physical examination, and an analysis of the patient's laboratory data. Numerous invasive and noninvasive diagnostic procedures may be performed to assist in the identification of the patient's disorder. This chapter focuses on clinical assessments, laboratory studies, and diagnostic procedures for the critically ill patient with a neurological dysfunction.

CLINICAL ASSESSMENT

A thorough clinical assessment of the patient with neurological dysfunction is imperative for the early identification and treatment of neurological disorders. The completed assessment is used for developing the management plan for the patient. The assessment process can be brief or can involve a detailed history and examination, depending on the nature and immediacy of the patient's situation.

HISTORY

Neurological assessment encompasses a wide variety of applications and a multitude of techniques. This chapter focuses on the type of assessment performed in a critical care environment. Common to all neurological assessments is the need to obtain a comprehensive history of events preceding hospitalization. An adequate neurological history includes information about clinical manifestations, associated complaints, precipitating factors, progression, and familial occurrences. If the patient is incapable of providing this information, family members or significant others should be contacted as soon as possible. An ideal historian is able to provide detailed information with emphasis on the chronology of events.

Valuable information is gained through medical history that assists the patient's clinical assessment. When someone other than the patient is the source of the history, it should be an individual who was in contact with the patient on a daily basis. Frequently, valuable information is gained that directs the caregiver to focus on certain aspects of the patient's clinical assessment.[1]

PHYSICAL EXAMINATION

Five major components make up the neurological evaluation of the critically ill patient. **Nursing assessment priorities focus on evaluating (1) level of consciousness, (2) motor function, (3) pupillary function, (4) respiratory function, and (5) vital signs.** A complete neurological examination requires assessment of all five components.[1]

Level of Consciousness

Assessment of the level of consciousness is the most important aspect of the neurological examination. In most situations, a patient's level of consciousness deteriorates before any other neurological changes are noticed. These deteriorations often are subtle and must be monitored carefully. **Nursing priorities in assessment of level of consciousness focus on (1) evaluating arousal or alertness and (2) appraising consciousness or awareness.**[1] Although universally accepted definitions for various levels of consciousness do not exist, the categories outlined in Box 17-1 are often used to describe the patient's level of consciousness.[1-4]

Evaluating Arousal

Assessment of the arousal component of consciousness is an evaluation of the reticular activating system and its connection with the thalamus and the cerebral cortex. Arousal is the lowest level of consciousness, and observation centers on the patient's ability to respond to verbal or noxious stimuli in an appropriate manner. To stimulate the patient, the nurse should begin with verbal stimuli in a normal tone. If the patient does not respond, the nurse should increase the stimuli by shouting at the patient. If the patient still does not respond, the nurse should further increase the stimuli by shaking the patient. Noxious stimuli should follow if previous attempts to arouse the patient are unsuccessful. To assess arousal, central stimulation should be used (Box 17-2).

Appraising Awareness

Content of consciousness is a higher-level function, and appraisal of awareness is concerned with assessment of the patient's orientation to person, place, and time. Assessment of content of consciousness requires the patient to give appropriate answers to a variety of questions. Changes in the patient's answers that indicate increasing degrees of confusion and disorientation may be the first sign of neurological deterioration.[1,3,4]

Glasgow Coma Scale

The most widely recognized level of consciousness assessment tool is the Glasgow Coma Scale (GCS).[5] This scored scale is based on evaluation of three categories: eye opening, verbal response, and best motor response (Table 17-1). The best possible score on the GCS is 15, and the lowest score is 3. A score of 8 or less on the GCS usually indicates coma. Originally, the scoring system was developed to assist in general communication concerning the severity of neurological injury. Recent testing of the GCS revealed a moderate to high agreement rating among physicians and nurses.[6,7] Several points should be kept in mind when the GCS is used for serial assessment. It provides data about level of consciousness only, and it never should be considered a

---

BOX 17-1	CATEGORIES OF CONSCIOUSNESS
Alert	Patient responds immediately to minimal external stimuli.
Confused	Patient is disoriented to time or place but usually oriented to person, with impaired judgment and decision making and decreased attention span.
Delirious	Patient is disoriented to time, place, and person with loss of contact with reality and often has auditory or visual hallucinations.
Lethargic	Patient displays a state of drowsiness or inaction in which the patient needs an increased stimulus to be awakened.
Obtunded	Patient displays dull indifference to external stimuli, and response is minimally maintained. Questions are answered with a minimal response.
Stuporous	Patient can be aroused only by vigorous and continuous external stimuli. Motor response is often withdrawal or localizing to stimulus.
Comatose	Vigorous stimulation fails to produce any voluntary neural response.

From Barker E: *Neuroscience nursing: a spectrum of care,* ed 3, St Louis, 2008, Mosby.

BOX 17-2	STIMULATION TECHNIQUES IN PATIENT AROUSAL

Central Stimulation
- *Trapezius pinch:* Squeeze trapezius muscle between thumb and first two fingers.
- *Sternal rub:* Apply firm pressure to sternum with knuckles, using a rubbing motion.

Peripheral Stimulation
- *Nail bed pressure:* Apply firm pressure, using object such as a pen, to nail bed.
- *Pinching of inner aspect of arm or leg:* Firmly pinch small portion of patient's tissue on sensitive inner aspect of arm or leg.

TABLE 17-1	GLASGOW COMA SCALE	
CATEGORY	**SCORE**	**RESPONSE**
Eye opening	4	Spontaneous: eyes open spontaneously without stimulation
	3	To speech: eyes open with verbal stimulation but not necessarily to command
	2	To pain: eyes open with noxious stimuli
	1	None: no eye opening regardless of stimulation
Verbal response	5	Oriented: accurate information about person, place, time, reason for hospitalization, and personal data
	4	Confused: answers not appropriate to question, but use of language is correct
	3	Inappropriate words: disorganized, random speech, no sustained conversation
	2	Incomprehensible sounds: moans, groans, and incomprehensible mumbles
	1	None: no verbalization despite stimulation
Best motor response	6	Obeys commands: performs simple tasks on command; able to repeat performance
	5	Localizes to pain: organized attempt to localize and remove painful stimuli
	4	Withdraws from pain: withdraws extremity from source of painful stimuli
	3	Abnormal flexion: decorticate posturing spontaneously or in response to noxious stimuli
	2	Extension: decerebrate posturing spontaneously or in response to noxious stimuli
	1	None: no response to noxious stimuli; flaccid

complete neurological examination. It is not a sensitive tool for evaluation of an altered sensorium, nor does it account for possible aphasia. The GCS is also a poor indicator of lateralization of neurological deterioration.[7] Lateralization involves decreasing motor response on one side or unilateral changes in pupillary reaction.

Motor Function

Nursing priorities in assessment of motor function focus on (1) evaluating muscle size and tone and (2) estimating muscle strength. Each side should be assessed individually and then compared with the other.[1,8]

Evaluating Muscle Size and Tone

Initially, the muscles should be inspected for size and shape. The presence of atrophy is noted. Muscle tone is assessed by evaluating the opposition to passive movement. The patient is instructed to relax the extremity while the nurse performs passive range-of-motion movements and evaluates the degree of resistance. Muscle tone is appraised for signs of flaccidity (no resistance), hypotonia (little resistance), hypertonia (increased resistance), spasticity, or rigidity.[8]

Estimating Muscle Strength

Having the patient perform a number of movements against resistance assesses muscle strength. The strength of the movement is then graded on a 6-point scale (Box 17-3). Ask the patient to extend both arms with the palms turned upward and to hold that position with the eyes closed. If the patient has a weaker side, that arm will drift downward and pronate. The lower extremities are tested by asking the patient to push and pull the feet against resistance or to elevate the legs.[9,10]

Abnormal Motor Responses

If the patient is incapable of comprehending and following a simple command, noxious stimuli are necessary to determine motor responses. The stimulus is applied to each extremity

BOX 17-3	MUSCLE STRENGTH GRADING SCALE

0–No movement or muscle contraction
1–Trace contraction
2–Active movement with gravity eliminated
3–Active movement against gravity
4–Active movement with some resistance
5–Active movement with full resistance

BOX 17-4	CLASSIFICATION OF ABNORMAL MOTOR FUNCTION

Spontaneous	Occurs without regard to external stimuli and may not occur by request
Localization	Occurs when the extremity opposite the extremity receiving pain crosses midline of the body in an attempt to remove the noxious stimulus from the affected limb
Withdrawal	Occurs when the extremity receiving the painful stimulus flexes normally in an attempt to avoid the noxious stimulus
Decortication	Abnormal flexion response that may occur spontaneously or in response to noxious stimuli (Figure 17-1, *A* and *C*)
Decerebration	Abnormal extension response that may occur spontaneously or in response to noxious stimuli (Figure 17-1, *B* and *C*)
Flaccid	No response to painful stimuli

separately to allow evaluation of individual extremity function. Peripheral stimulation is used to assess motor function (see Box 17-2).[1,2] Motor responses elicited by noxious stimuli are interpreted differently from those elicited by voluntary demonstration. These responses may be classified as shown in Box 17-4.[8]

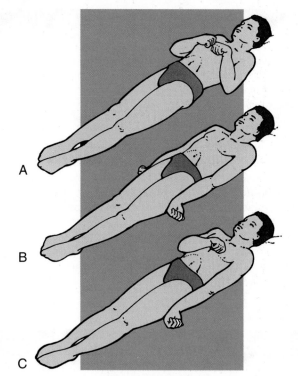

FIGURE 17-1 Abnormal Motor Responses. *A,* Decorticate posturing. *B,* Decerebrate posturing. *C,* Decorticate posturing on right side and decerebrate posturing on left side of body.

Abnormal flexion also is known as decorticate posturing (see Figure 17-1, *A*). In response to painful stimuli, the upper extremities exhibit flexion of the arm, wrist, and fingers with adduction of the limb. The lower extremity exhibits extension, internal rotation, and plantar flexion. Abnormal flexion occurs with lesions above the midbrain, located in the region of the thalamus or cerebral hemispheres. Abnormal extension also is known as decerebrate rigidity or posturing (see Figure 17-1, *B*); when the patient is stimulated, teeth clench, and the arms are stiffly extended, adducted, and hyperpronated. The legs are stiffly extended with plantar flexion of the feet. Abnormal extension occurs with lesions in the area of the brainstem. Because abnormal flexion and extension appear similar in the lower extremities, the upper extremities are used to determine the presence of these abnormal movements. It is possible for the patient to exhibit abnormal flexion on one side of the body and extension on the other (see Figure 17-1, *C*).[1-3] Outcome studies indicate that abnormal flexion or decorticate posturing has a less serious prognosis than does extension, or decerebrate posturing. Onset of posturing or a change from abnormal flexion to abnormal extension requires immediate physician notification.[3]

Pupillary Function

Nursing priorities in assessment of pupillary function focus on (1) estimating pupil size and shape, (2) evaluating pupillary reaction to light, and (3) assessing eye movements. Pupillary function is an extension of the autonomic nervous system. Parasympathetic control of the pupil occurs through innervation of the oculomotor nerve (CN III), which exits from the brainstem in the midbrain area. When the parasympathetic fibers are stimulated, the pupil constricts. Sympathetic control originates in the hypothalamus and travels down the entire length of the brainstem. When the sympathetic fibers are stimulated, the pupil dilates. Pupillary changes provide a valuable assessment tool because of pathway locations. The oculomotor nerve lies at the junction of the midbrain and the tentorial notch. Any increase of pressure that exerts force down through the tentorial notch compresses the oculomotor nerve. Oculomotor nerve compression results in a dilated, nonreactive pupil. Sympathetic pathway disruption occurs with involvement in the brainstem. Loss of sympathetic control leads to pinpoint, nonreactive pupils. Control of eye movements occurs with interaction of three cranial nerves: oculomotor (CN III), trochlear (CN IV), and abducens (CN VI). The pathways for these cranial nerves provide integrated function through the internuclear pathway of the medial longitudinal fasciculus (MLF) located in the brainstem. The MLF provides coordination of eye movements with the vestibular nerve (CN VIII) and the reticular formation.[3]

Estimating Pupil Size and Shape

Pupil diameter should be documented in millimeters with the use of a pupil gauge to reduce the subjectivity of description. Most people have pupils of equal size, between 2 and 5 mm. A discrepancy up to 1 mm between the two pupils is normal; it is called anisocoria and occurs in 16% to 17% of the human population.[11] Change or inequality in pupil size, especially in patients who previously have not shown this discrepancy, is a significant neurological sign. It may indicate impending danger of herniation and should be reported immediately. With the location of the oculomotor nerve (CN III) at the notch of the tentorium, pupil size and reactivity play a key role in the physical assessment of intracranial pressure (ICP) changes and herniation syndromes. In addition to CN III compression, changes in pupil size occur for other reasons. Large pupils can result from the instillation of cycloplegic agents, such as atropine or scopolamine, or can indicate extreme stress. Extremely small pupils can indicate opioid overdose, lower brainstem compression, or bilateral damage to the pons.[11,12]

Pupil shape is included in the assessment of pupils. Although the pupil is normally round, an irregularly shaped or oval pupil may be observed in patients who have undergone eye surgery. Initial stages of CN III compression from elevated ICP can cause the pupil to have an oval shape.[1,11]

Evaluating Pupillary Reaction to Light

The pupillary light reflex depends on optic nerve (CN II) and oculomotor nerve (CN III) function (Figure 17-2).[3,11] The technique for evaluation of the pupillary light response involves use of a narrow-beamed bright light shined into the pupil from the outer canthus of the eye. If the light is shined directly onto the pupil, glare or reflection of the light may prevent the assessor's proper visualization. Pupillary reaction to light is identified as brisk, sluggish, or nonreactive or fixed.[1] Each pupil should be evaluated for direct light response and for consensual response. The consensual pupillary response is constriction in response to a light shined into the opposite eye. This reflex occurs as a result of the crossing of nerve fibers at the optic chiasm.[1] Evaluation of consensual response is necessary to rule out optic nerve dysfunction as a cause for lack of a direct light reflex. Because the optic nerve is the afferent pathway for the light reflex, shining a light into a blind eye produces neither a direct light response in that eye nor a consensual response in the opposite eye. A consensual response in the blind eye produced by shining a light into

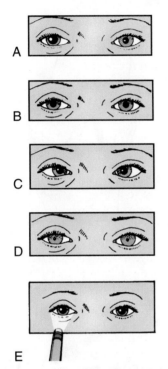

FIGURE 17-2 Abnormal Pupillary Responses. *A*, Oculomotor nerve compression. *B*, Bilateral diencephalon damage. *C*, Midbrain damage. *D*, Pontine damage. *E*, Dilated, nonreactive pupils.

the opposite eye demonstrates an intact oculomotor nerve. Oculomotor compression associated with transtentorial herniation affects the direct light response and the consensual response in the affected pupil.[1,2,11,12]

Assessing Eye Movement

In the conscious patient, the function of the three cranial nerves of the eye and their MLF innervation can be assessed by asking the patient to follow a finger through the full range of eye motion. If the eyes move together into all six fields, extraocular movements are intact (Figure 17-3).[1]

In the unconscious patient, assessment of ocular function and innervation of the MLF is performed by eliciting the doll's eyes reflex. If the patient is unconscious as a result of trauma, the nurse must ascertain the absence of cervical injury before performing this examination. To assess the oculocephalic reflex, the nurse holds the patient's eyelids open and briskly turns the head to one side while observing the eye movements and then briskly turns the head to the other side and observes. If the eyes deviate to the opposite direction in which the head is turned, the doll's eyes reflex is present, and the oculocephalic reflex arc is intact (Figure 17-4, *A*). If the oculocephalic reflex arc is not intact, the reflex is absent. This lack of response, in which the eyes remain midline and move with the head, indicates significant brainstem injury (Figure 17-4, *C*). The reflex may also be absent in severe metabolic coma. An abnormal oculocephalic reflex is present when the eyes rove or move in opposite directions from each other (Figure 17-4, *B*). Abnormal oculocephalic reflex indicates some degree of brainstem injury.[1-3]

The oculovestibular reflex is performed by a physician, often as one of the final clinical assessments of brainstem function. After confirmation that the tympanic membrane is intact, the head is raised to a 30-degree angle, and 20 to 100 mL of ice water is injected into the external auditory canal. The normal eye movement response is a conjugate, slow, tonic nystagmus deviating toward the irrigated ear and lasting 30 to 120 seconds. This response indicates brainstem integrity. Rapid nystagmus returns the eyes back to the midline only in a conscious patient with cortical functioning

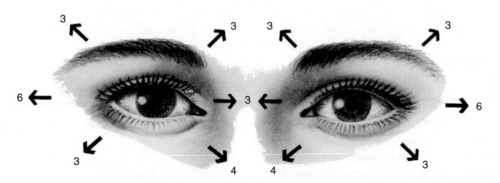

FIGURE 17-3 The Six Cardinal Directions of Gaze with Each Associated Cranial Nerve Supply. (From Seidel, HM et al: *Mosby's physical examination handbook*, ed 7, St Louis, 2010, Mosby.)

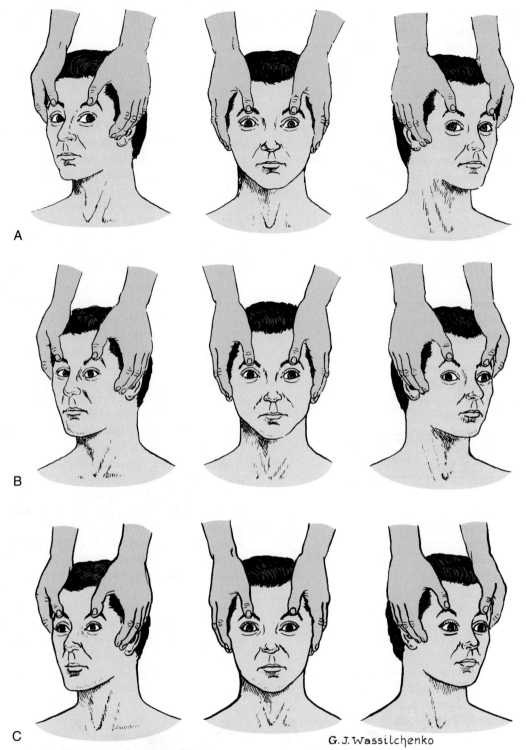

G.J.Wassilchenko

FIGURE 17-4 Oculocephalic Reflex (Doll's Eyes). *A*, Normal. *B*, Abnormal. *C*, Absent.

(Figure 17-5).[1] An abnormal response is disconjugate eye movement, which indicates a brainstem lesion, or no response, which indicates little or no brainstem function. The oculo-vestibular reflex may be temporarily absent in reversible metabolic encephalopathy.[3] This test is an extremely noxious stimulation and may produce a decorticate or decerebrate posturing response in a comatose patient. In the conscious patient, this procedure may produce nausea, vomiting, or dizziness.[1,12]

Respiratory Function

Nursing priorities in assessment of respiratory function focus on (1) observing respiratory pattern and (2) evaluating airway status. The activity of respiration is a highly

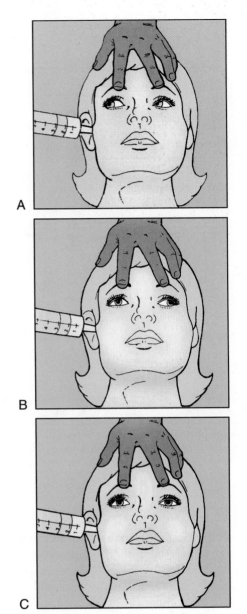

FIGURE 17-5 Oculovestibular Reflex (Cold Caloric Test). *A,* Normal. *B,* Abnormal. *C,* Absent.

TABLE 17-2	**RESPIRATORY PATTERNS**	
PATTERN OF RESPIRATION	**DESCRIPTION OF PATTERN**	**SIGNIFICANCE**
Cheyne-Stokes	Rhythmic crescendo and decrescendo of rate and depth of respiration; includes brief periods of apnea	Usually seen with bilateral deep cerebral lesions or some cerebellar lesions
Central neurogenic hyperventilation	Very deep, very rapid respirations with no apneic periods	Usually seen with lesions of the midbrain and upper pons
Apneustic	Prolonged inspiratory and/or expiratory pause of 2-3 sec	Usually seen in lesions of the middle to lower pons
Cluster breathing	Clusters of irregular, gasping respirations separated by long periods of apnea	Usually seen in lesions of the lower pons or upper medulla
Ataxic respirations	Irregular, random pattern of deep and shallow respirations with irregular apneic periods	Usually seen in lesions of the medulla

integrated function that receives input from the cerebrum, brainstem, and metabolic mechanisms. In clinical assessment, correlations exist among altered levels of consciousness, the level of brain or brainstem injury, and the patient's respiratory pattern. Under the influence of the cerebral cortex and the diencephalon, three brainstem centers control respirations. The lowest center, the medullary respiratory center, sends impulses through the vagus nerve to innervate muscles of inspiration and expiration. The apneustic and pneumotaxic centers of the pons are responsible for the length of inspiration and expiration and the underlying respiratory rate.[1-3]

Observing Respiratory Pattern

Changes in respiratory patterns assist in identifying the level of brainstem dysfunction or injury. Evaluation of the respiratory pattern must include assessment of the effectiveness of gas exchange in maintaining adequate oxygen and carbon dioxide levels (Table 17-2). Hypoventilation is not uncommon in the patient with an altered level of consciousness. Alterations in oxygenation or carbon dioxide levels can result in further neurological dysfunction. ICP increases with hypoxemia or hypercapnia.[1-3]

Evaluating Airway Status

Evaluation of the respiratory function in a patient with a neurological deficit must include assessment of airway maintenance and secretion control. Cough, gag, and swallow reflexes responsible for protection of the airway may be absent or diminished.[13]

Vital Signs

Nursing priorities in assessment of vital signs focus on (1) evaluating blood pressure and (2) monitoring heart rate and rhythm. As a result of the brain and brainstem influences on cardiac, respiratory, and body temperature functions, changes in vital signs can indicate deterioration in neurological status.

Evaluating Blood Pressure

A common manifestation of intracranial injury is systemic hypertension. Cerebral autoregulation, responsible for the control of cerebral blood flow (CBF), frequently is lost with any type of intracranial injury. After cerebral injury, the body

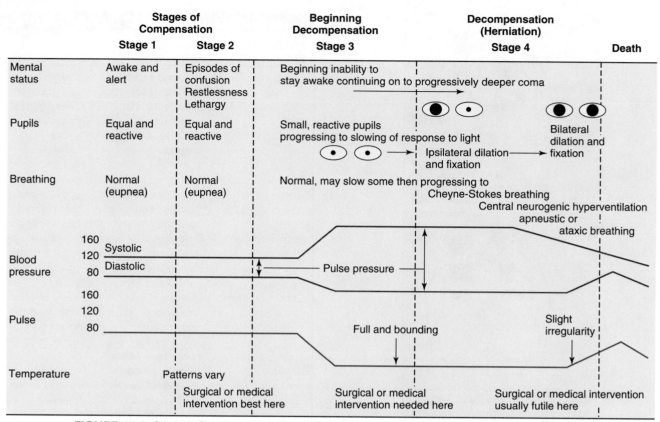

FIGURE 17-6 Clinical Correlates of Compensated and Decompensated Phases of Intracranial Hypertension. (From Beare PG, Myers JL: *Principles and practice of adult health nursing,* ed 3, St Louis, 1998, Mosby.)

often is in a hyperdynamic state (increased heart rate, blood pressure, and cardiac output) as part of a compensatory response. With the loss of autoregulation as blood pressure increases, CBF and cerebral blood volume increase, and ICP therefore increases. Control of systemic hypertension is necessary to stop this cycle, but caution must be exercised. The mean arterial pressure must be maintained at a level sufficient to produce adequate CBF in the presence of elevated ICP. Attention must also be paid to the pulse pressure because widening of this value may occur in the late stages of intracranial hypertension.[13]

Monitoring Heart Rate and Rhythm

The medulla and the vagus nerve provide parasympathetic control to the heart. When stimulated, this lower brainstem system produces bradycardia. Sympathetic stimulation increases the rate and contractility.[14] Various intracranial pathologies and abrupt ICP changes can produce bradycardia, premature ventricular contractions (PVCs), QT changes, and myocardial damage.[14,15]

Cushing's Triad

Cushing's triad is a set of three clinical manifestations (bradycardia, systolic hypertension, and widening pulse pressure) related to pressure on the medullary area of the brainstem.

These signs often occur in response to intracranial hypertension or a herniation syndrome. The appearance of Cushing's triad is a late finding that may be absent in patients with neurological deterioration. Attention should be paid to alteration in each component of the triad and intervention initiated accordingly.[3]

Neurological Changes Associated With Intracranial Hypertension

Assessment of the patient for signs of increasing ICP is an important responsibility of the critical care nurse. Increasing ICP can be identified by changes in level of consciousness, pupillary reaction, motor response, vital signs, and respiratory patterns (Figure 17-6).

LABORATORY STUDIES: LUMBAR PUNCTURE

The major laboratory study performed in the patient with neurological dysfunction is analysis of cerebrospinal fluid (CSF) obtained by a lumbar puncture or a ventriculostomy.[1-3] The main purpose of a lumbar puncture is to obtain CSF for analysis. CSF opening pressure may also be obtained. CSF samples are evaluated for the presence of subarachnoid blood or infection, or they are sent for laboratory analysis (Table 17-3).

TABLE 17-3	ANALYSIS OF CEREBROSPINAL FLUID		
CHARACTERISTIC	**NORMAL FINDINGS**	**ABNORMAL FINDINGS**	**POSSIBLE CAUSES AND COMMENTS**
Pressure	<200 mm H_2O	<60 mm H_2O	Faulty needle placement
			Dehydration
			Spinal block along subarachnoid space
			Block of foramen magnum
			Hydrocephalus
		>200 mm H_2O	Muscle tension
			Abdominal compression
			Brain tumor
			Subdural hematoma
			Brain abscess
			Brain cyst
			Cerebral edema (any cause)
Color	Clear, colorless	Cloudy or turbid	Cloudy as a result of microorganisms (e.g., WBCs)
			Turbid as a result of increased cell count
		Yellow (xanthochromic)	Breakdown of RBCs with RBC pigments, high protein count
		Smoky	RBCs
Blood	None	Red blood cells: blood tinged	Traumatic tap: bloody in first sample
		Grossly bloody	Traumatic tap: bloody in all samples
Volume	150 mL	Increase	Hydrocephalus
Specific gravity	1.007	Increase	Infection, presence of cells or protein
White blood cells (WBCs)	0-5 cells/mm^3	<500 cells/mm^3	Bacterial or viral infections of meninges, neurosyphilis, subarachnoid hemorrhage, infarction, abscess, tuberculous meningitis, metastatic lesions
		>500 cells/mm^3	Purulent infection
Glucose	50-75 mg/dL or 60%-70% of blood glucose	<40 mg/dL	Bacterial meningitis, tuberculosis, parasitic, fungal carcinomatous, subarachnoid hemorrhage
		>80 mg/dL	May not be of neurological significance
Chloride	700-750 mg/dL	Decreased (<625 mg/dL)	Meningeal infection, tuberculosis, meningitis, hypochloremia
		Increased (>800 mg/dL)	May not be of neurological significance; correlated with blood levels of chloride and not routine; done only on request
Culture and sensitivity	No organisms present	Neisseria or Streptococcus	Identify organisms to begin therapy; Gram stain for some cultures may take several weeks
Serology for syphilis	Negative	Positive	Syphilis
Protein	15-50 mg/dL	Increased (>60 mg/dL)	Bacterial meningitis, brain tumors (benign and malignant), complete spinal block, ALS, Guillain-Barré syndrome, subarachnoid hemorrhage, infarction, CNS trauma, CNS degenerative diseases, herniated disk, DM with polyneuropathy
		Decreased (<10 mg/dL)	May not be of neurological significance
Osmolality	295 Osm/L	Increased	Protein, WBCs, microorganisms, RBCs
Lactate	10-20 mg/dL	Increased	Bacterial, seizure activity, fungal meningitis, CNS trauma, coma related to toxic or metabolic causes

From Barker E: *Neuroscience nursing; a spectrum of care*, ed 3, St Louis, 2008, Mosby.
ALS, amyotrophic lateral sclerosis; *CNS*, central nervous system; *CSF*, cerebrospinal fluid; *DM*, diabetes mellitus; *RBC*, red blood cell; *WBC*, white blood cell.

DIAGNOSTIC PROCEDURES

Table 17-4 presents an overview of the various diagnostic procedures used to evaluate the patient with neurological dysfunction.

Nursing Management

The nursing management of a patient undergoing a diagnostic procedure involves a variety of interventions. **Nursing priorities are directed toward (1) preparing the patient psychologically and physically for the procedure, (2) monitoring**

TABLE 17-4   NEUROLOGICAL DIAGNOSTIC STUDIES

STUDY	PURPOSES	COMMENTS
Angiography	Visualizes extracranial and intracranial vasculature Identifies aneurysm, AVM, vasospasm, and vascular tumors Detects arterial occlusion and allows delivery of intraarterial therapy to restore blood flow	May cause local hematoma, vasospasm, vessel occlusion, allergic reaction to contrast media, and transient or permanent neurological dysfunction *Before test:* • Keep patient NPO for 4 hours and provide sedation before the study • Check for allergy to iodine • Evaluate renal function *After the test:* • Ensure hydration postprocedure (contrast medium used) • Maintain bed rest for 8-12 hours • Monitor arterial puncture point for hemorrhage or hematoma • Monitor neurovascular status of affected limb • Monitor for indications of systemic emboli • Reevaluate renal function
Cisternogram	Views CSF flow Identifies hydrocephalus Evaluates CSF leakage through a dural tear Evaluates abnormality of structures at the base of the brain and upper cervical cord region	Contraindicated in intracranial hypertension
CT computerized axial tomography	Views intracranial structures: size, shape, location, shifts Differentiates between tumors, hemorrhage, and infarction Identifies hydrocephalus, brain edema, infectious processes, trauma, aneurysm, hematoma, AVM, brain atrophy, and subacute and old brain infarction Evaluates arterial system if CT angiography studies performed	Patient must be cooperative Contrast media may be used; contrast media may be used after a noncontrast CT • Check for allergy to iodine or seafood before study • Patient will be NPO for 4-8 hours before the study • Sedation may be given • Monitor for signs of allergic reaction • Encourage fluid intake • Evaluate renal function when contrast media used
Digital subtraction angiography: brain; spine	Visualizes the vasculature, especially carotid and larger cerebral arteries Evaluates occlusive vascular disease Identifies tumors, aneurysms, AVM, vascular abnormalities	May be done IV or intraarterially • If IV, is less invasive with fewer complications than cerebral angiography • If intraarterially, care as for angiogram • Contrast media are used • Check for allergy to iodine, seafood before study • Patient will be NPO for 4-8 hours before the study • Monitor for signs of allergic reaction • Encourage fluid intake
Electroencephalography	Differentiates epilepsy from mass lesion Detects focus of seizure activity Evaluates drug intoxication Evaluates electrical function of the brain, which may be abnormal in the presence of cerebrovascular alterations Localizes tumor, abscess, and other mass lesions May be used in designation of brain death	Stimulants, anticonvulsants, tranquilizer, and antidepressants may be withheld for 24-48 hours before the study Hair shampooed before and after study
Electromyography; nerve conduction velocity studies	Detects muscle disease Identifies peripheral neuropathies, nerve compression Identifies nerve regeneration and muscle recovery	Patient must be cooperative Contraindicated in patients taking anticoagulants, with bleeding disorders, or skin infection May be uncomfortable for patient

TABLE 17-4	**NEUROLOGICAL DIAGNOSTIC STUDIES—cont'd**	
STUDY	**PURPOSES**	**COMMENTS**
Electronystagmography	Detects nystagmus, which may aid in identification of cerebellar or vestibular problem	
Evoked potential studies	Evaluates electrical potentials (responses) of brain to external stimuli; evaluate sensory and somatosensory neurological pathways	Hair shampooed before and after study
	Identifies neuromuscular disease, cerebrovascular disease, spinal cord injury, traumatic brain injury, peripheral nerve disease, and tumors	
	Determines prognosis in traumatic brain injury	
	Contributes to diagnosis of multiple sclerosis and brainstem injury	
Isotope ventriculography	Visualizes CSF circulation system	No CSF withdrawn
		May cause meningeal irritation and aseptic meningitis
Lumbar puncture or cisternal puncture	Obtains CSF for analysis	Cisternal puncture is higher risk but may be used if scar tissue prevents LP
	Measures CSF opening pressure (roughly equivalent to intracranial pressure for most patients if done recumbent and no blockage is present)	Patient must be cooperative
		Contraindicated in patients with intracranial hypertension because herniation may occur
		Contraindicated in bleeding disorders and in patients receiving anticoagulants
		Patient kept flat for 4-8 hours to prevent headache
		May cause headache, low back pain, meningitis, abscess, CSF leak, or puncture of spinal cord
Magnetic resonance angiography/magnetic resonance imaging	As for CT	Patient must be cooperative
	Visualizes tissue state (diffusion and perfusion) so that early ischemic changes are apparent (CT cannot visualize most early changes)	Contraindicated in patients with any implanted metallic device, including pacemakers
		Tends to overestimate degree of stenosis
	Identifies vascular lesions, tissue abnormalities, hemorrhage, infarction, epileptic foci, and multiple sclerosis	
	Identifies patency of large veins and venous sinuses	
	Identifies brainstem abnormalities	
	Identifies type, location, and extent of brain injury	
Myelography	Visualizes spinal subarachnoid space	If done with oil-based iophendylate (Pantopaque):
	Detects spinal cord lesions and cord or nerve root compression	• Patient must lie flat for 4-8 hours after study
	Detects pressure on spinal nerve roots	• May cause headache, nerve root irritation, allergic reaction, or adhesive arachnoiditis
		If done with water-soluble metrizamide (Amipaque):
		• Patient should have head of bed elevated
		• May cause headache, nausea, vomiting, backache and neck ache, chest pain, seizures, hallucinations, speech disorders, dysrhythmias, or allergic reaction
		Encourage fluid intake with either type of dye
Nerve conduction velocity studies	Identifies peripheral neuropathies and nerve compression	Needle electrodes are used
Oculoplethysmography	Indirectly measures ocular artery pressure	Contraindicated in patients who have undergone eye surgery within the last 6 months, who have had lens implants or cataracts, or who have had retinal detachment
	Reflects adequacy of cerebrovascular blood flow in the carotid artery retinal detachment	May cause conjunctival hemorrhage, corneal abrasions, or transient photophobia

TABLE 17-4   **NEUROLOGICAL DIAGNOSTIC STUDIES—cont'd**

STUDY	PURPOSES	COMMENTS
Pneumoencephalography	Visualizes ventricular system and subarachnoid space	Care as for LP
	Identifies intracranial tumors	Contraindicated in patients with intracranial hypertension
	Identifies brain atrophy	May cause headache, nausea, vomiting, autonomic dysfunction, herniation, subdural hematoma, air embolus, or seizures
		Keep patient flat for 12-24 hours after the study
Positron emission tomography or single-photon emission computed tomography	Evaluates oxygen and glucose metabolism	Patient must be cooperative
	Measures cerebral blood flow, which may be altered by traumatic brain injury, seizure, ischemia, stroke, or neoplasm	Contraindicated in pregnant and breastfeeding patients
	Also used to evaluate dementia, depression, schizophrenia, and Alzheimer's disease	
Radioisotope brain scan	Identifies tumors, cerebrovascular disease, infarction, trauma, infectious processes, and seizures	Generally replaced by CT scan
		Reassure patient that amount of radioactive material is minimal
		Patient must be cooperative
		Contraindicated in pregnant and breastfeeding patients
Regional cerebral blood flow (xenon [133Xe] inhalation)	Evaluates blood flow to the cerebral cortex	Assure patient that amount of radioactive is minimal material
	Identifies cerebrovascular disease	Contraindicated in pregnant and breastfeeding patients
	Detects regions of increased or decreased perfusion	
	Determines presence of collateral blood flow	
	Evaluates the effect of vasospasm on tissue perfusion	
Skull x-rays	Detects skull fracture, facial fracture, tumor, bone erosion, cranial anomalies, air-fluid level in sinuses, abnormal intracranial calcification, and radiopaque foreign bodies	Linear and basal fractures frequently missed by routine x-rays
		Contraindicated in pregnant patients
Somnography	Records electroencephalogram during sleep	
	Evaluates sleep and sleep disorders	
Spinal cord arteriography	Differentiates between spinal AVM, angioma, tumor, and ischemia	As for skull x-rays
		May cause thrombosis of spinal vessels and allergy to contrast agent
Spine x-rays	Detects vertebral dislocation or fracture, degenerative disease, tumor, bone erosion, or calcification	Care must be taken to prevent fracture displacement and spinal cord injury
	Identifies structural spinal deficits and rules out associated cervical spine injuries	C1-C2 view best obtained via open mouth; C6-C7 best obtained with arms pulled down
Suboccipital puncture	Obtains CSF for analysis	May cause trauma to the medulla
	Measures CSF pressure	
	Rarely performed but may be useful when LP is contraindicated	
Transcranial Doppler ultrasonography	Measures blood flow velocity through the cerebral arteries	Quality of findings and interpretation vary with user
	Identifies vasospasm, emboli, vascular stenosis, and brain death	Transtemporal window required (lacking in 14% of general population)
Ventriculography	Obtains CSF for analysis	May cause meningeal irritation, seizures, herniation, intracerebral or intraventricular hemorrhage
	Measures CSF pressure	
	Is used especially when intracranial hypertension contraindicates LP	

From Dennison RD: *Pass CCRN!*, ed 3, St Louis, 2007, Mosby.
AVM, Arteriovenous malformation; *CSF*, cerebrospinal fluid; *CT*, computed tomography; *IV*, intravenous; *LP*, lumbar puncture; *NPO*, nothing by mouth.

the patient's responses to the procedure, and (3) assessing the patient after the procedure. Preparation includes teaching the patient about the procedure, answering questions, and transporting and positioning the patient for the procedure. During the procedure, the nurse observes the patient for signs of pain, anxiety, or hemorrhage and monitors vital signs. After the procedure, the nurse observes for complications of the procedure and medicates the patient for any postprocedure discomfort. **Any evidence of increasing ICP should be immediately reported to the physician, and emergency measures to maintain circulation must be initiated.**

BEDSIDE MONITORING

Intracranial Pressure Monitoring

In the patient with suspected intracranial hypertension, a monitoring device may be placed within the cranium to quantify ICP. Under normal physiological conditions, mean ICP is maintained below 15 mm Hg. The device is used to monitor serial ICPs and assist with the management of intracranial hypertension. An increase in ICP can decrease blood flow to the brain, causing brain damage. It can also provide sterile access for draining excess CSF.[16]

Monitoring Sites

The four sites for monitoring ICP are the intraventricular space, the subarachnoid space, the epidural space, and the parenchyma (Figure 17-7). Each site has advantages and

disadvantages for monitoring ICP (Table 17-5). The type of monitor chosen depends on the suspected pathological condition and physician's preferences.[16,17] Nursing considerations for each type of device are discussed in Table 17-5.

Intraventricular Space. ICP monitoring is accomplished by placing a small catheter into the ventricular system; this procedure is known as a ventriculostomy. The catheter is inserted through a burr hole with the patient under local anesthesia, and it usually is placed in the anterior horn of the lateral ventricle. If possible, the side chosen for placement of the ventriculostomy is the nondominant hemisphere.[16,17]

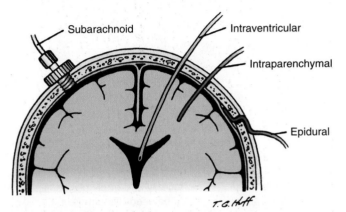

FIGURE 17-7 Intracranial Pressure Monitoring Sites. (From Lee KR, Hoff JT: *Youmans neurological surgery*, ed 4, Philadelphia, 1996, Saunders.)

TABLE 17-5	ADVANTAGES, DISADVANTAGES, AND NURSING CONSIDERATIONS OF ICP MONITORING TECHNIQUES		
MONITORING DEVICE	**ADVANTAGES**	**DISADVANTAGES**	**NURSING CONSIDERATIONS**
Intraventricular catheter (ventriculostomy)	Allows accurate ICP measurement Provides access to CSF for drainage or sampling Provides access for instillation of contrast media Allows reliable evaluation of intracranial compliances (volume-pressure relationships)	Provides an additional site for infection Is most invasive ICP monitoring technique Requires frequent transducer balancing or recalibration Catheter may be occluded by blood clot or tissue debris Insertion difficult if ventricles are small, compressed, or displaced Is associated with risk for CSF leakage around insertion site Is associated with increased risk for infection	Provide appropriate sedatives or analgesics during catheter insertion. Do baseline and serial neurological assessments. Measure patient's temperature at least every 4 hours. Notice character, amount, and turbidity of CSF drainage. Document ICP and CPP measurements, response to stimulation, and nursing care activities per hospital or unit protocol. Monitor quality of ICP waveform. Monitor system and tubing for air bubbles, and flush or purge system as appropriate. Drain CSF as indicated for treatment of ICP elevation. Notify physician if CSF drainage is not within prescribed parameters. Monitor insertion site for bleeding, drainage, swelling, and CSF leakage.

TABLE 17-5	ADVANTAGES, DISADVANTAGES, AND NURSING CONSIDERATIONS OF ICP MONITORING TECHNIQUES—cont'd		
MONITORING DEVICE	**ADVANTAGES**	**DISADVANTAGES**	**NURSING CONSIDERATIONS**
Subarachnoid bolt or screw	Is associated with lower infection rates than is ventriculostomy Is quickly and easily placed Can be used with small or collapsed ventricles Requires no penetration of brain tissue	Has potential for dampened waveform (cerebral edema, blood or tissue debris) Is less accurate at high ICP elevations Requires frequent balancing or recalibration (e.g., with position changes) Provides no access for CSF sampling	Zero or calibrate device per hospital or unit protocol. Level transducer at the foramen of Monro; external landmarks include the tragus of the patient's ear and the external auditory canal, among others; all ICP measurements should be made with the transducer at a consistent level relative to external landmarks. Administer sedatives or analgesics as appropriate to decrease risk of catheter being dislodged by patient's movements. Educate patient's family as indicated. Notify physician if ICP or CPP is not within specified parameters. Administer appropriate sedatives or analgesics during insertion. Do baseline and serial neurological assessments. Measure patient's temperature at least every 4 hours. Monitor insertion site for bleeding, drainage, swelling, and CSF leakage. Monitor quality of ICP waveform. Document ICP and CPP measurements and response to stimulation per hospital or unit protocol. Administer sedatives or analgesics as appropriate to decrease risk of catheter being dislodged by patient's movements.
Subdural or epidural catheter or sensor	Is least invasive Is associated with decreased risk of infection Is easily and quickly placed	Increase in baseline drift over time means possible loss of reliability or accuracy Provides no access for CSF drainage or sampling	Zero or calibrate device per hospital or unit protocol. Level transducer at the foramen of Monro; external landmarks include the tragus of the patient's ear and the external auditory canal, among others; all ICP measurements should be made with the transducer at a consistent level relative to external landmarks. Educate patient's family as indicated. Notify physician if ICP or CPP is not within specified parameters. Administer appropriate sedatives or analgesics during insertion. Do baseline and serial neurological assessments. Measure patient's temperature at least every 4 hours. Monitor insertion site for bleeding, drainage, and swelling.

TABLE 17-5	ADVANTAGES, DISADVANTAGES, AND NURSING CONSIDERATIONS OF ICP MONITORING TECHNIQUES—cont'd		
MONITORING DEVICE	**ADVANTAGES**	**DISADVANTAGES**	**NURSING CONSIDERATIONS**
			Monitor quality of ICP waveform and drift over time. Document ICP and CPP measurements and response to stimulation per hospital or unit protocol. Administer sedatives or analgesics as appropriate to decrease risk of catheter being dislodged or damaged by patient's movements. Educate patient's family as indicated. Notify physician if ICP or CPP is not within specified parameters.
Fiberoptic transducer-tipped catheter	Can be placed in subdural or subarachnoid space, in a ventricle, or directly within brain tissue Is easily transported Requires zeroing only once (during insertion) Has baseline drift of up to 1 mm Hg per day Is associated with decreased risk for infection when brain tissue is not penetrated Provides good-quality ICP waveforms (fewer artifacts than with other devices) Requires no adjustment in level of transducer with patient's change of position	Provides no access for CSF sampling or drainage Cannot be recalibrated after placement Requires periodic replacement of probe Is easily damaged	Administer appropriate sedatives or analgesics during insertion. Do baseline and serial neurological assessments. Measure patient's temperature at least every 4 hours. Monitor insertion site for bleeding, drainage, swelling, and CSF leakage. Monitor quality of ICP waveform and drift over time. Document ICP and CPP measurements and response to stimulation per hospital or unit protocol. Administer sedatives or analgesics as appropriate to decrease risk of catheter being dislodged or damaged by patient's movements. Educate patient's family as indicated. Notify physician if ICP or CPP is not within specified parameters.

From Arbour R: Intracranial hypertension: monitoring and nursing assessment, *Crit Care Nurse* 24(5):19, 2004.
CPP, cerebral perfusion pressure; *CSF*, cerebrospinal fluid; *ICP*, intracranial pressure.

Subarachnoid Space. ICP monitoring is accomplished by placing a small hollow bolt or screw into the subarachnoid space. It is inserted through a burr hole, usually located in the front of the skull behind the hairline, with the patient under local anesthesia. Inserting this device is easier than inserting the ventriculostomy catheter.[16,17]

Epidural Space. ICP monitoring is accomplished by placing a small fiberoptic sensor into the epidural space. It is inserted through a burr hole while the patient is under local anesthesia. The physician strips the dura away from the inner table of the skull before inserting the epidural monitor.[16,17]

Intraparenchymal Site. ICP monitoring is accomplished by placing a small fiberoptic catheter into the parenchymal tissue. After placing a subarachnoid bolt (as previously described), a hole is punched in the dura, and the catheter is inserted approximately 1 cm into the brain's white matter.[16,17]

Intracranial Pressure Waves

The ICP pulse waveform is observed on a continuous, real-time pressure display, and it corresponds to each heartbeat. The waveform arises primarily from pulsations of the major intracranial arteries but also receives retrograde venous pulsations.[16,17]

Normal Intracranial Pressure Waveform. The normal ICP wave has three or more defined peaks (Figure 17-8). The first peak (P1) is called the percussion wave. Originating from the pulsations of the choroid plexus, it has a sharp peak and is fairly consistent in its amplitude. The second peak (P2) is called the tidal wave. The tidal wave varies more in shape and amplitude, ending on the dicrotic notch. The P2 portion of the pulse waveform has been most directly linked to the state of decreased compliance. When the P2 component is equal to or higher than P1, decreased compliance occurs (Figure 17-9). Immediately after the dicrotic notch is the third wave (P3), which is called the dicrotic wave. After the dicrotic wave, the pressure usually tapers down to the diastolic position, unless retrograde venous pulsations add a few more peaks.[16-19]

A, B, and C pressure waves are not true waveforms (Figure 17-10). Rather, they are the graphically displayed trend data of ICP over time. These waves reflect spontaneous alterations in ICP associated with respiration, systemic blood pressure, and deteriorating neurological status.

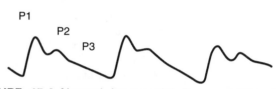

FIGURE 17-8 Normal Intracranial Pressure Waveform. (From Bader MK, Littlejohns LR: *AANN core curriculum for neuroscience nursing*, ed 4, St Louis, 2004, Elsevier.)

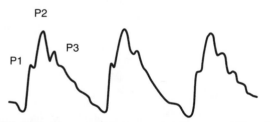

FIGURE 17-9 Abnormal Intracranial Pressure Waveform. (From Bader MK, Littlejohns LR: *AANN core curriculum for neuroscience nursing*, ed 4, St Louis, 2004, Elsevier.)

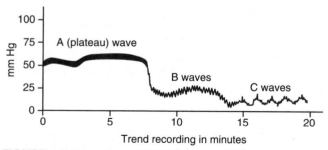

FIGURE 17-10 Intracranial Pressure Waves. Composite diagram of A (plateau) waves, B (sawtooth) waves, and C (small rhythmic) waves. (From Barker E: *Neuroscience nursing: a spectrum of care*, ed 3, St Louis, 2008, Mosby.)

A Waves. Also called plateau waves because of their distinctive shape, A waves are the most clinically significant of the three types. They usually occur in an already elevated baseline ICP (>20 mm Hg) and are characterized by sharp increases in ICP of 30 to 69 mm Hg, which plateau for 2 to 20 minutes and then return to baseline. The cause of A waves is unknown, but they may result from vasodilation and increased CBF, decreased venous outflow (and therefore increased cerebral blood volume), fluctuations in Pa_{CO_2} (and therefore changes in cerebral blood volume), or decreased CSF absorption. B waves often precede A waves. Plateau waves are considered significant because of the reduced cerebral perfusion pressure associated with ICP, in the range of 50 to 100 mm Hg. Transient signs of intracranial hypertension, such as a decreased level of consciousness, bradycardia, pupillary changes, or respiratory changes, may accompany these waves. Some research suggests that prolonged increases in ICP associated with plateau waves may result in transient and permanent cell damage from ischemia.[2,17]

B Waves. B waves are sharp, rhythmic oscillations with a sawtooth appearance that occur every 30 seconds to 2 minutes and that can raise the ICP from 5 to 70 mm Hg. They are a normal physiological phenomenon that can occur in any patient, but they are amplified in states of low intracranial compliance. B waves appear to reflect fluctuations in cerebral blood volume. Decompensation of normal intracranial volume compensatory capacity is indicated by B waves with a high amplitude (>15 mm Hg pressure change from peak to trough of the wave).[2,17]

C Waves. C waves are small, rhythmic waves that occur every 4 to 8 minutes at normal levels of ICP. They are related to normal fluctuations in respiration and systemic arterial pressure. C waves are considered clinically insignificant.[2,17]

Cerebral Perfusion Pressure

Measuring CBF in the clinical setting is difficult, but at the bedside, an estimated pressure of cerebral perfusion can be derived. Cerebral perfusion pressure (CPP) is the blood pressure gradient across the brain, and it is calculated as the difference between the incoming mean arterial pressure (MAP) and the opposing ICP on the arteries (see Appendix B).

The CPP in the average adult is approximately 80 to 100 mm Hg, with a range of 60 to 150 mm Hg. The CPP must be maintained near 80 mm Hg to provide adequate blood supply to the brain. If the CPP drops below this point, ischemia may develop. A sustained CPP of 30 mm Hg or less usually results in neuronal hypoxia and cell death. When the mean systemic arterial pressure equals the ICP, CBF may cease.[1-3]

Cerebral Oxygenation Monitoring
Cerebral Metabolism

The measurements of CBF and CPP do not address the brain's metabolic need for oxygen. Active neurons require greater amounts of oxygen than those that are inactive. The determination that CBF matches the brain's metabolic needs is expressed as cerebral metabolic rate (CMR_{O_2}), the normal value of which is 3.4 mL per 100 g of brain tissue per minute. Neuronal demand for oxygen is governed by the metabolic rate. For technical reasons, this value is not easily attained, although it can be calculated. It is the product of the measured CBF and calculated arteriojugular oxygen difference (AJDo$_2$) (see Appendix B).[20]

CBF can be measured using a variety of complex techniques (e.g., PET, SPECT). Most recently, continuous bedside monitoring of regional cerebrocortical blood flow has become available.[8] Arteriojugular oxygen difference is the amount of oxygen extracted by the brain, and it is reflected in the difference between the arterial oxygen content and the jugular venous oxygen content. The normal value is 5.0 to 7.5 vol%.[20]

Jugular Venous Oxygen Saturation

One method of measuring CBF allows continuous measurement of oxygenation within the jugular venous system through the use of the jugular bulb monitor. Jugular venous oxygen saturation (Sjvo$_2$) can be used to reflect cerebral oxygen supply-and-demand balance. Any disorder that increases CMRo$_2$ or decreases oxygen delivery may decrease Sjvo$_2$, and conversely, any disorder that that decreases CMRo$_2$ or increases oxygen delivery may increase Sjvo$_2$.[20,21]

To measure Sjvo$_2$ a fiberoptic catheter is placed retrograde through the internal jugular vein into the jugular bulb and attached to a bedside monitor. The normal value is 60% to 80%. Patients with values less than 50% and 55% are hypoxemic or oligemic (low CBF compared with metabolic rate). Oligemia occurs as a result of decreased blood flow due to hypotension, vasospasm, or intracranial hypertension or as a result of increased brain metabolic requirements due to fever or seizures.[20,21] Sjvo$_2$ values below 45% are indicative of severe cerebral hypoxia.[20] Patients with values above 75% to 80% are considered hyperemic (high CBF compared with metabolic need). Sjvo$_2$ also increases if the brain is so severely injured the neurons are unable to extract oxygen.[20,21]

Sjvo$_2$ monitoring has several limitations. Sjvo$_2$ is a global measure of cerebral oxygenation, and a normal Sjvo$_2$ value does not rule out localized areas of cerebral ischemia.[20,21] Readings are affected by the movement of the patient's head.[21] Up to 50% of low Sjvo$_2$ readings are false, which may be caused by technical issues with the catheter, particularly catheter migration.[22] For accurate reading, the tip of the catheter must be within 1 cm of the jugular bulb.[21]

Brain Tissue Oxygen Pressure

Over the past few years, a new device has become available to measure the partial pressure of oxygen within brain tissue (Pbto$_2$). The device consists of a monitoring probe on the end of a catheter, which is inserted into the brain parenchyma and attached to a bedside monitor. The probe may be inserted into the damaged portion of the brain to measure regional oxygenation or inserted into the undamaged portion of the brain to measure global oxygenation. One risk associated with insertion of the catheter is bleeding with hematoma formation.[23] Although there is no consensus on normal values because they vary from device to device, it has been concluded that the probability of death increases with prolonged periods of Pbto$_2$ less than 15 mm Hg and any episode of Pbto$_2$ less than 6 mm Hg.[23]

In the head-injured patient, the goal of treatment is to maintain the Pbto$_2$ greater than 20 mm Hg. Factors that decrease Pbto$_2$ include tissue hypoxia, hypocapnia, hypovolemia, decreased blood pressure, low hemoglobin levels, intracranial hypertension, and hyperthermia.[24] Treatment is directed at the underlying cause.

REFERENCES

1. Barker E: The adult neurological assessment. In Barker E, editor: *Neuroscience nursing: a spectrum of care*, ed 3, St Louis, 2008, Mosby.
2. Bader MK, Littlejohns LR: *AANN core curriculum for neuroscience nursing*, ed 4, St Louis, 2004, Elsevier.
3. Goetz CG: *Textbook of clinical neurology*, ed 3, St Louis, 2007, Saunders.
4. Haymore J: A neuron in a haystack: advanced neurologic assessment, *AACN Clin Issues* 15(4):568, 2004.
5. Teasdale G, Jennett B: Assessment of coma and impaired consciousness. A practical scale, *Lancet* 2(7872):81, 1974.
6. Holdgate A, et al: Variability in agreement between physicians and nurses when measuring the Glasgow Coma Scale in the emergency department limits its clinical usefulness, *Emerg Med Australas* 18(4):379, 2006.
7. Fischer J, Mathieson C: The history of the Glasgow Coma Scale: implications for practice, *Crit Care Nurs Q* 23(4):52, 2001.
8. Barnwell P: Assessing motor and sensory function – a focused survey, *Aust Emerg Nurs J* 2(3):16, 1999.
9. O'Hanlon-Nichols T: Neurologic assessment, *Am J Nurs* 99(6):44, 1999.
10. Seidel HM, et al: *Mosby's guide to physical examination*, ed 7, St Louis, 2010, Mosby.
11. Adoni A, McNett M: The pupillary response in traumatic brain injury: a guide for trauma nurses, *J Trauma Nurs* 14(4):191, 2007.
12. Bishop BS: Pathologic papillary signs: self-learning module, Part 2, *Crit Care Nurse* 11(7):58, 1991.
13. Chesnut RM: Management of brain and spine injuries, *Crit Care Clin* 20(1):25, 2004.
14. Keller C, Williams A: Cardiac dysrhythmias associated with central nervous system dysfunction, *J Neurosci Nurs* 25(6):349, 1993.
15. Samuels MA: The brain-heart connection, *Circulation* 116(1):77, 2007.
16. March K, Madden L: Intracranial pressure management. In Littlejohns LR, Bader MK, editors: *AACN-AANN protocols for practice: monitoring technologies in critically ill neuroscience patients*, Sudbury, Mass., 2009, Jones & Bartlett.
17. Arbour R: Intracranial hypertension: monitoring and nursing assessment, *Crit Care Nurse* 24(5):19, 2004.

18. Rangel-Castillo L, Robertson CS: Management of intracranial hypertension, *Crit Care Clin* 22(4):713, 2006.
19. Bhatia A, Gupta AK: Neuromonitoring in the intensive care unit. I. Intracranial pressure and cerebral blood flow monitoring, *Intensive Care Med* 33(7):1263, 2007.
20. Smith M: Perioperative uses of transcranial perfusion monitoring, *Anesthesiol Clin* 25(3):557, 2007.
21. Stevens WJ: Multimodal monitoring: head injury management using SjvO$_2$ and LICOX, *J Neurosci Nurs* 36(6):332, 2004.
22. Blissitt PA: Brain oxygen monitoring. In Littlejohns LR, Bader MK, editors: *AACN-AANN protocols for practice: monitoring technologies in critically ill neuroscience patients*, Sudbury, Mass., 2009, Jones & Bartlett.
23. Bader MK: Recognizing and treating ischemic insults to the brain: the role of brain tissue oxygen monitoring, *Crit Care Nurs Clin North Am* 18(2):243, 2006.
24. Wartenberg KE, et al: Multimodality monitoring in neurocritical care, *Crit Care Clin* 23(3):507, 2007.

18

Neurological Disorders and Therapeutic Management

Kathleen M. Stacy

⊖volve WEBSITE

Be sure to check out the bonus material, including free self-assessment exercises, on the Evolve web site at
http://evolve.elsevier.com/Urden/priorities/.

OBJECTIVES

- Describe the etiology and pathophysiology of selected neurological disorders.
- Identify the clinical manifestations of selected neurological disorders.
- Explain the treatment of selected neurological disorders.

- Discuss the nursing priorities for managing a patient with selected neurological disorders.
- Discuss the concept of cerebral autoregulation.
- Describe the therapies commonly used to treat intracranial hypertension.
- List the four supratentorial herniation syndromes.

To accurately anticipate and plan nursing interventions, the critical care nurse must have an understanding of the disease pathology, determine the areas of focused assessment, and be well acquainted with the medical management of the neurological patient. Fortunately, despite a wide array of neurological disorders, only a few routinely require the critical care environment.

COMA

Normal consciousness requires awareness and arousal. Awareness is the combination of cognition (mental and intellectual) and affect (mood) that can be construed based on the patient's interaction with the environment.[1] Alterations of consciousness may be the result of deficits in awareness, arousal, or both.[2] There are four discrete disorders of consciousness: coma, vegetative state, minimally conscious state, and locked-in syndrome. Coma is characterized by the absence of both wakefulness and awareness, whereas a vegetative state is characterized by the presence of wakefulness with the absence of awareness. In the minimally conscious state, wakefulness is presence and awareness is severely diminished but not absent. Locked-in syndrome is characterized by the presence of wakefulness and awareness, but with quadriplegia and the inability to communicate verbally; thus the patient appears to be unconscious.[3] Box 18-1 lists the disorders of consciousness in descending order of wakefulness.

Coma is the deepest state of unconsciousness; arousal and awareness are lacking.[1-3] The patient cannot be aroused and does not demonstrate any purposeful response to the surrounding environment.[4] Coma is a symptom rather than a disease, and it occurs as a result of some underlying process.[1,2] The incidence of coma is difficult to ascertain because a wide variety of conditions can induce coma.[1,2] This state of unconsciousness is unfortunately very common in critical care, and it is the focus of the following discussion.

Etiology

The causes of coma can be divided into two general categories: structural or surgical and metabolic or medical. Structural causes of coma include ischemic stroke, intracerebral hemorrhage (ICH), trauma, and brain tumors.[5] Metabolic causes of coma include drug overdose, infectious diseases, endocrine disorders, and poisonings.[5] Coma demands immediate attention, resulting in a high percentage of admissions to all hospital services.[6] Table 18-1 provides a list of the possible causes of coma.

Pathophysiology

Consciousness involves arousal, or wakefulness, and awareness. Neither of these functions is present in the patient in coma. Ascending fibers of the reticular activating system (ARAS) in the pons, hypothalamus, and thalamus maintain arousal as an autonomic function. Neurons in the cerebral

359

BOX 18-1 DISORDERS OF CONSCIOUSNESS

Consciousness
↓
Locked-in syndrome
↓
Minimally conscious state
↓
Vegetative state
↓
Coma

TABLE 18-1 CAUSES OF COMA

STRUCTURAL OR SURGICAL COMA	METABOLIC OR MEDICAL COMA
Trauma	Infection
Epidural hematoma	Meningitis
Subdural hematoma	Encephalitis
	Metabolic encephalopathy
Diffuse axonal injury	Metabolic conditions
	Hypoglycemia
Brain contusion	Hyperglycemia
Intracerebral hemorrhage	Hyperosmolar states
	Uremia
Subarachnoid hemorrhage	Hepatic encephalopathy
	Hypertensive encephalopathy
Posterior fossa hemorrhage	Hypoxic encephalopathy
	Hyponatremia
Supratentorial hemorrhage	Hypercalcemia
	Myxedema
Hydrocephalus	Intoxication
Ischemic stroke	Opioid overdose
Tumor	Alcohol
Other causes	Poisonings
	Psychogenic causes

cortex are responsible for awareness. Diffuse dysfunction of both cerebral hemispheres and diffuse or focal dysfunction of the reticular activating system can produce coma.[1,6,7] Structural causes usually produce compression or dysfunction in the area of the ARAS, whereas most medical causes lead to general dysfunction of both cerebral hemispheres.[8] Trauma, hemorrhage, and tumor can damage the ARAS, leading to coma. Destruction of large regions of bilateral cerebral hemispheres can be the result of seizures or viral agents. Toxic drugs, toxins, or metabolic abnormalities can suppress cerebral function.[5-7]

Assessment and Diagnosis

The clinical diagnosis of the coma state is readily established by assessment of the level of consciousness. However, determining the full nature and cause of coma requires a thorough history and physical examination. A medical history is essential, because events immediately preceding the change in level of consciousness can often provide valuable clues to the origin of the coma. When limited information is available and the coma is profound, the response of the patient to emergency treatment may provide clues to the underlying diagnosis; for example, the patient who becomes responsive with the administration of naloxone can be presumed to have ingested some type of opiate.[6]

Detailed serial neurological examinations are essential for all patients in coma. Assessment of pupillary size and reaction to light (normal, sluggish, or fixed), extraocular eye movements (normal, asymmetrical, or absent), motor response to pain (normal, decorticate, decerebrate, or flaccid), and breathing pattern yields important clues for determining whether the cause of the coma is structural or metabolic.[1,6]

The areas of the brainstem that control consciousness and pupillary responses are anatomically adjacent. The sympathetic and parasympathetic nervous systems control pupillary dilation and constriction, respectively. The anatomic directions of these pathways are known, and changes in pupillary responses can help identify where a lesion may be located. For example, if damage occurs in the midbrain region, pupils are slightly enlarged and unresponsive to light. Lesions that compress the third nerve result in a fixed and dilated pupil on the same side as the neurological insult. Pupillary responses are usually preserved when the cause of the coma is metabolic in origin. Pupillary light responses are often the key to differentiating between structural and metabolic causes of coma.[1,6,7,9]

Areas of the brainstem adjacent to those responsible for consciousness also control the oculomotor eye movement. The ability to maintain conjugate gaze requires preservation of the internuclear connections of cranial nerves III, VI, and VIII by means of the medial longitudinal fasciculus (MLF).[9] As with pupillary responses, structural lesions that impinge on these pathways cause oculomotor dysfunction such as a disconjugate gaze. Deficits in extraocular eye movements usually accompany a structural cause.[1,5,9]

Focal or asymmetric motor deficits usually indicate structural lesions.[1,5] Abnormal motor movements may also help pinpoint the location of a lesion. Decorticate posturing (abnormal flexion) can be seen with damage to the diencephalon. Decerebrate posturing (abnormal extension) can be seen with damage to the midbrain and pons. Flaccid posturing is an ominous sign and can be seen with damage to the medulla.[9]

Abnormal breathing patterns may also assist in differentiating structural from metabolic causes of coma. Cheyne-Stokes respirations are seen in patients with cerebral hemispheric dysfunction or metabolic suppression. Central neurogenic hyperventilation, or Kussmaul breathing, occurs with metabolic acidosis or damage to the midbrain and upper pons. Apneustic breathing may occur with damage to the pons, hypoglycemia, and anoxia. Ataxic breathing occurs with damage to the medulla. Agonal breathing occurs with failure of the respiratory centers in the medulla.[6,9]

In addition to physical assessment, laboratory studies and diagnostic procedures are done. Structural causes of coma are usually readily apparent with computed tomography (CT) or magnetic resonance imaging (MRI).[4,8] Evoked potentials are also useful in facilitating a differential diagnosis between the disorders of consciousness and in evaluating a patient's prognosis.[3] Generally a patient in a coma with an absence of brainstem auditory evoked responses (BAERs) is considered to have a poor prognosis of recovery.[3] Laboratory studies are also used to identify metabolic or endocrine abnormalities.[7] Occasionally, the cause of coma is never clearly determined.

Medical Management

The goal of medical management of the patient in a coma is identification and treatment of the underlying cause of the condition. Initial medical management includes emergency measures to support vital functions and prevent further neurological deterioration. Protection of the airway and ventilatory assistance are often needed. Administration of thiamine (at least 100 mg), glucose, and an opioid antagonist is suggested when the cause of coma is not immediately known.[1,6] Thiamine is administered before glucose, because the coma produced by thiamine deficiency, Wernicke's encephalopathy, can be precipitated by a glucose load.[1]

The patient who remains in a coma after emergency treatment requires supportive measures to maintain physiological body functions and prevent complications. Intubation for continued airway protection and nutritional support are essential. Fluid and electrolyte management is often complex because of alterations in the neurohormonal system. Anticonvulsant therapy may be necessary to prevent further ischemic damage to the brain.[1,5,6]

The health care team and the patient's family make decisions jointly regarding the level of medical management to be provided. Family members require informational support in terms of probable cause of the coma and prognosis for recovery of consciousness and function. Prognosis depends on the cause of the coma and the length of time unconsciousness persists. Only 15% of patients in nontraumatic coma make a satisfactory recovery.[7] Metabolic coma usually has a better prognosis than coma caused by a structural lesion, and traumatic coma usually has a better outcome than nontraumatic coma.[5,7]

Nursing Management

Nursing management of the patient in a coma incorporates a variety of nursing diagnoses (Nursing Diagnosis Priorities box on Coma) and is directed by the specific cause of the coma, although some common interventions are used. The patient in a coma totally depends on the health care team. **Nursing priorities are directed toward (1) monitoring for changes in neurological status and clues to the origin of the coma, (2) supporting all body functions, (3) maintaining surveillance for complications, (4) providing comfort and emotional support, and (5) initiating rehabilitation measures.** Measures to support body functions include promoting pulmonary hygiene, maintaining skin integrity, initiating range-of-motion exercises, managing bowel and bladder functions, and ensuring adequate nutritional support.[1]

Eye Care

The blink reflex is often diminished or absent in the comatose patient. The eyelids may be flaccid and may depend on body positioning to remain in a closed position, and edema may prevent complete closure. Loss of these protective mechanisms results in drying and ulceration of the cornea, which can lead to permanent scarring and blindness.[1]

Two interventions that are commonly used to protect the eyes are instilling saline or methylcellulose lubricating drops and taping the eyelids in the shut position. Evidence suggests that an alternative technique may be more effective in preventing corneal epithelial breakdown. In addition to instillation of saline drops every 2 hours, a polyethylene film is taped over the eyes, extending beyond the orbits and eyebrows. The film creates a moisture chamber around the cornea and assists in keeping the eyes moist and in the closed position. This technique also prevents damage to the eyes that results from placement of tape or gauze directly on the delicate skin of the eyelids.[10]

Collaborative management of the patient in a coma is outlined in the Collaborative Management box on Coma.

STROKE

Stroke is a descriptive term for the sudden onset of acute neurological deficit persisting for more than 24 hours and caused by the interruption of blood flow to the brain. Stroke is the third leading cause of death in the United States, preceded by heart disease and cancer, and the leading cause of adult disability.[11] Approximately 795,000 people have a stroke each year; 610,000 of these are first attacks, and 185,000 are recurrent attacks.[11]

Strokes are classified as ischemic or hemorrhagic (Concept Map on Stroke). Hemorrhagic strokes can be further categorized as subarachnoid hemorrhages (SAHs) and intracerebral hemorrhages. Approximately 87% of all strokes are ischemic, 10% are ICHs, and 3% are SAHs.[11] Although less common, hemorrhagic strokes (ICHs and SAHs) have a higher mortality rate than ischemic strokes. Approximately 8% to 12% of ischemic strokes and 37% to 45% of hemorrhagic strokes result in death within 30 days.[11] The annual cost for care and loss of productivity was estimated to be $73.7 billion in 2009.[11]

Ischemic Stroke

Ischemic stroke results from interruption of blood flow to the brain and accounts for 80% to 85% of all strokes. The interruption can be the result of a thrombotic or embolic event. Thrombosis can form in large vessels (large-vessel thrombotic strokes) or small vessels (small-vessel thrombotic strokes). Embolic sources include the heart (cardioembolic strokes) and atherosclerotic plaques in larger vessels (atheroembolic strokes). In 30% of the cases, the underlying cause of the stroke is unknown (cryptogenic strokes).[12]

Strokes are preventable. Most thrombotic strokes are the result of the accumulation of atherosclerotic plaque in the vessel lumen, especially at bifurcations or curves of the vessel. The pathogenesis of cerebrovascular disease is identical to that of coronary vasculature disease. The greatest risk factor for ischemic stroke is hypertension.[12,13] Other risk factors are dyslipidemia, diabetes, smoking, and carotid atherosclerotic disease.[11,14] Common sites of atherosclerotic plaque are the bifurcation of the common carotid artery, the origins of the middle and anterior cerebral arteries, and the origins of the vertebral arteries.[13] Ischemic strokes resulting from vertebral artery dissection have been reported after chiropractic manipulation of the cervical spine.[15]

Etiology

An embolic stroke occurs when an embolus from the heart or lower circulation travels distally and lodges in a small vessel, obstructing the blood supply. At least 20% of ischemic strokes are attributed to a cardioembolic phenomenon.[12] The most common cause of cardiac emboli is atrial fibrillation. It is responsible for about 50% of all cardiac emboli.[16] Other sources of cardiac emboli are mitral stenosis, mechanical valves, atrial myxoma, endocarditis, and recent myocardial infarction.[13] Researchers hypothesize that a patent foramen ovale or atrial septal aneurysms may be the cause of cryptogenic stroke.[17]

Pathophysiology

Ischemic stroke is a cerebral hemodynamic insult. When cerebral blood flow is reduced to a level insufficient to maintain neuronal viability, ischemic injury occurs. In focal stroke, an area of hypoperfused tissue, the ischemic penumbra, surrounds a core of ischemic cells. The ischemic penumbra can be salvaged with return of blood flow. However, sustained anoxic insult initiates a chain of biochemical events leading to apoptosis, or cellular death.[18]

The phenomenon of a focal ischemic stroke is identical to that associated with myocardial infarction, which is why *brain attack* is used in public education strategies. Often, a history of transient ischemic attacks (TIAs), brief episodes of neurological symptoms that last less than 24 hours, offers a warning that stroke is likely to occur. Sudden onset indicates embolism as the final insult to flow.[12,13] The size of the stroke depends on the size and location of the occluded vessel and the availability of collateral blood flow.[12] Global ischemia results when severe hypotension or cardiopulmonary arrest provokes a transient drop in blood flow to all areas of the brain.[18]

Cerebral edema sufficient to produce clinical deterioration develops in 10% to 20% of patients with ischemic stroke and can result in intracranial hypertension. The edema results from a loss of normal metabolic function of the cells and peaks at 4 days.[12] This process is commonly the cause of death during the first week after a stroke.[19] Secondary hemorrhage at the site of the stroke lesion, known as hemorrhagic conversion,[19] and seizures[20] are the two other major acute neurological complications of ischemic stroke.

Assessment and Diagnosis

The characteristic sign of an ischemic stroke is the sudden onset of focal neurological signs persisting for more than 24 hours.[12] These signs usually occur in combination. Box 18-2 lists common patterns of neurological symptoms associated with an ischemic stroke. Hemiparesis, aphasia, and hemianopia are common. Changes in the level of consciousness usually occur only with brainstem or cerebellar involvement, seizure, hypoxia, hemorrhage, or elevated intracranial pressure (ICP). These changes may be exhibited as stupor, coma, confusion, and agitation.[1] The reported frequency of seizures in patients with ischemic stroke ranges from 3% to 8%. If seizures occur, they are usually seen within 24 hours of an insult.[20]

The National Institutes of Health Stroke Scale (NIHSS) is often used as the basis of the focused neurological examination. The score ranges from 0 to 42 points; the higher the score, the more neurologically impaired the patient. A change of 4 points on the scale indicates significant neurological change. The components of the NIHSS include level of consciousness (LOC); LOC questions; LOC commands; gaze; visual fields; face, arm, and leg strength; sensation; limb ataxia; and language function.[12] A copy of the NIHSS

Concept Map: Stroke

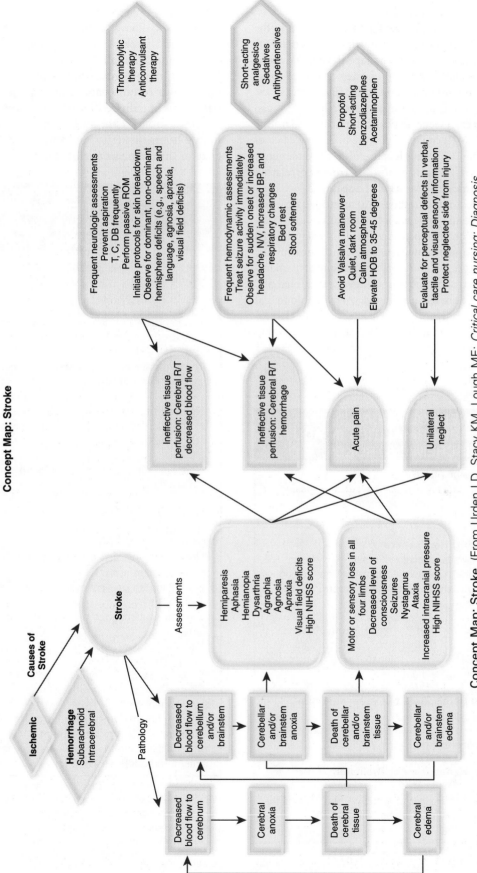

Concept Map: Stroke. (From Urden LD, Stacy KM, Lough ME: *Critical care nursing: Diagnosis and management*, ed 6, St. Louis, 2010, Mosby.)

with complete instructions can be retrieved at http://www.ninds.nih.gov/disorders/stroke/strokescales.htm.

Confirmation of the diagnosis of ischemic stroke is the first step in the emergency evaluation of these patients. Differentiation from intracranial hemorrhage is vital. Noncontrast CT scanning is the method of choice for this purpose and is considered the most important initial diagnostic study. In addition to excluding intracranial hemorrhage, CT can assist in identifying early neurological complications and the cause of the insult.[12] MRI can demonstrate infarction of cerebral tissue earlier than CT but is less useful in the emergency differential diagnosis.[21] Because of the strong correlation between acute ischemic stroke and heart disease, 12-lead electrocardiography, chest radiography, and continuous cardiac monitoring are suggested to detect a cardiac cause or coexisting condition. Echocardiography is valuable in identifying a cardioembolic phenomenon when a sufficient index of suspicion warrants its use.[1] Laboratory evaluation of hematological function, electrolyte and glucose levels, and renal and hepatic function is also recommended. Arterial blood gas analysis is performed if hypoxia is suspected, and an electroencephalogram is obtained if seizures are suspected. Lumbar puncture is performed only if SAH is suspected and the CT appearance is normal.[1]

BOX 18-2 **NEUROLOGICAL ABNORMALITIES IN ACUTE ISCHEMIC STROKES**

Left (Dominant) Hemisphere
Aphasia, right hemiparesis, right-sided sensory loss, right visual field defect, poor right conjugate gaze, dysarthria, difficulty in reading, writing, or calculating

Right (Nondominant) Hemisphere
Neglect of the left visual space, left visual field defect, left hemiparesis, left-sided sensory loss, poor left conjugate gaze, extinction of left-sided stimuli, dysarthria, spatial disorientation

Brainstem, Cerebellum, and Posterior Hemisphere
Motor or sensory loss in all four limbs, crossed signs, limb or gait ataxia, dysarthria, disconjugate gaze, nystagmus, amnesia, bilateral visual field defects

Small Subcortical Hemisphere or Brainstem (Pure Motor Stroke)
Weakness of face and limbs on one side of the body without abnormalities of higher brain function, sensation, or vision

Small Subcortical Hemisphere or Brainstem (Pure Sensory Stroke)
Decreased sensation of face and limbs on one side of the body without abnormalities of higher brain function, motor function, or vision

From Adams HP Jr, Brott TG, Crowell RM, et al: Guidelines for the management of patients with acute ischemic stroke. A statement for healthcare professionals from a special writing group of the Stroke Council, American Heart Association, *Circulation* 90(3):1588, 1994.

Medical Management

Major changes have taken place in the medical management of ischemic stroke since 1996. On the basis of results of the National Institute of Neurologic Disorders and Stroke (NINDS) rtPA Stroke Study, thrombolytic therapy with intravenous recombinant tissue-type plasminogen activator (rtPA) was initially recommended within 3 hours of onset of ischemic stroke. This time frame has now been expanded from 3 hours to 4.5 hours.[22] Patients who should be considered for thrombolysis are listed in Box 18-3. Confirmation of

---

BOX 18-3 **CHARACTERISTICS OF PATIENTS WITH ISCHEMIC STROKE WHO COULD BE TREATED WITH rtPA**

Diagnosis of ischemic stroke causing measurable neurological deficit.

The neurological signs should not be clearing spontaneously.

The neurological signs should not be minor and isolated. Caution should be exercised in treating a patient with major deficits.

The symptoms of stroke should not be suggestive of subarachnoid hemorrhage.

Onset of symptoms <3 hours before beginning treatment.

No head trauma or prior stroke in previous 3 months.

No myocardial infarction in the previous 3 months.

No gastrointestinal or urinary tract hemorrhage in previous 21 days.

No major surgery in the previous 14 days.

No arterial puncture at a noncompressible site in the previous 7 days.

No history of previous intracranial hemorrhage.

Blood pressure not elevated (systolic <185 mm Hg and diastolic <110 mm Hg).

No evidence of active bleeding or acute trauma (fracture) on examination.

Not taking an oral anticoagulant or, if anticoagulant being taken, INR ≤1.7.

If receiving heparin in previous 48 hours, aPTT must be in normal range.

Platelet count ≥100 000 mm³.

Blood glucose concentration ≥50 mg/dL (2.7 mmol/L).

No seizure with postictal residual neurological impairments.

CT does not show a multilobar infarction (hypodensity >1/3 cerebral hemisphere).

The patient or family members understand the potential risks and benefits from treatment.

INR indicates international normalized ratio; aPTT, activated partial thromboplastin time.

From Adams HP Jr, del Zoppo G, Alberts MJ, et al. Guidelines for the early management of adults with ischemic stroke: a guideline from the American Heart Association/American Stroke Association Stroke Council, Clinical Cardiology Council, Cardiovascular Radiology and Intervention Council, and the Atherosclerotic Peripheral Vascular Disease and Quality of Care Outcomes in Research Interdisciplinary Working Groups: the American Academy of Neurology affirms the value of this guideline as an educational tool for neurologists, *Stroke* 38(5):1655, 2007.

diagnosis with CT must be accomplished before rtPA administration. The recommended dose of rtPA is 0.9 mg/kg up to a maximum dose of 90 mg. Ten percent of the total dose is administered as an initial intravenous bolus, and the remaining 90% is administered by intravenous infusion over 60 minutes.[17,21]

The desired result of thrombolytic therapy is to dissolve the clot and reperfuse the ischemic brain. The goal is to reverse or minimize the effects of stroke. The major risk and complication of rtPA therapy is bleeding, especially intracranial hemorrhage. Unlike thrombolytic protocols for acute myocardial infarction, subsequent therapy with anticoagulant or antiplatelet agents is not recommended after rtPA administration in ischemic stroke. Patients receiving thrombolytic therapy for stroke should not receive aspirin, heparin, or warfarin for at least 24 hours after treatment.[12,17]

The major barriers to effective application of thrombolytic therapy for ischemic stroke are prehospital and in-hospital delays. To help decrease delays, the public needs to be educated about stroke symptoms and activation of the emergency medical system (EMS). EMS responders need adequate education and training on managing a patient with an acute ischemic stroke, focusing on stabilization and quick transport of the patient to the emergency department. The receiving hospital should ideally be primary stroke certified and have expert staff and the infrastructure to care for the complex stroke patient.[21]

Other emergency care of the patient with ischemic stroke must include airway protection and ventilatory assistance to maintain adequate tissue oxygenation.[19] Hypertension is often present in the early period as a compensatory response, and in most cases, blood pressure (BP) must not be lowered (Table 18-2). For the patient who has not received thrombolytic therapy, antihypertensive therapy is considered only if the diastolic blood pressure is greater than 120 mm Hg or the systolic blood pressure is greater than 220 mm Hg.[12] Criteria are different for patients who have received rtPA. Their blood pressure is kept below 180/105 mm Hg to prevent intracranial hemorrhage. Intravenous labetalol or nicardipine is used to achieve blood pressure control. If these agents are not effective, nitroprusside, hydralazine, or enalaprilat should be considered.[12] Body temperature and glucose levels also must be normalized.[12,19]

Medical management also includes the identification and treatment of acute complications such as cerebral edema and seizure activity. Prophylaxis for these complications is not

TABLE 18-2	**BLOOD PRESSURE MANAGEMENT FOR STROKE ACCORDING TO THE AMERICAN STROKE ASSOCIATION GUIDELINES**
BLOOD PRESSURE*	**TREATMENT**
Nonthrombolytic Candidates	
DBP >140 mm Hg	Sodium nitroprusside (0.5 mcg/kg/min); aim for 10%-20% reduction in DBP
SBP >220 mm Hg, DBP 121-140 mm Hg, or MAP† >130 mm Hg	10-20 mg of labetalol‡ given by IVP over 1-2 min; may repeat or double labetalol every 20 min to a maximum dose of 300 mg
SBP <220 mm Hg, DBP = 120 mm Hg, or MAP† <130 mm Hg	Emergency antihypertensive therapy is deferred in the absence of aortic dissection, acute myocardial infarction, severe congestive heart failure, or hypertensive encephalopathy
Thrombolytic Candidates	
Pretreatment	
SBP >185 mm Hg or DBP >110 mm Hg	1-2 inches of nitroglycerine paste (Nitropaste) or 1-2 doses of 10-20 mg of labetalol‡ given by IVP; if BP is not reduced and maintained to <185/110 mm Hg, the patient should not be treated with tPA
During and After Treatment	
Monitor BP	BP is monitored every 15 min for 2 hr, then every 30 min for 6 hr, and then hourly for 16 hr
DBP >140 mm Hg	Sodium nitroprusside (0.5 mcg/kg/min)
SBP >230 mm Hg or DBP 121-140 mm Hg	10 mg of labetalol‡ given by IVP over 1-2 min; may repeat or double labetalol every 10 min to a maximum dose of 300 mg or give initial labetalol bolus and then start a labetalol drip at 2-8 mg/min If BP not controlled by labetalol, consider sodium nitroprusside
SBP 180-230 mm Hg or DBP 105-120 mm Hg	10 mg of labetalol‡ given by IVP; may repeat or double labetalol every 10-20 min to a maximum dose of 300 mg or give initial labetalol bolus and then start a labetalol drip at 2-8 mg/min

*All initial blood pressures should be verified before treatment by repeating reading in 5 minutes.
†As estimated by one third of the sum of systolic and double diastolic pressure.
‡Labetalol should be avoided in patients with asthma, cardiac failure, or severe abnormalities in cardiac conduction. For refractory hypertension, alternative therapy with sodium nitroprusside or enalapril may be considered.
DBP, diastolic blood pressure; *IVP*, intravenous push; *MAP*, mean arterial pressure; *SBP*, systolic blood pressure.
From Bader MK, Littlejohns LR: *AANN core curriculum for neuroscience nursing*, ed 4, St Louis, 2004, Elsevier.

recommended. Deep vein thrombosis (DVT) prophylaxis, however, should be initiated to decrease the risk of pulmonary embolism.[12] One study demonstrated that improved outcomes for ischemic stroke patients can be achieved by managing swallowing issues, initiating DVT prophylaxis, and treating hypoxemia.[23] Surgical decompression is recommended if a large cerebellar infarction compresses the brainstem.[19]

Subarachnoid Hemorrhage

Subarachnoid hemorrhage is bleeding into the subarachnoid space, which usually is caused by rupture of a cerebral aneurysm or arteriovenous malformation (AVM).[19] At the time of autopsy, approximately 4% of the population has been found to have one or more aneurysms.[24] Aneurysmal SAH is associated with a mortality rate of 25% to 50%, with most patients dying on the first day after the insult.[24] Hemorrhage due to AVM rupture has a better chance of survival and is associated with an overall mortality rate of 10% to 15%.[25]

Etiology

Cerebral aneurysm rupture accounts for approximately 85% of all cases of spontaneous SAH.[24] An aneurysm is an outpouching of the wall of a blood vessel that results from weakening of the wall of the vessel (Table 18-3).[24] Ninety percent of aneurysms are congenital—the cause of which is unknown. The other 10% can be the result of traumatic injury (that stretches and tears the muscular middle layer of the arterial vessel) or infectious material (most often from infectious vegetation on valves of the left side of the heart after bacterial endocarditis) that lodges against a vessel wall and erodes the muscular layer, or they are of undetermined cause.[26] Multiple aneurysms occur in approximately 30% of the cases and often are bilateral, occurring in the same location on both sides of the cerebral vascular system.[27]

AVM rupture is responsible for roughly 6% of all SAHs.[27] An arteriovenous malformation is a tangled mass of arterial and venous blood vessels that shunt blood directly from the arterial side into the venous side, bypassing the capillary system. They may be small, focal lesions or large, diffuse lesions that occupy almost an entire hemisphere.[26] AVMs are always congenital, although the exact embryonic cause for these malformations is unknown. They also occur in the spinal cord and the renal, gastrointestinal, and integumentary systems.[27] In contrast to SAH from aneurysm, which occurs in the middle-aged population, SAH from an AVM usually occurs in the second to fourth decades of life.[27]

Pathophysiology

The pathophysiology of the two most common causes of SAH is distinctly different.

Cerebral Aneurysm. As the individual with a congenital cerebral aneurysm matures, blood pressure rises, and more stress is placed on the poorly developed and thin vessel wall. Ballooning of the vessel occurs, giving the aneurysm a berry-like appearance. Most cerebral aneurysms are saccular or berry-like with a stem or neck. Aneurysms are usually small,

2 to 7 mm in diameter, and often occur at the base of the brain on the circle of Willis.[28] Figure 18-1 illustrates the usual distribution between the vessels. Most cerebral aneurysms occur at the bifurcations of blood vessels.[24,25,28]

The aneurysm becomes clinically significant when the vessel wall becomes so thin that it ruptures, sending arterial blood at a high pressure into the subarachnoid space. For a brief moment after the aneurysm ruptures, ICP is thought to approach mean arterial pressure (MAP), and cerebral perfusion decreases.[28] In other situations, the unruptured aneurysm expands and places pressure on surrounding structures. This is particularly true with posterior communicating artery aneurysms, because they put pressure on the oculomotor nerve (cranial nerve III), causing ipsilateral pupil dilation and ptosis.[27]

Arteriovenous Malformation. The pathophysiologic features of an AVM are related to the size and location of the malformation. One or more cerebral arteries, also known as *feeders,* supply an AVM. These feeder arteries tend to enlarge over time, increasing both the volume of blood shunted through the malformation and the overall mass effect. Large, dilated, tortuous draining veins develop as a result of increasing arterial blood flow being delivered at a higher than normal pressure. Normal vascular flow has an MAP of 70 to 80 mm Hg, a mean arteriole pressure of 35 to 45 mm Hg, and a mean capillary pressure that drops from 35 to 10 mm Hg as it connects with the venous side. Lack of this capillary bridge allows blood with an MAP of 35 to 45 mm Hg to flow into the venous system. Unlike arteries, veins have no muscular layer, and the veins become extremely engorged and rupture easily. Some patients with AVMs also have cerebral atrophy. It is the result of chronic ischemia because of the shunting of blood through the AVM and away from normal cerebral circulation.[29]

Assessment and Diagnosis

The patient with an SAH characteristically has an abrupt onset of pain, described as the "worst headache of my life." A brief loss of consciousness, nausea, vomiting, focal neurological deficits, and a stiff neck may accompany the headache.[24,26-28] The SAH may result in coma or death.

The patient's history may reveal one or more incidences of sudden onset of headache with vomiting in the weeks preceding a major SAH. These are small "warning leaks" of an aneurysm in which small amounts of blood ooze from the aneurysm into the subarachnoid space. The presence of blood is an irritant to the meninges, particularly the arachnoid membrane, and the irritation causes headache, stiff neck, and photophobia. These warning leaks seldom are detected because the condition is not severe enough for the patient to seek medical attention.[28] If a neurological deficit, such as third cranial nerve palsy, develops before aneurysm rupture, medical intervention is sought, and the aneurysm may be surgically secured before the devastation of a rupture can occur. Symptoms of unruptured AVM—headaches with dizziness or syncope or fleeting neurological deficits—also may be found in the history.[27]

TABLE 18-3 ANEURYSM CLASSIFICATION ACCORDING TO TYPE, SHAPE, LOCATION, AND COMMON CHARACTERISTICS

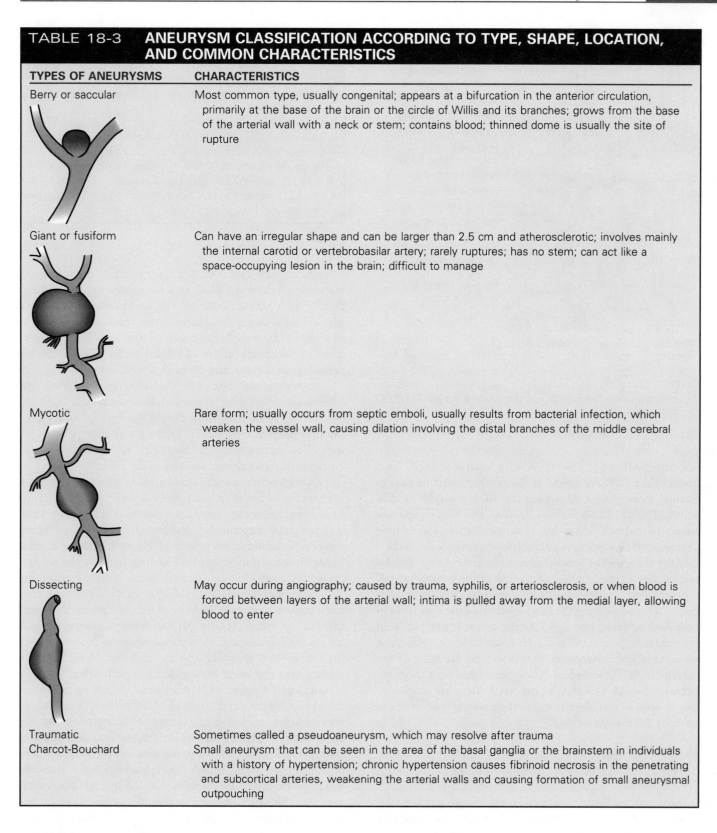

TYPES OF ANEURYSMS	CHARACTERISTICS
Berry or saccular	Most common type, usually congenital; appears at a bifurcation in the anterior circulation, primarily at the base of the brain or the circle of Willis and its branches; grows from the base of the arterial wall with a neck or stem; contains blood; thinned dome is usually the site of rupture
Giant or fusiform	Can have an irregular shape and can be larger than 2.5 cm and atherosclerotic; involves mainly the internal carotid or vertebrobasilar artery; rarely ruptures; has no stem; can act like a space-occupying lesion in the brain; difficult to manage
Mycotic	Rare form; usually occurs from septic emboli, usually results from bacterial infection, which weaken the vessel wall, causing dilation involving the distal branches of the middle cerebral arteries
Dissecting	May occur during angiography; caused by trauma, syphilis, or arteriosclerosis, or when blood is forced between layers of the arterial wall; intima is pulled away from the medial layer, allowing blood to enter
Traumatic	Sometimes called a pseudoaneurysm, which may resolve after trauma
Charcot-Bouchard	Small aneurysm that can be seen in the area of the basal ganglia or the brainstem in individuals with a history of hypertension; chronic hypertension causes fibrinoid necrosis in the penetrating and subcortical arteries, weakening the arterial walls and causing formation of small aneurysmal outpouching

Diagnosis of SAH is based on clinical presentation, CT findings, and lumbar puncture results. Noncontrast CT is the cornerstone of definitive SAH diagnosis. In 95% of the cases, CT can demonstrate blood in the subarachnoid space if performed within 48 hours of the hemorrhage.[24,28] On the basis of the appearance and the location of the SAH, diagnosis of the cause—aneurysm or AVM—may be made from the CT scan.[26] MRI is not routinely used, but it may provide greater sensitivity for detecting areas of SAH clot and potential location of bleed.[28]

If the initial CT finding is negative, a lumbar puncture is performed to obtain cerebrospinal fluid (CSF) for analysis.

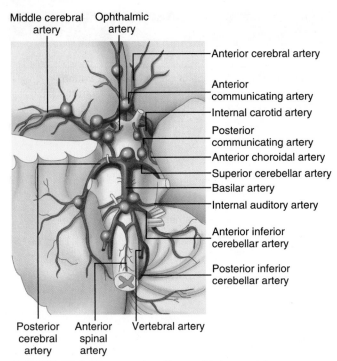

FIGURE 18-1 Common locations of intracranial aneurysms. (From Goldman L, Ausiello D: *Cecil medicine,* ed 23. St Louis, 2008, Saunders.)

- Grade I: asymptomatic or minimal headache and slight nuchal rigidity
- Grade II: moderate to severe headache, nuchal rigidity, but no neurological deficit other than cranial nerve palsy
- Grade III: drowsiness, confusion, or mild focal deficit
- Grade IV: stupor, moderate to severe hemiparesis, possible early decerebrate rigidity, and vegetative disturbances
- Grade V: deep coma, decerebrate rigidity, moribund appearance

CSF after SAH appears bloody and has a red blood cell count greater than 1000 cells/mm[3]. If the lumbar puncture is performed more than 5 days after the SAH, the CSF fluid is xanthochromic (dark amber) because the blood products have broken down.[29] Cloudy CSF usually indicates some type of infectious process, such as bacterial meningitis, not SAH.[28]

After the SAH has been documented, cerebral angiography is necessary to identify the exact cause of the hemorrhage. If a cerebral aneurysm rupture is the cause, angiography is essential for identifying the exact location of the aneurysm in preparation for surgery.[27,29,30] After the aneurysm has been located, it is graded using the Hunt and Hess classification scale. This scale categorizes the patient on the basis of the severity of the neurological deficits associated with the hemorrhage (Box 18-4).[31] If AVM rupture is the cause, angiography is necessary to identify the feeding arteries and draining veins of the malformation.[26]

Medical Management

SAH is a medical emergency, and time is of the essence. Preservation of neurological function is the goal, and early diagnosis is crucial. Initial treatment must always support vital functions. Airway management and ventilatory assistance may be necessary.[19] A ventriculostomy is performed to control ICP if the patient's level of consciousness is depressed.[30]

Evidence suggests that only 19% of the deaths attributable to aneurysmal SAH are related to the direct effects of the initial hemorrhage.[32] Rebleeding accounts for 22% of deaths from aneurysmal SAH, cerebral vasospasm for 23%, and nonneurological medical complications for 23%.[32] Principal nonneurological causes of death are systemic inflammatory response syndrome (SIRS) and secondary organ dysfunction.[33] After initial intervention has provided necessary support for vital physiologic functions, medical management of acute SAH is aimed primarily toward prevention and treatment of the complications of SAH that can produce further neurological damage and death.[28]

Rebleeding. Rebleeding is the occurrence of a second SAH in an unsecured aneurysm or, less commonly, an AVM.[6] The incidence of rebleeding during the first 24 hours after the first bleed is 4%, with a 1% to 2% chance per day for the following month. The mortality rate associated with aneurysmal rebleeding is approximately 70%.[26,27]

Historically, conservative measures to prevent rebleeding have included blood pressure control and SAH precautions (see "Nursing Management"). An elevation in blood pressure is a normal compensatory response to maintain adequate cerebral perfusion after a neurological insult. In the belief that hypertension contributes to rebleeding, intravenous antihypertensive agents are used to maintain a systolic blood pressure no greater than 140 mm Hg.[28] Individualized guidelines must be determined on the basis of the clinical condition and preexisting values of the patient. Evidence suggests that rebleeding has more to do with variations in blood pressure than it does with absolute values and that blood pressure control does not lower the incidence of rebleeding.[30]

Surgical Clipping of Aneurysms. Definitive treatment for the prevention of rebleeding is surgical clipping or endovascular coiling with complete obliteration of the aneurysm.[27,28] Timing of the operation is a key medical management issue. Since the introduction of microsurgery and improved surgical techniques, patients are commonly taken to the operating room within the first 48 hours after rupture.[28] This early surgical intervention to secure the aneurysm eliminates the risk of rebleeding and allows more aggressive therapy to be used in the postoperative period for the treatment of vasospasm.[26] Early surgery also allows the neurosurgeon to flush out the excess blood and clots from the basal cisterns (reservoir of CSF around the base of the brain and circle of Willis) to reduce the risk of vasospasm.[33] Careful consideration of the patient's clinical situation is necessary in determining the optimal time for surgery.

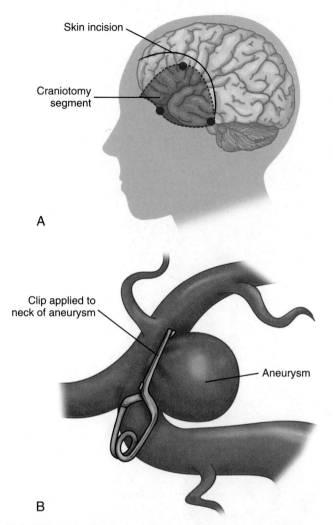

FIGURE 18-2 Clipping of a posterior communicating artery aneurysm. *A,* The *solid curved line* shows the typical skin incision, and the *dashed lines* show the craniotomy location. *B,* Application of the clip to the aneurysm.

The surgical procedure involves a craniotomy to expose and isolate the area of aneurysm. A clip is placed over the neck of the aneurysm to eliminate the area of weakness (Figure 18-2). This is a technically difficult procedure that requires the skill of an experienced neurosurgeon. It is not uncommon, particularly in early surgery, for the clot to break away from the aneurysm as it is surgically exposed. Extensive hemorrhage into the craniotomy site results, and cessation of the hemorrhage often causes increased neurological deficits. Deficits also may occur as a result of surgical manipulation to gain access to the site of the aneurysm.[28]

Surgical Excision of Arteriovenous Malformations. Management of AVMs has traditionally involved surgical excision or conservative management of such symptoms as seizures and headache. The decision for surgical excision depends on the location and size of the AVM. Some malformations are located so deep in the cerebral structures (thalamus or midbrain) that attempts to remove the AVM would cause severe neurological deficits. History of a previous hemorrhage and the patient's age and overall condition are also taken into account in the decision regarding surgical intervention.[28]

Surgical excision of large AVMs includes the risk of reperfusion bleeding. As feeding arteries of the AVM are clamped off, the arterial blood that usually flowed into the AVM is diverted into the surrounding circulation. In many cases, the surrounding tissue has been in a state of chronic ischemia, and the arterial vessels feeding these areas are maximally dilated. As arterial blood begins to flow at a higher volume and pressure into these dilated arteries, blood may seep from the vessels. Evidence of reperfusion bleeding in the operating room is an indication that no more arterial blood can be diverted from the AVM without risk of serious ICH. In the postoperative phase, a low blood pressure is maintained to prevent further reperfusion bleeding. For large AVMs, two to four stages of surgery may be required over 6 to 12 months.[28]

Embolization. Embolization is used to secure a cerebral aneurysm or AVM that is surgically inaccessible because of size or location or because of the medical instability of the patient. Embolization involves several new interventional neuroradiology techniques. All of the techniques use a percutaneous transfemoral approach in a manner similar to an angiogram. Under fluoroscopic guidance, the catheter is threaded up to the internal carotid artery. Specially developed microcatheters are then manipulated into the area of the vascular anomaly, and embolic materials are placed endovascularly. Three embolization techniques are used, depending on the underlying pathologic derangement.[26]

The first type of embolization is used to embolize an AVM. Small polymeric silicone (Silastic) beads or glue is slowly introduced into the vessels feeding the AVM. Blood flow carries the material to the site, and embolization is achieved. This procedure may be used in combination with surgery. One to three sessions of embolization of the feeding vessels are performed to reduce the size of the lesion before a craniotomy is performed for total excision. The primary risk of this procedure is lodging of the embolic substance in a vessel that feeds normal tissue, which creates an embolic stroke with the immediate onset of neurological symptoms.[26]

The second type of embolization involves placement of one or more detachable coils into an aneurysm to produce an endovascular thrombus (Figure 18-3). The advantage of this technique is that an electrical current creates a positive charge on the coil, which induces electrothrombosis. Complications include embolic stroke, coil migration, overproduction of the clot, subtotal occlusion and intraprocedural rupture of the vasculature, and death.[26]

Cerebral Vasospasm. The presence or absence of cerebral vasospasm significantly affects the outcome of aneurysmal SAH. This complication does not occur with SAH resulting from AVM rupture. Cerebral vasospasm is a narrowing of the lumen of the cerebral arteries, possibly in response to subarachnoid blood clots coating the outer surface of the blood vessels. Because aneurysms usually occur at the circle of Willis, the major vessels responsible for feeding the cerebral circulation are affected by vasospasm. Depending on the arterial

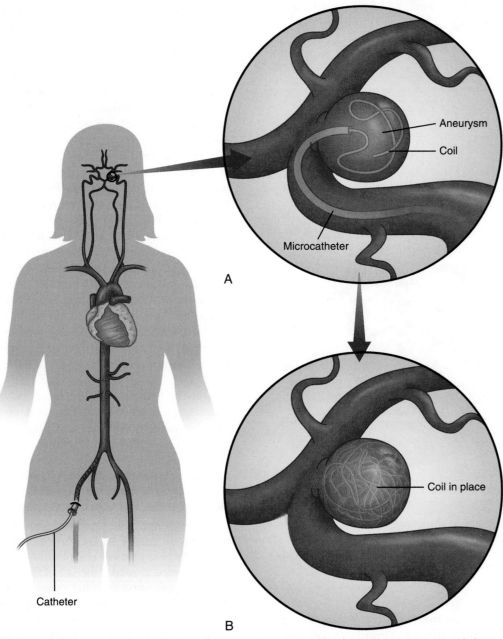

Aneurysm

Coil

Microcatheter

A

Coil in place

B

Catheter

FIGURE 18-3 Endovascular occlusion of a posterior communicating artery aneurysm. *A,* Insertion of the microcatheter into the aneurysm through the right femoral artery, aorta, and left carotid artery. *B,* Occlusion of the aneurysm with coils.

vessels involved in the vasospasm reaction, decreased arterial flow occurs in large areas of the cerebral hemispheres.[6]

It is estimated that vasospasm, which is demonstrable by angiography, develops in 70% of all patients with SAH.[34] Thirty-two percent of these patients have symptomatic vasospasm, resulting in ischemic stroke or death for up to 23% of them despite the use of maximal therapy.[34] The onset of vasospasm is usually 3 to 12 days after the initial hemorrhage.[19] Three treatments are commonly used: induced hypertensive, hypervolemic, hemodilution (HHH) therapy; oral nimodipine; and transluminal cerebral angioplasty.[34]

Hypertensive, Hypervolemic, Hemodilution Therapy. HHH therapy involves increasing the patient's blood pressure and cardiac output with vasoactive medications and diluting the patient's blood with fluid and volume expanders. The goal of the therapy is to maintain systolic blood pressure between 150 and 160 mm Hg. The increase in volume and pressure forces blood through the vasospastic area at higher pressures. Hemodilution facilitates flow through the area by reducing blood viscosity.[26] The Stroke Council of the American Heart Association (AHA) has recommended this therapy for prevention and treatment of vasospasm.[30]

The obvious deterrent to the use of induced hypertension is the risk of rebleeding in an unsecured aneurysm. Securing the aneurysm before HHH therapy is preferred. Cerebral edema, elevated ICP, cardiac failure, and electrolyte imbalance are also risks of HHH therapy. Careful monitoring of the patient's neurological status, hemodynamic parameters, ICP, and serum electrolytes is necessary.[28]

Nimodipine. Nimodipine is strongly recommended to reduce the poor outcomes associated with vasospasm. The exact nature of the effect of nimodipine is not clear, but use of the drug has demonstrated consistently positive effects on outcome without any demonstrable effect on the incidence or severity of vasospasm.[30,34] A dose of 60 mg of nimodipine is given orally every 4 hours for 14 to 21 days. Nimodipine may produce hypotension, especially when administered concurrently with other antihypertensive agents.[34]

Cerebral Angioplasty. Cerebral angioplasty is used when pharmacological management of cerebral vasospasm has failed. It is performed only when CT or MRI provides evidence that infarction has not occurred. An interventional neuroradiologist performs the procedure, and a local, general, or neuroleptic analgesia is used. The technique of cerebral angioplasty is very similar to that used in the coronary vasculature. Risks include intimal perforation or rupture, cerebral artery thrombosis or embolism, recurrence of stenosis, and severe, diffuse vasospasm unresponsive to therapy. Hemorrhage at the femoral site also may occur. This procedure is recommended when conventional therapy is unsuccessful.[30,34]

Hyponatremia. Hyponatremia develops in 10% to 43% of patients with SAH as the result of a central salt-wasting syndrome. It usually occurs during the same period as vasospasm, several days after the initial hemorrhage.[26] The use of fluid restriction to treat hyponatremia in the patient with SAH is associated with a poor outcome. The AHA Stroke Council strongly recommends that fluid restriction not be used in this instance and instead recommends sodium replenishment with isotonic fluids.[30]

Hydrocephalus. Hydrocephalus is a late complication that occurs in approximately 25% of patients after SAH.[30] Blood that has circulated in the subarachnoid space and has been absorbed by the arachnoid villi may obstruct the villi and reduce the rate of CSF absorption. Over time, increasing volumes of CSF in the intracranial space produce communicating hydrocephalus. Treatment consists of placing a drain to remove CSF. This can be accomplished temporarily by insertion of a ventriculostomy[24] or permanently by placement of a ventriculoperitoneal shunt.[27,30]

Intracerebral Hemorrhage

Intracerebral hemorrhage is bleeding directly into cerebral tissue.[35] ICH destroys cerebral tissue, causes cerebral edema, and increases ICP. The source of intracerebral bleeding is usually a small artery, but it can result also from rupture of an AVM or aneurysm. The most important cause of spontaneous ICH is hypertension, and this discussion concentrates on spontaneous hypertensive ICH.[36]

Spontaneous ICH accounts for at least 10% of all stroke admissions.[35] The likelihood of death or disability is higher with ICH than with ischemic stroke or SAH. The mortality rate for hemorrhagic stroke is up to 50% within 1 month.[37] Only 20% of patients with ICH return to a functional life at 6 months.[37] The key risk factors for ICH are age-associated cerebral amyloid angiopathy and hypertension.[35]

Etiology

ICH is most often caused by hypertensive rupture of a cerebral vessel, resulting from a long-standing history of hypertension.[35] Other possible causes of spontaneous ICH are anticoagulation or thrombolytic therapy, coagulation disorders, drug abuse, and hemorrhage into cerebral infarct or brain tumors.[27,38] Often on questioning, the patient with a hypertensive hemorrhage admits to having discontinued antihypertensive medication 2 to 3 weeks before the hemorrhage.

Pathophysiology

The pathophysiology of ICH is caused by continued elevated blood pressure exerting force against smaller arterial vessels that have become damaged from arteriosclerotic changes. Eventually, these arteries break, and blood bursts from the vessels into the surrounding cerebral tissue, creating a hematoma. ICP rises precipitously in response to the increase in overall intracranial volume.[38]

Assessment and Diagnosis

Initial assessment usually reveals a critically ill patient who often is unconscious and requires ventilatory support. History from a relative or significant other describes a sudden onset of focal deficit often accompanied by severe headache, nausea, vomiting, and rapid neurological deterioration.[39] Signs and symptoms vary depending on the location of the ICH.[38] One third of the patients have maximal symptoms at onset. Assessment of vital signs usually reveals a severely elevated blood pressure (200/100 to 250/150 mm Hg). Signs of increased ICP are often present by the time the patient arrives in the emergency department. Diagnosis is established with CT. Angiography is recommended for patients considered surgical candidates without a clear cause of hemorrhage.[35-39]

Medical Management

ICH is a medical emergency. Initial management requires attention to airway, breathing, and circulation. Intubation is usually necessary. Blood pressure management must be based on individual factors. Reduction in blood pressure is usually necessary to decrease ongoing bleeding, but lowering blood pressure too much or too rapidly may compromise cerebral perfusion pressure (CPP), especially in the patient with elevated ICP. National guidelines recommend keeping the *mean* arterial blood pressure below 130 mm Hg in patients with a history of hypertension by means of moderate blood pressure reduction to a mean arterial pressure below 110 mm Hg.[39] Vasopressor therapy after fluid replenishment is recommended if systolic blood pressure falls below 90 mm Hg.[36]

Increased ICP is common with ICH and is a major contributor to mortality. Recommended management includes mannitol when indicated, hyperventilation, and neuromuscular blockade with sedation. Steroids are avoided. The CPP must be kept higher than 70 mm Hg.[36,37]

The goal for fluid management is euvolemia, with a recommended pulmonary artery occlusion pressure (PAOP) of 10 to 14 mm Hg. Body temperature is maintained at less than 38.5° C through the use of acetaminophen or cooling blankets. Euglycemia, a blood glucose level less than 140 mg/dL, is maintained with insulin therapy, but hypoglycemia should be avoided. Use of short-acting benzodiazepines or propofol is recommended to treat agitation or hyperactivity. Pneumatic compression devices are used to decrease risk of pulmonary embolism. Anticonvulsant therapy is initiated if the patient experiences seizures. Coagulation disorders should be treated, and any anticoagulation medications should be withheld.[36,39]

The benefit of surgical treatment of spontaneous ICH is unclear. Recommendations for surgical removal of the clot depend on the size and location of the hematoma, the patient's ICP, and other neurological symptoms.[39] Surgical evacuation of the clot is recommended for patients with cerebellar hemorrhage greater than 3 cm with neurological deterioration or hydrocephalus with brainstem compression, as well as for young patients with moderate or large lobar hemorrhage with clinical deterioration. Numerous techniques are being investigated to lessen the risk of brain damage associated with craniotomy for ICH.[39]

Evidence-based guidelines for the management of the patient with ICH are listed in the Evidence-Based Practice box on Spontaneous Intracerebral Hemorrhage Management Guidelines.

Nursing Management

Nursing management of the patient with stroke incorporates a variety of nursing diagnoses (Nursing Diagnoses Priorities box on Stroke). **Nursing priorities are directed toward (1) monitoring for changes in neurological and hemodynamic status, (2) maintaining surveillance for complications, (3) providing comfort and emotional support, and (4) educating the patient and family.**

NURSING DIAGNOSIS PRIORITIES

Stroke

- Ineffective Cerebral Tissue Perfusion related to decreased cerebral blood flow, p. A-29
- Ineffective Cerebral Tissue Perfusion related to hemorrhage, p. A-29
- Acute Pain related to transmission and perception of cutaneous, visceral, muscular, or ischemic impulses, p. A-5
- Unilateral Neglect related to perceptual disruption, p. A-37
- Impaired Verbal Communication related to cerebral speech center injury, p. A-25
- Impaired Swallowing related to neuromuscular impairment, fatigue, and limited awareness, p. A-24
- Risk for Aspiration, p. A-35
- Risk for Infection, p. A-36
- Anxiety related to threat of biological, psychological, or social integrity, p. A-7
- Disturbed Body Image related to actual change in body structure, function, or appearance, p. A-16
- Compromised Family Coping related to critically ill family member, p. A-9
- Deficient Knowledge: Discharge Regimen related to lack of previous exposure to information (see Patient Education box on Stroke), p. A-15

EVIDENCE-BASED COLLABORATIVE PRACTICE

Spontaneous Intracerebral Hemorrhage Management Guidelines

The following are class 1 recommendations from the American Heart Association and American Stroke Association. Class 1 recommendations are conditions for which there is evidence for and/or general agreement that the procedure or treatment is useful and effective.

- Rapid neuroimaging with CT or MRI is recommended to distinguish ischemic stroke from ICH.
- Patients with a severe coagulation factor deficiency or severe thrombocytopenia should receive appropriate factor replacement therapy or platelets, respectively.
- In patients with ICH whose INR is elevated owing to OAC-therapy, warfarin should be withheld, and they should be given therapy to replace vitamin K–dependent factors and correct the INR and should receive intravenous vitamin K.
- Patients with ICH should receive intermittent pneumatic compression for prevention of venous thromboembolism in addition to elastic stockings.

- Initial monitoring and management of patients with ICH should take place in an intensive care unit, preferably one with physician and nursing neuroscience intensive care expertise.
- Blood glucose levels should be monitored and normoglycemia is recommended.
- Patients with clinical seizures should be treated with antiepileptic drugs. Patients with a change in mental status who are found to have electrographic seizures on EEG should be treated with antiepileptic drugs.
- Patients with cerebellar hemorrhage who are deteriorating neurologically or who have brainstem compression and/or hydrocephalus from ventricular obstruction should undergo surgical removal of the hemorrhage as soon as possible.
- After the acute ICH, absent medical contraindications, BP should be well controlled, particularly for patients with ICH location typical of hypertensive vasculopathy.

EEG, electroencephalogram; *OAC*, oral anticoagulants.
Modified from Morgenstern LB, Hemphill JC 3rd, Anderson C, et al; American Heart Association Stroke Council and Council on Cardiovascular Nursing: Guidelines for the management of spontaneous intracerebral hemorrhage: A Guideline for Healthcare Professionals From the American Heart Association/American Stroke Association, *Stroke* 41(9):2108, 2010.

Monitoring for Changes in Neurological and Hemodynamic Status

The goal of frequent assessments is early recognition of neurological or hemodynamic deterioration. Close monitoring of the patient's neurological signs and vital signs is essential and requires almost continuous observation. Automatic noninvasive devices such as a blood pressure cuff and a pulse oximeter are helpful. Seizure activity must be identified and treated immediately. It is essential that all personnel working with the patient be aware of the desired hemodynamic and neurological parameters set by the physician and that the physician be notified at the first sign of any changes.

Maintaining Surveillance for Complications

The patient with stroke should be monitored closely for signs of bleeding, vasospasm, and increased ICP. Other complications of stroke include aspiration, malnutrition, pneumonia, DVT, pulmonary embolism, pressure ulcers, contractures, and joint abnormalities.[29] Nursing measures to prevent these complications are well known.

Additional complications that may be seen in the patient with stroke are related to the area of the brain that has been damaged. Damage to the temporoparietal area can create a variety of disturbances that affect the patient's ability to interpret sensory information. Damage to the dominant hemisphere (usually left) produces problems with speech and language and abstract and analytic skills. Damage to the nondominant hemisphere (usually right) produces problems with spatial relationships. The resulting deficits include agnosia, apraxia, and visual field defects. Perceptual deficits are not as readily noticeable as motor deficits but may be more debilitating and can lead to the inability to perform skilled or purposeful tasks. The patient also may have impaired swallowing.[26,29]

Bleeding and Vasospasm. Sudden onset of or an increase in headache and nausea and vomiting, increased blood pressure, and changes in respiration herald the onset of rebleeding and indicate a second SAH in an unsecured aneurysm. The first indication of vasospasm is usually the appearance of new focal or global neurological deficits.

SAH precautions must be implemented to prevent any stress or straining that could potentially precipitate rebleeding. Precautions include blood pressure control; bed rest; a dark, quiet environment; and stool softeners. Short-acting analgesics and sedatives are used to relieve pain and anxiety. The patient must be kept calm. Limb restraints cause straining and must be avoided. The head of the bed should be elevated to 35 to 45 degrees at all times. The patient is taught to avoid any activities that correspond to performance of the Valsalva maneuver, such as pushing with the legs to move up in bed, straining for a bowel movement, or holding his or her breath during procedures or discomfort. DVT precautions are routinely implemented. Collaboration with the patient and family is used to establish a visitation plan to meet patient and family needs. Often,

family members at the bedside can help the patient remain calm.[26,28,29]

Increased Intracranial Pressure. Numerous signs and symptoms of increased ICP can be observed. A change in the level of consciousness is the most sensitive indicator. Others include unequal pupil size, decreased pupillary response to light, headache, projectile vomiting, altered breathing patterns, Cushing's triad (bradycardia, systolic hypertension, and bradypnea), diminished brainstem reflexes, papilledema, and abnormal extension (decerebrate posturing) or flexion (decorticate posturing).[26,28,29]

Impaired Swallowing. Normal swallowing occurs in four phases that are controlled by the cranial nerves. Damage to the brain, brainstem, or cranial nerves can result in a variety of swallowing deficits that can place the patient at risk for aspiration. The stroke patient is observed for signs of dysphagia, including drooling; difficulty handling oral secretions; absence of gag, cough, or swallowing reflex; moist, gurgling voice quality; decreased mouth and tongue movements; and the presence of dysarthria. A speech therapy consultation is initiated if any of these signs is present, and the patient must not be orally fed. In the absence of these warning signs, the patient may be fed, as ordered by the physician, although he or she must be continually monitored for signs of aspiration.[26,28,29]

Educating the Patient and Family

Rehabilitation starts in the critical care area, with a multidisciplinary team designing and implementing an individualized plan to maximize the patient's potential for neurological rehabilitation. Early in the patient's hospital stay, the patient and family must be taught about stroke, its causes, and its treatment. As the patient moves toward discharge, teaching focuses on the interventions necessary for preventing the recurrence of the event and on maximizing the patient's rehabilitation potential. The patient's family must be encouraged to participate in the patient's care; learn how to feed, dress, and bathe the patient; and learn some basic rehabilitation techniques. The importance of participating in a neurological rehabilitation program or a support group, or both, must be stressed (Patient Education box on Stroke).

PATIENT EDUCATION

Stroke

- Pathophysiology of disease
- Specific cause
- Risk factor modification
- Importance of taking medications
- Activities of daily living
- Measures to prevent injuries of impaired limbs
- Measures to compensate for residual deficits
- Basic rehabilitation techniques
- Importance of participating in neurological rehabilitation program or support group

Collaborative management of the patient with a stroke is outlined in the Collaborative Management box on Stroke.

COLLABORATIVE MANAGEMENT
Stroke

- Differentiate the cause of the stroke:
  - Ischemic
  - Subarachnoid hemorrhage
  - Cerebral aneurysm
  - AVM
  - Intracerebral bleed
- Implement treatment according to cause of bleed:
  - Ischemic:
    - Thrombolytic therapy
    - Blood pressure control
  - Subarachnoid hemorrhage:
    - Surgical aneurysm clipping or AVM excision
    - Embolization
  - Intracerebral bleed:
    - Blood pressure control
  - Protect patient's airway.
  - Provide ventilatory assistance as required.
  - Perform frequent neurological assessments.
  - Maintain surveillance for complications.
  - Cerebral edema:
    - Cerebral ischemia/vasospasm
    - Rebleeding
    - Impaired swallowing
  - Neurological deficits
- Provide comfort and emotional support.
- Design and implement appropriate rehabilitation program.
- Educate patient and family.

GUILLAIN-BARRÉ SYNDROME

Guillain-Barré syndrome (GBS), once thought to be a single entity characterized by inflammatory peripheral neuropathy, is a combination of clinical features with various forms of presentation and multiple pathological processes. A full discussion of this complex condition is beyond the scope of this chapter. Most cases of GBS do not require admission to a critical care unit. However, the prototype of GBS, known as *acute inflammatory demyelinating polyradiculoneuropathy* (AIDP), involves a rapidly progressive, ascending peripheral nerve dysfunction leading to paralysis that may produce respiratory failure. Because of the need for ventilatory support, AIDP is one of the few peripheral neurological diseases that necessitates care in a critical care environment.[40] In this discussion, all references to GBS pertain to the AIDP prototype.

The annual incidence of GBS is 1.2 to 2.3 cases per 100,000 persons.[41] It occurs more often in males and is the most commonly acquired demyelinating neuropathy.[41] Occasionally, clusters of cases are reported, such as occurred following the 1977 swine flu vaccinations.[42]

Etiology

The precise cause of GBS remains unknown, but the syndrome involves an immune-mediated response involving cell-mediated immunity and development of immunoglobulin G (IgG) antibodies. Most patients report a viral infection 1 to 3 weeks before the onset of clinical manifestations, usually involving the upper respiratory tract.[41]

Numerous antecedent causes, or triggering events, have been associated with GBS. They include viral infections (e.g., influenza; cytomegalovirus; hepatitis A, B, or C; Epstein-Barr virus; human immunodeficiency virus), bacterial infections (e.g., gastrointestinal *Campylobacter jejuni*, *Mycoplasma pneumoniae*), vaccines (e.g., rabies, tetanus, influenza), lymphoma, surgery, and trauma.[41]

Pathophysiology

GBS affects the motor and sensory pathways of the peripheral nervous system as well as the autonomic nervous system functions of the cranial nerves. The major finding in AIDP-type GBS is a segmental demyelination process of the peripheral nerves. GBS is thought to be an autoimmune response to antibodies formed in response to a recent physiological event. T cells migrate to the peripheral nerves, resulting in edema and inflammation. Macrophages then invade the area and break down the myelin. Inflammation around this demyelinated area causes further dysfunction. Some axonal damage also occurs.[41]

The myelin sheath of the peripheral nerves is generated by Schwann cells and acts as an insulator for the peripheral nerve. Myelin promotes rapid conduction of nerve impulses by allowing the impulses to jump along the nerve by means of the nodes of Ranvier. Disruption of the myelin fiber slows and may eventually stop the conduction of impulses along the peripheral nerves. In GBS, the more thickly myelinated fibers of motor pathways and the cranial nerves are more severely affected than are the thinly myelinated sensory fibers of cutaneous pain, touch, and temperature.[41]

After the temporary inflammatory reaction stops, myelin-producing cells begin the process of reinsulating the demyelinated portions of the peripheral nervous system. When remyelination occurs, normal neurological function should return. In some instances, the axon may be damaged during the inflammatory process. The degree of axonal damage is responsible for the degree of neurological dysfunction that persists after recovery.[41]

Assessment and Diagnosis

Symptoms of GBS include motor weakness, paresthesias and other sensory changes, cranial nerve dysfunction (especially oculomotor, facial, glossopharyngeal, vagal, spinal accessory, and hypoglossal), and some autonomic dysfunction. The usual course of GBS begins with an abrupt onset of lower extremity weakness that progresses to flaccidity and ascends over a period of hours to days. Motor loss usually is symmetric, bilateral, and ascending. In the most severe cases, complete flaccidity of all peripheral nerves, including spinal and cranial nerves, occurs.[40,41,43]

The patient is admitted to the hospital when lower extremity weakness prevents mobility. Admission to the critical care unit is necessary when progression of the weakness threatens respiratory muscles. As the patient's weakness progresses, close observation is essential. Frequent assessment of the respiratory system, including ventilatory parameters such as inspiratory force and tidal volume, is necessary. The most common cause of death of patients with GBS is respiratory arrest. As the disease progresses and respiratory effort weakens, intubation and mechanical ventilation are necessary. Frequent assessment of neurological deterioration is continued until the patient reaches the peak of the disease, and a plateau occurs.[41,43]

The diagnosis of GBS is based on clinical findings plus the results of CSF analysis and nerve conduction studies. The diagnostic finding is elevated CSF protein with normal cell count.[44] The increased protein count usually occurs after the first week but does not occur in approximately 10% of all cases. Nerve conduction studies that test the velocity at which nerve impulses are conducted show significant reduction, as the demyelinating process of the disease suggests.[43]

Medical Management

With no curative treatment available, the medical management of GBS is limited. The disease must run its course, which is characterized by ascending paralysis that advances over 1 to 3 weeks and then remains at a plateau for 2 to 4 weeks.[41] The plateau stage is followed by descending paralysis and return to normal or near-normal function. The main focus of medical management is the support of bodily functions and the prevention of complications.[41]

Plasmapheresis and intravenous immune globulin (IVIG) are used to treat GBS.[41] They have been shown to be equally effective.[45] Plasmapheresis involves the removal of venous blood through a catheter, separation of plasma from blood cells, and reinfusion of the blood cells plus autologous plasma or another replacement solution. Although the number of exchanges may vary, the usual regimen is five exchanges over a 5-day period.[41] IVIG has emerged as the preferred therapy because of convenience and availability. The usual dose is 0.4 mg/kg for five days.[43]

Nursing Management

The nursing management of the patient with GBS incorporates a variety of nursing diagnoses and interventions (Nursing Diagnoses Priorities box on Guillain-Barré syndrome). The goal of nursing management is to support all normal body functions until the patient can do so on his or her own. Although the condition is reversible, the patient with GBS requires extensive long-term care, because recovery can be a long process. **Nursing priorities are directed toward (1) maintaining surveillance for complications, (2) initiating rehabilitation, (3) facilitating nutritional support, (4) providing comfort and emotional support, and (5) educating the patient and family.**

NURSING DIAGNOSIS PRIORITIES
Guillain-Barré Syndrome

- Ineffective Breathing Pattern related to musculoskeletal fatigue or neuromuscular impairment, p. A-27
- Acute Pain related to transmission and perception of cutaneous, visceral, muscular, or ischemic impulses, p. A-4
- Activity Intolerance related to prolonged immobility or deconditioning, p. A-7
- Risk for Aspiration, p. A-35
- Imbalanced Nutrition: Less Than Body Requirements related to lack of exogenous nutrients or increased metabolic demand, p. A-22
- Risk for Infection, p. A-36
- Anxiety related to threat of biological, psychological, or social integrity, p. A-7
- Powerlessness related to lack of control over current situation or disease progression, p. A-7
- Ineffective Coping related to situational crisis and personal vulnerability, p. A-30
- Compromised Family Coping related to critically ill family member, p. A-9
- Deficient Knowledge: Discharge Regimen related to lack of previous exposure to information (see Patient Education box on Guillain-Barré syndrome) , p. A-15

Maintaining Surveillance for Complications

Continuous assessment of the progressive paralysis associated with GBS is essential to timely intervention and the prevention of respiratory arrest and further neurological insult. After the patient is intubated and started on mechanical ventilation, close observation for pulmonary complications, such as atelectasis, pneumonia, and pneumothorax, is necessary. Autonomic dysfunction (dysautonomia) in the GBS patient can produce variations in heart rate and blood pressure that can reach extreme values.[40,41,46] Hypertension and tachycardia may require beta-blocker therapy. All patients with GBS must be observed for this phenomenon.

Initiating Rehabilitation

In patients with GBS, immobility may last for months. The usual course of the disease involves an average of 10 days of symptom progression and 10 days of maximal level of dysfunction, followed by 2 to 48 weeks of recovery. Although GBS usually is completely reversible, the patient requires physical and occupational rehabilitation because of the problems of long-term immobility. Rehabilitation starts in the critical care area, with a multidisciplinary team designing and implementing an individualized plan to maximize the patient's potential for rehabilitation.[46]

Facilitating Nutritional Support

Nutritional support is implemented early in the course of the disease. Because recovery from GBS is a long process, adequate nutritional support will be a problem for an extended period. Nutritional support is usually accomplished through the use of enteral feeding.

Providing Comfort and Emotional Support

Pain control is another important component in the care of the patient with GBS. Although patients may have minimal to no motor function, most sensory functions remain, causing patients considerable muscle aching and pain. Because of the duration of this illness, a safe, effective, long-term solution to pain management must be identified.[46] These patients also require extensive psychological support. Although the illness is almost 100% reversible, lack of control over the situation, constant pain or discomfort, and the long-term nature of the disorder create coping difficulties for the patient. GBS does not affect the level of consciousness or cerebral function. Patient interaction and communication are essential elements of the nursing management plan.

Educating the Patient and Family

Early in the patient's hospital stay, the patient and family must be taught about GBS and its different treatments. As the patient moves toward discharge, teaching focuses on the interventions to maximize the patient's rehabilitation potential. The patient's family must be encouraged to participate in the patient's care and to learn some basic rehabilitation techniques. The importance of participating in a neurological rehabilitation program (if necessary) must be stressed (Patient Education box on Guillain-Barré Syndrome).[46]

PATIENT EDUCATION

Guillain-Barré Syndrome

- Pathophysiology of disease
- Importance of taking medications
- Measures to compensate for residual deficits
- Basic rehabilitation techniques
- Importance of participating in neurological rehabilitation program, if necessary

---

Collaborative management of the patient with Guillain-Barré syndrome is outlined in the Collaborative Management box on Guillain-Barré syndrome.

CRANIOTOMY

A craniotomy is performed to gain access to portions of the central nervous system (CNS) inside the cranium, usually to allow removal of a space-occupying lesion such as a brain tumor (Table 18-4). Common procedures include tumor resection or removal, cerebral decompression, evacuation of hematoma or abscess, and clipping or removal of an aneurysm or AVM. Most patients who undergo craniotomy for tumor resection or removal do not require care in a critical care unit. Patients who do usually need intensive monitoring or are at greater risk for complications because of underlying cardiopulmonary dysfunction or the surgical approach used. Box 18-5 provides definitions of common neurosurgical terms.[47]

Preoperative Care

Protection of the integrity of the CNS is a major priority of care for the patient awaiting a craniotomy. Optimal arterial oxygenation, hemodynamic stability, and cerebral perfusion are essential for maintaining adequate cerebral oxygenation. Management of seizure activity is essential for controlling metabolic needs.[44]

Detailed assessment and documentation of the patient's preoperative neurological status are imperative for accurate postoperative evaluation. Attention is focused on identifying and describing the nature and extent of any preoperative neurological deficits. When pituitary surgery is planned, a thorough evaluation of endocrine function is necessary to prevent major intraoperative and postoperative complications.[45]

Trends in health care demand judicious use of routine preoperative studies. Depending on the type of surgery to be performed and the general health of the patient, preoperative screening may include a complete blood cell count (CBC); tests for blood urea nitrogen (BUN), creatinine, and fasting blood glucose (FBG); a chest radiograph; and an electrocardiogram. Blood type and crossmatch may also be ordered.

Preoperative teaching is necessary to prepare the patient and family for what to expect in the postoperative period. A description of the intravascular lines and intracranial catheters used during the postoperative period allows the family to focus on the patient, rather than be overwhelmed by masses of tubing. Some or all of the patient's hair is shaved

---

COLLABORATIVE MANAGEMENT

Guillain-Barré Syndrome

- Support bodily functions:
  - Protect airway.
  - Provide ventilatory assistance, as required.
- Initiate treatments to limit duration of the syndrome:
  - Plasmapheresis
  - Intravenous immunoglobulin
- Initiate nutritional support.
- Maintain surveillance for complications:

- Infections
- Cardiac dysrhythmias
- Blood pressure alterations
- Temperature alterations
- Provide comfort and emotional support.
- Design and implement appropriate rehabilitation program.
- Educate patient and family.

TABLE 18-4 TUMOR TYPES AND CHARACTERISTICS

TUMOR	CLINICAL FEATURES	TREATMENT/PROGNOSIS
Glioblastoma multiforme	Often manifests with nonspecific complaints and increased ICP As tumor grows, focal deficits develop	Rapidly progressive course, with poor prognosis Total surgical removal usually not possible; response to radiation poor
Astrocytoma	Presentation similar to that of glioblastoma multiforme, but course more protracted, often over several years; cerebellar astrocytoma, especially in children, may have more benign course	Variable prognosis By diagnosis, total excision usually impossible; tumor often not radiosensitive In cerebellar astrocytoma, total excision often possible
Medulloblastoma	Glioma most often seen in children Usually arises from roof of fourth ventricle and leads to increased ICP, with brainstem and cerebellar signs; may seed subarachnoid space	Treatment consists of surgery with radiation therapy and chemotherapy
Ependymoma	Glioma arising from ependyma of ventricle, especially fourth; leads early to signs of increased ICP; arises also from central canal of spinal cord	Tumor not radiosensitive and best treated surgically, if possible
Oligodendroglioma	Slow-growing glioma; usually arises in cerebral hemisphere in adults Calcification may be visible on radiograph	Treatment is surgical and usually successful
Brainstem glioma	Manifests in childhood with cranial nerve palsies, then long-tract signs in limbs; signs of increased ICP occur late in course	Tumor is inoperable Treatment with irradiation and with shunt for increased ICP
Cerebellar hemangioblastoma	Manifests with dysequilibrium, ataxia of trunk or limbs, and signs of increased ICP; sometimes familial; may be associated with retinal and spinal lesions, polycythemia, and hypernephroma	Treatment is surgical
Pineal tumor	Manifests with increased ICP, sometimes associated with impaired upward gaze (Parinaud's syndrome) and other deficits indicating midbrain lesion	Ventricular decompression by shunting, followed by surgical approach to tumor Irradiation if tumor malignant Prognosis depends on histopathological findings and tumor extent
Craniopharyngioma	Originates from remnants of Rathke's pouch above sella turcica, depressing optic chiasm May manifest at any age but usually in childhood with endocrine dysfunction and bitemporal field deficits	Treatment is surgical, but total removal may not be possible
Acoustic neuroma	Most common initial symptom is ipsilateral hearing loss; subsequent symptoms may include tinnitus, headache, vertigo, facial weakness or numbness, and long-tract signs May be familial and bilateral when related to neurofibromatosis Most sensitive screening tests are magnetic resonance imaging and brainstem auditory-evoked potentials	Treatment is by excision using a translabyrinthine approach, craniectomy, or combination Prognosis usually good
Meningioma	Originates from dura mater or arachnoid; compresses rather than invades adjacent neural structures Increasingly common with advancing age Tumor size varies greatly; symptoms vary with tumor site* Tumor usually benign; readily detected by computed tomography; may lead to calcification and bone erosion visible on plain skull radiographs	Treatment is surgical Tumor may recur if removal is incomplete; patient may receive irradiation with incomplete excision to decrease risk of recurrence
Primary central lymphoma	Associated with AIDS and other immunodeficiency states May manifest with focal deficits or disturbances of cognition and consciousness; may be indistinguishable from cerebral toxoplasmosis	Treatment is by whole-brain irradiation Chemotherapy may have adjunctive role Prognosis depends on CD4 cell count at diagnosis

*For example, unilateral exophthalmos (sphenoidal ridge), anosmia, and optic nerve compression (olfactory groove).

AEP, auditory-evoked potential; *AIDS,* acquired immunodeficiency syndrome; *GM,* glioblastoma multiforme.

From Gawlinski A, Hamwi D, editors: *Acute care nurse practitioner: clinical curriculum and certification review,* Philadelphia, 1999, Saunders.

BOX 18-5 OPERATIVE TERMS

Burr hole: hole made into the cranium using a special drill
Craniotomy: surgical opening of the skull
Craniectomy: removal of a portion of the skull without replacing it
Cranioplasty: plastic repair of the skull
Supratentorial: above the tentorium, separating the cerebrum from the cerebellum
Infratentorial: below the tentorium; includes the brainstem and the cerebellum; an infratentorial surgical approach may be used for temporal or occipital lesions

off in the operating room, and a large, bulky, turban-like craniotomy dressing is applied. Most patients experience some degree of postoperative eye or facial swelling and periorbital ecchymosis. An explanation of these temporary changes in appearance helps alleviate the shock and fear many patients and families experience in the immediate postoperative period.

All patients undergoing craniotomy require instruction to avoid activities known to provoke sudden changes in ICP. These activities include bending, lifting, straining, and the Valsalva maneuver. Patients commonly elicit the Valsalva maneuver during repositioning in bed by holding the breath and straining with a closed epiglottis. Teaching the patient to continue to breathe deeply through the mouth during all position changes is an effective deterrent.

The patient undergoing transsphenoidal surgery requires preparation for the sensations associated with nasal packing. The patient often awakens with alarm because of the inability to breathe through the nose. Preoperative instruction in mouth breathing and avoidance of coughing, sneezing, and blowing of the nose facilitates postoperative cooperation.

The psychosocial issues associated with the prospect of neurosurgery cannot be overemphasized. Few procedures are as threatening as those involving the brain or spinal cord. For some patients, the fear of permanent neurological impairment may be as ominous as or more so than the fear of death. Steps to meet the needs of the patient and the family include collaboration with clergy and social services personnel, patient-controlled visitation, and provision of as much privacy as the patient's condition permits. The patient and family must be given the opportunity to express their fears and concerns jointly and apart from each other.[47]

Surgical Considerations

Whereas the emphasis in the surgical approach for most other types of surgery is to gain adequate exposure of the surgical site, the neurosurgeon must select a route that also produces the least amount of disruption to the intracranial contents. Neural tissue is unforgiving. A significant portion of neurological trauma and postoperative deficits is related to the surgical pathway through the brain tissue, rather than to the procedure performed at the site of pathology. Depending on the location of the lesion and the surgical route chosen, a transcranial or a transsphenoidal approach is used to open the skull.

Transcranial Approach

In the transcranial approach, a scalp incision is made, and a series of burr holes is drilled into the skull to form an outline of the area to be opened (Figure 18-4). A special saw is then used to cut between the holes. In most cases, the bone flap is left attached to the muscle to create a hinge effect. In some cases, the bone flap is removed completely and stored for later retrieval and implantation or discarded and replaced with synthetic material. Next, the dura is opened and retracted. After the intracranial procedure, the dura and the bone flap are closed, the muscles and scalp are sutured, and a turban-like dressing is applied.[44,47]

Transsphenoidal Approach

The transsphenoidal approach is the technique of choice for removal of a pituitary tumor without extension into the intracranial vault (Figure 18-5).[44,45] This approach involves making a microsurgical entrance into the cranial vault through the nasal cavity. The sphenoid sinus is entered to reach the anterior wall of the sella turcica. The sphenoid bone and the dura are then opened to gain intracranial access. After removal of the tumor, the surgical bed is packed with a small section of adipose tissue grafted from the patient's abdomen or thigh. After closure of the intranasal structures, nasal splints and soft packing or nasal tampons impregnated with antibiotic ointment are placed in the nasal cavities. Occasionally, epistaxis balloons are used instead. A nasal drip pad or mustache-type dressing is placed at the base of the nose to catch surgical drainage.[47]

The patient may be placed in a supine, prone, or sitting position for a craniotomy procedure. A skull clamp connected to skull pins is used to position and secure the patient's head throughout the operation. During a transsphenoidal approach or a transcranial approach into the infratentorial area, the patient's head is elevated during surgery. This position puts the patient at risk for an air embolism. Air can enter the vascular system through the edges of the dura or a venous opening. Continuous monitoring of the patient's heart sounds by Doppler ultrasonography signal allows immediate recognition of this complication. If it occurs, an attempt may be made to withdraw the embolus from the right atrium through a central line. Flooding the surgical field with irrigation fluid and placing a moistened sterile surgical sponge over the surgical site creates an immediate barrier to any further air entrance.[44,47]

Postoperative Medical Management

Definitive management of the postoperative neurosurgical patient varies, depending on the underlying reason for the craniotomy. During the initial postoperative period, management is usually directed toward the prevention of complications. Complications associated with a craniotomy include intracranial hypertension, surgical hemorrhage, fluid imbalance, CSF leak, and DVT.

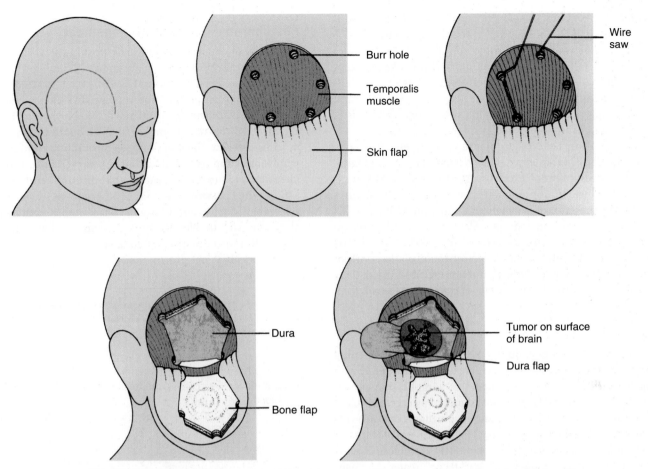

FIGURE 18-4 Craniotomy. (From Beare PG, Myers JL: *Principles and practice of adult health nursing*, ed 2, St Louis, 1994, Mosby.)

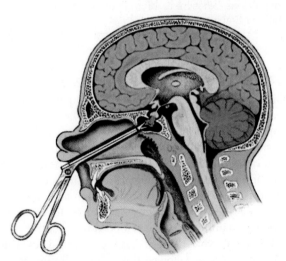

FIGURE 18-5 Transsphenoidal hypophysectomy.

Intracranial Hypertension

Postoperative cerebral edema is expected to peak 48 to 72 hours after surgery. If the bone flap is not replaced at the time of surgery, intracranial hypertension produces bulging at the surgical site. Close monitoring of the surgical site is important so that integrity of the incision can be maintained. Postcraniotomy management of intracranial hypertension is usually accomplished through CSF drainage, patient positioning, and steroid administration.[44]

Surgical Hemorrhage

Surgical hemorrhage after a transcranial procedure can occur in the intracranial vault and is manifested by signs and symptoms of increasing ICP. Hemorrhage after a transsphenoidal craniotomy may be evident from external drainage, the patient's complaint of persistent postnasal drip, or excessive swallowing. Loss of vision after pituitary surgery indicates an evolving hemorrhage. Postoperative hemorrhage requires surgical reexploration.[45]

Fluid Imbalance

Fluid imbalance in the postcraniotomy patient usually results from a disturbance in production or secretion of antidiuretic hormone (ADH). ADH is secreted by the posterior pituitary (neurohypophysis) gland. It stimulates the renal tubules and collecting ducts to retain water in response to low circulating blood volume or increased serum osmolality. Inoperative trauma or postoperative edema of the pituitary gland or hypothalamus can result in insufficient ADH secretion. The outcome is unabated renal water loss even when blood volume is low and serum osmolality is high. This condition is known as *diabetes insipidus* (DI). The polyuria associated with DI is often more than 200 mL/hour. Urine specific gravity of 1.005 or less and elevated serum osmolality provide evidence of insufficient ADH. The loss of volume may provoke hypotension and inadequate cerebral perfusion. DI is usually self-limiting, and fluid replacement is the only required therapy. In some cases, however, it may be necessary to administer vasopressin intravenously to control the loss of fluid.[44]

The syndrome of inappropriate antidiuretic hormone [secretion] (SIADH) commonly occurs with neurological insult and results from excessive ADH secretion. SIADH is manifested by inappropriate water retention with hyponatremia in the presence of normal renal function. Urine specific gravity is elevated, and urine osmolality is greater than serum osmolality. The dangers associated with SIADH include circulating volume overload and electrolyte imbalance, both of which may impair neurological functioning. SIADH is usually self-limiting, with the mainstay of treatment being fluid restriction.[44]

Cerebrospinal Fluid Leak

Leakage of cerebrospinal fluid (CSF) results from an opening in the subarachnoid space, as evidenced by clear fluid draining from the surgical site. When this complication occurs after transsphenoidal surgery, it is signified by excessive, clear drainage from the nose or persistent postnasal drip. To differentiate CSF drainage from postoperative serous drainage, a specimen is tested for glucose content. A CSF leak is confirmed by glucose values of 30 mg/dL or greater. Management of the patient with a CSF leak includes bed rest and head elevation. Lumbar puncture or placement of a lumbar subarachnoid catheter may be used to reduce CSF pressure until the dura heals. The risk of meningitis associated with CSF leak often necessitates surgical repair to reseal the opening.[44,45]

Deep Vein Thrombosis

Research has demonstrated that neurosurgical patients have a higher risk for development of a DVT than non-neurosurgical patients. This difference is due to numerous additional risk factors significantly associated with neurosurgery, including preoperative leg weakness, longer preoperative critical care unit stay, longer recovery room time, longer postoperative critical care unit stay, more days of bed rest, and delay of postoperative mobility and activity.[48] Clinical manifestations of DVT include leg or calf pain, edema, localized tenderness, and pain with dorsiflexion or plantar flexion (Homans' sign). Unfortunately, the patient with a DVT is often asymptomatic and the diagnosis is not made until the patient experiences a pulmonary embolus.

The primary treatment for DVT is prophylaxis. In the neurosurgery patient, sequential (intermittent) pneumatic compression boots or stockings are effective in reducing the incidence of DVT. Effectiveness is enhanced when these devices are initiated in the preoperative period. Low-dose unfractionated heparin or low-molecular-weight heparin may also be used prophylactically in high-risk patients.[44]

Postoperative Nursing Management

The nursing management of the neurosurgical patient incorporates a variety of nursing diagnoses (Nursing Diagnosis Priorities box on Craniotomy). As in preoperative care, the primary goal of postcraniotomy nursing management is protection of the integrity of the CNS. **Nursing priorities are directed toward (1) preserving adequate CPP, (2) promoting arterial oxygenation, (3) providing comfort and emotional support, (4) maintaining surveillance for complications, (5) initiating early rehabilitation, and (6) educating the patient and family.** Frequent neurological assessment is necessary to evaluate accomplishment of these objectives and to identify problems and quickly intervene if complications do arise. Often, a ventriculostomy is placed to facilitate ICP monitoring and CSF drainage.

NURSING DIAGNOSIS PRIORITIES
Craniotomy

- Decreased Intracranial Adaptive Capacity related to failure of normal intracranial compensatory mechanisms, p. A-12
- Ineffective Cerebral Tissue Perfusion related to decreased blood flow, p. A-29
- Ineffective Cerebral Tissue Perfusion related to hemorrhage, p. A-29
- Acute Pain related to transmission and perception of cutaneous, visceral, muscular, or ischemic impulses, p. A-4
- Disturbed Body Image related to actual change in body structure, function, or appearance, p. A-16
- Deficient Knowledge: Discharge Regimen related to lack of previous exposure to information (see Patient Education box on Craniotomy) , p. A-15

Preserving Adequate Cerebral Perfusion

Nursing interventions to preserve cerebral perfusion include patient positioning, fluid management, and avoidance of postoperative vomiting and fever.

Positioning. Patient positioning is an important component of care for the craniotomy patient. The head of the bed should be elevated 30 to 45 degrees at all times to reduce the incidence of hemorrhage, facilitate venous drainage, and control ICP. Other positioning measures to control ICP include maintaining the patient's head in a neutral position at all times and avoiding neck and hip flexion. These rules of positioning must be followed throughout all nursing activities, including linen changes and transporting of the patient for diagnostic evaluation. Most craniotomy patients can be turned from side to side within these restrictions, using pillows for support, except in some cases of extensive tumor removal, cranioplasty, and when the bone flap is not replaced. Specific orders from the surgeon must be obtained in these instances. The patient with an infratentorial incision may be restricted to only a very small pillow under the head to prevent strain on the incision. Avoidance of anterior and lateral neck flexion also protects the integrity of this type of incision.

Fluid Management. Fluid management is another important component of postcraniotomy care. Hourly monitoring of fluid intake and output facilitates early identification of fluid imbalance. Urine specific gravity must be measured if DI is suspected. Fluid restriction may be ordered as a routine measure to lessen the severity of cerebral edema or as treatment for the fluid and electrolyte imbalances associated with SIADH.

Vomiting and Fever. Postoperative vomiting must be avoided to prevent sharp spikes in ICP and possibly surgical hemorrhage. Antiemetics are administered as soon as nausea is apparent. Early resumption of nutrition in the neurosurgical patient is beneficial. If the patient is unable to eat, enteral hyperalimentation delivered through a feeding tube is the preferred method of nutritional support and can be initiated as early as 24 hours after surgery.[50] Postoperative fever may also adversely affect ICP and increase the metabolic needs of the brain. Acetaminophen is administered orally, rectally, or through a feeding tube. External cooling measures, such as a hypothermia blanket, may be necessary.

Promoting Arterial Oxygenation

Routine pulmonary care is used to maintain airway clearance and prevent pulmonary complications. To prevent dangerous elevations in ICP, this care must be performed with the use of proper technique and at time intervals that are adequately spaced from other patient care activities. If pulmonary complications do arise, consideration must be given to maintaining adequate oxygenation during repositioning. It may be necessary to restrict turning the patient to only the side that places the good lung down.

Providing Comfort and Emotional Support

Pain management in the postcraniotomy patient primarily involves control of headache. Small doses of intravenous morphine are used in the critical care setting. As soon as oral analgesics can be tolerated, acetaminophen with codeine is used. Both analgesics cause constipation. Administration of stool softeners and initiation of a bowel program are important components of postcraniotomy care. Constipation is hazardous, because straining to have a bowel movement can create significant elevations in blood pressure and ICP.

Maintaining Surveillance for Complications

The postoperative neurosurgical patient is at risk for infection, corneal abrasions, and injury from falls or seizures.

Infection. Care of the incision and surgical dressings is specific to the institution and physician. The rule of thumb for a craniotomy dressing is to reinforce it as needed and change it only with a physician's order. Often, a drain is left in place to facilitate decompression of the surgical site. If a ventriculostomy is present, it is treated as a component of the surgical site. All drainage devices must be secured to the dressing to prevent unintentional displacement with patient movement. Sterile technique is required to prevent infection and resultant meningitis.

Corneal Abrasions. Routine eye care may be necessary to prevent corneal drying and ulceration. Periorbital edema interferes with normal blinking and eyelid closure, which are essential to adequate corneal lubrication. Saline drops are instilled every 2 hours. If the patient remains in a coma state, covering the eyes with a polyethylene film extending over the orbits and eyebrows may be beneficial.[10]

Injury. The postcraniotomy patient may experience periods of altered mentation. Protection from injury may require the use of restraint devices. The side rails of the bed must be padded to protect the patient from injury. Having a family member stay at the bedside or use of music therapy is often helpful to keep the patient calm during periods of restlessness. In rare circumstances, neuromuscular blockade and sedation may be necessary to control patient activity and metabolic needs on a short-term basis.

Initiating Early Rehabilitation

Increased activity, including ambulation, is begun as soon in the postoperative period as tolerated by the patient. Rehabilitation measures and discharge planning may begin in the critical care unit but are beyond the scope of this chapter. Transfer to a general care or rehabilitation unit is usually accomplished as soon as the patient is considered to be stable and free of complications.

Educating the Patient and Family

Preoperatively, the patient and family should be taught about the precipitating event necessitating the need for the craniotomy and its expected outcome. The severity of the disease and the need for critical care management postoperatively must be stressed. As the patient moves toward discharge, teaching focuses on medication instructions; incisional care, including the signs of infection; and the signs and symptoms of increased ICP. If the patient has neurological deficits, teaching focuses on the interventions to maximize the patient's rehabilitation potential, and the patient's family members must be encouraged to participate in the patient's care and to learn some basic rehabilitation techniques. The importance of participating in a neurological rehabilitation program must be stressed (Patient Education box on Craniotomy).

PATIENT EDUCATION

Craniotomy

Before Surgery
- Pathophysiology and expected outcome of underlying disease
- Need for intensive care management after surgery
- Routine preoperative surgical care

Continued

INTRACRANIAL HYPERTENSION

Pathophysiology

The intracranial space comprises three components: brain substance (80%), CSF (10%), and blood (10%). Under normal physiological conditions, the mean ICP is maintained below 15 mm Hg.[29,49] Essential to understanding the pathophysiology of ICP, the Monro-Kellie hypothesis proposes that an increase in volume of one intracranial component must be compensated by a decrease in one or more of the other components so that total volume remains fixed. This compensation, although limited, includes displacing CSF from the intracranial vault to the lumbar cistern, increasing CSF absorption, and compressing the low-pressure venous system.[50,51] Pathophysiological alterations that can elevate ICP are outlined in Table 18-5.

Volume-Pressure Curve

When capable of compliance, the brain can tolerate significant increases in intracranial volume without much increase in ICP. The amount of intracranial compliance, however, does have a limit. After this limit has been reached, a state of decompensation with increased ICP results. As the ICP rises, the relationship between volume and pressure changes, and small increases in volume may cause major elevations in ICP (Figure 18-6).[29,50] The exact configuration of the volume-pressure curve and the point at which the steep rise in pressure occurs vary among patients. The configuration of this curve is also influenced by the cause and the rate of volume increases within the intracranial vault; for example, neurological deterioration occurs more rapidly in a patient with an acute epidural hematoma than in a patient with a meningioma of the same size.[49] Regardless of how fast the pressure increases, intracranial hypertension occurs when ICP is greater than 20 mm Hg.[50]

Cerebral Blood Flow and Autoregulation

Cerebral blood flow (CBF) corresponds to the metabolic demands of the brain and is normally 50 mL/100 g of brain tissue/min. Although the brain makes up only 2% of body weight, it requires 15% to 20% of the resting cardiac output and 15% of the body's oxygen demands. The normal brain has a complex capacity to maintain constant CBF, despite wide ranges in systemic arterial pressure—an effect known as *autoregulation.* A mean arterial pressure of 50 to 150 mm Hg does not alter CBF when autoregulation is functioning. Outside the limits of this autoregulation, CBF becomes passively dependent on the perfusion pressure.[50]

TABLE 18-5	MECHANISMS OF INTRACRANIAL PRESSURE ELEVATION	
PATHOPHYSIOLOGY	**EXAMPLE**	**TREATMENT**
Disorders of CSF Space		
Overproduction of CSF	Choroid plexus papilloma	Diuretics, surgical removal
Communicating hydrocephalus from obstructed arachnoid	Old subarachnoid hemorrhage	Surgical drainage from lumbar drain
Noncommunicative hydrocephalus	Posterior fossa tumor obstructing aqueduct	Surgical drainage by ventricular drain
Interstitial edema	Any of above	Surgical drainage of CSF
Disorders of Intracranial Blood		
Intracranial hemorrhage causing increased ICP	Epidural hematoma	Surgical drainage
Vasospasm	Subarachnoid hemorrhage	Hypervolemia and hypertensive therapy
Vasodilation	Elevated $PaCO_2$	Hyperventilation
Increasing cerebral blood volume and ICP	Hypoxia	Adequate oxygenation
Disorders of Brain Substance		
Expanding mass lesion with local vasogenic edema causing increased ICP	Brain tumor	Steroids Surgical removal
Ischemic brain injury with cytotoxic edema increasing ICP	Anoxic brain injury from cardiac or respiratory arrest	Resistant to therapy
Increased cerebral metabolic rate increasing cerebral blood flow and ICP	Seizures, hyperthermia	Anticonvulsant medications to control fever

Modified from Helfaer MA, Kirsch JR: Intracranial vault pathophysiology, *Crit Care Rep* 1:12, 1989.

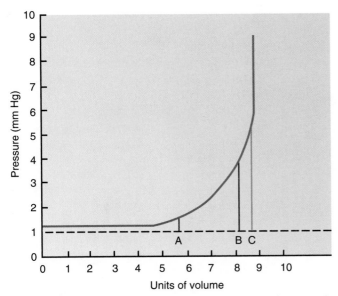

FIGURE 18-6 Intracranial volume-pressure curve. Pressure is normal (A) and increases in intracranial volume are tolerated without increases in intracranial pressure. Increases in volume (B) may cause increases in pressure. Small increases in volume (C) may cause larger increases in pressure.

Factors other than arterial blood pressure that affect CBF are conditions that result in acidosis, alkalosis, and changes in metabolic rate. Conditions that cause acidosis (e.g., hypoxia, hypercapnia, ischemia) result in cerebrovascular dilation. Conditions causing alkalosis (e.g., hypocapnia) result in cerebrovascular constriction. Normally, a reduction in metabolic rate (e.g., from hypothermia or barbiturates) decreases CBF, and rises in metabolic rate (e.g., from hyperthermia) increase CBF.[49,52]

Arterial blood gases exert a profound effect on CBF. Carbon dioxide, which affects the pH of the blood, is a potent vasoactive substance. Carbon dioxide retention (hypercapnia) leads to cerebral vasodilation, with increased cerebral blood volume, whereas hypocapnia leads to cerebral vasoconstriction and a reduction in cerebral blood volume. Prolonged hypocapnia, however, can lead to cerebral ischemia.[53] Low arterial partial pressure of oxygen (Pao_2) levels, especially below 40 mm Hg, lead to cerebral vasodilation, which increases the intracranial blood volume and can contribute to increased ICP. High Pao_2 levels have not been shown to affect CBF in either direction.[49,52]

Assessment and Diagnosis

The numerous signs and symptoms of increased ICP include decreased level of consciousness, Cushing's triad, diminished brainstem reflexes, papilledema, decerebrate posturing (abnormal extension), decorticate posturing (abnormal flexion), unequal pupil size, projectile vomiting, decreased pupillary reaction to light, altered breathing patterns, and headache.[29] Patients may exhibit one or all of these symptoms, depending on the underlying cause of the elevation in ICP. One of the earliest and most important signs of increased

ICP is a decrease in the level of consciousness. This change must be reported immediately to the physician.[52]

In the patient with suspected intracranial hypertension, a monitoring device may be placed within the cranium to quantify ICP. Under normal physiological conditions, the mean ICP is maintained below 15 mm Hg. The device is used to monitor ICP serially and assist with the management of intracranial hypertension. An increase in ICP can decrease blood flow to the brain, causing brain damage. The monitoring device can also provide a sterile access for draining excess CSF. The four sites for monitoring ICP are the intraventricular space, the subarachnoid space, the epidural space, and the parenchyma. Each site has advantages and disadvantages for monitoring ICP. The type of monitor chosen depends on the suspected pathological condition and the physician's preferences.[49,51,52,54] Chapter 17 provides a more detailed discussion of ICP monitoring.

Medical and Nursing Management

After intracranial hypertension is documented, therapy must be prompt to prevent secondary insults (Concept Map on Intracranial Hypertension). Although the exact pressure level denoting intracranial hypertension remains uncertain, most current evidence suggests that ICP generally must be treated when it exceeds 20 mm Hg.[49,52] All therapies are directed toward reducing the volume of one or more of the components (e.g., blood, brain, CSF) that lie within the intracranial vault. A major goal of therapy is to determine the cause of the elevated pressure and, if possible, to remove the cause.[49,55] In the absence of a surgically treatable mass lesion, intracranial hypertension is treated medically. **Nursing priorities focus on (1) rapid assessment and (2) implementation of appropriate therapies for reducing ICP.**

Positioning and Other Nursing Activities

Positioning of the patient is a significant factor in the prevention and treatment of intracranial hypertension. Head elevation has long been advocated as a conventional nursing intervention to control ICP, presumably by increasing venous return. However, this may decrease CPP. Close monitoring of ICP and CPP should be done with positioning, which should be customized to maximize CPP and minimize ICP.[51]

Positions that impede venous return from the brain cause elevations in ICP. Obstruction of jugular veins or an increase in intrathoracic or intraabdominal pressure is communicated as increased pressure throughout the open venous system, thereby impeding drainage from the brain and increasing ICP. Positions that decrease venous return from the head (e.g., Trendelenburg position, prone position, extreme flexion of the hips, angulation of the neck) must be avoided if possible. If changes to positions such as Trendelenburg are necessary to provide adequate pulmonary care, critical care nurses must closely monitor ICP and vital signs.[49]

Some routine nursing activities do affect ICP and can be harmful. Use of positive end-expiratory pressures (PEEP) greater than 20 cm H_2O, coughing, suctioning, tight tracheostomy tube ties, and the Valsalva maneuver have been

Concept Map: Intracranial Hypertension

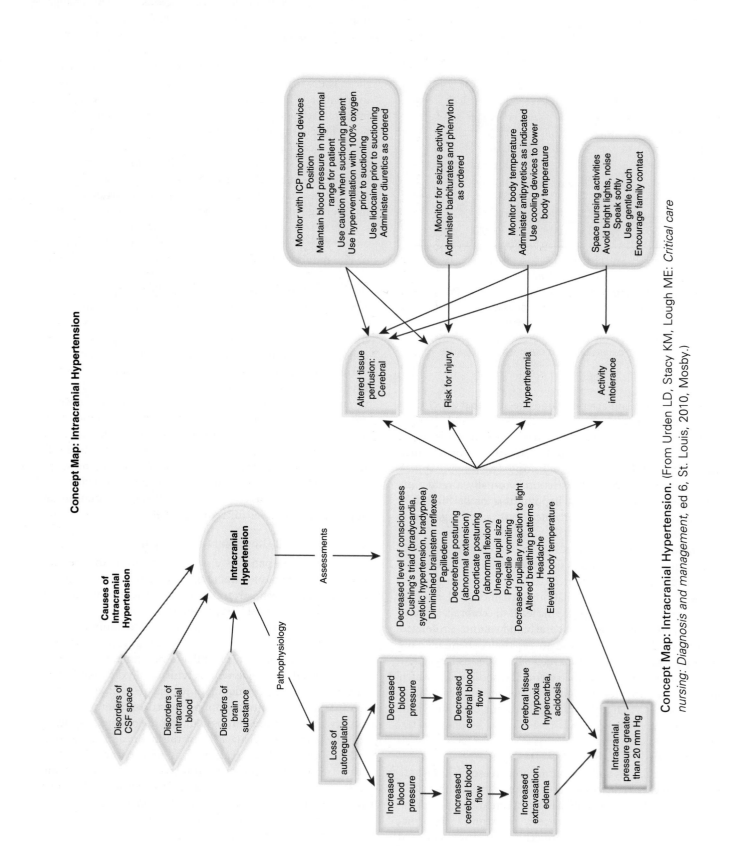

Concept Map: Intracranial Hypertension. (From Urden LD, Stacy KM, Lough ME: *Critical care nursing: Diagnosis and management*, ed 6, St. Louis, 2010, Mosby.)

associated with increases in ICP. Cumulative increases in ICP have been reported when care activities are performed one after another. Conversely, family contact and gentle touch have been associated with decreases in ICP.[49]

Hyperventilation

Controlled hyperventilation has been an important adjunct of therapy for the patient with increased ICP. The rationale employed in hyperventilation is that if the $Paco_2$ can be reduced from its normal level of 35 to 40 mm Hg to a range of 25 to 30 mm Hg in the patient with intracranial hypertension, vasoconstriction of cerebral arteries, reduction of CBF, and increased venous return will result. This practice is being reexamined. Additional research has indicated that severe or prolonged hyperventilation can reduce cerebral perfusion and lead to cerebral ischemia and infarction. The current trend is to maintain $Paco_2$ levels on the lower side of normal (35 ± 2 mm Hg) by carefully monitoring arterial blood gas measurements and by adjusting ventilator settings.[53,55]

Although hypoxemia must be avoided, excessively high levels of oxygen offer no benefits, and increasing inspired oxygen concentrations above 60% may lead to toxic changes in lung tissue. The use of pulse oximetry has led to greater awareness of the circumstances, such as pain and anxiety, that can cause oxygen desaturation and therefore elevate ICP.[29,49]

Temperature Control

Directly proportional to body temperature, cerebral metabolic rate increases 10% per 1° C of increase in body temperature.[51] This fact is significant because as the cerebral metabolic rate increases, blood flow to the brain must increase to meet the tissue demands. To avoid the increase in blood volume associated with a greater cerebral metabolic rate, nurses must prevent hyperthermia in the patient with a brain injury. Antipyretics and cooling devices must be used when appropriate while the source of the fever is being determined.[51,52]

Blood Pressure Control

Maintenance of arterial blood pressure in the high-normal range is essential in the brain-injured patient. Inadequate perfusion pressure decreases the supply of nutrients and oxygen requirements for cerebral metabolic needs. However, a blood pressure that is too high increases cerebral blood volume and may raise ICP.[52] Figure 18-7 shows the relationship between blood pressure and ICP.

Control of systemic hypertension may require nothing more than the administration of a sedative agent. Small, frequent doses may be sufficient to blunt noxious stimuli and prevent them from triggering increases in blood pressure. When sedation proves inadequate in controlling systemic arterial hypertension, antihypertensive agents are used. Care must be taken in choosing these agents because many of the peripheral vasodilators (e.g., nitroprusside, nitroglycerin) also are cerebral vasodilators. All antihypertensives are believed to cause some degree of cerebral vasodilation. To reduce this vasodilating effect, concurrent treatment with beta-blockers (e.g., metoprolol, labetalol) may be beneficial.[49,52]

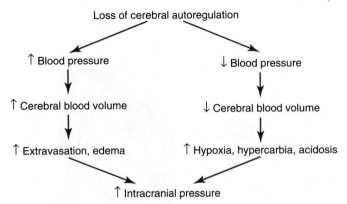

FIGURE 18-7 Loss of pressure autoregulation.

Systemic hypotension should be treated aggressively with fluids to maintain a systolic blood pressure greater than 90 mm Hg. Crystalloids, colloids, and blood products can be used, depending on the patient's condition. Studies have demonstrated a positive effect on ICP and CPP with hypertonic saline. If fluids fail to adequately elevate the patient's blood pressure, the use of inotropic agents may be necessary.[49]

Seizure Control

The incidence of posttraumatic seizures in the head-injured population has been estimated at 15% to 20%. Because of the risk of a secondary ischemic insult associated with seizures, many physicians prescribe anticonvulsant medications prophylactically. Seizures cause metabolic requirements to increase, resulting in elevation of CBF, cerebral blood volume, and ICP, even in paralyzed patients. If blood flow cannot match demand, ischemia develops, cerebral energy stores are depleted, and irreversible neuronal destruction occurs. The usual anticonvulsant regimen for seizure control includes phenytoin or phenobarbital, or both, in therapeutic doses.[52] Fast-acting, short-duration agents such as lorazepam may be indicated for breakthrough seizures until therapeutic levels of the longer-acting drugs can be achieved.

Cerebrospinal Fluid Drainage

CSF drainage for intracranial hypertension may be used with other treatment modalities (Figures 18-8 and 18-9). CSF drainage is accomplished by the insertion of a pliable catheter into the anterior horn of the lateral ventricle (ventriculostomy), preferably on the nondominant side. This drainage can help support the patient through periods of cerebral edema by controlling spikes in ICP. One of the major advantages of the ventriculostomy is its dual role as a monitoring device and a treatment modality. Care should be taken to avoid infection. However, cleansing ointment such as bacitracin or povidone is not recommended.[56]

Hyperosmolar Therapy

Osmotic diuretics and hypertonic saline have also been used to reduce increased ICP. In the presence of an intact blood-brain barrier, hyperosmolar therapy is used to draw water

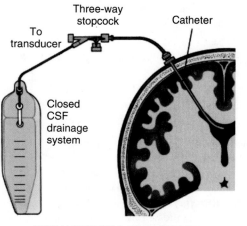

INTRAVENTRICULAR CATHETER

FIGURE 18-8 Intermittent drainage system. Intermittent drainage involves draining cerebrospinal fluid (CSF) through a ventriculostomy when intracranial pressure (ICP) exceeds the upper pressure parameter set by the physician. Intermittent drainage is achieved by opening the three-way stopcock to allow CSF to flow into the drainage bag for brief periods (30 to 120 seconds) until the pressure is below the upper pressure parameter. (From Barker E: *Neuroscience nursing,* ed 3, St Louis, 2008, Mosby.)

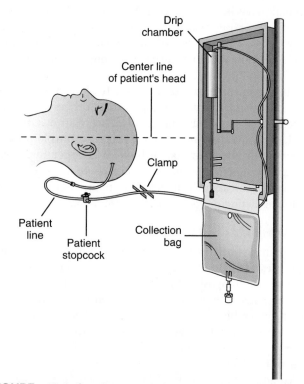

FIGURE 18-9 Continuous drainage system. Continuous drainage involves placing the drip chamber of the drainage system at a specified level above the foramen of Monro (usually 15 cm). The system is left open to allow continuous drainage of cerebrospinal fluid (CSF) into the chamber (which drains into a collection bag) against a pressure gradient that prevents excessive drainage and ventricular collapse. (Courtesy Codman & Shurtleff, Inc., Raynham, MA.)

from brain tissue into the intravascular compartment. The direction of flow is from the hypoconcentrated tissue to the hyperconcentrated cerebral vasculature.[52]

The most widely used osmotic diuretic is mannitol, a large-molecule agent that is retained almost entirely in the extracellular compartment and has little or none of the rebound effect observed with other osmotic diuretics. Administration of mannitol increases cerebral blood flow and thus induces cerebral vasoconstriction as part of the brain's autoregulatory response to maintain blood flow constant.[52]

Two major complications associated with osmotic diuretics are electrolyte disturbances and dehydration. Careful attention must be paid to body weight and fluid and electrolyte stability. Serum osmolality should be kept between 300 and 320 mOsm/L. Hypernatremia and hypokalemia often are associated with repeated administration of osmotic agents. Central venous pressure readings should be monitored to assess for hypovolemia. Smaller doses of mannitol simplify fluid and electrolyte management, and their use is encouraged whenever possible.[49,52]

Hypertonic saline, given in concentrations ranging from 3% to 23.4%, can also be used to treat increased ICP. Hypertonic saline can be used in hypovolemic patients when mannitol is contraindicated.[52] Adverse effects include electrolyte abnormalities,[52] hypotension, pulmonary edema, acute renal failure, hemolysis, central pontine myelinolyisis, coagulopathy, and dysrhythmias.[57]

Control of Metabolic Demand

Any treatment modality that increases the incidence of noxious stimulation to the patient carries with it the potential for increasing ICP. Noxious stimuli include pain, the presence of an endotracheal tube, coughing, suctioning, repositioning, bathing, and many other routine nursing interventions. Agents used to reduce metabolic demands include the use of benzodiazepines such as midazolam and lorazepam, intravenous sedative-hypnotics such as propofol, opioid narcotics such as fentanyl and morphine, and neuromuscular blocking agents such as vecuronium and atracurium. These agents may be administered separately or in combination by continuous drip or as an intravenous bolus on an as-needed basis.[49]

The preferred treatment regimen begins with the administration of benzodiazepines for sedation and narcotics for analgesia. If these agents fail to blunt the patient's response to noxious stimuli, propofol or a neuromuscular blocking agent is added. The use of these medications is recommended only in patients with an ICP monitor in place, because sedatives, opioids, and neuromuscular blocking agents affect the reliability of neurological assessment. The use of neuromuscular blocking agents without sedation is not recommended because these agents can cause skeletal muscle paralysis and because they have no analgesic effect and do not adequately protect the patient from pain and the physiological responses that can occur from pain-producing procedures.[58] If these agents fail to control the patient's ICP, barbiturate therapy is considered.[52]

Barbiturate Therapy. Barbiturate therapy is a treatment protocol developed for the management of uncontrolled intracranial hypertension that has not responded to the conventional treatments previously described.[52] The two most commonly used drugs in high-dose barbiturate therapy are pentobarbital and thiopental. The goal with either drug is a reduction of ICP to 15 to 20 mm Hg, while a mean arterial pressure of 70 to 80 mm Hg is maintained. Patients are maintained on high-dose barbiturate therapy until ICP has been controlled within the normal range for 24 hours. Barbiturates must never be stopped abruptly; they are tapered slowly over approximately 4 days. Despite the theoretical reasons for barbiturate use, clinical trials of its use have not shown improved outcome.[49]

Complications of high-dose barbiturate therapy can be disastrous unless a specific and organized approach is used. The most common complications are hypotension, hypothermia, and myocardial depression. If any complications occur and are allowed to persist unchecked, they may cause secondary insults to an already damaged brain. Hypotension, the most common complication, results from peripheral vasodilation and can be compounded in an already dehydrated patient who has received large doses of an osmotic diuretic in an attempt to control ICP. Careful monitoring of fluid status by central venous pressure or a pulmonary artery catheter can help prevent this complication. Myocardial depression results from cardiac muscle suppression and can be avoided by frequent monitoring of fluid status, cardiac output, and serum drug levels. If an adequate cardiac output cannot be maintained in the presence of normothermia, barbiturate doses must be reduced, regardless of serum levels.[49,52]

Collaborative management of the patient's intracranial hypertension is outlined in the Collaborative Management box on Intracranial Hypertension.

COLLABORATIVE MANAGEMENT
Intracranial Hypertension

- Position patient to achieve maximal ICP reduction.
- Reduce environmental stimulation.
- Maintain normothermia.
- Control ventilation to ensure a normal PaCO$_2$ level (35 ± 2 mm Hg).
- Administer diuretic agents, anticonvulsants, sedation, analgesia, paralytic agents, and vasoactive medications to ensure (CPP >70 mm Hg).
- Drain cerebrospinal fluid for ICP >20 mm Hg.

Herniation Syndromes

The goal of neurological evaluation, ICP monitoring, and treatment of increased ICP is to prevent herniation. Herniation of intracerebral contents results in the shifting of tissue from one compartment of the brain to another and places pressure on cerebral vessels and vital function centers of the brain. If unchecked, herniation rapidly causes death as a result of the cessation of CBF and respirations.[49]

Supratentorial Herniation

The four types of supratentorial herniation syndrome are uncal; central, or transtentorial; cingulate; and transcalvarial (Figure 18-10).

Uncal Herniation. Uncal herniation is the most common herniation syndrome. In uncal herniation, a unilateral, expanding mass lesion, usually of the temporal lobe, increases ICP, causing lateral displacement of the tip of the temporal lobe (uncus). Lateral displacement pushes the uncus over the edge of the tentorium, puts pressure on the oculomotor nerve (cranial nerve III) and the posterior cerebral artery ipsilateral to the lesion, and flattens the midbrain against the opposite side. Clinical manifestations of uncal herniation include ipsilateral pupil dilation, decreased level of consciousness, respiratory pattern changes leading to respiratory arrest, and contralateral hemiplegia leading to decorticate or decerebrate posturing. If no intervention occurs, uncal herniation results in fixed and dilated pupils, flaccidity, and respiratory arrest.[49,59]

Central Herniation. In central, or transtentorial, herniation, an expanding mass lesion of the midline, frontal, parietal, or occipital lobe results in downward displacement of the hemispheres, basal ganglia, and diencephalon through the tentorial notch. Central herniation often is preceded by uncal and cingulate herniation. Clinical manifestations of central herniation include loss of consciousness; small, reactive pupils progressing to fixed, dilated pupils; respiratory changes leading to respiratory arrest; and decorticate posturing progressing to flaccidity. In the late stages, uncal and central herniation syndromes affect the brainstem similarly.[49,59]

Cingulate Herniation. Cingulate herniation occurs when an expanding lesion of one hemisphere shifts laterally and forces the cingulate gyrus under the falx cerebri. Cingulate herniation occurs often. When a lateral shift is observed on the CT scan, cingulate herniation has occurred. Little is known about the effects of cingulate herniation, and there are no accompanying clinical manifestations that assist in its diagnosis. Cingulate herniation is not in itself a life-threatening condition, but if the expanding mass lesion that

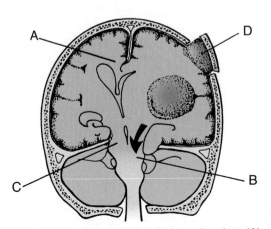

FIGURE 18-10 Supratentorial herniation: cingulate (A), uncal (B), central (C), and transcalvarial (D).

TABLE 18-6 PHARMACOLOGICAL MANAGEMENT NEUROLOGICAL DISORDERS

DRUG	DOSAGE	ACTIONS	SPECIAL CONSIDERATIONS
Anticonvulsants			
Phenytoin (Dilantin)	Loading dose: 10-20 mg/kg IV Maintenance dose: 100 mg q6-8h IV	Prevents the influx of sodium at the cell membrane	Monitor serum levels closely; therapeutic level is 10-20 mg/L (if hypoalbuminuria, monitor free phenytoin serum levels: therapeutic level of 0.1–0.2 mg/L) Infuse phenytoin no faster than 50 mg/min; administer with normal saline only because it precipitates with other solutions
Fosphenytoin (Cerebyx)	Loading dose: 15-20 mg/kg IV Maintenance dose: 4-6m g/kg/24 hr IV	Prevents the influx of sodium at the cell membrane	Monitor serum levels closely; therapeutic level is 10-20 mg/L Dosage, concentration, and infusion rate of fosphenytoin are expressed as phenytoin sodium equivalents (PE)
Barbiturates			
Phenobarbital	Loading dose: 6-8 mg/kg IV Maintenance dose: 1-3 mg/kg/24 hr IV	Produces central nervous system depression and reduces the spread of an epileptic focus	May depress cardiac and respiratory function Administer phenobarbital at a rate of 60 mg/min; monitor serum level closely; therapeutic level is 15-40 mg/L
Pentobarbital	Loading dose: 3-10 mg/kg over 30 min Maintenance dose: 0.5-3 mg/kg/hr IV	Induces barbiturate coma	Monitor serum level of pentobarbital closely; therapeutic level for coma is 15-40 mg/L
Osmotic Diuretics			
Mannitol	1-2 g/kg IV	Treats cerebral edema by pulling fluid from the extravascular space into the intravascular space; requires intact blood-brain barrier	Side effects include hypovolemia and increased serum osmolality Monitor serum osmolality and notify the physician if >310 mOsm/L Warm and shake before administering to ensure crystals are dissolved
Calcium Channel Blockers			
Nimodipine (Nimotop)	60 mg q4h NG or PO for 21 days	Decreases cerebral vasospasm	Side effects include hypotension, palpitations, headache, and dizziness Monitor blood pressure frequently when implementing therapy
Local Anesthetics			
Lidocaine	50-10 0mg IV or 2 mL of 4% solution	Blunts the effects of tracheal stimulation on intracranial pressure	Must be administered not longer than 5 minutes before suctioning
Thrombolytics			
Tissue-type plasminogen activator (tPA)	0.9 mg/kg total, with 10% of the dose administered as IV bolus over 1 min and 90% of the dose administered as continuous IV infusion over 1 hr	Converts plasminogen to plasmin to dissolve clot	Treatment must start within 3 hr of the onset of the symptoms Do not exceed 90 mg Do not use anticoagulants during the first 24 hr Monitor patient for bleeding

IV, intravenous; *NG*, nasogastric; *PO*, by mouth.

caused cingulate herniation is not controlled, uncal or central herniation will follow.[49,59]

Transcalvarial Herniation. Transcalvarial herniation is the extrusion of cerebral tissue through the cranium. In the presence of severe cerebral edema, transcalvarial herniation occurs through an opening from a skull fracture or craniotomy site.[49]

Infratentorial Herniation

The two infratentorial herniation syndromes are upward transtentorial herniation and downward cerebellar herniation.

Upward Transtentorial Herniation. Upward transtentorial herniation occurs when an expanding mass lesion of the cerebellum causes protrusion of the vermis (central area) of the cerebellum and the midbrain upward through the tentorial notch. Compression of the third cranial nerve and

diencephalon occurs. Blockage of the central aqueduct and distortion of the third ventricle obstruct CSF flow. Deterioration progresses rapidly.[49,59]

Downward Cerebellar Herniation. Downward cerebellar herniation occurs when an expanding lesion of the cerebellum exerts pressure downward, sending the cerebellar tonsils through the foramen magnum. Compression and displacement of the medulla oblongata occur, rapidly resulting in respiratory and cardiac arrest.[49,59]

PHARMACOLOGICAL AGENTS

Many pharmacological agents are used in the care of patients with neurological disorders. Table 18-6 reviews the various agents used and any special considerations necessary for administering them.[60]

CASE STUDY   PATIENT WITH A NEUROLOGICAL PROBLEM

Answers to the Case Study Questions can be found on the Evolve web site at http://evolve.elsevier.com/Urden/priorities/.

Brief Patient History

Mr. P is a 24-year-old man. While he was water skiing, he was hit by a boat. He was rescued from the water by friends. He was immobilized and transported to the hospital by paramedics called to the scene.

Clinical Assessment

Mr. P is admitted to the emergency department with abrasions and bruising to his head and shoulders. He is having difficulty breathing and is unable to move his extremities. He complains of neck pain, and a cervical collar is in place. He has urinary and fecal incontinence. There is no response to motor, sensory, or deep tendon reflexes from the neck to the feet. He is awake and able to talk.

Diagnostic Procedures

The admission MRI showed an incomplete spinal cord transection. Baseline vital signs include the following: blood

pressure of 85/60 mm Hg, heart rate of 48 beats/min (sinus bradycardia), respiratory rate of 8 breaths/min, temperature of 99.3° F, and O_2 saturation of 88%. The Glasgow Coma Scale score was 10.

Medical Diagnosis

Mr. P is diagnosed with an incomplete spinal cord transection and neurogenic shock.

Questions

1. What major outcomes do you expect to achieve for this patient?
2. What problems or risks must be managed to achieve these outcomes?
3. What interventions must be initiated to monitor, prevent, manage, or eliminate the problems and risks identified?
4. What interventions should be initiated to promote the optimal functioning, safety, and well-being of the patient?
5. What possible learning needs do you anticipate for this patient?
6. What cultural and age-related factors may have a bearing on the patient's plan of care?

REFERENCES

1. Barker E: Altered states of consciousness and sleep. In Barker E, editor: *Neuroscience nursing: a spectrum of care*, ed 3, St Louis, 2008, Mosby.
2. Hoesch RE et al: Coma after global ischemic brain injury: pathophysiology and emerging therapies, *Crit Care Clin* 24:25, 2008.
3. Gawryluk JR, D'Arcy RC, Connolly JF, Weaver DF: Improving the clinical assessment of consciousness with advances in electrophysiological and neuroimaging techniques, *BMC Neurol* 10:11, 2010.
4. Rosenberg RN: Consciousness, coma, and brain death 2009, *JAMA* 301:1172, 2009.
5. Stevens RD, Bhardwaj A: Approach to the comatose patient, *Crit Care Med* 34:31, 2006.
6. Fauce K et al: *Harrison's principles of internal medicine*, ed 17, Philadelphia, 2008, McGraw-Hill.
7. Bleck TP: Levels of consciousness and attention. In Goetz CG, editor: *Textbook of clinical neurology*, ed 3, St Louis, 2007, Saunders.
8. Berger JR: Stupor and coma. In Bradley WG, Daroff RB, Jankovic J, Fenichel G, et al, editors: *Neurology in clinical practice*, ed 5, Boston, 2008, Butterworth-Heinemann.
9. Boss BJ: Alterations in cognitive systems, cerebral hemodynamics, and motor function. In McCance KL, Huether SE, editors: *Pathophysiology: the biologic basis for disease in adults and children*, ed 6, St Louis, 2010, Mosby.
10. Cortese D, Capp L, McKinley S: Moisture chamber versus lubrication for the prevention of corneal epithelial breakdown, *Am J Crit Care* 4:425, 1995.

11. Writing Group Members: Heart disease and stroke statistics—2010 update: A report from the American Heart Association, *Circulation* 121:e46, 2010.

12. American Association of Neuroscience Nurses: *Guide to the care of the patient with hospitalized patient with ischemic stroke: AANN clinical practice guideline series*, ed 2, Chicago, 2009, The Association.

13. Bill J: Vascular diseases of the nervous system. In Bradley WG, Daroff RB, Jankovic J, Fenichel G, et al, editors: *Neurology in clinical practice*, ed 5, Boston, 2008, Buterworth-Heinemann.

14. Romano JG, Sacco RL: Progress in secondary stroke prevention, *Ann Neurol* 63:418, 2008.

15. Murphy DR: Current understanding of the relationship between cervical manipulation and stroke: what does it mean for the chiropractic profession? *Chiropr Osteopat* 18:22, 2010.

16. Babarro EG, Rego AR, González-Juanatey JR: Cardioembolic stroke: Call for a multidisciplinary approach, *Cerebrovasc Dis* 27:(1 suppl)82, 2009.

17. Albers GW, Amarenco P, Easton JD, et al: Antithrombotic and thrombolytic therapy for ischemic stroke: American College of Chest Physicians Evidence-Based Clinical Practice Guidelines (8th Edition), *Chest* 133:(6 suppl)630, 2008.

18. Boss BJ: Disorders of central and peripheral nervous system and the neuromuscular junction. In McCance KL, Huether SE, editors: *Pathophysiology: the biologic basis for disease in adults and children*, ed 6, St Louis, 2010, Mosby.

19. Seder DB, Mayer SA: Critical care management of subarachnoid hemorrhage and ischemic stroke, *Clin Chest Med* 30:103, 2009.

20. Szaflarski JP, Rackley AY, Kleindorfer DO, et al: Incidence of seizures in the acute phase of stroke: a population-based study, *Epilepsia* 49:974, 2008.

21. Alexandrov AW: Hyperacute ischemic stroke management: Reperfusion and evolving therapies, *Crit Care Nurs Clin N Am* 21:451, 2009.

22. Del Zoppo GJ, Saver JL, Jauch EC, et al: Expansion of the time window for treatment of acute ischemic stroke with intravenous tissue plasminogen activator: a science advisory from the American Heart Association/American Stroke Association, *Stroke* 40:2945, 2009.

23. Bravata DM, Wells CK, Lo AC, et al: Processes of care associated with acute stroke outcomes, *Arch Intern Med* 170:804, 2010.

24. Anderson T: Current and evolving management of subarachnoid hemorrhage, *Crit Care Nurs Clin N Am* 21: 529, 2009.

25. Fahy BG, Sivaraman V: Current concepts in neurocritical care, *Anesthesiol Clin North Am* 20:441, 2002.

26. Pillai P, et al: Management of aneurysms, subarachnoid hemorrhage, and arteriovenous malformations. In Barker E, editor: *Neuroscience nursing: a spectrum of care*, ed 3, St Louis, 2008, Mosby.

27. Lindsay KW, Bone I, Fuller G: *Neurology and neurosurgery illustrated*, ed 5, London, 2010, Churchill Livingstone.

28. American Association of Neuroscience Nurses: *Care of the patient with aneurysmal subarachnoid hemorrhage: AANN clinical practice guideline series*, Chicago, 2009, The Association.

29. Bader MK, Littlejohns LR: *AANN core curriculum for neuroscience nursing*, ed 4, St Louis, 2004, Elsevier.

30. Benderson JB, Connolly ES Jr, Batjer HH, et al: Guidelines for the management of aneurysmal subarachnoid hemorrhage: a statement for healthcare professionals from a special writing group of the Stroke Council, American Heart Association, *Circulation* 40:994, 2009.

31. Hunt WE, Hess RM: Surgical risks as related to time of intervention in the repair of intracranial aneurysms, *J Neurosurg* 28:14, 1968.

32. Solenski NJ, Haley EC Jr, Kassell NF, et al: Medical complications of aneurysmal subarachnoid hemorrhage: a report of the multicenter, cooperative aneurysm study, *Crit Care Med* 23:1007, 1995.

33. Claassen J, Vu A, Kreiter KT, et al: Effect of acute physiologic derangements on outcome after subarachnoid hemorrhage, *Crit Care Med* 32:832, 2004.

34. Keyrouz SG, Diringer MN: Clinical review: Prevention and therapy vasospasm in subarachnoid hemorrhage, *Crit Care* 11:220, 2007.

35. Rincon F, Mayer SA: Clinical review: critical care management of spontaneous intracerebral hemorrhage, *Crit Care* 12:237, 2008.

36. Hsieh PC, Awad IA, Getch CC, et al: Current updates in perioperative management of intracerebral hemorrhage, *Neurol Clin* 24:745, 2006.

37. Naval NS, Nyquist PA, Carhuapoma JR: Management of spontaneous intracerebral hemorrhage, *Neurol Clin* 26:373, 2008.

38. Zivin JA: Hemorrhagic cerebrovascular disease. In Goldman L, Ausiello D, editors: *Cecil medicine*, ed 23, St Louis, 2008, Saunders.

39. Morgenstern LB, Hemphill JC 3rd, Anderson C, et al; American Heart Association Stroke Council and Council on Cardiovascular Nursing: Guidelines for the management of spontaneous intracerebral hemorrhage: A Guideline for Healthcare Professionals From the American Heart Association/American Stroke Association, *Stroke* 41:2108, 2010.

40. Shah DN: The spectrum of Guillain-Barré syndrome, *Dis Mon*, 56:262, 2010.

41. van Doorn PA, Ruts L, Jacobs BC: Clinical features, pathogenesis, and treatment of Guillain-Barré syndrome, *Lancet Neurol* 7:939, 2008.

42. Randall DP: Guillain-Barré syndrome and immunizations, *Dis Mon*, 56:293, 2010.

43. Randall DP: Guillain-Barré syndrome, *Dis Mon*, 56:256, 2010.

44. Delaune A et al: Cranial surgery. In Barker E, editor: *Neuroscience nursing: a spectrum of care*, ed 3, St Louis, 2008, Mosby.

45. Vance ML: Perioperative management of patients undergoing pituitary surgery, *Endocrinol Metab Clin North Am* 32:355, 2003.

46. Mullings KR, Alleva JT, Hudgins TH: Rehabilitation of Guillain-Barré syndrome, *Dis Mon* 56:288, 2010.

47. Rothrock JC: *Alexander's care of the patient in surgery*, ed 13, St Louis, 2007, Mosby.

48. Smith SF, Biggs MT, Sekhon LH: Risk factors and prophylaxis for deep venous thrombosis in neurosurgery, *Surg Technol Int* 14:69, 2005.

49. Barker E: Intracranial pressure and monitoring. In Barker E, editor: *Neuroscience nursing: a spectrum of care*, ed 3, St Louis, 2008, Mosby.

50. Eigsti J, Henke K: Anatomy and physiology of neurological compensatory mechanisms, *Dimens Crit Care Nurs* 25:197, 2006.

51. March K, Madden L: Intracranial pressure management. In Littlejohns LR, Bader MK, editors: *AACN-ANNA protocols for practice: monitoring technologies in critically ill neuroscience patients*, Sudbury, MA, 2009, Jones & Bartlett.

52. Rangel-Castilla L, Gopinath S, Robertson CS: Management of intracranial hypertension, *Neurol Clin* 26:521, 2008.

53. Curley G, Kavanagh BP, Laffey JG: Hypocapnia and the injured brain: more harm than benefit, *Crit Care Med* 38:1348, 2010.

54. Bhatia A, Gupta AK: Neuromonitoring in the intensive care unit. I. Intracranial pressure and cerebral blood flow monitoring, *Intensive Care Med* 33:1263, 2007.

55. Rauen CA, Chulay M, Bridges E, et al: Seven evidence-based practice habits: putting some sacred cows out to pasture, *Crit Care Nurse* 28(2):98, 2008.

56. Leeper B, Lovasik D: Cerebrospinal drainage systems: external ventricular and lumbar drains. In Littlejohns LR, Bader MK, editors: *AACN-ANNA protocols for practice: monitoring technologies in critically ill neuroscience patients*, Sudbury, MA, 2009, Jones & Bartlett.

57. Koenig MA, Bryan M, Lewin JL 3rd, et al: Reversal of transtentorial herniation with hypertonic saline, *Neurology* 70:1023, 2008.

58. Cook AM, Weant KA: Pharmacologic strategies for the treatment of elevated intracranial pressure: focus on metabolic suppression, *Adv Emerg Nurs J* 29:309, 2007.

59. Morrison CAM: Brain herniation syndromes, *Crit Care Nurs* 7:(5)34, 1987.

60. Gahart BL, Nazareno AR: 2011 Intravenous medications, ed 27, St Louis, 2011, Mosby.

CHAPTER

19

Renal Clinical Assessment and Diagnostic Procedures

Mary Schira

evolve WEBSITE

Be sure to check out the bonus material, including free self-assessment exercises, on the Evolve web site at *http://evolve.elsevier.com/Urden/priorities/*.

OBJECTIVES

- Describe the priorities of the nursing assessment to detect acute kidney injury (AKI).
- Identify ways in which alterations of hemoglobin and hematocrit levels can signal fluid volume deficit or excess.
- Explain why elevation of blood urea nitrogen (BUN) and serum creatinine signal kidney dysfunction.

A history of acute kidney injury begins with a description stated in the patient's own words, including the onset, location, duration, and factors or strategies that lessen or aggravate the problem.[1] A careful history that explores symptoms fully is an essential component of the clinical assessment.

Predisposing factors for acute kidney dysfunction include the use of over-the-counter medicines, recent infections requiring antibiotic therapy, antihypertensive medicines, and any diagnostic procedures performed using a radiopaque contrast agent.[2] The history may be significant for the recent onset of nausea and vomiting, appetite loss caused by taste changes (uremia often causes a metallic taste), or rapid fluid volume gains. For example, weight gain of more than 2 pounds per day, sleeping on additional pillows, and sitting in a chair to sleep are signals of volume overload and potential cardiopulmonary stress related to kidney dysfunction.

PHYSICAL EXAMINATION

In the critical care area, nursing assessment does not routinely include a full physical examination of the kidneys and urologic system. Although a thorough kidney assessment is rarely performed in the depth described in the following sections, the critical care nurse must be aware of how to perform one if needed in patients with kidney dysfunction.

Inspection

Nursing priorities for inspection of the patient with acute kidney injury focus on (1) bleeding, (2) volume depletion or overload, and (3) edema.

Bleeding

Visual inspection related to the kidneys focuses on the patient's flank and abdomen. Kidney trauma is suspected if a purplish discoloration is present on the flank (Grey Turner's sign) or near the posterior 11th or 12th ribs.[1] Bruising, abdominal distention, and abdominal guarding may also signal kidney trauma or a hematoma around a kidney. Individuals who have experienced a traumatic injury are carefully assessed for signs of kidney trauma.

Volume

Fluid volume assessment begins with an inspection of the patient's jugular neck veins as described in Chapter 11. The supine position facilitates normal jugular venous distention. An absence of distention (flat neck veins) indicates hypovolemia. Assessment continues with the head of the bed elevated 45 to 90 degrees.[1] Fluid overload exists when the neck veins remain distended more than 2 cm above the sternal notch when the bed is at 45 degrees.[3]

Inspection of hand veins for venous distention when the hand is held in the dependent position is a component of volume assessment. Venous filling that takes longer than 5 seconds suggests hypovolemia. When the hand is elevated, the distention should disappear within 5 seconds. If distention does not disappear within 5 seconds after the hand is elevated, fluid overload is suspected.

To assess skin turgor, the examiner picks up skin over the forearm and then releases it. Normal elasticity and fluid status allow an almost immediate return to shape after the skin is released. In fluid volume deficit, the skin remains raised and does not return to its normal position for several seconds. Because of the loss of skin elasticity in older adults, skin turgor assessment is not an accurate fluid assessment for this age group.

Inspection of the oral cavity provides clues to fluid volume deficit as the mucous membranes of the mouth can become dry. However, mouth breathing and some medicines (e.g., antihistamines) can also dry the oral mucous membranes. The most accurate way to assess the oral cavity is to inspect the mouth using a tongue blade.[3]

Edema

Edema is the presence of excess volume in the interstitial space. Edema may develop in dependent areas of the body, such as the feet and legs of an ambulatory person or the sacrum of an individual confined to bed.

The presence of edema does not always indicate fluid volume overload. A loss of albumin from the vascular space can also cause peripheral edema. A key feature that identifies edema due to excess volume or hypoalbuminemia is that the edema does not reverse with elevation of the extremity.

Presence of pitting edema is assessed by application of fingertip pressure on the swollen area over a bony prominence, such as the ankles, pretibial areas (shins), and sacrum. If the indentation made by the fingertip does not disappear within 15 seconds, pitting edema exists. Pitting edema indicates increased interstitial volume, and it usually is not evident until significant weight gain has occurred.[4] Edema also may appear in the hands, around the eyes, in the cheeks, and in dependent areas, such as the feet and sacrum. One way of estimating edema is by using a subjective 1 to 4 scale, with

1 indicating only minimal pitting and 4 indicating severe pitting (Table 19-1).[1]

Auscultation

Nursing priorities in auscultation of the patient with acute kidney injury focus on (1) the heart, (2) blood pressure, and (3) the lungs.

Heart

Auscultation of the heart requires assessing the rate and rhythm and listening for extra heart sounds. Fluid overload is often accompanied by a third or fourth heart sound, which is auscultated with the bell of the stethoscope.[1] Increased heart rate alone provides little information about fluid volume, but combined with a low blood pressure, it may suggest hypovolemia.

The heart is auscultated for the presence of a pericardial friction rub. A rub can best be heard at the third intercostal space to the left of the sternal border while the individual leans slightly forward.[1] A pericardial friction rub indicates pericarditis, and it may result from uremia in a patient with kidney failure.

Blood Pressure

Blood pressure (BP) and heart rate (HR) changes are useful in assessing fluid volume deficit. In stable critically ill patients or in patients on a telemetry unit, orthostatic vital sign measurements provide clues to blood loss, dehydration, unexplained syncope, and the effects of some antihypertensive medications.[4,5] A drop in systolic BP of 20 mm Hg or more, a drop in diastolic BP of 10 mm Hg or more, or a rise in pulse rate of more than 15 beats/min from lying to sitting or from sitting to standing indicate orthostatic hypotension. Box 19-1 describes how to assess for orthostatic hypotension.

Lungs

Lung assessment is essential in gauging fluid status. Crackles indicate fluid overload. Dyspnea with mild exertion, dyspnea at night that prevents sleeping in a flat position (orthopnea), or dyspnea that awakens the individual from sleep (paroxysmal nocturnal dyspnea) may indicate pooling of fluid in the lungs.

TABLE 19-1	PITTING EDEMA SCALE
RATING	**APPROXIMATE EQUIVALENT**
+1	2-mm depth
+2	4-mm depth (lasting up to 15 sec)
+3	6-mm depth (lasting up to 60 sec)
+4	8-mm depth (lasting longer than 60 sec)

BOX 19-1   ORTHOSTATIC HYPOTENSION ASSESSMENT

1. Take BP and HR with patient lying down.
2. Assist patient to sitting position.
   a. Monitor patient for complaints of dizziness or imbalance.
   b. Take BP and HR immediately and record.
   c. Take BP and HR after 3 minutes and record.
3. Assist patient to a standing position (if patient is not dizzy or imbalanced).
   a. Assess as above.

Percussion

Nursing priorities in percussion of the patient with acute kidney injury focus on (1) the kidneys and (2) the abdomen. Percussion is performed to detect pain in the area of a kidney or to determine excess accumulation of air, fluid, or solids around the kidneys. Neither palpation nor percussion of the kidneys is a routine part of a nursing assessment in critical care.

Kidneys

Percussion of a kidney is performed with the patient in a side-lying or sitting position, with the examiner's hand placed over the costovertebral angle (lower border of the rib cage on the flank).[1] Striking the back of the hand with the other fist produces a dull thud, which is normal. Pain may indicate kidney infection, or injury resulting from trauma. Traumatic injury to the kidneys should be assessed in the presence of a penetrating abdominal wound, with blunt abdominal trauma, or with a fractured pelvis or ribs.[6,7] Mortality is increased when AKI is a complication of traumatic injury.[7]

Abdomen

Observation and percussion of the abdomen may help in assessing fluid status. Percussing the abdomen with the patient in the supine position generally yields a dull sound (solid bowel contents or fluid) or a hollow sound (gaseous bowel).[1]

Ascites, or excess fluid accumulation and distention of the abdominal cavity, is an important observation in determining fluid overload. Differentiating ascites from distortion caused by solid bowel contents is accomplished by producing a fluid wave. A fluid wave is elicited by exerting pressure to the abdominal midline while one hand is placed on the right or left flank.[1,4] Tapping the opposite flank produces a wave in the accumulated fluid that can be felt under the examiner's hands (Figure 19-1). Other signs of ascites include a protuberant, rounded abdomen and abdominal striae.[1]

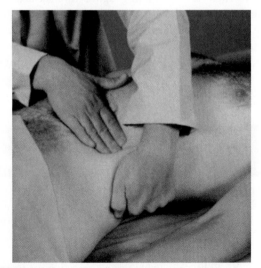

FIGURE 19-1 Test for the presence of a fluid wave. (From Barkauskas V, Baumann LC, Darl CS: *Health & physical assessment*, ed 3, St Louis, 2002, Mosby.)

FLUID BALANCE ASSESSMENT

Nursing priorities for the patient undergoing fluid balance assessment focus on (1) weight, (2) intake and output, and (3) hemodynamic monitoring.

Weight

In the critical care unit, weight is monitored daily and is an important vital signs measurement. Significant fluctuations in body weight over a 1- to 2-day period indicate fluid gains and losses. Rapid weight gains or losses of more than 2 pounds per day usually indicate fluid rather than nutritional factors. One liter of fluid equals 1 kg, or approximately 2.2 pounds.

The weight is obtained at the same time each day, with the patient wearing the same amount of clothing and using the same scale. The individual's weight is of critical importance to the dialysis nurse caring for a patient with acute or chronic kidney failure. The differences in weight from day to day are used to calculate the amount of fluid to remove during a dialysis treatment.[8]

Intake and Output

Intake and output are monitored for every patient in the critical care unit and can be compared with the patient's weight to more accurately evaluate fluid gains or losses. Urinary output plus insensible fluid losses (perspiration, stool, and water vapor from the lungs) can vary by 750 to 2400 mL/day. When intake exceeds output (e.g., excessive intravenous fluid, decreased urine output), a positive fluid balance exists.

Conversely, if output exceeds intake (e.g., fever, increased respiration, profuse sweating, vomiting, diarrhea, gastric suction, diuretic therapy), a negative fluid balance exists, and volume deficit results. During a 24-hour period, fever can increase skin and respiratory losses by as much as 75 mL per 1° F increase in temperature.

Individuals with acute kidney injury (AKI) often exhibit a decrease in urine output, or oliguria (<0.5 mL/kg/hr in adults). Although urine output is a sensitive indicator, kidney function cannot be accurately determined by urine output alone.

In the maintenance of daily records of intake and output, all gains or losses must be recorded. A standard list of the fluid volumes held in various containers (e.g., milk cartons, juice containers) expedites this process. Discussions about the importance of accurate intake and output with the patient and family or friends can improve the accuracy of intake and output volumes assessment.

Hemodynamic Monitoring

Body fluid status is accurately reflected in measurements of cardiovascular hemodynamics. Measurements such as central venous pressure (CVP), pulmonary artery occlusion pressure (PAOP), cardiac index (CI), and mean arterial pressure (MAP) provide a clear picture of the increases or decreases in vascular volume returning to and being ejected from the heart.[9] Volume depletion and volume overload are monitored by use of central venous and arterial catheters, from which pressure measurements are obtained (Table 19-2).

A central venous catheter often is inserted to evaluate fluid volume status and to measure the CVP. The CVP represents the filling pressure of the right atrium and is a measurement of right ventricular preload. The CVP changes with fluctuations in volume status. A normal CVP is 2 to 5 mm Hg.

If the patient has coexisting cardiopulmonary disease or if more information about hemodynamic function is required, a pulmonary artery catheter may be inserted. This catheter provides information about left ventricular filling pressures and cardiac output. The normal PAOP, or "wedge" pressure, is 5 to 12 mm Hg. In fluid volume excess, the PAOP increases. In fluid volume deficit, the PAOP is low.[9] Pulmonary artery catheters are not routinely used to diagnose AKI but may be inserted when the patient is hemodynamically unstable from other conditions, such as heart failure, trauma, and sepsis.

Severe sepsis and septic shock are common precursors of AKI in the critically ill.[10] Sepsis may present with hypotension, and prolonged hypotensive episodes increase risk of AKI and increase mortality.[10] Hemodynamic monitoring with skillful nursing interpretation of trends provides essential information about the effectiveness of treatment.

LABORATORY ASSESSMENT

Acute kidney injury often leads to electrolyte and acid-base imbalances that result from retention of metabolic waste products. Box 19-2 summarizes important aspects that should be considered during assessment. Retention of waste products and inability to buffer hydrogen ions contribute to the acidosis that occurs with kidney failure.

Lethargy, decreased attention or memory, coma, and confusion may result from electrolyte imbalance and retained waste products (see Box 19-2). Patients with kidney failure and the accompanying systemic increases in electrolytes, fluids, and nitrogenous waste products may exhibit a range of symptoms from restlessness and confusion to apathy and withdrawal.[2] The speed of onset depends on how rapidly or slowly kidney failure progresses and alters homeostasis.

Serum Components
Blood Urea Nitrogen

Blood urea nitrogen is a by-product of protein and amino acid metabolism.[11] The normal value for BUN is 5 to 25 mg/dL. This value rises as kidney function deteriorates.[12] BUN elevation represents a decrease in the glomerular filtration rate (GFR) and resultant decrease in urea excretion. Elevations in the BUN correlate with the clinical manifestations of uremia.[2] Many conditions result in BUN elevation, including dehydration,[13] nephrotoxic drugs, excessive protein intake, and catabolism.[11] The BUN level also rises from hematoma resorption, gastrointestinal bleeding, excessive licorice ingestion, or steroid or tetracycline therapy.

A decrease in the BUN level may indicate volume overload, liver damage, severe malnutrition from depleted protein stores, use of phenothiazines, or pregnancy.[12]

TABLE 19-2	HEMODYNAMIC ASSESSMENT OF FLUID STATUS	
MEASUREMENT	**VALUE WITH VOLUME DEPLETION**	**VALUE WITH VOLUME OVERLOAD**
CVP (mm Hg)	<2	>5
PAOP (mm Hg)	<5	>12
CI (L/min/m²)	<2.2	>4
MAP	Decreased	Increased

BOX 19-2	FLUID AND ELECTROLYTE ASSESSMENT

Fluid Status
- Skin turgor
- Mucous membranes
- Intake and output
- Presence of edema or ascites
- Neck and hand vein engorgement
- Lung sounds (crackles)
- Dyspnea
- CVP <2 mm Hg or >5 mm Hg
- PAOP <5 mm Hg or >12 mm Hg
- Tachycardia
- Hypertension, hypotension
- CI <2.2 L/min/m²
- S_3, S_4 heart sounds
- Headache
- Blurred vision
- Vertigo on rising
- Papilledema
- Mental changes
- Serum osmolality

Electrolyte and Waste Product Status
- Complete blood cell count (CBC)
- Serum electrolyte levels
- BUN
- Electrocardiogram tracings (potassium, calcium, magnesium levels)
- Behavioral and mental changes (sodium, BUN levels)
- Chvostek's and Trousseau's signs (calcium levels)
- Changes in peripheral sensation (numbness, tremor—sodium, potassium, calcium levels)
- Muscle strength (potassium, BUN)
- Gastrointestinal changes (nausea and vomiting—BUN)
- Itching (calcium, phosphorus, BUN)
- Therapies that can alter electrolyte status (gastrointestinal suction, diuretics, antihypertensives, calcium channel blockers)

Creatinine

Creatinine is a by-product of muscle and normal cell metabolism, and it appears in serum in amounts generally proportional to the body muscle mass. Although slightly higher in males than females, the normal serum creatinine level is about 0.5 to 1.5 mg/dL.[12] Creatinine is freely filtered by the glomerulus, easily excreted by the renal tubules, and minimally resorbed or secreted in the tubules.[2] Creatinine levels are fairly constant and are affected by fewer factors than BUN. Consequently, the serum creatinine level is a more sensitive and specific indicator of kidney function.

Elevated creatinine values may occur in muscle growth disorders such as acromegaly with skeletal muscle destruction (e.g., rhabdomyolysis in a trauma patient), and with some medications that decrease creatinine removal (e.g., trimethoprim, cimetidine) in the absence of acute kidney injury.[14]

Another useful diagnostic parameter in acute kidney injury is the ratio of BUN to creatinine. The usual ratio is 10 to 1, and a change in the ratio may indicate kidney dysfunction.[12,15]

Creatinine Clearance

The creatinine clearance is a measure of how effectively the kidneys remove creatinine. Because of the relatively constant rate at which creatinine is produced and the nearly complete removal of creatinine by normal kidneys, the ability to remove (clear) creatinine from the blood is an indication of how well the glomeruli and tubules are working. The normal value for creatinine clearance is 110 to 120 mL/min; values less than 50 mL/min indicate significant kidney dysfunction. The creatinine clearance is best measured using a 12-hour or 24-hour urine collection and blood sample. In critical care, a smaller-volume urine specimen and blood sample is generally used.

Creatinine clearance can also be estimated from the serum creatinine level.[15] (Box 19-3). The estimated or calculated creatinine clearance is widely used to determine changes in drug dosing with kidney dysfunction because many medications are excreted by the kidneys.[15] To adjust drug dosages, the critical care nurse should use the Cockcroft-Gault formula for estimating creatinine clearance.[15,16]

OSMOLALITY

The serum osmolality reflects the concentration or dilution of vascular fluid and measures the dissolved particles in the serum. The normal serum osmolality is 275 to 295 mOsm/L.[3] An elevated osmolality value indicates hemoconcentration or dehydration, and a decreased osmolality value indicates hemodilution or volume overload. Sodium accounts for 85% to 95% of the serum osmolality value. Multiplying the serum sodium level by 2 gives an estimate of the serum osmolality level in healthy individuals.[12] A more precise estimation of serum osmolality can be calculated from the following formula:

$$(2 \times Na) + \left(\frac{BUN}{3}\right) + \left(\frac{Glucose}{18}\right)$$

BOX 19-3   CREATININE CLEARANCE CALCULATIONS

Measured

Calculation of clearance from a 24-hour urine sample*:

$$\frac{(Urine\ creatinine \times Volume\ of\ urine)}{Serum\ creatinine}$$

Estimated

In Adults

Cockcroft-Gault Formula

$$\frac{[(140 - Age) \times Body\ weight\ (kg)]}{[72 \times Plasma\ creatinine\ (mg/dL)]}$$

For women, multiply the result by 0.85.

Modified Modification of Diet in Renal Disease (MDRD) Formula

$$186 \times (Plasma\ creatinine)$$
$$-1.154 \times (Age\ in\ years) - 0.203$$

For women, multiply the result by 0.742.
For African Americans, multiply the result by 1.210.[†]

In Children

Weight ≤10 kg: $\dfrac{0.45 \times Height\ (cm)}{Serum\ creatinine\ (mg/dL)}$

Weight >10 but < 70 kg: $\dfrac{0.55 \times Height\ (cm)}{Serum\ creatinine\ (mg/dL)}$

Weight ≥70 kg: $\dfrac{[1.55 \times Age\ (yr)] + 0.5 \times Height\ (cm)}{Serum\ creatinine\ (mg/dL)}$

*Calculations available from the National Kidney Foundation (www.kidney.org/professionals).
†Both risk factor assessments apply for African American women. The number would be multiplied by both 0.742 (woman) and 1.210 (African American).

The calculated serum osmolality level is a useful tool during the wait for full laboratory results. Measured serum osmolality is a useful parameter in determining fluid replacement therapy for critically ill patients.

Anion Gap

The *anion gap* is a calculation of the difference between the measurable extracellular plasma anions (chloride and bicarbonate) and the measurable cations (sodium and potassium).[3] In plasma, chloride is the predominant anion and sodium is the predominant cation. Generally, potassium is not included in the formula because the value is so small. This leaves the following equation for calculation of the anion gap:

$$[Na^+] - ([Cl^-] + [HCO_3^-])$$

The normal anion gap is 8 to 16 mEq. The 'gap' represents the unmeasurable ions present in the extracellular fluid (phosphates, sulfates, ketones, lactate). An increased anion gap usually reflects overproduction of acid products and indicates metabolic acidosis.

Acute kidney injury and chronic kidney failure can increase the anion gap because of retention of acids and altered bicarbonate resorption. The anion gap is also increased in diabetic ketoacidosis (DKA) caused by ketone production. The measurement of a high anion gap is a rapid method for identifying acid-base imbalance but cannot be used to pinpoint the source of the acid-base disturbance specifically.

Hemoglobin and Hematocrit

The hemoglobin and hematocrit levels can indicate increases or decreases in intravascular fluid volume.[11] An increase in the hematocrit value may occur with fluid volume deficit that produces hemoconcentration. Conversely, a decreased hematocrit can indicate fluid volume excess because of the dilutional effect of the extra fluid load.

Hemoglobin is decreased as a result of anemia, blood loss, liver damage, or hemolytic reactions.[12] In individuals with acute kidney failure, anemia may occur early in the disease.

Urinalysis

Analysis of the urine provides excellent information about the patient's kidney function and condition relative to fluids and electrolytes. Specific tests and abnormal indications are presented in Table 19-3.[12,17-24] In many cases, urinalysis in the critically ill patient aids in locating the site of kidney damage or disease and therefore guides therapeutic management of the patient's care.

TABLE 19-3	**URINALYSIS RESULTS**		
TEST	**NORMAL VALUE/RANGE**	**POSSIBLE CAUSES FOR INCREASED VALUES**	**ACIDOSIS**
pH	4.5-8.0	Alkalosis	Acidosis Intrarenal AKI
Specific gravity	1.003-1.030*	Volume deficit Glycosuria Proteinuria Prerenal AKI (>1.020)	Volume overload Intrarenal AKI
Osmolality	300-1200 mOsm/kg	Volume deficit Prerenal AKI (urine osmolality > serum osmolality)	Volume excess Intrarenal AKI (urine osmolality < serum osmolality)
Protein	30-150 mg/24 hr†	Trauma Infection Intrarenal AKI Transient with exercise Glomerulonephritis	
Sodium	40-220 mEq/24 hr	High-sodium diet Intrarenal AKI	Prerenal AKI
Creatinine	1-2 g/24 hr		Intrarenal AKI Chronic kidney failure
Urea	6-17 g/24 hr		Intrarenal AKI Chronic kidney failure
Myoglobin	Absent	Crush injury Rhabdomyolysis	
RBCs	0-5 per low-power field	Trauma Intrarenal AKI Infection Strenuous exercise Renal artery thrombus	
WBCs	0-5 per low-power field	Infection	
Bacteria	None to few	Infection	
Casts	None to few	RBC: glomerular disease WBC: pyelonephritis Glomerular disease Nephrotic syndrome Epithelial: glomerular disease	

RBC, red blood cell; *WBC*, white blood cell.
*Adult value.
†Higher values usually apply for persons after exercise; lower values apply for persons at rest.

TABLE 19-4	KIDNEY IMAGING TESTS
TEST	**COMMENTS**
Kidney-ureter-bladder (KUB) radiograph	Flat-plate x-ray film of the abdomen; determines position, size, and structure of the kidneys, urinary tract, and pelvis; useful for evaluating the presence of calculi and masses; usually followed by additional tests
Intravenous pyelogram (IVP)	Intravenous injection of contrast with radiography; allows visualization of internal kidney tissues
Angiography	Injection of contrast into arterial blood perfusing the kidneys; allows visualization of renal blood flow; may also visualize stenosis, cysts, clots, trauma, and infarctions
Computed tomography (CT)	Radioisotope is administered by intravenous route and absorbed by the kidneys; scintillation photography is then performed in several planes; spiral or helical CT allows rapid imaging; density of the image helps evaluate kidney vessels, perfusion, tumors, cysts, stones/calculi, hemorrhage, necrosis, and trauma
Ultrasound	High-frequency sound waves are transmitted to the kidneys and urinary tract, and the image is viewed on an oscilloscope; noninvasive; identifies fluid accumulation or obstruction, cysts, stones/calculi, and masses; useful for evaluating kidney before biopsy
Magnetic resonance imaging (MRI)	A scanner produces three-dimensional images in response to the application of high-energy radiofrequency waves to the tissues; produces clear images; density of the image may indicate trauma, cysts, masses, malformation of the vessels or tubules stones/calculi, and necrosis

DIAGNOSTIC PROCEDURES

Imaging Studies

Although laboratory assessment is used most often in diagnosing kidney problems in the critically ill patient, imaging studies can confirm or clarify causes of particular disorders. Imaging includes the use of ultrasound and radiologic techniques. Kidney ultrasound is especially useful in determining the size, shape, and contour of the kidneys, the presence of masses or cysts, and the presence of renal artery stenosis.[25,26] Radiological assessment ranges from basic to more complex (Table 19-4) and provides information about abnormal masses, abnormal fluid collections, obstructions, vascular supply alterations, and other disorders of the kidneys and urinary tract.[2,24-26]

Some radiologic studies require the use of a contrast agent or injection of a radiopaque dye. Because many of the dyes used in radiology are potentially nephrotoxic, they must be used carefully in patients with AKI or chronic kidney disease. An individual with AKI undergoing a test using a contrast agent may experience deterioration of kidney function caused by the dye. To prevent nephrotoxicity, adequate hydration before and after the test and careful monitoring of kidney function are indicated any time a contrast agent is used.

Kidney Biopsy

Kidney biopsy is the definitive tool for diagnosing disease processes of the kidney. Two methods are used: closed biopsy and open biopsy. Percutaneous needle biopsy (closed method) involves inserting a needle through the flank to obtain a specimen of cortical and medullary kidney tissue. An open biopsy is a surgical procedure and is rarely done in critically ill patients. In either case, biopsy is often the last choice for diagnostic assessment in the critically ill patient because of the postprocedural risks of bleeding, hematoma formation, and infection.

REFERENCES

1. Seidel HM, Ball JW, Dains JE, et al: *Mosby's guide to physical examination*, ed 5, St Louis, 2003, Mosby.
2. Schira M, section editor: Assessment of kidney structure and function. In Counts C, editor: *Core curriculum for nephrology nursing*, ed 5, Pitman, NJ, 2008, American Nephrology Nurses Association.
3. Parker K: Alterations in fluid, electrolyte, and acid-base balance. In Molzahn A, Butera E, editors: *Contemporary nephrology nursing: principles and practice*, ed 2, Pitman, NJ, 2006, American Nephrology Nurses Association.
4. Ejaz AA, Haley WE, Wasiluk A, et al: Characteristics of 100 consecutive patients presenting with orthostatic hypotension, *Mayo Clin Proc* 79(7):890, 2004.
5. Irvin D: The importance of accurately assessing orthostatic hypotension, *Geriatr Nurs* 25(2):99, 2004.
6. Bozeman C, Zabari G, Caldito G, et al: Selective operative management of major blunt renal trauma, *J Trauma* 57(2):305, 2004.
7. Bagshaw S, George C, Gibney RT, et al: A multi-center evaluation of early acute kidney injury in critically ill trauma patients, *Renal Failure* 30(6):581, 2008.
8. Purcell W, Manias E, Williams A, et al: Accurate dry weight assessment: reducing the incidence of hypertension and cardiac disease in patients on hemodialysis, *Nephrol Nurs J* 31(6):631, 2004.
9. Subramanian S, Ziedalski TM: Oliguria, volume overload, Na balance, and diuretics, *Crit Care Clin* 21(20): 291, 2005.

10. Bagshaw S, Gibney RT: Acute kidney injury in septic shock: clinical outcomes and impact of duration of hypotension prior to initiation of antimicrobial therapy, *Intensive Care Med* 35(5):871, 2009.

11. Robinson BE, Weber H: Dehydration despite drinking: beyond the BUN/creatinine ratio, *J Am Med Dir Assoc* 5(2 suppl):S67, 2004.

12. Kee J: *Laboratory & diagnostic tests with nursing implications*, ed 7, Upper Saddle River, NJ, 2006, Pearson Prentice-Hall.

13. Thomas DR, Tariq SH, Makhdomm S, et al: Physician misdiagnosis of dehydration in older adults, *J Am Med Dir Assoc* 5(2 suppl):S30, 2004.

14. Bagshaw S, Gibney N: Conventional markers of kidney function, *Crit Care Med* 36(4 suppl):S152, 2008.

15. Dong K, Quan D: Appropriately assessing renal function for drug dosing, *Nephrol Nurs J* 37(3):304, 2010.

16. Pequignot R, et al: Renal function in older hospital patients is more accurately estimated using the Cockcroft-Gault formula than the modification diet in renal disease formula, *J Am Geriatr Soc* 57(9):1638, 2009.

17. Greenberg A: Urinalysis. In Greenberg A, editor: *Primer on kidney diseases*, ed 4, Philadelphia, 2005, Saunders.

18. Hanson K: Laboratory studies in the evaluation of urologic disease. Part I, *Urol Nurs* 23(6):400, 2004.

19. Cabellon A: Art and science of urinalysis. In Windus D, editor: *The Washington manual nephrology subspecialty consult*, ed 2, Philadelphia, 2008, Lippincott Williams & Wilkins.

20. Glassock R: Hematuria and proteinuria. In Greenberg A, editor, *Primer on kidney diseases*, ed 4, Philadelphia, 2005, Saunders.

21. Mwintshi K: Approach to proteinuria. In Windus D, editor: *The Washington manual nephrology subspecialty consult*, ed 2, Philadelphia, 2008, Lippincott Williams & Wilkins.

22. Madison J, Spies C, Schatz IJ, et al: Proteinuria and risk for stroke and coronary heart disease during 27 years of follow-up: The Honolulu heart program, *Arch Intern Med* 166(8):884, 2006.

23. Russell T: Acute renal failure related to rhabdomyolysis: pathophysiology, diagnosis, and collaborative management, *Nephrol Nurs J* 32(4):409, 2005.

24. Hanson K: Diagnostic tests and tools in the evaluation of urologic disease. Part II, *Urol Nurs* 23(6):405, 2004.

25. Higgins T, et al: Kidney imaging techniques. In Greenberg A, editor: *Primer on kidney diseases*, ed 4, Philadelphia, 2005, Saunders.

26. Pregerson B: Imaging options for patients with acute abdominal pain, Cortland Forum August: 21. 2010. Available at http://www.cortlandtforum.com/imaging-options-for-patients-with-acute-abdominal-pain/article/176680/.

CHAPTER 20

Renal Disorders and Therapeutic Management

Mary E. Lough

℮volve WEBSITE

Be sure to check out the bonus material, including free self-assessment exercises, on the Evolve web site at *http://evolve.elsevier.com/Urden/priorities/.*

OBJECTIVES

- List three etiologies of acute kidney injury.
- Identify the priorities of nursing management in acute kidney injury.
- Discuss the differences between hemodialysis and continuous renal replacement therapy.
- Explain the differences between a living-donor and a deceased-donor kidney transplant.
- Describe the priorities of nursing management for the kidney transplant recipient.

ACUTE KIDNEY INJURY

Acute kidney injury (AKI) describes the spectrum of acute-onset kidney failure that can occur with critical illness; it replaces the traditional terms acute renal failure (ARF)[1] and acute tubular necrosis (ATN). Severe AKI is characterized by a sudden decline in glomerular filtration rate (GFR), with subsequent retention of products in the blood that are normally excreted by the kidneys; this disrupts electrolyte balance, acid-base homeostasis, and fluid volume equilibrium.[1,2] A transition to greater use of the word kidney rather than renal reflects a trend in the nephrology literature that emphasizes the vulnerability of the kidney during critical illness.

Critical Illness and Acute Kidney Injury

The estimated incidence of AKI is between 2000 and 3000 cases per 1 million people per year.[3] Researchers estimate that AKI accounts for 1% of acute hospital admissions and complicates more than 7% of inpatient episodes, especially for older individuals and those with preexistent chronic kidney disease.[2]

Critical care patients with AKI have a longer length of hospital stay and more complications.[3] After AKI has occurred in the critically ill patient, the risk of death rises dramatically.[3,4] The mortality rate ranges from 38% to 80%.[5] One of the reasons for the high mortality rate is that critical care patients often have coexisting nonrenal health problems that increase their susceptibility to the development of AKI. High-risk conditions include heart failure, shock, respiratory failure, and sepsis, and this situation has altered the spectrum of AKI.[4,5] An observational study that examined the incidence and course of severe AKI that resulted in ARF in six academic medical centers in the United States found that AKI was accompanied by multiorgan failure in most patients, even those who did not require dialysis.[4] In this study of 618 patients with ARF, 64% of patients required dialysis, the in-hospital mortality rate was 37%, and the permanent loss of kidney function or death was 50%.[4] The clinicians' conclusion is that death of the critically ill patient with AKI-related ARF is related to the severity of coexisting nonrenal diseases.[4] Mortality rates exceeded 50% when four or more body systems had failed.[4]

Cohort studies suggest that the incidence of AKI is increasing, whereas the mortality rate is declining.[6] Patients with AKI often have associated multiple organ dysfunction syndrome (MODS) and have more complex illnesses and comorbidities than patients 40 years ago, and more critical care patients are receiving dialysis therapies in the critical care unit.

Typically, a patient is not admitted to the critical care unit with a diagnosis of AKI alone; there is always coexisting hemodynamic, cardiac, pulmonary, or neurologic compromise. Many individuals come into the hospital with underlying changes in kidney function, such as an elevated serum creatinine (Cr) level, although the patient is not symptomatic and is often unaware of the compromised kidney.[7] The lack of kidney reserve places the patient at increased risk for AKI if complications occur in any of the other major organ systems. As a result, the picture of AKI in the modern critical care unit has changed to encompass patients with kidney injury who also have multisystem dysfunction that complicates their clinical course.[3]

Definitions of Acute Kidney Injury and Acute Renal Failure

One of the challenges of estimating the incidence of AKI or ARF in the critical care unit has been the wide variation in definitions that have been used.[8] Measurement of kidney function is necessarily indirect, and the diagnosis of AKI is predominantly derived from changes in urine output (UO) and serum creatine level, with the assumption that changes in these values reflect changes in the GFR.[8] Urine output is sometimes a problematic measure to use because diuretics artificially increase the urine output but do not alter the course of kidney failure. The clinical insult may have direct effects on the kidney, such as the inflammation associated with sepsis, which accounts for 50% of the AKI seen in critical care units.[9]

RIFLE Criteria

The risk of development of AKI in critically ill patients has been classified by a multinational group of nephrologists.[10] The classification uses the acronym RIFLE (*r*isk, *i*njury, *f*ailure, *l*oss, and *e*nd-stage kidney disease [ESKD]).[11] The RIFLE system classifies AKI into three categories of increasing severity (R, I, F) and two outcome criteria (L, E) based on GFR status reflected by the change in urine output or loss of kidney function[11] (Table 20-1). If AKI is superimposed on a

TABLE 20-1	RIFLE CRITERIA FOR ACUTE KIDNEY DYSFUNCTION	
RIFLE CRITERIA	**SERUM CREATININE CRITERIA***	**URINE OUTPUT CRITERIA**
Risk	Serum Cr increased 1.5 times above normal *or* Serum Cr increase ≥0.3 mg/dL	UO <0.5 mL/kg/hr for 6 hr
Injury	Serum Cr increased 2 times above normal	UO <0.5 mL/kg/hr for 12 hr
Failure	Serum Cr increased 3 times above normal *or* Serum Cr ≥4 mg/dL *or* Serum Cr acute rise ≥0.5 mg/dL	UO <0.3 mL/kg/hr for 24 hr or anuria for 12 hr (oliguria)
Loss	Persistent AKI = complete loss of kidney function for >4 wk	
ESKD	End-stage kidney disease	

*All serum creatinine references are based on changes from baseline.
Data from Kellum JA, Bellomo R, Ronco C: Definition and classification of acute kidney injury, *Nephron Clin Pract* 109(4): c182, 2008.

kidney that is already compromised, the term chronic is added to the RIFLE criteria to denote the cause as acute-on-chronic kidney failure.[11]

Acute Kidney Injury Network Criteria

The Acute Kidney Injury Network (AKIN) criteria are listed in Box 20-1. These criteria are similar to those proposed by the RIFLE group, and both groups intend to make the point that in the acutely ill patient, small changes in the serum creatinine level and urine output may signal important declines in the GFR and kidney function. A conceptual model that combines the features of the RIFLE criteria and AKIN criteria are shown in Figure 20-1.[11]

Etiology of Acute Kidney Injury

Previously, AKI was predominantly classified by the location of the insult relative to the kidney: prerenal (before), intrarenal (within), and postrenal (after) (Box 20-2). This remains a useful way to imagine the relationship between anatomy and functional insults to the kidney when one is learning about

---

BOX 20-1   ACUTE KIDNEY INJURY NETWORK (AIKN) CRITERIA FOR THE DIAGNOSIS OF ACUTE KIDNEY INJURY

Definition: Acute kidney injury (AKI) is an abrupt (within 48 hours) reduction in kidney function defined as:
- An absolute increase in the serum creatinine level of more than or equal to 0.3 mg/dL (=26.4 µmol/L)
- A percentage increase in serum creatinine of more than or equal to 50% (1.5-fold from baseline)
- A reduction in urine output (documented oliguria of less than 0.5 mL/kg/hr for more than 6 hours)

Explanatory Notes

Serum creatinine: These criteria include an absolute and a percentage change in creatinine to accommodate variations related to age, gender, and body mass index and to reduce the need for a baseline creatinine level, but they do require at least two serum creatinine values within 48 hours.

Urine output: The urine output criterion was included based on the predictive importance of this measure but with the awareness that urine outputs may not be measured routinely in nonintensive care unit settings. It is assumed that the diagnosis based on the urine output criterion alone will require exclusion of urinary tract obstructions that reduce urine output or of other easily reversible causes of reduced urine output.

Clinical context: These criteria should be used in the context of the clinical presentation and after adequate fluid resuscitation when applicable. Many acute kidney diseases exist, and some may result in AKI. Because diagnostic criteria are not documented, some cases of AKI may not be diagnosed.

Physiologic state: AKI may be superimposed on or lead to chronic kidney disease.

Data from Mehta RL, Kellum JA, Shah SV, et al, for the Acute Kidney Injury Network: Acute Kidney Injury Network: Report of an initiative to improve outcomes in acute kidney injury. *Crit Care* 11(2):R31, 2007.

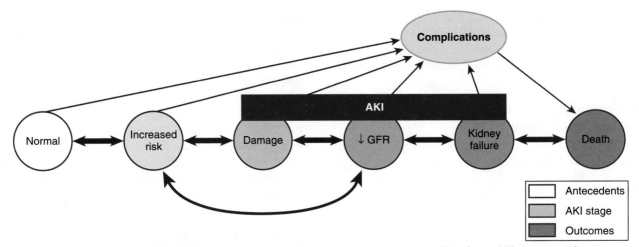

FIGURE 20-1 Model of the components of acute kidney injury. (Modified from AKI conceptual model developed by AKIN [the Acute Kidney Injury Network] at the Vancouver Summit 2006; available at http://www.akinet.org).

BOX 20-2   ACUTE KIDNEY INJURY

Prerenal Acute Kidney Injury
- Prolonged hypotension (sepsis, vasodilation)
- Prolonged low cardiac output (heart failure, cardiogenic shock)
- Prolonged volume depletion (dehydration, hemorrhage)
- Renovascular thrombosis (thromboemboli)

Intrarenal Acute Kidney Injury
- Kidney ischemia (advanced stage of prerenal acute kidney injury)
- Endogenous toxins (rhabdomyolysis, tumor lysis syndrome)
- Exogenous toxins (radiocontrast dye, nephrotoxic drugs)
- Infection (acute glomerulonephritis, interstitial nephritis)

Postrenal Acute Kidney Injury
- Obstruction (urethra, prostate, or bladder)
- Rare as a cause of acute kidney injury in critical care

AKI, although deleterious effects on the kidney are unlikely to be restricted to only one anatomical section at a time.[11]

Prerenal Acute Kidney Injury

Any condition that decreases blood flow, blood pressure (BP), or kidney perfusion before arterial blood in the renal artery enters the kidney may be anatomically described as prerenal AKI. When arterial hypoperfusion due to low cardiac output, hemorrhage, vasodilation, thrombosis, or other cause reduces the blood flow to the kidney, glomerular filtration and, consequently, urine output decrease (see Box 20-2). This is a major reason that the critical care nurse monitors the urine output on an hourly basis. Initially, in prerenal states, the integrity of the kidney's nephron structure and function may be preserved. If normal perfusion and cardiac output are restored quickly, the kidney will not suffer permanent injury. However, if the prerenal insult is not corrected, the GFR will decline, the blood urea nitrogen (BUN) concentration will rise (prerenal azotemia),[9] oliguria will develop, and the patient will be at risk for significant kidney damage. Oliguria

(urine output <400 mL/day) is a classic finding in AKI.[5] Prerenal AKI is seen frequently in the critically ill. In a study of hospitalized older patients with kidney failure, prerenal AKI occurred in 58%.[5] This compares with rates of 34% for intrarenal AKI and 8% for postrenal AKI in the same study.[5]

Intrarenal Acute Kidney Injury

Any condition that produces an ischemic or toxic insult directly at the site of the nephron places the patient at risk for development of intrarenal AKI (see Box 20-2).

Ischemic damage to the kidney can also damage internal structures from prolonged hypotension or low cardiac output. In the multicenter study of critical care patients with AKI by Mehta and colleagues,[4] 50% of the patients had ischemic injury, which was largely precipitated by hypotension (20%) and sepsis (19%).

Toxins that damage kidney tubular endothelium include medications that are administered to treat a coexisting condition[12] as well as radiopaque (contrast) dye administered during an interventional or diagnostic radiological study. Complications from the contrast dye cause AKI in 9% to 14% of patients.[4] In affected patients, the serum creatinine levels typically begin to rise 48 to 72 hours after the study, peak at 3 to 5 days, and return to baseline within another 3 to 5 days.[13] Kidney dysfunction can persist up to 3 weeks after the procedure. Although patients with normal kidney function are not considered to be at risk, those with elevated serum creatinine levels, diabetes, or microvascular disease are highly vulnerable.[13]

Postrenal Acute Kidney Injury

Any obstruction that hinders the flow of urine from beyond the kidney through the remainder of the urinary tract may lead to postrenal AKI. This is not a common cause of kidney failure in the critically ill. When monitoring of the urine output reveals a sudden decrease in the patient's urine output from the urinary catheter, a blockage may be responsible. Sudden development of anuria (urine output <100 mL/24 hr) should prompt verification that the urinary catheter is not occluded.

continue

BOX 20-3 ISCHEMIC VERSUS TOXIC ACUTE KIDNEY INJURY

Ischemic Injury
- Advanced stage of prerenal injury
- Massive hemorrhage
- Severe volume loss
- Severe dehydration
- Severe, prolonged hypotension
- Shock: cardiogenic, hypovolemic, septic
- Sepsis
- Anaphylaxis

Nephrotoxic Injury
Endogenous Nephrotoxins
- Rhabdomyolysis
- Tumor lysis syndrome

*Exogenous Nephrotoxins**
- Radiopaque contrast dye

Nephrotoxic Antimicrobials
- Aminoglycosides: gentamicin, tobramycin, amikacin, vancomycin
- Cephalosporins: cefazolin
- Antifungals: amphotericin B
- Antivirals: acyclovir

Nephrotoxic Immunosuppressants
- Cyclosporin
- Tacrolimus (FK506)

Nephrotoxic Chemotherapeutics
- 5-Azacitidine
- Cisplatin
- Methotrexate

Nephrotoxic Street Drugs
- Heroin
- Amphetamines
- Phencyclidine (PCP)

Nephrotoxic Analgesics
- Nonsteroidal antiinflammatory drugs (NSAIDs)

*Represents only a partial list of potential nephrotoxic medications.

Azotemia

The term azotemia is used to describe an acute rise in the BUN level.[9] Uremia is another term used to describe an elevated BUN value.

Phases of Acute Kidney Injury

AKI can result from nephrotoxic or ischemic injury that damages the kidney tubular epithelium. In severe cases, the injury extends to the collagen of the basement membrane (Box 20-3).

Onset Phase

The onset (initiating) phase of AKI is the period from the initial insult until cell injury occurs. Ischemic injury is evolving during this time. The GFR is decreased because of impaired blood flow to the kidney and decreased glomerular ultrafiltration pressure. The GFR decrease disrupts the integrity of the tubular epithelium. This phase lasts hours to days, depending on the severity of the injury. If treatment is initiated during this time, irreversible damage may be alleviated. A longer course of recovery reflects the presence of more extensive tubular injury.

Oliguric or Anuric Phase

The oliguric or anuric phase, the second phase of AKI, lasts 5 to 8 days in the nonoliguric patient and 10 to 16 days in the oliguric patient.[14] The accumulation of necrotic cellular debris in the tubular space blocks the flow of urine and causes damage to the tubular wall and basement membranes. Back-leak occurs because damage in the tubular wall causes the glomerular filtrate to flow passively into the kidney tissue rather than to be passed out as urine through the ureters and bladder. Oliguria is encountered more often in ischemic damage and is a sign that the damage is extensive and severe. During the oliguric or anuric phase, the GFR is greatly reduced, leading to increased levels of BUN (azotemia), elevated serum creatinine values, electrolyte abnormalities (hyperkalemia, hyperphosphatemia, hypocalcemia), and metabolic acidosis.

Diuretic Phase

The third phase, the diuretic phase of AKI, may last 7 to 14 days and is characterized by an increase in the GFR. During the diuretic phase, the tubular obstruction has passed, but edema and scarring remain. In this situation, the GFR returns and the kidneys can clear fluid volume but not solutes.

Recovery Phase

Critically ill patients with AKI have a high mortality on long-term follow-up.[15] Kidney function may return to normal, or near normal, with a GFR that is 70% to 80% of normal within 1 to 2 years.[16] However, if significant kidney parenchymal damage has occurred, BUN and creatinine levels may never return to normal. Of the patients who survive AKI, approximately 62% eventually recover normal kidney function, 33% have residual kidney damage, and at least 5% require long-term hemodialysis.[16]

Laboratory Assessment

After acute kidney disease is suspected, the presence or degree or AKI is assessed using urinalysis and blood analysis. Table 20-2 lists the initial urinalysis findings for patients with AKI. Most serum electrolyte values become increasingly elevated as AKI develops (Tables 20-3 and 20-4). Normal and abnormal urinalysis findings are summarized in Chapter 19.

Acidosis

Acidosis (pH <7.35) is one of the trademarks of severe AKI.[17] Metabolic acidosis occurs from accumulated metabolic waste products. The acid waste products consist of strong negative ions (anions), elevated serum phosphorus values (hyperphosphatemia), and other normally unmeasured ions (e.g., sulfate, urate, lactate) that decrease the serum pH.[17] A low serum albumin concentration, which often occurs in AKI, has a slight alkalinizing effect, but it is not enough to offset the metabolic acidosis.[17] Even respiratory compensation and

TABLE 20-2	INITIAL URINE LABORATORY ANALYSIS FINDINGS IN ACUTE KIDNEY INJURY*			
ASSESSMENT	**PRERENAL**[†]	**INTRARENAL**[‡]		**POSTRENAL**[§]
Urine volume	Normal	Oliguria or nonoliguria		Oliguria to anuria
Urine specific gravity	>1.020	1.010		1.000-1.010
Urine osmolality (mOsm/kg)	>350	<300		300-400
Urine sodium (mEq/L)	<20	>30		20-40
FENa (%)	<1	>2-3		1-3
BUN/Cr ratio	20:1	Ischemic: 20:1		10:1
		Toxic: 10:1		
Urine microscopy (sediment)	Normal	AKI: dark granular casts, hyaline casts, kidney epithelial cells		Normal

*Results of urine laboratory tests are valid only in the absence of diuretics.
[†]Urine in prerenal failure is concentrated, with low sodium.
[‡]Urine in intrarenal failure shows kidney damage because the nephron cannot concentrate urine or conserve sodium, and evidence of kidney damage (casts) is seen.
[§]Urine test results in postrenal failure vary because the findings initially depend on the hydration status of the patient rather than the status of the kidney.
Anuria, urine volume less than 100 mL/24 hr; *oliguria*, urine volume of 100-400 mL/24 hr.

TABLE 20-3	NORMAL SERUM ELECTROLYTE VALUES
ELECTROLYTE	**NORMAL VALUE**
Sodium	135-145 mEq/L
Potassium	3.5-4.5 mEq/L
Chloride	98-108 mEq/L
Calcium	8.5-10.5 mg/dL or 4.5-5.8 mEq/L
Phosphorus	2.7-4.5 mg/dL
Magnesium	1.5-2.5 mEq/L
Bicarbonate	24-28 mEq/L

mechanical ventilatory support are rarely sufficient to reverse the metabolic acidosis. Information on acidosis and arterial blood gas interpretation is found in Chapter 14. Anion gap measurement is discussed in Chapter 19.

Blood Urea Nitrogen

The BUN level is not a reliable indicator of kidney damage.[9,18] The BUN concentration is changed by protein intake, blood in the gastrointestinal (GI) tract, and cell catabolism, and it is diluted by fluid administration. An elevated BUN-to-creatinine ratio may signal early AKI. The BUN-to-creatinine ratio is most useful in diagnosing prerenal AKI (often described as prerenal azotemia), in which the BUN value is greatly elevated relative to the serum creatinine value.

Serum Creatinine

Creatinine is a by-product of muscle metabolism that is formed from nonenzymatic dehydration of creatine in the liver[18]; 98% of creatine is in the muscles,[18] and it is almost totally excreted by the kidney tubules. If the kidneys are not working, the serum creatinine level will increase. When the serum creatinine values doubles (e.g., from 0.75 to 1.5 mg/dL), the increase reflects a decrease of approximately 50% in the GFR.[18] Serum creatinine level is assessed daily to follow the trend of kidney function and to determine whether kidney function is stable, getting better, or getting worse.[18]

Creatinine Clearance

If the patient is making sufficient urine, the urinary creatinine clearance can be measured. A normal urinary creatinine clearance rate is 120 mL/min, but this value decreases with kidney failure. Critical care patients with severe AKI are oliguric, and the urinary creatinine clearance rate is infrequently measured.

Fractional Excretion of Sodium

The fractional excretion of sodium (FENa) in the urine is measured early in the AKI course to differentiate between a prerenal condition and AKI (intrarenal). A FENa value below 1% (in the absence of diuretics) suggests prerenal compromise, because resorption of almost all the filtered sodium is an appropriate response to decreased perfusion to the kidneys. If diuretics are being administered, however, results of the test would be meaningless. A FENa value above 2% implies that the kidney cannot concentrate the sodium and that AKI has occurred.

Urinary sodium is measured in milliequivalents per liter (mEq/L). The interpretation of results is similar to that for FENa. A urinary sodium concentration less than 10 mEq/L (low) suggests prerenal AKI. A urinary sodium level greater than 40 mEq/L (with an elevated serum creatinine in the absence of a high salt load) suggests that intrarenal damage has occurred. As with other urinalysis tests, the use of diuretics invalidates any results.

AT-RISK DISEASE STATES AND ACUTE KIDNEY INJURY

Many patients come into the critical care unit with disease states that predispose them to the development of AKI. Many others already have kidney damage but are unaware of this condition.[7]

TABLE 20-4 SERUM ELECTROLYTES IN ACUTE KIDNEY FAILURE

ELECTROLYTE DISTURBANCE	SERUM VALUE	CLINICAL FINDINGS
Potassium		
Hypokalemia	<3.5 mEq/L	Muscular weakness
		Cardiac irregularities on ECG
		Abdominal distention and flatulence
		Paresthesia
		Decreased reflexes
		Anorexia
		Dizziness, confusion
		Increased sensitivity to digitalis
Hyperkalemia	>4.5 mEq/L	Irritability and restlessness
		Anxiety
		Nausea and vomiting
		Abdominal cramps
		Weakness
		Numbness and tingling (fingertips and circumoral)
		Cardiac irregularities on ECG
Sodium		
Hyponatremia	<135 mEq/L	Disorientation
		Muscle twitching
		Nausea, vomiting, abdominal cramps
		Headaches, dizziness
		Seizures, postural hypotension
		Cold, clammy skin
		Decreased skin turgor
		Tachycardia
		Oliguria
Hypernatremia	>145 mEq/L	Extreme thirst
		Dry, sticky mucous membranes
		Altered mentation
		Seizures (later stages)
Calcium		
Hypocalcemia	<8.5 mg/dL or <4.5 mEq/L	Irritability
		Muscular tetany, muscle cramps
		Decreased cardiac output (decreased contractions)
		Bleeding (decreased ability to coagulate)
		Changes on ECG
		Positive Chvostek's or Trousseau's sign
Hypercalcemia	>10.5 mg/dL or >5.8 mEq/L	Deep bone pain
		Excessive thirst
		Anorexia
		Lethargy, weakened muscles
Magnesium		
Hypomagnesemia	<1.4 mEq/L	Choroid or athetoid muscle activity
		Facial tics, spasticity
		Cardiac dysrhythmias
Hypermagnesemia	>2.5 mEq/L	CNS depression
		Respiratory depression
		Lethargy
		Coma
		Bradycardia
		Changes on ECG

TABLE 20-4	SERUM ELECTROLYTES IN ACUTE KIDNEY FAILURE—cont'd	
ELECTROLYTE DISTURBANCE	**SERUM VALUE**	**CLINICAL FINDINGS**
Phosphate		
Hypophosphatemia	<3.0 mg/dL	Hemolytic anemias
		Depressed white blood cell function
		Bleeding (decreased platelet aggregation)
		Nausea, vomiting
		Anorexia
Hyperphosphatemia	>4.5 mg/dL	Tachycardia
		Nausea, diarrhea, abdominal cramps
		Muscle weakness, flaccid paralysis
		Increased reflexes
Chloride		
Hypochloremia	<98 mEq/L	Hyperirritability
		Tetany or muscular excitability
		Slow respirations
Hyperchloremia	>108 mEq/L	Weakness, lethargy
		Deep, rapid breathing
		Possible unconsciousness (later stages)
Albumin		
Hypoalbuminemia	<3.8 g/dL	Muscle wasting
		Peripheral edema (fluid shift)
		Decreased resistance to infection
		Poorly healing wounds

CNS, central nervous system; *ECG*, electrocardiogram.

TABLE 20-5	DECREASED KIDNEY FUNCTION BY STAGE IN ADULT U.S. POPULATION		
STAGE*	**POPULATION AFFECTED***	**GFR AND DIAGNOSIS***	**PERCENTAGE WHO KNOW THEY HAVE KIDNEY DYSFUNCTION (%)[†]**
1	9 million (3.3%)	Normal; persistent albuminuria	40.5
2	5.3 million (3.0%)	60-89; persistent albuminuria	29.3
3	7.6 million (4.3%)	30-59	22.0
4	400,000 (0.2%)	15-29	44.5
5	300,000 (0.2%)	<15: ESKD	100

*Data from Coresh J et al: Prevalence of chronic kidney disease and decreased kidney function in the adult US population: Third National Health and Nutrition Examination Survey, *Am J Kidney Dis* 41(1):1-12, 2003. GFR is measured as mL/min/1.73 m² of body surface area.
[†]Data from Nickolas TL et al: Awareness of kidney disease in the US population: findings from the National Health and Nutrition Examination Survey (NHANES) 1999 to 2000, *Am J Kidney Dis* 44(2):185-197, 2004.

Underlying Chronic Kidney Disease

The incidence of chronic kidney disease (CKD) in the United States is estimated to be 11% (19.2 million adults).[19] Clinical practice guidelines for the management of end-stage kidney disease (ESKD) categorizes kidney dysfunction in five stages.[20] Because of the large numbers of adults with kidney dysfunction (diagnosed or not), kidney function must be assessed in all critically ill patients at risk for fluid and electrolyte imbalance. The GFR associated with each stage and the numeric population estimates for each stage of kidney dysfunction are shown in Table 20-5.

Most people in the early stages of kidney disease are unaware of their condition.[7] A national health survey queried individuals about whether they had ever been told by their physician that they had 'weak or failing kidneys'. The answer to this question was correlated with each patient's GFR and the presence of albumin in the urine was used to stratify the patients according to the five stages of CKD (see Table 20-5). The results showed that more than one half of the respondents were unaware that they had kidney dysfunction until their disease had reached stage 5 or ESKD, when they would become dialysis dependent.[7] The results categorized by stage of CKD are listed in Table 20-5.

Older Age and Acute Kidney Injury

Older age appears to be a risk factor for CKD, because 11% of individuals older than 65 years without hypertension or diabetes have stage 3 or worse CKD.[19] In the presence of diabetes or hypertension, the risk for CKD increases substantially.

Heart Failure and Acute Kidney Injury

There is a strong association between kidney failure and cardiovascular disease. In studies of critically ill patients with acute kidney failure, 54%[4] to 63%[5] have acute kidney failure and heart failure. Hypertension, a major contributor to the development of heart failure, is also a major risk factor for the development of CKD.[21] Unfortunately, people with hypertension and diabetes are at increased risk for CKD and premature death.[21] As a patient's GFR declines, the risks of cardiovascular disease, myocardial infarction, and death increase, especially for the patient with stage 3 or worse CKD.[22,23]

Respiratory Failure and Acute Kidney Injury

There is a significant association between respiratory failure and kidney failure. In studies of critically ill patients with kidney failure, 54% to 88% have respiratory failure.[4,5] The range in values reflects how the kidney failure was classified. For example, in one study, 57% had respiratory and kidney failure but were not treated with dialysis,[4] and in another study, 88% had respiratory and kidney failure and were given dialysis treatment with continuous renal replacement therapy (discussed later).[5]

The process of mechanical ventilation affects the kidney, although it is not known whether the effect is deleterious.[24] Positive-pressure ventilation reduces blood flow to the kidney, lowers the GFR, and decreases urine output.[24] These effects are intensified with the addition of positive end-expiratory pressure (PEEP).[24] AKI increases inflammation, causes the lung vasculature to become more permeable, and contributes to the development of acute respiratory failure.[25] Prolonged mechanical ventilation in critical illness is associated with an increased incidence of AKI and dialysis.[26]

Sepsis and Acute Kidney Injury

Sepsis is the most common cause of AKI in the critically ill.[9] Sepsis and septic shock create hemodynamic instability and reduce perfusion to the kidney. Immunologic, toxic, and inflammatory factors may alter the function of the kidney microvasculature and tubular cells.[27] Sepsis caused 19% of AKI in one study[4] and 55% of AKI in a population of older hospitalized patients.[5] Clinical guidelines for hemodynamic support in sepsis emphasize the need for adequate fluid resuscitation, because in 40% to 50% of cases, reversal of hypotension and restoration of hemodynamic stability can be achieved with fluids alone.[28] Unfortunately, in severely septic patients, inflammation increases vascular permeability, and much of the fluid may move into the third space (interstitial space). If the blood pressure remains low, the use of vasopressors is recommended to raise refractory low blood pressure after volume resuscitation.[28] Vasopressors raise blood pressure and increase systemic vascular resistance (SVR), but they also may raise the vascular resistance within the kidney microvasculature. Other practices aimed at reversing the deleterious effects of sepsis include maintaining the patient's hemoglobin level

at 7 to 9 g/dL and blood glucose level below 150 mg/dL and ensuring optimal hydration as evidenced by a central venous pressure (CVP) above 8 mm Hg.[28]

Trauma and Acute Kidney Injury
Trauma Admissions

Trauma patients have different demographics from those of other critical care populations. They are always emergency admissions, are younger, are more often male, and have fewer coexisting illnesses.[29] A 5-year retrospective study of 9449 trauma admissions to critical care units in Australia and New Zealand used the RIFLE criteria to determine incidence of AKI in the first 24 hours after admission; AKI developed in 18% of trauma patients.[29] However, if patients were older or had preexisting comorbid illnesses, their risk of AKI rose to 35%.[29] Although these AKI numbers are high, they likely underestimate the true incidence because the study did not include patients in whom AKI developed more than 24 hours after admission to the critical care unit.[29]

Rhabdomyolysis

Trauma patients with major crush injuries have an elevated risk of kidney failure because of the release of creatine and myoglobin from damaged muscle cells, a condition called rhabdomyolysis.[30] Myoglobin in large quantities is toxic to the kidney. Overall survival from rhabdomyolysis is 77%.[30]

The level of creatine kinase (CK), a marker of systemic muscle damage, increases in patients with rhabdomyolysis. One trauma service reported that of 2083 trauma patients admitted to critical care, 85% had elevated CK values, and acute kidney failure resulting from rhabdomyolysis developed in 10%.[31] A CK level of 5000 units/L was the lowest abnormal value in patients in whom AKI associated with rhabdomyolysis developed.[31]

Volume resuscitation is the primary treatment for preservation of adequate kidney function and prevention of AKI. In many hospitals, the intravenous (IV) fluids are alkalinized by the addition of sodium bicarbonate, and the urine output is increased by intravenous administration of the diuretic mannitol.[30] A bicarbonate and mannitol regimen is instituted to prevent acidosis and hyperkalemia, because both are frequent complications of rhabdomyolysis. Close attention is paid to urine output, CK levels, increases in serum creatinine levels, and any signs of compartment syndrome in all patients admitted with this diagnosis.

Contrast-Induced Acute Kidney Injury

More than one million radiologic studies or procedures that involve use of intravenous radiopaque contrast are performed every year.[13] Approximately 1% of the patients undergoing those studies require dialysis as a result of contrast-induced nephrotoxicity,[32] with prolongation of the hospital stay to an average of 17 days.[13] Patients at risk are those with chronic kidney dysfunction, baseline serum creatinine levels more than 1.5 mg/dL, and known diabetes, heart failure, or volume depletion.[33,34] A clinical definition of contrast-induced nephrotoxicity is an increase in serum creatinine concentration of 0.5 mg/dL or more or a 25% increase from the patient's baseline value within 48 to 72 hours of contrast medium exposure.[13,33] The effects of reversible, contrast-induced AKI may not be limited to the immediate hospitalization; it has been linked to a higher mortality in the 5-year period after the reversible AKI than in similar patients who did not have kidney injury.[34]

Limit Radiopaque Contrast

High-molecular-weight contrast medium is a potential cause of nephrotoxicity.[13,35] Kidney-protection strategies include identification of patients at high risk and use of alternative imaging modalities that do not involve contrast. If radiopaque contrast use is inevitable, smaller contrast volumes should be used for each study, and low-osmolar, or iso-osmolar (iohexol), contrast media that are less nephrotoxic should be selected.[35,36]

Promote Hydration and Avoid Dehydration

The best method of prevention is aggressive hydration with intravenous normal saline during and after the procedure.[37,38] After some diagnostic intravascular catheterization procedures, the alert patient is asked to drink several liters of water over a 12-hour period to protect the kidney. Avoiding dehydration is vital. In research studies, the addition of sodium bicarbonate or N-acetylcysteine did not confer additional protection to the vulnerable kidney beyond hydration with normal saline only.[37-39]

Medications

Several medications have been investigated to mitigate the risk of AKI in at-risk patients who undergo diagnostic studies involving radiopaque contrast agents. The agents include oral N-acetylcysteine, intravenous sodium bicarbonate, and an intravenous infusion of fenoldopam.[37-40] In randomized, controlled trials, N-acetylcysteine has not lived up to its early promise.[37-40] For sodium bicarbonate, the picture is mixed, with some studies reporting a benefit[39,41] and other studies reporting no effect.[37,38] Because N-acetylcysteine and sodium bicarbonate are inexpensive and have almost no side effects, many physicians prescribe them on an empirical basis, even though the research evidence is not yet conclusive.

In summary, the mainstay measures to protect the kidney from contrast-induced AKI are to use the smallest dose of low- or iso-osmolar contrast media possible, provide vigorous fluid volume expansion, stop all nephrotoxic drugs, and avoid repeat contrast media injections within 48 hours.[42]

Hemodynamic Monitoring and Fluid Balance

Hemodynamic monitoring is important for the analysis of fluid volume status in the critically ill patient with AKI.

Hemodynamic Monitoring

Hemodynamic monitoring includes surveillance of the CVP, pulmonary artery occlusion pressure, cardiac output, and cardiac index.[43] A less high-tech method that is also important consists of a daily weight and focused physical assessment.

Daily Weight

The daily weight, combined with accurate intake and output monitoring, is a powerful indicator of fluid gains or losses over 24 hours. A 1-kg weight gain over 24 hours represents 1000 mL (1 liter) of additional fluid retention.

Physical Assessment

Physical signs and symptoms are used to assess fluid balance. Signs that suggest extracellular fluid (ECF) depletion include thirst, decreased skin turgor, and lethargy. Signs that imply intravascular fluid volume overload include pulmonary congestion, increasing heart failure, and rising blood pressure. The patient with untreated AKI is edematous. The following factors contribute to this state:
- Fluid retention caused by inadequate urine output.
- Low serum albumin levels create a lower oncotic pressure in the vasculature, and more fluid seeps out into the interstitial spaces to cause peripheral edema.
- Inflammation associated with AKI or a coexisting non-renal disease increases vascular permeability, facilitating fluid movement from the vessels into interstitial spaces.

In critical illness, even though there is peripheral edema and the patient may have gained 8 L of fluid over his or her "dry-weight" baseline, the patient may remain "intravascularly dry" and hemodynamically unstable, because the retained fluid is not inside a vascular compartment and cannot contribute to maintenance of hemodynamic stability. The patient with AKI is assessed frequently for pitting edema over bony prominences and in dependent body areas.

Electrolyte Balance

Potassium

Electrolyte levels require frequent observation, especially in the critical phases of AKI (Table 20-4). Potassium may quickly reach levels of 6.0 mEq/L or higher. Specific electrocardiographic changes are associated with hyperkalemia: peaked T waves, a widening of the QRS interval, and ultimately, ventricular tachycardia or fibrillation. If hyperkalemia is identified, all potassium supplements are stopped.[44] If the patient is producing urine, intravenous diuretics can be administered. Acute hyperkalemia can be treated temporarily by IV administration of insulin and glucose. An infusion of 50 mL of 50% dextrose accompanied by 10 units of regular insulin forces potassium out of the serum and into the cells.

Sodium polystyrene sulfonate (Kayexalate), a cation-exchange resin, is mixed in water and sorbitol and given orally, rectally, or through a nasogastric tube. The resin binds potassium in the bowel, which eliminates it in the feces. Kayexalate and dialysis are the only permanent methods of potassium removal.[44]

Sodium

Dilutional hyponatremia, associated with kidney failure, is an expected finding in AKI (see Table 20-4). It can be corrected over a few days with fluid restriction. Sodium levels may be raised more rapidly during dialysis by changing the amount of sodium in the dialysate bath.

Calcium and Phosphorus

Serum calcium levels are reduced (hypocalcemia) in kidney failure (see Table 20-4). This reduction results from multiple factors, including hyperphosphatemia. Long-term elevations of serum phosphorus (>5.5 to 6.5 mEq/L) are associated with higher mortality rates for patients in kidney failure.[20,45,46] Calcium and phosphorus are regulated in part by parathyroid hormone (PTH). Normally, PTH helps calcium be resorbed back into the bloodstream at the proximal tubule and distal nephron, and it promotes excretion of phosphorus by the kidney to maintain homeostasis. In kidney failure, this mechanism is nonfunctional; the serum phosphorus level rises, and the serum calcium level falls.

Calcium Replacement

Most calcium in the bloodstream is bound to protein. Calcium levels can be measured in two ways: total calcium (tCa) or ionized calcium (iCa).[46] Unfortunately, protein-calcium binding confounds the measurement of accurate calcium levels. In the past, calculations were used to estimate the amounts of protein-bound versus unbound calcium, but these calculations have been shown to produce inaccurate results.[47] The metabolically active, non–protein-bound portion is known as the ionized calcium and is the preferred method of measurement.[47] Without adequate levels of serum calcium, a compensatory mechanism 'steals' calcium from the bones, making the patient with kidney failure more vulnerable to fractures.[48] Maintaining adequate calcium stores in the body is important and is achieved by administration of calcium supplements, vitamin D preparations, and synthetic calcitriol.[49]

Dietary Phosphorus–Binding Drugs

A second method used in tandem with calcium supplements to achieve normal calcium levels is to lower the level of phosphorus in the bloodstream.[46] Phosphorus occurs in many foods, and eliminating all phosphorus-containing foods from the diet would make it unpalatable.[50] Foods that contain particularly high levels of phosphorus include dairy products, processed meats, some carbonated drinks, and nuts.[50] After these foods are eaten, free phosphorus passes from the GI tract into the bloodstream and raises the serum level. Medications that bind dietary phosphorus in the gastrointestinal tract are administered orally or by nasogastric tube. The binding agent must be taken at the same time as a meal.[50] After the dietary phosphorus is bound to the binding substance in the bowel, it is eliminated from the intestine with stool. This lowers the serum phosphorus level.

The types of dietary-phosphorus binders used have changed over the years. The original binders were aluminum salts (aluminum hydroxide) that bound dietary phosphorus effectively in the gastrointestinal tract but conferred aluminum toxicity because some of the aluminum metal was also absorbed.[50] For this reason, aluminum binders have largely been abandoned.[50]

The second generation of dietary phosphorus–binding agents that are most widely prescribed use calcium salts (calcium carbonate; calcium acetate [PhosLo]) to bind dietary phosphorus in the gastrointestinal tract. Calcium-based drugs are safer, but elevated serum calcium values and calcium deposits in other areas of the body (extraosseous calcification) are a problem.[50] This category of drugs remains in widespread use.

A third generation of dietary phosphorus–binding medications is available. They are not aluminum- or calcium-based. They include sevelamer hydrochloride (RenaGel) and lanthanum carbonate (Fosrenol).[50]

Medical Management
Treatment Goals

Treatment goals for patients with AKI focus on prevention, compensation for the deterioration of kidney function, and regeneration of the remaining kidney functional capacity. Over the past 4 decades, the mortality rate for AKI has remained at more than 50%.[4,5] Key areas that are evaluated include prevention strategies, fluid balance, anemia, medications, and electrolyte imbalance.

Prevention

The only truly effective remedy for AKI is prevention. Effective prevention requires assessment of the patient's risk for AKI. Knowledge of the most frequent causes of AKI in the critically ill is essential if prevention strategies are to be enacted. The critical care team collaborates closely with the clinical pharmacist to avoid drugs with nephrotoxic side effects in patients with AKI or CKD.[19,20] Nonsteroidal anti-inflammatory drugs (NSAIDs) for pain relief are avoided in patients with elevated creatinine values.[2] The use of intravascular contrast dye is preferably delayed until the patient is fully rehydrated.[42]

Fluid Resuscitation

Prerenal failure is caused by decreased perfusion and flow to the kidney. It is often associated with trauma, hemorrhage, hypotension, and major fluid losses. If contrast dye is used, aggressive fluid resuscitation with normal saline (NaCl) is recommended. Fluid replacement is the only treatment shown to prevent kidney tubular injury.[51] The objectives of volume replacement are to replace fluid and electrolyte losses and to prevent ongoing loss. Maintenance intravenous fluid therapy is initiated when oral (PO) fluid intake is inadvisable. Maintenance fluids are calculated with consideration for individual body surface area. Adults require approximately 1500 mL/m^2/24 hr; fever, burns, and trauma significantly increase fluid requirements. Other important criteria in the calculation of fluid volume replacement include baseline metabolism, environmental temperature, and humidity. The rate of replacement depends on cardiopulmonary reserve, adequacy of kidney function, urine output, fluid balance, ongoing loss, and type of fluid replaced.

Crystalloids and Colloids. Crystalloids and colloids are two different types of intravenous fluids used for volume

TABLE 20-6   FREQUENTLY USED INTRAVENOUS SOLUTIONS

SOLUTION	ELECTROLYTE COMPONENTS, PH, OXMOLALITY	INDICATIONS
Crystalloids*		
Dextrose in water (D₅W), isotonic	None	Maintain volume Replace mild loss Provide minimal calories
Normal saline solution (0.9% NaCl)	Sodium: 154 mEq/L Chloride: 154 mEq/L Osmolality: 308 mEq/L	Maintain volume Replace mild loss Correct mild hyponatremia
Half-strength saline solution (0.45% NaCl)	Sodium: 77 mEq/L Chloride: 77 mEq/L	Free water replacement Correct mild hyponatremia Free water and electrolyte replacement (fluid- and electrolyte-restricted conditions)
Lactated Ringer's solution	Sodium: 130 mEq/L Potassium: 4 mEq/L Calcium: 2.7 mEq/L Chloride: 107 mEq/L Lactate: 27 mEq/L pH: 6.5	Fluid and electrolyte replacement (contraindicated for patients with kidney or liver disease or in lactic acidosis)
Colloids		
5% Albumin (Albumisol)	Albumin: 50 g/L Sodium: 130-160 mEq/L Potassium: 1 mEq/L Osmolality: 300 mOsm/L Osmotic pressure: 20 mm Hg pH: 6.4 to 7.4	Volume expansion Moderate protein replacement Achievement of hemodynamic stability in shock states
25% Albumin (salt-poor)	Albumin: 240 g/L Globulins: 10 g/L Sodium: 130-160 mEq/L Osmolality: 1500 mOsm/L pH: 6.4-7.4	Concentrated form of albumin sometimes used with diuretics to move fluid from tissues into the vascular space for diuresis
Hetastarch	Sodium: 154 mEq/L Chloride: 154 mEq/L Osmolality: 310 mOsm/L Colloid osmotic pressure: 30-35 mm Hg	Synthetic polymer (6% solution) used for volume expansion Hemodynamic volume replacement after cardiac surgery, burns, sepsis
Low-molecular-weight dextran (LMWD)	Glucose polysaccharide molecules with average molecular weight of 40,000; no electrolytes	Volume expansion and support (contraindicated for patients with bleeding disorders)
High-molecular-weight dextran (HMWD)	Glucose polysaccharide molecules with average molecular weight of 70,000; no electrolytes	Used prophylactically in some cases to prevent platelet aggregation; available in saline and glucose solutions

*For crystalloid solutions that contain electrolytes, specific concentrations of electrolytes and pH vary according to the manufacturer.

management in critically ill patients. These intravenous solutions are used on all types of patients, not just those with acute kidney failure. Adequacy of intravenous fluid replacement depends on strict, ongoing evaluation and frequent adjustment. Frequent monitoring of serum electrolyte levels is required, and strictly regulated intake and output are correlated with daily weight records. In septic shock, hemodynamic readings are frequently undertaken. After a fluid challenge, a merely minimal increase in CVP implies that additional fluid replacement is required. Continued decreases in CVP, pulmonary artery occlusion pressure, and the cardiac index indicate ongoing volume losses.

Which intravenous fluid to select to most successfully resuscitate hemodynamically unstable patients has been a controversial topic in critical care. The major debate centers on the differences between crystalloid and colloid solutions.

Crystalloids. Crystalloid solutions, which are balanced salt solutions, are in widespread use for maintenance infusion and replacement therapy. Crystalloid fluids include normal saline solution (0.9 NaCl), half-strength saline solution (0.45 NaCl), and lactated Ringer's (LR) solution (Table 20-6). LR solution usually is avoided in patients with kidney failure because it contains potassium. A noncrystalloid solution that may be infused is dextrose (5% or 10%) in water (D₅W, D₁₀W).

Colloids. Colloids are solutions containing oncotically active particles that are used to expand intravascular volume to achieve and maintain hemodynamic stability. Albumin

(5% and 25%) and hetastarch are colloid solutions (see Table 20-6). Colloids expand intravascular volume, and the effect can last as long as 24 hours. The goal is to optimize the pulmonary artery occlusion pressure (PAOP), raise mean arterial pressure (MAP), and increase cardiac output and the cardiac index to a therapeutic level.

The controversy over whether colloids or crystalloid intravenous fluids are most effective for volume resuscitation appears to have been put to rest by a series of randomized clinical trials and meta-analytic reviews. The SAFE study (saline versus albumin fluid evaluation) was a randomized, prospective, double-blind trial that examined whether the selection of resuscitation fluid in the critical care unit affected survival at 28 days. This was a huge study, with almost 7000 critical care patients randomly assigned to two similar treatment groups. One group received 4% albumin, and the other group received 0.9 normal saline (NaCl) for fluid resuscitation. The patients in the two groups were similar in terms of organ dysfunction, mechanical ventilator support (64% of patients), and renal replacement therapy (1% of patients). The SAFE results showed that there was no difference in the mortality rate, time in the critical care unit, ventilator days, or renal replacement therapy days between the treatment groups. The researchers concluded that albumin and saline should be considered clinically equivalent treatments for intravascular volume expansion in critically ill patients.[52] The exception was for patients with traumatic brain injury (TBI), in whom albumin was associated with a higher mortality rate.[53]

The findings of the SAFE study investigators have been validated by a systematic review of randomized trials of crystalloids versus colloids that reported no difference in mortality rates for the critically ill and injured based on resuscitation fluid.[54] Consequently, colloids are not favored because of their higher cost, and crystalloids are the recommended fluid to use for resuscitation in critical care.

Fluid Restriction. Fluid restriction constitutes a large part of the medical treatment for acute kidney failure. Fluid restriction is used to prevent circulatory overload and the development of interstitial edema when the kidneys cannot remove excess volume. The fluid requirements are calculated on the basis of daily urine volumes and insensible losses. Obtaining daily weight measurements and keeping accurate intake and output records is essential. Patients with kidney failure are usually restricted to 1 L of fluid per 24 hours if the urine output is 500 mL or less. Insensible losses range from 500 to 750 mL/day.

Fluid Removal. Acute kidney failure promotes increased amounts of water, solutes, and potential toxins in the circulation, and prompt measures are needed to decrease their levels. Diuretics are used to stimulate the urine output. However, renal replacement therapy (hemodialysis or hemofiltration) is the treatment of choice, particularly if volume overload exacerbates acute lung injury and heart failure.

Pharmacologic Management

The first step is to eliminate all nephrotoxic medications. Second, if drugs are eliminated through the kidneys, it is important to decrease the frequency of administration (e.g.,

from every 6 hours to every 12 or 24 hours) or to decrease the dose and to monitor the serum concentration by measuring serum drug levels.[55]

Diuretics

Diuretics are used to stimulate urinary output in the fluid overloaded patient with functioning kidneys. Care must be taken in their use to avoid the creation of secondary electrolyte abnormalities (Table 20-7). Diuretics reduce volume overload and are helpful for symptoms such as pulmonary edema, but they have not been shown to prevent AKI.[56] Diuretics are used in many patient populations other than those with incipient kidney failure.

Loop Diuretics. The loop diuretic furosemide (Lasix) is the most frequently used diuretic in critical care patients. It may be prescribed as a bolus dose or as a continuous infusion.[56] Electrolytic abnormalities are frequently encountered with the use of furosemide, and close monitoring of serum potassium, magnesium, and sodium values is essential.[57,58]

The optimal use of furosemide and other diuretics in critical illness is being actively investigated. Mehta and colleagues published an observational study showing that for critically ill patients with established AKI and oliguria, loop diuretics increased the mortality rate and delayed kidney recovery.[59] A subsequent study found that furosemide helped maintain urine output but had no more impact on survival and recovery of kidney function than a placebo.[60] A third research trial found that furosemide neither helped nor worsened AKI in the critically ill.[61] The debate and research studies will continue, but for now, it appears that loop diuretics increase the urine output and reduce volume overload, but have no impact on the outcome of established oliguric AKI.[56,62] Studies are under way to determine the optimal use of furosemide in critical illness.[63]

Thiazide Diuretics. Diuretics may be prescribed in combination. A thiazide diuretic such as chlorothiazide (Diuril), hydrochlorothiazide (HydroDiuril), or the thiazine-like diuretic or metolazone (Zaroxolyn) may be administered and followed by a loop diuretic to take advantage of the fact that these drugs work on different parts of the nephron. The diuretic efficacy of chlorothiazide and hydrochlorothiazide is reduced when creatine clearance is less than 30 mL/minute.

Osmotic Diuretics. Osmotic diuretics (e.g., mannitol) are used to decrease fluid overload and improve urine output. It is important to use an in-line 5-micron filter when administering this drug. Mannitol is frequently administered to patients with brain injury and increased intracranial pressure (ICP). More information on the use of mannitol in this population can be found in Chapter 17.

Heart Failure. For patients with heart failure, two of the natriuretic peptides (atrial natriuretic peptide [ANP] and brain natriuretic peptide [BNP], which acts on the ventricles) may be prescribed. These drugs work by stimulating natriuretic receptors in the atrium (ANP) and ventricular myocardium (BNP). The potassium-sparing diuretic Aldactone (spironolactone) is also used in heart failure management,

TABLE 20-7	PHARMACOLOGIC MANAGEMENT: KIDNEY-RELATED MEDICATIONS		
DRUG	**DOSAGE**	**ACTIONS**	**SPECIAL CONSIDERATIONS**
Diuretics			
Bumetanide	20-80 mg/day (Lasix)	Acts on loop of Henle to inhibit sodium and chloride	May cause ototoxicity if administered too rapidly or with other ototoxic drugs
Furosemide	0.5-2 mg/day (Bumex)		Monitor intake and output, hydration; watch for hypotension
Thiazide Diuretics			
Chlorothiazide (Diuril)	500 mg-1 g/day	Inhibits sodium, chloride resorption in distal tubule	Enhanced with low-sodium diet
			Synergistic effect with loop diuretics
Potassium-Sparing Diuretics			
Aldactone	100 mg/day for 5 days	Exerts effects on collecting tubule; reduces potassium and hydrogen, and increases sodium	Weak diuretic effect, so given with other diuretics
			Potassium supplements not required; monitor for hyperkalemia
			Used as an aldosterone blocker to treat heart failure
Osmotic Diuretics			
Mannitol	0.25-1.0 g/kg IV infusion as a 15%-20% solution over 30-90 min	Increases urine output because higher plasma osmolality increases flow of water from tissues, raising GFR	Often used in head injury to decrease cerebral edema
			Can be used to promote urinary secretion of toxic substances
		Increases serum sodium, potassium levels	At low temperatures mannitol may crystallize; use in-line 5-micron IV filter with >15% (>15 g/100 mL) solutions

ECG, electrocardiogram.

not as a diuretic but primarily as an aldosterone antagonist to lower aldosterone levels. Eplerenone (INSPRA) is a newer aldosterone antagonist used to treat chronic heart failure. Most heart failure patients and hypertensive patients require loop diuretics as part of their medication regimen to control fluid volume overload. More information on the use of diuretics in heart failure management is provided in Chapters 12 and 13.

Dopamine

Low-dose dopamine (2 to 3 mcg/kg/min), previously known as renal-dose dopamine, is infused to stimulate blood flow to the kidney. Dopamine is effective in increasing urine output in the short term, but tolerance of the dopamine renal receptor to the drug is theorized to develop in the critically ill patients who are most at risk for AKI.[64] A meta-analysis of related research studies determined that renal-dose dopamine did not prevent onset of AKI and did not decrease the need for dialysis or reduce mortality.[65] At this point, the support for routine use of low-dose dopamine for the prevention of AKI remains anecdotal only.[66] See Table 13-16 and the Priority Medications Box: Dopamine in Chapter 13 for more information on dopamine.

Acetylcysteine

N-Acetylcysteine (Mucomyst, Mucosil) is an N-acetyl derivative of the amino acid L-cysteine. It has been used for many years as a mucolytic agent to assist with expectoration of thick

pulmonary secretions. It is also frequently prescribed for patients with mildly elevated serum creatinine values before a radiologic study using contrast dye.[67] In research trials, the addition of N-acetylcysteine to normal saline hydration has not showed a reduction in the incidence of contrast-induced AKI.[37,39,67] In clinical trials enrolling cardiac surgery patients, prophylactic use of N-acetylcysteine did not decease the rate of AKI.[67,68] Most studies suggest that N-acetylcysteine does not prevent AKI during radiologic procedures or after cardiac surgery.

Fenoldopam

Fenoldopam mesylate (Corlopam) is a dopamine 1 (D_1) receptor agonist similar in structure to dopamine and dobutamine. It is used to lower blood pressure. Claims that this drug would prevent contrast-induced nephrotoxicity in high-risk patients have not been supported by clinical trial results.[40]

Dietary Phosphorus Binders

Many patients with kidney failure are prescribed a dietary phosphorus–binding medication (see earlier "Dietary-Phosphorus Binding Drugs").[50] Many dietary phosphorus–binding drugs are available, and some important issues concern all of them. The dietary phosphorus binder must be taken at the time of the meal. If it is taken 2 hours later, it will increase only the level of the binding substance (e.g., calcium) in the bloodstream and will not lower the serum phosphorus level. Related issues such as the quantity of phosphorus in the diet should be discussed with a clinical nutritionist (dietitian).

Nutrition

Diet or nutritional supplementation for the patient with AKI in the critical care unit is designed to account for the diminished excretory capacity of the kidney. The recommended energy intake is between 20 and 30 kilocalories/kg per day, with 1.2 to 1.5 g/kg of protein per day to control azotemia (increased BUN level).[69] Oral nutrition is preferred, and if the patient cannot eat, enteral nutrition is recommended over parenteral (intravenous) nutrition. Fluids are limited, and tight glucose control is recommended.[69] The electrolytes potassium, sodium, and phosphorus are strictly limited.

Nursing Management

Nursing management of the patient with AKI involves a variety of nursing diagnoses (see Nursing Diagnosis Priorities box on Acute Kidney Dysfunction). 'Prevention is the best cure' is an old saying that captures the role of the critical care nurse, who evaluates all patients for level of kidney function, risk of infection, fluid imbalance, electrolyte disturbances, anemia, readiness to learn, and need for education.

NURSING DIAGNOSIS PRIORITIES

Acute Kidney Dysfunction

- Excess Fluid Volume related to kidney dysfunction, p. A-19
- Ineffective Renal Tissue Perfusion related to decreased renal blood flow, p. A-33
- Anxiety related to threat to biologic, psychological, or social integrity, p. A-7
- Decreased Cardiac Output related to decrease in preload, p. A-10
- Risk for Infection, p. A-36
- Disturbed Body Image related to functional dependence on life-sustaining technology, p. A-16
- Ineffective Coping related to situational crisis and personal vulnerability, p. A-30
- Disturbed Sleep Pattern related to fragmented sleep, p. A-17
- Deficient Knowledge related to lack of previous exposure to information, p. A-15

Risk Factors for Acute Kidney Injury

Some individuals are at increased risk for AKI as a complication during hospitalization, and the alert critical care nurse recognizes potential risk factors and acts as a patient advocate.[19,20] Patients at risk include older persons because their GFR may be decreased,[5] dehydrated patients with kidney hypoperfusion, patients who have increased creatinine values before hospitalization, and patients undergoing a radiologic procedure involving contrast dye.

Infectious Complications

The critical care patient with infectious complications is at risk for AKI. Signs of infection such as an increased white blood cell (WBC) count, redness at a wound or intravenous line site, or increased temperature are always a cause for concern. A urinary catheter is inserted to facilitate accurate urine measurement and patient comfort. However, any indwelling catheter is a potential source for infection. When the patient no longer makes large quantities of urine and is hemodynamically stable, the catheter must be removed promptly. If the patient cannot void urine spontaneously, a scheduled straight catheterization is performed to minimize the risk of infection from an indwelling catheter and drainage system. This method allows the patient's bladder to be emptied, but the urinary catheter does not remain in place.

Fluid Balance

Intravascular fluid balance is often assessed on an hourly basis for the critically ill patient in whom hemodynamic lines have been inserted. Hemodynamic values (heart rate, blood pressure, CVP, PAOP, cardiac output, and cardiac index) and daily weight measurements are correlated with the intake and output. Urine output is measured hourly by means of a urinary catheter and drainage bag throughout all phases of AKI, particularly in response to diuretics. Any fluid removed with dialysis is included in the daily fluid balance. Recognition of the clinical signs and symptoms of fluid overload is important. Excess fluid moves from the vascular system into the peripheral tissues (dependent edema), abdomen (ascites), and lungs (crackles, pulmonary edema, and pulmonary effusions); around the heart (pericardial effusions); and into the brain (increased intracranial swelling).

Electrolyte Imbalance

Hyperkalemia, hypocalcemia, hyponatremia, hyperphosphatemia, and acid-base imbalances occur during AKI (see Table 20-4). Clinical manifestations of these electrolyte imbalances must be prevented and their associated side effects controlled. The more likely imbalances are hyperkalemia and hypocalcemia, which can result in life-threatening cardiac dysrhythmias. Dilutional hyponatremia may develop as fluid overload worsens in the patient with oliguria. Monitoring the serum sodium level is important to prevent this complication. Hyperphosphatemia results in severe pruritus. Nursing care is directed at soothing the itching by performing frequent skin care with emollients, discouraging scratching, and administering phosphate-binding medications.[50] The acid-base imbalances that occur with AKI are monitored by arterial blood gas (ABG) analyses. The goal of treatment is to maintain the pH within the normal range.

Preventing Anemia

Anemia is an expected side effect of kidney failure that occurs because the kidney no longer produces the hormone erythropoietin.[70] As a result, the bone marrow is not stimulated to produce red blood cells (RBCs). Decreased RBC production by the bone marrow also occurs as a consequence of critical illness.[71] Care is taken to prevent blood loss in the patient with AKI, and blood withdrawal is minimized as much as possible. Irritation of the GI tract from metabolic waste accumulation is expected, and stress ulcer prophylaxis must be prescribed. Gastrointestinal bleeding remains a possibility. Stool, nasogastric tube drainage, and emesis are routinely tested for occult blood. Anemia may be treated pharmacologically by the administration of recombinant human erythropoietin (rhEPO), epoetin alfa (Procrit, Epogen), to stimulate erythrocyte production by the bone marrow and if required by RBC transfusion. Treatment of anemia early in the course of AKI (before dialysis) appears to slow the progression of the kidney failure and delays the initiation or renal replacement therapies.[72] Even in anemic, critically ill patients without kidney failure, administration of rhEPO weekly significantly decreases the number of blood transfusions.[73] However, this therapy is not recommended for anemia related to sepsis in the critically ill.[28]

Patient Education

Accurate and uncomplicated information must be provided to the patient and family about AKI, including its prognosis, treatment, and possible complications.[7] Education of the patient can be challenging because elevations of BUN and creatinine can negatively affect the level of consciousness. Sleep-rest disorders and emotional upset often occur as complications of AKI and can disrupt short-term memory. Encouraging the patient and family to voice concerns, frustrations, or fears and allowing the patient to control aspects of the acute care environment and treatment are essential.

RENAL REPLACEMENT THERAPY: DIALYSIS

Two types of renal replacement therapy are available for the treatment of AKI. They are intermittent hemodialysis (IHD) therapy and continuous renal replacement therapy (CRRT).

Hemodialysis

Hemodialysis roughly translates as 'separating from the blood.' Indications and contraindications for hemodialysis are listed in Box 20-4. As a treatment, hemodialysis separates and removes from the blood the excess electrolytes, fluids, and toxins by means of a hemodialyzer (Figure 20-2). Although hemodialysis is efficient in removing solutes, it does not remove all metabolites. Levels of electrolytes, toxins, and fluids increase between treatments, necessitating hemodialysis on a regular basis. Hemodialysis therapy is always intermittent; each dialysis treatment takes 3 to 4 hours. In the acute phases of kidney failure, dialysis is performed daily.[74] The dialysis frequency gradually decreases to three times per week as the patient moves into a more chronic phase of kidney failure.

Hemodialyzer

Hemodialysis works by circulating blood outside the body through synthetic tubing to a dialyzer, which consists of hollow-fiber tubes. The dialyzer is sometimes described as an

---

> ### BOX 20-4 INDICATIONS AND CONTRAINDICATIONS FOR HEMODIALYSIS
>
> **Indications**
> - Blood urea nitrogen (BUN) level exceeds 90 mg/dL
> - Serum creatinine level of 9 mg/dL
> - Hyperkalemia
> - Drug toxicity
> - Intravascular and extravascular fluid overload
> - Metabolic acidosis
> - Symptoms of uremia
> - Pericarditis
> - Gastrointestinal bleeding
> - Changes in mentation
> - Contraindications to other forms of dialysis
>
> **Contraindications**
> - Hemodynamic instability
> - Inability to anticoagulate
> - Lack of access to circulation

---

artificial kidney (Figure 20-3). While the blood flows through the membranes, which are semipermeable, a fluid (dialysate bath) bathes the membranes and, through osmosis and diffusion, performs exchanges of fluid, electrolytes, and toxins from the blood to the bath, where toxins and dialysate then pass out of the artificial kidney. The blood and the dialysate bath are shunted in opposite directions (countercurrent flow) through the dialyzer to match the osmotic and chemical gradients at the most efficient level for effective dialysis.

Ultrafiltration

To remove fluid, a positive hydrostatic pressure is applied to the blood, and a negative hydrostatic pressure is applied to the dialysate bath. The two forces together, called transmembrane pressure, pull and squeeze the excess fluid from the blood. The difference between the two values (expressed in millimeters of mercury [mm Hg]) represents the transmembrane pressure and results in fluid extraction, known as ultrafiltration, from the vascular space.

Anticoagulation

Heparin or sodium citrate is added to the system just before the blood enters the dialyzer to anticoagulate the blood within the dialysis tubing. Without an anticoagulant, the blood clots because its passage through the foreign tubular substances of the dialysis machine activates the clotting mechanism. Heparin can be administered by bolus injection or intermittent infusion. It has a short half-life, and its effects subside within 2 to 4 hours. If necessary, the effects of heparin are easily reversed with the antidote protamine sulfate. When there is concern about the development of heparin-induced thrombocytopenia (HIT),[75] alternative anticoagulants can be used. Citrate (trisodium citrate) can be infused as an anticoagulant by intermittent bolus or continuous infusion.[76]

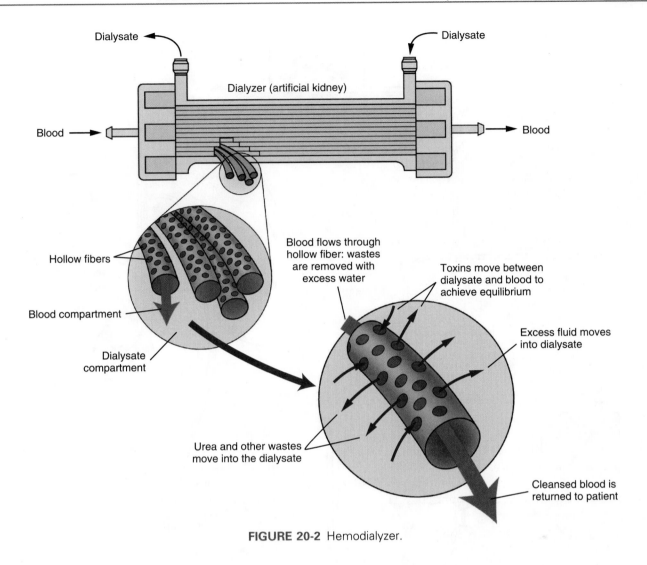

Dialysate

Dialysate

Dialyzer (artificial kidney)

Blood

Blood

Hollow fibers

Blood flows through hollow fiber: wastes are removed with excess water

Toxins move between dialysate and blood to achieve equilibrium

Blood compartment

Excess fluid moves into dialysate

Dialysate compartment

Urea and other wastes move into the dialysate

Cleansed blood is returned to patient

FIGURE 20-2 Hemodialyzer.

Vascular Access

Hemodialysis requires access to the bloodstream. Various types of temporary and permanent devices are in clinical use. It is important for patient safety that the nurse be able to recognize these different vascular access devices and properly care for them. The following section discusses temporary vascular access catheters used in the acute care hospital environment and permanent methods used for long-term hemodialysis.

Temporary Acute Access. Subclavian and femoral veins are catheterized when short-term access is required or when vascular access is nonfunctional in a patient requiring immediate hemodialysis. Subclavian and femoral catheters are routinely inserted at the bedside. Most temporary catheters are venous lines only. Blood flows out toward the dialyzer and flows back to the patient through the same vein. A dual-lumen venous catheter is most commonly used. It has a central partition running the length of the catheter. The outflow catheter section pulls the blood flow through openings that are proximal to the inflow openings on the opposite side (Figure 20-4). This design helps prevent dialyzing the same blood just returned to the area (recirculation), which

would severely reduce the procedure's efficiency. A silicone rubber, dual-lumen catheter with a polyester cuff designed to decrease catheter-related infections is also available.

Permanent Vascular Access. The common denominator in permanent vascular access devices is a connection to the arterial circulation and a return conduit to the venous circulation.

Arteriovenous Fistula. The arteriovenous fistula is created by surgically exposing a peripheral artery and vein, creating a side-by-side opening in the artery and the vein that joins the two vessels together. The high arterial flow creates a swelling of the vein, or a pseudoaneurysm, at which point (when healed) a large-bore needle can be inserted to obtain arterial outflow to the dialyzer. Inflow is accomplished through a second large-bore needle inserted into a peripheral vein distal to the fistula (Figure 20-5). If the patient's vessels are adequate, fistulas are the preferred mode of access because of the durability of blood vessels, relatively few complications, and less need for revision in comparison with other access methods.[20] An initial disadvantage of a fistula concerns the time required for development of sufficient arterial flow to enlarge the new access. The minimum reported length of

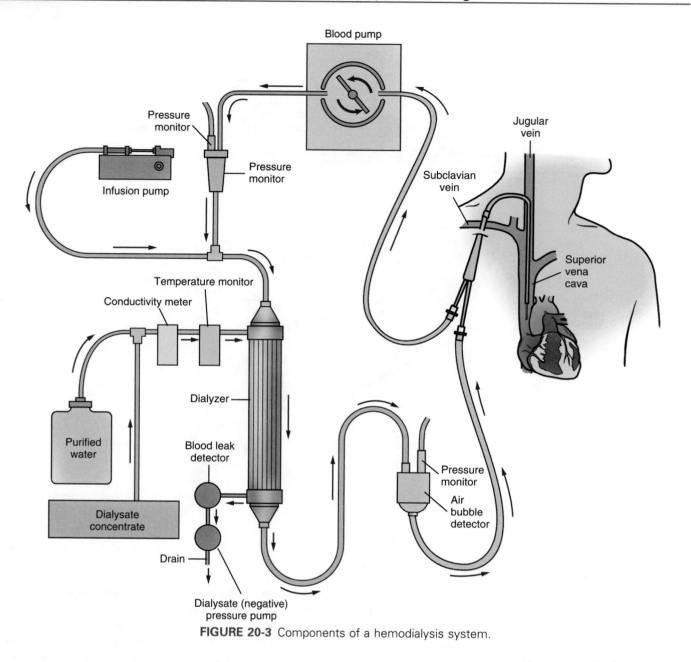

FIGURE 20-3 Components of a hemodialysis system.

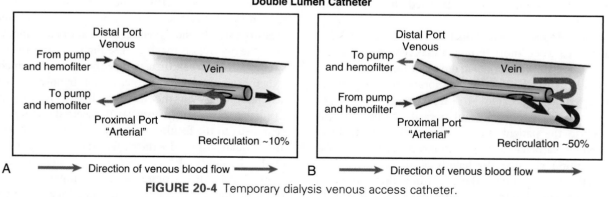

FIGURE 20-4 Temporary dialysis venous access catheter.

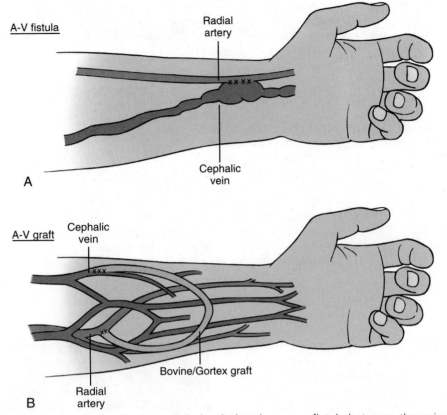

FIGURE 20-5 Methods of vascular access for hemodialysis. *A,* Arteriovenous fistula between the vein and artery. *B,* Internal synthetic graft corrects the artery and vein.

time before a fistula can be cannulated for dialysis is 14 days,[77] but the time lag for many patients is longer, as much as weeks or months.[78]

In the care of a patient with a fistula, some important nursing priorities ensure the ongoing viability of the vascular access and safety of the limb (Table 20-8). The critical care nurse frequently assesses the quality of blood flow through the fistula. A patent fistula has a thrill when palpated gently with the fingers and has a bruit if auscultated with a stethoscope. The extremity should be pink and warm to the touch. No blood pressure measurements, intravenous infusions, or laboratory phlebotomy procedures are performed on the arm with the fistula.[79]

The arteriovenous fistula is the preferred long-term access for hemodialysis.[20] However, in the United States, only 27% of hemodialysis patients have an arteriovenous fistula; 47% have a synthetic graft; and 23% have a tunneled hemodialysis catheter.[80] An arteriovenous fistula provides the most favorable long-term patency for hemodialysis access and is recommended if patients require long-term hemodialysis.[20]

Arteriovenous Grafts. Arteriovenous grafts are vascular access devices for treating chronic kidney failure. The graft is a tube made of synthetic material that is surgically implanted inside the limb. The area is surgically opened, and an artery and a vein are located. A tunnel is created in the tissue where the graft is placed. Anastomoses are made with the graft ends connected to the artery and vein. The blood is allowed to flow through the graft, and the surgical area is closed. The graft creates a raised area that looks like a large peripheral vein just under the skin and peripheral tissue layers (see Figure 20-5). Two large-bore needles are used for outflow from and inflow to the graft. For grafts and fistulas, after needle removal at the end of the hemodialysis treatment, firm pressure must be applied to stop any bleeding (see Table 20-8).

Tunneled Catheters. While waiting for the fistula or graft to mature to be ready for access, some patients with CKD may have a tunneled, cuffed catheter placed.[81] The cuff and tunneling are physical barriers to reduce central venous catheter infections. Modern catheters are made of silicone or polyurethane, tunneled under the skin, and inserted through the jugular or subclavian vein into the superior vena cava.[77,81]

Medical Management

Medical management involves the decision to place a vascular access device and then to choose the most appropriate type and location for each patient. Patients in the critical care setting who require vascular access for hemodialysis typically use a temporary hemodialysis catheter. The exact quantity of fluid and solute removal to be achieved by hemodialysis is determined individually for each patient by clinical examination and review of all relevant laboratory results.

Nursing Management

A noncritical care nurse who is specially trained in dialysis manages the IHD. The dialysis nurse typically comes to the patient's bedside with the hemodialysis machine. During the

TABLE 20-8	COMPLICATIONS AND NURSING MANAGEMENT OF ARTERIOVENOUS FISTULA OR GRAFT	
TYPE	**COMPLICATIONS**	**NURSING MANAGEMENT**
Fistula	Thrombosis	Teach patients to avoid wearing constrictive clothing on limbs containing access.
	Infection	Teach patients to avoid sleeping on and bending accessed limb for prolonged periods.
	Pseudoaneurysm	Use aseptic technique when cannulating access.
	Vascular steal syndrome	Avoid repetitious cannulation of one segment of access.
	Venous hypertension	Offer comfort measures, such as warm compresses and ordered analgesics, to
	Carpal tunnel syndrome	lessen pain of vascular steal.
	Inadequate blood flow	Teach patients to develop blood flow in the fistulas through exercises (squeezing a rubber ball) while applying mild impedance to flow just distal to the access (at least once per day for 10-15 min).
		Avoid too-early cannulation of new access.
Graft	Bleeding	Teach patients to avoid wearing constrictive clothing on accessed limbs.
	Thrombosis	Avoid repeated cannulation of one segment of access.
	False aneurysm formation	Use aseptic technique when cannulating access.
	Infection	Monitor for changes in arterial or venous pressure while patients are on dialysis.
	Arterial or venous stenosis	Provide comfort measures to reduce the pain of vascular steal (e.g., warm
	Vascular steal syndrome	compresses, analgesics as ordered).

acute phase of treatment, hemodialysis occurs daily. The frequency is reduced to 3 days per week as the patient becomes hemodynamically stable. The essential role of the critical care nurse during dialysis is to monitor the patient's hemodynamic status and ensure that the patient remains hemodynamically stable. The AKI patient undergoing hemodialysis depends on a viable venous access catheter. When not in use, the catheter is 'heparin-locked' to preserve patency. The critical care nurse provides education about the disease process and treatment plan to patient and family.

Continuous Renal Replacement Therapy

CRRT is a newer mode of dialysis that has many similarities to traditional hemodialysis. CRRT is a continuous therapy that is monitored by the critical care nurse, and it may continue over many days. The venous blood is circulated through a highly porous hemofilter. As with traditional hemodialysis, access and return of blood are achieved through a large venous catheter (venovenous). The CRRT system allows the continuous removal of fluid from the plasma. The patient's blood flow is 100 to 200 mL/min, and the dialysate flow is 17 to 40 mL/min.[82] The fluid removal rate varies depending on the particular CRRT method used and removal of solutes (urea, creatinine, and electrolytes), as listed in Table 20-9. The removed fluid is described as ultrafiltrate. In an ideal situation, the hydrostatic pressure exerted by an MAP greater than 70 mm Hg would propel a continuous flow of blood through the hemofilter to remove fluid and solute. However, because many critically ill patients are hypotensive and cannot provide adequate flow through the hemofilter, an electric roller pump 'milks' the tubing to augment flow. If large amounts of fluid are to be removed, intravenous replacement solutions are infused. Indications and contraindications for CRRT are described in Box 20-5.

Controversy exists about when CRRT should be started, what the optimal dialysis dose is, which patients can derive

---

BOX 20-5   INDICATIONS AND CONTRAINDICATIONS FOR CONTINUOUS RENAL REPLACEMENT THERAPY

Indications
- Need for large fluid volume removal in hemodynamically unstable patient
- Hypervolemic or edematous patients showing no response to diuretic therapy
- Patients with multiple organ dysfunction syndrome
- Ease of fluid management in patients requiring large daily fluid volume
- Replacement for oliguria
- Administration of total parenteral nutrition
- Contraindication to hemodialysis and peritoneal dialysis
- Inability to be anticoagulated

Contraindications
- Hematocrit >45%
- Terminal illness

---

the greatest benefit, and when CRRT should be discontinued.[83-86] The debate over the optimal "dose" of dialysis is likely to continue because the multicenter Veterans Administration and National Institutes of Health trial showed no difference in mortality between critically ill patients receiving intensive and those receiving nonintensive dialysis regimens.[87] Other studies have confirmed that a high CRRT "dose" does not improve mortality.[88]

Because controlled removal and replacement of fluid are possible over many hours or days with CRRT, hemodynamic stability is maintained. This makes CRRT highly advantageous for use in the hemodynamically unstable patient with multisystem problems. The following modes of CRRT are used in critical care units[85,86]:

TABLE 20-9   COMPARISON OF CONTINUOUS RENAL REPLACEMENT THERAPY METHODS

TYPE	ULTRAFILTRATION RATE	FLUID REPLACEMENT	METHOD OF SOLUTE REMOVAL	INDICATION
SCUF	100-300 mL/hr	None	None	Fluid removal
CVVH	500-800 mL/hr	Predilution or postdilution, calculating hourly net loss	Convection	Fluid removal, moderate solute removal
CVVHD	500-800 mL/hr	Predilution or postdilution, subtracting dialysate, then calculating hourly net loss	Diffusion	Fluid removal, maximum solute removal
CVVHDF		Predilution or postdilution, subtracting dialysate, then calculating hourly net loss	Convection and diffusion	Maximal fluid removal, maximal solute removal

TABLE 20-10   SIZE OF MOLECULES CLEARED BY CONTINUOUS RENAL REPLACEMENT THERAPY

TYPE OF MOLECULE	SIZE OF MOLECULE	SOLUTES	SOLUTE REMOVAL METHOD
Small	<500 daltons	Urea, creatinine	Convection, diffusion
Middle	500-5000 daltons	Vancomycin	Convection better than diffusion
Low-molecular-weight (small) proteins	5000-50,000 daltons	Cytokines, complement	Convection or absorption onto hemofilter
Large proteins	>50,000 daltons	Albumin	Minimal removal

- Slow continuous ultrafiltration (SCUF)
- Continuous venovenous hemofiltration (CVVH)
- Continuous venovenous hemodialysis (CVVHD)
- Continuous venovenous hemodiafiltration (CVVHDF)

The decision about which type of therapy to initiate is based on clinical assessment, metabolic status, severity of uremia, whether a particular treatment modality is available at that institution, and other factors.

Terminology for Continuous Renal Replacement Therapy

In CRRT, solutes are removed from the blood by diffusion or convection. Both processes remove fluid, and the two methods remove molecules of different sizes.

Diffusion. Diffusion describes the movement of solutes along a concentration gradient from a high concentration to a low concentration across a semipermeable membrane. This is the main mechanism used in hemodialysis. Solutes such as creatinine and urea cross the dialysis membrane from the blood to the dialysis fluid compartment.

Convection. Convection occurs when a pressure gradient is set up so that the water is pushed or pumped across the dialysis filter and carries the solutes from the bloodstream with it. This method of solute removal is known as solvent drag, and it is commonly employed in CRRT.

Absorption. The filter attracts solute, and molecules attach (adsorb) to the dialysis filter. The size of solute molecules is measured in daltons. The different sizes of molecules that can be removed by convection or diffusion methods are shown in Table 20-10. Tiny molecules such as urea and creatinine are removed by diffusion and convection (all

methods). As the molecular size increases above 500 daltons, convection is the more efficient method.

Ultrafiltrate Volume. The fluid that is removed each hour is not called urine; it is known as ultrafiltrate.

Replacement Fluid. Typically, some of the ultrafiltrate is replaced through the CRRT circuit by a sterile replacement fluid. The replacement fluid can be added before the filter (prefilter dilution) or after the filter (postfilter dilution). The purpose is to increase the volume of fluid passing through the hemofilter and improve convection of solute.

Anticoagulation. Because the blood outside the body is in contact with artificial tubing and filters, the coagulation cascade and complement cascades are activated. To prevent the hemofilter from becoming obstructed by clotting, or clotting off, low-dose anticoagulation must be used.[89] The dose should be low enough to have no effect on patient anticoagulation parameters. Systemic anticoagulation is not the goal. Typical anticoagulant choices include unfractionated heparin (UFH) and sodium citrate.[76,89] Citrate is an effective prefilter anticoagulant, which has the side effect that it chelates (binds to and removes) calcium from the blood. Consequently, ionized calcium levels are verified, and calcium is replaced per protocol when sodium citrate is the anticoagulant.

Methods of Continuous Renal Replacement

Because of the design of the CRRT machine, it is not possible to look at the outside and follow the flow of blood and, if used, dialysate. Each of the CRRT methods is described here, and diagrams are employed to clarify the mode of CRRT that is used (Figure 20-6, *A-D*).

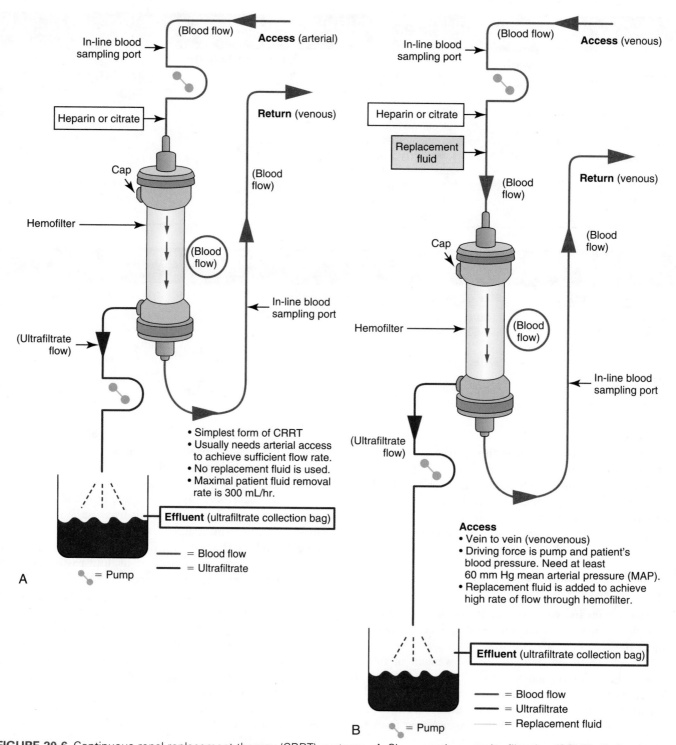

FIGURE 20-6 Continuous renal replacement therapy (CRRT) systems. *A,* Slow, continuous ultrafiltration (SCUF). *B,* Continuous venovenous hemofiltration (CVVH).
Continued

Slow Continuous Ultrafiltration. SCUF slowly removes fluid (100 to 300 mL/hr) through a process of ultrafiltration (see Figure 20-6, *A*). It consists of a movement of fluid across a semipermeable membrane. SCUF has minimal impact on solute removal. Because this process removes small amounts of fluid, it was initially hoped that it would be a suitable choice for edematous patients with acute heart failure and diminished kidney perfusion. However, SCUF is an infrequent clinical choice because it requires both arterial and venous access and is more likely to thrombose (clot off) than other CRRT methods that use higher flows.

Continuous Venovenous Hemofiltration. CVVH is indicated when the patient's clinical condition warrants removal of significant volumes of fluid and solutes (see Figure 20-6, *B*). Fluid is removed by ultrafiltration in volumes of 5 to 20 mL/min or up to 7 to 30 L/24 hr. Removal of solutes such

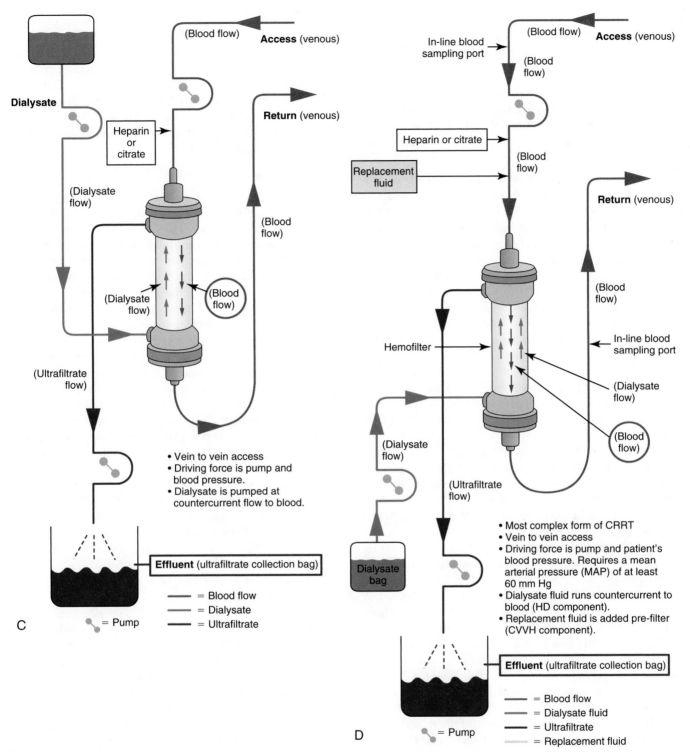

FIGURE 20-6, cont'd *C,* Continuous venovenous hemofiltration dialysis (CVVHD). *D,* Continuous venovenous hemodiafiltration (CVVHDF).

as urea, creatinine, and other small non-protein-bound toxins is accomplished by convection. The replacement fluid rate of flow through the CRRT circuit can be altered to achieve desired fluid and solute removal without causing hemodynamic instability.

As with other CRRT systems, the blood outside the body is anticoagulated, and the ultrafiltrate is drained off by gravity or by the addition of negative-pressure suction into a large drainage bag. Because large volumes of fluid may be removed in CVVH, some of the removed ultrafiltrate volume must be replaced hourly with a continuous infusion (replacement fluid) to avoid intravascular dehydration. Replacement fluids may consist of standard solutions of bicarbonate, potassium-free LR solution, acetate, or dextrose. Electrolytes such as potassium, sodium, calcium chloride, magnesium sulfate, and sodium bicarbonate may be added. The formula used to calculate the volume removed from the patient follows with an example:

$$\text{Ultrafiltrate in bag} + \text{Other output} -$$
$$(\text{CVVH replacement fluid} + \text{intravenous/}$$
$$\text{oral/nasogastric tube intake}) = \text{Output}$$
$$1000\ \text{mL} - 800\ \text{mL} = 200\ \text{mL/hr output}$$

Continuous Venovenous Hemodialysis. CVVHD is technically like traditional hemodialysis, and it removes solute by diffusion because of a slow (15 to 30 mL/min) countercurrent drainage flow on the membrane side of the hemofilter (see Figure 20-6, *C*). Blood and fluid move by countercurrent flow through the hemofilter. Countercurrent means the blood flows in one direction and the dialysate flows in the opposite direction. As with other types of CRRT and hemodialysis, although arterial access is always possible, venovenous vascular access is the most common choice.

CVVHD is indicated for patients who require large-volume removal for severe uremia or critical acid-base imbalances or for those who are resistant to diuretics. An MAP of at least 70 mm Hg is desirable for effective volume removal and dialysis, and it is most effective when used over days, not hours. The use of replacement fluid is optional and depends on the patient's clinical condition and plan of care. The critical care nurse is responsible for calculating the hourly intake and output, identifying fluid trends, and replacing excessive losses. This therapy is ideal for hemodynamically unstable patients in the critical care setting because they do not experience the abrupt fluid and solute changes that can accompany standard hemodialysis treatments.

Continuous Venovenous Hemodiafiltration. Another CRRT option is CVVHDF, which combines two of the previously described methods (CVVH and CVVHD) to achieve maximal fluid and solute removal (see Figure 20-6, *D*). A strong transmembrane pressure is applied to the hemofilter to push water across the filter, and a negative pressure is applied at the other side to pull fluid across the membrane and produce large volumes of ultrafiltrate and to create a "solvent drag" (CVVH method). The blood and the dialysate are circulated in a countercurrent flow pattern to remove fluid and solutes by diffusion (hemodialysis method). CVVHDF can remove large volumes of fluid and solute because it employs diffusion gradients and convection.

Complications

Potential problems associated with CRRT and appropriate nursing interventions are listed in Table 20-11. Complications are often related to the rate of flow through the system. If the patient becomes hypotensive or the access lines remain kinked, the ultrafiltration rate will decrease. This can lead to increased clot formation within the hemofilter. As the surface of the hemofilter becomes more clotted, it will not provide effective fluid or solute clearance, and CRRT will be stopped; a new CRRT circuit must then be set up. The critical care

nurse keeps track of the pressures displayed on the CRRT machine screen to monitor the positive pressure of fluid going into the hemofilter (inflow) and the pressures coming out of the hemofilter to ensure that that resistance to the negative-pressure pull of the fluid across the hemofilter membrane has not developed. Other patient-related complications include fluid and electrolyte alterations, bleeding because of anticoagulation, and problems with the access site, such as dislodgement and infection.

Medical Management

The choice of the method of blood purification to use to treat AKI is a medical decision. There is no clear clinical or research consensus about whether IHD or CRRT is the most beneficial. Age, gender, and preexisting chronic conditions are of little help in determining the need for hemofiltration or hemodialysis. Often, the acute clinical diagnosis, physician's preference, availability of the CRRT machine, and knowledgeable physicians and nurses at the hospital are the deciding factors. Infectious complications are associated with a grave prognosis. Dialysis is prescribed for almost anyone who develops severe AKI, unless the patient is clearly dying.

IHD or CCRT is usually begun before the BUN level exceeds 90 mg/dL or the creatinine level exceeds 9 mg/dL. In many hospitals, the threshold to begin treatment is considerably lower. Whether daily treatment is more effective than treatment every other day is controversial. The patient's serum creatinine concentration, BUN level, and fluid volume status are the deciding factors. CCRT is often prescribed when the BUN level is approximately 60 mg/dL. CRRT is more effective in the early stages of AKI. If the patient has severe electrolyte imbalance or fluid overload, even earlier intervention may be required.

Nursing Management

Critical care nurses play a vital role in monitoring the patient receiving CRRT. In many critical care units, the CRRT system is set up by the dialysis staff but is run on a 24-hour basis by critical care nurses with additional training. Complications may be related to the CRRT circuit, the CRRT pump, or to the patient, as shown in Box 20-6. The critical care nurse monitors fluid intake and output, prevents and detects potential complications (e.g., bleeding, hypotension), identifies trends in electrolyte laboratory values, supervises safe operation of the CRRT equipment, and provides patient and family education about the patient's condition and the use of CRRT.

KIDNEY TRANSPLANTATION

When the kidney to be transplanted is procured from the donor, whether living or cadaveric, the ureter, renal vein, and renal artery are dissected, leaving as much length as possible.

Living Donor Surgery

Living kidney donors are typically related to the person who will receive the kidney. The procurement can be a laparoscopic procedure or an open procedure. After the kidney is

TABLE 20-11	COMPLICATIONS ASSOCIATED WITH CONTINUOUS RENAL REPLACEMENT THERAPY		
PROBLEM	**CAUSE**	**CLINICAL MANIFESTATIONS**	**NURSING MANAGEMENT**
Decreased ultrafiltration rate	Hypotension Dehydration Kinked lines Bending of catheters Clotting of filter	Ultrafiltration rate decreased Minimal flow through blood lines	Observe filter and arteriovenous system. Control blood flow. Control coagulation time. Position patient on back. Lower height of collection container.
Filter clotting	Obstruction Insufficient heparinization	Ultrafiltration rate decreased, despite height of collection container being lower	Control anticoagulation (heparin/citrate). Maintain continuous system anticoagulation. Call physician. Remove system. Prime catheters with anticoagulated solution. Prime new system; connect it. Start predilution with 1000 mL saline 0.9% solution per hour. Do not use three-way stopcocks.
Hypotension	Increased ultrafiltration rate Blood leak Disconnection of one of lines	Bleeding Call physician	Control amount of ultrafiltration. Control access sites. Clamp lines.
Fluid and electrolyte changes	Too much or too little removal of fluid Inappropriate replacement of electrolytes Inappropriate dialysate	Changes in mentation ↑ or ↓ CVP ↑ or ↓ PAOP ECG change ↑ or ↓ BP and heart rate Abnormal electrolyte levels	Observe for: • Changes in CVP or PAOP • Changes in vital signs • ECG changes resulting from electrolyte abnormalities Monitor output values every hour. Control ultrafiltration.
Bleeding	System disconnection ↑ Heparin dose	Oozing from catheter insertion site or connection	Monitor ACT no less than once every hour (heparin). Adjust heparin dose within specifications to maintain ACT. Monitor serum calcium if using citrate as an anticoagulant. Observe dressing on vascular access for blood loss. Observe for blood in filtrate (filter leak).
Access dislodgement or infection	Catheter or connections not secured Break in sterile technique Excessive patient movement	Bleeding from catheter site or connections Inappropriate flow or infusion Fever Drainage at catheter site	Observe access site at least once every 2 hours. Ensure that clamps are available within easy reach at all times. Observe strict sterile technique when dressing vascular access.

ACT, activated coagulation time; *ECG*, electrocardiogram; ↑, increased; ↓, decreased.

secured, it is flushed with a cold electrolyte preservative solution until the venous return is clear.[90] This usually requires 100 to 200 mL of solution.[90] The kidney is then transported to the operating room to be transplanted.

Deceased Donor Surgery

If the kidney is from a deceased donor, it is flushed with a cold electrolyte preservative solution and simultaneously cooled externally as quickly as possible. It can be transported on a kidney perfusion machine or packed in an iced preservation solution. After it is procured and placed in the hypothermic solution, it can be maintained for 48 to 72 hours before it must be transplanted.[90] Most transplant centers attempt to transplant an organ within 24 hours after procurement, to

minimize the risk of kidney injury.[90] At the time of procurement, the kidney is assessed in situ for color, shape, and form. It is palpated to determine firmness, and often a biopsy specimen is taken to rule out undiagnosed kidney dysfunction.

Recipient Surgery

The patient is anesthetized in the usual manner, and a urinary catheter is placed. A curvilinear incision is made 3 to 4 cm above the symphysis pubis and extended to the iliac crest (Figure 20-7, *A*). The kidney will be placed in the extraperitoneal space of the right or left iliac fossa. The muscles and fascia are divided and retracted medially to expose the iliac vessels. The renal artery is anastomosed to the external iliac artery, using an end-to-side or an end-to-end anastomosis,

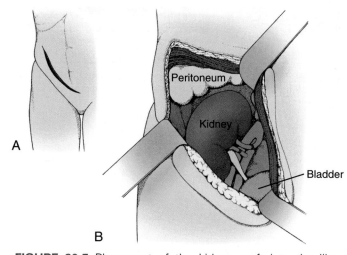

FIGURE 20-7 Placement of the kidney graft into the iliac fossa. *A,* The incision in the right side of the abdomen is used for graft implantation in the right iliac fossa. *B,* The iliac vessels are exposed. (Modified from Smith SL: *AACN tissue and organ transplantation: implications for professional nursing practice,* St Louis, 1990, Mosby.)

and the vein is sutured to the common iliac vein in a similar manner (Figure 20-7, *B*).[90]

During the procedure, a CVP ranging from 8 to 16 mm Hg must be maintained, and a systolic BP at least as high as the patient's baseline value should be maintained to ensure adequate perfusion of the transplanted kidney.

Postoperative Medical Management and Nursing Care

After the transplantation is completed and the patient is stable and ready for discharge from the recovery room, most transplant centers admit the patient directly to the organ transplantation unit or to the critical care unit. Serious complications can occur in the immediate postoperative period, and a sound knowledge base of medical/surgical nursing, kidney function, anatomy, and immunosuppressive medications is imperative.

Fluid Status

If the transplanted organ is working well, the patient's fluid status, as monitored by observations of CVP, weight, and vital signs, must be regulated very closely. Adequate hydration is an absolute necessity for continued graft function in the immediate postoperative period. Hypovolemia can lead to compromised blood flow to the kidney, acute kidney injury, and possible graft failure. The new kidney will be producing large amounts of urine, and fluid replacement, usually maintained in a 1:1 ratio, must be sustained.

Electrolytes

Electrolyte balance is also of grave concern. Because of the large volumes of urine produced, the potential exists for hypokalemia, hypomagnesemia, and hypocalcemia, leading to possible cardiac compromise.[91] Electrolytes must be monitored at least every 4 to 6 hours and replaced as necessary. Assessment of the BUN and the creatinine concentration also is necessary every 4 to 6 hours to monitor graft function and determine the need for dialysis.

Postoperative Complications

The complete blood count and platelet count should be monitored every 4 to 6 hours. Blood loss during the operation is minimal, usually 500 mL or less. Abrupt decreases or continuously falling counts may indicate hemorrhage at an anastomosis site, which requires a return to the operating room for repair. Even with minimal blood loss during surgery, transfusion of blood products after the surgery is often necessary. Frequent observation and assessment of the surgical incision are needed to evaluate for drainage and swelling. Urine output volume and color should be monitored at least every 30 minutes. The bladder anastomosis is fragile, and it is not uncommon for clots to occlude the catheter. The bladder must remain decompressed for several days to promote proper healing. If clots occlude the end of the catheter, gentle irrigation or aspiration may be necessary. If the clot cannot be dislodged or aspirated out, the catheter may have to be changed. Painful bladder spasms also can occur, and opiates, usually in the form of a belladonna and opium suppository, may be required to relax the bladder.

Immunosuppression

Initiation of induction immunosuppressant therapy begins at the time of transplantation, usually in the form of a polyclonal antithymocyte/antilymphocyte intravenous compound or an intravenous monoclonal antibody compound. These compounds remove the lymphocytes from the patient's system, preventing rejection and suppressing the immune system until oral drugs can be safely administered and blood drug levels are sufficient to allow discontinuation of the intravenous agent. Because the patient is now immunocompromised, strict aseptic technique is required to prevent infection.

Infection Risk

Thorough hand washing, aseptic dressing changes, discontinuation of any unnecessary invasive lines, and limiting the number of visitors are necessary protective measures. Because of the patient's immunocompromised status, subtle changes in the temperature, WBC count, or wound drainage can signal an active infection. Patients also are susceptible to infection by opportunistic native organisms such as *Candida*, *Pneumocystis* pneumonia, cytomegalovirus, Epstein-Barr virus, and herpes simplex virus.

The average length of stay in the hospital after uncomplicated kidney transplantation is 5 to 7 days.[92] During the first few days, the patient must learn self-care related to the new organ. Medication regimens are very complicated, and most centers initiate a self-medication program at the patient's bedside as a training tool. Patients are taught the signs and symptoms of infection and graft rejection, the protocols of the transplant clinic, and new dietary limitations. Frequent transplant clinic visits to check the functioning of the organ and to adjust down the doses of immunosuppressant medications are necessary for the first few months after transplantation.[92]

Rejection

Rejection of the transplanted kidney represents an ongoing concern for all transplant patients. The graft function is monitored closely, and if rejection is suspected, a biopsy is performed. If the biopsy reveals acute rejection, rescue therapy is initiated. This therapy can be given in the form of high-dose intravenous steroids for mild rejection or intravenous monoclonal antibody for moderate to severe rejection. If the biopsy reveals chronic rejection, the oral immunosuppressant medications are increased or returned to the higher doses used immediately after transplantation. No two patients' immune systems are exactly alike, and the immunosuppressant medication regimen required to prevent rejection must be tailored to each patient individually. The goal is to create a balance among medications that allows the patient to fight off most infections but avoid rejection of the transplanted organ.

Patient adherence to the complicated medical regimen that is required to maintain a transplanted organ is of major concern. Adequate education of the patient and family as to the importance of taking the medications as instructed is of paramount importance. Patients are reluctant to take the medications appropriately if they are experiencing severe or disfiguring side effects. Decreasing the doses of the medications can often alleviate these side effects but may lead to a rejection episode. The goal is to create a balance so that medications allow the patient to fight off most infections and yet avoid rejection of the transplanted kidney.

CASE STUDY   PATIENT WITH A KIDNEY PROBLEM

Answer to the Case Study Questions can be found on the Evolve web site at http://www.evolve.elsevier.com/Urden/priorities/.

Brief Patient History
Ms. L is a 32-year-old woman who was found lying down in the street near the hospital. She is awake but confused. She unable to give any medical history and has no idea how long she has been in the street.

Clinical Assessment
Ms. L is admitted to the critical care unit with muscle pain and minimal dark urine output. She continues to be confused, but her neurologic examination results are otherwise normal. She repeatedly tells the nurses that she is tired, has pain everywhere, and just wants to sleep. She is able to move all her extremities and has no signs of injury on skin examination.

Diagnostic Procedures
Laboratory tests show the following results: creatinine phosphokinase (CPK) level of 40,400 U/L, serum myoglobin level of 2.5 mg/L, urinary myoglobin level of 300 mg/L, and serum potassium level of 4.8 mEq/dL. Baseline vital signs were as follows: blood pressure of 85/60 mm Hg, heart rate of 128 beats/min (sinus tachycardia), respiratory rate of 18 breaths/min, temperature of 101.3° F, and O₂ saturation of 98%.

The toxicology screen showed that the patient tested positive for cocaine. The Glasgow Coma Scale score was 14.

Medical Diagnosis
Ms. L is diagnosed with rhabdomyolysis.

Questions
1. What major outcomes do you expect to achieve for this patient?
2. What problems or risks must be managed to achieve these outcomes?
3. What interventions must be initiated to monitor, prevent, manage, or eliminate the problems and risks identified?
4. What interventions should be initiated to promote the optimal functioning, safety, and well-being of this patient?
5. What possible learning needs do you anticipate for this patient?
6. What cultural and age-related factors may have a bearing on this patient's plan of care?

REFERENCES

1. Kellum JA: Acute kidney injury, *Crit Care Med* 36(4 suppl): S141, 2008.
2. Brincat S, Hilton R: Prevention of acute kidney injury, *Br J Hosp Med (Lond)* 69(8):450, 2008.
3. Kellum JA, Hoste EA: Acute kidney injury: epidemiology and assessment, *Scand J Clin Lab Invest Suppl* 241:6, 2008.
4. Mehta RL, Pascual MT, Soroko S, et al: Program to Improve Care in Acute Renal Disease: Spectrum of acute renal failure in the intensive care unit: the PICARD experience, *Kidney Int* 66(4):1613, 2004.
5. Sesso R, Roque A, Vicioso B, et al: Prognosis of ARF in hospitalized elderly patients, *Am J Kidney Dis* 44(3):401-419, 2004.
6. Ponte B, Felipe C, Muriel A, et al: Long-term functional evolution after an acute kidney injury: a 10-year study, *Nephrol Dial Transplant* 23(12):3859, 2008.
7. Nickolas TL, Frisch GD, Opotowsky AR, et al: Awareness of kidney disease in the US population: findings from the National Health and Nutrition Examination Survey (NHANES) 1999 to 2000, *Am J Kidney Dis* 44(2):185, 2004.
8. Brochard L, Abroug F, Brenner M, et al: An Official ATS/ERS/ESICM/SCCM/SRLF Statement: Prevention and Management of Acute Renal Failure in the ICU Patient: an international consensus conference in intensive care medicine. *Am J Respir Crit Care Med* 181(10):1128, 2010.
9. Bellomo R, et al: Pre-renal azotemia: a flawed paradigm in critically ill septic patients? *Contrib Nephrol* 156:1, 2007.
10. Bellomo R, et al: Acute renal failure-definition, outcome measures, animal models, fluid therapy and information technology needs: the Second International Consensus Conference of the Acute Dialysis Quality Initiative (ADQI) Group, *Crit Care* 8(4):R204-212, 2004.
11. Kellum JA, Bellomo R, Ronco C: Definition and classification of acute kidney injury, *Nephron Clin Pract* 109(4):c182, 2008.
12. Bentley ML, Corwin HL, Dasta J: Drug-induced acute kidney injury in the critically ill adult: recognition and prevention strategies *Crit Care Med* 38(6):S169, 2010.
13. Asif A, Epstein M: Prevention of radiocontrast-induced nephropathy, *Am J Kidney Dis* 44(1):12, 2004.
14. Sheridan AM, Bonventre JV: Cell biology and molecular mechanisms of injury in ischemic acute renal failure, *Curr Opin Nephrol Hypertens* 9(4):427, 2000.
15. Van Berendoncks AM, Elseviers MM, Lins RL, SHARF Study Group: Outcome of acute kidney injury with different treatment options, *Clin J Am Soc Nephrol* 5(10):1755, 2010.
16. Liano F, Junco E, Pascual J, et al: The spectrum of acute renal failure in the intensive care unit compared with that seen in other settings. The Madrid Acute Renal Failure Study Group, *Kidney Int Suppl* 66:S16, 1998.
17. Rocktaeschel J, Morimatsu H, Uchino S, et al: Acid-base status of critically ill patients with acute renal failure: analysis based on Stewart-Figge methodology, *Crit Care* 7(4):R60, 2003.
18. Bellomo R, Kellum JA, Ronco C: Defining acute renal failure: physiological principles, *Intensive Care Med* 30(1):33, 2004.
19. Coresh J, Astor BC, Greene T, et al: Prevalence of chronic kidney disease and decreased kidney function in the adult US population: Third National Health and Nutrition Examination Survey, *Am J Kidney Dis* 41(1):1, 2003.

20. K/DOQI clinical practice guidelines for chronic kidney disease: evaluation, classification, and stratification, *Am J Kidney Dis* 39(2 suppl 1):S1, 2002.
21. K/DOQI clinical practice guidelines on hypertension and antihypertensive agents in chronic kidney disease, *Am J Kidney Dis* 43(5 suppl 1):S1, 2004.
22. Go AS, Chertow GM, Fan D, et al: Chronic kidney disease and the risks of death, cardiovascular events, and hospitalization, *N Engl J Med* 351(13):1296, 2004.
23. Anavekar NS, McMurray JJ, Velazquez EJ, et al: Relation between renal dysfunction and cardiovascular outcomes after myocardial infarction, *N Engl J Med* 351(13):1285, 2004.
24. Pannu N, Mehta RL: Mechanical ventilation and renal function: an area for concern? *Am J Kidney Dis* 39(3):616, 2002.
25. Scheel PJ, Liu M, Rabb H: Uremic lung: new insights into a forgotten condition, *Kidney Int* 74(7):849, 2008.
26. Vieira JM Jr, Castro I, Curvello-Neto A, et al: Effect of acute kidney injury on weaning from mechanical ventilation in critically ill patients, *Crit Care Med* 35(1):184, 2007.
27. Wan L, May CN, Gobe G, et al: Pathophysiology of septic acute kidney injury: what do we really know? *Crit Care Med* 36(4 suppl):S198, 2008.
28. Dellinger RP, Levy MM, Carlet JM, et al: Surviving Sepsis Campaign: international guidelines for management of severe sepsis and septic shock: 2008, *Crit Care Med* 36(1):296, 2008.
29. Bagshaw SM, George C, Gibney RT, et al: A multi-center evaluation of early acute kidney injury in critically ill trauma patients, *Ren Fail* 30(6):581, 2008.
30. Criddle LM: Rhabdomyolysis: pathophysiology, recognition, and management, *Crit Care Nurse* 23(6):14, 2003.
31. Brown CV, Rhee P, Chan L, et al: Preventing renal failure in patients with rhabdomyolysis: do bicarbonate and mannitol make a difference? *J Trauma* 56(6):1191, 2004.
32. Weisbord SD, Hartwig KC, Sonel AF, et al: The incidence of clinically significant contrast-induced nephropathy following non-emergent coronary angiography, *Catheter Cardiovasc Interv* 71(7):879, 2008.
33. Kandzari DE, Rebeiz AG, Wang A, et al: Contrast nephropathy: an evidence-based approach to prevention, *Am J Cardiovasc Drugs* 3(6):395, 2003.
34. Goldenberg I, Chonchol M, Guetta V: Reversible acute kidney injury following contrast exposure and the risk of long-term mortality, *Am J Nephrol* 29(2):136, 2008.
35. Aspelin P, Aubry P, Fransson SG, et al: Nephrotoxicity in High-Risk Patients Study of Iso-Osmolar and Low-Osmolar Non-Ionic Contrast Media Study Investigators: Nephrotoxic effects in high-risk patients undergoing angiography, *N Engl J Med* 348(6):491, 2003.
36. Kuhn MJ, Scialfa G, Gao PY, et al: The PREDICT study: a randomized double-blind comparison of contrast-induced nephropathy after low- or iso-osmolar contrast agent exposure, *AJR Am J Roentgenol* 191(1):151, 2008.
37. Maioli M, Toso A, Leoncini M, et al: Sodium bicarbonate versus saline for the prevention of contrast-induced nephropathy in patients with renal dysfunction undergoing coronary angiography or intervention, *J Am Coll Cardiol* 52(8):599, 2008.
38. Brar SS, Shen AY, Jorgensen MB, et al: Sodium bicarbonate vs sodium chloride for the prevention of contrast medium-induced nephropathy in patients undergoing coronary angiography: a randomized trial, *JAMA* 300(9):1038, 2008.

39. Ozcan EE, Guneri S, Akdeniz B, et al: Sodium bicarbonate, N-acetylcysteine, and saline for prevention of radiocontrast-induced nephropathy: A comparison of 3 regimens for protecting contrast-induced nephropathy in patients undergoing coronary procedures. A single-center prospective controlled trial, *Am Heart J* 154(3):539, 2007.

40. Stone GW, McCullough PA, Tumlin JA, et al: Fenoldopam mesylate for the prevention of contrast-induced nephropathy: a randomized controlled trial, *JAMA* 290(17):2284, 2003.

41. Kanbay M, Covic A, Coca SG, et al: Sodium bicarbonate for the prevention of contrast-induced nephropathy: a meta-analysis of 17 randomized controlled trials. *Int Urol Nephrol* 41(3):617, 2009.

42. Thomsen HS, Morcos SK, Barrett BJ: Contrast-induced nephropathy: the wheel has turned 360 degrees, *Acta Radiol* 49(6):646, 2008.

43. McGee WT, Mailloux P, Jodka P, et al: The pulmonary artery catheter in critical care, *Semin Dial* 19(6):480, 2006.

44. Ahee P, Crowe AV: The management of hyperkalaemia in the emergency department, *J Accid Emerg Med* 17(3): 188, 2000.

45. Levey AS, Coresh J, Balk E, et al: National Kidney Foundation practice guidelines for chronic kidney disease: evaluation, classification, and stratification, *Ann Intern Med* 139(2):137, 2003.

46. K/DOQI clinical practice guidelines for bone metabolism and disease in chronic kidney disease, *Am J Kidney Dis* 42 (4 suppl 3):S1, 2003.

47. Gauci C, Moranne O, Fouqueray B, et al; NephroTest Study Group: Pitfalls of measuring total blood calcium in patients with CKD, *J Am Soc Nephrol* 19(8):1592, 2008.

48. Leavey SF, Weitzel WF: Endocrine abnormalities in chronic renal failure, *Endocrinol Metab Clin North Am* 31(1):107, 2002.

49. McCann L: Calcium in chronic kidney disease: recommended intake and serum targets, *Adv Chronic Kidney Dis* 14(1):75, 2007.

50. Emmett M: A comparison of clinically useful phosphorus binders for patients with chronic kidney failure, *Kidney Int Suppl* (90):S25, 2004.

51. Mehta RL, Clark WC, Schetz M: Techniques for assessing and achieving fluid balance in acute renal failure, *Curr Opin Crit Care* 8(6):535, 2002.

52. The SAFE Study Investigators: A comparison of albumin and saline for fluid resuscitation in the intensive care unit, *N Engl J Med* 350(22):2247, 2004.

53. The SAFE Study Investigators: Saline or albumin for fluid resuscitation in patients with traumatic brain injury, *N Engl J Med* 357(9):874, 2007.

54. Perel P, Roberrts I: Colloids versus crystalloids for fluid resuscitation in critically ill patients, *Cochrane Database Syst Rev* (4):CD000567, 2007.

55. Schetz M, Dasta J, Goldstein S, et al: Drug-induced acute kidney injury, *Curr Opin Crit Care* 11(6):555, 2005.

56. Karajala V, Mansour W, Kellum JA: Diuretics in acute kidney injury, *Minerva Anestesiol* 75(5):251, 2009.

57. Joshua L, Devi P, Guido S: Adverse drug reactions in medical intensive care unit of a tertiary care hospital. *Pharmacoepidemiol Drug Saf* 18(7):639, 2009.

58. Baldwin KA, Budzinski CE, Shapiro, CJ: Acute Sensorineural Hearing Loss: Furosemide Ototoxicity Revisited. *Hosp Pharm* 43(12):982, 2008.

59. Mehta RL, Pascual MT, Soroko S, et al: Diuretics, mortality, and nonrecovery of renal function in acute renal failure, *JAMA* 288(20):2547, 2002.

60. Cantarovich F, Rangoonwala B, Lorenz H, et al: High-Dose Furosemide in Acute Renal Failure Study Group: High-dose furosemide for established ARF: a prospective, randomized, double-blind, placebo-controlled, multicenter trial, *Am J Kidney Dis* 44(3):402, 2004.

61. Uchino S, Doig GS, Bellomo R, et al: Beginning and Ending Supportive Therapy for the Kidney (B.E.S.T. Kidney) Investigators: Diuretics and mortality in acute renal failure, *Crit Care Med* 32(8):1669, 2004.

62. van der Voort PH, Boerma EC, Koopmans M, et al: Furosemide does not improve renal recovery after hemofiltration for acute renal failure in critically ill patients: a double blind randomized controlled trial. *Crit Care Med* 37(2):533, 2009.

63. Bagshaw SM, Gibney RT, McAlister FA, et al: The SPARK Study: a phase II randomized blinded controlled trial of the effect of furosemide in critically ill patients with early acute kidney injury. *Trials* 11:50, 2010.

64. Ichai C, Passeron C, Carles M, et al: Prolonged low-dose dopamine infusion induces a transient improvement in renal function in hemodynamically stable, critically ill patients: a single-blind, prospective, controlled study, *Crit Care Med* 28(5):1329, 2000.

65. Kellum JA, Decker JM: Use of dopamine in acute renal failure: a meta-analysis, *Crit Care Med* 29(8):1526, 2001.

66. Bellomo R, Chapman M, Finfer S, et al: Low-dose dopamine in patients with early renal dysfunction: a placebo-controlled randomised trial. Australian and New Zealand Intensive Care Society (ANZICS) Clinical Trials Group, *Lancet* 356(9248):2139, 2000.

67. Sisillo E, Ceriani R, Bortone F, et al: N-acetylcysteine for prevention of acute renal failure in patients with chronic renal insufficiency undergoing cardiac surgery: a prospective, randomized, clinical trial, *Crit Care Med* 36(1):81, 2008.

68. Haase M, Haase-Fielitz A, Bagshaw SM, et al: Phase II, randomized, controlled trial of high-dose N-acetylcysteine in high-risk cardiac surgery patients, *Crit Care Med* 35(5):1324, 2007.

69. Casaer MP, Mesotten D, Schetz MR, et al: Bench-to-bedside review: metabolism and nutrition, *Crit Care* 12(4):222, 2008.

70. KDOQI Clinical Practice Guidelines and Clinical Practice Recommendations for Anemia in Chronic Kidney Disease, *Am J Kidney Dis.* 47(5) Suppl 3:S11–145, 2006.

71. Corwin HL, Eckardt KU: Erythropoietin in the critically ill: what is the evidence? *Nephrol Dial Transplant* 20(12):2605, 2005.

72. Gouva C, Nikolopoulos P, Ioannidis JP, et al: Treating anemia early in renal failure patients slows the decline of renal function: a randomized controlled trial, *Kidney Int* 66(2): 753, 2004.

73. Corwin HL, Gettinger A, Pearl RG, et al: EPO Critical Care Trials Group: Efficacy of recombinant human erythropoietin in critically ill patients: a randomized controlled trial, *JAMA* 288(22):2827, 2002.

74. Baldwin I, Bellomo R, Naka T, et al: A pilot randomized controlled comparison of continuous veno-venous haemofiltration and extended daily dialysis with filtration: effect on small solutes and acid-base balance, *Intensive Care Med* 33(5):830, 2007.

75. Warkentin TE, Greinacher A, Koster A, et al: Treatment and prevention of heparin-induced thrombocytopenia: American College of Chest Physicians Evidence-Based Clinical Practice Guidelines (8th Edition), *Chest* 133(6 suppl):340S, 2008.

76. Fealy N, Bellomo R, Naka T, et al: A pilot randomized controlled crossover study comparing regional heparinization to regional citrate anticoagulation for continuous venovenous hemofiltration, *Int J Artif Organs* 30(4):301, 2007.

77. Rayner HC, Pisoni RL, Gillespie BW, et al: Creation, cannulation and survival of arteriovenous fistulae: data from the Dialysis Outcomes and Practice Patterns Study, *Kidney Int* 63(1):323, 2003.

78. Beathard GA, Arnold P, Jackson J, et al: Aggressive treatment of early fistula failure, *Kidney Int* 64(4):1487, 2003.

79. McCann M, Einarsdóttir H, Van Waeleghem JP, et al: Vascular access management 1: an overview, *J Ren Care* 34(2):77, 2008.

80. Asif A, Leclercq B, Merrill D, et al: Arteriovenous fistula creation: should US nephrologists get involved? *Am J Kidney Dis* 42(6):1293, 2003.

81. Bagul A, Brook NR, Kaushik M, et al: Tunnelled catheters for the haemodialysis patient, *Eur J Vasc Endovasc Surg* 33(1):105, 2007.

82. O'Reilly P, Tolwani A: Renal replacement therapy III: IHD, CRRT, SLED, *Crit Care Clin* 21(2):367, 2005.

83. Gibney N, Uchino S, Bellomo R, et al: Beginning and Ending Supportive Therapy for the Kidney (BEST Kidney) Investigators: Timing of initiation and discontinuation of renal replacement therapy in AKI: unanswered key questions, Clin *J Am Soc Nephrol* 3(3):876, 2008.

84. Bagshaw SM, Gibney RT: Ideal determinants for the initiation of renal replacement therapy: timing, metabolic threshold or fluid balance? *Acta Clin Belg Suppl* 2007(2): 357, 2007.

85. Chrysochoou G, Marcus RJ, Sureshkumar KK, et al: Renal replacement therapy in the critical care unit, *Crit Care Nurs Q* 31(4):282, 2008.

86. Dirkes S, Hodge K: Continuous renal replacement therapy in the adult intensive care unit: history and current trends, *Crit Care Nurse* 27(2):61, 2007.

87. VA/NIH Acute Renal Failure Trial Network, Palevsky PM, Zhang JH, O'Connor TZ, et al: Intensity of renal support in critically ill patients with acute kidney injury, *N Engl J Med* 359(1):7, 2008.

88. Casey ET, Gupta BP, Erwin PJ, et al: The dose of continuous renal replacement therapy for acute renal failure: a systematic review and meta-analysis *Ren Fail* 3(5):555, 2010.

89. Joannidis M, Oudemans-van Straaten HM: Clinical review: patency of the circuit in continuous renal replacement therapy, *Crit Care* 11(4):218, 2007.

90. Forsythe LR, editor: *Transplantation: a companion to specialist surgical practice*, ed 3, Philadelphia, 2005, Elsevier.

91. Holechek MJ, Armstrong G: Kidney transplantation. In Ohler L, Cupples S, editors: *Core Curriculum for Transplant Nurses*, Philadelphia, 2008, Mosby Elsevier.

92. Danovich GM: *Handbook of kidney transplantation*, ed 4, Philadelphia, 2005, Lippincott Williams & Wilkins.

UNIT 7

Gastrointestinal Alterations

21

Gastrointestinal Clinical Assessment and Diagnostic Procedures

Kathleen M. Stacy

℮volve WEBSITE

Be sure to check out the bonus material, including free self-assessment exercises, on the Evolve web site at *http://evolve.elsevier.com/Urden/priorities/*.

OBJECTIVES

- Identify the components of a gastrointestinal history.
- Describe inspection, palpation, percussion, and auscultation of the patient with gastrointestinal dysfunction.
- Delineate the clinical significance of selected laboratory tests used in the assessment of gastrointestinal disorders.

- Identify key diagnostic procedures used in assessment of the patient with gastrointestinal dysfunction.
- Discuss the nursing management of a patient undergoing a gastrointestinal diagnostic procedure.

Assessment of the critically ill patient with gastrointestinal dysfunction includes a review of the patient's history, a thorough physical examination, and analysis of the patient's laboratory data. Numerous invasive and noninvasive diagnostic procedures may also be performed to help identify the disorder.

CLINICAL ASSESSMENT

A thorough clinical assessment of the patient with gastrointestinal dysfunction is imperative for the early identification and treatment of gastrointestinal disorders. The completed assessment serves as the foundation for developing the management plan for the patient. The assessment process can be brief or can involve a detailed history and examination, depending on the nature and immediacy of the patient's situation.[1]

HISTORY

Taking a thorough and accurate history is extremely important to the assessment process. The patient's history provides the foundation and direction for the rest of the assessment. The overall goal of the patient interview is to expose key clinical manifestations that will facilitate the identification of the underlying cause of the illness. This information can then assist in the development of an appropriate management plan.[2]

The initial presentation of the patient determines the rapidity and direction of the interview. For a patient in acute distress, the history should be curtailed to a few questions about the patient's chief complaint and the precipitating events. For a patient in no obvious distress, the history should focus on four different areas: (1) review of the patient's present illness; (2) overview of the patient's general

429

gastrointestinal status including previous GI diagnostic studies or interventional procedures; (3) examination of the patient's personal and social history, including dietary habits, nutritional status, bowel characteristics (stool descriptions), alcohol intake, and dependence on laxatives or enemas; and (4) survey of the patient's family history, including metabolic disorders, malabsorption syndromes, and cancer of the GI tract.[3,4]

PHYSICAL EXAMINATION

The physical examination helps to establish baseline data about the physical dimensions of the patient's situation.[3] The abdomen is divided into four quadrants (left upper, right upper, left lower, and right lower), with the umbilicus as the middle point, to help specify the location of examination findings (Figure 21-1 and Box 21-1). The assessment should proceed when the patient is as comfortable as possible and in the supine position; however, the position may need readjustment if it elicits pain. To prevent stimulation of gastrointestinal activity, the order for the assessment should be changed to inspection, auscultation, percussion, and palpation.[4]

Inspection

Inspection of the patient focuses on three priorities: (1) observation of the oral cavity, (2) assessment of the skin over the abdomen, and (3) evaluation of the shape of the abdomen. The examination should be performed in a warm, well-lighted environment with the patient in a comfortable position and with the abdomen exposed.

Observation of the Oral Cavity

Although assessment of the gastrointestinal system classically begins with inspection of the abdomen, the patient's oral cavity also must be inspected to determine any unusual

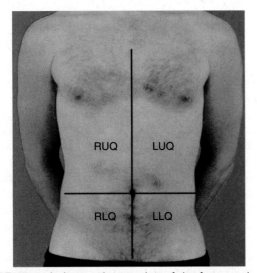

FIGURE 21-1 *A,* Anatomic mapping of the four quadrants of the abdomen. *B,* Auscultation for bowel sounds. (From Barkauskas V, et al: *Health & physical assessment,* ed 3, St Louis, 2002, Mosby.)

findings. Abnormal findings of the mouth include joint tenderness, inflammation of the gums, missing teeth, dental caries, ill-fitting dentures, and mouth odor.[5]

Assessment of the Skin over the Abdomen

Observe the skin for pigmentation, lesions, striae, scars, petechiae, signs of dehydration, and venous pattern. Pigmentation may vary considerably and still be within normal limits because of race and ethnic background, although the abdomen usually is a lighter color than other exposed areas of the skin. Abnormal findings include jaundice, skin lesions, and a tense and glistening appearance of the skin. Old striae (stretch marks) usually are silver, whereas pinkish purple

---

BOX 21-1 **ANATOMIC CORRELATES OF THE FOUR QUADRANTS OF THE ABDOMEN**

Right Upper Quadrant
- Liver and gallbladder
- Pylorus
- Duodenum
- Head of pancreas
- Right adrenal gland
- Portion of right kidney
- Hepatic flexure of colon
- Portion of ascending and transverse colon

Right Lower Quadrant
- Lower pole of right kidney
- Cecum and appendix
- Portion of ascending colon
- Bladder (if distended)
- Ovary and salpinx
- Uterus (if enlarged)
- Right spermatic cord
- Right ureter

Left Upper Quadrant
- Left lobe of liver
- Spleen
- Stomach
- Body of pancreas
- Left adrenal gland
- Portion of left kidney
- Splenic flexure of colon
- Portions of transverse and descending colon

Left Lower Quadrant
- Lower pole of left kidney
- Sigmoid colon
- Portion of descending colon
- Bladder (if distended)
- Ovary and salpinx
- Uterus (if distended)
- Left spermatic cord
- Left ureter

From Barkauskas V, et al: *Health & physical assessment,* ed 3, St Louis, 2002, Mosby.

striae may indicate Cushing's syndrome.[4] A bluish discoloration of the umbilicus (Cullen's sign) and of the flank (Grey Turner's sign) indicates retroperitoneal bleeding.[1]

Evaluation of the Shape of the Abdomen

Observe the abdomen for contour, noting whether it is flat, slightly concave, or slightly round; observe for symmetry and for movement. Marked distention is an abnormal finding. In particular, ascites may cause generalized distention and bulging flanks. Asymmetric distention may indicate organ enlargement or a mass. Peristaltic waves should not be visible except in very thin patients. In the case of intestinal obstruction, hyperactive peristaltic waves may be observed. Pulsation in the epigastric area is often a normal finding, but increased pulsation may indicate an aortic aneurysm. Symmetric movement of the abdomen with respirations is usually seen in men.[4,5]

Auscultation

Auscultation of the patient focuses on two priorities: (1) evaluation of bowels sounds and (2) assessment of bruits. Auscultation of the abdomen provides clinical data regarding the status of the bowel's motility. Initially, listen with the diaphragm of the stethoscope below and to the right of the umbilicus. The examination proceeds methodically through all four quadrants, lifting and then replacing the diaphragm of the stethoscope lightly against the abdomen (see Figure 21-1).

Evaluation of Bowel Sounds

Normal bowel sounds include high-pitched, gurgling sounds that occur approximately every 5 to 15 seconds or at a rate of 5 to 34 times per minute. Colonic sounds are low-pitched and have a rumbling quality. A venous hum may be audible sometimes.[6,7] Table 21-1 provides a list of abnormal abdominal sounds.

Abnormal findings include the absence of bowel sounds throughout a 5-minute period, extremely soft and widely separated sounds, and increased sounds with a high-pitched, loud rushing sound (peristaltic rush). Absent bowel sounds may result from inflammation, ileus, electrolyte disturbances, and ischemia. Bowels sounds may be increased with diarrhea and early intestinal obstruction.[6,7]

Assessment of Bruits

The abdomen should be auscultated for the presence of bruits, using the bell of the stethoscope. Bruits are created by turbulent flow over a partially obstructed artery and are always considered an abnormal finding. The aorta, the right and left renal arteries, and the iliac arteries should be auscultated.[5-7]

Percussion

Percussion of the patient focuses on one priority: (1) assessment of the deep organs. Percussion is used to elicit information about deep organs, such as the liver, spleen, and pancreas. Because the abdomen is a sensitive area, muscle tension may

TABLE 21-1	ABNORMAL ABDOMINAL SOUNDS
SOUND	**CAUSE**
Hyperactive bowel sounds (borborygmi), loud and prolonged	Hunger, gastroenteritis, or early intestinal obstruction
High-pitched, tinkling sounds	Intestinal air and fluid under pressure; characteristic of early intestinal obstruction
Decreased (hypoactive) bowel sounds, infrequent and abnormally faint sounds	Possible peritonitis or ileus
Absence of bowel sounds (confirmed only after auscultation of all four quadrants and continuous auscultation for 5 min)	Temporary loss of intestinal motility, as occurs with complete ileus
Friction rubs, high-pitched sounds heard over liver and spleen (RUQ and LUQ), synchronous with respiration	Pathological conditions such as tumors or infection that cause inflammation of organ's peritoneal covering
Bruits, audible swishing sounds that may be heard over aortic, iliac, renal, and femoral arteries	Abnormality of blood flow (requires additional evaluation to determine specific disorder)
Venous hum, low-pitched, continuous sound	Increased collateral circulation between portal and systemic venous systems

From Doughty DB, Jackson DB: *Gastrointestinal disorders*, St Louis, 1993, Mosby.
LUQ, left upper quadrant; *RUQ*, right upper quadrant.

interfere with this part of the assessment. Percussion often helps relax tense muscles, and it is performed before palpation. Percussion in the absence of disease helps to delineate the position and size of the liver and spleen, and it assists in the detection of fluid, gaseous distention, and masses in the abdomen.[5]

Assessment of Deep Organs

Percussion should proceed systematically and lightly in all four quadrants. Normal findings include tympany over the stomach when empty, tympany or hyperresonance over the intestine, and dullness over the liver and spleen. Abnormal areas of dullness may indicate an underlying mass. Solid masses, enlarged organs, and a distended bladder also produce areas of dullness. Dullness over both flanks may indicate ascites and necessitates further assessment.[6]

Palpation

Palpation of the patient focuses on one priority: (1) detection of abdominal pathological conditions. Both light and deep palpation of each organ and quadrant should be completed. Light palpation, which has a palpation depth of

TABLE 21-2	SELECTED LABORATORY STUDIES OF GASTROINTESTINAL FUNCTION	
TEST	**NORMAL FINDINGS**	**CLINICAL SIGNIFICANCE OF ABNORMAL FINDINGS**
Stool studies	Resident microorganisms: clostridia, enterococci, *Pseudomonas*, a few yeasts	Detection of *Salmonella typhi* (typhoid fever), *Shigella* (dysentery), *Vibrio cholerae* (cholera), *Yersinia* (enterocolitis), *Escherichia coli* (gastroenteritis), *Staphylococcus aureus* (food poisoning), *Clostridium botulinum* (food poisoning), *Clostridium perfringens* (food poisoning), *Aeromonas* (gastroenteritis)
	Fat: 2-6 g/24 hr	Steatorrhea (increased values) can result from intestinal malabsorption or pancreatic insufficiency.
	Pus: none	Large amounts of pus are associated with chronic ulcerative colitis, abscesses, and anorectal fistula.
	Occult blood: none (ortho-toluidine or guaiac test)	Positive test results associated with bleeding
	Ova and parasites: none	Detection of *Entamoeba histolytica* (amebiasis), *Giardia lamblia* (giardiasis), and worms
D-Xylose absorption	5-hr urinary excretion: 4.5 g/L Peak blood level: >30 mg/dL	Differentiation of pancreatic steatorrhea (normal D-xylose absorption) from intestinal steatorrhea (impaired D-xylose absorption)
Gastric acid stimulation	11-20 mEq/hr after stimulation	Detection of duodenal ulcers, Zollinger-Ellison syndrome (increased values), gastric atrophy, gastric carcinoma (decreased values)
Manometry*	Values vary at different levels of the intestine	Inadequate swallowing, motility, sphincter function
Culture and sensitivity of duodenal contents	No pathogens	Detection of *Salmonella typhi* (typhoid fever)

From McCance KL, et al, editors: *Pathophysiology: The biologic basis for disease in adults and children*, ed 6, St Louis, 2010, Mosby.
*Use of water-filled catheters connected to pressure transducers passed into the esophagus, stomach, colon, or rectum to evaluate contractility.

approximately 1 cm, assesses to the depth of the skin and fascia. Deep palpation assesses the *rectus abdominis* muscle and is performed bimanually to a depth of 4 to 5 cm. Deep palpation is most helpful in detecting abdominal masses. Areas in which the patient complains of tenderness should be palpated last.[6]

Detection of Abdominal Pathological Conditions

Normal findings include no areas of tenderness or pain, no masses, and no hardened areas. Persistent involuntary guarding may indicate peritoneal inflammation, particularly if it continues even after relaxation techniques are used. Rebound tenderness, in which pain increases with quick release of a palpated area, indicates an inflamed peritoneum.[4]

LABORATORY STUDIES

The value of various laboratory studies used to diagnose and treat diseases of the gastrointestinal system has been emphasized often. However, no single study provides an overall picture of the various organs' functional state, and no single value is predictive by itself. Laboratory studies used in the assessment of gastrointestinal function, liver function, and pancreatic function are found in Tables 21-2, 21-3, and 21-4, respectively.

DIAGNOSTIC PROCEDURES

Table 21-5 presents an overview of the various diagnostic procedures used to evaluate the patient with GI dysfunction.

Nursing Management

The nursing management of a patient undergoing a diagnostic procedure involves a variety of interventions. **Nursing priorities include (1) preparing the patient psychologically and physically for the procedure, (2) monitoring the patient's responses to the procedure, and (3) assessing the patient after the procedure.** Preparing the patient includes teaching the patient about the procedure, answering any questions, and transporting and positioning the patient for the procedure. Monitoring the patient's responses to the procedure includes observing the patient for signs of pain, anxiety, or hemorrhage and monitoring vital signs. Assessing the patient after the procedure includes observing for complications of the procedure and medicating the patient for any postprocedural discomfort. **Any evidence of gastrointestinal bleeding should be immediately reported to the physician, and emergency measures to maintain circulation must be initiated.**[8]

TABLE 21-3   COMMON LABORATORY STUDIES OF LIVER FUNCTION

TEST	NORMAL VALUE	INTERPRETATION
Serum Enzymes		
Alkaline phosphatase	13-39 units/mL	Increases with biliary obstruction and cholestatic hepatitis
Aspartate aminotransferase (AST; formerly serum glutamate oxaloacetate transaminase [SGOT])	5-40 units/mL	Increases with hepatocellular injury
Alanine aminotransferase (ALT; formerly serum glutamate pyruvate transaminase [SGPT])	5-35 units/mL	Increases with hepatocellular injury
Lactate dehydrogenase (LDH)	200-500 units/mL	Isoenzyme LD_5 is elevated with hypoxic and primary liver injury
5'-Nucleotidase	2-11 units/mL	Increases with increase in alkaline phosphatase and cholestatic disorders
Bilirubin Metabolism		
Serum bilirubin		
• Indirect (unconjugated)	<0.8 mg/dL	Increases with hemolysis (lysis of red blood cells)
• Direct (conjugated)	0.2-0.4 mg/dL	Increases with hepatocellular injury or obstruction
Total	<1.0 mg/dL	Increases with biliary obstruction
Urine bilirubin	0	Decreases with biliary obstruction
Urine urobilinogen	0-4 mg/24 hr	Increases with hemolysis or shunting or portal blood flow
Serum Proteins		
Albumin	3.3-5.5 g/dL	Reduced with hepatocellular injury
Globulin	2.5-3.5 g/dL	Increases with hepatitis
Total	6-7 g/dL	
Albumin-to-globulin (A/G) ratio	1.5-2.5:1	Ratio reverses with chronic hepatitis or other chronic liver disease
Transferrin	250-300 µg/dL	Liver damage with decreased values, iron deficiency with increased values
Alpha-fetoprotein	6-20 ng/mL	Elevated values in primary hepatocellular carcinoma
Blood Clotting Functions		
Prothrombin time	11.5-14 sec or 90%-100% of control	Increases with chronic liver disease (cirrhosis) or vitamin K deficiency
Partial thromboplastin time	25-40 sec	Increases with severe liver disease or heparin therapy
Bromsulphalein (BSP) excretion	<6% retention in 45 min	Increased retention with hepatocellular injury

From McCance KL, et al, editors: *Pathophysiology: The biologic basis for disease in adults and children*, ed 6, St Louis, 2010, Mosby.

TABLE 21-4   COMMON LABORATORY STUDIES OF PANCREATIC FUNCTION

TEST	NORMAL VALUE	CLINICAL SIGNIFICANCE
Serum amylase	60-180 Somogyi units/mL	Elevated levels with pancreatic inflammation
Serum lipase	1.5 Somogyi units/mL	Elevated levels with pancreatic inflammation (may be elevated with other conditions; differentiates with amylase, isoenzyme study)
Urine amylase	35-260 Somogyi units/hr	Elevated levels with pancreatic inflammation
Secretin test	Volume 1.8 mL/kg/hr Bicarbonate concentration: >80 mEq/L Bicarbonate output: >10 mEq/L/30 sec	Decreased volume with pancreatic disease because secretin stimulates pancreatic secretion
Stool fat	2-5 g/25 hr	Measures fatty acids: decreased pancreatic lipase increases stool fat

From McCance KL, et al, editors: *Pathophysiology: The biologic basis for disease in adults and children*, ed 6, St Louis, 2010, Mosby.

TABLE 21-5 GASTROINTESTINAL DIAGNOSTIC STUDIES

STUDY	EVALUATES	COMMENTS

Angiography: celiac or mesenteric	• Evaluates portal vasculature
	• Diagnoses source of GI bleeding
	• Evaluates cirrhosis, portal hypertension, vascular damage resulting from trauma, intestinal ischemia, and tumors
	• May be used to treat GI bleeding using vasopressin
		• Perform bowel preparation (e.g., cathartics) as prescribed.
		• Keep patient NPO for 8 hours before the study.
		• Sedative usually is prescribed before the procedure.
		• Contrast media used:
		  • Check for allergy to iodine before the study.
		  • Monitor for allergic reaction following procedure.
		  • Ensure hydration following procedure.
		Postprocedure
		• Keep extremity in which catheter was placed immobilized in a straight position for 6-12 hours.
		• Monitor arterial puncture point for hemorrhage or hematoma.
		• Monitor neurovascular status of affected limb.
		• Monitor for indications of systemic emboli.

Barium enema (also called *lower GI series*) NOTE: Meglumine diatrizoate (Gastrografin) may be used especially if bowel perforation is suspected.	• Visualizes the movement, position, and filling of various segments of the colon after instillation of barium by enema • Diagnoses colorectal lesions, diverticulitis, inflammatory bowel disease, strictures, fistulae • Evaluates colon size, length, and patency	• Maintain low-fiber diet for 1 to 3 days before the study. • Perform bowel preparation with bowel irrigation (e.g., GoLYTELY) and cathartics. • Keep patient NPO for 8-12 hours before study. • Cathartics must be given after study. • Contraindicated if bowel perforation or obstruction exists.
Barium swallow, upper GI series, and small bowel follow-through NOTE: Tests are ordered according to which area or areas need to be evaluated, such as the upper GI with small bowel follow-through evaluates stomach, pylorus, duodenum; barium swallow with upper GI evaluates esophagus, stomach, pylorus. NOTE: Meglumine diatrizoate (Gastrografin) may be used especially if bowel perforation is suspected.	• Visualizes the position, shape, and activity of the esophagus, stomach, duodenum, and jejunum • Diagnoses esophageal lesions, varices, or esophageal motility disorders, hiatal hernia, gastric ulcers and tumors, small bowel obstruction, small bowel lesions, Crohn's disease • Evaluates gastric and small bowel motility	• Perform preparation with bowel irrigation (e.g., GoLYTELY) and cathartics. • Keep patient NPO for 8-12 hours before study. • Cathartics must be given after study. • Contraindicated if bowel perforation or obstruction exists.
Cholecystography (oral, IV, intravenous, percutaneous transhepatic, or common bile duct)	• Assesses gallbladder function, patency of the biliary system, and presence of gallstones • Diagnoses extrahepatic or intrahepatic jaundice, biliary calculi, biliary obstruction, and common bile duct injury	• Percutaneous transhepatic cholangiography is contraindicated in patients with bleeding disorders. • May have a fatty meal the day before the study, but the evening meal is fat free. • Enema may be given the evening before the study. • Keep patient NPO 8-12 hours before the study.

TABLE 21-5   GASTROINTESTINAL DIAGNOSTIC STUDIES—cont'd

STUDY	EVALUATES	COMMENTS

		• Contrast medium is administered orally the evening before the study, administered IV immediately before the study, injected percutaneously into the bile duct, or injected directly into the common bile duct during surgery.
		   • Check for allergy to iodine before the study.
		   • Monitor for allergic reaction following procedure.
		   • Ensure hydration following procedure.
		• Monitor for clinical indications of bile leakage, hemorrhage, or peritonitis after percutaneous transhepatic cholangiography.

Computed tomography scan of abdomen	• Diagnoses tumors, pancreatic cancer or cysts, pancreatitis, biliary tract disorders, obstructive versus nonobstructive jaundice, cirrhosis, liver metastases, ascites, lymph node metastases, and aneurysm
	• Evaluates vasculature and focal points found on nuclear scans
	• Used to direct biopsy of tumors or aspiration of abscess
		• No special preparation required.
		• Contrast medium may be used; if used:
		   • Check for allergy to iodine before the study.
		   • Monitor for allergic reaction postprocedure.
		   • Ensure hydration postprocedure.

Endoscopic retrograde cholangiopancreatography	• Diagnoses biliary stones, ductal stricture, ductal compression, and neoplasms of the pancreas and biliary system • Evaluates patency of biliary and pancreatic ducts, jaundice, pancreatitis, cholecystitis, and hepatitis	• Same as for esophagogastroduodenoscopy. • Contraindicated if patient is uncooperative or if bilirubin is greater than 3.5 mg/dL. • Monitor for clinical indications of pancreatitis (most common complication) after study. • Monitor for clinical indications of sepsis.
Endoscopy • Esophagogastroduodenoscopy • Colonoscopy • Proctosigmoidoscopy	• Directly visualizes mucosa of areas of the GI tract • Esophagogastroduodenoscopy can be extended to visualize the pancreas and gallbladder • Esophagogastroduodenoscopy is used to diagnose esophagitis, esophageal ulcers, esophageal strictures, esophageal varices, hiatal hernia, gastritis, gastric ulcers, pyloric obstruction, pernicious anemia, foreign bodies, and duodenal inflammation or ulcers; it evaluates esophageal or gastric motility, bleeding, lesions, and status of surgical anastomoses • Esophagoscopy or gastroscopy also may be used therapeutically for sclerosis of varices • Proctosigmoidoscopy diagnoses rectosigmoid cancer, strictures, polyps, inflammatory processes, and hemorrhoids; it evaluates bleeding from rectosigmoid and surgical anastomoses • Colonoscopy diagnoses diverticular disease, obstruction, strictures, radiation injury, polyps, neoplasms, bleeding, and ischemia	• Sedation may be prescribed, especially for colonoscopy. • Bowel preparation with gastric irrigation (e.g., GoLYTELY) and cathartics required before lower GI endoscopy. • Keep patient NPO 4-8 hours before study. • Keep patient NPO until gag reflex returns if sedation used. • Monitor closely after procedure for clinical indications of perforation or hemorrhage.

Continued

TABLE 21-5　**GASTROINTESTINAL DIAGNOSTIC STUDIES—cont'd**

STUDY	EVALUATES	COMMENTS
	• Colonoscopy or sigmoidoscopy may be used therapeutically for removal of polyps • Biopsies may be taken during any endoscopy	
Flat plate of abdomen (may also be referred to as KUB)	• Diagnoses perforated viscus, paralytic ileus, mechanical obstruction, and intraabdominal mass • Evaluates the distribution of visceral gas (and identifies free air in the peritoneum indicative of bowel perforation) • Evaluates organ size	• No preparation required.

Liver biopsy	• Obtains tissue specimen for microscopic evaluation
	• Diagnoses liver disease or malignancy
		• May be performed open or closed.
		  • Open is done in surgery.
		  • Closed biopsy may be done at bedside.
		• Clotting profile is evaluated preprocedure.
		  • Closed biopsy is contraindicated if platelet count is less than 100,000 platelets/mm^3.
		• Patient must be cooperative because he or she must take a deep breath and hold it for closed biopsy.
		• Type and crossmatch for 2 units of blood preprocedure.
		• Keep patient NPO for 4-8 hours before study.
		Postprocedure
		• Position patient on right side for 2 hours.
		• Pressure dressing is applied, and the patient is on bed rest for 24 hours.
		• Observe for the following:
		  • Hemorrhage: hypotension, dyspnea (subphrenic hematoma)
		  • Pneumothorax: dyspnea; chest pain; diminished breath sounds on right; hypoxemia
		• Sepsis: fever; leukocytosis; rebound tenderness

Liver scan	• Diagnoses cirrhosis, hepatitis, tumors, abscesses, cysts, and tuberculosis	• No preparation required.
Magnetic resonance imaging	• Evaluates liver, biliary tree, pancreas, and spleen • Differentiation between cyst and solid mass • Diagnoses hepatic metastasis • Evaluates abscesses, fistulae, and source of GI bleeding • Used for staging of colorectal cancer	• Cannot be used in patients with any implanted metallic device, including pacemakers. • No special preparation required. • Cannot be done on a patient being mechanically ventilated.
Paracentesis	• Analysis of fluid removed during peritoneal tap • Diagnoses intraperitoneal bleeding with diagnostic peritoneal lavage	• Monitor for peritoneal leakage after tap. • Monitor for clinical indications of infection or peritonitis after tap.
Percutaneous transhepatic portography	• Diagnoses esophageal varices and visualizes portal venous circulation	• As for angiography
Percutaneous transhepatic cholangiography	• Diagnoses extrahepatic or intrahepatic jaundice, biliary calculi, bile duct obstruction, and bile duct injury • Evaluates the patency of the biliary ductal system	• Contraindicated in uncorrected coagulopathy, allergy to iodine, severe ascites, or cholangitis. • Monitor closely for clinical indications of bleeding. • Monitor closely for clinical indications of peritonitis.

TABLE 21-5	**GASTROINTESTINAL DIAGNOSTIC STUDIES—cont'd**	
STUDY	**EVALUATES**	**COMMENTS**
Radionuclide imaging (hepatobiliary scintigraphy) • HIDA scan • PIPIDA scan	• Diagnoses hepatocellular disease, hepatic metastasis, biliary disease, lower GI bleeding, gastric reflux	• Keep patient NPO 2 hours before study.
Schilling test	• Evaluates ileal absorption of vitamin B_{12} • Diagnoses pernicious anemia caused by intrinsic factor and inadequate ileal absorption of intrinsic factor-vitamin B_{12} complex	• Intramuscular injections of vitamin B_{12} and oral radioactive B_{12} are given, and 24-hour urine specimen is collected.
Ultrasound of abdomen	• Evaluates the pancreas, biliary ducts, gallbladder, and liver • Identifies tumor, abdominal abscesses, hepatocellular disease, splenomegaly, and pancreatic or splenic cysts • Differentiates obstructive from nonobstructive jaundice	• All barium must have been cleared from the GI tract before ultrasonography. • Keep patient NPO for 8 hours before study. • If for evaluation of gallbladder: fat-free meal the evening before study.

From Dennison RD: *Pass CCRN!*, ed 3, St Louis, 2007, Mosby.
GI, Gastrointestinal; *IV,* intravenous; *NPO,* nothing by mouth.

REFERENCES

1. O'Toole MT: Advanced assessment of the abdomen and gastrointestinal problems, *Nurs Clin North Am* 25(4):771, 1990.
2. Baid H: The process of conducting a physical assessment: a nursing perspective, *Br J Nurs* 15(13):710, 2006.
3. Seidel HM, et al: *Mosby's guide to physical examination*, ed 7, St Louis, 2010, Mosby.
4. Barkauskas V, et al: *Health & physical assessment*, ed 3, St Louis, 2002, Mosby.
5. Thompson JM, et al: *Mosby's clinical nursing*, ed 5, St Louis, 2002, Mosby.
6. O'Hanlon-Nicholas T: Basic assessment series: gastrointestinal system, *Am J Nurs* 98(4):48, 1998.
7. Baid H: A critical review of auscultating bowel sounds, *Br J Nurs* 18(18):1125, 2009.
8. Society of Gastroenterology Nurses and Associates Core Curriculum Committee: *Gastroenterology nursing: a core curriculum*, ed 3, St Louis, 2003, Mosby.

22

Gastrointestinal Disorders and Therapeutic Management

Sheryl E. Leary

evolve WEBSITE

OBJECTIVES

- Describe the etiology and pathophysiology of the major gastrointestinal (GI) disorders seen in the critical care unit.
- Identify the clinical manifestations of GI disorders.
- Explain the treatment of GI disorders.
- Discuss the nursing priorities for managing a patient with GI dysfunction.
- Outline the use and care of GI tubes.
- Depict the postoperative nursing management of a patient undergoing GI surgery or liver transplantation.

Understanding the pathology of a disease, the areas of assessment on which to focus, and the usual medical management allows the critical care nurse to accurately anticipate and plan nursing interventions. This chapter focuses on gastrointestinal disorders commonly seen in the critical care environment.

ACUTE GASTROINTESTINAL HEMORRHAGE

Gastrointestinal hemorrhage is a potentially life-threatening emergency that remains a common complication of critical illness[1] and results in 400,000 hospital admissions yearly.[2] Despite advances in medical knowledge and nursing care, the mortality rate for patients with acute gastrointestinal bleeding remains at 10%.[1,3]

Etiology

Gastrointestinal hemorrhage occurs from bleeding in the upper or lower gastrointestinal tract. The ligament of Treitz is the anatomic division used to differentiate between the two areas. Bleeding proximal to the ligament is considered to be upper gastrointestinal in origin, and bleeding distal to the ligament is considered to be lower gastrointestinal in origin.[1,4] The various causes of acute gastrointestinal hemorrhage are listed in Box 22-1.[4,5] Only the three main causes of gastrointestinal hemorrhage commonly seen in the intensive care unit (ICU) are discussed further.

Peptic Ulcer Disease

Peptic ulcer disease (gastric and duodenal ulcers), which results from the breakdown of the gastromucosal lining, is the leading cause of upper gastrointestinal hemorrhage, accounting for approximately 21% of cases.[4] Normally, protection of the gastric mucosa from the digestive effects of gastric secretions is accomplished in several ways. First, the gastroduodenal mucosa is coated by a glycoprotein mucous barrier that protects the surface of the epithelium from hydrogen ions and other noxious substances present in the gut lumen.[6,7] Adequate gastric mucosal blood flow is necessary to maintain this mucosal barrier function. Second, gastroduodenal epithelial cells are protected structurally against damage from acid and pepsin because they are connected by tight junctions that help prevent acid penetration. Third, prostaglandins and nitric oxide protect the mucosal barrier by stimulating mucus and bicarbonate secretion and inhibiting the secretion of acid.[7]

Peptic ulceration occurs when these protective mechanisms cease to function, allowing gastroduodenal mucosal breakdown. After the mucosal lining is penetrated, gastric secretions autodigest the layers of the stomach or duodenum, leading to injury of the mucosal and submucosal layers. This results in damaged blood vessels and subsequent hemorrhage. The two main causes of disruption of gastroduodenal mucosal resistance are nonsteroidal antiinflammatory drugs and the bacterial action of *Helicobacter pylori*.[4,8,9]

Stress-Related Mucosal Disease

Stress-related mucosal disease (SRMD) is an acute erosive gastritis that covers both types of mucosal lesions that are often found in the critically ill patient: stress-related injury and discrete stress ulcers.[10,11] These abnormalities develop within hours of admission.[10] They range from superficial mucosal erosions to deep focal lesions and usually affect the upper gastrointestinal tract.[10] SRMD occurs by means of the same pathophysiological mechanisms as peptic ulcer disease, but the main cause of disruption of gastric mucosal resistance is increased acid production and decreased mucosal blood flow, resulting in ischemia and degeneration of the mucosal lining.[10,11] Patients at risk include those in situations of high physiological stress, such as occur with mechanical ventilation, extensive burns, severe trauma, major surgery, shock, sepsis, coagulopathy, or acute neurological disease.[10,11] Gastroduodenal lesions are estimated to occur in 75% to 100% of ICU patients within 24 hours of admission.[10] SRMD is a leading cause of upper gastrointestinal hemorrhage, accounting for approximately 15% of cases.[11]

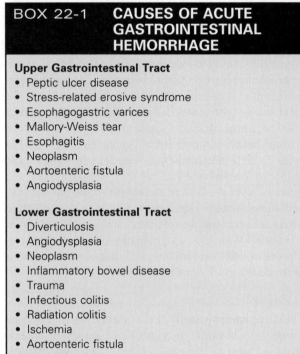

BOX 22-1 **CAUSES OF ACUTE GASTROINTESTINAL HEMORRHAGE**

Upper Gastrointestinal Tract
- Peptic ulcer disease
- Stress-related erosive syndrome
- Esophagogastric varices
- Mallory-Weiss tear
- Esophagitis
- Neoplasm
- Aortoenteric fistula
- Angiodysplasia

Lower Gastrointestinal Tract
- Diverticulosis
- Angiodysplasia
- Neoplasm
- Inflammatory bowel disease
- Trauma
- Infectious colitis
- Radiation colitis
- Ischemia
- Aortoenteric fistula
- Hemorrhoids

Esophagogastric Varices

Esophagogastric varices are engorged and distended blood vessels of the esophagus and proximal stomach that develop as a result of portal hypertension caused by hepatic cirrhosis, a chronic disease of the liver that results in damage to the liver sinusoids (Figure 22-1). Without adequate sinusoid function, resistance to portal blood flow is increased, and pressures within the liver are elevated. This leads to increased portal venous pressure (portal hypertension), causing collateral circulation to divert portal blood from areas of high pressure within the liver to adjacent areas of low pressure outside the liver, such as into the veins of the esophagus, the spleen, the intestines, and the stomach. The tiny, thin-walled vessels of the esophagus and proximal stomach that receive this diverted blood lack sturdy mucosal protection. The vessels become engorged and dilated, forming esophagogastric varices that are vulnerable to damage from gastric secretions and that may result in subsequent rupture and massive hemorrhage.[12] The risk of variceal bleeding increases with disease severity and variceal size, but overall, bleeding occurs in up to 30% of patients with medium or large varices, and only 50% of patients stop bleeding spontaneously.[12,13]

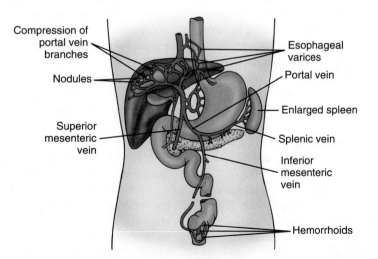

FIGURE 22-1 Esophageal varices caused by cirrhosis. (Modified from Powell LW, Piper DW: *Fundamentals of gastroenterology,* Sydney, 1991, McGraw-Hill. Reproduced with permission of the McGraw-Hill Companies.)

Pathophysiology

Gastrointestinal hemorrhage is a life-threatening disorder that is characterized by acute, massive bleeding. Regardless of the cause, acute gastrointestinal hemorrhage results in hypovolemic shock, initiation of the shock response, and development of multiple organ dysfunction syndrome if left untreated (Concept Map on Acute Gastrointestinal Hemorrhage).[7] However, the most common cause of death in cases of gastrointestinal hemorrhage is exacerbation of the underlying disease, not intractable hypovolemic shock.

Assessment and Diagnosis

The initial clinical presentation of the patient with acute gastrointestinal hemorrhage is that of a patient in hypovolemic shock, and the clinical presentation depends on the amount of blood lost (Table 22-1).[7] Hematemesis (bright red or brown, coffee grounds emesis), hematochezia (bright red stools), and melena (black, tarry, or dark red stools) are the hallmarks of gastrointestinal hemorrhage.[1,4,5]

Hematemesis

The patient who is vomiting blood is usually bleeding from a source above the duodenojejunal junction; reverse peristalsis is seldom sufficient to cause hematemesis if the bleeding point is below this area. The hematemesis may be bright red or look like coffee grounds, depending on the amount of gastric contents at the time of bleeding and the length of time the blood has been in contact with gastric secretions. Gastric acid converts bright red hemoglobin to brown hematin, accounting for the coffee grounds appearance of the emesis. Bright red emesis results from profuse bleeding with little contact with gastric secretions.[1]

Hematochezia and Melena

The presence of blood in the gastrointestinal tract results in increased peristalsis and diarrhea. Hematochezia (bright red stool) occurs from massive lower gastrointestinal hemorrhage and, if rapid enough, upper gastrointestinal hemorrhage. Melena (black, tarry, or dark red stool) occurs from digestion of blood from an upper gastrointestinal hemorrhage and may take several days to clear after the bleeding has stopped.[2,4]

Laboratory Studies

Laboratory tests can help to determine the extent of bleeding, although the patient's hemoglobin level and hematocrit are poor indicators of the severity of blood loss if the bleeding is acute. As whole blood is lost, plasma and red blood cells are lost in the same proportion; if the patient's hematocrit is 45% before a bleeding episode, it will be 45% several hours later.[7] It may take as long as 72 hours for the redistribution of plasma from the extravascular space to the intravascular space to occur and cause the patient's hemoglobin level and hematocrit value to decrease.[14]

Diagnostic Procedures

To isolate and treat the source of bleeding, an urgent fiberoptic endoscopy is usually undertaken. If performed within 12 hours of the bleeding event, endoscopy therapy has a 90% effectiveness rate in achieving hemostasis and reducing mortality.[1,2] Before endoscopy, the patient must be hemodynamically stabilized.[15] Tagged red blood cell scanning or angiography, or both, may be done to assist with localizing and treating a bleeding lesion in the gastrointestinal tract when it is impossible to clearly view the gastrointestinal tract because of continued active bleeding.[1,5]

Medical Management

To reduce mortality related to gastrointestinal hemorrhage, patients at risk should be identified early, and interventions should be implemented to reduce gastric acidity and support the gastric mucosal defense mechanisms. Management of the patient at risk for gastrointestinal hemorrhage should include prophylactic administration of pharmacological agents for gastric acid neutralization. These agents include antacids, histamine-2 (H_2) antagonists, cytoprotective agents, and proton-pump inhibitors (PPIs).[10,11]

Priorities in the medical management of the patient with gastrointestinal hemorrhage include airway protection, fluid resuscitation to achieve hemodynamic stability, correction of comorbid conditions (e.g., coagulopathy), therapeutic procedures to control or stop bleeding, and diagnostic procedures to determine the exact cause of the bleeding.[1,2,15]

Stabilization

The initial treatment priority is the restoration of adequate circulating blood volume to treat or prevent shock. This is accomplished with the administration of intravenous infusions of crystalloids, blood, and blood products.[13,15,16] Hemodynamic monitoring can help to guide fluid replacement therapy,[8] particularly in patients at risk for cardiac failure. Supplemental oxygen therapy is initiated to increase oxygen delivery and improve tissue perfusion.[2,5] Intubation may be necessary in the patient at risk for aspiration or to facilitate gastric lavage.[15] A large nasogastric tube may be inserted to confirm the diagnosis of active bleeding and to prepare the esophagus, stomach, and proximal duodenum for endoscopic evaluation.[1,2] A urinary drainage catheter should be inserted to monitor urine output.[14]

Controlling the Bleeding

Interventions to control bleeding are the second priority for the patient with gastrointestinal hemorrhage.

Peptic Ulcer Disease. In the patient with gastrointestinal hemorrhage related to peptic ulcer disease, bleeding hemostasis may be accomplished by endoscopic injection therapy in conjunction with thermal or hemostatic clips.[2,17] Endoscopic thermal therapy uses heat to cauterize the bleeding vessel, and endoscopic injection therapy uses a variety of agents such as hypertonic saline, epinephrine, ethanol, and sclerosants to induce localized vasoconstriction of the

Concept Map: Acute Gastrointestinal Hemorrhage

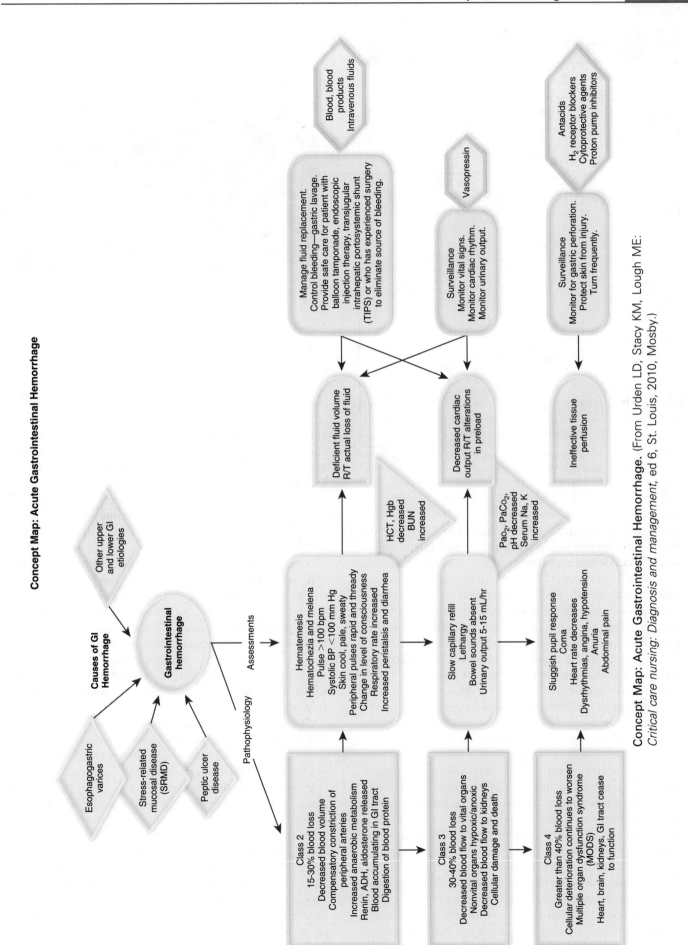

Concept Map: Acute Gastrointestinal Hemorrhage. (From Urden LD, Stacy KM, Lough ME: *Critical care nursing: Diagnosis and management*, ed 6, St. Louis, 2010, Mosby.)

TABLE 22-1		CLINICAL CLASSIFICATION OF HEMORRHAGE
CLASS	**BLOOD LOSS (%)**	**CLINICAL SIGNS AND SYMPTOMS**
1	≤15	Pulse rate: normal or <100 beats/min (supine) Capillary refill <3 sec Urine output: adequate (30-35 mL/hr) Orthostatic hypotension Apprehensive
2	15-30	Pulse rate: increased (>100 beats/min) Capillary refill: sluggish Pulse pressure: decreased Blood pressure: normal (supine) Tachypnea Urine output: low (25-30 mL/hr)
3	30-40	Pulse rate: 120+ beats/min (supine) Hypotension Skin: cool, pale Confused Hyperventilating Urine output: low (5-15 mL/hr)
4	≥40	Profoundly hypotensive Pulse rate: 140+ beats/min Confused, lethargic Urine output minimal

From Klein DG: Physiologic response to traumatic shock, *AACN Clin Issues Crit Care Nurs* 1(3):505, 1990.

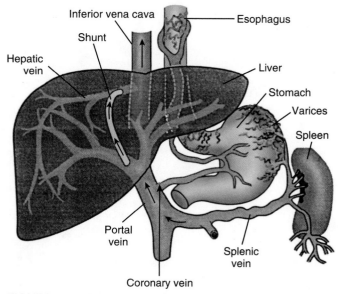

FIGURE 22-2 Anatomic location of the transjugular intrahepatic portosystemic shunt (TIPS). (From Vargas HE, et al: Management of portal hypertension-related bleeding, *Surg Clin North Am* 79[1]:1, 1999.)

bleeding vessel.[1,2,17] Intraarterial infusion of vasopressin into the gastric artery or intraarterial injection of an embolizing agent (e.g., Gelfoam pledgets, polyvinyl alcohol particles, coils) can be performed during arteriography to control bleeding after the site has been identified.[2]

Stress-Related Mucosal Disease. In the patient with gastrointestinal hemorrhage caused by SRMD, bleeding hemostasis may be accomplished by intraarterial infusion of vasopressin and intraarterial embolization. Endoscopic therapies provide minimal benefit because of the diffuse nature of the disease.[15]

Esophagogastric Varices. In acute variceal hemorrhage, control of bleeding may be initially accomplished through the use of pharmacological agents and endoscopic variceal ligation.[13] Intravenous vasopressin, somatostatin, and octreotide can reduce portal venous pressure and slow variceal hemorrhaging by constricting the splanchnic arteriolar bed.[18] Endoscopic variceal ligation is the preferred endoscopic therapy for controlling acute gastrointestinal bleeding related to varices. Bands are placed around the varices to create an obstruction to stop the bleeding.[13]

If these initial therapies fail, transjugular intrahepatic portosystemic shunting (TIPS) or esophagogastric balloon tamponade may be necessary. In a TIPS procedure, a channel between the systemic and portal venous systems is created to redirect portal blood, thereby reducing portal hypertension

and decompressing the varices to control bleeding (Figure 22-2).[1,13] Balloon tamponade tubes (Sengstaken-Blakemore, Linton, and Minnesota tubes) stop hemorrhaging by applying direct pressure against bleeding vessels while decompressing the stomach.[19] This therapy is rarely needed anymore given the success rate of the other therapies.

Surgical Intervention

The patient who remains hemodynamically unstable despite volume replacement may need urgent surgery.

Peptic Ulcer Disease. The operative procedure of choice to control bleeding from peptic ulcer disease is a vagotomy and pyloroplasty. During this procedure, the vagus nerve to the stomach is severed, eliminating the autonomic stimulus to the gastric cells and reducing hydrochloric acid production. Because the vagus nerve also stimulates motility, a pyloroplasty is performed to provide for gastric emptying.[9]

Stress-Related Mucosal Disease. Several operative procedures can be used to control bleeding from SRMD. A total gastrectomy is performed when bleeding is generalized. The ulcers are oversewn when bleeding is localized.[20] Total gastrectomy involves the complete removal of the stomach with anastomosis of the esophagus to the jejunum. During an oversew of the ulcers, the bleeding vessel is ligated, and the ulcer crater is closed.[16,20]

Esophagogastric Varices. Operative procedures to control bleeding gastroesophageal varices include portacaval shunt, mesocaval shunt, and splenorenal shunt (Figure 22-3).[20] These shunt procedures are also referred to as decompression procedures, because they result in the diversion of portal blood flow away from the liver and decompression

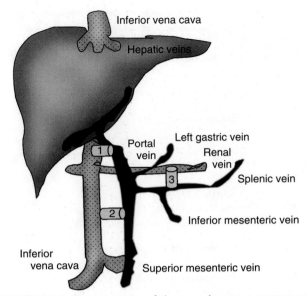

FIGURE 22-3 The anatomy of the portal venous system and the sites in which surgical anastomoses are made to shunt blood from the portal *(dark)* to the systemic *(light)* venous circulation. Several sites are used for surgical portal decompression: (1) portacaval shunt; (2) mesocaval shunt; (3) splenorenal shunt. (From Luketic VA, Sanyal AJ: Esophageal varices. II. TIPS (transjugular intrahepatic portosystemic shunt) and surgical therapy, *Gastroenterol Clin North Am* 29[2]:387, 2000.)

of the portal system. The portacaval shunt procedure has two variations. An end-to-side portacaval shunt procedure involves the ligation of the hepatic end of the portal vein with subsequent anastomosis to the vena cava. During a side-to-side portacaval shunt procedure, the side of the portal vein is anastomosed to the side of the vena cava. A mesocaval shunt procedure involves the insertion of a graft between the superior mesenteric artery and the vena cava. During a distal splenorenal shunt procedure, the splenic vein is detached from the portal vein and anastomosed to the left renal vein.[20]

Nursing Management

All critically ill patients should be considered at risk for stress ulcers and therefore gastrointestinal hemorrhage. Patients at risk also should be assessed for the presence of bright red or coffee grounds emesis; bloody nasogastric aspirate; and bright red, black, or dark red stools. Any signs of bleeding should be promptly reported to the physician.

Nursing management of a patient experiencing acute gastrointestinal hemorrhage incorporates a variety of nursing diagnoses (Nursing Diagnosis Priorities Box on Acute Gastrointestinal Hemorrhage). **Nursing priorities are directed toward (1) administering volume replacement, (2) controlling the bleeding, (3) providing comfort and emotional support, (4) maintaining surveillance for complications, and (5) educating the patient and family.**

Administering Volume Replacement

Measures to facilitate volume replacement include obtaining intravenous access and administering prescribed fluids and blood products. Two large-diameter peripheral intravenous catheters should be inserted to facilitate the rapid administration of prescribed fluids.[13]

Controlling the Bleeding

One measure to control active bleeding is gastric lavage. It is used to decrease gastric mucosal blood flow and evacuate blood from the stomach. Gastric lavage is performed by inserting a large-bore nasogastric tube into the stomach and irrigating it with normal saline or water until the returned solution is clear. It is important to keep accurate records of the amount of fluid instilled and aspirated to ascertain the true amount of bleeding.[1] Historically, iced saline was favored as a lavage irrigant. Research has shown, however, that low-temperature fluids shift the oxyhemoglobin dissociation curve to the left, decrease oxygen delivery to vital organs, and prolong bleeding time and prothrombin time. Iced saline also may further aggravate bleeding; therefore room-temperature water or saline is the preferred irrigant for use in gastric lavage.[21]

Maintaining Surveillance for Complications

The patient should be continuously observed for signs of gastric perforation. Although a rare complication, gastric perforation constitutes a surgical emergency. Signs and symptoms include sudden, severe, generalized abdominal pain with significant rebound tenderness and rigidity. Perforation should be suspected when fever, leukocytosis, and tachycardia persist despite adequate volume replacement.[9]

Educating the Patient and Family

Early in the hospital stay, the patient and family should be taught about acute gastrointestinal hemorrhage and its causes and treatments. As the patient moves toward discharge, teaching should focus on the interventions necessary for preventing the recurrence of the precipitating disorder. If an alcohol abuser, the patient should be encouraged to stop drinking and be referred to an alcohol cessation program (Patient Education Box on Acute Gastrointestinal Hemorrhage). Collaborative management of the patient is outlined in the Box on Collaborative Management of Acute Gastrointestinal Hemorrhage.

PATIENT EDUCATION

Acute Gastrointestinal Hemorrhage

- Gastrointestinal hemorrhage
- Specific cause
- Precipitating factor modification
- Interventions to reduce further bleeding episodes
- Importance of taking medications
- Lifestyle changes
- Stress management
- Diet modifications
- Alcohol cessation
- Smoking cessation

COLLABORATIVE MANAGEMENT

Acute Gastrointestinal Hemorrhage

- Initiate fluid resuscitation to achieve hemodynamic stability.
  - Crystalloids
  - Colloids
  - Blood and blood products
- Determine the cause of the bleeding.
  - Gastric lavage
- Control bleeding.
  - Endoscopic interventions
  - Vasopressin, somatostatin, octreotide
  - Transjugular intrahepatic portosystemic shunting
  - Surgery
- Provide comfort and emotional support.
- Maintain surveillance for complications.
  - Hypovolemic shock
  - Gastric perforation

ACUTE PANCREATITIS

Acute pancreatitis is an inflammation of the pancreas that produces exocrine and endocrine dysfunction that may also involve surrounding tissues and/or remote organ systems. The clinical course can range from a mild, self-limiting disease to a systemic process characterized by organ failure, sepsis, and death. In approximately 80% of patients, it takes the milder form of *edematous interstitial pancreatitis,* whereas the other 20% develop severe *acute necrotizing pancreatitis.*[22] Reported mortality rates for acute pancreatitis range from 2% to 15% overall and from 20% to 50% for patients with severe disease.[22,23] Several prognostic scoring systems have been

---

BOX 22-2 **RANSON'S CRITERIA FOR ESTIMATING THE SEVERITY OF ACUTE PANCREATITIS**

At Admission
- Age >55 years
- Hypotension
- Abnormal pulmonary findings
- Abdominal mass
- Hemorrhagic or discolored peritoneal fluid
- Increased serum LDH levels (>350 units/L)
- AST >250 units/L
- Leukocytosis (>16,000/mm^3)
- Hyperglycemia (>200 mg/dL; no diabetic history)
- Neurological deficit (confusion, localizing signs)

During Initial 48 Hours of Hospitalization
- Fall in hematocrit >10% with hydration or hematocrit <30%
- Necessity for massive fluid and colloid replacement
- Hypocalcemia (<8 mg/dL)
- Arterial Po$_2$ <60 mm Hg with or without acute respiratory distress syndrome
- Hypoalbuminemia (<3.2 mg/dL)
- Base deficit >4 mEq/L
- Azotemia

From Latifi R, et al: Nutritional management of acute and chronic pancreatitis, *Surg Clin North Am* 71(3):579, 1991.
AST, aspartate aminotransferase; *LDH,* lactate dehydrogenase; *PO$_2$,* partial pressure of oxygen.

---

developed to predict the severity of acute pancreatitis. One of the most commonly used is Ranson's criteria (Box 22-2). If the patient has 0 to 2 factors present, the predicted mortality rate is 2%; with 3 to 4 factors, the rate is 15%; with 5 to 6 factors, the rate is 40%; and with 7 to 8 factors, predicted mortality rate is 100%.[22,24]

Etiology

The two most common causes of acute pancreatitis are gallstones and alcoholism. Together, they account for approximately 80% of cases. Less common causes are quite diverse and include surgical trauma, hypercalcemia, various toxins, ischemia, infections, and the use of certain drugs (Box 22-3). In 10% to 20% of patients with acute pancreatitis, no etiologic factor can be determined.[23]

Pathophysiology

In acute pancreatitis, the normally inactive digestive enzymes become prematurely activated within the pancreas itself, leading to autodigestion of pancreatic tissue. The enzymes become activated through various mechanisms, including obstruction of or damage to the pancreatic duct system, alterations in the secretory processes of the acinar cells, infection, ischemia, and other unknown factors.[8,22]

Trypsin is the enzyme that becomes activated first. It initiates the autodigestion process by triggering the secretion of proteolytic enzymes such as kallikrein, chymotrypsin, elastase, phospholipase A, and lipase. Release of kallikrein and

BOX 22-3 CAUSES OF ACUTE PANCREATITIS

- Toxins (ethyl alcohol, methyl alcohol, scorpion venom, parathion)
- Biliary disease (stones, sludge, common bile duct obstruction)
- Drugs (sulfonamides, thiazide diuretics, furosemide, estrogens, tetracycline, pentamidine, procainamide, salicylates, steroids, cyclosporine, amphetamines, nonsteroidal antiinflammatory agents, valproic acid, azathioprine, allopurinol)
- Hypercalcemia (hyperparathyroidism)
- Hyperlipidemia
- Tumors
- Infections (bacterial, viral, parasitic)
- Trauma (abdominal, surgical, endoscopic)
- Ischemia
- Graft-versus-host disease
- Vasculitis
- Pregnancy
- Hypothermia
- Sphincter of Oddi dysfunction
- Systemic lupus erythematosus
- Ampullary stenosis
- Idiopathic cause

Data from Steer ML: Acute pancreatitis. In Taylor MB, editor: *Gastrointestinal emergencies*, Baltimore, 1992, Williams & Wilkins.

BOX 22-4 PRESENTING CLINICAL MANIFESTATIONS OF ACUTE PANCREATITIS

Mild Disease
- Pain
- Vomiting
- Nausea
- Fever
- Abdominal distention
- Abdominal guarding
- Abdominal tympany
- Hypoactive or absent bowel sounds

Severe Disease
- Peritoneal signs
- Ascites
- Jaundice
- Palpable abdominal mass
- Grey-Turner's sign
- Cullen's sign
- Signs of hypovolemic shock

From Krumberger JM: Acute pancreatitis, *Crit Care Nurs Clin North Am* 5(1):185, 1993.

chymotrypsin results in increased capillary membrane permeability, leading to leakage of fluid into the interstitium and the development of edema and relative hypovolemia. Elastase is the most harmful enzyme in terms of direct cell damage. It dissolves the elastic fibers of blood vessels and ducts, leading to hemorrhage. Phospholipase A, in the presence of bile, destroys the phospholipids of cell membranes, causing severe pancreatic and adipose tissue necrosis. Lipase flows into the damaged tissue and is absorbed into the systemic circulation, resulting in fat necrosis of the pancreas and surrounding tissues.[8,22]

The extent of injury to the pancreatic cells determines the type of acute pancreatitis that develops. If injury to the pancreatic cells is mild and without necrosis, edematous pancreatitis develops. The acinar cells appear structurally intact, and blood flow is maintained through small capillaries and venules. This form of acute pancreatitis is self-limiting. If injury to the pancreatic cells is severe, acute necrotizing pancreatitis develops.[22,23] Cellular destruction in pancreatic injury results in the release of toxic enzymes and inflammatory mediators into the systemic circulation and causes injury to vessels and other organs distant from the pancreas; this may result in systemic inflammatory response syndrome (SIRS), multiorgan failure, and death.[22,23] Local tissue injury results in infection, abscess and pseudocyst formation, disruption of the pancreatic duct, and severe hemorrhage with shock.[22]

Assessment and Diagnosis

The clinical manifestations of acute pancreatitis range from mild to severe and often mimic those of other disorders (Box 22-4). Acute onset of abdominal pain is a hallmark symptom.[23]

Epigastric to periumbilical pain may vary from mild and tolerable to severe and incapacitating. Many patients report a twisting or knifelike sensation that radiates to the low dorsal region of the back. The patient may obtain some comfort by leaning forward or assuming a semifetal position. Nausea and vomiting are common.[23] Other clinical findings include fever, diaphoresis, weakness, tachypnea, hypotension, and tachycardia. Depending on the extent of fluid loss and hemorrhage, the patient may exhibit signs of hypovolemic shock.[22,23,25]

Physical Examination

The results of physical assessment usually reveal hypoactive bowel sounds and abdominal tenderness, guarding, distention, and tympany. Findings that may indicate pancreatic hemorrhage include Grey Turner's sign (gray-blue discoloration of the flanks) and Cullen's sign (discoloration of the umbilical region); however, they are rare and usually seen several days into the illness.[22] A palpable abdominal mass indicates the presence of a pseudocyst or abscess.[26]

Laboratory Studies

Assessment of laboratory data usually demonstrates elevated levels of serum amylase and lipase. Serum lipase is more pancreas-specific than amylase and a more accurate marker for acute pancreatitis. Amylase is present in other body tissues, and other disorders (e.g., intraabdominal emergencies, renal insufficiency, salivary gland trauma, liver disease) may contribute to an elevated level. Unlike other serum enzymes, however, amylase is excreted in urine, and this clearance increases with acute pancreatitis. Measurement of urinary versus serum amylase should be considered in light

TABLE 22-2 LABORATORY TESTS AND DIAGNOSTIC PROCEDURES FOR ACUTE PANCREATITIS

STUDY	FINDING IN PANCREATITIS
Laboratory Studies	
Serum amylase	Elevated
Serum isoamylase	Elevated
Urine amylase	Elevated
Serum lipase (if available)	Elevated
Serum triglycerides	Elevated
Glucose	Elevated
Calcium	Decreased
Magnesium	Decreased
Potassium	Decreased
Albumin	Decreased or increased
White blood cell count	Elevated
Bilirubin	May be elevated
Liver enzymes	May be elevated
Prothrombin time	Prolonged
Arterial blood gases	Hypoxemia, metabolic acidosis
Diagnostic Procedures	
Abdominal ultrasonography	
Computed tomography scan	
Magnetic resonance imaging	
Endoscopic retrograde cholangiopancreatography	
Abdominal radiographs (flat plate and upright or decubitus)	
Chest radiographs (posteroanterior and lateral)	

Modified from Krumberger JM: Acute pancreatitis, *Crit Care Nurs Clin North Am* 5(1):185, 1993.

of the patient's creatinine clearance. The serum amylase level may be elevated for only 3 to 5 days; if the patient delays seeking treatment, a normal level (false-negative result) may be detected. Leukocytosis, hypocalcemia, hyperglycemia, hyperbilirubinemia, and hypoalbuminemia may also be present (Table 22-2).[8,22,23]

Diagnostic Procedures

An abdominal ultrasound scan is obtained as part of the diagnostic evaluation to determine the presence of biliary stones. A contrast-enhanced computed tomography (CT) scan is considered the gold standard for diagnosing pancreatitis and for ascertaining the overall degree of pancreatic inflammation and necrosis.[22,23]

Medical Management

Initial management of the patient with severe acute pancreatitis includes ensuring adequate fluid and electrolyte replacement, providing nutritional support, and correcting metabolic alterations.[23] Careful monitoring for systemic and local complications is critical.[22,24,25]

Fluid Management

Because pancreatitis if often associated with massive fluid shifts, intravenous crystalloids and colloids are administered immediately to prevent hypovolemic shock and maintain hemodynamic stability. In severe forms of acute pancreatitis, a pulmonary artery catheter may be used to guide ongoing fluid management.[25] Electrolytes are monitored closely, and abnormalities such as hypocalcemia, hypokalemia, and hypomagnesemia are corrected.[22,25] If hyperglycemia develops, exogenous insulin may be required.[25]

Nutritional Support

Over the past 3 decades, nutritional support has shifted. Previously, conventional nutritional management was to place the patient on a no oral intake (NPO) regimen and institute intravenous hydration. The rationale was to rest the inflamed pancreas and prevent enzyme release. Oral feeding was initiated only when the attack had subsided and enzymes had normalized. Total parenteral nutrition (TPN) was started for patients anticipated to have oral feedings held for more than 5 days. Randomized clinical trials have demonstrated that enteral feeding (gastric or jejunal) is safe and cost-effective and that it is associated with fewer septic and metabolic complications than other methods.[27,28] Enteral feeding enhances immune modulation and maintenance of the intestinal barrier, and it avoids complications associated with parental nutrition.[27-29] Early initiation of enteral feeding is preferred over TPN.[27-29] However, TPN still has a role for the critically ill patient with acute pancreatitis who does not tolerate enteral feeding or when nutritional goals are not reached within 2 days.[23,27] In the past, nasogastric suction was also recommended, but this intervention has not been shown to be of benefit and should be instituted only if the patient has persistent vomiting, obstruction, or gastric distention.[22]

Systemic Complications

Acute pancreatitis can affect every organ system, and recognition and treatment of systemic complications are crucial to management of the patient (Box 22-5). The most serious complications are hypovolemic shock, acute lung injury (ALI), acute renal failure (ARF), and gastrointestinal hemorrhage. Hypovolemic shock is the result of relative hypovolemia resulting from third spacing of intravascular volume and vasodilation caused by the release of inflammatory immune mediators. These mediators also contribute to the development of ALI and ARF. Other possible pulmonary complications include pleural effusions, atelectasis, and pneumonia.

Local Complications

Local complications include the development of infected pancreatic necrosis and pancreatic pseudocyst.[23,27] The necrotic areas of the pancreas can lead to development of a widespread pancreatic infection (infected pancreatic necrosis), which significantly increases the risk of death.[27]

BOX 22-5 COMPLICATIONS OF ACUTE PANCREATITIS

Respiratory
- Early hypoxemia
- Pleural effusion
- Atelectasis
- Pulmonary infiltration
- Acute lung injury
- Mediastinal abscess

Cardiovascular
- Hypotension
- Pericardial effusion
- ST-T changes

Renal
- Acute tubular necrosis
- Oliguria
- Renal artery or vein thrombosis

Hematological
- Disseminated intravascular coagulation
- Thrombocytosis
- Hyperfibrinogenemia

Endocrine
- Hypocalcemia
- Hypertriglyceridemia
- Hyperglycemia

Neurological
- Fat emboli
- Psychosis
- Encephalopathy

Ophthalmic
- Purtscher's retinopathy (sudden blindness)

Dermatological
- Subcutaneous fat necrosis

Gastrointestinal or Hepatic
- Hepatic dysfunction
- Obstructive jaundice
- Erosive gastritis
- Paralytic ileus
- Duodenal obstruction
- Pancreatic
  - Pseudocyst
  - Phlegmon
  - Abscess
  - Ascites
- Bowel infarction
- Massive intraperitoneal bleed
- Perforation
  - Stomach
  - Duodenum
  - Small bowel
  - Colon

Prophylactic antibiotics reduce sepsis and mortality and are initiated in patients suspected of having necrotizing pancreatitis.[27] After the patient develops infected necrosis, however, surgical débridement is necessary.[23,27] The procedure of choice is a minimally invasive necrosectomy, which entails careful débridement of the necrotic tissue in and around the pancreas. A pancreatic pseudocyst is a collection of pancreatic fluid enclosed by a nonepithelialized wall.[26] Cyst formation may result from liquefaction of a pancreatic fluid collection or from direct obstruction in the main pancreatic duct.[24] A pancreatic pseudocyst may (1) resolve spontaneously; (2) rupture, resulting in peritonitis; (3) erode a major blood vessel, resulting in hemorrhage; (4) become infected, resulting in abscess; or (5) invade surrounding structures, resulting in obstruction.[24] Treatment involves drainage of the pseudocyst surgically,[30] endoscopically, or percutaneously.[23,27]

Nursing Management

Nursing management of the patient with pancreatitis incorporates a variety of nursing diagnoses (Nursing Diagnosis Priorities Box on Acute Pancreatitis). **Nursing priorities are directed toward (1) providing pain relief and emotional support, (2) maintaining surveillance for complications, and (3) educating the patient and family.**

NURSING DIAGNOSIS PRIORITIES
Acute Pancreatitis

- Acute Pain related to transmission and perception of cutaneous, visceral, muscular, ischemia impulses, p. A-4
- Deficient Fluid Volume related to relative fluid loss, p. A-14
- Decreased Cardiac Output related to alterations in preload, p. A-10
- Ineffective Breathing Pattern related to decreased lung expansion, p. A-27
- Imbalanced Nutrition: Less Than Body Requirements related to lack of exogenous nutrients or increased metabolic demand, p. A-22
- Anxiety related to threat to biological, psychological, and/or social integrity, p. A-7
- Compromised Family Coping related to critically ill family member, p. A-9
- Deficient Knowledge related to lack of previous exposure to information (see the Patient Education box on Acute Pancreatitis) , p. A-15

Providing Comfort and Emotional Support

Pain management is a major priority in acute pancreatitis. Administration of analgesics to achieve pain relief is essential. For years, meperidine (Demerol) was considered to be the preferred agent in the patient with acute pancreatitis because morphine produced spasms at the sphincter of Oddi. However, studies have demonstrated that all opioids have a spasmogenic effect on the sphincter of Oddi. There is no evidence to indicate that morphine is contraindicated for use in acute pancreatitis, and it may provide more effective

BOX 22-6   SIGNS AND SYMPTOMS OF PANCREATIC INFECTION

Symptoms
- Persistent abdominal pain
- Abdominal tenderness

Signs
- Prolonged fever
- Abdominal distention
- Palpable abdominal mass
- Vomiting

Diagnostics
- Laboratory findings
  - Increased white blood cell count
  - Persistent elevation of serum amylase
  - Hyperbilirubinemia
  - Elevated alkaline phosphatase level
  - Positive culture and Gram's stain
- Radiography or computed tomography findings
  - Pancreatic inflammation or enlargement
  - Necrosis
  - Cystic or mass lesions
  - Fluid accumulations
  - Pseudocyst abscess

Modified from Krumberger JM: Acute pancreatitis, *Crit Care Nurs Clin North Am* 5(1):185, 1993.

PATIENT EDUCATION
Acute Pancreatitis

- Pancreatitis
- Specific cause
- Precipitating factor modification
- Interventions to reduce further episodes
- Importance of taking medications
- Lifestyle changes
- Diet modification
- Stress management
- Alcohol cessation
- Diabetes management, if needed

COLLABORATIVE MANAGEMENT
Acute Pancreatitis

- Ensure adequate circulating volume.
- Provide nutritional support.
- Correct metabolic alterations.
- Minimize pancreatic stimulation.
- Provide comfort and emotional support.
- Maintain surveillance for complications.
  - Multiple organ dysfunction syndrome

analgesia with fewer side effects than meperidine.[22,27] Relaxation techniques and positioning the patient in the knee-chest position can also assist in pain control.

Maintaining Surveillance for Complications

The patient must be routinely monitored for signs of local or systemic complications (see Box 22-5). Intensive monitoring of each of the organ systems is imperative, because organ failure is a major indicator of the severity of the disease.[31] The patient must be closely monitored for signs and symptoms of pancreatic infection, which include increased abdominal pain and tenderness, fever, and increased white blood cell count (Box 22-6).[22]

Educating the Patient and Family

Early in the patient's hospital stay, the patient and family should be taught about acute pancreatitis and its causes and treatment. As the patient moves toward discharge, teaching should focus on the interventions necessary for preventing the recurrence of the precipitating disorder. If there is sustained, permanent damage to the pancreas, the patient will require teaching specific to diet modification and supplemental pancreatic enzymes. Diabetes education may also be necessary. If an alcohol abuser, the patient should be encouraged to stop drinking and be referred to an alcohol cessation program (Patient Education Box on Acute Pancreatitis).[25] Collaborative management of the patient is outlined in the Box on Collaborative Management of Acute Pancreatitis.

ACUTE LIVER FAILURE

Description

Acute liver failure (ALF) is a life-threatening condition characterized by severe and sudden liver cell dysfunction, coagulopathy, and hepatic encephalopathy.[32,33] Although uncommon, ALF is associated with a mortality rate as high as 33%, and it usually occurs in patients without preexisting liver disease.[33,34] Because liver transplantation is one of the few definitive treatments, the patient with ALF should be transferred to a critical care unit and strongly considered for referral to a major medical center where transplantation services are available.[32-34]

Etiology

The causes of ALF include infections, drugs, toxins, hypoperfusion, metabolic disorders, and surgery (Box 22-7); however, viral hepatitis and drug-induced liver damage are the predominant causes in North America. Patients are usually healthy before the onset of symptoms because ALF tends to occur in patients with no known liver history. A thorough medication and health history is imperative to determine a possible cause. The patient should be questioned about exposure to environmental toxins, hepatitis, intravenous drug use, and sexual history. Viral hepatitis, drug toxicity, poisoning, and vascular and metabolic disorders such as Reye's syndrome and Wilson's disease should be considered.[32]

Pathophysiology

ALF is a syndrome characterized by the development of acute liver failure over 1 to 3 weeks, followed by the development of hepatic encephalopathy within 8 weeks, in a patient with a previously healthy liver. The interval between the failure of the liver and the onset of hepatic encephalopathy usually is less than 2 weeks. The underlying cause is massive necrosis of the hepatocytes.[32,33]

Acute liver failure results in a number of derangements, including impaired bilirubin conjugation, decreased production of clotting factors, depressed glucose synthesis, and decreased lactate clearance. This results in jaundice, coagulopathies, hypoglycemia, and metabolic acidosis. Other effects of acute liver failure include increased risk of infection and altered carbohydrate, protein, and glucose metabolism. Hypoalbuminemia, fluid and electrolyte imbalances, and acute portal hypertension contribute to the development of ascites.[33,34] Hepatic encephalopathy is thought to result from failure of the liver to detoxify various substances in the bloodstream, and it may be worsened by metabolic and electrolyte imbalances.[33]

The patient may experience a variety of other complications, including cerebral edema, cardiac dysrhythmias, acute respiratory failure, sepsis, and acute renal failure. Cerebral edema and increased intracranial pressure (ICP) develop as a result of breakdown of the blood-brain barrier and astrocyte swelling. Circulatory failure that mimics sepsis is common in ALF and may exacerbate low cerebral perfusion pressure (CPP).[34] Hypoxemia, acidosis, electrolyte imbalances, and cerebral edema can precipitate the development of cardiac dysrhythmias. Acute respiratory failure, progressing to ALI, can result from pulmonary edema, aspiration pneumonia, and atelectasis. ARF may be caused by acute tubular necrosis, hypotension, or hemorrhage.[33,34]

Assessment and Diagnosis

Early recognition of ALF is essential. The diagnosis should include potentially reversible conditions (e.g., autoimmune hepatitis) and should differentiate ALF from decompensating chronic liver disease. Prognostic indicators such as coma grade, serum bilirubin, prothrombin time, coagulation factors, and pH should be assessed and potential causes investigated.[33,34]

Signs and symptoms of ALF include headache, hyperventilation, jaundice, mental status changes, palmar erythema, spider nevi, bruises, and edema. The patient should be evaluated for the presence of asterixis or "liver flap," best described as the inability to voluntarily sustain a fixed position of the extremities. Asterixis is best demonstrated by having the patient extend the arms and dorsiflex the wrists, resulting in downward flapping of the hands. Hepatic encephalopathy is assessed using a grading system that stages the encephalopathy according to the patient's clinical manifestations (Box 22-8).[33,34] Diagnostic findings include elevated levels of serum bilirubin, aspartate aminotransferase (AST), alkaline phosphatase, and serum ammonia and decreased levels of serum albumin. Arterial blood gases (ABGs) reveal respiratory alkalosis or metabolic acidosis, or both. Hypoglycemia, hypokalemia, and hyponatremia also may be present.[33,34]

BOX 22-7   CAUSES OF ACUTE LIVER FAILURE

Infections
- Hepatitis A, B, C, D, E, non-A, non-B, non-C
- Herpes simplex virus (types 1 and 2)
- Epstein-Barr virus
- Varicella zoster
- Dengue fever virus
- Rift Valley fever virus

Drugs or Toxins
- Industrial substances (chlorinated hydrocarbons, phosphorus)
- *Amanita phalloides* (mushrooms)
- Aflatoxin (a toxic metabolite of fungus)
- Medications (isoniazid, rifampin, halothane, methyldopa, tetracycline, valproic acid, monoamine oxidase inhibitors, phenytoin, nicotinic acid, tricyclic antidepressants, isoflurane, ketoconazole, trimethoprim-sulfamethoxazole, sulfasalazine, pyrimethamine, octreotide)
- Acetaminophen toxicity
- Cocaine

Hypoperfusion
- Venous obstructions
- Budd-Chiari syndrome
- Veno-occlusive disease
- Ischemia

Metabolic Disorders
- Wilson's disease
- Tyrosinemia
- Heat stroke
- Galactosemia

Surgery
- Jejunoileal bypass
- Partial hepatectomy
- Liver transplant failure

Other Causes
- Reye's syndrome
- Acute fatty liver of pregnancy
- Massive malignant infiltration
- Autoimmune hepatitis

BOX 22-8   STAGING OF HEPATIC ENCEPHALOPATHY

I	Euphoria or depression, mild confusion, slurred speech, disordered sleep rhythm; slight asterixis and normal electroencephalogram (EEG)
II	Lethargy, moderate confusion; marked asterixis and abnormal EEG
III	Marked confusion, incoherent speech, sleeping but arousable; asterixis present and abnormal EEG
IV	Coma; initially responsive to noxious stimuli, later unresponsive; asterixis absent and abnormal EEG

Factors I (fibrinogen), II (prothrombin), V, VII, IX, and X are produced exclusively by the liver. Prothrombin time may be the most useful of tests of these in the evaluation of ALF because levels may be 40 to 80 seconds above control values. Test results show decreased levels of plasmin and plasminogen and increased levels of fibrin and fibrin-split products. Platelet counts may be less than 100,000/mm[3].[33]

Medical Management

Medical interventions are directed toward management of the multiple system impact of ALF.

Ammonia Levels

Neomycin or lactulose is administered to remove or decrease production of nitrogenous wastes in the large intestine. Neomycin, given orally or rectally, reduces bacterial flora of the colon. This aids in decreasing ammonia formation by decreasing bacterial action on protein in the feces. Side effects include renal toxicity and hearing impairment. Lactulose, a synthetic ketoanalogue of lactose split into lactic acid and acetic acid in the intestine, is given orally through a nasogastric tube or as a retention enema. The result is the creation of an acidic environment that decreases bacterial growth. Lactulose also traps ammonia and has a laxative effect that promotes expulsion.[34]

Complications

Bleeding is best controlled through prevention. Because these patients are at risk for acute gastrointestinal hemorrhage, stress ulcer prophylaxis is essential.[35] If an invasive procedure (e.g., central line placement, ICP monitor) will be performed or the patient develops active bleeding, vitamin K, fresh-frozen plasma (to maintain a reasonable prothrombin time), and platelet transfusions are necessary.[34] Metabolic disturbances such as hypoglycemia, metabolic acidosis, hypokalemia, and hyponatremia should be monitored and treated appropriately. Prophylactic antibiotic administration may be initiated because the patient is at high risk for an infection.[33,34]

The development of cerebral edema necessitates ICP monitoring. Mannitol is the only treatment shown to be of benefit in managing increased ICP in the patient with ALF, but it must be used with caution in patients with renal failure.[35] Other interventions to control intracranial hypertension include elevating the head of the bed (HOB) to 30 degrees, treating fever and hypertension, minimizing noxious stimulation, and correcting hypercapnia and hypoxemia.[35] Various experimental therapies to prevent or treat cerebral edema, such as induction of hypothermia, prophylactic phenytoin, and induction of hypernatremia, have been studied but have not improved survival.[35] If renal failure develops, continuous renal replacement therapy (CRRT) should be initiated.[35] Intubation and mechanical ventilation may be necessary as the inability to protect the airway and hypoxemia develops.[34] Hemodynamic instability is a common complication necessitating fluid administration and vasoactive medications to prevent prolonged episodes of hypotension. A pulmonary artery catheter may be used to guide clinical management.[34]

If ALF continues and the patient shows no immediate signs of improvement or reversal, the patient should be considered for a liver transplant. Prompt referral to a transplantation center should be a high priority for patients experiencing ALF.[33-35]

Nursing Management

Nursing management of the patient with ALF incorporates a variety of nursing diagnoses (Nursing Diagnosis Priorities Box on Acute Liver Failure). **Nursing priorities are directed toward (1) protecting the patient from injury, (2) providing comfort and emotional support, (3) maintaining surveillance for complications, and (4) educating the patient and family.**

NURSING DIAGNOSIS PRIORITIES
Acute Liver Failure

- Ineffective Breathing Pattern related to decreased lung expansion, p. A-27
- Impaired Gas Exchange related to ventilation/perfusion mismatching or intrapulmonary shunting, p. A-22
- Decreased Cardiac Output related to alterations in preload, p. A-10
- Decreased Cardiac Output related to alterations in heart rate, p. A-11
- Decreased Intracranial Adaptive Capacity related to failure of normal compensatory mechanisms, p. A-12
- Ineffective Renal Tissue Perfusion related to decreased renal blood flow, p. A-33
- Risk for Infection, p. A-36
- Imbalanced Nutrition: Less Than Body Requirements related to lack of exogenous nutrients or increased metabolic demand, p. A-22
- Disturbed Body Image related to actual change in body structure, function, or appearance, p. A-16
- Compromised Family Coping related to critically ill family member, p. A-9
- Deficient Knowledge related to lack of previous exposure to information (see the Patient Education box on Acute Liver Failure) , p. A-15

Protecting the Patient from Injury

Use of benzodiazepines and other sedatives is discouraged in the ALF patient because pertinent neurological changes may be masked and hepatic encephalopathy may be exacerbated.[34] These patients are often very difficult to manage because they may be extremely agitated and combative. Physical restraint may be necessary to prevent patient injury.

Maintaining Surveillance for Complications

As the neurological condition worsens, respiratory depression and arrest can occur quickly. Continuous pulse oximetry monitoring and ABG analysis are helpful in assessing adequacy of respiratory efforts. A thorough neurological assessment should be performed at least every hour.

Educating the Patient and Family

Early in the patient's hospital stay, the patient and family should be taught about ALF and its causes and treatment. As the patient moves toward discharge, teaching should focus on the interventions necessary for preventing the recurrence of the precipitating cause. If the patient is considered a candidate for liver transplantation, the patient and family will need specific information regarding the procedure and care. Liver transplant evaluation may include screening for medical contraindications, human immunodeficiency virus (HIV) serology, anticipated compliance, and assessment of the social support system. Psychiatric and other specialty team consultations are necessary for a thorough evaluation of the patient's suitability for a liver transplant (Patient Education Box on Acute Liver Failure). Collaborative management of the patient with ALF is outlined in the Collaborative Management Box on Acute Liver Failure.

THERAPEUTIC MANAGEMENT

Gastrointestinal Intubation

Because gastrointestinal intubation is used so often in critical care units, it is important for nurses to know the clinical indications and responsibilities inherent in tube use. The four categories of gastrointestinal tubes are based on function: nasogastric suction tubes, long intestinal tubes, feeding tubes, and esophagogastric balloon tamponade tubes (Patient Safety Priorities Box on Tubing Misconnections).

PATIENT EDUCATION

Acute Liver Failure

- Specific cause
- Precipitating factor modification
- Interventions to reduce further episodes
- Importance of taking medications
- Lifestyle changes
- Diet modification
- Alcohol cessation

COLLABORATIVE MANAGEMENT

Acute Liver Failure

- Decrease ammonia levels.
- Control bleeding.
- Correct metabolic alterations.
- Prevent infection.
- Prepare patient for liver transplantation, if necessary.
- Protect patient from injury.
- Provide comfort and emotional support.
- Maintain surveillance for complications:
  - Cerebral edema
  - Renal failure

⚡ PATIENT SAFETY PRIORITIES

Tubing Misconnections – A Persistent and Potentially Deadly Occurrence

Tubing and catheter misconnection errors are an important and underreported problem in health care organizations. These errors often are caught and corrected before any injury to the patient occurs. Given the reality of and potential for life-threatening consequences, increased awareness and analysis of these errors—including averted errors—can lead to dramatic improvement in patient safety.

Nine cases involving tubing misconnections have been reported to The Joint Commission's Sentinel Event Database. These errors resulted in eight deaths and one instance of permanent loss of function, and they affected seven adults and two infants. Reports in the media and to organizations such as the ECRI Institute, the U.S. Food and Drug Administration (FDA), the Institute for Safe Medication Practices (ISMP), and the United States Pharmacopeia (USP) indicate that misconnection errors occur with significant frequency and, in a number of instances, lead to deadly consequences.

Types of Misconnections

The types of tubes and catheters involved in the cases reported to The Joint Commission included central intravenous (IV) catheters, peripheral IV catheters, nasogastric (NG) feeding tubes, percutaneous enteric feeding tubes, peritoneal dialysis catheters, tracheostomy cuff inflation tubes, and automatic blood pressure cuff insufflation tubes. The specific misconnections involved an enteric tube feeding into an IV catheter (4 cases); injection of barium sulfate (gastrointestinal contrast medium) into a central venous catheter (1 case); an enteric tube feeding into a peritoneal dialysis catheter (1 case); a blood pressure insufflator tube connected to an IV catheter (2 cases); and injection of IV fluid into a tracheostomy cuff inflation tube (1 case).

A review by the USP of more than 300 cases reported to its databases found misconnection errors involving the following:

- IV infusions connected to epidural lines and epidural solutions (intended for epidural administration) connected to peripheral or central IV catheters
- Bladder irrigation solutions using primary IV tubing connected as secondary infusions to peripheral or central IV catheters
- Infusions intended for IV administration connected to an indwelling bladder (Foley) catheter
- Infusions intended for IV administration connected to NG tubes
- IV solutions administered with blood administration sets and blood products transfused with primary IV tubing
- Primary IV solutions administered through various other functionally dissimilar catheters, such as external dialysis catheters, a ventriculostomy drain, an amnio-infusion catheter, and the distal port of a pulmonary artery catheter

Continued

⚡ PATIENT SAFETY PRIORITIES—cont'd
Tubing Misconnections – A Persistent and Potentially Deadly Occurrence

Many of the misconnection cases involved Luer connectors, which are small devices used in the connection of many medical components and accessories. There are two types of Luer connectors: slips and locks. A Luer slip connector consists of a tapered "male" fitting that slips into a wider "female" fitting to create a secure connection. The Luer lock connector has a threaded collar on the male fitting and a flange on the female fitting that screw together to create a more secure connection. Examples of misconnections involving Luer connectors include the following:

- Capnography sampling tube to an IV cannula
- Enteral feeding set to a central venous catheter
- Enteral feeding set to a hemodialysis line
- Noninvasive blood pressure (NIBP) insufflation tube to a needleless IV port
- Oxygen tubing to a needleless IV port
- Sequential compression device (SCD) hose to a needleless "piggy-back" port of an IV administration set

Root Causes Identified
The basic lesson from these cases is that if it *can* happen, it *will* happen. Luer connectors are implicated in or contribute to many of these errors because they enable functionally dissimilar tubes or catheters to be connected. Other causes include the routine use of tubes or catheters for unintended purposes, such as using IV extension tubing for epidurals, irrigation, drains, and central lines; using them to extend enteric feeding tubes; and positioning functionally dissimilar tubes used in patient care close to one another. In the cases reported to the Sentinel Event Database, contributing factors included movement of the patient from one setting or service to another and staff fatigue associated with working consecutive shifts.

Risk Reduction Strategies
There are no published standards that specifically restrict the use of Luer connectors to certain medical devices. Consequently, a broad range of medical devices, which have different functions and access the body through different routes, are often outfitted with Luer fittings that can be easily misconnected. Organizations in Europe and the United States are developing standards to restrict the types of devices that use Luer fittings in an attempt to mitigate misconnection hazards. According to Jim Keller, vice president of Health Technology Evaluation and Safety for the ECRI Institute, and Stephanie Joseph, project engineer for the ECRI Institute, the solution to reducing or eliminating misconnection errors lies in engineering controls respecting how products and devices are designed ("incompatibility by design") and in re-engineering work practices.

"A well-designed device should prevent misconnections and should prompt the user to take the correct action," explained Joseph, author of a guidance article published in the March 2006 issue of the ECRI Institute's *Health Devices* journal. As a first step in prevention, Joseph urges hospitals to avoid buying non-IV equipment (e.g., nebulizers, NIBP devices, enteral feeding sets) that can mate with the Luer connectors on patient IV lines. Joseph also emphasizes that the single most important work practice solution for clinicians is to trace all lines back to their origin before connecting or disconnecting any devices or infusions.

Other solutions include specific education and training regarding this problem for all clinicians and having practitioners take simple precautions such as turning on the light in a darkened room before connecting or reconnecting tubes or devices. The risk of waking a sleeping patient is minimal by comparison. Errors have occurred when patients or family members attempted to disconnect and reconnect equipment themselves. Staff should emphasize to all patients the importance of contacting a clinical staff member for assistance when there is an identified need to disconnect or reconnect devices.

Some approaches to reducing the risk of misconnections have significant potential for unintended consequences:

- Labeling all tubes and catheters may not always be practical and may therefore lead to inconsistent implementation. However, labeling certain high-risk catheters (e.g., epidural, intrathecal, arterial) should always be done.
- Color-coding tubes and catheters can lead users to rely on the color coding rather than having a clear understanding of which tubes and catheters are connected correctly to which body inlets. Training or educating all staff (including temporary agency and travel staff) about the institution's color-coding system requires ongoing attention. Color-coding schemes often vary across institutions in the same community, creating increased risk when agency and travel staff are used.

Joint Commission Recommendations
The Joint Commission offers the following recommendations and strategies to health care organizations to reduce tubing misconnection errors:

1. Do not purchase non-IV equipment that is equipped with connectors that can physically mate with a female Luer IV line connector.
2. Conduct acceptance testing (for performance, safety, and usability) and, as appropriate, risk assessment (e.g., failure mode and effect analysis) on new tubing and catheter purchases to identify the potential for misconnections, and take appropriate preventive measures.
3. Always trace a tube or catheter from the patient to the point of origin before connecting any new device or infusion.
4. Recheck connections, and trace all patient tubes and catheters to their sources on the patient's arrival to a new setting or service as part of the hand-off process. Standardize this "line reconciliation" process.
5. Route tubes and catheters having different purposes in different, standardized directions (e.g., IV lines routed toward the head; enteric lines toward the feet). This is especially important in the care of neonates.
6. Inform nonclinical staff, patients, and their families that they must get help from clinical staff whenever there is a real or perceived need to connect or disconnect devices or infusions.
7. For certain high-risk catheters (e.g., epidural, intrathecal, arterial), label the catheter, and do not use catheters that have injection ports.

Tubing Misconnections – A Persistent and Potentially Deadly Occurrence

8. Never use a standard Luer syringe for oral medications or enteric feedings.
9. Emphasize the risk of tubing misconnections in orientation and training curricula.
10. Identify and manage conditions and practices that may contribute to health care worker fatigue, and take appropriate action.

The Joint Commission also urges product manufacturers to implement "designed incompatibility," as appropriate, to prevent dangerous misconnections of tubes and catheters.

Resources

The ECRI Institute: Fatal air embolism caused by the misconnection of medical device hoses to needleless Luer ports on IV administration sets [hazard report], Health Devices 33(6):223, 2004.

The ECRI Institute: Misconnected flowmeter leads to two deaths [special report], Health Devices Alerts January 25, 2003.

The ECRI Institute: Preventing misconnections of lines and cables, Health Devices 35(3):81, 2006.

Safe systems, safe patients: common connectors pose a threat to safe practice, Texas Board Nurs Bull 37(2):6, 2006.

U.S. Food and Drug Administration: FDA patient safety news, Show #31, September 2004; Show #20, October 2003; Show #46 December 2005 Available at www.accessdata.fda.gov/psn/index.cfm (accessed May 2009).

Modified from The Joint Commission: Sentinel Event Alert, no. 36 April 3, 2006 Available at http://www.jointcommission.org/sentinel_event_alert_issue_36_tubing_misconnections-a_persistent_and_potentially_deadly_occurrence/ (accessed May 2009)

Nasogastric Suction Tubes. Nasogastric tubes remove fluid regurgitated into the stomach, prevent accumulation of swallowed air, may partially decompress the bowel, and reduce the patient's risk for aspiration. Nasogastric tubes also can be used for collecting specimens, assessing the presence of blood, and administering tube feedings. The most common nasogastric tubes are the single-lumen Levin tube and the double-lumen Salem sump. The Salem sump has one lumen that is used for suction and drainage and another that allows air to enter the patient's stomach and prevents the tube from adhering to the gastric wall and damaging the mucosa. The tube is passed through the nose into the nasopharynx and then down through the pharynx into the esophagus and stomach. The length of time the nasogastric tube remains in place depends on its use. The tube is then placed to gravity, or low continuous suction, and in rare instances, it is clamped.[36,37]

Nursing management focuses on preventing complications common to this therapy, such as ulceration and necrosis of the nares, esophageal reflux, esophagitis, esophageal erosion and stricture, gastric erosion, and dry mouth and parotitis from mouth breathing. Interference with ventilation and coughing, aspiration, and loss of fluid and electrolytes can be critical problems. Interventions include irrigating the tube every 4 hours with normal saline, ensuring the blue air vent of the Salem sump is patent and maintained above the level of the patient's stomach, and providing frequent mouth and nares care.[36]

Long Intestinal Tubes

Miller-Abbott, Cantor, and Andersen tubes are examples of long, weighted-tip intestinal tubes that are placed preoperatively or intraoperatively. The long length allows removal of contents from the intestine to treat an obstruction that cannot be managed by a nasogastric tube. These tubes can decompress the small bowel and can splint the small bowel

intraoperatively or postoperatively. Because progression of the tubes depends on bowel peristalsis, their use is contraindicated in patients with paralytic ileus and severe mechanical bowel obstructions. Older devices such as the Cantor and Miller-Abbott tubes are rarely used today because the balloon and the distal end is filled with mercury; the newer Andersen tube has a preweighted tungsten tip and is a safer option.[36]

Interventions used in the care of the patient with a long intestinal tube are similar to those with a nasogastric tube. The patient should be observed for (1) gaseous distention of the balloon section, which makes removal difficult; (2) rupture of the balloon or spillage of mercury into the intestine; (3) overinflation of the balloon, which can lead to intestinal rupture; and (4) reverse intussusception if the tube is removed rapidly. Intestinal tubes should be removed slowly; usually 6 inches of the tube is withdrawn every hour.[36]

Feeding Tubes. Small-diameter (8- to 12-Fr) flexible feeding tubes, such as Dobhoff tubes, are commonly placed at the bedside for patients who cannot take nourishment orally. The feeding tube may be inserted orally or nasally so that the tip ends up in the stomach or duodenum. To facilitate passage into the gastrointestinal tract, these tubes have a weighted tungsten tip, and a guidewire is needed to prevent them from curling up in the back of the patient's throat. An x-ray film must be obtained to verify correct placement of the tube before initiating feeding.[36-39] The tube should also be marked with indelible ink where it exits the mouth or nares so that the nurse can later verify that the tube has not been dislodged.[39]

Nursing management of the patient with a feeding tube includes prevention of complications and monitoring the tolerance of feeding. Tracheobronchial aspiration of gastric contents is a serious potential complication.[38] Before administering medications or feedings, it is important to ensure that the tube is in the patient's stomach or duodenum. Assessing the exit point marked on the tube helps to determine whether the tube has maintained the same position. Looking for coiling in the mouth or throat can help detect upward displacement that may have occurred as a result of vomiting. The traditional practice of confirming placement by auscultating air inserted through the tube over the epigastrium is not reliable and is not recommended.[37-39] If there is any doubt about the tube's position, a repeat radiograph should be obtained. During feedings, the head of bed should be elevated at least 30 degrees to minimize the risk of aspiration, and gastric residuals should be checked at least every 4 to 6 hours.[38] Large gastric residuals, cramping, and abdominal distention may indicate intolerance of feeding, and the physician should be notified.[38] Other interventions include nares and oral care and flushing the tube with normal saline or water to maintain patency.[36,37]

Endoscopic Injection Therapy

Endoscopic injection therapy is used to control bleeding of varices and ulcers. It may be performed emergently, electively, or prophylactically. An endoscope is introduced through the patient's mouth, and endoscopy of the esophagus and stomach is performed to identify the bleeding varices or ulcers. An injector with a retractable 23- to 25-gauge needle is introduced through the biopsy channel of the endoscope. The needle then is inserted in or around the varices or into the area around the ulcer, and a liquid agent is injected. The most commonly used agent is epinephrine, which results in localized vasoconstriction and enhanced platelet aggregation. Sclerosing agents such as ethanolamine, alcohol, and polidocanol also may be used. These agents cause an inflammatory reaction in the vessel that results in thrombosis and eventually produces a fibrous band. Repeated sclerotherapy results in the development of supportive scar tissue around the varices. Other agents used include fibrinogen and thrombin, which when injected together react to form an active fibrin clot, and cyanoacrylate glue, which is used as a sealant to stop the bleeding.[17,18]

Endoscopic injection therapy controls acute variceal bleeding in as many as 80% of patients.[40] Complications can vary from mild to severe and include esophageal perforation, extravasation of the injection agent, and strictures of the esophagus. This procedure is contraindicated in patients with severe coagulopathies.[3]

Endoscopic Variceal Ligation

Endoscopic variceal ligation involves applying bands or metal clips around the circumference of the bleeding varices to induce venous obstruction and control bleeding. Between 1 and 2 days after the procedure, necrosis and scar formation promote band and tissue sloughing. Fibrinous deposits within the healing ulcer potentiate vessel obliteration. Band ligation is accomplished through endoscopy, with 5 to 8 bands placed per session.[40] The procedure may be repeated on an inpatient or outpatient basis over 2 to 3 weeks until all the varices are obliterated.[13]

Endoscopic variceal ligation controls bleeding approximately 80% to 90% of the time.[13] This procedure is reported to require fewer endoscopic treatment sessions and has a lower rebleeding rate and fewer complications than endoscopic sclerotherapy. The most common complication of endoscopic variceal ligation is the development of superficial mucosal ulcers. Systemic complications are rare.[40]

Transjugular Intrahepatic Portosystemic Shunt

Transjugular intrahepatic portosystemic shunting (TIPS) is an angiographic interventional procedure for decreasing portal hypertension. TIPS is advocated for (1) patients with portal hypertension who are also experiencing active bleeding or have poor liver reserve, (2) transplant recipients, and (3) patients with other operative risks. The TIPS procedure is usually performed by a gastroenterologist, vascular surgeon, or interventional radiologist.

Portal hypertension is confirmed by direct measurement of the pressure in the portal vein (gradient greater than 10 mm Hg). Cannulation is achieved through the internal jugular vein, and an angiographic catheter is advanced into the middle or right hepatic vein. The mid-hepatic vein is then catheterized, and a new route is created connecting the portal and hepatic veins using a needle and guidewire with a dilating balloon. An expandable stainless steel stent is then placed in the liver parenchyma to maintain that connection (Figure 22-4). The increased resistance in the liver is bypassed.[41]

TIPS may be performed on patients with bleeding varices, with refractory bleeding varices, or as a bridge to liver transplantation if the candidate becomes hemodynamically unstable. Postprocedural care should include observation for overt (cannulation site) or covert (intrahepatic site) bleeding, hepatic or portal vein laceration (resulting in rapid loss of blood volume), and inadvertent puncture of surrounding organs. Other complications include bile duct trauma, stent migration, and stent thrombosis.[41] Portal hypertension recurs almost universally after TIPS, whereas shunt dysfunction occurs in 50% to 60% of patients within 6 months.[42]

Gastrointestinal Surgery
Types of Surgery

Gastrointestinal surgery refers to a wide variety of surgical procedures that involve the esophagus, the stomach, the intestine, the liver, the pancreas, or the biliary tract. Indications for gastrointestinal surgery are numerous and include bleeding or perforation from peptic ulcer disease, obstruction, trauma, inflammatory bowel disease, and malignancy. Patients may be admitted to the critical care unit for monitoring after gastrointestinal surgery as a result of their underlying medical condition; however, this portion of the chapter focuses only on several surgical procedures that commonly require postoperative critical care.

Esophagectomy. Esophagectomy is usually performed for cancer of the distal esophagus and gastroesophageal junction. The technically difficult procedure involves the removal of part or the entire esophagus, part of the stomach, and lymph nodes in the surrounding area. The stomach is then pulled

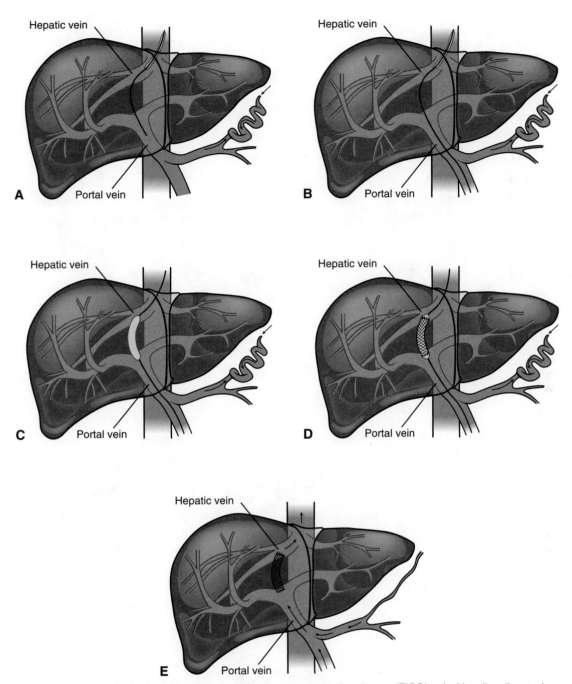

FIGURE 22-4 Transjugular intrahepatic portosystemic shunt (TIPS). *A,* Needle directed though liver parenchyma to portal vein. *B,* Needle and guidewire passed down to midportal vein. *C,* Balloon dilation. *D,* Deployment of stent. *E,* Intrahepatic shunt from portal to hepatic vein.

up into the chest and connected to the remaining part of the esophagus. If the entire esophagus and stomach must be removed, part of the bowel may be used to form the esophageal replacement (Figures 22-5 and 22-6).[43,44]

Pancreaticoduodenectomy. The standard operation for pancreatic cancer is a pancreaticoduodenectomy, also called a *Whipple procedure.* In the Whipple procedure, the pancreatic head, the duodenum, part of the jejunum, the common bile duct, the gallbladder, and part of the stomach are

removed. The continuity of the gastrointestinal tract is restored by anastomosing the remaining portion of the pancreas, the bile duct, and the stomach to the jejunum (Figure 22-7).[44,45]

Bariatric Surgery. Bariatric surgery refers to surgical procedures of the gastrointestinal tract that are performed to induce weight loss. Bariatric procedures are divided into three broad types: restrictive, malabsorptive, and combined restrictive and malabsorptive.[46] Restrictive procedures such

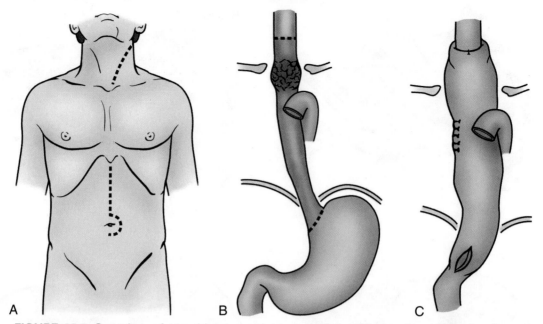

FIGURE 22-5 Overview of transhiatal esophagectomy. *A,* With gastric mobilization *B,* and gastric pull-up *C,* for cervical-esophagogastric anastomosis. (*A to C,* Modified from Ellis F: Esophagogastrectomy for carcinoma: technical considerations based on anatomic location of lesion, *Surg Clin North Am* 60[2]:265, 1980.)

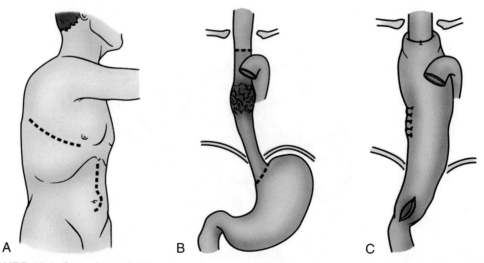

FIGURE 22-6 Overview of right thoracotomy. *A,* With esophageal resection, gastric mobilization *B,* and intrathoracic anastomosis *C,* for a midesophageal tumor. (*A to C,* Modified from Ellis FH: Esophagogastrectomy for carcinoma: technical considerations based on anatomic location of lesion, *Surg Clin North Am* 60[2]:265, 1980.)

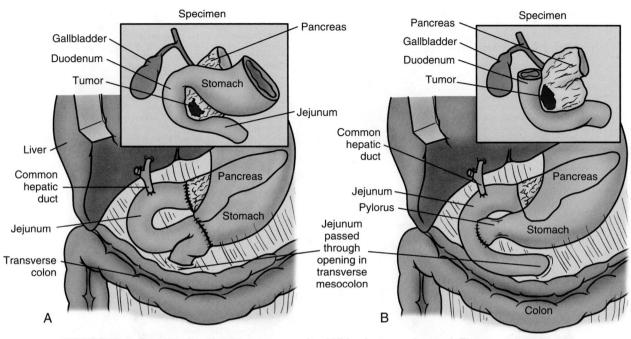

FIGURE 22-7 Standard and pylorus-preserving Whipple procedures. *A,* The standard Whipple procedure involves resection of the gastric antrum, head of pancreas, distal bile duct, and entire duodenum with reconstruction as shown. *B,* The pylorus-preserving Whipple procedure does not include resection of the distal stomach, pylorus, or proximal duodenum. (From Cameron JL: Current status of the Whipple operation for periampullary carcinoma, *Surg* Rounds 77, 1988.)

as vertical banded gastroplasty (VBG) (Figure 22-8, *A*) and gastric banding (Figure 22-8, *B*) reduce the capacity of the stomach and limit the amount of food that can be consumed. Malabsorptive procedures such as the biliopancreatic diversion (BPD) (Figure 22-8, *C*) alter the gastrointestinal tract to limit the digestion and absorption of food. The Roux-en-Y gastric bypass (RYGBP) (Figure 22-8, *D*) combines both strategies by creating a small gastric pouch and anastomosing the jejunum to the pouch. Food then bypasses the lower stomach and duodenum, resulting in decreased absorption of digestive materials.[46,47]

Preoperative Care

A thorough preoperative evaluation should be conducted to evaluate the patient's physical status and identify risk factors that may affect the postoperative course. Because obesity is associated with a higher incidence of comorbidities such as cardiovascular disease, hypertension, diabetes, gastroesophageal reflux, obstructive sleep apnea, and heart failure, an extensive workup may be required for the bariatric patient.[47] Before esophagectomy or pancreaticoduodenectomy, the patient may undergo multiple diagnostic tests, such as CT, positron emission tomography (PET), and endoscopic ultrasound (EUS), to determine the invasiveness of the tumor.[43]

Surgical Considerations

Two approaches may be used for esophageal resection: transhiatal or transthoracic (see Figures 22-6 and 22-7). In both approaches, the stomach is mobilized through an abdominal incision and then transposed into the chest. The anastomosis

of the stomach to the esophagus is performed in the chest (transthoracic) or in the neck (transhiatal). The approach selected depends on the location of the tumor, the patient's overall health and pulmonary function, and the experience of the surgeon. After surgery, the patient has a nasogastric tube in place that should not be manipulated because of the potential to damage the anastomosis. Those who undergo transthoracic esophagectomy have one or more chest tubes.[43,44]

Most bariatric procedures can be performed using an open or laparoscopic surgical technique. Although laparoscopic approaches are more technically difficult to perform, they have largely replaced open procedures because they are associated with decreased pulmonary complications, less postoperative pain, reduced length of hospital stay, fewer wound complications (e.g., infections, incisional hernia), and an earlier return to full activity.[46,48] Open procedures are performed on patients who have had prior upper abdominal surgery, are morbidly obese, or who may not be able to tolerate the increased abdominal pressure associated with laparoscopic procedures.[44]

Complications and Medical Management

Several complications are associated with gastrointestinal surgery, including respiratory failure, atelectasis, pneumonia, anastomotic leak, deep vein thrombosis, pulmonary embolus, and bleeding. The morbidly obese patient is at even greater risk for many postoperative complications.[46,47]

Pulmonary Complications. The risk for pulmonary complications is substantial after gastrointestinal surgery, and adverse respiratory events such as atelectasis and pneumonia

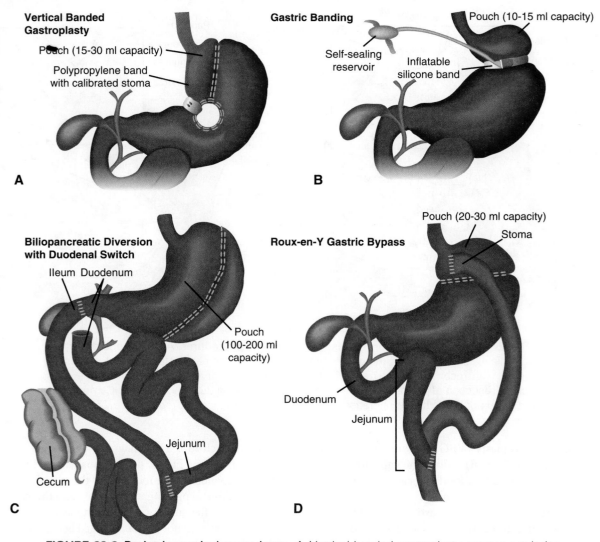

FIGURE 22-8 Bariatric surgical procedures. *A,* Vertical banded gastroplasty creates a tubular stomach that is restrictive. *B,* Gastric banding systems are adjustable and reversible, and they can be placed laparoscopically. *C,* Biliopancreatic diversion with duodenal switch and vertical gastroplasty/sleeve gastrectomy. *D,* Roux-en-Y proximal gastric bypass. (From Lewis et al: *Medical surgical nursing: Assessment and management of clinical problems,* ed 7, St Louis, 2007, Mosby. Redrawn from Price SA, Wilson LM: *Pathophysiology: Clinical concepts of disease processes,* ed 6, St Louis, 2003, Mosby.)

are twice as likely to occur in the obese patient.[46] Aggressive pulmonary exercise should be initiated in the immediate postoperative period. Early ambulation and adequate pain control assist in reducing the risk of atelectasis development. Suctioning, chest physiotherapy, or bronchodilators may be needed to optimize pulmonary function. Patients should be closely monitored for the development of oxygenation problems. Treatment should be aimed at supporting adequate ventilation and gas exchange. Mechanical ventilation may be required in the event of respiratory failure.

Anastomotic Leak. An anastomotic leak is a severe complication of gastrointestinal surgery. It occurs when there is a breakdown of the suture line in a surgical anastomosis and results in leakage of gastric or intestinal contents into the abdomen or mediastinum (transthoracic esophagectomy).[43,46,47] The clinical signs and symptoms of a leak can be

subtle and often go unrecognized. They include tachycardia, tachypnea, fever, abdominal pain, anxiety, and restlessness.[46,47] In the patient with an esophagectomy, a leak of the esophageal anastomosis may manifest as subcutaneous emphysema in the chest and neck.[43] If undetected, a leak can result in sepsis, multiorgan failure, and death. Patients with progressive tachycardia and tachypnea should have a radiological study (upper gastrointestinal study with Gastrografin or CT scan with contrast) to rule out an anastomotic leak.[47] The type of treatment depends on the severity of the leak. If the leak is small and well contained, it may be managed conservatively by maintaining the NPO status, administering antibiotics, and draining the fluid percutaneously. If the patient is deteriorating rapidly, an urgent laparotomy is indicated to repair the defect.[49]

Deep Vein Thrombosis and Pulmonary Embolism. Pulmonary embolism (PE) is a very serious complication of any surgical procedure. Deep vein thrombosis (DVT) prophylaxis should be initiated before surgery and continue until the patient is fully ambulatory to reduce the risk of clot development. Typically, a combination of sequential compression devices and subcutaneous unfractionated heparin or low-molecular-weight heparin is used. Patients determined to be at high risk for PE may benefit from prophylactic inferior vena cava filter placement.[43,46,48]

Bleeding. Upper gastrointestinal bleeding is an uncommon but life-threatening complication of gastrointestinal surgery. Early bleeding typically occurs at the site of the anastomosis and can usually be treated through endoscopic intervention. Surgical revision may be needed for persistent, uncontrolled bleeding. Late bleeding is usually a result of ulcer development. Medical therapy is aimed at the prevention of this complication through administration of H_2-antagonists or PPIs.[43]

Postoperative Nursing Management

Nursing care of the patient who has had gastrointestinal surgery incorporates a number of nursing diagnoses (Nursing Diagnosis Priorities Box on Gastrointestinal Surgery). **Nursing priorities are directed toward (1) optimizing oxygenation and ventilation, (2) providing comfort and emotional support, and (3) maintaining surveillance for complications.**

NURSING DIAGNOSIS PRIORITIES
Gastrointestinal Surgery

- Ineffective Breathing Pattern related to decreased lung expansion, p. A-27
- Impaired Gas Exchange related to alveolar hypoventilation, p. A-22
- Decreased Cardiac Output related to alterations in preload, p. A-10
- Acute Pain related to transmission and perception of cutaneous, visceral, muscular, or ischemic impulses, p. A-4
- Anxiety related to threat to biological, psychological, or social integrity, p. A-7
- Disturbed Body Image related to actual change in body structure, function, or appearance, p. A-16
- Deficient Knowledge related to lack of previous exposure to information, p. A-15

Optimizing Oxygenation and Ventilation. Nursing interventions in the postoperative period are focused on promoting ventilation and adequate oxygenation and preventing complications such as atelectasis and pneumonia. After the patient is extubated, deep-breathing exercises and incentive spirometry should be initiated and then performed regularly. Early ambulation is encouraged to promote maximal lung inflation and thereby reduce the risk of pulmonary complications and to reduce the potential for pulmonary embolus.

Providing Comfort and Emotional Support. It is imperative to appropriately manage the patient's pain after gastrointestinal surgery. Adequate analgesia is necessary to promote

mobility of the patient and decrease pulmonary complications. Initial pain management may be accomplished by intravenous opioid (morphine, hydromorphone) administration by means of a patient-controlled analgesia (PCA) pump, or through continuous epidural infusion of an opioid and local anesthetic (bupivacaine).[44,46,47] Oral pain medications can be started after an anastomosis leak is ruled out. Nonpharmacological interventions such as positioning, application of heat or cold, and distraction may also be used. If the patient's pain is not being sufficiently relieved, the pain management service should be consulted.[43,47]

Liver Transplantation
Indications and Selection

Liver transplantation must be considered for any patient who suffers from irreversible acute or chronic liver disease that is progressive and for which there is no therapy of established efficacy. Diseases of the liver may be categorized as chronic, vascular, acute liver failure, and include inborn errors of metabolism and hepatic malignancies. Box 22-9 lists the most common diseases seen in patients who undergo

---

BOX 22-9 END-STAGE LIVER DISEASES COMMONLY TREATED WITH LIVER TRANSPLANTATION

Cholestatic Liver Diseases
- Biliary atresia
- Primary sclerosing cholangitis
- Primary biliary cirrhosis

Chronic Hepatocellular Diseases
- Viral hepatitis (types A, B, C, D, E)
- Alcoholic liver disease (Laënnec disease)
- Autoimmune hepatitis
- Cryptogenic cirrhosis
- Drug-induced liver disease

Vascular Diseases
- Budd-Chiari syndrome
- Veno-occlusive disease

Acute Liver Failure
- Viral hepatitis (types A, B, C, D, E)
- Drug-induced liver failure (acetaminophen, isoniazid overdoses)
- Wilson's disease

Inborn Metabolic Disorders
- Wilson's disease
- α_1-Antitrypsin deficiency
- Hemochromatosis
- Tyrosinemia
- Glycogen storage disease, types I and II

Primary Hepatic Malignancies
- Hepatocellular carcinoma
- Hemangioendothelioma
- Hepatoblastoma

liver transplantation. In the United States, the single most common indication for liver transplantation in adults is chronic viral hepatitis C.[50]

Candidate selection is an important aspect of transplantation. Given the shortage of available organs, the transplantation team must have reasonable assurance of a successful outcome. The timing of transplantation is of utmost importance. The patient must not be so ill as to be unable to survive the surgery but yet be experiencing deterioration in the quality of life. Body mass index (BMI) plays a role in posttransplantation survival. Patients who are underweight (BMI < 20) or morbidly obese (BMI > 40) are at greater risk for death after transplantation.[51] In general, liver transplantation is not to be offered to persons in the following groups:

- Those who would not be likely to survive major surgery
- Those who would not survive the effects of long-term immunosuppression
- Those who have a disease that is likely to recur quickly and fatally after transplantation
- Those who are not willing to comply with long-term and sometimes difficult and demanding medical regimens

The absolute contraindications listed in Box 22-10 fall under these four specific categories.

Having one relative contraindication may not rule out transplantation, but having several predicts poor outcome. Chronological age is less important than physiological age. Reports of transplantation in older patients describe favorable results.[52] Certain diseases can recur after transplantation, including viral hepatitis,[53] sclerosing cholangitis,[54] and biliary malignancies.[55] In the case of viral hepatitis, serologic indicators of viral replication are monitored closely. In the presence of aggressively replicating virus and in certain malignancies, it is in the patient's best interest not to proceed to transplantation, because it would actually hasten death. Multicenter protocols are important in evaluating the outcomes and efficacies of transplantations in patients with diseases that recur. The decision to offer liver transplantation to any patient must be based on evaluation criteria, which vary among institutions and are modified as advances in technical ability, immunosuppression, and perioperative management continue. In the absence of complications, the average hospital stay after liver transplantation is 7 to 14 days.

Recipient Evaluation

The candidate for liver transplantation undergoes a thorough evaluation to determine the cause and severity of the liver disease, to establish the need for transplantation rather than other interventions, and to identify objective indications and contraindications. Evaluation begins with a carefully elicited patient history (Box 22-11). A comprehensive approach includes laboratory, radiographic, and diagnostic testing and multidisciplinary consultations (Box 22-12). Not every patient undergoes every test and consultation. Careful history taking and a good physical examination direct the initial diagnostic testing. For instance, a patient with a past history of malignancy would undergo extensive testing to rule out metastases, whereas a patient with acute liver failure may have a more abbreviated workup that is focused on determining the cause and potential for hepatic recovery.[56]

During the workup, the candidate's support systems are evaluated by the entire transplantation team, which includes the surgeon, the hepatologist, the clinical transplantation nurse coordinator, the social worker, the dietitian, and the financial counselor. Other services, such as cardiology, nephrology, psychiatry, gynecology, anesthesia, infectious disease, endocrinology, hematology, rheumatology, and oral surgery or dentistry, may also be included in the evaluation. Ideally, all immunizations are brought up to date in an attempt to minimize postoperative infections. The patient and family receive education regarding the evaluation, waiting list, surgery, postoperative management including immunosuppression, and long-term follow-up. At the

---

BOX 22-10 CONTRADICTIONS TO LIVER TRANSPLANTATION

Absolute Contraindications
- Brain death
- Metastatic malignancy
- Extrahepatic malignancy
- Active drug or alcohol abuse
- Advanced cardiopulmonary disease
- Acquired immunodeficiency syndrome
- Extrahepatic sepsis

Relative Contraindications
- Physiological age
- Advanced renal disease
- Multiple hepatic malignancies
- Moderate cardiopulmonary disease
- Peripheral vascular disease
- Psychosocial behaviors indicating noncompliance with medical regimens
- Human immunodeficiency virus infection

BOX 22-11 PRETRANSPLANTATION HISTORY FOR A PATIENT WITH END-STAGE LIVER DISEASE

- Risk factors for viral hepatitis: transfusions, intravenous drug abuse, tattoos, other parenteral exposure
- Family history of liver disease
- Associated disorders: hypothyroidism, osteoporosis, infertility, arthritis
- Onset, duration, and description of symptoms and complications: jaundice, lethargy, bleeding disorders, pruritus, confusion, ascites, edema, melenic stools, abdominal pain, bone pain or fractures, chronic diarrhea, gynecomastia (in men), amenorrhea (in women)
- Current and past medical history: hospitalizations, surgeries
- Social history: exposure to alcohol, drugs, toxins, tobacco products
- Status of immunizations

BOX 22-12 SAMPLE EVALUATION BEFORE LIVER TRANSPLANTATION

Laboratory Tests

- Liver function profile: transaminases (AST, ALT, GGT), alkaline phosphatase, bilirubin, albumin, prothrombin time, partial thromboplastin time, clotting factors, cholesterol, triglycerides
- Kidney function profile with electrolytes: blood urea nitrogen, creatinine, sodium, potassium, carbon dioxide, chloride
- Hematology: CBC, reticulocytes, ESR
- Thyroid function: T_3RIA; T_4RIA; thyroid-stimulating hormone; T_4 and T_3 uptake
- Serology studies for hepatic viruses and other infectious diseases: viral hepatitis (A, B, C, D, E); cytomegalovirus, Epstein-Barr virus, herpes virus I and II, parvovirus, HIV; RPR
- Blood type and antibody screen
- Immunological profiles: antinuclear antibody; antimitochondrial antibody; anti-smooth muscle antibody; immunoglobulins (A, G, M)
- Nutritional profiles: vitamin levels (A, D, E, B_{12}, folate); iron studies with ferritin
- Tumor markers: α-fetoprotein, CEA, PSA,
- Miscellaneous: ceruloplasmin, α_1-antitrypsin level and phenotype

Urine

- 24-hour protein and electrolytes, cultures, creatinine clearance, urinalysis, copper

Stool

- Ova, cysts, parasites, occult blood, 48-hour fecal fat, cultures

Gastrointestinal Workup

- Endoscopy, colonoscopy, endoscopic retrograde cholangiopancreatography, liver biopsy

Pulmonary Profile

- Arterial blood gases, pulmonary function studies

Radiographic and Diagnostic Tests

- Chest radiograph, ultrasound studies of liver including vascular studies

Optional Tests

- Doppler studies; sinus radiography; computed tomography (abdomen, chest, head); electrocardiography; echocardiography; cardiac stress test; cardiac catheterization; mammography; peripheral vascular studies; carotid ultrasonography; abdominal angiography; percutaneous cholangiography; bone mineral density

ALT, alanine aminotransferase; *AST*, aspartate transaminase; *CBC*, complete blood cell count; *CEA*, carcinoembryonic agents; *ESR*, erythrocyte sedimentation rate; *GGT*, γ-glutamyltransferase; *HIV*, human immunodeficiency virus; *PSA*, prostate-specific antigen; *RPR*, rapid plasma reagin; *T_3RIA*, serum triiodothyronine (T_3) radioimmunoassay; *T_4RIA*, serum triiodothyronine (T_4) radioimmunoassay.

conclusion of the evaluation, one of several outcomes is possible: (1) the patient is deemed a transplant candidate, (2) the patient is deemed not a candidate, or (3) the patient may be a candidate sometime in the future if certain criteria are met. These criteria may be of a physical nature (e.g., it is too early in the disease process to list now, in which case the patient will be re-evaluated at set intervals), or they may be of a psychosocial nature (e.g., the patient must attend a formal alcohol or drug rehabilitation program or undergo treatment of depression).[56]

After candidacy has been determined and the patient is ready for transplantation, his or her social security number is entered into the national computer system operated by United Network for Organ Sharing (UNOS). Objective criteria are used to place a patient on the waiting list. These data are used in a formula to determine the patient's score, which is directly associated with the patient's risk of death within 3 months (the higher the score, the higher the risk).

Model for End-Stage Liver Disease. The Model for End-Stage Liver Disease (MELD) formula is used in all U.S. transplant centers to calculate risk of mortality in patients 12 years old or older. The MELD objective criteria include serum total bilirubin, serum creatinine, prothrombin time, and international normalized ratio.[57]

Placement on the waiting list is determined by blood type, weight, and patient urgency. Patients with acute liver failure are considered to be in most urgent need and are placed at the top of the list. Patients with chronic end-stage liver disease are prioritized by their MELD score. Those with higher scores are placed higher on the list. The duration of waiting time is used only as a tie-breaker for patients with equal scores. Each UNOS region has special exception cases that must be voted on by the regional review board (comprising one member from each transplant center in the region). In these cases, the board may be asked to assign higher-than-calculated scores for patients with special problems that are not addressed by the use of only objective criteria, such as children with intractable pruritus, ascites, hemorrhage, or infectious complications and patients with hepatocellular carcinoma.[58]

The frequency of recalculation of the MELD score is determined by the score itself. MELD scores greater than 25, between 19 and 24, and between 11 and 18 are evaluated every 7, 30, and 90 days, respectively.[59] A score of less than 10 is recalculated yearly barring any exacerbation of the liver disease or patient condition.[59]

Next, one of the most difficult phases begins: the waiting period. It is not possible to anticipate when an appropriate organ will become available. The patient may feel that his or her life is being put "on hold." Because of the shortage of donors, it is not uncommon for patients in critical care units to die while awaiting transplantation. And knowing that another person must die so that he or she may live can cause feelings of guilt as the patient hopes for a liver to become available. Patients with end-stage liver disease know that the only alternative to transplantation is death. By understanding the basic social processes that patients experience while awaiting transplantation, nurses can facilitate health-promotion activities. It is important for the patient and family to receive ongoing psychosocial assessment and to attend pretransplantation support groups, which are available at most transplant centers.[60]

Pretransplantation Phase

The patient with end-stage liver disease who is awaiting a transplant may pose one of the greatest care challenges in the critical care unit. Hepatic encephalopathy, coagulopathies, portal hypertension, severe fluid and electrolyte imbalances, cardiac compromise, and renal deterioration are not uncommon. Frequent mental status assessments are important in determining the patient's continued candidacy for transplantation. Hepatic encephalopathy may improve with the administration of antibiotics and laxatives, or the patient may proceed to stage IV coma. Protection of the airway is especially important in an encephalopathic patient who is not intubated. In these circumstances, if hematemesis or vomiting occurs, intubation and use of paralytic agents may be necessary to protect the patient's airway. Diagnostic studies may be needed to evaluate the possibility of an intracranial bleed. The head of the patient's bed is maintained at 30 to 45 degrees to avoid even slight increases in intracranial pressure. Patients who have chronic liver disease also have nutritional deficits. They require supplements of the fat-soluble vitamins (A, D, E, and K), may be on protein restriction to reduce serum ammonia levels, and may experience severe muscle wasting.[33]

Consequences of portal hypertension must be corrected. Gastrointestinal hemorrhage from varices may respond to administration of propranolol or to procedures such as banding and sclerotherapy. Portal hypertension may be reduced by transjugular intrahepatic portosystemic shunting (TIPS) in interventional radiology. Rarely, the patient may need to undergo surgical intervention with a vascular shunt created between the portacaval system and the mesangial, splenic, or renal vascular system. Patients with massive ascites usually have total body fluid overload but are intravascularly contracted and require sodium restriction and administration of colloidal fluids (e.g., albumin) along with diuretics.

Careful documentation of fluid intake and output, daily weight determinations, and frequent measurement of vital signs are needed to monitor fluid status. Ascites can interfere with lung expansion and can compromise oxygenation. Patients with large, distended abdomens also find adequate oral nutrition difficult. Use of diuretics to control ascites is common but can compromise kidney function or even worsen hepatorenal syndrome. Paracentesis (removal of ascites) may be required for intractable ascites. However, frequent large-volume paracentesis procedures can contribute to renal demise and cardiovascular compromise related to fluid volume shifts.

Spontaneous bacterial peritonitis can be manifested in the patient with end-stage liver disease by an acute decline in the hepatic and renal function accompanied by fever, abdominal pain, and hepatic encephalopathy. The paracentesis fluid shows increased white blood cells with or without a positive

culture. Patients are treated aggressively with antibiotics and are temporarily deferred from transplantation during treatment for and recovery from bacterial peritonitis.

Determining Donor Suitability

The two criteria necessary for matching a donor liver to a recipient are blood type and body size. Human leukocyte antigen (HLA) tissue typing is not used in the matching of donor livers, because it has not been shown to significantly affect patient outcomes. Donors are carefully screened for infectious diseases and metastatic carcinomas, because these can be transmitted to the recipient. The transplant center is notified by the regional organ procurement organization that a liver is available. If the organ is accepted, a member of the transplantation team contacts the patient.

In very urgent situations, the donor blood type (e.g., type A) may not be compatible with that of the recipient (e.g., type O). Despite this incompatibility, such liver transplantations can be successful. There may be some early postoperative complications, such as mild hemolysis, higher incidence of acute cellular rejection, and increased postoperative hepatic vascular and biliary complications, but innovative use of immunosuppressive regimens and plasmapheresis have improved graft survival of patients with recipient-donor ABO incompatibility.[61] Extended-criteria donor livers that are otherwise unremarkable—such as those with a cold ischemia time longer than 12 hours or those from donors older than 60 years—are expanding the donor pool and shortening waiting times.[62]

Living Donor Liver Transplantation

Living Donor Liver Transplantation (LDLT) began in 1989 with adult-to-child donations, commonly from a parent to his or her infant. The left lateral hepatic lobe is resected, leaving the donor with the larger mass of liver remaining.[63] In such cases, the risks to the healthy donor are thought to be outweighed by the benefits of having a healthy child.[64] Adult-to-adult LDLT donation began in the 1990s. The whole left hepatic lobe or right hepatic lobe is resected, taking 30% to 60% of the liver mass from the live donor.[63] Complications for the donor after partial hepatectomy are usually of low severity. The most common ones are bile leak, bacterial infection, incisional hernia, pleural effusion, neuropraxia (temporary nerve dysfunction), wound infection, and abdominal abcess.[59,64] More serious potential complications for the liver donor include portal vein thrombosis, inferior vena cava thrombosis, and death.[59,64] Critical care nurses play an important role in caring for these donors and must be vigilant in assessing for complications and initiating early interventions.

Liver Transplantation Surgical Procedure

Liver transplantation surgery is lengthy and technically difficult, often lasting 4 to 12 hours. The procedure involves the combined efforts of surgeons, anesthesiologists, nurse anesthetists, operating room nurses and technicians, perfusionists, and personnel from the blood bank and laboratory and radiology departments, among others. The patient is taken to the operating room for anesthesia induction, insertion of large-bore intravenous catheters that allow high-volume fluid infusion, and insertion of a pulmonary artery catheter for hemodynamic monitoring. Continuous renal replacement may be continued or initiated in the operating room by a filter-trained critical care or dialysis nurse. Other devices, such as an arterial line, a nasogastric tube, and a urinary drainage catheter, are also inserted. The patient is positioned on the operating room table in such a way as to minimize pressure that could cause ischemia and chronic injury to tissue and peripheral nerves. Liver transplantation surgery can be divided into three stages: (1) recipient hepatectomy, (2) vascular anastomoses with donor liver, and (3) biliary anastomosis.[65]

Recipient Hepatectomy. Stage 1 is the longest and most difficult part of the surgery, because it involves removal of the native liver. It is complicated even more by coagulopathies, adhesions, portal hypertension, and venous collaterals. Before completion of this stage, the patient may be placed on venovenous bypass (Figure 22-9), although not all patients require this procedure. A centrifugal pump cycles the blood out through iliac and portal vein cannulas and returns it to the central circulation through the axillary or subclavian vein. Advances in surgical techniques, anesthesia, and fluid management have shortened the length of surgery enough to warrant elimination of venovenous bypass in some cases.[66]

Vascular Anastomoses with a Donor Liver. Stage 2 comprises the four vascular anastomoses: suprahepatic inferior vena cava, infrahepatic vena cava, hepatic artery, and portal vein. Many variations and adaptations, such as vascular patches, may be used, depending on the anatomy of the donor and recipient. If venovenous bypass is used, it is removed after the infrahepatic vena cava anastomosis and before the hepatic artery anastomosis.[66]

Biliary Anastomosis. Stage 3 can be achieved by choledochojejunostomy (bile duct to jejunum) or by choledochocholedochostomy (bile duct to bile duct). Choledochojejunostomy is performed in patients who have diseased bile ducts, such as those with biliary atresia or sclerosing cholangitis. It is also known as a Roux-en-Y procedure and is shown in Figure 22-10. The choledochocholedochostomy is performed in patients who have a healthy and intact common bile duct and is shown in Figure 22-11. The patient returns from surgery with or without an external stent or T-tube that is connected to a bag into which bile drains. Patients who do not have external biliary tubes may have an internal stent inserted in the bile duct across the biliary anastomosis. Eventually, the internal stent moves and is passed with the stool.[66]

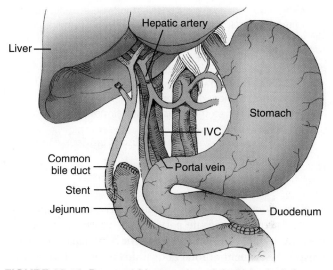

FIGURE 22-10 Roux-en-Y procedure (choledochojejunostomy). *IVC,* inferior vena cava.

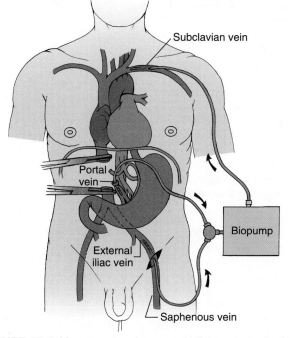

FIGURE 22-9 Venovenous bypass during removal of the native liver. The portal and iliac veins are cannulated, and blood is circulated by a centrifugal pump to the subclavian vein.

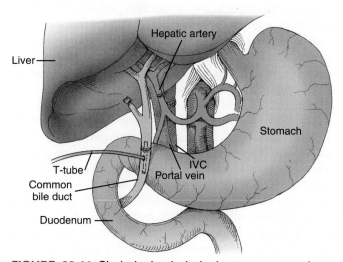

FIGURE 22-11 Choledochocholedochostomy procedure. *IVC,* inferior vena cava.

Postoperative Medical and Nursing Management

The common nursing diagnoses associated with liver transplantation are listed in the Nursing Diagnosis Priorities Box on Liver Transplantation. After surgery, some patients are extubated before they arrive in the critical care unit, but most arrive unreversed from anesthesia and remain intubated for 12 to 24 hours. **Immediate priorities include (1) reestablishment of normal body temperature, (2) hemodynamic stabilization, and (3) maintenance of an effective airway.** Postoperative hypothermia is common after orthotopic liver transplantation (OLT). The critical care nurse must achieve rewarming safely by the use of methods such as warming blankets and head covers.

NURSING DIAGNOSIS PRIORITIES

Liver Transplantation

- Risk for Infection: immunosuppressive drugs required to prevent rejection of the transplanted liver, p. A-36
- Imbalanced Nutrition: Less Than Body Requirements related to lack of exogenous nutrients or increased metabolic demand, p. A-22
- Deficient Fluid Volume related to absolute loss, p. A-13
- Disturbed Body Image related to actual change in body structure, function, or appearance, p. A-16
- Anxiety related to threat to biological, psychological, and social integrity, p. A-7
- Deficient Knowledge related to lack of previous exposure to information, p. A-15

Hemodynamics. Hemodynamic stabilization is a particular challenge, because the patient may arrive hypervolemic, euvolemic, or hypovolemic and may be hypertensive or hypotensive. Assessment of total body fluids compared with intravascular fluid status is important. Because of inherent presurgical problems with decreased serum albumin, some centers tend to keep the patient "dry." Hypervolemia often results in third spacing, with resultant ascites and a leaking wound. Accurate measurements of hemodynamic function, such as arterial blood pressure, peripheral blood pressure, central venous pressure, pulmonary artery pressure, pulmonary artery occlusion pressure, urinary output, patency of drains, and bile totals are assessed frequently to evaluate true volume status. Choice of replacement fluids and pharmacological agents for correction of volume and blood pressure abnormalities is specific to the transplant center. These protocols vary in their use of albumin or fresh-frozen plasma, and in the use of intravenous renal-dose dopamine or prostaglandin, as well as other agents and solutions. Still, the goals are the same: optimize tissue perfusion and deliver oxygen to all tissues, especially the newly transplanted graft.

Electrolytes. Electrolyte abnormalities can occur after OLT. Disturbances in potassium and magnesium levels are common. High serum levels of electrolytes are usually associated with renal impairment; low levels can be the result of

drug side effects (e.g., diuretic therapy). The presence of hypernatremia or hyponatremia complicates the correction of volume status and fluid replacement.

Pulmonary Management. Ventilatory support of the patient is maintained until the anesthetic agent has been metabolized and cleared by the new liver and the patient awakens. Frequent measurement of arterial blood gas levels, continuous pulse oximetry, and assessment of breath sounds are needed. The patient may require changes in ventilatory settings, suctioning to remove secretions, or administration of pharmacological agents to correct acid-base imbalances. Pulmonary complications are common, as listed in Box 22-13. While the patient is on ventilatory support, pneumonia can be avoided by maintaining the head of bed elevated at 30 degrees, turning the patient frequently, providing good oral care, and brushing the patient's teeth. After extubation, patients must be encouraged to perform incentive spirometry exercises and to turn and deep-breathe frequently to help prevent atelectasis and pneumonia.

Coagulopathy Risk. Management of coagulopathies is important in the early postoperative phase. Close monitoring of drainage tubes and incisions is required along with other nursing assessments of blood loss, such as identifying signs of hypovolemia, tachypnea, tachycardia, or poor peripheral oxygenation. Sanguineous nasogastric output, and black, tarry stools are hallmarks of bleeding problems and must be reported immediately. Laboratory monitoring during the

BOX 22-13   COMMON COMPLICATIONS AFTER LIVER TRANSPLANTATION

Pulmonary Complications
Pleural effusion
Pulmonary edema
Pneumonia
Pneumothorax or hemothorax
Atelectasis
Paralysis of right diaphragm

Biliary Complications
Leaks
Strictures
Obstruction
Infection (cholangitis)
Breakdown of anastomosis

Gastrointestinal Complications
Bleeding and ulceration
Gastrointestinal infections (cytomegalovirus, *Candida*, *Clostridium difficile*)
Bowel perforations

Vascular Complications
Hepatic artery thrombosis
Portal vein thrombosis
Vena caval thrombosis
Peripheral and central line sepsis
Hepatic vein thrombosis

first 24 hours after surgery is necessary to assess blood loss and coagulopathies and includes hematocrit, hemoglobin, platelet count, prothrombin time, partial thromboplastin time, fibrinogen, and fibrin split products. Reversal of coagulopathies is done judiciously, with consideration for the potential to thrombose newly anastomosed blood vessels in the liver. Blood products such as platelets, fresh-frozen plasma, and specific factors can be given along with pharmacological agents such as vitamin K.

Neurological Status. Neurological assessment of the patient is important in the early postoperative phase to determine mental status and graft function. Patients who were encephalopathic preoperatively are usually slower to clear mentally. Nevertheless, with good liver function, the patient should be alert and oriented within 1 to 2 days. The improved mental status is a reflection of a functional new liver. Certain pharmacological agents, including immunosuppressants, can cause peripheral and central neurological side effects that may alter neurological status. Induction therapy may be used to delay the initiation of immunosuppressant medications associated with neurological and nephrogenic side effects.[66,67]

Pain Management. The critical care nurse must always be aware of the potential for intracranial bleeds in a patient who has coagulopathies, serum sodium imbalances, and hemodynamic instability. All of these conditions can interfere with pain management, because the pharmacological agents used for pain can mask deterioration in mental status. Medications to relieve pain are administered, but other nonpharmacological nursing interventions also must be used.

Glucose Control. Intensive blood glucose control (<150 mg/dL) during liver transplantation surgery has been associated with a significant decrease in the infection rate at 30 days and in the mortality rate at 1 year.[68] In the intensive care setting, insulin therapy is used to support the newly transplanted liver during the fluctuations in blood glucose related to the patient's immunosuppressant regimen.

Kidney Function. Liver transplantation can alter kidney function by several mechanisms, including cyclosporine or tacrolimus administration, acute tubular necrosis, intrinsic kidney disease, and poor liver function. Some studies estimate that 48% to 94% of OLT patients develop renal failure.[69] Patients are managed with attention to fluid and electrolyte imbalances, by avoidance of nephrotoxic drugs, and occasionally with ultrafiltration, continuous renal replacement therapy, or intermittent hemodialysis. With good liver function, kidney function usually improves. However, certain immunosuppressive agents and antimicrobials can deleteriously affect kidney function. Adjustments in dose or avoidance of use must be balanced with assessment of kidney and liver function. Daily monitoring of cyclosporine or tacrolimus serum levels is vital to determining adequate immunosuppression, and daily serum creatinine levels are necessary to watch for renal impairment. As the patient's condition continues to improve, the frequency of laboratory testing may decrease.[69]

Infection Risk. Immunosuppressive therapy places the transplant recipient at an increased risk for infection. Infectious complications are common and continue to be the leading cause of death among OLT patients. The potential for infection is greatest when patients receive high doses of immunosuppressants.[66] All persons who come into contact with the transplant recipient throughout the hospitalization must practice good hand hygiene techniques and standard precautions to prevent the transmission of infection.[60] Infections are treated with appropriate antimicrobials specific to the invading organism. Prophylactic therapies are commonly used as well.[59]

Bile Drains. Careful attention to any external biliary drain line is important. If the patient has an external biliary drain, the critical care nurse documents color, character, and amount of drainage and reports any changes. Biliary complications can occur after OLT. Posttransplantation complications, including biliary ones, are listed in Box 22-13.

Nutrition. The nasogastric tube is removed when its output is minimal, bowel sounds have returned, and the patient is extubated. If the patient will be intubated longer than several days, total parenteral nutrition may be started. Consultation with a nutritionist (dietitian) should be sought after the patient is stable. Prealbumin levels may be measured to assess nutritional status. Otherwise, nutrition may begin orally or through a feeding tube as soon as bowel function returns. The diet is slowly advanced as tolerated.

Liver Function Tests. The standard laboratory biomarkers used to monitor graft function are serum aspartate aminotransferase (AST), alanine aminotransferase (ALT), alkaline phosphatase, and γ-glutamyltransferase (GGT); serum bilirubin; and prothrombin time. The serum levels of these markers are measured frequently during the first few postoperative days and may continue to rise before peaking and subsequently falling. As liver function improves, the frequency of laboratory testing decreases, but the critical care nurse can anticipate performing these liver function tests daily after the initial postoperative period.

Liver Graft Nonfunction. The patient with suspected primary nonfunction of a liver graft demonstrates (1) hemodynamic instability, (2) progressive deterioration of kidney function, (3) coagulopathies and abnormal serum liver function laboratory tests, (4) hypoglycemia, (5) continued ventilatory dependence, and (6) an inability to awaken from anesthesia. Continued nonfunction of the graft necessitates relisting the patient for another donor liver. Early signs of optimal graft function include improving kidney function, mental alertness, a high to normal serum glucose concentration, and early extubation. The serum ALT, AST, GGT, and alkaline phosphatase levels may peak on the third or fourth day but later decrease. The serum bilirubin concentration may take a week before beginning to fall, and there may be a mild elevation when the external biliary drainage tube is clamped or after a blood transfusion. Early mobilization and physical therapy are encouraged.

Rejection Surveillance. Acute rejection in OLT is a cellular-mediated event and should be suspected if the serum liver function laboratory tests, especially AST and ALT, become elevated compared with previous levels. Such elevations usually precede any other sign of acute rejection of the liver allograft. Sometimes, the patient also exhibits fever, a drop in bile output (if a T-tube is still connected to a drainage bag), and a change in the color and viscosity of the bile. At first the patient may not have any other physical symptoms, but eventually late signs of rejection may occur, including malaise, dark urine, and clay-colored stools. Certain infections, such as CMV, can also cause liver function test values to increase.

Rejection is suspected when liver function test values increase, but other reasons for these elevations need to be ruled out. Mechanical and vascular complications are ruled out by Doppler ultrasonography and angiography. Endoscopic retrograde cholangiopancreatography, hepatobiliary iminodiacetic acid (HIDA) scanning, or transhepatic cholangiography may reveal biliary obstruction or leakage. A liver biopsy may be indicated to determine the cause of liver dysfunction if the other tests are inconclusive. Acute rejection can occur at any time after transplantation, but most commonly it occurs during the first few months and even as early as the first week after surgery. Most liver transplant recipients experience at least one acute rejection episode. Treatment of acute rejection requires increasing immunosuppression (i.e., an increase in tacrolimus or steroid dose and possibly an addition of monoclonal or polyclonal antilymphocyte antibodies or other newer pharmacological agents). Immunosuppressant protocols vary from center to center and are usually successful at reversing acute rejection.

Chronic rejection is a humoral event and is progressive and nonreversible. Chronic rejection in a liver transplant recipient usually requires retransplantation if the patient is still a candidate.

Transfer Out of Critical Care.
After the patient is stable and the transplanted liver is functional, catheters and drains are removed before the patient is transferred out of the critical care unit. Central venous catheters and arterial lines are removed. The urinary catheter is removed as soon as the patient is awake enough to be continent. Drain lines are removed as drainage outputs become minimal. As the patient begins to participate in self-care, plans are made for transfer out of the critical care unit to the transplantation nursing unit.

On the transplantation unit, laboratory data and vital signs continue to be monitored on a routine basis. Self-care is promoted. Increasing levels of physical therapy are encouraged, diet is advanced, and much of the nurse's effort is directed toward teaching the patient and family.

Patient Education.
Considerable attention is focused on patient education and discharge planning. Discharge booklets are helpful in the education process. It is important for the patient to learn how to self-administer medications, monitor vital signs, care for the incision and the T-tube (if present), prevent infections, and identify problems that must promptly receive medical attention. Because it is not uncommon for patients to be discharged within 2 weeks after OLT, it is important for discharge instructions to begin as soon as the patient is mentally alert. Patients discharged early may require home health nurse referrals to assist with follow-up

of incision care, intravenous therapies, and other procedures. Education must be provided about rejection surveillance, signs and symptoms of infection, lifestyle changes as needed, long-term medication considerations, and the follow-up visit schedule.

Long-Term Follow-Up.
OLT patients who do not live in the same city in which their surgery was performed usually remain in the immediate area of the transplant center after discharge before returning home. During this period, they may be monitored by a home health nurse and be seen in the clinic several times a week by the transplantation team. Continued serologic testing is done to monitor graft function, to determine blood levels of certain immunosuppressive agents, and to identify postoperative complications. Although many of these complications can be managed successfully in the outpatient setting, readmissions do occur. Because rejections, readmissions, grieving for the donor, and pharmacological side effects can create anxiety for the family and the patient, they are encouraged to attend transplantation support groups if offered by the center. After patients return home, they are encouraged to resume a close relationship with their local primary care physician and gastroenterologist.

OLT patients need long-term follow-up surveillance for hypertension, kidney failure, obesity, dyslipidemias, biliary and infectious complications, and malignancies.[59] Early intervention affects the quality and length of life. Behavior modifications and therapeutic lifestyle changes should be frequently reinforced to positively affect long-term health. Financial concerns are a major source of stress in this patient population. Many transplant recipients suffered from chronic liver disease before their surgery. They often were disabled for some time and already have experienced financial stressors related to illness. As these patients live longer with liver transplants, issues of insurability, continued disability, and even the ability to obtain work will have to be addressed.

Pharmacological Agents

Many pharmacological agents are used in the care of patients with gastrointestinal disorders. Table 22-3 reviews the various agents and any special considerations necessary for administering them.

Antiulcer Agents

A number of different antiulcer agents are commonly used in the critical care setting, including H_2-antagonists, gastric PPIs, and gastric mucosal agents.[70] H_2-antagonists are used to decrease the volume and concentration of gastric secretions and control gastric pH, decreasing the incidence of stress-related upper gastrointestinal bleeding. These agents work by blocking histamine stimulation of the H_2-receptors on the gastric parietal cells, reducing acid production. Although these drugs may be administered orally, intramuscularly, or intravenously, they usually are given intravenously in the critical care setting. Proton-pump inhibitors decrease gastric acid secretion by binding to the proton pump, blocking the release of acid from the gastric parietal cells. PPIs are potent

TABLE 22-3	PHARMACOLOGICAL MANAGEMENT: GASTROINTESTINAL DISORDERS		
MEDICATION	**DOSAGE**	**ACTIONS**	**SPECIAL CONSIDERATIONS**
Antacids	30-90 mL q1-2h PO or NG; possibly titrated to NG pH	Used to buffer stomach acid and raise gastric pH	Can cause diarrhea or constipation and electrolyte disturbances. Irrigate NG tube with water after administration because antacids can clog tube.
Histamine$_2$-(H$_2$) Antagonists			
Cimetidine (Tagamet)	300 mg q6h IV or PO	Used to reduce volume and concentration of gastric secretions	Side effects include CNS toxicity (confusion or delirium) and thrombocytopenia. Separate administration of antacids and histamine blocking agents by 1 hour.
Ranitidine (Zantac)	150 mg q12h PO or 50 mg q8h IV		
Famotidine (Pepcid)	40 mg daily PO or 20 mg q12h IV		
Nizatidine (Axid)	150 mg q12h PO or 300 mg q24h		
Gastric Mucosal Agents			
Sucralfate (Carafate)	1 g q6h NG or PO, given 1 hour before meals and at bedtime	Forms an ulcer-adherent complex with proteinaceous exudates Covers the ulcer and protects against acid, pepsin, and bile salts	Requires an acid medium for activation; do not administer within 30 minutes of an antacid. May cause severe constipation. May cause decreased absorption of certain drugs.
Gastric Proton-Pump Inhibitors			
Omeprazole (Prilosec)	20-40 mg q12h PO	Inactivates acid, or hydrogen, acid pump, blocking secretion of hydrochloric acid by gastric parietal cells	Capsules should be swallowed intact. May increase levels of phenytoin, diazepam, warfarin. May administer concomitantly with antacids.
Lansoprazole (Prevacid)	15-30 mg q24h PO 30 mg over 30 min q24h IV		
Rabeprazole (AcipHex)	20-40 mg q24h PO		
Esomeprazole (Nexium)	40 mg q12-24h PO 20-40 mg q24h IV		
Pantoprazole (Protonix)	20-40 mg q24h PO 80 mg q8-12h IV		
Vasopressin (Pitressin Synthetic)	Loading dose of 20 units over 20 min IV, followed by 0.2-0.4 unit/min IV infusion Doses can be increased to 0.9 unit/min if necessary	Decreases splanchnic blood flow, reducing portal pressure	Side effects include coronary, mesenteric, and peripheral vasoconstriction. May be administered concurrently with nitroglycerin to minimize side effects.
Octreotide (Sandostatin)	Bolus dose of 25-50 mcg followed by IV infusion of 25-50 mcg/hr for 48 hours	Decreases splanchnic blood flow, reducing portal pressure	May cause hyperglycemia or hypoglycemia when initiating the drip and changing dosages.

CNS, central nervous system; *IV*, intravenous; *NG*, nasogastric; *PO*, by mouth.

acid inhibitors and have greater suppressive ability than the H_2-agonists.[71,72]

Unlike H_2-antagonists or PPIs, sucralfate does not affect gastric acid concentration but rather exerts its action locally. Sucralfate reacts with hydrochloric acid to form a sticky, paste-like substance that adheres to the surface of the ulcer and shields it from pepsin, acid, and bile. Sucralfate predominantly binds to damaged gastrointestinal mucosa, with minimal adherence to normal tissue.[72] It is administered orally or through a gastric tube. Sucralfate should not be crushed but may be dissolved in 10 mL of water to form a slurry. It is also available as a suspension.

Vasopressin

Vasopressin is used to control gastric ulcer and variceal bleeding. It is administered intraarterially, through a catheter inserted into the right or left gastric artery (through the femoral artery, aorta, and celiac trunk) or intravenously. It causes splanchnic and systemic vasoconstriction, subsequently reducing portal blood flow and pressure.[71] A major side effect of the drug is systemic vasoconstriction, which can result in cardiac ischemia, chest pain, hypertension, acute heart failure, dysrhythmias, phlebitis, bowel ischemia, and cerebrovascular accident. These side effects can be offset with concurrent administration of nitroglycerin. Other complications include bradycardia and fluid retention. Nursing responsibilities associated with the use of this therapy include maintenance of a patent infusion line and continuous monitoring for vasoconstrictive complications of therapy.[18]

Somatostatin and Octreotide

Somatostatin is a peptide that is administered parenterally in the acutely bleeding, cirrhotic patient. It reduces splanchnic vasodilation and portal pressure through the inhibition of secretion of various vasodilator hormones, and it is as effective as vasopressin in treating variceal bleeding with minimal side effects. Octreotide is a commonly used, long-acting synthetic analogue of somatostatin.[18,71]

CASE STUDY   PATIENT WITH GASTROINTESTINAL ISSUES

Answers to the Case Study Questions can be found on the Evolve web site at http://evolve.elsevier.com/Urden/priorities/.

Brief Patient History
Mrs. S is a 70-year-old woman with a long history of chronic back pain. She has been taking nonsteroidal antiinflammatory drugs (NSAIDs) for several years. She was recently started on warfarin for atrial fibrillation.

Clinical Assessment
Mrs. S is admitted to the intensive care unit because she is vomiting bright red blood. She is pale and diaphoretic and complains of epigastric pain.

Diagnostic Procedures
Mrs. S's vital signs include the following: blood pressure of 70/40 mm Hg, heart rate of 130 beats/min (sinus tachycardia), respiratory rate of 30 breaths/min, and temperature of 101.3° F. Her urine output is 15 mL/hr, hemoglobin level is 9 g/dL, and international normalized ratio (INR) is 5.3.

Medical Diagnosis
Mrs. S is diagnosed with upper gastrointestinal bleeding.

Questions
1. What major outcomes do you expect to achieve for this patient?
2. What problems or risks must be managed to achieve these outcomes?
3. What interventions must be initiated to monitor, prevent, manage, or eliminate the problems and risks identified?
4. What interventions should be initiated to promote optimal functioning, safety, and well-being of the patient?
5. What possible learning needs do you anticipate for this patient?
6. What cultural and age-related factors may have a bearing on the patient's plan of care?

REFERENCES

1. Tariq SH, Mekhjian G: Gastrointestinal bleeding in older adults, *Clin Geriatr Med* 23(4):769, 2007.
2. Gralnek IM, et al: Management of acute bleeding from a peptic ulcer, *N Engl J Med* 359(9):928, 2008.
3. Barkun AN, et al: International consensus recommendations on the management of patients with nonvariceal upper gastrointestinal bleeding, *Ann Intern Med* 152(2):101, 2010.
4. Cappell MS, Friedel D: Acute nonvariceal upper gastrointestinal bleeding: endoscopic diagnosis and therapy, *Med Clin North Am* 92(3):511, 2008.
5. Manning-Dimmitt LL, et al: Diagnosis of gastrointestinal bleeding in adults, *Am Fam Physician* 71(7):1339, 2005.
6. Schubert ML: Gastric secretion, *Curr Opin Gastroenterol* 26(6):598, 2010.
7. Huether SE: Alterations of digestive function. In McCance KL, et al, editors: *Pathophysiology: the biologic basis for disease in adults and children*, ed 6, St Louis, 2010, Mosby.
8. Napolitano L: Refractory peptic ulcer disease, *Gastroenterol Clin North Am* 38(2):267, 2009.
9. Ramakrishnan K, Salinas RC: Peptic ulcer disease, *Am Fam Physician* 76(7):1005, 2007.
10. Ali T, Harty RF: Stress-induced ulcer bleeding in critically ill patients, *Gastroenterol Clin North Am* 38(2):245, 2009.
11. Sesler JM: Stress-related mucosal disease in the intensive care unit: an update on prophylaxis, *AACN Adv Crit Care* 18(2):119, 2007.

12. Garcia-Tsao G, Bosch J: Management of varices and variceal hemorrhage in cirrhosis, *N Engl J Med* 362(9):823, 2010.

13. Toubia N, Sanyal AJ: Portal hypertension and variceal hemorrhage, *Med Clin North Am* 92(3):551, 2008.

14. Dutton RP: Current concepts in hemorrhagic shock, *Anesthesiol Clin* 25(1):23, 2007.

15. Cheung FK, Lau JY: Management of massive peptic ulcer bleeding, *Gastroenterol Clin N Am* 38(2):231, 2009.

16. Wilmot LA: Shock: early recognition and management, *J Emerg Nurs* 36(2):134, 2010.

17. Park WG, et al: Injection therapies for nonvariceal bleeding disorders of the GI tract, *Gastrointest Endosc* 66(2):343, 2007.

18. Cat TB, Liu-DeRyke X: Medical management of variceal hemorrhage, *Crit Care Nurs Clin North Am* 22(3):381, 2010.

19. Christensen T: The treatment of oesophageal varices using a Sengstaken-Blakemore tube: considerations for nursing practice, *Nurs Crit Care* 9(2):58, 2004.

20. de Caestecker J, Straus J: Upper gastrointestinal bleeding: surgical treatment, 2009. Available at http://emedicine. medscape.com/article/196561-overview (accessed April 2011).

21. Gilbert DA, Saunders DR: Iced saline lavage does not slow bleeding from experimental canine gastric ulcers, *Dig Dis Sci* 26(12):1065, 1981.

22. Holcomb SS: Stopping the destruction of acute pancreatitis, *Nursing* 37(6):42, 2007.

23. Carroll JK, et al: Acute pancreatitis: diagnosis, prognosis, and treatment, *Am Fam Physician* 75(10):1513, 2007.

24. Whitcomb DC: Clinical practice. Acute pancreatitis, *N Engl J Med* 354(20):2142, 2006.

25. Cappell MS: Acute pancreatitis: etiology, clinical presentation, diagnosis, and therapy, *Med Clin North Am* 92(4):889, 2008.

26. Habashi S, Draganov PV: Pancreatic pseudocyst, *World J Gastroenterol* 15(1):38, 2009.

27. O'Keefe SJ, Sharma S: Nutritional support in severe acute pancreatitis, *Gastroenterol Clin North Am* 36(2):297, 2007.

28. Al-Omran M, et al: Enteral versus parenteral nutrition for acute pancreatitis, Cochrane Database Syst Rev Jan 20;(1):CD002837, 2010.

29. Lugli AK, et al: The importance of nutrition status assessment: the case of severe acute pancreatitis, *Nutr Rev* 65(7):329, 2007.

30. Gourgiotis S, et al: Surgical management of chronic pancreatitis, *Hepatobiliary Pancreat Dis Int* 6(2):121, 2007.

31. Munsell MA, Buscaglia JM: Acute pancreatitis, *J Hosp Med* 5(4):241, 2010.

32. Fontana RJ: Acute liver failure including acetaminophen overdose, *Med Clin North Am* 92(4):761, 2008.

33. Stravitz RT: Clinical management decisions in patients with acute liver failure, *Chest* 134(5):1092, 2008.

34. Stravitz RT, et al: Intensive care of patients with acute liver failure: recommendations of the U.S. Acute Liver Failure Study Group, *Crit Care Med* 35(11):2498, 2007.

35. O'Grady J: Modern management of acute liver failure, *Clin Liver Dis* 11(2):291, 2007.

36. Noble KA: Name that tube, *Nursing* 33(3):56, 2003.

37. May S: Testing nasogastric tube positioning in the critically ill: exploring the evidence, *Br J Nurs* 16(7):414, 2007.

38. Metheny NA: Preventing respiratory complications of tube feedings: evidence-based practice, *Am J Crit Care* 15(4):360, 2006.

39. American Association of Critical-Care Nurses: Practice alert: Verification of feeding tube placement, *AACN News* 22(5):4, 2005.

40. Cappell MS: Therapeutic endoscopy for acute upper gastrointestinal bleeding, *Nat Rev Gastroenterol Hepatol* 7(4):214, 2010.

41. Kalva SP, et al: Transjugular intrahepatic portosystemic shunt for acute variceal hemorrhage, *Tech Vasc Interv Radiol* 12(2):92, 2009.

42. Cura M, et al: Causes of TIPS dysfunction, *AJR Am J Roentgenol* 191(6):1751, 2008.

43. Mackenzie DJ, et al: Care of patients after esophagectomy, *Crit Care Nurse* 24(1):16, 2004.

44. Smith CE: Gastrointestinal surgery. In Rothrock JC, editor: *Alexander's care of the patient in surgery*, ed 13, St Louis, 2007, Mosby.

45. Wente MN, et al: Pancreaticojejunostomy versus pancreaticogastrostomy: systematic review and meta-analysis, *Am J Surg* 193(2):171, 2007.

46. Barth MM, Jenson CE: Postoperative nursing care of gastric bypass patients, *Am J Crit Care* 15(4):378, 2006.

47. Harrington L: Postoperative care of patients undergoing bariatric surgery, *Medsurg Nurs* 15(6):357, 2006.

48. Leslie D, et al: Bariatric surgery primer for the internist: keys to the surgical consultation, *Med Clin North Am* 91(3):353, 2007.

49. Bell BJ, et al: Management of complications after laparoscopic Roux-en-Y gastric bypass, *Minerva Chir* 64(3):265, 2009.

50. Ahmed A, Keeffe EB: Current indications and contraindications for liver transplantation, *Clin Liver Dis* 11(2):227, 2007.

51. Pelletier SJ, et al: Effect of body mass index on the survival benefit of liver transplantation, *Liver Transpl* 13(12):1678, 2007.

52. Lipshutz GS, Busuttil RW: Liver transplantation in those of advancing age: the case for transplantation, *Liver Transpl* 13(10):1355, 2007.

53. Jiang L, Yan LN: Current therapeutic strategies for recurrent hepatitis B virus infection after liver transplantation, *World J Gastroenterol* 16(20):2468, 2010.

54. Mottershead M, Neuberger J: Transplantation in autoimmune liver diseases, *World J Gastroenterol* 14(21):3388, 2008.

55. Rosen CB, et al: Surgery for cholangiocarcinoma: the role of liver transplantation, *HPB(Oxford)* 10(3):186, 2008.

56. Dawwas MF, Gimson AE: Candidate selection and organ allocation in liver transplantation, *Semin Liver Dis* 29(1):40, 2009.

57. Mascarenhas R, Gurakar A: Recent advances in liver transplantation for the practicing gastroenterologist, *Gastroenterol Hepatol (N Y)* 5(6):443, 2009.

58. Mathews SB, et al: Liver transplant considerations for evaluation, CTP, and MELD, *Crit Care Nurs Clin North Am* 22(3):403, 2010.

59. Bufton S, et al: Liver transplantation. In Ohler L, Cupples S, editors: *Core curriculum for transplant nurses*, St Louis, 2008, Elsevier.

60. Watanabe A, Inoue T: Transformational experiences in adult-to-adult living-donor liver transplant recipients, *J Adv Nurs* 66(1):69, 2010.

61. Abbasoglu O: Liver transplantation: yesterday, today and tomorrow, *World J Gastroenterol* 14(20):3117, 2008.

62. Heffron T, et al: Successful ABO-incompatible pediatric liver transplantation utilizing standard immunosuppression with selective postoperative plasmapheresis, *Liver Transpl* 12(6):972, 2006.

63. Rudow DL, Goldstein MJ: Critical care management of the liver transplant recipient, *Crit Care Nurs Q* 31(3): 232, 2008.

64. Ghobrial RM, et al: Donor morbidity after living donation for liver transplantation, *Gastroenterology* 135(2):468, 2008.

65. Neil JA: Surgery of the liver, biliary tract, pancreas, and spleen. In Rothrock JC, editor: *Alexander's care of the patient in surgery,* ed 13, St Louis, 2007, Mosby.

66. Koffron A, Stein JA: Liver transplantation: indications, pretransplant evaluation, surgery, and posttransplant complications, *Med Clin North Am* 92(4):861, 2008.

67. Campara M, et al: Interleukin-2 receptor blockade with humanized monoclonal antibody for solid organ transplantation, *Expert Opin Biol Ther* 10(6):959 2010.

68. Ammori JB, et al: Effect of intraoperative hyperglycemia during liver transplantation, *J Surg Res* 140(2):227, 2007.

69. Yalavarthy R, et al: Acute renal failure and chronic kidney disease following liver transplantation, *Hemodial Int* 11 (Suppl 3):S7, 2007.

70. Quenot JP, et al: When should stress ulcer prophylaxis be used in the ICU? *Curr Opin Crit Care* 15(2):139, 2009.

71. Gahart BL, Nazareno AR: *2011 Intravenous medications*, ed 27, St Louis, 2011, Mosby.

72. Singh H, et al: Gastrointestinal prophylaxis in critically ill patients, *Crit Care Nurs Q* 31(4):291, 2008.

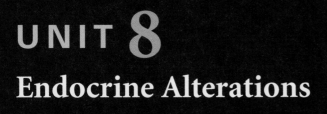

Endocrine Clinical Assessment and Diagnostic Procedures

Mary E. Lough

evolve WEBSITE

Be sure to check out the bonus material, including free self-assessment exercises, on the Evolve web site at *http://evolve.elsevier.com/Urden/priorities/*.

OBJECTIVES

- Identify the components of an endocrine history.
- Describe clinical findings in patients with pancreatic and posterior pituitary dysfunction.
- Explain the clinical significance of laboratory and diagnostic tests of pancreatic dysfunction.
- Explain the clinical significance of laboratory and diagnostic tests of posterior pituitary dysfunction.

Assessment of the patient with endocrine dysfunction is a systematic process that incorporates the history and the physical examination. Most of the endocrine glands are deeply encased in the human body. Although the placement of the glands provides security, their inaccessibility limits clinical examination. The location of the endocrine glands, with the hormones they produce, target cells or organs, and hormonal actions, is presented in Figure 23-1. This chapter describes clinical and diagnostic evaluation of the pancreas and posterior pituitary gland.

HISTORY

The initial presentation of the patient determines the rapidity and direction of the interview. For a patient in acute distress, the history is curtailed to only a few questions about the patient's chief complaint and precipitating events. For the patient without obvious distress, the endocrine history focuses on five areas: current health status, description of the current illness, medical history, general endocrine status, and family history.

PANCREAS

Physical Assessment

Nursing priorities for physical assessment of the patient with pancreatic dysfunction focus on (1) hyperglycemia and (2) hypoglycemia.

Insulin, which is produced by the pancreas, is responsible for glucose metabolism. The clinical assessment provides information about pancreatic functioning. Hyperglycemia is the clinical manifestation of abnormal glucose metabolism.[1,2] Patients with hyperglycemia may ultimately be diagnosed with type 1 or type 2 diabetes[1,2] or be hyperglycemic in association with a severe critical illness.[1,3] Hypoglycemia is often a complication of intensive insulin therapy. These conditions have specific identifying features as described in further detail in Chapter 24. Data collection for diabetic complications is outlined in Box 23-1.

Hyperglycemia

Because severe hyperglycemia affects a variety of body systems, all systems are assessed. The patient may complain of blurred vision, headache, weakness, fatigue, drowsiness,

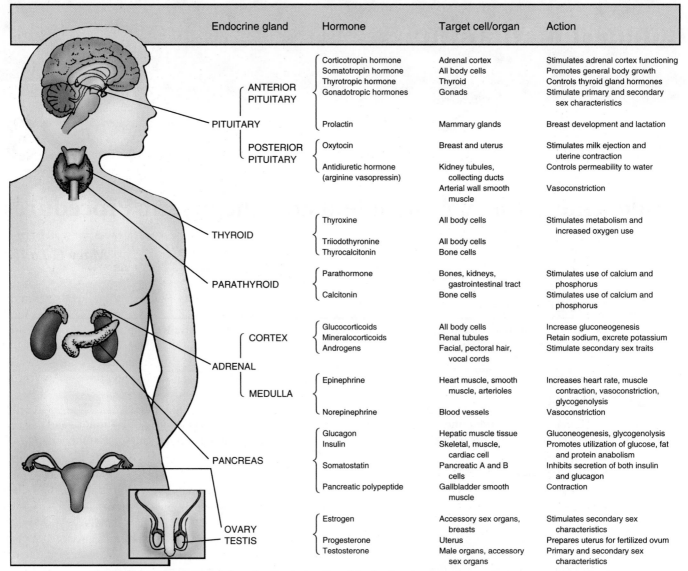

Endocrine gland		Hormone	Target cell/organ	Action
PITUITARY	ANTERIOR PITUITARY	Corticotropin hormone	Adrenal cortex	Stimulates adrenal cortex functioning
		Somatotropin hormone	All body cells	Promotes general body growth
		Thyrotropic hormone	Thyroid	Controls thyroid gland hormones
		Gonadotropic hormones	Gonads	Stimulate primary and secondary sex characteristics
		Prolactin	Mammary glands	Breast development and lactation
	POSTERIOR PITUITARY	Oxytocin	Breast and uterus	Stimulates milk ejection and uterine contraction
		Antidiuretic hormone (arginine vasopressin)	Kidney tubules, collecting ducts	Controls permeability to water
			Arterial wall smooth muscle	Vasoconstriction
THYROID		Thyroxine	All body cells	Stimulates metabolism and increased oxygen use
		Triiodothyronine	All body cells	
		Thyrocalcitonin	Bone cells	
PARATHYROID		Parathormone	Bones, kidneys, gastrointestinal tract	Stimulates use of calcium and phosphorus
		Calcitonin	Bone cells	Stimulates use of calcium and phosphorus
ADRENAL	CORTEX	Glucocorticoids	All body cells	Increase gluconeogenesis
		Mineralocorticoids	Renal tubules	Retain sodium, excrete potassium
		Androgens	Facial, pectoral hair, vocal cords	Stimulate secondary sex traits
	MEDULLA	Epinephrine	Heart muscle, smooth muscle, arterioles	Increases heart rate, muscle contraction, vasoconstriction, glycogenolysis
		Norepinephrine	Blood vessels	Vasoconstriction
PANCREAS		Glucagon	Hepatic muscle tissue	Gluconeogenesis, glycogenolysis
		Insulin	Skeletal, muscle, cardiac cell	Promotes utilization of glucose, fat and protein anabolism
		Somatostatin	Pancreatic A and B cells	Inhibits secretion of both insulin and glucagon
		Pancreatic polypeptide	Gallbladder smooth muscle	Contraction
OVARY TESTIS		Estrogen	Accessory sex organs, breasts	Stimulates secondary sex characteristics
		Progesterone	Uterus	Prepares uterus for fertilized ovum
		Testosterone	Male organs, accessory sex organs	Primary and secondary sex characteristics

FIGURE 23-1 Location of endocrine glands with the hormones they produce, target cells or organs, and hormonal actions.

anorexia, nausea, and abdominal pain. On *inspection,* the patient has flushed skin, polyuria, polydipsia, vomiting, and evidence of dehydration. Progressive deterioration in the level of consciousness, from alert to lethargic or comatose, is observed as the hyperglycemia exacerbates. If ketoacidosis occurs, the patient's breathing becomes deep and rapid (Kussmaul respirations), and the breath may have a fruity odor. *Auscultation* of the abdomen may reveal hypoactive bowel sounds. *Palpation* elicits abdominal tenderness. *Percussion* may reveal diminished deep tendon reflexes. Because hyperglycemia results in osmotic diuresis, the patient's fluid volume status is assessed. Signs of dehydration include tachycardia, orthostatic hypotension, and poor skin turgor. The key laboratory tests that confirm the assessment of hyperglycemia are discussed under laboratory studies.

Hypoglycemia

Patients with hypoglycemia may experience symptoms of tiredness, extreme hunger, headache, dizziness or blurred vision. On *inspection,* the skin may be diaphoretic, cool and clammy, or sweaty. Hands may be shaky with decreased coordination. Deterioration in the level of consciousness, from alert to disorientated, lethargic to coma occur. Seizures can occur with hypoglycemia. Although hypoglycemia can be suspected from physical signs and symptoms, a blood glucose level, as described under laboratory studies, is required to confirm this suspicion.

Laboratory Studies

Pertinent laboratory tests for pancreatic function measure short-term and long-term blood glucose levels, which can identify and diagnose diabetes.

BOX 23-1 TAKING A HEALTH HISTORY FOR DIABETIC COMPLICATIONS

Current Health Status

The body may not be able to adjust to increased insulin needs resulting from sudden physiological changes such as infection, injury, or surgery. The nurse assesses whether the patient has a severe infection, surgical wound, or traumatic injury.

- Recent or current signs and symptoms
- Unexplained changes in weight, thirst, hunger
- Headache, blurred vision
- Long-standing, unhealed infection
- Vaginitis, pruritus
- Leg pain, numbness
- Unexplained change in urinary patterns (e.g., daytime and nighttime, frequency, volume)
- Energy or stamina changes
  - Endurance level
  - Weakness
  - Unexplained, excessive fatigue
- Behavior or mental changes (also ask family member or significant other for input)
  - Memory loss
  - Orientation

Assessment of Current Illness: Onset, Characteristics, and Course

- Chronic illness—physiological or psychological stress can increase endogenous glucose
- Recent treatments that could be a source of exogenous glucose
  - Hyperalimentation
  - Peritoneal dialysis
  - Hemodialysis
- Medications, including prescription and over-the-counter preparations—pharmacological agents can alter pancreatic function by increasing or decreasing the release of endocrine hormones. Drugs also may interfere with hormonal action at the receptor site on the target cell.

Patient's Medical History: Questions

- Have you had prior pancreatic surgery?
- Have you ever been told that any of the following applied to you?
  - Too much sugar in the urine?
  - Too much sugar in the blood?
  - Will probably develop too much sugar later in life?
  - Are prediabetic?
- If you answered yes to any of these questions, what treatment, if any, was prescribed?
- Are you currently following such a treatment?

Family History: Questions

- Has a family member ever been diagnosed with diabetes or "sugar in the blood"?
- If so, how did he or she treat the condition?

Blood Glucose

The fasting plasma glucose (FPG) level is assessed by a simple blood test after the person has not eaten for 8 hours.[1] A normal FPG level is between 70 and 100 mg/dL.[1] A fasting glucose level between 100 and 125 mg/dL identifies a person who is *prediabetic*. Even prediabetic individuals are at increased risk for complications of diabetes such as coronary heart disease and stroke. An FPG level of 126 mg/dL (7 mmol/L) or higher is diagnostic of diabetes (Table 23-1). In non-urgent settings, the test is repeated on another day to ensure the result is accurate. In a patient with classic symptoms of hyperglycemia as described above, a non-fasting blood glucose level above 200 mg/dL (11.1 mmol\L) suggests diabetes.[1,2] After a meal, the concentration of glucose will increase in the bloodstream. Postprandial glucose levels should never exceed 180 mg/dL (10 mmol/L).[4]

All hospitalized patients must have their blood glucose levels monitored frequently while in the hospital.[1] Clinical practice guidelines from the American Association of Clinical Endocrinologists (AACE) and the American Diabetes Association (ADA) recommend a target blood glucose level of 140 to 180 mg/dL in the critically ill.[5] This range was selected to increase patient safety while on continuous insulin infusions by decreasing the risk of hypoglycemia.

When a continuous insulin infusion is administered, point-of-care blood glucose testing is performed hourly or according to hospital protocol by the critical care nurse to achieve and maintain the blood glucose within the target range.[1,5]

Hypoglycemia is defined as a blood glucose level below 70 mg/dL (3.9 mmol/L).[1,5,6] Severe hypoglycemia is defined as a blood glucose level below 40 mg/dL. Not all patients with hypoglycemia experience symptoms such as fatigue, hunger, diaphoresis, and dizziness. With severe hypoglycemia, mental status changes leading to coma can occur. A complication of intensive glucose control is that hypoglycemic episodes may occur more frequently.[5-7] Critically ill patients at risk of hypoglycemia are usually placed on a regimen of routine blood glucose checks using bedside point-of-care testing.

TABLE 23-1 BLOOD GLUCOSE LEVELS

PATIENT STATUS LEVEL	(mg/dL)	LEVEL (mmol/L)
Hypoglycemia	<70	<3.9
Normal FPG level	70-100	≥3.9-5.6
Impaired FPG level pre-diabetes*	100-125	5.6-6.9
Fasting FPG level diagnostic of diabetes	≥126	≥7.0
Non-FPG level diagnostic of diabetes	≥200	≥11.1

Data from American Diabetes Association: Standards of medical care in diabetes—2010, *Diabetes Care* 33(Suppl 1):S11, 2010.
FPG, fasting plasma glucose.
*Intermediate group whose FPG levels do not meet the criteria for diabetes but are too high to be considered normal.

Before discharge to home, diabetic patients should be taught to monitor their blood glucose levels.[1,4,7] Maintaining blood glucose within the normal range is associated with fewer types of diabetes-related complications and a lower rate of complications of diabetes.[4] Laboratory tests and point-of-care or self-monitoring of blood glucose represent the standard of care for management of diabetes. Unfortunately, home monitoring of blood glucose is not the norm, despite research evidence that maintaining blood glucose levels as close to normal as possible prolongs life and reduces complications. Only 40% of patients with type 1 diabetes and 26% of patients with type 2 diabetes monitor their blood glucose levels at least once daily.[4]

Urine Glucose

Testing the urine for glucose is not recommended for diabetic patients because there is too much variation in the renal threshold for glucose when diabetes-related kidney damage has occurred.[4] Urine glucose measurements are affected by variation in fluid intake, reflect an average glucose level, and not a specific point in time, and are altered by some drugs. Urine glucose testing does not offer any help in the identification of hypoglycemia.[4] For all of these reasons, urine testing is not recommended.

Glycated Hemoglobin

Blood testing of glucose is useful for daily management of diabetes. However, a different blood test is used to achieve an objective measure of blood glucose over an extended period. The glycated hemoglobin test (also known as glycosylated hemoglobin [HbA_{1C} or A_{1C}]) provides information about the average amount of glucose that has been present in the patient's bloodstream over the previous 3 to 4 months.[4] During the 120-day life span of red blood cells (erythrocytes), the hemoglobin within each cell binds to the available blood glucose through a process known as *glycosylation*. Typically, 4% to 6% of hemoglobin contains the glucose group A_{1C}. A normal HbA_{1C} value is 4% to 6%. HbA_{1C} values above 6.5% are diagnostic for diabetes.[1] For individuals with established diabetes, below 7% is the suggested HbA_{1C} target to decrease the risk of microvascular and cardiac complications.[1] The HbA_{1C} value correlates with specific blood glucose levels as shown in Table 23-2.[1] Not all clinical laboratories use the same analytic techniques to measure the glycated hemoglobin A_{1C}, and methods to standardize the reporting of results worldwide are being developed.[4,8] The American Diabetes Association recommends use of the HbA_{1C} value both during initial assessment of diabetes mellitus, and for follow-up to monitor treatment effectiveness.[1]

Blood Ketones

Ketones (acetoacetate, β-hydroxybutyrate, and acetone) are by-products of fat metabolism. In most cases, when the body uses carbohydrate as its main source of energy, the liver completes fat metabolism, and minimal or no ketones are found in the blood. Ketone levels in the blood rise in acute illness,

TABLE 23-2	CORRELATION BETWEEN HEMOGLOBIN A_{1C} CONCENTRATION AND PLASMA GLUCOSE LEVEL	
HbA$_{1C}$ (%)	MEAN PLASMA GLUCOSE LEVEL (mg/dL)	MEAN PLASMA GLUCOSE LEVEL (mmol/L)
6	126	7.0
7	154	8.6
8	183	10.2
9	212	11.8
10	240	13.4
11	269	14.9
12	298	16.5

Data from American Diabetes Association: Standards of medical care in diabetes—2010, *Diabetes Care* 33(Suppl 1):S11, 2010.

fasting, and with sustained elevation of blood glucose in type 1 diabetes when there is insufficient insulin. Home monitors to test capillary blood for elevated ketones (generally β-hydroxybutyrate) are recommended for type 1 diabetics in times of illness or stress.[4]

Elevated levels of ketones (ketonemia) are also detected by a fruity, sweet-smelling odor on the exhaled breath. This distinctive breath odor derives from the elimination of acetone as part of the compensatory response to maintain a normal pH. Ketones are also eliminated in the urine.

Urine Ketones

Urine ketone monitoring is important for critically ill patients with type 1 diabetes.[4] The presence of ketones in urine is retrospective and indicates that blood ketones were elevated. In diabetic ketoacidosis (DKA), fat breakdown (lipolysis) occurs so rapidly that fat metabolism is incomplete, and ketone bodies (acetone, β-hydroxybutyric acid, and acetoacetic acid) accumulate in the blood (ketonemia) and are excreted in the urine (ketonuria). It is recommended that all diabetic patients self-test or have their blood or urine tested for the presence of ketones during any acute illness or stress with a blood glucose level greater than 250 mg/dL, with symptoms of nausea, vomiting, or abdominal pain; and for women during pregnancy.

Normally, in healthy non-fasting individuals, only minute quantities of ketones are present in the urine, and these low levels are below the threshold of detection with routine testing methods.[4] In fasting and starvation states, ketones may be present in the urine.[4]

PITUITARY GLAND

The pituitary gland, recessed in the base of the cranium, is not accessible to physical assessment. One essential hormone formed in the hypothalamus but secreted through the posterior pituitary gland is *antidiuretic hormone* (ADH), also known as *vasopressin*.

Physical Assessment

Nursing priorities for physical assessment of the patient with pituitary gland dysfunction focus on (1) hydration status, (2) vital signs, and (3) accurate intake and output.

ADH controls the amount of fluid lost and retained within the body. Acute dysfunction of the posterior pituitary or the hypothalamus can result in insufficient or excessive ADH production. The clinical signs of posterior pituitary dysfunction often manifest as fluid volume deficit (insufficient ADH production) or fluid volume excess (excessive ADH production).

Hydration Status

The nurse determines the effectiveness of ADH production by conducting a hydration assessment. A hydration assessment includes observations of skin integrity, skin turgor, and buccal membrane moisture. Moist, shiny buccal membranes indicate satisfactory fluid balance. Skin turgor that is resilient and returns to its original position in less than 3 seconds after being pinched or lifted indicates adequate skin elasticity. Skin over the forehead, clavicle, and sternum is the most reliable for testing tissue turgor because it is less affected by aging and more easily assessed for changes related to fluid balance. A well-hydrated patient has skin in the groin and axilla that is slightly moist to touch. In older patients, these typical assessment findings may be absent. Older persons, especially women, experience as much as a 50% decrease in total-body water content by age 75.[9]

Other indicators that the patient's hydration status is adequate for metabolic demands include a balanced intake and output and absence of thirst. Absence of thirst, however, is not a reliable indicator of dehydration in the older adult or in critically ill patients. Indicators of normal hydration include absence of edema, stable weight, and normal urine specific gravity that falls within the normal range (1.005 to 1.030).

Vital Signs

Changes in heart rate, blood pressure, and central venous pressure (when available) are useful adjuncts to changes in fluid volume status. Blood pressure and pulse are monitored frequently. Decreased blood pressure with increased pulse is characteristic of hypovolemia, whereas elevated blood pressure and a rapid, bounding pulse may indicate hypervolemia. Orthostatic hypotension, which occurs when intravascular fluid volume decreases, is identified by a drop in systolic blood pressure of 20 mm Hg or a drop in diastolic blood pressure of 10 mm Hg when the patient changes position from lying to standing.

Weight Changes and Intake and Output

Daily weight changes coincide with fluid retention and fluid loss. Sudden changes in weight can result from a change in fluid balance; 1 L of fluid lost or retained is equal to approximately 2.2 pounds, or 1 kg, of weight gained or lost. To use weight as a true determinant of the fluid balance, all extraneous variables are eliminated, and the same scale is used at the same time each day. Precise measurement and notation of intake and output are used as criteria for fluid replacement therapy.

Laboratory Assessment

No single diagnostic test identifies dysfunction of the posterior pituitary gland. Diagnosis is made through an array of laboratory tests combined with the clinical profile of the patient.

Serum Antidiuretic Hormone

The result of a blood test for normal levels of serum ADH is 1 to 5 pg/mL.[9] To prepare the patient for the test, all drugs that may alter the release of ADH are withheld for a minimum of 8 hours. Common medications that affect ADH levels include morphine sulfate, lithium carbonate, chlorothiazide, carbamazepine, oxytocin, and selective serotonin reuptake inhibitors (SSRIs).[10] Nicotine, alcohol, positive-pressure and negative-pressure ventilation, and emotional stress also influence ADH levels and must be considered in the interpretation of values.

The test, which is read by comparing serum ADH levels with the blood and urine osmolality, is helpful in differentiating the *syndrome of inappropriate antidiuretic hormone* (SIADH) from central *diabetes insipidus* (DI). Increased ADH levels in the bloodstream compared with a low serum osmolality and elevated urine osmolality confirms the diagnosis of SIADH. Reduced levels of serum ADH in a patient with high serum osmolality, hypernatremia, and reduced urine concentration signal central DI. Chapter 18 provides more information about SIADH and DI.

Urine and Serum Osmolality

Values for serum osmolality in the bloodstream range from 275 to 295 mOsm/kg H_2O. *Osmolality* measurements determine the concentration of dissolved particles in a solution. In a healthy person, a change in the concentration of solutes triggers a chain of events to maintain adequate serum dilution. Urine osmolality in the person with normal kidneys depends on fluid intake. With high fluid intake, particle dilution is low but will increase if fluids are restricted, and the expected range for urine osmolality therefore is wide, ranging from 50 to 1400 mOsm/kg.

Increased serum osmolality stimulates the release of ADH, which reduces the amount of water lost through the kidney. Body fluid thereby is retained to dilute the particle concentration in the bloodstream. Decreased serum osmolality inhibits the release of ADH, the kidney tubules increase their permeability, and fluid is eliminated from the body in an attempt to regain normal concentration of particles in the bloodstream. The most accurate measures of the body's fluid balance are obtained when urine and blood samples are collected simultaneously.

Antidiuretic Hormone Test

The ADH test is used to differentiate *neurogenic* DI (central) from *nephrogenic* (kidney) DI. The patient is challenged with 0.05 to 1.0 mL of intranasally administered ADH in the form of desmopressin (1-deamino-8-D-arginine vasopressin [DDAVP]).[11] An intravenous line is inserted before ADH administration, and urine volume and osmolality are measured every 30 minutes for 2 hours before and after the ADH challenge. The patient with normal posterior pituitary function responds to the exogenous ADH by resorbing water at the kidney tubule and raising the urine osmolality slightly. In cases of severe central DI, in which the pituitary is affected, the urine osmolality shows a significant increase (becomes more concentrated), which indicates that the cell receptor sites on the kidney tubules are responsive to vasopressin.

Test results in which urine osmolality remains unchanged indicate nephrogenic DI, suggesting kidney dysfunction because the kidneys are no longer responsive to ADH. This test is rarely performed in the critical care unit because of the unstable hemodynamic and volume status of most patients.[11]

DIAGNOSTIC PROCEDURES

In addition to laboratory tests, radiographic examination, computed tomography (CT), and magnetic resonance imaging (MRI) are used to diagnose structural lesions such as cranial bone fractures, tumors, or blood clots in the region of the pituitary. Although these procedures do not diagnose DI or SIADH, they are useful in uncovering the likely underlying cause.[11,12]

Radiographic Examination

A basic x-ray examination of the inferior skull views the sella turcica and surrounding bone formation. Bone fractures or tissue swelling at the base of the brain, which are apparent on a radiograph, suggest interference with the vascular supply and nerve impulses to the hypothalamic-pituitary system. Dysfunction can occur if the hypothalamus, infundibular stalk, or pituitary is impaired.

Computed Tomography

CT of the base of the skull identifies pituitary tumors, blood clots, cysts, nodules, or other soft tissue masses. This rapid procedure causes no discomfort except that it requires the patient to lie perfectly still. CT studies can be performed with radiopaque contrast (sodium iodine solution) or without contrast. The contrast dye is given intravenously to highlight the hypothalamus, infundibular stalk, and pituitary gland. This dye may cause allergic reactions in iodine-sensitive persons, and the patient must be carefully questioned about iodine allergy before the test. The size and shape of the sella turcica and the position of the hypothalamus, infundibular stalk, and pituitary are identified.

Magnetic Resonance Imaging

MRI enables the radiologist to visualize internal organs and cellular characteristics of specific tissues. MRI uses a magnetic field rather than radiation to produce high-resolution, cross-sectional images. The soft brain tissue and surrounding cerebrospinal fluid (CSF) make the brain especially suited to MRI. Although not a definitive diagnostic test for posterior pituitary hormonal imbalance, MRI may identify anatomic disruption of the gland and the surrounding area to uncover a primary cause of DI or SIADH.

REFERENCES

1. American Diabetes Association: Standards of medical care in diabetes – 2010, *Diabetes Care* 33(Suppl 1):S11, 2010.
2. American Diabetes Association: Diagnosis and classification of diabetes mellitus, *Diabetes Care* 33(Suppl 1):S62, 2010.
3. ACE/ADA Task Force on Inpatient Diabetes: American College of Endocrinology and American Diabetes Association Consensus statement on inpatient diabetes and glycemic control, *Diabetes Care* 29(8):1955, 2006.
4. Goldstein DE, et al: Tests of glycemia in diabetes, *Diabetes Care* 27(7):1761, 2004.
5. Moghissi ES, et al: American Association of Clinical Endocrinologists and American Diabetes Association consensus statement on inpatient glycemic control, *Endocr Pract* 15(4):353, 2009.
6. Cryer PE, et al: Evaluation and management of adult hypoglycemic disorders: An Endocrine Society clinical practice guideline, *J Clin Endocrinol Metab* 94(3):709, 2009.
7. Funnell MM, et al: National standards for diabetes self-management education, *Diabetes Care* 32(Suppl 1):S87, 2009.
8. Weykamp C, et al: The IFCC Reference Measurement System for HbA1c: a 6-year progress report, *Clin Chem* 54(2):240, 2008.
9. Janicic N, Verbalis JG: Evaluation and management of hypo-osmolality in hospitalized patients, *Endocrinol Metab Clin North Am* 32(2):459, 2003.
10. Rottmann CN: SSRIs and the syndrome of inappropriate antidiuretic hormone secretion, *Am J Nurs* 107(1):51, 2007.
11. Holcomb SS: Diabetes insipidus, *Dimens Crit Care Nurs* 21(3):94, 2002.
12. Hadjizacharia P, et al: Acute diabetes insipidus in severe head injury: a prospective study, *J Am Coll Surg* 207(4):477, 2008.

24

Endocrine Disorders and Therapeutic Management

Mary E. Lough

OBJECTIVES

- Summarize the role of the hypothalamic-pituitary-adrenal axis, liver, pancreas and thyroid in response to the stress of critical illness.
- Discuss the assessment and management of adrenal dysfunction in critical illness.
- Describe the management of hyperglycemia in critical illness.
- Compare and contrast etiology and management of type 1 and type 2 diabetes.
- Describe the use of intensive insulin therapy in the critical care unit.
- Compare and contrast management of diabetic ketoacidosis and hyperglycemic hyperosmolar syndrome.
- Discuss the nursing priorities for managing a patient with diabetes insipidus.
- List three causes of the syndrome of inappropriate secretion of antidiuretic hormone.

The endocrine system is almost invisible when it functions well, but it causes widespread upset when an organ is overly suppressed, stimulated, or under physiological stress. This results in a wide spectrum of possible disorders; some are rare, and others are frequently encountered in the critical care unit. This chapter focuses on the neuroendocrine stress associated with critical illness, and disorders of the pancreas.

NEUROENDOCRINOLOGY OF STRESS AND CRITICAL ILLNESS

Major neurological and endocrine changes occur when an individual is confronted with physiological stress caused by any critical illness,[1,2] sepsis,[3-5] trauma, major surgery, or underlying cardiovascular disease.[5,6] The normal "fight-or-flight" response that is initiated in times of physiological or psychological stress is exacerbated in critical illness through activation of the neuroendocrine system, specifically the hypothalamic-pituitary-adrenal axis (HPA),[3,7] thyroid,[8] and pancreas.[1,2] The influence of the HPA on the course of critical illness is just beginning to be understood. Hormonal neuroendocrine output is active at the beginning of a critical insult but greatly diminishes if the critical illness is prolonged.[9,10]

All endocrine organs are affected by acute critical illness, as shown in Table 24-1.

Acute Neuroendocrine Response to Critical Illness

The fight-or-flight acute response to physiological threat is a rapid discharge of the catecholamines *norepinephrine* and *epinephrine* into the bloodstream.[6] Norepinephrine is released from the nerve endings of the sympathetic nervous system (SNS).[6]

Hypothalamic-Pituitary-Adrenal Axis in Acute Stress

Epinephrine (adrenalin) is released from the medulla of the adrenal glands. Epinephrine increases cerebral blood flow and cerebral oxygen consumption and may be the trigger for recruitment of the hypothalamic-pituitary axis.[6]

The pituitary gland has two parts (anterior and posterior) that function under control of the hypothalamus, as described in Figure 23-1 in Chapter 23. As a response to stress, the *posterior pituitary gland* releases antidiuretic hormone (ADH), also known as *vasopressin* (pitressin). This hormone is an antidiuretic with a powerful vasoconstrictive effect on blood vessels.[6] The combination of epinephrine and vasopressin raises blood pressure quickly; it also decreases gastric

TABLE 24-1		ENDOCRINE RESPONSES TO STRESS
GLAND OR ORGAN	**HORMONE**	**RESPONSE OR PHYSICAL EXAMINATION**
Adrenal cortex	Cortisol	↑ Insulin resistance → ↑ glycogenolysis → ↑ glucose circulation
		↑ Hepatic gluconeogenesis → ↑ glucose available
		↑ Lipolysis
		↑ Protein catabolism
		↑ Sodium → ↑ water retention to maintain plasma osmolality by movement of extravascular fluid into the intravascular space
		↓ Connective tissue fibroblasts → poor wound healing
	Glucocorticoid	↓ Histamine release → suppression of immune system
		↓ Lymphocytes, monocytes, eosinophils, basophils
		↑ Polymorphonuclear leukocytes → ↑ infection risk
		↑ Glucose
		↓ Gastric acid secretion
	Mineralocorticoids	↑ Aldosterone → ↓ sodium excretion → ↓ water excretion → ↑ intravascular volume
		↑ Potassium excretion → hypokalemia
		↑ Hydrogen ion excretion → metabolic acidosis
Adrenal medulla	Epinephrine	↑ Endorphins → ↓ pain
	Norepinephrine	↑ Metabolic rate to accommodate stress response
		↑ Live glycogenolysis → ↑ glucose
		↑ Insulin (cells are insulin resistant)
		↑ Cardiac contractility
		↑ Cardiac output
		↑ Dilation of coronary arteries
		↑ Blood pressure
		↑ Heart rate
		↑ Bronchodilation → ↑ respirations
		↑ Perfusion to heart, brain, lungs, liver, and muscle
		↓ Perfusion to periphery of body
		↓ Peristalsis
	Norepinephrine	↑ Peripheral vasoconstriction
		↑ Blood pressure
		↑ Sodium retention
		↑ Potassium excretion
Pituitary	All hormones	↑ Endogenous opioids → ↓ pain
Anterior pituitary	Corticotropin	↑ Aldosterone → ↓ sodium excretion → ↓ water excretion → ↑ intravascular volume
		↑ Cortisol → ↑ blood volume
	Growth hormones	↑ Protein anabolism of amino acids to protein
		↑ Lipolysis → ↑ gluconeogenesis
Posterior pituitary	Antidiuretic hormone	↑ Vasoconstriction
		↑ Water retention → restoration of circulating blood volume
		↓ Urine output
		↑ Hypoosmolality
Pancreas	Insulin	↑ Insulin resistance → hyperglycemia
	Glucagon	↑ Glycolysis (directly opposes action of insulin)
		↑ Glucose for fuel
		↑ Glycogenolysis
		↑ Gluconeogenesis
		↑ Lipolysis
Thyroid	Thyroxine	↓ Routine metabolic demands during stress
Gonads	Sex hormones	Energy and oxygen supply diverted to brain, heart, muscles, and liver

↑, Increased; →, causes; ↓, decreased.

motility.[6] Epinephrine increases heart rate, causes ventricular dysrhythmias in susceptible patients, and provides some analgesia or lack of pain awareness during acute physical stress.[6]

The *anterior pituitary gland* is under the control of the hypothalamus (see Figure 23-1 in Chapter 23). In acute physiological stress, "pulses" of growth hormone (GH) are released from the anterior pituitary gland to boost serum GH levels.[10] In critical illness, the anterior pituitary actively secretes GH hormone, but the quantity may be insufficient for extreme physiological needs. A different problem is that peripheral tissues may be resistant and unable to use the anabolic GH.[11] The anterior pituitary gland also produces *corticotropin* (also called ACTH), which stimulates release of *cortisol* from the adrenal cortex.[12] Cortisol release is an important protective response, and serum levels increase sixfold with normal adrenal function.[12]

Liver and Pancreas in Acute Stress

The liver releases the hormone *glucagon* to stimulate the liver to pour additional glucose into the bloodstream. This greatly raises blood glucose levels.[3] Paradoxically, the pancreas does not produce more insulin, and serum insulin levels remain normal, even with the increased metabolic demand associated with critical illness or sepsis. Peripheral tissues become *insulin resistant*.[3] In other words, the tissues are unable to use the available insulin to transport glucose inside the cells for normal metabolism. This raises blood glucose levels, causing persistent hyperglycemia. There is an alternative glucose transport system that enables insulin to enter the cell by means of specialized *glucose transporters*, usually abbreviated as *GLUT*. Although insulin-independent *glucose transporters* (GLUT-1, GLUT-2, and GLUT-3) are active during physiological stress, they cannot keep up with the massive increase in glucose production by the liver.[13]

Thyroid Gland in Acute Stress

Within 2 hours after trauma or surgery, serum levels of triiodothyronine (T_3) decrease.[10] The greater the decrease of T_3 in the first 24 hours, the more severe the critical illness.[8] Thyroid-stimulating hormone (TSH) and thyroxine (T_4) briefly increase and then return to normal levels. In the acute phase of critical illness, a low serum T_3 is associated with a poor prognosis.[10]

Systemic illnesses that do not directly involve the thyroid gland but alter thyroid gland metabolism are referred to as *nonthyroidal illness syndromes* or *sick euthyroid syndromes*.[14] The significance of altered thyroid function in critical illness is unknown.[14,15]

Prolonged Neuroendocrine Response to Critical Illness

If critical illness is prolonged, the neuroendocrine response changes dramatically. The initially high hormonal levels are reduced, and output decreases from all endocrine glands.

Hypothalamic-Pituitary-Adrenal Axis in Prolonged Stress

If critical illness is prolonged for more than 7 to 10 days, the production of hormones from the pituitary gland is significantly lessened.

Adrenal dysfunction is a frequent finding if critical illness lasts longer than 7 to 10 days. A 20-fold increase in adrenal failure has been reported in critically ill patients older than 50 years who spend more than 14 days in a critical care unit.[10] If the critical illness is prolonged and the patient remains hypotensive, vasopressor-dependent, and mechanically ventilated, adequacy of adrenal function must be evaluated. Older patients are particularly susceptible to adrenal failure.[16]

Liver-Pancreas in Prolonged Stress

Hyperglycemia is often persistent. Gluconeogenesis (the metabolism of glucose from fat or protein) and proteolysis (protein breakdown) continue throughout the catabolic phase of critical illness.[11] Critically ill patients can lose up to 10% of their lean body mass per week.[11] The addition of adequate supplemental nutrition is recommended, in addition to an intravenous insulin infusion, to reduce hyperglycemia and provide additional substrate other than the patient's own body tissues.[1,2] Insulin is an anabolic hormone and can improve protein synthesis and reduce protein breakdown.[11] While the critical illness is ongoing, nutrition and insulin seem to limit rather than stop the loss of lean body mass.

Thyroid Gland in Prolonged Stress

The thyroid gland appears to follow a pattern similar to that of the pituitary gland when critical illness is prolonged. The serum levels of T_3, T_4, and TSH are greatly reduced, and the normal pulses of TSH are flattened.[10]

Adrenal Dysfunction in Critical Illness

Diminished adrenal gland function may result from one or more causes during critical illness:

- *Primary adrenal failure* is rare and occurs in only 0.01% to 3% of critically ill patients.[17,18]
- *Critical illness-related corticosteroid insufficiency* (CIRCI) describes a situation in which the adrenal gland produces glucocorticosteroids but the quantity is insufficient for the disease process. Estimates of the frequency of CIRCI range from about 20% in medical patients to 60% in septic patients.[19]
- *Peripheral cortisol resistance* is thought to occur in severe sepsis and septic shock.[7,17] In septic patients, inflammatory cytokines induce cellular resistance to cortisol; low-dose, short-term replacement corticosteroids may be provided to patients with CIRCI.[7,17]

Assessment of Adrenal Function

Clinical assessment of adrenal dysfunction is difficult in the critically ill, and a specialized laboratory assay is necessary for an accurate diagnosis. First, a baseline serum cortisol level is obtained. Adrenal failure is likely if the cortisol level is less than 10 mcg/dL.[7]

Cosyntropin Stimulation Test

Further confirmation of adrenal dysfunction may be obtained by performance of a corticotropin stimulation test (*cosyntropin test*). Cosyntropin is a medication made from the first 24 amino acids of corticotropin.[12] In the test, 250 mcg cosyntropin is administered by the intravenous route, and serum blood levels are measured 30 minutes later. A serum cortisol rise from baseline of less than 9 mcg/dL after 30 minutes denotes inability of the adrenal gland to respond to a stress stimulus (nonresponder).[7,12] If the cortisol rise is greater than 9 mcg/dL in response to corticotropin stimulation, the adrenal glands are functioning normally (responder).[7] Corticosteroids are given only to nonresponders. The combination of a low baseline cortisol value (<10 mcg/dL) with minimal or no rise (<9 mcg/dL) after cosyntropin stimulation is evidence of corticosteroid deficiency.[7]

Corticosteroid Replacement

Clinical practice guidelines[7] recommend short-term provision of low-dose hydrocortisone for patients who have a diagnosis of septic shock with refractory vasopressor-dependent hypotension. Hydrocortisone is the recommended replacement because it is the pharmacological steroid that most resembles endogenous cortisol.

The guidelines recommend use of the cosyntropin stimulation test as described previously. However, the test is not recommended as a stand-alone method to identify patients who might receive low-dose steroids. This apparent contradiction is explained by the fact that several clinical trials of low-dose steroid replacement in sepsis have demonstrated a faster resolution of the shock symptoms but no difference in overall mortality compared with placebo.[7] The controversy continues. The most recently published randomized control trial of low-dose steroids versus placebo in 499 patients with septic shock did not show any mortality benefit, even among responders to the cosyntropin stimulation test. Nor was there any difference in survival between those who responded to the 250 mcg cosyntropin and received steroids and those who responded and received a placebo.[20]

High-dose steroid replacement is never recommended in the management of sepsis. Corticosteroids are never discontinued abruptly and must be tapered gradually over several days.[7]

Hyperglycemia in Critical Illness

Normal fasting blood glucose levels range between 70 and 100 mg/dL in a healthy person. Critically ill patients frequently have much higher blood glucose levels, and several retrospective analyses have reported that hyperglycemic patients have a higher mortality rate than patients with normal blood glucose values.[21] In 2001 a landmark prospective, randomized study showed a significant reduction in morbidity and mortality among critically ill surgical patients whose blood glucose concentration was maintained between 80 and 110 mg/dL with a continuous insulin infusion, compared with those whose blood glucose was only treated if it was greater than 180 mg/dL.[1] A study of medical critical care patients by the same group with the same protocol demonstrated a mortality benefit after 3 days of tight glucose control with an insulin infusion.[2] These initial studies were greeted with tremendous enthusiasm and many critical care units adopted stringent glucose-control standards to reduce hyperglycemia-associated morbidity and mortality. However, these earlier studies have now been challenged.

The NICE-SUGAR trial was a prospective randomized trial of 6,014 critically ill patients.[22] It compared continuous insulin infusion to achieve tight glucose control (target 80 to 108 mg/dL) with a conventional glucose-control range (target below 180 mg/dL).[22] In the tight glucose-control group, 6.8% had episodes of severe hypoglycemia (below 40 mg/dL); in the conventional control group, only 0.5% experienced severe hypoglycemia.[22] There was a 2.6% higher risk of death in the intensive glucose-control group (27.5% died) compared with the conventional control group (24.9% died).[22] Other prospective, randomized trials[23,24] and meta-analysis[25] were unable to demonstrate a reduction in mortality with tight glucose control. These research studies suggest that the risks of hypoglycemia with the use of intensive insulin protocols outweigh the benefits of tight glucose control in the critically ill.[22-25]

Clinical Practice Guidelines Related to Blood Glucose Management in Critically Ill Patients

As a result of the studies just described, the American Association of Clinical Endocrinologists (AACE) and the American Diabetes Association (ADA) developed clinical practice guidelines that recommend the use of continuous insulin infusions to maintain blood glucose in critical care patients between 140 to 180 mg/dL, with frequent monitoring of blood glucose.[5] The 140 to 180 mg/dL level was selected to minimize the risk of hypoglycemia.

Other glucose-control guidelines relevant to critical illness have also been published. The Society of Critical Care Medicine (SCCM) Surviving Sepsis guidelines recommend maintaining blood glucose concentration lower than 150 mg/dL in critically ill septic patients after initial stabilization.[4] The American Heart Association recommends a target range of 90 to 140 mg/dL while avoiding hypoglycemia.[26] The American College of Physicians (ACP) recommends a target blood glucose range of 140 to 200 mg/dL for ICU patients whether diabetic or nondiabetic.[27] More liberal blood glucose ranges for critically ill patients are now recommended in clinical guidelines.[4,5,26,27]

Hyperglycemia and the Cardiovascular System

Many patients who are admitted to the hospital with acute complications of atherosclerotic disease are diabetic. Risk of coronary artery disease is two to three times higher in diabetics compared with nondiabetics.[28] Hyperglycemia is present in 25% to 50% of patients with acute coronary syndrome (ACS) who are admitted to the hospital, and the higher the blood glucose level, the greater the risk of death.[26] Diabetic patients who were admitted to the hospital for an acute myocardial infarction and had an admission blood glucose level greater than 180 mg/dL had a 70% relative increase in the risk of in-hospital death compared with similar patients who had a normal glucose value on admission.[26] Retrospective analyses of blood glucose levels of cardiac surgery patients show a higher in-hospital mortality rate for patients with elevated blood glucose concentrations.[29,30] Patients who were unaware of their diabetes before hospital admission and nondiabetic patients who were hyperglycemic during their critical illness also had higher mortality rates.[31,32]

Hypoglycemia and Brain Injury

The brain does not store glucose and is dependent on a continuous supply of glucose from the peripheral bloodstream. It is essential to avoid hypoglycemia in any brain-injured patient. However, there are no published guidelines as what the correct target glucose range should be for this population. Experts favor a less restrictive target, because blood glucose concentrations lower than 135 mg/dL (6 mmol/L) have been shown to increase brain metabolic distress.[33]

Insulin Management in the Critically Ill

A profound shift in the management of the hyperglycemic critically ill ventilated patient has recently taken place. As a result of the research that has highlighted the deleterious effects of hyperglycemia in critical illness, most hospitals have developed an institution-specific tight glucose-control algorithm to lower blood glucose into the targeted range. The vigilance of the critical care nurse is pivotal to the success of any intervention to lower blood glucose using a continuous insulin infusion. As discussed earlier, many glucose-control protocols are becoming less restrictive due to concerns about iatrogenic hypoglycemia.

Some clinical interventions increase the likelihood that the patient will receive exogenous insulin. Infusion of total parental nutrition (TPN) typically requires a continuous insulin infusion to normalize blood glucose. In a study of critically ill surgical patients with preexisting type 2 diabetes who did not previously require insulin, 77% of patients needed insulin to control blood sugar while receiving TPN.[34] Some enteral nutrition formulas are high in carbohydrates and increase blood sugar in the same way. In this situation, the composition of the enteral feeding is altered, or the insulin dosage is increased to achieve target blood glucose levels. It is important to provide nutrition, and insulin can be a powerful adjunct to nutritional support.

Frequent Blood Glucose Monitoring

Monitoring blood glucose with a point-of-care glucometer is the basis of targeted glucose control. As part of the comprehensive initial assessment, the blood sugar is measured by a standard laboratory sample or by a finger-stick capillary blood sample. In many institutions, if the blood sugar is greater than 180 mg/dL (an initial value that may vary among hospitals), the patient is started on a continuous intravenous insulin infusion. In critically ill catabolic patients, the initial blood glucose level can be well above 200 mg/dL. While the glucose is elevated, blood sample measurements are usually obtained hourly, to allow titration of the insulin drip to lower blood glucose. After the patient is stable, blood glucose measurements can be spaced approximately every 2 hours, based on individual hospital protocols.[21]

Several different blood-sampling methods are available. A capillary finger-stick is perhaps the easiest initial option, although the fingers can become noticeably marked if there are numerous sticks over several days. Trauma to the fingers is also exacerbated if peripheral perfusion is diminished. If a central venous catheter (CVC) or an arterial line with a blood conservation system attached is in place, this can be a highly efficient system for sampling, because there is no blood wastage. If a blood conservation setup is not attached, use of the venous or arterial catheter for access is unacceptable because of the amount of waste blood that would be discarded.

Continuous Insulin Infusion

Many hospitals use insulin infusion protocols that are implemented by the critical care nurse for management of stress-induced hyperglycemia.[5] Effective glucose protocols gauge the insulin infusion rate based on two parameters: (1) the immediate blood glucose result and (2) the rate of change in the blood glucose level since the last hourly measurement. The following three examples illustrate this concept:

- Patient A receives 3 units of continuous intravenous regular insulin per hour and has a blood glucose measurement of 110 mg/dL, but 1 hour ago it was 190 mg/dL; the insulin rate must be decreased to avoid sudden hypoglycemia.
- Patient B receives 3 units of continuous IV regular insulin per hour and has a blood glucose measurement of 120 mg/dL, but 1 hour ago it was 122 mg/dL; in this situation, no change is made in the insulin infusion rate.
- Patient C receives 3 units of continuous intravenous regular insulin per hour and has a blood glucose measurement of 190 mg/dL, and 1 hour ago it was 197 mg/dL; the insulin rate must be increased to more rapidly move the patient's blood sugar toward the targeted glucose range (i.e., 140 to 180 mg/dL, although this range will vary by hospital and protocol).

The important point to emphasize is that the *rate of change* of the blood glucose is as important as the *most recent* blood glucose measurement. Each of the patients described in the examples may have the same insulin infusion rate, depending on their catabolic state, but individualization among patients with different diagnoses can be safely achieved as long as the rate of change is also considered.

A person's insulin requirement often fluctuates over the course of an illness. This occurs in response to changes in the clinical condition, such as development of an infection, caloric alterations caused by stopping or starting enteral nutrition or TPN, administration of therapeutic steroids, or because the person is less catabolic.[34] A method to allow for corrective incremental changes (up or down) to adapt to the reality of clinical developments and maintain the glucose within the target range is essential.[34] Some protocols alter only the infusion rate, whereas others incorporate bolus insulin doses if the glucose concentration is greater than a preestablished threshold (e.g., 180 mg/dL). Typically, after the blood glucose has remained within the target range for a number of hours (4 to 12 hours, depending on the hospital protocol), the time interval between measurements for blood glucose monitoring is extended to every 2 hours.

Transition from Continuous to Intermittent Insulin Coverage

The transition from a continuous insulin infusion to intermittent insulin coverage must be handled with care to avoid large fluctuations in blood glucose levels. Before the conversion, the regular insulin infusion should be at a stable and preferably low rate, and the patient's blood glucose level should be maintained consistently within the target range. The transition from intravenous to subcutaneous administration depends on numerous factors, especially whether the patient is able to eat a normal diet.[34]

Clinicians use various methods to calculate the quantity of insulin to prescribe during the transition from intravenous to subcutaneous insulin to maintain stable blood glucose levels. Figure 24-1 depicts hypothetical examples of how a

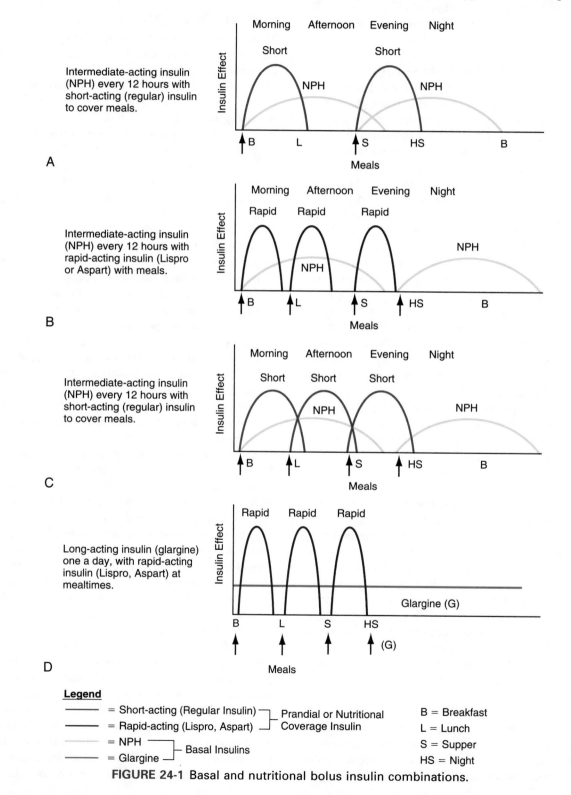

FIGURE 24-1 Basal and nutritional bolus insulin combinations.

combination of basal and bolus insulin regimens (prandial insulin) can work in clinical practice.[21,35] The following paragraphs describe the application of one calculation method for a 67-year-old patient, Alice Smith, who is recovering from critical illness and has recently been extubated.

1. Ms. Smith is in stable condition on a regular insulin drip at 1 unit per hour. She is ready to be transitioned to subcutaneous insulin and will be taking food and liquids by mouth. Her total insulin requirement over the previous 24 hours was 30 units. Ms. Smith will now require basal coverage (provided by subcutaneous intermediate or long-acting insulin) and nutritional coverage for mealtimes (provided by short-acting subcutaneous insulin).

2. The 30 units of insulin infused during the previous 24 hours is Ms. Smith's required daily insulin dose. To transition to subcutaneous insulin, a proportion of this amount (i.e., 75%-80%) will be divided between basal and prandial components.[5] In this situation, 80% of the 30 units = 24 units. Half of this amount (12 units) will be administered subcutaneously as intermediate or long-acting insulin; the other half will be administered as short-acting insulin to coincide with meals (i.e., 4 units with each of three meals).

3. The options for insulin administration for Ms. Smith are as follows:[34-36]
   - *Basal insulin:* 12 units of glargine once daily, *or* 6 units twice daily of Neutral Protamine Hagedorn (NPH) administered subcutaneously
   - *Prandial/nutritional insulin:* 4 units regular insulin given subcutaneously before each meal (short-acting), *or* 4 units Lispro or Aspart given subcutaneously with each meal (ultra-short-acting insulin); verify current blood glucose level.
   - *Supplemental correction dosages:* A supplemental correction scale can be used to cover any hyperglycemia above the target range, and administration can be combined with scheduled blood glucose measurements; verify current blood glucose level.

After the transition to subcutaneous insulin, the dosage is adjusted to the individual patient's needs. In a stable *insulin-sensitive* patient, 1 unit of short-acting insulin will lower the blood glucose by 50 to 100 mg/dL.[21] In a critical care patient, more insulin is typically required to reduce blood glucose levels, because of the physiological stress of the critical illness.[36]

Table 24-2 describes the various types of insulin available for use. These include ultra-short-acting, short-acting, intermediate-acting, long-acting, and combination insulin replacement options. Even after the transition to subcutaneous insulin is completed, blood glucose is monitored frequently to maintain blood glucose within the target range and detect hyperglycemia or hypoglycemia.

Intermittent Insulin Coverage

A patient may be prescribed supplemental "correctional" doses of insulin in addition to the basal/prandial insulin combination. The use of the trio of basal, prandial, and correctional insulin is designed to eliminate the use of the traditional sliding scale.[35] A frequent criticism of sliding-scale therapy is that the dosages are rarely reevaluated or adjusted once established.[34] A second criticism is that the scales treat hyperglycemia only after it has occurred; they are not proactive in the manner of continuous insulin infusions.[34]

Hypoglycemia Management

It is important to have a protocol for the management of hypoglycemia. The major drawback to use of intensive insulin protocols, as described earlier, is the potential for hypoglycemia. Whenever hypoglycemia is detected, it is important to *stop* any continuous infusion of insulin. An example of one protocol to reverse hypoglycemia follows:
- *Blood glucose level lower than 40 mg/dL:* administer 50 mL dextrose (50%) in water ($D_{50}W$) as an intravenous bolus.
- *Blood glucose level between 40 and 70 mg/dL:* administer 25 mL of $D_{50}W$ as an intravenous bolus.

In all cases of hypoglycemia, the blood glucose concentration is monitored every 15 to 20 minutes until the blood sugar has risen into a safe range. The ADA recommends incorporation of level of consciousness plus the blood glucose result as a guide to glucose replacement to treat hypoglycemia.[37] Administer 15 to 20 g of glucose to the conscious hypoglycemic patient. A different protocol suggests the following response to a blood glucose concentration of less than 60 mg/dL:[36]
- *Blood glucose level lower than 60 mg/dL and patient is awake and responsive:* administer intravenous push of 25 mL of $D_{50}W$.
- *Blood glucose level lower than 60 mg/dL and patient is unresponsive:* administer intravenous push of 50 mL of $D_{50}W$.

Nursing Management

Nursing management of the patient with neuroendocrine stress resulting from critical illness incorporates a variety of nursing diagnoses. **Nursing priorities are directed toward (1) monitoring blood glucose levels, insulin therapy, and avoiding hypoglycemia; (2) providing nutrition; and (3) providing education to the patient and family.**

Monitoring Hyperglycemic Side Effects of Vasopressor Therapy

Two vasopressors frequently used as continuous infusions to counteract hypotension in the critically ill also raise blood glucose. Epinephrine and, to a lesser extent, norepinephrine stimulate an increase in gluconeogenesis (creation of new glucose), an increase of skeletal muscle and hepatic glycogenolysis (increased glucose production), an increase in lipolysis (increased fat breakdown), direct suppression of insulin secretion, and an increase in peripheral insulin resistance.[13] All of these

TABLE 24-2 PHARMACOLOGICAL MANAGEMENT: INSULIN*

INSULIN	ROUTE†	ACTION	ONSET/PEAK/DURATION	SPECIAL CONSIDERATIONS
Ultra-Short-Acting Insulins				
Aspart (NovoLog)	SQ & IV	Insulin replacement, rapid onset	5-15 min/30-90 min/<5 hr	Insulin analogue almost *immediately* absorbed; must be taken with food. Insulin appearance should be clear. Must be used in combination with intermediate-acting or long-acting basal insulin regimen. See Figure 24-1.
Lispro (Humalog)	SQ	Insulin replacement, rapid onset	5-15 min/30-90 min/<5 hr	First available synthetic insulin (analogue); almost *immediately* absorbed; must be taken with food. Shorter duration of action than regular insulin; should be used with basal longer-acting insulin. See Figure 24-1.
Glulisine (Apidra)	SQ & IV	Insulin replacement, rapid onset	5-15 min/30-90 min/<5 hr	New insulin analog
Short-Acting Insulin				
Regular	IV or SQ	Insulin replacement therapy	IV: <15 min SQ: 30-60 min/2-3 hr/5-8 hr	Only type of insulin suitable for IV continuous infusion or bolus administration.
Intermediate-Acting Basal Insulin				
Neutral Protamine Hagedorn (NPH)	SQ	Insulin replacement, intermediate action	2-4 hr/4-10 hr/10-16 hr	
Long-Acting Basal Insulins				
Glargine (Lantus)	SQ	Long-acting basal insulin analog; longer-acting than NPH or Ultralente	2-4 hr until steady state/no peak; concentration relatively constant over 20-24 hr	Synthetic insulin (analog); differs from human insulin by three amino acids, slowing release over 24 hr; no peak. Decrease dose by 20% if switching from NPH to glargine. Must not be diluted or mixed with other insulins. See Figure 24-1.
Detemir (Levemir)	SQ	Long-acting basal analog	3-8 hr until steady state/no peak/5-23 hr	
Combination (Premixed) Insulins				
Various	SQ	Rapid plus intermediate or long-acting insulin combination	Varies according to combination used	Many combinations exist; examples (long-acting component/short-acting component) include 70/30 regular (70% NPH with 30% regular), NovoLog mix 70/30 (70% aspart protamine suspension with 30% aspart), and Humalog mix 75/25 (75% lispro protamine suspension with 25% lispro).

Data from Rodbard HW, et al: American Association of Clinical Endocrinologists medical guidelines for clinical practice for the management of diabetes mellitus, *Endocr Pract* 13(Suppl 1):3, 2007.
*Dosages are individualized according to patient's age and size.
†Only regular insulin is suitable for intravenous use.
IV, intravenous; *SQ*, subcutaneous.

actions serve to raise the serum glucose level in the bloodstream.

Monitoring Blood Glucose Levels, Insulin Therapy, Avoiding Hypoglycemia

The critical care nurse is responsible for the hourly monitoring of blood glucose and titration of the insulin infusion according to the hospital's established protocol while the patient is hyperglycemic. The use of standardized protocols makes possible a systematic approach to the control of blood glucose. This results in improved glycemic control and lower rates of hypoglycemia. It is essential and recommended that nurses receive effective and ongoing education about the anabolic impact of insulin therapy in critical illness.[5] Hospital protocols to minimize development of hypoglycemia, such as using the 140 to 180 mg/dL target range,[5] and rapid reversal of any occurrence of severe hypoglycemia (below 40 mg/dL) by provision of intravenous dextrose ($D_{50}W$) are mandatory.

Providing Nutrition

Whenever an insulin infusion is started to lower blood glucose, nutritional support (enteral or TPN) should be considered. In the absence of nutrition, a 10% dextrose solution may temporarily be infused. The 10% dextrose offers the advantage of carbohydrate calories for metabolism, limits fluctuations in the blood sugar, and reduces the risk of hypoglycemia. After the patient's metabolic condition is stable, introduction of non-glucose nutrition (protein and fat) is recommended.[38]

Providing Patient Education

When the patient is acutely ill, the majority of the educational interventions are directed to the family and supportive friends at the bedside. Numerous explications are required to describe the IV medications, the nutritional needs, the purpose of insulin, the role of other medications, and the ongoing nursing care to provide comfort and prevent complications.

Collaborative Management

It is well established that standardized protocols designed to manage the complications of critical illness result in lower morbidity and mortality for patients. Optimally, all disciplines concerned with the endocrine status of the patient will have participated in the design of these guidelines in each critical care area. The guideline that applies to most patients relates to targeted glucose control. Many professional organizations have endorsed the importance of monitoring blood glucose in the critically ill patient, as described in the Evidence-Based Collaborative Practice Box on Hyperglycemia Management in Critical Illness.[5,34]

EVIDENCE-BASED COLLABORATIVE PRACTICE

Hyperglycemia Management in Critical Illness

Summary of evidence and evidence-based recommendations for controlling hyperglycemic symptoms related to physiological stress of critical illness

Strong Evidence to Support

- Initiate insulin therapy for persistent hyperglycemia beginning at a threshold of no greater than 180 mg/dL.
- Once a continuous insulin infusion is initiated, maintain the target blood glucose level between 140 and 180 mg/dL.
- Frequent blood glucose monitoring to avoid hypoglycemia (hypoglycemia is defined as a blood glucose below 70 mg/dL; severe hypoglycemia <40 mg/dL).
- For patients who are eating, maintain preprandial blood glucose below 110 mg/dL; maintain 2-hour postprandial blood glucose below 140 mg/dL.
- A multidisciplinary team approach to implement institutional guidelines, protocols, and standardized order-sets results in fewer hypoglycemic and hyperglycemic events.

Data from ACE/ADA task force on inpatient diabetes: American College of Endocrinology and American Diabetes Association consensus statement on inpatient diabetes and glycemic control, *Endocr Pract* 12(4):458, 2006; Moghissi ES, et al: American Association of Clinical Endocrinologists and American Diabetes Association consensus statement on inpatient glycemic control, *Endocr Pract* 15(4):353, 2009.

DIABETES MELLITUS

Diabetes mellitus is a progressive endocrinopathy associated with carbohydrate intolerance and insulin dysregulation.

Morbidity and Mortality Associated with Diabetes Mellitus

According to the U.S. Centers for Disease Control and Prevention (CDC), diabetes is the sixth most common cause of death among U.S. adults. Heart disease and stroke are the first and third leading causes of death among U.S. adults.[39] These data must be interpreted in light of the knowledge that adults with diabetes have a risk for dying from cardiovascular diseases that is two to four times greater than in adults without diabetes. Diabetes is also associated with an increased risk of cancer. Malignant neoplasms are the second leading cause of death in the United States.[39] The CDC reports that diabetes is also an independent predictor of mortality from cancer of the colon, the pancreas, the female breast and, in men, the liver and the bladder.[40] The annual cost for hospital care per capita for persons with diabetes is $6,309, compared with $2,971 for persons without diabetes.[34] This represents a cost ratio of 2:1.[34]

Diagnosis of Diabetes

Diabetes mellitus is diagnosed by measurement of the fasting plasma glucose (FPG) laboratory test. The blood glucose may also be called a fasting blood glucose (FBG) or fasting blood sugar (FBS) level. The benchmarks for a normal FPG value have been progressively lowered as more knowledge has been gained about the benefits of maintaining the plasma glucose level as close to normal as possible.

The current values endorsed by the American Diabetes Society are as follows:[41]

- An FPG level of 70 to 100 mg/dL (5.6 mmol/L) signifies normal fasting glucose.
- An FPG level between 100 and 125 mg/dL (5.6 and 6.9 mmol/L) denotes impaired fasting glucose (IFG).
- An FPG level greater than 126 mg/dL (7 mmol/L) provides a diagnosis of diabetes (result is verified by testing more than once).

Two FPG values of 126 mg/dL or higher confirm the diagnosis of diabetes. For the acutely ill patient, hyperglycemia is actively treated with insulin to lower the blood sugar to a safe target range.[5] There are differences in the values of plasma versus whole blood glucose measurements. Plasma glucose values are 10% to 15% higher than whole blood glucose values, and it is essential that health care clinicians and people with diabetes know whether their monitor and strips provide whole blood or plasma results, especially when results from more than one setting (laboratory or monitor) are being compared. Although most laboratories measure plasma glucose levels, most home-monitoring units and point-of-care units measure glucose using whole blood from capillary blood obtained by a finger-stick.[42]

The benefit and importance of maintaining blood glucose at levels as close to normal as possible has been conclusively demonstrated in patients with type 1 and type 2 diabetes.[42] The Diabetes Control and Complications Trial (DCCT) of 1995 on type 1 diabetes, and the United Kingdom Prospective Diabetes Study (UKPDS), published in 1998, on type 2 diabetes, demonstrated that lifestyle changes and use of medications that lead to consistently normal glucose levels reduce microvascular diabetes-related complications and decrease mortality.[42]

Glycated Hemoglobin

For individuals with diabetes, maintenance of blood glucose within a tight normal range is fundamental to avoid the development of microvascular and neuropathic secondary conditions. Although the FPG produces a snapshot of the blood glucose concentration at a single point in time, the *glycated hemoglobin* (HbA$_{1C}$), also known as *glycosylated hemoglobin*, identifies the percentage of glucose that the red cells have absorbed from the plasma over the previous 3-month period. A normal HbA$_{1c}$ falls between 4% and 6%.[41] The target for diabetic patients is an A$_{1C}$ value lower than 6.5%.[41,43] The HbA$_{1C}$ value is also used to diagnose diabetes.[43]

Types of Diabetes

Two distinct types of diabetes are discussed in this chapter:[41]

- Type 1 diabetes results from beta-cell destruction, usually leading to absolute insulin deficiency.
- Type 2 diabetes results from a progressive insulin secretory defect in addition to insulin resistance.

The two diseases are different in nature, cause, treatment, and prognosis.[41] A further category of *prediabetes* has more recently been added to describe patients with impaired fasting glucose (FPG between 100 and 125 mg/dL) who are likely to develop diabetes at some time in the future and are at increased risk for coronary artery disease and stroke.[41] Other conditions, such as gestational diabetes, are not discussed in this chapter.

Type 1 Diabetes

Type 1 diabetes mellitus accounts for only about 5% to 10% of the diabetic population.[37] Older names for this condition included insulin-dependent diabetes (IDDM) and juvenile diabetes. Type 1 diabetes is a cellular-mediated autoimmune disease that causes progressive destruction of the beta cells of the islets of Langerhans in the pancreas. Autoantibodies falsely identify the patient's own pancreas as "foreign" and destroy the native pancreatic tissue. Many responsible autoantibodies contribute to pancreatic destruction, including autoantibodies to the islet cell, to insulin, to glutamic acid decarboxylase (GAD65), and to the tyrosine phosphatases IA-2 and IA-2β.[37] One or more of these autoantibodies are present in 85% to 90% of individuals with type 1 diabetes when fasting hyperglycemia is initially detected.[37] Over time, the autoantibodies render the pancreatic beta cells incapable of secreting insulin and regulating intracellular glucose. In type 1 diabetes, the rate of beta-cell destruction is highly variable. It occurs rapidly in some individuals (mainly children) and slowly in others (mainly adults). Some patients, particularly children and adolescents, may have ketoacidosis as the first manifestation of their disease.

Genetic predisposition and unknown environmental factors are also believed to play an important role.[37] Patients with type 1 diabetes are prone to development of other autoimmune disorders such as Graves' disease (hyperthyroidism), Hashimoto's thyroiditis, Addison's disease, autoimmune hepatitis, myasthenia gravis, and pernicious anemia.[37] Lack of insulin impairs carbohydrate, protein, and fat metabolism.

Management of Type 1 Diabetes. Patients with type 1 diabetes must receive intravenous (IV) or subcutaneous (SC) insulin therapy. Treatment with exogenous insulin replacement restores normal entry of glucose into the cells. The range of insulin replacements available is expanding, and it is essential that critical care nurses be knowledgeable about this class of medications (see Table 24-2). Without insulin, the rapid breakdown of noncarbohydrate substrate, particularly fat, leads to ketonemia, ketonuria, and diabetic ketoacidosis (DKA), a life-threatening complication associated with type 1 diabetes (see later discussion).

Type 2 Diabetes

An estimated 8.7% of the population in the United States has diabetes; almost all of them have type 2.[44] Most individuals are older and obese and have a condition known as *cardiometabolic syndrome*.[45] However, the number of adolescents and young adults with type 2 diabetes is also rising.[41] Up to one third of people with diabetes remain undiagnosed.

Patients at high risk for type 2 diabetes include those who meet the following criteria:[44-46]

- A family history of type 2 diabetes in a first-degree relative
- Member of racial or ethnic groups known to be at greater risk for type 2 diabetes (American Indians, African Americans, Hispanic Americans, Asians/South Pacific Islanders)
- Signs of *insulin resistance syndrome* or conditions associated with insulin resistance, such as hypertension, dyslipidemia, polycystic ovary syndrome, and metabolic syndrome

In type 2 diabetes, pancreatic beta cells are present and functioning; however, the amount of insulin they produce varies greatly among patients:

- In some patients, the pancreatic beta cells do not produce sufficient insulin to meet the metabolic need. In these patients, there is evidence that the beta cells may have been in decline for years before the appearance of clinical symptoms. This is called an *inadequate insulin response.*
- In some patients, the pancreas may produce sufficient insulin or even more than is needed (hyperinsulinemia), but the tissues are resistant to the effects of the insulin. This is known as *insulin resistance syndrome.*[47]
- Some patients have a combination of conditions—a lower-than-normal level of insulin production and a heightened insulin resistance at the cellular level.

Insulin resistance describes a complex metabolic situation in which organ and tissue cells deny entry to insulin and glucose. This creates the clinical paradox in which elevated serum insulin levels and hyperglycemia are present at the same time. Obesity increases insulin resistance.[41] Insulin resistance has a strong association with type 2 diabetes.[45,47]

Cardiometabolic Syndrome. The major known stimuli for development of metabolic syndrome are obesity and disorders of insulin resistance.[45] Specific measurable factors are diagnostic of metabolic syndrome. These include abdominal adiposity, as demonstrated by a waist measurement greater than 40 inches in men or 35 inches in women; triglyceride levels higher than 150 mg/dL; high-density lipoprotein (L) cholesterol levels lower than 40 mg/dL in men or 35 mg/dL in women; blood pressure higher than 130/85 mm Hg; and an FPG value higher than 100 mg/dL. The ADA uses the FPG cutoff point of 100 mg/dL to identify individuals who are prediabetic.[45]

Screening for Type 2 Diabetes. The ADA recommends screening individuals who are at risk for type 2 diabetes at 3-year intervals, beginning at 45 years of age, especially those who are overweight (defined as a body mass index [BMI] ≥25 kg/m^2) or obese (BMI ≥30 kg/m^2).[44] With the rise of obesity in the United States, the incidence of type 2 diabetes in children and adolescents has also increased dramatically in the last decade.[41]

Lifestyle Management for Type 2 Diabetes. Most adults with type 2 diabetes are overweight or obese based on their BMI. For most patients with type 2 diabetes, a program of weight reduction, increased physical exercise, and a change in diet pattern are recommended. Diets that contain large quantities of carbohydrate are discouraged.[48] The diet should contain less than 30% of calories from fat; reduced sugar intake; low levels of saturated and trans fats; and an increased quantity of whole grains, vegetables, and fruits. Crash diets are discouraged, and a gradual program of weight loss and increased exercise, if needed, is recommended.[48,49]

Pharmacological Management of Type 2 Diabetes. If lifestyle changes are unsuccessful in reversing the pattern of type 2 diabetes, oral antihyperglycemic medications are prescribed. These drugs are not oral forms of insulin, because insulin would be destroyed by gastric juices. Oral antidiabetic drugs lower plasma glucose levels by several different mechanisms that include increasing insulin secretion, increasing sensitivity to insulin, or delaying carbohydrate absorption.[49-53]

A serious complication of type 2 diabetes that often requires admission to a critical care unit is *hyperglycemic hyperosmolar state* (HHS).[54] This severe, sustained elevation of glucose levels leads to a serum hyperosmolality, and if left untreated, it progresses toward cellular dehydration, coma, and death (discussed later).

DIABETIC KETOACIDOSIS

Epidemiology and Etiology

Diabetic ketoacidosis (DKA) is a life-threatening hyperglycemic crisis associated with diabetes mellitus. Type 1 diabetics who are dependent on insulin are typically affected. The diagnostic criteria for DKA are as follows:[54]

- Blood glucose >250 mg/dL
- pH <7.3
- Serum bicarbonate <15 mEq/L
- Moderate or severe ketonemia or ketonuria

Infection is a major reason that diabetic patients progress to DKA. Symptoms of fatigue and polyuria may precede full-blown DKA, which can develop in less than 24 hours in a person with type 1 diabetes. In an undiagnosed diabetic patient, it is unknown how long it may take for DKA to develop as the pancreatic beta cells gradually fail. About 20% of hospital admissions for DKA are related to diagnosis of new-onset type 1 diabetes.[55] With current management, the mortality rate for adults with type 1 diabetes in DKA is less than 1%,[54] although a mortality rate of greater than 5% has been reported in older adults and in patients with life-threatening critical illness.[54]

Changes in the type of insulin, change in dosage, or increased metabolic demand can precipitate DKA in individuals with type 1 diabetes.[54] Life-cycle changes, such as growth spurts in the adolescent, require an increase in insulin intake, as do surgery, infection, and trauma. In young persons with diabetes, psychological problems combined with eating disorders are a contributing factor in up to 20% of cases of DKA.[54]

Ketoacidosis also occurs with acute pancreatitis. In addition to elevated glucose and acidosis, the serum amylase and lipase are abnormally high, which helps to establish the diagnosis as separate from type 1 diabetes.[55] Other nondiabetes causes of ketoacidosis are starvation and alcoholism. These cases are distinguished from classical DKA by clinical history and usually by a plasma glucose concentration of less than 250 mg/dL.[54]

Pathophysiology
Insulin Deficiency
Insulin is the metabolic key to the transfer of glucose from the bloodstream into the cell, where it can be used immediately for energy or stored for use at a later time. Without insulin, glucose remains in the bloodstream, and cells are deprived of their energy source. A complex pathophysiological chain of events follows (Figure 24-2).[54] The release of glucagon from the liver is stimulated when insulin is ineffective in providing the cells with sufficient glucose for energy. Glucagon increases the amount of glucose in the bloodstream by breaking down stored glucose, a process known as glycogenolysis. Noncarbohydrates (fat and protein) are converted into glucose, by a process known as gluconeogenesis. The breakdown of protein is termed proteolysis. The breakdown of fat (lipid) is known as lipolysis.

Blood glucose levels for the patient in DKA typically range from 300 to 800 mg/dL of blood. The reason the plasma glucose concentration is not higher is because of the short time period during which DKA develops in a patient with established type 1 diabetes. Elevated serum glucose levels alone do not define DKA; the major determining factor is an elevation in the total blood concentration of ketones[54] and often the presence of ketoacidosis.

Hyperglycemia
Hyperglycemia increases the plasma osmolality, and the blood becomes hyperosmolar. Cellular dehydration occurs as the hyperosmolar extracellular fluid draws the more dilute intracellular and interstitial fluid into the vascular space in an attempt to return the plasma osmolality to normal.

Dehydration stimulates catecholamine production in an effort to provide emergency support. Catecholamine output stimulates further lipolysis, glycogenolysis, and gluconeogenesis, pouring glucose into the bloodstream (see Figure 24-2). *Counterregulatory hormones*, such as glucagon and epinephrine, govern this physiological process. These hormones are normally released with hypoglycemia. In DKA, although the plasma glucose is elevated, the interior of the cells are starved of glucose, and the lack of intracellular glucose initiates the physiological processes described in Figure 24-2. DKA presentation is described as mild, moderate, or severe, depending on the plasma blood glucose (Table 24-3). As the blood glucose rises, acidosis develops and the level of consciousness decreases.

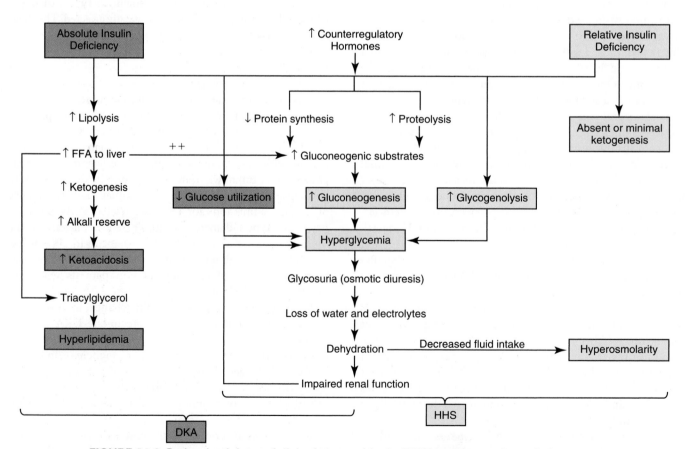

FIGURE 24-2 Pathophysiology of diabetic ketoacidosis (DKA) and hyperglycemic hyperosmolar state (HHS). (From Kitabchi AE, et al: Hyperglycemic crises in adult patients with diabetes: a consensus statement of the American Diabetes Association, *Diabetes Care* 32[7]:1335, 2009.)

TABLE 24-3	DIAGNOSTIC CRITERIA FOR DIABETIC KETOACIDOSIS (DKA) AND HYPERGLYCEMIC HYPEROSMOLAR SYNDROME (HHS)			
	DKA			**HHS**
	MILD (PLASMA GLUCOSE >250 mg/dL)	**MODERATE (PLASMA GLUCOSE >250 mg/dL)**	**SEVERE (PLASMA GLUCOSE >250 mg/dL)**	**PLASMA GLUCOSE >600 mg/dL**
Arterial pH	7.25-7.30	7.00 to <7.24	<7.00	>7.30
Serum bicarbonate (mEq/L)	15-18	10 to <15	<10	>18
Urine ketone*	Positive	Positive	Positive	Small
Serum ketone*	Positive	Positive	Positive	Small
Effective serum osmolality†	Variable	Variable	Variable	>320 mOsm/kg
Anion gap‡	>10	>12	>12	Variable
Mental status	Alert	Alert/drowsy	Stupor/coma	Stupor/coma

Data from Kitabchi AE, et al: Hyperglycemic crises in adult patients with diabetes: a consensus statement from the American Diabetes Association, *Diabetes Care* 32(7):1335, 2009.
*Nitroprusside reaction method.
†Effective serum osmolality: 2[measured Na+(mEz/L)] + glucose (mg/dL)18.
‡Anion gap: (Na+) − (Cl− + HCO3−) mEq/L.

Fluid Volume Deficit

Polyuria (excessive urination) and *glycosuria* (sugar in the urine) occur as a result of the osmotic particle load that occurs with DKA. The excess glucose, filtered at the glomeruli, cannot be resorbed at the renal tubule and spills into the urine. The unresorbed solute exerts its own osmotic pull in the renal tubules, and less water is returned to circulation through the collecting ducts. As a result, large volumes of water, along with sodium, potassium, and phosphorus, are excreted in the urine, causing a fluid volume deficit. The serum sodium concentration may be decreased because of the movement of water from the intracellular to the extracellular (vascular) space.[54]

Ketoacidosis

In the healthy individual, the presence of insulin in the bloodstream suppresses the manufacture of ketones. In insulin deficiency states, fat is rapidly converted into glucose (gluconeogenesis). Ketoacidosis occurs when free fatty acids are metabolized into ketones: acetoacetate, β-hydroxybutyrate, and acetone are the three ketone bodies that are produced.[56] During normal metabolism, the ratio of β-hydroxybutyrate to acetoacetate is 1:1, with acetone present in only small amounts. In insulin deficiency, the quantities of all three ketone bodies increase substantially, and the ratio of β-hydroxybutyrate to acetoacetate increases to as much as 10:1.[56] β-Hydroxybutyrate and acetoacetate are the ketones responsible for acidosis in DKA. Acetone does not cause acidosis and is safely excreted in the lungs, causing the characteristic fruity odor.

Ketones are measurable in the bloodstream (ketonemia). Blood tests that measure the quantity of β-hydroxybutyric acid, the predominant ketone body in the blood, are the most useful.[54] Because ketones are excreted by the kidney, they are also measurable in the urine *(ketonuria)*. Ketone blood tests are preferred over urine tests for diagnosis and monitoring of DKA in critical care. When the blood and urine become clear of ketones, the DKA is resolved.

Acid-Base Balance

The acid-base balance varies depending on the severity of the DKA. The patient with mild DKA typically has a pH between 7.25 and 7.30. In moderate to severe DKA, the pH can drop below 7.00.[54] Acid ketones dissociate and yield hydrogen ions (H+), which accumulate and precipitate a fall in serum pH. The level of serum bicarbonate also decreases, consistent with a diagnosis of metabolic acidosis. Breathing becomes deep and rapid—a respiratory pattern known as Kussmaul respirations—to release carbonic acid in the form of carbon dioxide. Acetone is exhaled, giving the breath its characteristic fruity odor.

Assessment and Diagnosis
Clinical Manifestations

DKA has a predictable clinical presentation. It is usually preceded by patient complaints of malaise, headache, polyuria (excessive urination), polydipsia (excessive thirst), and polyphagia (excessive hunger). Nausea, vomiting, extreme fatigue, dehydration, and weight loss follow. Central nervous system depression, with changes in the level of consciousness, can lead quickly to coma.[41,54]

The patient with DKA may be stuporous or unresponsive, depending on the degree of fluid-balance disturbance. The physical examination reveals evidence of dehydration, including flushed dry skin, dry buccal membranes, and skin turgor that takes longer than 3 seconds to return to its original position after the skin has been lifted. Often "sunken eyeballs," resulting from lack of fluid in the interstitium of the eyeball, are observed. Tachycardia and hypotension may signal profound fluid losses. Kussmaul respirations are present, and the fruity odor of acetone may be detected.

Laboratory Studies

Considering the complexity and potential seriousness of DKA, the laboratory diagnosis is straightforward. With a known diabetic patient, the presence of urine ketones and hyperglycemia on bedside finger-stick samples provides rapid diagnostic confirmation of DKA. If a blood gas sample is obtained, it can confirm the acid-base imbalance. Other clues may be gleaned from the venous blood chemistry panel. CO_2, if measured, is low in the presence of uncompensated metabolic acidosis, and the anion gap is elevated. Serum sodium may be low because water moves from the intracellular space into the extracellular (vascular) space.[54] The serum potassium level may be elevated, as potassium moves from inside the cell to the extracellular space.[54]

Medical Management

Diagnosis of DKA is based on the combination of presenting symptoms, patient history, medical history (type 1 diabetes), precipitating factors (if known), and results of serum glucose and urine ketone testing. After diagnosis, DKA requires aggressive clinical management to prevent progressive decompensation. The goals of treatment are to reverse dehydration, replace insulin, reverse ketoacidosis, and replenish electrolytes.

Reversing Dehydration

The patient with DKA is dehydrated and may have lost 5% to 10% of body weight in fluids. A fluid deficit of up to 6 L can exist in severe dehydration. Aggressive fluid replacement is provided to rehydrate the intracellular and extracellular compartments and prevent circulatory collapse (Figure 24-3).[54] Assessment of hydration is an important first step in the treatment of DKA.

Intravenous isotonic normal saline (0.9% NaCl) is infused to replenish the vascular deficit and to reverse hypotension. For the severely dehydrated patient, 1 L of normal saline is infused immediately. Laboratory assessment of serum osmolality and the serum sodium concentration can help guide the subsequent interventions.

After the serum glucose level decreases to 200 mg/dL, the infusing solution is changed to a 50/50 mix of hypotonic saline (0.45% NaCl) and 5% dextrose, infused at 150 to 250 mL/hour.[54] Dextrose is added to replenish depleted cellular glucose as the circulating serum glucose level falls. Dextrose infusion also prevents unexpected hypoglycemia when the insulin infusion is continued but the patient cannot take in sufficient carbohydrate from an oral diet.

Replacing Insulin

In moderate to severe DKA, an initial intravenous (IV) bolus of regular insulin at 0.1 unit for each kilogram of body weight is administered.[54] Subsequently, a continuous infusion of regular insulin at 0.1 unit/kg/hr is infused simultaneously with intravenous fluids (see Figure 24-3).[54] The plasma glucose concentration is expected to fall by 50 to 75 mg/dL per hour with this regimen. The glucose measurement should be rechecked and the hydration status of the patient re-evaluated. Figure 24-3 is a diagrammatic representation of intravenous and subcutaneous insulin administration options in DKA.

Frequent assessment of the patient's blood glucose concentration is mandatory in moderate to severe DKA. Initially, blood glucose tests are performed hourly. The frequency then decreases to every 2 to 4 hours as the patient's blood glucose level stabilizes and approaches normal. After the level has decreased to 200 mg/dL, the acidosis has been corrected, and rehydration has been achieved, the insulin IV infusion rate may be decreased to 0.02–0.05 unit/kg/hr.[54] It is important to verify that the serum potassium concentration is not lower than 3.3 mEq/L and to replace potassium if necessary, before administering the initial insulin bolus.[54]

Reversing Ketoacidosis

Replacement of fluid volume and insulin interrupts the ketotic cycle and reverses the metabolic acidosis. In the presence of insulin, glucose enters the cells, and the body ceases to convert fats into glucose.

Adequate hydration and insulin replacement usually correct the acidosis, and this treatment is sufficient for many patients with DKA. As shown in Figure 24-3, replacement of bicarbonate is no longer routine except for the severely acidotic patient with a serum pH value lower than 7.0.[54] An indwelling arterial line provides access for hourly sampling of arterial blood gases (ABGs) to evaluate pH, bicarbonate, and other laboratory values in the patient with severe DKA. If an arterial line is not available, the venous pH can be used.[54]

Hyperglycemia usually resolves before the ketoacidemia does. In one clinical report, patients with previously diagnosed type 1 diabetes in DKA took an average of 21 hours after being started on an intravenous insulin protocol to clear ketones from the urine; the infusion was continued for 36 hours until the patients could tolerate an oral diet; and the patients received a total of 9.5 L of normal saline for rehydration.[55] Patients who are newly diagnosed with type 1 diabetes take longer to clear urine ketones and require more insulin to achieve normal glycemic control, compared with long-term diabetics.[55]

Replenishing Electrolytes

Low serum potassium (hypokalemia) occurs as insulin promotes the return of potassium into the cell and metabolic acidosis is reversed. Replacement of potassium by administration of potassium chloride (KCl) begins as soon as the

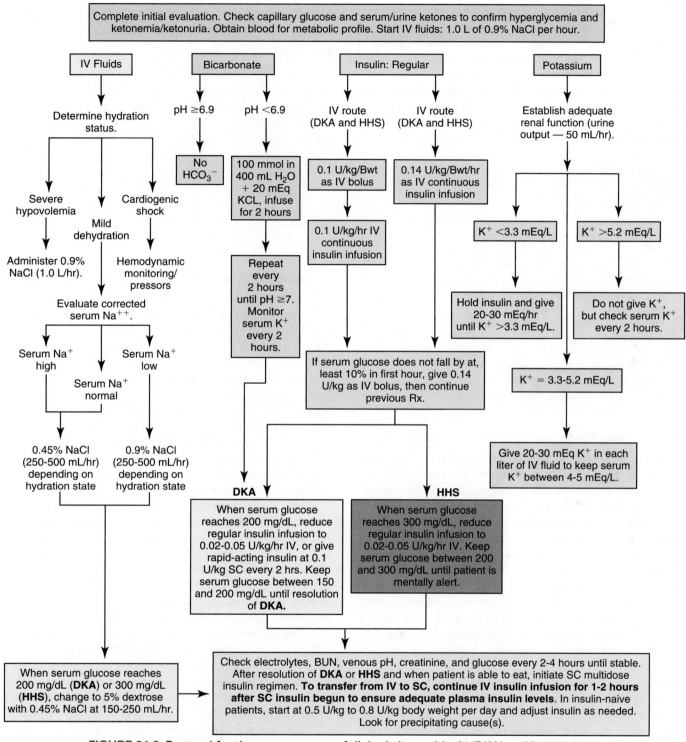

FIGURE 24-3 Protocol for the management of diabetic ketoacidosis (DKA) and hyperosmolar hyperglycemic state (HHS) in adult patients. (From Kitabchi AE, et al: Hyperglycemic crises in adult patients with diabetes: a consensus statement of the American Diabetes Association, *Diabetes Care* 32[7]:1335, 2009.)

serum potassium falls below normal. Frequent verification of the serum potassium concentration is required for the DKA patient receiving fluid resuscitation and insulin therapy.

The serum phosphate level is sometimes low (hypophosphatemia) in DKA. Insulin treatment may make this more obvious as phosphate is returned to the interior of the cell. If the serum phosphate level is less than 1 mg/dL, phosphate replacement is recommended.[54] See Figure 24-3 for further information about potassium replacement options.

Nursing Management

Nursing management of the patient with DKA incorporates a variety of nursing diagnoses (Nursing Diagnoses Priorities Box on Diabetic Ketoacidosis). **Nursing priorities are directed toward (1) administering fluids, insulin, and electrolytes; (2) monitoring response to therapy; (3) surveillance for complications; and (4) providing patient education.**

NURSING DIAGNOSIS PRIORITIES

Diabetic Ketoacidosis

- Decreased Cardiac Output related to alterations in preload, p. A-10
- Deficient Fluid Volume related to absolute loss, p. A-13
- Anxiety related to threat to biological, psychological, and social integrity, p. A-7
- Disturbed Body Image related to functional dependence on life-sustaining technology, p. A-16
- Ineffective Coping related to situational crisis and personal vulnerability, p. A-30
- Powerlessness related to lack of control over current situation and/or disease progression, p. A-33
- Deficient Knowledge: Discharge Regimen related to lack of previous exposure to information, p. A-15

Administering Fluids, Insulin, and Electrolytes

Rapid intravenous fluid replacement requires the use of a volumetric pump. Insulin is administered intravenously to patients who are severely dehydrated or have poor peripheral perfusion, to ensure effective absorption. Patients with DKA are kept on NPO status (nothing by mouth) until the hyperglycemia is under control. Throughout the insulin therapy, the patient's response and the laboratory data are assessed for changes relating to blood glucose levels. The critical care nurse is responsible for monitoring the rate of plasma glucose decline in response to insulin. The goal is to achieve a fall in glucose levels of approximately 50 to 75 mg/dL each hour.[54] The coordination involved in monitoring blood glucose, potassium, and often blood gases on an hourly basis is considerable.

When the blood glucose level falls to 200 mg/dL, a 5% dextrose solution (D_5W) with 0.45% NaCl solution is infused to prevent hypoglycemia.[54] At this time, it is likely that the insulin dose per hour will also be decreased. The regular insulin drip is not discontinued until the ketoacidosis subsides, as identified by absence of ketones and a normal pH by arterial or venous blood gas analysis.[54]

Insulin is given subcutaneously after glucose levels, dehydration, hypotension, and acid-base balance are normalized and the patient is in stable condition and taking an oral diet.

Monitoring Response to Therapy

Accurate intake and output (I&O) measurements must be maintained to monitor reversal of dehydration. Hourly urine output is an indicator of kidney function and provides

---

BOX 24-1 HYDRATION ASSESSMENT

- Hourly intake
- Blood pressure changes
  - Orthostatic hypotension
  - Pulse pressure
  - Pulse rate, character, rhythm
- Neck vein filling
- Skin turgor
- Skin moisture
- Body weight
- Central venous pressure
- Pulmonary arterial occlusion pressure
- Hourly output
- Complaints of thirst

---

information to prevent overhydration or underhydration. Vital signs, especially heart rate (HR), hemodynamic values, and blood pressure (BP), are continuously monitored to assess response to the fluid replacement. Evidence that fluid replacement is effective includes normal central venous pressure (CVP), decreased HR, and normal BP. Box 24-1 lists the standard features to be included in an assessment of hydration status. More invasive hemodynamic monitoring, such as a pulmonary artery catheter, is rarely needed. Further evidence of hydration improvement includes a change from a previously weak pulse to a pulse that is strong and full, and a change from hypotension to a gradual elevation of systolic BP. Respirations are assessed frequently for changes in rate, depth, and presence of the fruity acetone odor.

Blood glucose is measured each hour in the initial period. Sometimes, potassium is measured just as frequently. The serum osmolality and serum sodium concentration are evaluated, and blood urea nitrogen (BUN) and creatinine levels are assessed for possible kidney impairment related to decreased renal perfusion. The purpose of these frequent assessments is to determine that the patient's clinical status is improving. After the patient has stable laboratory indicators and is awake and alert, the transition to subcutaneous insulin and an oral diet can be made. Hypoglycemia is a risk during the transition period. For example, in anticipation of discontinuing the insulin and intravenous dextrose infusion, a patient receives a subcutaneous dose of insulin and is expected to eat a meal. However, if the patient is then unable to eat an adequate amount, hypoglycemia results from the administration of subcutaneous insulin without adequate glucose.[55]

The markers for resolution of DKA include a blood glucose level lower than 200 mg/dL, absence of ketones in the blood, a serum bicarbonate level greater than 18 mEq/L, and a venous pH level greater than 7.3.[54]

Surveillance for Complications

The patient in DKA can experience a variety of complications, including fluid volume overload, hypoglycemia, hypokalemia or hyperkalemia, hyponatremia, cerebral edema, and infection.

Fluid Volume Overload. Fluid overload from rapid volume infusion is a serious complication that can occur in the patient with a compromised cardiopulmonary system or kidneys. Neck vein engorgement, dyspnea without exertion, and pulmonary crackles on auscultation signal circulatory overload. Reduction in the rate and volume of infusion, elevation of the head of the bed, and provision of oxygen may be required to manage the increased intravascular volume. Hourly urine measurement is mandatory to assess renal output and adequacy of fluid replacement.

Hypoglycemia. Hypoglycemia is defined as a serum glucose level lower than 70 mg/dL.[41] Most acute care hospitals have specific procedures for management of the hypoglycemic patient. For example, if hypoglycemia is detected by finger-stick point-of-care testing at the bedside, a blood sample is sent to the laboratory for verification, the physician is notified immediately, and replacement glucose is given intravenously or orally, depending on the patient's clinical condition, diagnosis, and level of consciousness.

Unexpected behavior change or decreased level of consciousness, diaphoresis, and tremors are physical warning signs that the patient has become hypoglycemic. These symptoms are especially important to recognize if the frequency of glucose testing has lengthened to 2- to 4-hour intervals. A comparison between the physical symptoms expected with hypoglycemia and those of hyperglycemia is provided in Box 24-2.

Hypokalemia and Hyperkalemia. Hypokalemia can occur within the first 4 hours of rehydration and insulin treatment. Continuous cardiac monitoring is required, because low serum potassium (hypokalemia) can cause ventricular dysrhythmias.

Hyperkalemia occurs with acidosis or with overaggressive administration of potassium replacement in patients with compromised kidney function. Severe hyperkalemia is demonstrated on the cardiac monitor by a large, peaked T-wave; flattened P-wave; and widened QRS complex. See Figure 11-45 in Chapter 11. Ventricular fibrillation can follow if the hyperkalemia is not corrected.

Hyponatremia. Sodium elimination from the body results from the osmotic diuresis and is compounded by the vomiting and diarrhea that occur during DKA. Clinical manifestations of hyponatremia include abdominal cramping, apprehension, postural hypotension, and unexpected behavioral changes. Sodium chloride is infused as the initial intravenous solution. Maintenance of the saline infusion depends on clinical manifestations of sodium imbalance and serum laboratory values.

Risk for Cerebral Edema. Changes in the patient's neurological status may be insidious. Alterations in level of consciousness, pupil reaction, and motor function may be the result of fluctuating glucose levels and cerebral fluid shifts. Confusion and sudden complaints of headache are ominous signs that may signal cerebral edema. These observations require immediate action to prevent neurological damage. Neurological assessments are performed every hour or as needed during the acute phase of hyperglycemia and rehydration. Assessment of level of consciousness (LOC) is the index of the brain's response to rehydration therapy.

Skin Integrity. Skin care takes on new dimensions for the patient with DKA. Dehydration, hypovolemia, and hypophosphatemia interfere with oxygen delivery at the cell site and contribute to inadequate perfusion and tissue breakdown. Patients must be repositioned frequently to relieve capillary pressure and promote adequate perfusion to body tissues. The typical patient with type 1 diabetes is of normal weight or underweight. Bony prominences must be assessed for tissue breakdown, and the patient's body weight must be repositioned every 1 to 2 hours. Irritation of skin from adhesive tape, shearing force, and detergents should be avoided. Maintenance of skin integrity prevents unwanted portals of entry for microorganisms. Diabetic patients are at high risk of microvascular complications that decrease circulation to the legs and feet. This can result in diabetic ulcers and foot infections that require specialized wound care assessment and treatment.

Oral care, including tooth brushing and use of lip balm, helps keep lips supple and prevents cracking. Prepared sponge sticks or moist gauze pads can be used to moisten oral membranes of the unconscious patient. Swabbing the mouth moistens the tissue and displaces the bacteria that collect when saliva, which has a bacteriostatic action, is curtailed by dehydration. The conscious patient must be provided the

---

BOX 24-2   CLINICAL MANIFESTATIONS OF HYPOGLYCEMIA AND HYPERGLYCEMIA

HYPOGLYCEMIA	HYPERGLYCEMIA
• Restlessness	• Excessive thirst
• Apprehension	• Excessive urination
• Irritability	• Hunger
• Trembling	• Weakness
• Weakness	• Listlessness
• Diaphoresis	• Mental fatigue
• Pallor	• Flushed, dry skin
• Paresthesia	• Itching
• Headache	• Headache
• Hunger	• Nausea
• Difficulty thinking	• Vomiting
• Loss of coordination	• Abdominal cramps
• Difficulty walking	• Dehydration
• Difficulty talking	• Weak, rapid pulse
• Visual disturbances	• Postural hypotension
• Blurred vision	• Hypotension
• Double vision	• Acetone breath odor
• Tachycardia	• Kussmaul respirations
• Shallow respirations	• Rapid breathing
• Hypertension	• Changes in level of consciousness
• Changes in level of consciousness	• Stupor
• Seizures	• Coma
• Coma	

means to self-remove oral bacteria by tooth brushing and frequent oral rinsing.

Risk for Infection. Strict sterile technique is used to maintain all intravenous systems. All venipuncture sites are checked every 4 hours for signs of inflammation, phlebitis, or infiltration. Strict surgical asepsis is used for all invasive procedures. Sterile technique is used if urinary catheterization is necessary to obtain urine samples for testing. Urinary catheter care is provided per hospital protocol.

Providing Patient Education

It is important to be aware of the knowledge level and compliance history of patients with previously diagnosed diabetes to formulate an appropriate teaching plan. Learning objectives include a discussion of target glucose levels, definition of hyperglycemia and its causes, harmful effects, symptoms, and how to manage insulin and diet when one is unwell and unable to eat.[55] Additional objectives include a definition of DKA and its causes, symptoms, and harmful consequences. The patient and family are also expected to learn the principles of diabetes management. Universal precautions must be emphasized for all family caregivers.[34] The patient and family must also learn the warning signs to report to the attention of a health care practitioner. Education of the patient, family, or other support persons is crucial to achieve knowledge-based, independent self-management of blood glucose level and avoidance of diabetes-related complications, which are the ultimate goals of the teaching process.

Collaborative Management

In all aspects of patient care management, health care professionals work as a team with the major collaborative goal of providing the best possible outcome for each patient. Current guidelines related to collaborative management of patients with hyperglycemia crisis are in the Evidence-Based Collaborative Practice Box on Diabetic Ketoacidosis.

EVIDENCE-BASED COLLABORATIVE PRACTICE

Diabetic Ketoacidosis

Summary of evidence and evidence-based recommendations for controlling symptoms related to diabetic ketoacidosis (DKA)

Strong Evidence to Support
- Unless the DKA is mild, regular insulin by continuous infusion is recommended.
- Replace serum potassium if level is lower than 3.3 mEq/L.
- Replace serum phosphate if level is lower than 1.0 mg/dL.

Very Little Evidence to Support
- No support for use of routine bicarbonate to correct low serum pH; use may be considered if pH is below 7.0.

Data from Kitabchi AE, et al: Hyperglycemic crises in adult patients with diabetes: a consensus statement from the American Diabetes Association, *Diabetes Care* 32(7):1335, 2009.

HYPERGLYCEMIC HYPEROSMOLAR STATE

Epidemiology and Etiology

HHS is a potentially lethal hyperglycemic complication of type 2 diabetes. The hallmarks of HHS are extremely high levels of plasma glucose with resultant elevation in hyperosmolality causing osmotic diuresis. Ketosis is absent or mild (see Table 24-3). Inability to replace fluids lost through diuresis leads to profound dehydration and changes in level of consciousness. The mortality rate from HHS is 5% to 20%.[54] However, because patients with HHS have type 2 diabetes as an underlying disorder, they are older and have associated illnesses, which increase their mortality risk. When the mortality rate for diabetic patients is stratified by age, there is no difference based on the underlying hyperglycemic crisis (HHS or DKA). For HHS patients younger than 75 years, the mortality rate is 10%; for those age 75 to 84 years, it is 19%; and for those older than 85 years, it is 35%.[56]

The diagnostic criteria for HHS are as follows:[54]
- Blood glucose >600 mg/dL
- Arterial pH >7.3
- Serum bicarbonate >15 mEq/L
- Serum osmolality >320 mOsm/kg H_2O (320 mmol/kg)
- Absent or mild ketonuria

Most patients with this level of metabolic disruption experience visual changes, mental status changes, and potentially hypovolemic shock.

HHS occurs when the pancreas produces a relatively insufficient amount of insulin for the high levels of glucose that flood the bloodstream. HHS primarily affects older, obese persons with underlying cardiovascular conditions. Infection is the primary reason that type 2 diabetics develop HHS; the most common infections are pneumonia and urinary tract infections. The patient may have type 2 diabetes treated with diet and oral hypoglycemic agents that is destabilized by an infection. Other precipitating causes of HHS include stroke, myocardial infarction, trauma, burns, and the stress of a major illness. Many classes of medications have been associated with the development of HHS, including corticosteroids, phenytoin, thiazide diuretics, beta-blockers, dobutamine, terbutaline, and antipsychotics.[54,55]

Differences between Hyperglycemic Hyperosmolar State and Diabetic Ketoacidosis

Clinically, HHS is distinguished from DKA by the presence of extremely elevated serum glucose, more profound dehydration, and minimal or absent ketosis (see Table 24-3). Another major difference is that protein and fats are not used to create new supplies of glucose in HHS as they are in DKA; as a result, the ketotic cycle is never started or does not occur until the glucose level is extremely elevated. Patients with type 1 diabetes do not develop HHS, whereas some patients with type 2 diabetes do develop DKA.[54,55]

Pathophysiology

HHS represents a deficit of insulin and an excess of glucagon (see Figure 24-2). Reduced insulin levels prevent the movement of glucose into the cells, allowing glucose to accumulate in the plasma. The decreased insulin triggers glucagon release from the liver, and hepatic glucose is poured into the circulation. As the number of glucose particles increases in the blood, serum hyperosmolality increases. In an effort to decrease the serum osmolality, fluid is drawn from the intracellular compartment (inside the cells) into the vascular bed. Profound intracellular volume depletion occurs if the patient's thirst sensation is absent or decreased. HHS may evolve over days or even weeks.[54]

Hemoconcentration persists despite removal of large amounts of glucose in the urine (glycosuria). The glomerular filtration and elimination of glucose by the kidney tubules is ineffective in reducing the serum glucose level sufficiently to maintain normal glucose levels. The hyperosmolality and reduced blood volume stimulate release of ADH to increase the tubular resorption of water. ADH, however, is powerless to overcome the osmotic pull exerted by the glucose load. Excessive fluid volume is lost at the kidney tubule, with simultaneous loss of potassium, sodium, and phosphate in the urine. This chain of events results in progressively worsening hypovolemia.

Hypovolemia reduces renal perfusion and oliguria develops. Although this process conserves water and preserves the blood volume, it prevents further glucose loss, and hyperosmolality increases. Ketosis is absent or mild in HHS. However, the patient with HHS who has an extremely elevated serum glucose level (>1000 mg/dL) can develop a metabolic acidosis from dehydration, poor tissue perfusion, and lactic acid accumulation.

The SNS reacts to the body's stress response to try to restore homeostasis. Epinephrine, a potent stimulus for gluconeogenesis, is released, and additional glucose is added to the bloodstream.

Unless the glycemic diuresis cycle is broken by aggressive fluid replacement and insulin administration, intracellular dehydration negatively affects fluid and oxygen transport to the brain cells. Central nervous system dysfunction may result and may lead to coma. Hemoconcentration increases the blood viscosity, which may result in clot formation, thromboemboli, and cerebral, cardiac, and pleural infarcts.

Assessment and Diagnosis
Clinical Manifestations

HHS has a slow, subtle onset and develops over several days. Initially, the symptoms may be nonspecific and may be ignored or attributed to the patient's concurrent disease processes. History reveals malaise, blurred vision, polyuria, polydipsia (depending on the patient's thirst sensation), weight loss, and advancing weakness.[56] Medical attention may

not be obtained for these nonspecific, nonacute symptoms until the patient is unable to take sufficient fluids to offset the fluid losses. Progressive dehydration follows and leads to mental confusion, convulsions, and eventually coma, especially in older patients.

The physical examination may reveal a profound fluid deficit. Signs of severe dehydration include longitudinal wrinkles in the tongue, decreased salivation, and decreased CVP, with increases in HR and rapid respirations (Kussmaul air hunger does not occur). In older patients, assessment of clinical signs of dehydration is challenging. Neurological status is affected as the serum glucose climbs, especially at levels greater than 1500 mg/dL. Without intervention, obtundation and coma occur.

Laboratory Studies

Laboratory findings are used to establish the definitive diagnosis of HHS. Plasma glucose levels are strikingly elevated (>600 mg/dL). Serum osmolality is greater than 320 mOsm/kg. Acidosis is absent (arterial pH >7.3), and the serum bicarbonate concentration is greater than 18 mEq/L. Ketonuria is absent or mild.[54] The patient may have an elevated hematocrit and depleted potassium and phosphorus levels.

Point-of-care finger-stick or arterial-line testing of glucose at the bedside is the usual method for frequent monitoring of the serum blood glucose. Insulin replacement is then prescribed according to the blood glucose result. Some electrolytes also can be tested at the bedside (potassium, sodium, ionized calcium), but usually an arterial line is required for frequent blood access. If point-of-care testing is not available, traditional serial laboratory tests keep the clinician apprised of the fluctuating serum electrolyte levels and provide the basis for electrolyte replacement. Intracellular potassium and phosphate levels usually are depleted as a result of dehydration.

Medical Management

The goals of medical management are rapid rehydration, insulin replacement, and correction of electrolyte abnormalities, specifically potassium replacement. The underlying stimulus of HHS must be discovered and treated. The same basic principles used to treat DKA are used for the patient with HHS.

Rapid Rehydration

The primary intervention for HHS is rapid rehydration to restore the intravascular volume. The fluid deficit may be as much as 15 to 20 mL/kg/hour. The average 150-pound adult can lose more than 7 to 10 L of fluid.

The total body deficit of sodium and potassium may be as high as 500 to 700 mEq. Physiological saline solution (0.9%) is infused at 1 L/hr, especially for the patient in hypovolemic shock. Between 6 and 10 L of fluid replacement in the first 10 hours may be required to achieve a BP and CVP within normal range. This may necessitate an initial infusion rate of 250 to 500 mL/hour with infusion volumes adjusted according to the patient's hydration state and sodium level (see Figure 24-3).[54]

The serum sodium concentration is the parameter that is monitored to determine whether to change from isotonic (0.9%) to hypotonic (0.45%) saline. For example, patients with sodium levels equal to or less than 140 mEq/L may be given 0.9% normal saline solution, whereas those with levels greater than 140 mEq/L are given 0.45% saline solution (see Figure 24-3). In reality, it is difficult to assess the serum sodium level in the presence of hemoconcentration. Another recommendation is to calculate a *corrected sodium value.* This involves adding 1.6 mEq to the sodium laboratory value for each 100 mg/dL plasma glucose above normal.[54] Sodium input should not exceed the amount required to replace the losses. Careful monitoring of the serum sodium level is recommended to avoid a sodium-water imbalance and hemolysis as hemoconcentration is reduced.

To prevent hypoglycemia, when the serum glucose decreases to 300 mg/dL, change the hydrating solution to D_5W with 0.45% NaCl to infuse at 150 to 250 mL/hr.[54]

Insulin Administration

Volume resuscitation lowers the serum glucose level and improves symptoms even without insulin administration.[56] However, insulin replacement is recommended in the treatment of HHS because of clinical reports that acidosis can develop if insulin is withheld.[56] Insulin is given to facilitate the cellular use of glucose.

Methods to lower the blood glucose level vary. One method is to administer an intravenous bolus of regular insulin (0.1 unit/kg of body weight) initially, followed by a continuous insulin drip. Regular insulin, infusing at an initial rate calculated as 0.1 unit/kg hourly (e.g., 7 units/hr for a person weighing 70 kg) should lower the plasma glucose concentration by 50 to 75 mg/dL per hour. If the measured glucose level does not decrease by at least 10%, 0.14 insulin unit/hour may be given as a bolus.[54] The goal is to reduce the blood glucose by 50 to 75 mg/dL per hour.[54]

Insulin Resistance. Patients with HHS have underlying type 2 diabetes; many have metabolic syndrome and exhibit signs of insulin resistance.[48] In critical illness, the presence of *counter-regulatory hormones,* also known as *stress hormones* (cortisol, glucagon, GH, epinephrine), increases glucose production and also induces insulin resistance.[56] Patients with HHS may initially require supraphysiological doses of insulin to overcome the hyperglycemia and insulin resistance.[56] Hourly serial monitoring of the blood glucose level permits safe glycemic management and avoids the most common complication, which is hypoglycemia caused by overzealous insulin administration.[54] After the patient is over the hyperglycemic crisis and insulin has been discontinued, oral agents designed to decrease insulin resistance in type 2 diabetics are prescribed.

Electrolyte Replacement

Increasing the circulating levels of insulin with therapeutic doses of intravenous insulin promotes the rapid return of potassium and phosphorus into the cell. Serial laboratory tests keep the clinician apprised of the serum electrolyte levels and provide the basis for electrolyte replacement. Potassium typically is added to the intravenous infusion (see Figure 24-3). If the serum potassium concentration is lower than 3.3 mEq/L, it is essential to replenish the serum potassium before giving insulin.[54] Many hospitals have potassium replacement algorithms that are used to treat hypokalemia. Serum phosphate levels are carefully monitored, and phosphate replaced if the level is lower than 1.0 mg/dL.[54]

Nursing Management

Nursing management of the patient with HHS incorporates a variety of nursing diagnoses (see the Nursing Diagnosis Priorities Box on Hyperglycemic Hyperosmotic State). **Nursing priorities are directed toward (1) administering fluids, insulin, and electrolytes; (2) monitoring response to therapy; (3) surveillance for complications; and (4) providing patient education.**

NURSING DIAGNOSIS PRIORITIES

Hyperglycemic Hyperosmolar State

- Decreased Cardiac Output related to alterations in preload, p. A-10
- Deficient Fluid Volume related to absolute loss, p. A-13
- Anxiety related to threat to biological, psychological, and social integrity, p. A-7
- Deficient Knowledge: Discharge Regimen related to previous lack of exposure to information, p. A-15

Administering Fluids, Insulin, and Electrolytes

Rigorous fluid replacement and continuous intravenous insulin replacement must be controlled with an electronic volumetric pump. Accurate I&O measurements are maintained to monitor fluid balance. I&O measurements include the total of all fluids administered minus hourly losses, typically urine output and sometimes emesis. Hemodynamic monitoring may include use of an arterial line and measurements of CVP if the patient manifests signs of hypovolemic shock. Arterial line access is very helpful in monitoring serial blood glucose and electrolyte values. The use of a blood conservation system on the arterial line is essential to avoid iatrogenic exsanguination of the patient. Most critical care units have developed protocols or guidelines to ensure that patients in hyperglycemic crisis are managed safely (see Figure 24-3). The major responsibility for delivery of insulin, hourly monitoring of blood glucose, and infusion of appropriate crystalloid solutions lies with the critical care nurse. Many hospitals mandate a double-check procedure for medications such as insulin that have the potential to cause harm if wrongly administered.

Monitoring Response to Therapy

The BP, HR, and CVP are monitored to evaluate the degree of dehydration, the effectiveness of hydration therapy, and the patient's fluid tolerance. Because patients with HHS have underlying type 2 diabetes and, if older, are likely to have preexisting illnesses such as heart failure and kidney failure, it is important to monitor for symptoms of circulatory overload. Symptoms to anticipate include elevated CVP, tachycardia, bounding pulse, dyspnea, tachypnea, lung crackles, and engorged neck veins. The astute critical care nurse is aware of the clinical manifestations of fluid overload and observes for potential complications when rehydrating the patient with HHS and cardiac, pulmonary, or renal disease.

The serum glucose level should decrease by 50 to 75 mg/dL per hour with insulin administration.[54] This decrease is monitored by hourly blood glucose determinations. Based on the glucose result, the critical care nurse can alter the infusion of insulin according to hospital protocol (see Figure 24-3).

Surveillance for Complications

The potential complications of HHS are similar to those described for DKA: hypoglycemia, hypokalemia or hyperkalemia, and infection. The patient with HHS is at risk for other complications specific to associated disease entities. A history of cardiovascular, pulmonary, or kidney disease, whether known or latent, places HHS patients at high risk for complications.

Providing Patient Education

As the patient's condition improves and the patient demonstrates readiness to learn, education about type 2 diabetes and avoiding a recurrence of HHS becomes a priority. Most teaching occurs after the patient has left the critical care unit. Teaching topics include a description of type 2 diabetes and how it relates to HHS, dietary restrictions, exercise requirements, medication protocols, home testing of blood glucose, signs and symptoms of hyperglycemia and hypoglycemia, foot care, and lifestyle modifications if cardiovascular disease is present.

Collaborative Management

Because HHS is an acute condition superimposed on the chronic health problem of type 2 diabetes, many health professionals provide care and work collaboratively to restore homeostasis for each patient (Evidence-Based Collaborative Practice Box on Hyperglycemic Hyperosmolar State).

EVIDENCE-BASED COLLABORATIVE PRACTICE

Hyperglycemic Hyperosmolar State

Summary of evidence and evidence-based recommendations for controlling symptoms related to hyperglycemic hyperosmolar state (HHS)

Strong Evidence to Support
- Regular insulin by continuous infusion is recommended to normalize blood glucose to 80 to 110 mg/dL (euglycemic levels).
- Replace serum phosphate if the level is less than 1 mg/dL.
- A multidisciplinary team approach to care reduces length of stay and improves clinical outcomes.
- Close follow-up after discharge is recommended to maintain glycosylated hemoglobin (HbA$_{1c}$) at less than 7% and to prevent diabetes-related complications.

Weak Evidence to Support
- Use of a sliding insulin scale alone is discouraged, because it is associated with poor glucose control, increasing risk of hyperglycemia and hypoglycemia in hospitalized patients.

Data from Clement S, et al: Management of diabetes and hyperglycemia in hospitals, *Diabetes Care* 27(2):553, 2004; Garber AJ, et al: American College of Endocrinology position statement on inpatient diabetes and metabolic control, *Endocr Pract* 10(Suppl 2):4, 2004; Kitabchi AE, et al: Hyperglycemic crises in adult patients with diabetes: a consensus statement from the American Diabetes Association, *Diabetes Care* 32(7):1335, 2009.

DIABETES INSIPIDUS

Diabetes insipidus (DI) is recognized by the vast quantities of very dilute urine not caused by administration of diuretics or a fluid challenge. In the critically ill patient, the extreme diuresis is most likely to be caused by a lack of ADH (vasopressin). Any patient who has head trauma or has undergone neurosurgery has an increased risk of developing DI. Ordinarily, ADH is produced in the hypothalamus and stored in the posterior pituitary gland. ADH is normally released in response to elevations in serum osmolality and secondarily in reaction to hypovolemia or hypotension.[57] DI can occur if (1) the hypothalamus produces insufficient ADH, (2) the posterior pituitary fails to release ADH, or (3) the kidney nephron is resistant (unresponsive) to ADH.[58]

Etiology

DI is divided into three types according to cause: central, nephrogenic, and psychogenic (Box 24-3). Only *central DI*, also known as *neurogenic DI* because of its association with the brain, is encountered with any frequency in the critical care unit.

Central Diabetes Insipidus

In central DI, there is an inability to secrete an adequate amount of arginine vasopressin in response to an osmotic or nonosmotic stimuli, resulting in inappropriately dilute

BOX 24-3 ETIOLOGY OF DIABETES INSIPIDUS (DI)

Central Diabetes Insipidus
Primary (Rare in Critical Care)
ADH deficiency from hypothalamic-hypophyseal malformation
- Congenital defect
- Idiopathic

Secondary (Most Common in Critical Care)
ADH deficiency from damage to the hypothalamic-hypophyseal system
- Trauma
- Infection
- Surgery
- Primary neoplasms
- Metastatic malignancies

Nephrogenic Diabetes Insipidus
Inability of kidney tubules to respond to circulating ADH
- Decrease or absence of ADH receptors
- Cellular damage to nephron, especially loop of Henle
- Kidney damage (e.g., hydronephrosis, pyelonephritis, polycystic kidney)
- Untoward response to drug therapy (e.g., lithium carbonate, demeclocycline)

Psychogenic Diabetes Insipidus
Rare form of water intoxication
- Compulsive water drinking

ADH, Antidiuretic hormone.

urine.[59,60] The synthesis of ADH is incomplete in the hypothalamus, or the release of ADH from the pituitary is interrupted. Central DI can be congenital or idiopathic. In critical care, the most likely acute cause of central DI is neurosurgery, traumatic head injury, tumors, increased intracranial pressure, brain death, and infections such as encephalitis or meningitis. Among patients undergoing surgery on the pituitary gland, DI occurs in approximately 12% and is permanent in 3%.[61] The degree of hormone replacement required after surgery depends on the quantity of pituitary tissue removed.[61] One prospective study reported the incidence of central DI to be 15% among patients with traumatic brain injury.[62]

Nephrogenic Diabetes Insipidus

Nephrogenic DI is a rare congenital or acquired disorder that occurs when the V_2 receptors on the kidney tubule become nonresponsive to the action of ADH. Some drugs cause nephrogenic DI by decreasing the responsiveness of the kidney tubules to ADH. Long-term use of lithium carbonate, prescribed for bipolar disorder, was a frequent culprit in the past.[63]

Psychogenic Diabetes Insipidus

Psychogenic DI is a rare form of the disease that occurs with compulsive drinking of more than 5 L of water daily. Long-standing psychogenic DI closely mimics nephrogenic DI

because the kidney tubules become less responsive to ADH as a result of prolonged conditioning to hypotonic urine. This condition is uncommonly seen in the critical care unit.

Pathophysiology

The purpose of ADH is to maintain normal serum osmolality and circulating blood volume. Normally, ADH binds to the V_2 receptors on the kidney collecting tubules, causing insertion of water channels, known as aquaporins, along the luminal surface.[57] Even small (1% to 2%) increases in plasma osmolality are sufficient to stimulate ADH release.[57] Although there are several types of DI, this discussion focuses on neurogenic (central) DI, the condition encountered in the critical care unit after neurosurgery or head injury[56] (Figure 24-4).

In DI, as free water is eliminated, the urine osmolality and specific gravity decrease (dilute urine). At the same time, in the bloodstream, the serum sodium concentration and serum osmolality rise above 290 mOsm per kilogram of H_2O (290 mmol/L).[57] Normally at 295 mOsm/kg H_2O, the thirst sensors are activated in the hypothalamus, which triggers the synthesis and release of ADH.[57] In central DI, however, no ADH is released, or the ADH released is insufficient. Without ADH, the kidney collecting tubules are incapable of concentrating urine and retaining water.

As extracellular dehydration ensues, hypotension and hypovolemic shock occur. If the person is alert, extreme thirst will drive the person to drinking lots of water. This excessive intake of water reduces the serum osmolality to a more normal level and prevents dehydration. In the person with decreased level of consciousness, the polyuria leads to severe hypernatremia, dehydration, decreased cerebral perfusion, seizures, loss of consciousness, and death.

Assessment and Diagnosis
Clinical Manifestations

The clinical diagnosis is made based on the dramatic increase in dilute urine output occurring in the absence of diuretics, a fluid challenge, or hyperglycemia. Central DI is anticipated in conditions in which the underlying disease process is likely to disrupt posterior pituitary function. Central DI that occurs because of increasing intracranial pressure is life-threatening. It is imperative that the underlying condition be recognized and treated. In this situation, medications that treat DI are not sufficient.

Laboratory Studies

The core diagnostic tests used to establish the presence of DI and that evaluate the body's ability to balance fluid and electrolytes are not specific to the endocrine system. The most common laboratory tests are serum sodium concentration, serum osmolality, and urine osmolality (Table 24-4). The combination of an obvious clinical picture with high volumes of hypotonic urine, in the presence of the following laboratory criteria, is sufficient to diagnose central DI:[60]
- Serum sodium level >145 mEq/L
- Serum osmolality >295 mOsm/kg H_2O (>295 mmol/L)

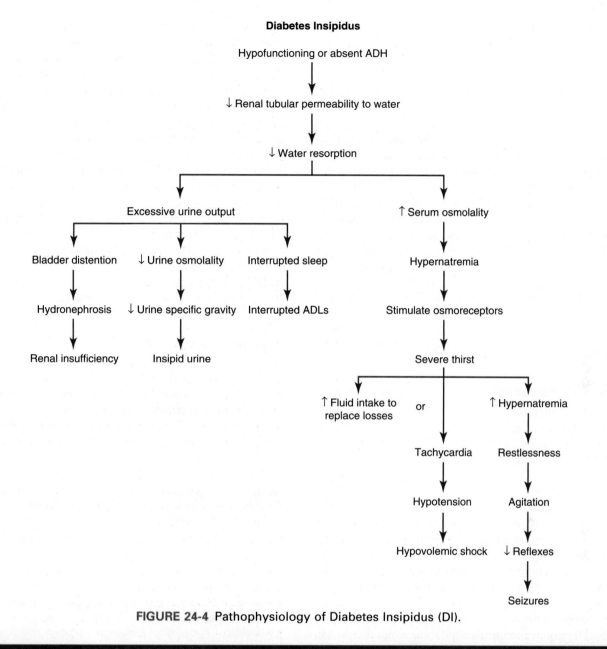

FIGURE 24-4 Pathophysiology of Diabetes Insipidus (DI).

TABLE 24-4	LABORATORY VALUES FOR PATIENTS WITH DIABETES INSIPIDUS (DI) AND SYNDROME OF INAPPROPRIATE ANTIDIURETIC HORMONE (SIADH)		
VALUE	**NORMAL**	**DI**	**SIADH**
Serum ADH	1-5 pg/mL	Decreased in central DI	Elevated
Serum osmolality (mOsm/L)	275-295*	>295*	<270
Serum sodium (mEq/L)	135-145	>145	<120
Urine osmolality (mOsm/L)	300-1400	<300	Increased
Urine specific gravity	1.005-1.030	<1.005	>1.030
Urine output	1.0-1.5 L/day	1.0-1.5 L/hr	Below normal

*Some hospitals use 280-300 mOsm/L as the normal reference value.
ADH, antidiuretic hormone; *DI,* diabetes insipidus; *SIADH,* syndrome of inappropriate antidiuretic hormone.

- Urine osmolality <200 mOsm/kg H_2O (<200 mmol/L)
- Urine specific gravity <1.005

Serum Sodium. The normal serum sodium concentration is 140 mEq/L (range, 135 to 145 mEq/L). In central DI, the serum sodium level can rise precipitously because of loss of free water. Hypernatremia is always associated with serum hyperosmolality.[64]

Serum Osmolality Test. Serum osmolality has a narrow normal range, 275 to 295 mOsm/kg. Severe DI can raise serum osmolality to greater than 320 mOsm/kg.[57]

Urine Osmolality. Urine osmolality is low, less than 300 mOsm/kg H_2O (300 mmol/L) in patients with central DI. For greatest accuracy, the urine sample should be collected and tested simultaneously with the blood sample.

Measurement of Antidiuretic Hormone. Measurement of the baseline serum ADH level is an additional diagnostic step. This is not typically performed in critical care if the clinical circumstances (e.g., head injury with raised intracranial pressure) make further testing unnecessary. Normal ADH levels range from 1 to 5 pg/mL. Most hydrated people have a morning fasting serum level lower than 4 pg/mL.[65]

To test for the underlying cause of DI, exogenous ADH may be administered. An ADH plasma concentration of approximately 1 pg/mL increases urinary concentration and decreases urine flow. Maximum antidiuresis occurs at an ADH concentration of approximately 5 pg/mL.[59] ADH administration (1 mcg of desmopressin (DDAVP) given subcutaneously) is used to distinguish between central DI and nephrogenic DI.[64] A urine output that is greatly decreased in response to ADH administration diagnoses central DI. A urine output that is unchanged in response to ADH administration suggests nephrogenic DI.

Medical Management

Immediate management of DI requires an aggressive approach. Treatment goals include restoration of circulating fluid volume, pharmacological ADH replacement, and treatment of the underlying condition.

Volume Restoration

Fluid replacement is provided in the initial phase of the treatment to prevent circulatory collapse. Patients who are able to drink are given voluminous amounts of fluid orally to balance output. For those who are unable to take sufficient fluids orally, hypotonic intravenous solutions are infused and carefully monitored to restore the hemodynamic balance.

Medications

Central DI requires immediate pharmacological management. Table 24-5 presents the medications most frequently prescribed to treat central DI and replace ADH.

Medications Used for Central Diabetes Insipidus. Patients with central DI who are unable to synthesize ADH require replacement with ADH *(vasopressin)* or an ADH analogue. The most commonly prescribed drug is the synthetic analogue of ADH, *desmopressin* (DDAVP). It is preferred over vasopressin (Pitressin) because it has a stronger antidiuretic action with little effect on blood pressure. DDAVP can be given intravenously, subcutaneously, or as a nasal spray. A typical DDAVP dose is 1 to 2 mcg given intravenously or subcutaneously every 12 hours.[66] Sometimes as little as 0.5 mcg is administered IV. The dosage is subsequently titrated according to the patient's antidiuretic response to the drug. To avoid a medication error, it is important to be aware that DDAVP is also used to control hemorrhage caused by platelet disorders and that the dose ranges for all of these conditions are different.

Vasopressin (Pitressin), 5 to 10 units given intramuscularly every 3 to 4 hours, produces a reduction in urine output.[66] Vasopressin acts on the V_1 receptors in vascular smooth muscle and can elevate systemic blood pressure. Water intoxication also can occur if the dosage is higher than the therapeutic level. Because of the risk of hypertension, this is not typically the first drug of choice for treating central DI. Vasopressin is also prescribed for septic shock states as an intravenous infusion and for cardiac arrest as an intravenous push. Dosages for these conditions are very different from that used to treat central DI. Extreme care must be taken to ensure that all drug dosages are accurate for each specific diagnosis.

Medications Used for Nephrogenic Diabetes Insipidus. The mainstay of therapy is to stop any medications that are inducing the ADH resistance. Nephrogenic DI is not a diagnosis frequently encountered in critical care. It is treated with hydrochlorothiazide, 12.5 to 25 mg administered once or twice daily. The dosage is then titrated according to the patient's antidiuretic response.

Nursing Management

Nursing management of the patient with DI incorporates a variety of nursing diagnoses (Nursing Diagnosis Priorities Box on Diabetes Insipidus). **Nursing priorities are directed toward (1) administering fluids and medications, (2) evaluating response to therapy, (3) maintaining surveillance for complications, and (4) providing patient education.**

NURSING DIAGNOSIS PRIORITIES
Diabetes Insipidus

- Deficient Fluid Volume related to decreased secretion of antidiuretic hormone (ADH), p. A-13
- Decreased Cardiac Output related to alterations in preload, p. A-10
- Anxiety related to threat to biological, psychological, and social integrity, p. A-7
- Deficient Knowledge: Discharge Regimen related to lack of previous exposure to information, p. A-15

Administrating Fluids and Medications

Rapid intravenous fluid replacement requires the use of a volumetric pump. Initially, a hypotonic intravenous solution is used to replace fluids lost and lower the serum hyperosmolality. ADH replacement is accomplished with extreme caution in the patient with a history of cardiac disease, because ADH may cause hypertension and overhydration. At the first signs of cardiovascular impairment, the drug is discontinued and fluid intake is restricted until urine specific gravity is less than 1.015 and polyuria resumes.

Evaluation of Response to Therapy

Critical assessment and management of fluid status are the most important initial concerns for the patient with DI. Monitoring of HR, BP, CVP, and pulmonary artery pressures

TABLE 24-5 PHARMACOLOGICAL MANAGEMENT: DIABETES INSIPIDUS (DI)

DRUG	DOSAGE*	ACTIONS	SPECIAL CONSIDERATIONS
Central Diabetes Insipidus			
DDAVP (available IV, as nasal spray, Rhinal tube, Rhinyle drops, Stimate)	Nasal: 10-40 mcg at bedtime or in divided doses Parenteral: 2-4 mcg twice daily	*Central DI* Antidiuretic Increases water resorption in nephron Prevents and controls polydipsia, polyuria	Few side effects Observe for nasal congestion, upper respiratory infection, allergic rhinitis. Monitor intake and output, urine osmolality, serum sodium level.
Vasopressin (Pitressin Synthetic, Pressyn)	Intramuscular, intravenous, subcutaneous, intra-arterial Topical: nasal mucosa	*Central DI* Antidiuretic Promotes resorption of water at kidney tubule Decreases urine output Increases urine osmolality Diagnostic aid Increases gastrointestinal peristalsis	Monitor fluid volume often, especially in older patients. Assess cardiac status. May precipitate angina, hypertension, or myocardial infarction if increased dose is given to patient with cardiac history. Parenteral extravasation can cause skin necrosis.
Lypressin (Diapid)	Intranasal: 1-2 sprays (7-14 mcg) in each nostril four times daily	*Central DI* Synthetic ADH Increases resorption of sodium and water in nephron	Proper instillation is important for absorption and action. Patient sits upright while holding bottle upright for administration. Repeat sprays (>2-3) are ineffective and wasteful; if dose is increased to 2-3 sprays, shorten time between dosing. Cough, chest tightness, shortness of breath
Nephrogenic Diabetes Insipidus			
Thiazide diuretics	Varies according to diuretic chosen, patient's size, and age	*Nephrogenic DI* Leads to mild fluid depletion Increases resorption of water and sodium in proximal nephron; less fluid travels to distal nephron, excreting less water	Varies according to diuretic chosen
Psychogenic Diabetes Insipidus			
Anti-compulsive disorder drugs, anxiolytics, psychopharmacological agents	Dosage varies	*Psychogenic DI*	Varies according to medication chosen

*Parenteral indicates intravenous or subcutaneous administration.
ADH, antidiuretic hormone; *DI*, diabetes insipidus; *DDAVP*, desmopressin acetate; *IV*, intravenous.

(if a pulmonary artery catheter is in place) provides early indications of response to fluid volume replacement. I&O measurement, condition of buccal membranes, skin turgor, daily weight measurements, presence of thirst, and temperature provide a basic assessment list that is vital for the patient who is unable to regulate fluid needs and losses. Placement of a urinary catheter is essential to accurately monitor the urinary output. Simultaneous urine and blood specimens for determination of osmolality and sodium and potassium levels are collected, and the results are relayed to the physician as necessary. The patient who is unable to satisfy sensations of thirst or to complete any task or self-care activity without the need to urinate may be confused and frightened. For patients who are able to verbalize their fears, having a caring nurse who is interested and nonjudgmental helps to reduce the emotional turmoil associated with their condition.

Surveillance for Complications

The most dangerous potential complication is hypertension and vasospasm of cardiac, cerebral, or mesenteric arterial vessels in response to vasopressin replacement. In most cases, DDAVP is selected for ADH replacement to avoid this complication. A less serious complication of DI is constipation due to fluid loss; it is treated with dietary fiber, stool softeners, or both. Conversely, diarrhea, abdominal cramping, and intestinal hyperactivity may accompany vasopressin therapy.

Untoward effects can be mitigated by modification of the vasopressin dose.

Patient Education

Educating the patient and the family about the disease process and how it affects thirst, urination, and fluid balance encourages patients to participate in their care. For most critical care patients, central DI is a temporary condition that resolves as the underlying medical condition (e.g., brain injury) improves. Patients who are discharged with DI are taught, along with their families, the signs and symptoms of dehydration and overhydration and procedures for accurate daily weight and urine specific gravity measurements. Printed information pertaining to drug actions, side effects, dosages, and timetable is provided, as well as an outline of factors that must be reported to the physician.

Collaborative Management

Central DI is a life-threatening condition. The collaborative assessment and clinical skills of all health care professionals and use of a clear plan of care are essential to achieve optimal outcomes for each patient.

SYNDROME OF INAPPROPRIATE SECRETION OF ANTIDIURETIC HORMONE

The opposing syndrome to DI is the syndrome of inappropriate secretion of antidiuretic hormone (SIADH), also known as the *syndrome of antidiuresis* (SIAD).[67] The patient with SIADH has an excess of ADH secreted into the bloodstream, more than the amount needed to maintain normal blood volume and serum osmolality. Excessive water is resorbed at the kidney tubule, leading to dilutional hyponatremia.

Etiology

Numerous causes of SIADH are observed in patients who are critically ill (Box 24-4). Central nervous system injury, tumors, and diseases that interfere with the normal functioning of the hypothalamic-pituitary system can cause SIADH.[67] A common cause is malignant bronchogenic small cell carcinoma.[68] This type of malignant cell is capable of synthesizing and releasing ADH regardless of the body's needs.[57,69] With much less frequency, other cancers that involve the brain, head and neck, gastroenteral, gynecological, and hematological systems are capable of autonomous production of ADH.[57] Levels of ADH rise with the use of positive-pressure ventilators that decrease venous return to the thorax, because they stimulate pulmonary baroreceptors to release and increase levels of circulating ADH.

Pathophysiology

ADH is a powerful, complex polypeptide compound. When released into the circulation by the posterior pituitary gland, ADH regulates water and electrolyte balance in the body. In SIADH, profound fluid and electrolyte disturbances result from the unsolicited, continuous release of the hormone into the bloodstream (Figure 24-5). Excessive ADH stimulates the kidney tubules to retain fluid regardless of need. This results in severe overhydration.

Excessive ADH dramatically alters the sodium balance in the extracellular vascular compartment. The overhydration causes a dilutional hyponatremia and reduces the sodium concentration to critically low levels. In the healthy adult, hyponatremia inhibits the release of ADH; in SIADH, however, the increased levels of circulating ADH are unrelated to the serum sodium concentration. Aldosterone production from the adrenal glands is also suppressed. Serum hypoosmolality leads to a shift of fluid from the extracellular fluid space into the intracellular fluid compartment (inside the cells) in an attempt to equalize osmotic pressure. Because minimal sodium is present in this fluid, edema usually does not result. Without ADH and aldosterone, water is retained, urine output is diminished, and further sodium is excreted in the urine. The urine has an increased osmolality from the decreased water excretion. Urinary concentration is also elevated by excess sodium in the urine. It is believed that, despite the serum hyponatremia, the increased release of ADH promotes sodium loss through the kidneys into the urine.

Assessment and Diagnosis
Clinical Manifestations

The clinical manifestations of SIADH relate to the excess fluids in the extracellular compartment and the proportionate dilution of the circulating sodium. Edema usually is not present, although slight weight gain may occur from the expanded extracellular fluid volume. Early clinical manifestations of dilutional hyponatremia include lethargy, anorexia, nausea, and vomiting. Severe neurological symptoms usually do not develop until the serum sodium concentration drops to less than 120 mEq/L.[70] Progressively deteriorating neurological signs of hyponatremia then predominate, and the patient is admitted to the critical care unit. Symptoms of severe hyponatremia include inability to concentrate, mental confusion, apprehension, seizures, decreased level of consciousness, coma, and death.

Laboratory Values

Patients with SIADH present with very concentrated urine output and very dilute serum. Laboratory values confirm this clinical picture. In SIADH, the serum is hypoosmolar (<275 mOsm/kg H_2O), with low serum sodium concentration and a urine osmolality greater than would be expected with such hypotonic blood (>100 mOsm/kg has been suggested).[67] A serum sodium concentration of less than 125 mEq/L (<120 mEq/L according to some experts) is associated with increasing severity of neurological symptoms.[64,70] An elevated urine sodium concentration, greater than 30 to 40 mEq/L, is congruent with the concentrated urine output of SIADH.[64,67,70] Use of diuretics negates the reliability of the urine sodium and urine osmolality levels.[70] Table 24-5 compares the typical laboratory values associated with SIADH with those of DI.

BOX 24-4 CAUSES OF SYNDROME OF INAPPROPRIATE SECRETION OF ANTIDIURETIC HORMONE

***Malignant disease* associated with autonomous production of ADH:**
- Bronchogenic small cell carcinoma
- Pancreatic adenocarcinoma
- Duodenal, bladder, ureter, and prostatic carcinomas
- Lymphosarcoma, Ewing's sarcoma
- Acute leukemia, Hodgkin's disease
- Cerebral neoplasm, thymoma

***Central nervous system diseases* that interfere with the hypothalamic-posterior pituitary system and increase the production or release of ADH:**
- Head injury
- Brain abscess
- Hydrocephalus
- Pituitary adenoma
- Subdural hematoma
- Subarachnoid hemorrhage
- Cerebral atrophy
- Guillain-Barré syndrome

***Neurogenic stimuli* capable of increasing ADH:**
- Decreased glomerular filtration rate
- Physical or emotional stress
- Pain
- Fear
- Trauma
- Surgery
- Myocardial infarction
- Acute infection
- Hypotension
- Hemorrhage
- Hypovolemia

***Pulmonary diseases* believed to stimulate the baroreceptors and increase ADH:**
- Pulmonary tuberculosis
- Viral and bacterial pneumonia
- Empyema

- Lung abscess
- Chronic obstructive lung disease
- Status asthmaticus
- Cystic fibrosis

***Endocrine disturbances* that hormonally influence ADH:**
- Myxedema
- Hypothyroidism
- Hypopituitarism
- Adrenal insufficiency—Addison's disease

***Medications* that mimic, increase the release of, or potentiate ADH:**
- Hypoglycemics
  - Insulin
  - Tolbutamide
  - Chlorpropamide
- Potassium-depleting thiazide diuretics
- Tricyclic antidepressants
  - Imipramine
  - Amitriptyline
- Phenothiazine
  - Fluphenazine
  - Thioridazine
- Thioxanthenes
  - Thiothixene
  - Chlorprothixene
- Chemotherapeutic agents
  - Vincristine
  - Cyclophosphamide
- Opiates
- Carbamazepine
- Clofibrate
- Acetaminophen
- Nicotine
- Oxytocin
- Vasopressin
- Anesthetics

ADH, antidiuretic hormone.

Medical Management

In the critical care unit, SIADH often occurs as a secondary disease. Ideally, recognition and treatment of the primary disease will reduce the production of ADH. If the patient is receiving any of the medications suspected of causing SIADH, discontinuing the drug may return ADH levels to normal. Some of the drugs that alter ADH levels are listed in Box 24-4. The goals of medical management are to restore fluid and sodium balance.

Fluid Restriction

The medical therapy that is the most effective (along with treatment of the primary disease) is simple reduction of fluid intake.[64] This is achieved most successfully in the patient with a moderate increase in body fluid volume and hyponatremia.

Although fluid restrictions are calculated on the basis of individual needs and losses, a general criterion is to restrict fluids to 500 mL less than average daily output.[57]

Sodium Replacement

Patients with severe hyponatremia (<125 mEq/L serum sodium) experience severe neurological symptoms, even seizures. How rapidly the sodium should be corrected and which sodium concentration to use remain controversial.[71] One recommended regimen is an intravenous rate that provides sufficient sodium to raise serum sodium levels by up to 12 mEq/day for the first 24 hours (no more than 0.5 mEq each hour), with a total rise of 18 mEq/L in the initial 48 hours.[64] Another option is to add furosemide (Lasix) to increase the diuresis of free water.

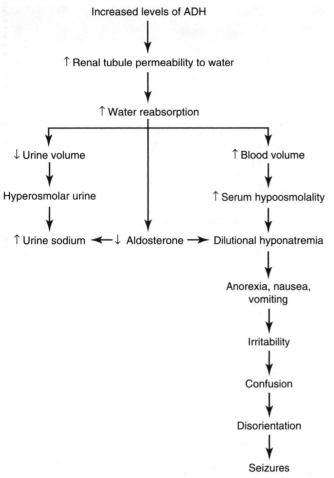

Increased levels of ADH

↑ Renal tubule permeability to water

↑ Water reabsorption

↓ Urine volume

↑ Blood volume

Hyperosmolar urine

↑ Serum hypoosmolality

↑ Urine sodium ← ↓ Aldosterone → Dilutional hyponatremia

Anorexia, nausea, vomiting

Irritability

Confusion

Disorientation

Seizures

FIGURE 24-5 Pathophysiology of Syndrome of Inappropriate Antidiuretic Hormone (SIADH).

If hyponatremia is severe (<120 mEq/L), an infusion of 3% hypertonic saline solution may be used to replenish the serum sodium without adding extra volume. It is imperative to be aware that hypertonic saline solution is dangerous if administered too quickly, and calculation of the quantity of sodium that will be administered is advised. An example of one sodium replacement regimen is an infusion of 3% saline infusion at 35 mL/hr in a 70-kg patient, which will increase the serum sodium level by approximately 0.5 mEq/L per hour (12 mEq/day).[64] Suggested end points at which to stop the acute sodium repletion include the following: (1) the patient's symptoms are abolished; (2) a safe serum sodium level is achieved (usually >120 mEq/L); (3) a total correction of 20 mEq/L is achieved.[64]

Too-rapid serum sodium correction must be avoided to reduce the risk of *osmotic demyelination,* previously known as *central pontine myelinolysis.* The demyelination occurs in the pons and in other areas of the brain's white matter.[57] The lesions may be detected on imaging studies (computed tomography and magnetic resonance imaging), and severe neurological damage or death can result.[57] Patients with a baseline serum sodium level lower than 120 mEq/L are most at risk.[57] Serum sodium levels must be evaluated at least every 4 hours during the acute phase of sodium replacement.[64]

Medications

Medications are prescribed only if water restriction is ineffective in correcting the SIADH. Certain drugs decrease the output of ADH from the pituitary gland, and others increase the action of ADH on the V_2 kidney tubule receptors so that more water is excreted.

Medications that Increase Kidney Water Excretion. Two classes of drugs are available to treat SIADH. Until recently, the only medication used to treat SIADH was demeclocycline, a derivative of tetracycline.[64] The dosage range is from 600 to 1200 mg per day, and several days of therapy are necessary to achieve maximal effects.[64] It is advisable to wait several days before changing the initial dose regimen.[64]

The arginine vasopressin receptor antagonists are a newer class of drugs, not yet in widespread use. Conivaptan (Vaprisol), at a dosage of 20 to 40 mg/day given IV, is approved for management of hypervolemic hyponatremia, such as SIADH. It is available in oral and IV forms and is approved for use only in hospitalized patients. Conivaptan is a nonselective vasopressin receptor antagonist, which means that it blocks V_1 receptors in the vasculature and V_2 receptors in the kidney.[67] The patient must be observed carefully to avoid hypotension (caused by V_1 receptor blockade), and hypovolemia is an absolute contraindication. New V_2 receptor antagonist medications collectively known as 'vaptans' are becoming available for treatment of chronic hyponatremia.[72,73] Vaptans block the antidiuretic effect of vasopressin by binding to V_2 receptors in the kidney. V_2 receptor blockade results in "water diuresis," otherwise known as aquaresis, which reduces body water content thus raising plasma sodium levels.[73]

Nursing Management

Nursing management of the patient with SIADH incorporates a variety of nursing diagnoses (Nursing Diagnosis Priorities Box on Syndrome of Inappropriate Secretion of Antidiuretic Hormone). **Nursing priorities are directed toward (1) restricting fluids, (2) maintaining surveillance for complications, and (3) providing patient education.**

NURSING DIAGNOSIS PRIORITIES

Syndrome of Inappropriate Secretion of Antidiuretic Hormone

- Excess Fluid Volume related to comprised regulation mechanism, p. A-19
- Anxiety related to lack of control over current situation or disease progression, p. A-7
- Deficient Knowledge: Discharge Regimen related to lack of previous exposure to information, p. A-15

Restricting Fluids

Thorough, astute nursing assessments are required for care of the patient with SIADH while an attempt is made to correct the fluid and sodium imbalance; the systemic effects of hyponatremia occur rapidly and can be lethal. Frequent assessment of the patient's hydration status is accomplished with serial measurements of urine output, serum sodium levels, and serum osmolality. Accurate measurement of I&O is required to calculate fluid replacement for the patient with SIADH. All fluids are restricted. Intake that equals urine output may be given until the serum sodium level returns to normal. Frequent mouth care (moistening of the buccal membrane) may give comfort during the period of fluid restriction. The patient is weighed daily to gauge fluid retention or loss. Weight gain signifies continual fluid retention, whereas weight loss indicates loss of body fluid.

Constipation is a frequent complication of decreased fluid intake. Cathartics or low-volume hypertonic enemas may be given to stimulate peristalsis. Tap water or hypotonic enemas should never be given, because the water in the enema solution may be absorbed through the bowel and potentiate water intoxication.

Maintaining Surveillance for Complications

The patient's neurological status, especially level of consciousness, should be evaluated on an hourly basis if the serum sodium level is critically low (<125 mEq/L). Seizure precautions for the patient with SIADH are provided regardless of the degree of hyponatremia. Serum sodium levels may fluctuate rapidly, and neurological impairment may occur with no apparent warning. The patient's altered neurological response also may be influenced by the acuteness of the primary disease (central nervous system disease) and not solely by the low sodium levels. Seizure precautions include nursing actions to protect the patient from injury (padded side rails, bed in low position when patient is unattended) and to provide an open airway (oral airway, head turned to the side without forcible restraint of the patient, suction apparatus). Oxygen may be required to maintain a saturation level greater than 92% if there is pulmonary congestion or edema that interferes with alveolar gas exchange.

Patient Education

Rapidly occurring changes in the patient's neurological status may worry visiting family members. Sensitivity to the family's unspoken fears can be shown by words that express empathy and by providing time for the patient and family to ask questions and express their concerns. The nurse may discuss the course of SIADH, its effect on water balance, and the reasons for fluid restrictions.

Collaborative Management

At this time, there are no published guidelines that discuss acute collaborative care management of the patient with SIADH. This is a complex condition, and effective clinical management requires the skills of many health care professionals working as a team, with goals that are clearly communicated to all team members.

CASE STUDY   PATIENT WITH AN ENDOCRINE DISORDER

Answers to the Case Study Questions can be found on the Evolve web site at http://evolve.elsevier.com/Urden/priorities/.

Brief Patient History
Ms. S is a 72-year-old woman with a history of hypertension treated with an angiotensin-converting enzyme (ACE) inhibitor and thiazide diuretics. She has a past 100-pack-year history of tobacco abuse but quit 2 years ago. Ms. S lives independently in a senior apartment and was brought to the hospital by friends because of a fall. Ms. S states that she has a severe headache but cannot recall whether she hit her head during the fall. She is also having difficulty recalling recent events.

Clinical Assessment
Ms. S is admitted to the intensive care unit from the emergency department because of nonspecific ECG changes suggestive of inferior wall ischemia and electrolyte abnormalities. She is awake; alert; oriented to person, time, place; and unable to recall the events leading to her hospitalization. She states that her headache is severe and feels like someone is hitting her head with a hammer. Her skin is warm and dry. Ms. S's gait is visibly unsteady.

Diagnostic Procedures
Ms. S's vital signs include the following: blood pressure of 180/92 mm Hg, heart rate of 100 beats/min (sinus rhythm), respiratory rate of 24 breaths/min, and temperature of 98.8° F.

Ms. S reports that her headache is a 10 on the Baker-Wong faces scale. Laboratory findings include the following: sodium level of 116 mmol/L, potassium level of 3.3 mmol/L, chloride level of 88 mmol/L, carbon dioxide level of 22 mEq/L, magnesium level of 1.8 mg/dL, urinary sodium level of 30 mmol/L, and urine osmolality value of 118 mOsm/L. The test result for troponin I on admission was negative. ECG testing shows a normal sinus rhythm, T-wave inversion in leads II, III, and AVF, and a change from prior ECG findings, suggestive of inferior wall ischemia. Chest radiography identified a mass in the right upper lobe that strongly suggested a neoplasm.

Medical Diagnosis
Ms. S is diagnosed with syndrome of inappropriate diuretic hormone (SIADH).

Questions
1. What major outcomes do you expect to achieve for this patient?
2. What problems or risks must be managed to achieve these outcomes?
3. What interventions must be initiated to monitor, prevent, manage, or eliminate the problems and risks identified?
4. What interventions should be initiated to promote optimal functioning, safety, and well-being of the patient?
5. What possible learning needs do you anticipate for this patient?
6. What cultural and age-related factors may have a bearing on the patient's plan of care?

REFERENCES

1. van den Berghe G, et al: Intensive insulin therapy in the critically ill patients, *N Engl J Med* 345(19):1359, 2001.
2. van den Berghe G, et al: Intensive insulin therapy in the medical ICU, *N Engl J Med* 354(5):449, 2006.
3. Marik PE, Raghavan M: Stress-hyperglycemia, insulin and immunomodulation in sepsis, *Intensive Care Med* 30(5):748, 2004.
4. Dellinger RP, et al: Surviving Sepsis Campaign: international guidelines for management of severe sepsis and septic shock: 2008, *Crit Care Med* 36(1):296, 2008.
5. Moghissi ES, et al: American Association of Clinical Endocrinologists and American Diabetes Association consensus statement on inpatient diabetes control, *Endocr Pract* 15(4):353, 2009.
6. Wortsman J: Role of epinephrine in acute stress, *Endocrinol Metab Clin North Am* 31(1):79, 2002.
7. Marik PE, et al: Recommendations for the diagnosis and management of corticosteroid insufficiency in critically ill adult patients: consensus statements from an international task force by the American College of Critical Care Medicine, *Crit Care Med* 36(6):1937, 2008.
8. Peeters RP, et al: Changes within the thyroid axis during critical illness, *Crit Care Clin* 22(1):41, 2006.
9. van den Berghe G: Neuroendocrine pathobiology of chronic critical illness, *Crit Care Clin* 18(3):509, 2002.
10. van den Berghe G: Endocrine evaluation of patients with critical illness, *Endocrinol Metab Clin North Am* 32(2):385, 2003.
11. Weekers F, van den Berghe G: Endocrine modifications and interventions during critical illness, *Proc Nutr Soc* 63(3):443, 2004.
12. Cooper MS, Stewart PM: Corticosteroid insufficiency in acutely ill patients, *N Engl J Med* 348(8):727, 2003.
13. Collier B, et al: Glucose control and the inflammatory response, *Nutr Clin Pract* 23(1):3, 2008.
14. Langton JE, Brent GA: Nonthyroidal illness syndrome: evaluation of thyroid function in sick patients, *Endocrinol Metab Clin North Am* 31(1):159, 2002.
15. Wyne KL: The role of thyroid hormone therapy in acutely ill cardiac patients, *Crit Care* 9(4):333, 2005.
16. Rivers EP, et al: Adrenal insufficiency in high-risk surgical ICU patients, *Chest* 119(3):889, 2001.
17. Keh D, Sprung CL: Use of corticosteroid therapy in patients with sepsis and septic shock: an evidence-based review, *Crit Care Med* 32(Suppl 11):S527, 2004.
18. Axelrod L: Perioperative management of patients treated with glucocorticoids, *Endocrinol Metab Clin North Am* 32(2):367, 2003.
19. Marik PE: Mechanisms and clinical consequences of critical illness associated adrenal insufficiency, *Curr Opin Crit Care* 13(4):363, 2007.
20. Sprung CL, et al: Hydrocortisone therapy for patients with septic shock, *N Engl J Med* 358(2):111, 2008.
21. Clement S: Better glycemic control in the hospital: beneficial and feasible, *Cleve Clin J Med* 74(2):111, 2007.
22. NICE-SUGAR Study Investigators: Intensive versus conventional glucose control in critically ill patients, *N Eng J Med* 360(13):1283, 2009.
23. De La Rosa G, et al: Strict glycaemic control in patients hospitalised in a mixed medical and surgical intensive care unit: a randomised clinical trial, *Crit Care* 12(5):R120, 2008.
24. Gandhi GY, et al: Intensive intraoperative insulin therapy versus conventional glucose management during cardiac surgery: a randomized trial, *Ann Intern Med* 146(4):233, 2007.
25. Wiener RS, et al: Benefits and risks of tight glucose control in critically ill adults: a meta-analysis, *JAMA* 300(8):933, 2008.
26. Deedwania P, et al: Hyperglycemia and acute coronary syndrome: a scientific statement from the American Heart Association Diabetes Committee of the Council on Nutrition, Physical Activity, and Metabolism, *Circulation* 117(12):1610, 2008.
27. Qaseem A, et al: Use of intensive insulin therapy for the management of glycemic control in hospitalized patients: A clinical practice guideline from the American College of Physicians, *Ann Intern Med* 154(4):260, 2011.
28. Rydén L, et al: Guidelines on diabetes, pre-diabetes, and cardiovascular diseases: executive summary. The Task Force on Diabetes and Cardiovascular Diseases of the European Society of Cardiology (ESC) and of the European Association for the Study of Diabetes (EASD), *Eur Heart J* 28(1):88, 2007.
29. Ascione R, et al: Inadequate blood glucose control is associated with in-hospital mortality and morbidity in diabetic and nondiabetic patients undergoing cardiac surgery, *Circulation* 118(2):113, 2008.
30. Jones KW, et al: Hyperglycemia predicts mortality after CABG: postoperative hyperglycemia predicts dramatic increases in mortality after coronary artery bypass graft surgery, *J Diabetes Complications* 22(6):365, 2008.
31. Whitcomb BW, et al: Impact of admission hyperglycemia on hospital mortality in various intensive care unit populations, *Crit Care Med* 33(12):2772, 2005.
32. Egi M, et al: Blood glucose concentration and outcome of critical illness: the impact of diabetes, *Crit Care Med* 36(8):2249, 2008.
33. Oddo M, et al: Glucose control after severe brain injury, *Curr Opin Clin Nutr Metab Care* 11(2):134, 2008.
34. Clement S, et al: Management of diabetes and hyperglycemia in hospitals, *Diabetes Care* 27(2):553, 2004.
35. Braithwaite SS: Inpatient insulin therapy, *Curr Opin Endocrinol Diabetes Obes* 15(2):159, 2008.
36. Moghissi E: Hospital management of diabetes: beyond the sliding scale, *Cleve Clin J Med* 71(10):801, 2004.
37. American Diabetes Association: Diagnosis and classification of diabetes mellitus, *Diabetes Care* 33(Suppl 1):S62, 2010.
38. American Diabetes Association: Nutrition recommendations and interventions for diabetes: a position statement of the American Diabetes Association, *Diabetes Care* 31 (Suppl 1):S61, 2008.
39. Heron MP: *Deaths: leading causes for 2004, National Vital Statistics Reports* 56(5), Hyattsville, Md., 2007, National Center for Health Statistics.
40. Coughlin SS, et al: Diabetes mellitus as a predictor of cancer mortality in a large cohort of US adults, *Am J Epidemiol* 159(12):1160, 2004.
41. American Diabetes Association: Standards of medical care in diabetes—2011, *Diabetes Care* 34(Suppl 1):S11, 2011.
42. Blake DR, Nathan DM: Point-of-care testing for diabetes, *Crit Care Nurs Q* 27(2):150, 2004.
43. American Diabetes Association: Diagnosis and classification of diabetes mellitus, *Diabetes Care* 34(Suppl 1):S62, 2011.
44. American Diabetes Association: Screening for type 2 diabetes, *Diabetes Care* 27(Suppl 1):S11, 2004.

45. Grundy SM, et al: Diagnosis and management of the metabolic syndrome: an American Heart Association/National Heart, Lung, and Blood Institute Scientific Statement, *Circulation* 112(17):2735, 2005.

46. Rosenzweig JL, et al: Primary prevention of cardiovascular disease and type 2 diabetes in patients at metabolic risk: an Endocrine Society clinical practice guideline, *J Clin Endocrinol Metab* 93(10):3671, 2008.

47. Einhorn D, et al: American College of Endocrinology position statement on the insulin resistance syndrome, *Endocr Pract* 9(Suppl 2):5, 2003.

48. Grundy SM, et al: Clinical management of metabolic syndrome: report of the American Heart Association/National Heart, Lung, and Blood Institute/American Diabetes Association conference on scientific issues related to management, *Circulation* 109(4):551, 2004.

49. Rodbard HW, et al: Statement by an American Association of Clinical Endocrinologists/American College of Endocrinology consensus panel on type 2 diabetes mellitus: an algorithm for glycemic control, *Endocr Pract* 15(6):540, 2009.

50. Krentz AJ, et al: New drugs for type 2 diabetes mellitus: what is their place in therapy? *Drugs* 68(15):2131, 2008.

51. Nathan DM, et al: Management of hyperglycemia in type 2 diabetes: a consensus algorithm for the initiation and adjustment of therapy: a consensus statement from the American Diabetes Association and the European Association for the Study of Diabetes, *Diabetes Care* 29(8):1963, 2006.

52. Nathan DM, et al: Management of hyperglycemia in type 2 diabetes: a consensus algorithm for the initiation and adjustment of therapy: update regarding thiazolidinediones: a consensus statement from the American Diabetes Association and the European Association for the Study of Diabetes, *Diabetes Care* 31(1):173, 2008.

53. Nesto RW, et al: Thiazolidinedione use, fluid retention, and congestive heart failure: a consensus statement from the American Heart Association and American Diabetes Association, *Circulation* 108(23):2941, 2003.

54. Kitabchi AE, et al: Hyperglycemic crises in adult patients with diabetes: a consensus statement from the American Diabetes Association, *Diabetes Care* 32(7):1335, 2009.

55. Newton CA, Raskin P: Diabetic ketoacidosis in type 1 and type 2 diabetes mellitus: clinical and biochemical differences, *Arch Intern Med* 164(17):1925, 2004.

56. Gaglia JL, et al: Acute hyperglycemic crisis in the elderly, *Med Clin North Am* 88(4):1063, 2004.

57. Janicic N, Verbalis JG: Evaluation and management of hypo-osmolality in hospitalized patients, *Endocrinol Metab Clin North Am* 32(2):459, 2003.

58. Holcomb SS: Diabetes insipidus, *Dimens Crit Care Nurs* 21(3):94, 2002.

59. Wong LL, Verbalis JG: Systemic diseases associated with disorders of water homeostasis, *Endocrinol Metab Clin North Am* 31(1):121, 2002.

60. Loh JA, Verbalis JG: Disorders of water and salt metabolism associated with pituitary disease, *Endocrinol Metab Clin North Am* 37(1):213, 2008.

61. Vance ML: Perioperative management of patients undergoing pituitary surgery, *Endocrinol Metab Clin North Am* 32(2):355, 2003.

62. Hadjizacharia P, et al: Acute diabetes insipidus in severe head injury: a prospective study, *J Am Coll Surg* 207(4):477, 2008.

63. Khanna A: Acquired nephrogenic diabetes insipidus, *Semin Nephrol* 26(3):244, 2006.

64. Verbalis JG: Disorders of body water homeostasis, *Best Pract Res Clin Endocrinol Metab* 17(4):471, 2003.

65. Holmes CL, et al: Science review: vasopressin and the cardiovascular system part 2—clinical physiology, *Crit Care* 8(1):15, 2004.

66. DDAVP. In *Mosby's Drug Consult*, St Louis, 2004, Mosby.

67. Ellison DH, Berl T: Clinical practice: the syndrome of inappropriate antidiuresis, *N Engl J Med* 356(20):2064, 2007.

68. Gustafsson BI, et al: Bronchopulmonary neuroendocrine tumors, *Cancer* 113(1):5, 2008.

69. Seute T, et al: Neurologic disorders in 432 consecutive patients with small cell lung carcinoma, *Cancer* 100(4):801, 2004.

70. Freda BJ, et al: Evaluation of hyponatremia: a little physiology goes a long way, *Cleve Clin J Med* 71(8):639, 2004.

71. Johnson AL, Criddle LM: Pass the salt: indications for and implications of using hypertonic saline, *Crit Care Nurse* 24(5):36, 2004.

72. Gassanov N, et al: Arginine vasopressin (AVP) and treatment with arginine vasopressin receptor antagonists (vaptans) in congestive heart failure, liver cirrhosis and syndrome of inappropriate antidiuretic hormone secretion (SIADH), *Eur J Clin Pharmacol* 67(4):333, 2011.

73. Robertson GL: Vaptans for the treatment of hyponatremia, *Nat Rev Endocrinol* 7(3):151, 2011.

CHAPTER

25

Trauma

Kara Snyder

evolve WEBSITE

Be sure to check out the bonus material, including free self-assessment exercises, on the Evolve web site at
http://evolve.elsevier.com/Urden/priorities/.

OBJECTIVES

- Compare and contrast injuries associated with blunt and penetrating trauma.
- Discuss mechanism of injury, pathophysiology, assessment findings, medical management, and nursing
- management of traumatic injuries to the head, spinal cord, heart, lungs, and abdomen.
- Use assessment findings to identify potential complications and sequelae of traumatic injuries.

Trauma is a leading cause of death for all age groups younger than 44 years. Injury costs the United States hundreds of billions of dollars annually. It is one of the most pressing health problems in the United States today.

Injury as a result of trauma is no longer considered to be an accident. The term *motor vehicle accident* (MVA) has been replaced with *motor vehicle crash* (MVC), and the term *accident* has been replaced with *unintentional injury*. A program for prevention, recognition, and treatment of intimate partner violence is described in Box 25-1.

Clinicians working with trauma patients, however, are uniquely poised to impact the person who presents to the trauma center following a traumatic event that may be related to drugs or alcohol. The American College of Surgeons Committee on Trauma recommends that all patients presenting to a trauma center be screened for alcohol use and history that could have contributed to the traumatic event that brought them to the trauma center.[1] The program of alcohol screening, brief interventions, and recommendations for rehabilitation (SBIRT) reduces recidivism and cost for trauma care.[2] There are several alcohol use screening tools available, including the **A**lcohol **U**se **D**isorders **I**dentification **T**est (AUDIT), and the CAGE tool, which is an acronym for **C**ut down, **A**nnoyed, **G**uilty, **E**ye opener morning alcoholic drink. The AUDIT is outlined in Table 25-1.

A patient who screens positive is recommended to undergo "brief interventions" for alcohol use. Brief interventions are by their very name short and are based upon motivational interviewing. Once a rapport is built with the patient, the following motivational-style interview questions may be used:[3] 1) What is a typical day like for you on a day when you drink? 2) How important is it to you to make a change in your drinking? 3) How confident are you that you can make a change? 4) What do you like and dislike about your drinking habits? 5) How would your life be different if you were to change your drinking? 6) What are some of the most important things to you? These questions serve to help the patient dichotomize the impact of drinking, both positively and negatively.

Major advances have been made in the management of patients with traumatic injuries. This chapter reviews selected critical care nursing management of patients with traumatic injuries.

MECHANISMS OF INJURY

Trauma occurs when an external force of energy impacts the body and causes structural or physiological alterations, or *injuries*. External forces can be radiation, electrical, thermal, chemical, or mechanical forms of energy. This chapter focuses on trauma from mechanical energy. Mechanical energy can produce blunt or penetrating traumatic injuries. Understanding the mechanism of injury helps health care providers anticipate and predict potential internal injuries.

Blunt Trauma

Blunt trauma is seen most often with MVCs, contact sports, blunt force injuries (e.g., trauma caused by a baseball bat), or falls. Injuries occur because of the forces sustained during a rapid change in velocity (deceleration). To estimate the amount of force sustained in an MVC, multiply the person's weight by the miles per hour (speed) the vehicle was traveling. A 130-pound woman in a vehicle traveling at 60 miles per hour that hits a brick wall, for example, would sustain 7800 pounds of force within milliseconds. As the body stops suddenly, tissues and organs continue to move forward. This sudden change in velocity causes injuries that result in lacerations or crush injuries of internal body structures.

Penetrating Trauma

Penetrating injuries occur with stabbings, firearms, or impalement—injuries that penetrate the skin and result in damage to internal structures. Damage is created along the path of penetration. Penetrating injuries can be misleading inasmuch as the condition of the outside of the wound does not determine the extent of internal injury. Bullets can create internal cavities 5 to 30 times larger than the diameter of the bullet.

Several factors determine the extent of damage sustained as a result of penetrating trauma. Different weapons cause different types of injuries. The severity of a gunshot wound depends on the type of gun, type of ammunition used, and the distance and angle from which the gun was fired. At close range, shotgun pellets expand on impact and cause multiple injuries to internal structures. From a distance, shotgun pellets cause only minor injuries. Handgun bullets usually damage what is directly in the bullet's path. Inside the body, the bullet can ricochet off bone and create further damage along its pathway. With penetrating stab wounds, factors that determine the extent of injury include the type and length of object used and the angle of insertion.

PHASES OF TRAUMA CARE

Care of trauma victims during wartime enhanced principles of triage and rapid transport of the injured to medical facilities. The military experience has demonstrated that decreasing the time from injury to definitive care saves more lives. It also has enhanced incentives and models for improvements in civilian trauma care, such as emergency medical service (EMS) systems and trauma care centers. The goal with critically injured patients is to minimize the time from initial insult to definitive care and to optimize prehospital care so that the patient arrives at the hospital alive.

Nursing management of the patient with traumatic injuries begins the moment a call for help is received and continues until the patient's death or return to the community. Care of the trauma patient is seen as a continuum that includes six phases: prehospital resuscitation, hospital resuscitation, definitive care and operative phase, critical care, intermediate care, and rehabilitation.

Prehospital Resuscitation

The goal of prehospital care is immediate stabilization and transportation. This is achieved through airway maintenance, control of external bleeding and shock, immobilization of the patient, and immediate transport (ground or air) to the closest appropriate medical facility.[4] Prehospital personnel should communicate information needed for triage at the hospital. Advanced planning for the injured patient is essential.

Emergency Department Resuscitation

The American College of Surgeons developed Advanced Trauma Life Support (ATLS) guidelines for rapid assessment, resuscitation, and definitive care for trauma patients in the emergency department.[4] The ATLS guidelines delineate a systematic approach to care of the trauma patient: rapid primary survey, resuscitation of vital functions, more detailed secondary survey, and initiation of definitive care. This process constitutes the ABCDEs of trauma care and assists in identifying injuries.

Primary Survey

On arrival of the trauma patient in the emergency department, the primary survey is initiated. During this assessment, life-threatening injuries are discovered and treated. The five steps in the trauma primary survey are performed in ABCDE sequence (Table 25-2):

TABLE 25-1	AUDIT ALCOHOL SCREENING QUESTIONNAIRE
QUESTION	**SCORE***
1. How often do you have a drink containing alcohol?	Never (1) Monthly or less (2) 2-4 times per month (3) 2-3 times per week (4) 4 or more times per week
2. How many standard drinks containing alcohol do you have on a typical day when drinking?	(0) 1 or 2 (1) 3 or 4 (2) 5 or 6 (3) 7 to 9 (4) 10 or more
3. How often do you have six or more drinks on one occasion?	(0) Never (1) Less than monthly (2) Monthly (3) Weekly (4) Daily or almost daily
4. During the past year, how often have you found that you were not able to stop drinking once you had started?	(0) Never (1) Less than monthly (2) Monthly (3) Weekly (4) Daily or almost daily
5. During the past year, how often have you failed to do what was normally expected of you because of drinking?	(0) Never (1) Less than monthly (2) Monthly (3) Weekly (4) Daily or almost daily
6. During the past year, how often have you needed a drink in the morning to get yourself going after a heavy drinking session?	(0) Never (1) Less than monthly (2) Monthly (3) Weekly (4) Daily or almost daily
7. During the past year, how often have you had a feeling of guilt or remorse after drinking?	(0) Never (1) Less than monthly (2) Monthly (3) Weekly (4) Daily or almost daily
8. During the past year, have you been unable to remember what happened the night before because you had been drinking?	(0) Never (1) Less than monthly (2) Monthly (3) Weekly (4) Daily or almost daily
9. Have you or someone else been injured as a result of your drinking?	(0) No (2) Yes, but not in the past year (4) Yes, during the past year
10. Has a relative or friend, doctor or other health worker been concerned about your drinking or suggested you cut down?	(0) No (2) Yes, but not in the past year (4) Yes, during the past year
Total Points	

*Scores for each question range from 0 to 4, with the first response for each question (never) scoring 0, the second (less than monthly) scoring 1, the third (monthly) scoring 2, the fourth (weekly) scoring 3, and the fifth response (daily or almost daily) scoring 4. For the last two questions, which only have three responses, the scoring is 0, 2, and 4. A score of 8 or more is associated with harmful or hazardous drinking, and a score of 13 or more by women or 15 or more by men is likely to indicate alcohol dependence.

Airway maintenance with cervical spine protection
Breathing and ventilation
Circulation with hemorrhage control
Disability and neurological status
Exposure or environmental control

Resuscitation Phase

Concurrent with the primary survey is the resuscitation phase. Hypovolemic shock is the most common type of shock that occurs in trauma patients.[4] Hemorrhage must be identified and treated rapidly. Two large-bore (14- to 16-gauge)

TABLE 25-2 PRIMARY SURVEY OF THE TRAUMA PATIENT

SURVEY COMPONENT	NURSING DIAGNOSIS	NURSING ASSESSMENT, CARE
Airway	Ineffective Airway Clearance related to obstruction or actual injury	Immobilize cervical spine. *Look* • Is there obvious airway trauma, tachypnea, accessory muscle use, tracheal shift? *Listen* • Stridor, hyperresonance, dullness to percussion? *Feel* • For air exchange over the mouth; insert finger sweep to clear foreign bodies. Secure airway. • Oropharyngeal • Nasopharyngeal • Endotracheal tube • Cricothyrotomy
Breathing	Ineffective Breathing Pattern related to actual injury Impaired Gas Exchange related to actual injury or disrupted tissue perfusion	Assess for: • Spontaneous breathing • Respiratory rate, depth, symmetry • Chest wall integrity For absent breathing: • Intubate, mechanical ventilation If breathing, but ineffective: • Assess life-threatening conditions (e.g., tension pneumothorax, flail chest). • Administer supplemental oxygen. • Initiate pulse oximetry.
Circulation	Decreased Cardiac Output related to actual injury Alteration in Tissue Perfusion related to actual injury or shock Deficient Fluid Volume related to actual loss of circulating volume	Assess pulse quality and rate. Use ECG monitoring. If no pulse: • Initiate ACLS. If pulse, but ineffective • Assess and treat life-threatening conditions (uncontrolled bleeding, shock). Initiate two large-bore IVs or central catheter; obtain serum samples for laboratory tests. Provide fluid replacement.
Disability	Ineffective Cerebral Tissue Perfusion Risk for Injury related to actual injury of brain or spinal cord	Determine Glasgow Coma Scale score. Assess pupil size and reactivity.
Exposure or environmental control	Risk for Imbalanced Body Temperature	Remove all clothing to inspect all body regions. Prevent hypothermia.

ACLS, advanced cardiac life support; *ECG,* electrocardiogram; *IV,* intravenous line.

peripheral intravenous catheters, a central venous catheter or intraosseous access is inserted. Management of hemorrhagic shock starts with IV fluids followed quickly by O-negative blood or type-specific blood.[4] Many trauma centers have developed massive transfusion protocols to make sure adequate blood products are available as needed. Fluid warmers are used to prevent hypothermia. Blood samples are also drawn (Box 25-2).

Placement of urinary and gastric catheters is part of the resuscitation phase. An indwelling urinary catheter can help evaluate urine output as an indicator of volume status and kidney perfusion. A gastric tube is inserted to reduce gastric distention and lower the risk of aspiration.

The resuscitation phase begins in the emergency department and may continue well into the critical care phase. During resuscitation from traumatic hemorrhagic shock, normalization of standard clinical parameters such as blood pressure, heart rate, and urine output are important but do not represent the end-point.[5] Optimal resuscitation goals are to improve oxygen tissue delivery and normalize base deficit, lactate, or gastric pH during the first 24 hours after injury.[6]

BOX 25-2 **SERUM SAMPLES TO OBTAIN WITH INTRAVENOUS PLACEMENT**

- Complete blood cell (CBC) count
- Electrolyte profile (Na^+, K^+, Cl^-, CO_2, glucose, blood urea nitrogen [BUN] creatinine [Cr])
- Coagulation parameters: prothrombin time (PT), partial thromboplastin time (PTT)
- Type and screen (ABO compatibility)
- Amylase
- Toxicology screens
- Liver function studies
- Pregnancy test (for females of childbearing age)
- Lactate

BOX 25-3 **HISTORY OF MECHANISM OF INJURY**

Penetrating Trauma
- Weapon used (handgun, shotgun, rifle, knife)
- Caliber of weapon
- Number of shots fired
- Gender of assailant
- Position of victim and assailant when injury occurred

Blunt Trauma
- Height of fall
- Motor vehicle crash extrication time
- Ejection
- Steering wheel deformation
- Location in automobile (passenger, driver, front seat, back seat)
- Restraint status (lap belt, shoulder harness, or combination; unrestrained)
- Speed of automobiles, direction of impact
- Occupants (number and morbidity status)

Secondary Survey

The secondary survey begins when the primary survey is completed, resuscitation is well established, and the patient is hemodynamically stable. During the secondary survey, a head-to-toe approach is used to thoroughly examine each body region. The history is one of the most important aspects of the secondary survey. Prehospital providers can usually provide vital information pertaining to the unintentional injury. Specific information that must be elicited about mechanism of injury is summarized in Box 25-3. The patient's pertinent past history can be assessed by use of the mnemonic AMPLE:

Allergies

Medications currently used

Past medical illnesses/pregnancy

Last meal

Events/environment related to the injury

During the secondary survey, the nurse ensures the completion of special procedures, such as an electrocardiogram (ECG), radiographic studies, and the FAST exam (Focused Assessment Sonography for Trauma). Throughout the secondary survey, the nurse continuously monitors the patient's vital signs and response to medical therapies. Emotional support to the patient and family is imperative.

Definitive Care and Operative Phase

After the secondary survey has been completed, specific injuries are diagnosed. Trauma is often referred to as a "surgical disease" because the nature and extent of injuries may require operative management. After surgery, depending on the patient's status, transfer to a critical care unit may be indicated.

Critical Care Phase

Critically ill trauma patients are admitted into the intensive care unit (ICU) as direct transfers from the emergency department or operating room. Information the ICU nurse must obtain from the emergency department, operating room nurse, or both, is summarized using the SBAR method: Situation, Background, Assessment, and Recommendation (Box 25-4). This information must be obtained before the

---

BOX 25-4 **NURSING REPORT FROM A REFERRING AREA USING THE SBAR METHOD**

S: Situation	Age
	Gender
	Mechanism of injury/injuries sustained
	Admission diagnosis/chief complaint; any loss of consciousness and its duration with current Glasgow Coma Scale score
	Diagnostic tests and procedures completed and results
	Laboratory results
	Medications administered (particularly opiates, sedatives)
	Current issues, including derangements in any physical assessments requiring acute interventions
B: Background	Significant medical and surgical history
	Home medications
A: Assessments	Current assessment findings, including vital signs, level of consciousness, established airway and mechanical ventilation settings
	Family members present and their assessment of coping and current knowledge of nature and extent of injuries and treatment plan
R: Recommendations	Description of the plan, including fluid volume and blood products

TABLE 25-3	EFFECTS OF TRAUMA RESUSCITATION
ASPECT OF INJURY OR RESUSCITATION	**EFFECT ON ICU COURSE**
Prolonged extrication time	Gives an indication of length of time patient may have been hypotensive and/or hypothermic before medical care
Period of respiratory or cardiac arrest	Effects of loss of perfusion to brain (anoxic injury), kidneys, and other vital organs
Time on backboard	Potentiates risk of sacral or occipital breakdown
Number of units of blood; whether any were not fully cross-matched; packed cells versus whole blood used	Potentiates risk of ARDS, MODS

ARDS, acute respiratory distress syndrome; *ICU*, intensive care unit; *MODS*, multiple organ dysfunction syndrome.

TABLE 25-4	FACTORS PREDISPOSING THE TRAUMA PATIENT TO IMPAIRED OXYGENATION
FACTOR	**IMPAIRMENT**
Impaired ventilation	Injury to airway structures, loss of central nervous system regulation of breathing, impaired level of consciousness
Impaired pulmonary gas diffusion	Pneumothorax, hemothorax, aspiration of gastric contents Shifts to the left of the oxyhemoglobin dissociation curve (can result from infusion of large volumes of banked blood, hypocarbia or alkalosis, or hypothermia)
Decreased oxygen supply	Reduced hemoglobin (from hemorrhage) Reduced cardiac output (cardiovascular injury, decreased preload)
Increased oxygen supply	Increased metabolic demands (associated with the stress response to injury)

patient's admission to the ICU to ensure availability of needed personnel, equipment, and supplies. This information also helps the nurse to assess the impact of trauma resuscitation on the patient's presentation and course. Table 25-3 summarizes the prehospital, emergency department, and operating room resuscitative measures that can affect the trauma patient's care in the ICU.

One of the most important nursing roles is assessment of the balance between oxygen delivery and oxygen demand. Oxygen delivery must be optimized to prevent further system damage. Assessment of circulatory status includes the use of noninvasive and invasive techniques. The trauma patient is at high risk for impaired oxygenation as a result of a variety of factors (Table 25-4). These risk factors must be promptly identified and treated to prevent life-threatening sequelae. Prevention and treatment of hypoxemia depend on accurate assessment of the adequacy of pulmonary gas exchange, oxygen delivery, and oxygen consumption.

Frequent and thorough nursing assessments of all body systems are important because these assessments are the cornerstone of the medical and nursing management of the critically ill trauma patient. The nurse can detect subtle changes and facilitate the implementation of timely therapeutic interventions to prevent complications often associated with trauma. The nurse must be knowledgeable about specific organ injuries and their associated sequelae.

TRAUMA INJURIES

Traumatic Brain Injuries

More than 1.7 million traumatic brain injuries (TBIs) occur annually, with approximately 275,000 patients hospitalized as a result of their injuries. Approximately 52,000 Americans die each year of TBI.[7] At least 5.3 million Americans are living with disabilities resulting from TBI.[8]

Mechanism of Injury

TBIs occur when mechanical forces are transmitted to brain tissue. Mechanisms of injury include penetrating or blunt trauma to the head. The leading causes of TBI include falls (35.2%), MVCs (17.3%), struck by or against events (16.5%), and assaults (10%).[7] Penetrating trauma can result from the penetration of a foreign object such as a bullet, which causes direct damage to cerebral tissue. Blunt trauma can be the result of deceleration, acceleration, or rotational forces. Deceleration causes the brain to crash against the skull after it has hit something such as the dashboard of a car. Acceleration injuries occur when the brain has been forcefully hit, such as with a baseball bat. Brian injury occurs when the brain moves toward the point of impact (acceleration) and then as the brain reverses direction (deceleration) it hits the other side of the skull. These injuries are described as *coup* and *contrecoup*; this injury is shown in Figure 25-1.

Pathophysiology

Review of the pathophysiology of a TBI can be divided into two categories: primary injury and secondary injury. The critical care nurse uses knowledge of this pathophysiology to provide interventions that reduce morbidity and mortality from secondary injury.

Primary Injury. The primary injury occurs at the moment of impact as a result of mechanical forces to the head. The extent of and recovery from injury are related to whether the primary injury was localized to an area or whether it was diffuse or widespread throughout the brain. Primary injuries may include direct damage to the parenchyma or injury to

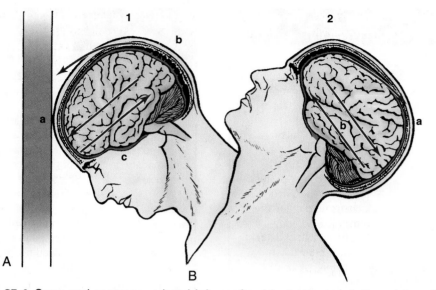

FIGURE 25-1 Coup and contrecoup head injury after blunt trauma. *A,* Coup injury: impact against object, showing the site of impact and direct trauma to brain (a), shearing of subdural veins (b), and trauma to the base of the brain (c). *B,* Contrecoup injury: impact within skull, showing the site of impact from brain hitting opposite side of skull (a) and shearing forces throughout brain (b). These injuries occur in one continuous motion; the head strikes the wall (coup) and then rebounds (contrecoup).

the vessels that causes hemorrhage, compressing nearby structures. Examples of primary injuries include contusion, laceration, shearing injuries, and hemorrhage. Primary injury may be mild, with little or no neurological damage, or severe, with major tissue damage. Immediately after the injury, a cascade of neural and vascular processes is activated.

Secondary Injury. Secondary injury is the biochemical and cellular response to the initial trauma that can exacerbate the primary injury and cause loss of brain tissue not originally damaged. Secondary injury can be caused by ischemia, hypercapnia, hypotension, cerebral edema, sustained hypertension, calcium toxicity, or metabolic derangements. Hypoxia or hypotension, the best known culprits for secondary injury, typically are the result of extracranial trauma.[9] A detrimental cycle may develop causing a focal primary injury to expand as a result of uncontrolled, refractory secondary injury.

Tissue ischemia occurs in areas of poor cerebral perfusion as a result of hypotension or hypoxia. The cells in ischemic areas become edematous. Extreme vasodilation of the cerebral vasculature occurs in an attempt to supply oxygen to the cerebral tissue. This increase in blood volume increases intracranial volume and raises intracranial pressure (ICP).

Significant hypotension causes inadequate perfusion to neural tissue. Hypotension rarely is associated with TBI. Hypotension typically is not caused by brain injury unless terminal medullary failure occurs.[10] If a trauma patient is unconscious and hypotensive, a detailed assessment of the chest, abdomen, and pelvis is performed to rule out internal injuries.

Hypercapnia (elevated CO_2) is a powerful vasodilator. Most often caused by hypoventilation in an unconscious patient, hypercapnia results in cerebral vasodilation and increased cerebral blood volume and ICP.

Cerebral edema occurs as a result of the changes in the cellular environment caused by contusion, loss of autoregulation, and increased permeability of the blood-brain barrier. Cerebral edema can be focal as it localizes around the area of contusion, or diffuse as a result of hypotension or hypoxia. Optimizing other aspects of secondary injury, such as oxygenation, ventilation, and perfusion can limit the extent of cerebral edema.

Initial hypertension in the patient with severe TBI is common. Because of the loss of autoregulation, increased blood pressure results in increased intracranial blood volume and ICP. The effects of increased ICP may be varied. As pressure increases inside the closed skull vault, cerebral perfusion decreases, which further compromises the brain. The combined effects of increasing pressure and decreasing perfusion precipitate a downward spiral of events.

Classification

Injuries of the brain are described by the functional changes or losses that occur. Some of the major functional abnormalities seen in head injury are described here.

Skull Fracture. Skull fractures are common, but they do not by themselves cause neurological deficits. Skull fractures can be classified as open (dura is torn) or closed (dura is not torn), or they can be classified as those of the vault or those of the base. Common vault fractures occur in the parietal and temporal regions. Basilar skull fractures usually are not visible on conventional skull films and a computed tomography (CT) scan is typically required. Assessment findings may include cerebral spinal fluid rhinorrhea (from nose) or otorrhea (from ear), Battle's sign (ecchymosis overlying the mastoid process behind the ear), "raccoon eyes" (subconjunctival and periorbital ecchymosis), or palsy of the seventh cranial nerve.

The significance of a skull fracture is that it identifies the patient with a higher probability of having or developing an intracranial hematoma. Open skull fractures require surgical intervention to remove bony fragments and to close the dura. The major complications of basilar skull fractures are cranial nerve injury and leakage of cerebrospinal fluid (CSF). CSF leakage may result in a fistula, which increases the possibility of bacterial contamination and resultant meningitis. Because fistula formation may be delayed, patients with a basilar skull fracture are admitted to the hospital for observation and possible surgical intervention.

Concussion. A concussion is a brain injury accompanied by a brief loss of neurological function, especially loss of consciousness. When loss of consciousness occurs, it may last for seconds to an hour. The neurological dysfunctions include confusion, disorientation, and sometimes a period of antegrade or retrograde amnesia. Other clinical manifestations that occur after concussion are headache, dizziness, nausea, irritability, inability to concentrate, impaired memory, and fatigue. The diagnosis of concussion is based on the loss of consciousness inasmuch as the brain remains structurally intact despite functional impairment.

Contusion. Contusion, or bruising of the brain, usually is related to acceleration-deceleration injuries, which result in hemorrhage into the superficial parenchyma, often the frontal and temporal lobes. Frontal or temporal contusions are most common and can be seen in a coup-contrecoup mechanism of injury (see Figure 25-1). Coup injury affects the cerebral tissue directly under the point of impact. Contrecoup injury occurs in a line directly opposite the point of impact.

The clinical manifestations of contusion are related to the location of the contusion, the degree of contusion, and the presence of associated lesions. Contusions can be small, in which localized areas of dysfunction result in a focal neurological deficit. Larger contusions can evolve over 2 to 3 days after injury as a result of edema and further hemorrhaging. A large contusion can produce a mass effect that can cause a significant increase in ICP.

Contusions of the tips of the temporal lobe are a common occurrence and are of particular concern. Because the inner aspects of the temporal lobe surround the opening in the tentorium where the midbrain enters the cerebrum, edema in this area can cause rapid deterioration of the patient's condition and can lead to herniation. Because of the location, this deterioration can occur with little or no warning at a deceptively low ICP.

Medical management of cerebral contusions may consist of medical or surgical therapies. Because a contusion can progress over 3 to 5 days after injury, secondary injury may occur. If contusions are small, focal, or multiple, they are treated medically with serial neurological assessments and possibly with ICP monitoring. Larger contusions that produce considerable mass effect require surgical intervention to prevent the increased edema and ICP as the contusion matures. Outcome of cerebral contusion varies, depending on the location and the degree of contusion.

Cerebral Hematomas. Extravasation of blood creates a space-occupying lesion within the cranial vault that can lead to increased ICP. Three types of hematomas are discussed here (Figure 25-2). The first two, epidural and subdural hematomas, are extraparenchymal (outside of brain tissue) and produce injury by pressure effect and displacement of intracranial contents. The third type, intracerebral hematoma, directly damages neural tissue and can produce further injury as a result of pressure and displacement of intracranial contents.

Epidural Hematoma. Epidural hematoma (EDH) is a collection of blood between the inner table of the skull and the outermost layer of the dura. EDHs are most often associated with patients with skull fractures and middle meningeal artery lacerations (two thirds of patients) or skull fractures with venous bleeding.[4] A blow to the head that causes a linear skull fracture on the lateral surface of the head may tear the middle meningeal artery. As the artery bleeds, it pulls the dura away from the skull, creating a pouch that expands into the intracranial space.

The incidence of EDH is relatively low. EDH can occur as a result of low-impact injuries (e.g., falls) or high-impact injuries (e.g., MVCs). EDH occurs from trauma to the skull and meninges rather than from the acceleration-deceleration forces seen in other types of head trauma.

The classic clinical manifestations of EDH include brief loss of consciousness followed by a period of lucidity. Rapid deterioration in the level of consciousness should be

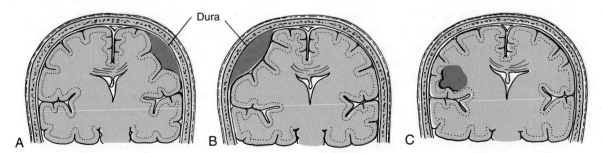

FIGURE 25-2 Types of hematomas. *A,* Subdural hematoma. *B,* Epidural hematoma. *C,* Intracerebral hematoma.

anticipated because arterial bleeding into the epidural space can occur quickly. A dilated and fixed pupil on the same side as the impact area is a hallmark of EDH.[4] The patient may complain of a severe, localized headache and may be sleepy. Diagnosis of EDH is based on clinical symptoms and evidence of a collection of epidural blood identified on the CT scan. Treatment of EDH involves surgical intervention to remove the blood and to cauterize the bleeding vessels.

Subdural Hematoma. Subdural hematoma (SDH), which is the accumulation of blood between the dura and the underlying arachnoid membrane, most often is related to a rupture in the bridging veins between the cerebral cortex and the dura. Acceleration-deceleration and rotational forces are the major causes of SDH, which often is associated with cerebral contusions and intracerebral hemorrhage. SDH is common, representing about 30% of severe head injuries. The three types of SDH—acute, subacute, and chronic—are based on the time frame from injury to clinical symptoms.

Acute Subdural Hematoma. Acute SDHs are hematomas that occur after a severe blow to the head. The clinical presentation of acute SDH is determined by the severity of injury to the underlying brain at the time of impact and the rate of blood accumulation in the subdural space. In other situations, the patient has a lucid period before deterioration. Careful observation for deterioration of the level of consciousness or lateralizing signs, such as inequality of pupils or motor movements, is essential. Rapid surgical intervention—including craniectomy, craniotomy, or burr hole evacuation—and aggressive intervention can reduce mortality.

Subacute Subdural Hematoma. Subacute SDHs are hematomas that develop symptomatically 2 days to 2 weeks after trauma. In subacute SDHs, the expansion of the hematoma occurs at a rate slower than that in acute SDH, and it takes longer for symptoms to become obvious. Clinical deterioration of the patient with a subacute SDH is slower than with an acute SDH, but treatment by surgical intervention, when appropriate, is identical.

Chronic Subdural Hematoma. Chronic SDH is diagnosed when symptoms appear days or months after injury. Most patients with chronic SDH are older or in late middle age. Patients at risk for chronic SDH include those with coordination or balance disturbances, older adults, and those receiving anticoagulation therapy. Clinical manifestations of chronic SDH are insidious. The patient may report a variety of symptoms, such as lethargy, absent-mindedness, headache, vomiting, stiff neck, and photophobia and may show signs of transient ischemic attack, seizures, pupillary changes, or hemiparesis. Because a history of trauma often is not significant enough to be recalled, chronic SDH seldom is seen as an initial diagnosis. CT evaluation can confirm the diagnosis of chronic SDH.

If surgical intervention is required, evacuation of the chronic SDH may occur by craniotomy, burr holes, or catheter drainage. Evacuation by burr hole involves drilling a hole in the skull over the site of the chronic SDH and draining the fluid. Drains or catheters are left in place for at least 24 hours to facilitate total drainage. Outcome after chronic SDH evacuation varies. Return of neurological status often depends on the degree of neurological dysfunction before removal. Because this condition is most common in older or debilitated patients, recovery is a slow process. Recurrence of chronic SDH is not infrequent.

Intracerebral Hematoma. Intracerebral hematoma (ICH) results when bleeding occurs within cerebral tissue. Traumatic causes of ICH include depressed skull fractures, penetrating injuries (bullet, knife), or sudden acceleration-deceleration motion. The ICH can act as a rapidly expanding lesion; late ICH into the necrotic center of a contused area also is possible. Sudden clinical deterioration of a patient 6 to 10 days after trauma may be the result of ICH.

Medical management of ICH may include surgical or nonsurgical treatment. Hemorrhages that do not cause significant ICP elevation are treated without surgery. Over time, the hemorrhage may be reabsorbed. If significant problems with ICH mass effect occur, surgical removal is necessary. The outcome of a patient with an ICH depends greatly on the location of the hemorrhage. Size, mass effect, and displacement of other intracranial structures also affect the outcome.

Missile Injuries. Missile injuries penetrate the skull and produce significant focal damage, but little acceleration-deceleration or rotational injury. The injury may be depressed, penetrating, or perforating (Figure 25-3). Depressed injuries are caused by fractures of the skull, with penetration of bone into cerebral tissue. A low-velocity penetrating injury (knife) may involve only focal damage and no loss of consciousness. A high-velocity missile (bullet) can produce shock waves that are transmitted throughout the brain in addition to the injury caused by the bullet. Perforating injuries are missile injuries that enter and then exit the brain. Perforating injuries have much less ricochet effect but are still responsible for significant injury.

Risk of infection and cerebral abscess is a concern in cases of missile injuries. If fragments of the missile are embedded within the brain, careful consideration of the location and risk of increasing neurological deficit is weighed against the risk of abscess or infection. The outcome after missile injury is based on the degree of penetration, the location of the injury, and the velocity of the missile.

Diffuse Axonal Injury. Diffuse axonal injury (DAI) is a term used to describe prolonged posttraumatic coma that is typically not caused by a mass lesion. DAI covers a wide range of brain dysfunction typically caused by acceleration-deceleration and rotational forces. DAI occurs as a result of damage to the axons or disruption of axonal transmission of the neural impulses.

The pathophysiology of DAI is related to the stretching and tearing of axons as a result of movement of the brain inside the cranium at the time of impact. The stretching and tearing of axons result in microscopic lesions throughout the brain, but especially deep within cerebral tissue and the base of the cerebrum. Disruption of axonal transmission of impulses results in loss of consciousness. Unless surrounding tissue areas are significantly injured, causing small

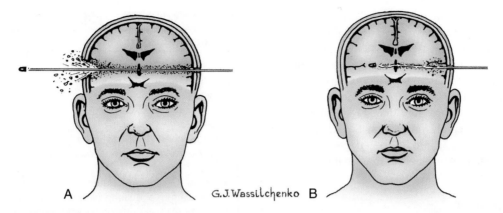

FIGURE 25-3 Bullet wounds of the head. A bullet wound or other penetrating missile wounds cause an open (compound) skull fracture and damage to brain tissue. Shock wave effects are transmitted throughout the brain. *A,* Perforating injury. *B,* Penetrating injury.

hemorrhages, DAI may not be visible on CT or magnetic resonance imaging (MRI). DAI can be classified as one of three grades based on the extent of lesions: mild, moderate, or severe. The patient with mild DAI may be in a coma for 24 hours and may exhibit periods of decorticate and decerebrate posturing. Patients with moderate DAI may be in a coma for longer than 24 hours and exhibit periods of decorticate and decerebrate posturing. Severe DAI usually manifests as a prolonged, deep coma with periods of hypertension, hyperthermia, and excessive sweating. Treatment of DAI includes support of vital functions and maintenance of ICP within normal limits. The outcome after severe DAI is poor because of the extensive dysfunction of cerebral pathways.

Neurological Assessment of Traumatic Brain Injury

The neurological assessment is the most important tool for evaluating the patient with a severe TBI, because it can indicate the severity of injury, provide prognostic information, and dictate the speed with which further evaluation and treatment must proceed. The cornerstone of the neurological assessment is the Glasgow Coma Scale (GCS),[4] although it is not a complete neurological examination. Pupils and motor strength assessment must be incorporated into the early and ongoing assessments. After injuries are specifically identified, a more thorough, focused neurological assessment, such as examination of the cranial nerves, is warranted. To assist with the initial assessment, TBIs are divided into three descriptive categories—mild, moderate, or severe—on the basis of the patient's GCS score and duration of the unconscious state.

Degree of Injury

Mild Injury. Mild TBI is described as a GCS score of 13 to 15, with a loss of consciousness that lasts up to 15 minutes. Patients with mild injury often are seen in the emergency department and discharged home with a family member who is instructed to evaluate the patient routinely and to bring the patient back to the hospital if any further neurological symptoms appear.

Moderate Injury. Moderate TBI is described as a GCS score of 9 to 12, with a loss of consciousness for up to 6 hours. Patients with this type of TBI usually are hospitalized. They are at high risk for deterioration from increasing cerebral edema and ICP, and serial clinical assessments are an important function of the nurse. Hemodynamic and ICP monitoring and ventilatory support may not be required for these patients unless other systemic injuries make them necessary. A CT scan usually is obtained on admission. Repeat CT scans are indicated if the patient's neurological status deteriorates.

Severe Injury. Patients with a GCS score of 8 or less after resuscitation or those who deteriorate to that level within 48 hours of admission have a severe TBI. Patients with severe TBI often receive ventilatory support along with ICP and hemodynamic monitoring. A CT scan is performed to rule out mass lesions that can be surgically removed. Patients are placed in a critical care setting for continual assessment, monitoring, and management.

Nursing Assessment of the Patient with Traumatic Brain Injury

As in all traumatic injuries, evaluation of the airway, breathing, and circulation (ABCs) is the first step in the assessment of the patient with TBI in the ICU. After stabilization of the ABCs is ensured, a neurological assessment is performed.

Level of consciousness, motor movements, pupillary response, respiratory function, and vital signs are all part of a complete neurological assessment in the patient with a TBI. Level of consciousness to assess wakefulness is elicited by obtaining the patient's response to verbal and painful stimuli. Determination of orientation to person, place, and time assesses mental alertness. Pupils are assessed for size, shape, equality, and reactivity. Pupil asymmetry must be reported immediately. Pupils are also assessed for constriction to a light source (parasympathetic innervation) or dilation (sympathetic innervation). A dilated or "blown" pupil can be caused by compression of the third ocular nerve or by transtentorial herniation.

Neurological assessments are ongoing as part of the initial shift assessment and as part of ongoing assessments to detect subtle deterioration. Serial assessments include hemodynamic status and ICP monitoring. The use of muscle relaxants and sedation for ICP control can mask neurological signs in the patient with a severe head injury. In these situations, observations for changes in pupils and vital signs become extremely important. Sedatives with a very short half-life, such as propofol, can be turned off, and within minutes, a neurological examination can be performed.

Diagnostic Procedures

The cornerstone of diagnostic procedures for evaluation of TBI is the CT scan. CT is a rapid, noninvasive procedure that can provide invaluable information about the presence of mass lesions and cerebral edema. Serial CT scans may be used over a period of several days to assess areas of contusion and ischemia and to detect delayed hematomas. A nurse must always remain with a TBI patient during a CT scan to provide continued observation and monitoring and during transport to and from the scanner. Transporting the patient, moving the patient from the bed to the CT table, and positioning the head flat during the CT scan are all stressful events and can cause severe increases in ICP. Continuous monitoring enables rapid intervention.

Medical Management

Surgical Management. If a lesion identified on CT is causing a shift of intracranial contents or increasing ICP, surgical intervention is necessary. Space-occupying hematomas such as EDH or SDH are removed via craniotomy. To alleviate excessive intracranial pressure and prevent herniation, a part of the skull may be removed (decompressive craniectomy). Patients who have had penetrating head trauma have an increased incidence of posttraumatic seizures, and may receive anticonvulsants.

Nonsurgical Management. Most of the TBI management occurs in the ICU. Nonsurgical management includes management of ICP, maintenance of adequate cerebral perfusion pressure and oxygenation, and treatment of any complications (e.g., pneumonia, infection). ICP monitoring may be required for patients with a GCS score less than 8 and abnormal findings on a head CT scan.[9]

Nursing Management

Nursing priorities in management of traumatic brain injury focus on (1) stabilizing vital signs, (2) preventing further injury, and (3) reducing increased ICP and maintaining adequate CPP.

Nursing diagnoses for the patient with TBI are listed in the Nursing Diagnosis Priorities Box on Traumatic Brain Injury. Ongoing nursing assessments are the cornerstone of the care of patients with TBI. These assessments are the primary mechanism for determining secondary brain injury from cerebral edema and increased ICP.

NURSING DIAGNOSIS PRIORITIES
Traumatic Brain Injury

- Ineffective Breathing Pattern related to musculoskeletal fatigue or neuromuscular impairment, p. A-27
- Risk for Aspiration, p. A-35
- Impaired Gas Exchange related to alveolar hypoventilation, p. A-23
- Imbalanced Nutrition: Less Than Body Requirements related to lack of exogenous nutrients and increased metabolic demand, p. A-22
- Acute Confusion related to sensory overload, sensory deprivation, and sleep pattern disturbance, p. A-2
- Powerlessness related to lack of control over current situation, p. A-33
- Decreased Intracranial Adaptive Capacity related to failure of decreased compensatory mechanisms, p. A-12
- Ineffective Cerebral Tissue Perfusion related to hemorrhage, p. A-29

BOX 25-5   **RECOMMENDATIONS FOR SUCTIONING PATIENTS WITH TRAUMATIC BRAIN INJURY**

- Pass the suction catheter for no longer than 10 seconds.
- Limit the number of suction catheter passes, preferably to no more than two passes per suctioning episode.
- Hyperoxygenate the patient before and after each passage of the suction catheter (e.g., deliver 4 ventilator breaths at 135% of the patient's tidal volume on 100% FiO_2, at a rate of 4 breaths in 20 seconds).
- Minimize airway stimulation (e.g., stabilize endotracheal tube, avoid passing the suction catheter all the way to the carina).

From McQuillan KA, Thurman P: Traumatic brain injuries. In McQuillan K, et al, editors: *Trauma nursing: from resuscitation through rehabilitation,* ed 4 Philadelphia 2009, WB Saunders.

Hemodynamic and fluid management are vital. Arterial blood pressure should be monitored because hypotension in a patient with TBI is rare and may indicate additional injuries. *Cerebral perfusion pressure* (CPP) should be maintained at a minimum of 60 mm Hg.[9] If secondary injury is to be prevented, the critical care nurse must respond immediately to hypotensive events and, in collaboration with physicians, maximize cerebral perfusion pressure through reduction of ICP and restoration of mean arterial pressure.[9]

Aggressive pulmonary care must be instituted. However, endotracheal suctioning can elevate ICP. Techniques to eliminate elevation in ICP with suctioning are outlined in Box 25-5. Cerebral oxygen consumption is increased during periods of increased body temperature, and therefore normothermia (36° to 37° C) is achieved with use of anti-pyretics and cooling measures.

In the early postinjury phase, the patient's environment must be controlled. Stimuli that produce pain, agitation, or discomfort can increase ICP. Analgesics and sedatives are administered, and patients are given rest periods.

After ICP stabilization, stimulation programs for patients in a coma may be employed. These programs provide stimulation to the tactile, kinesthetic, olfactory, gustatory, auditory, and visual senses. Several methods have been used to stimulate coma patients with various degrees of intensity:

- Intense Multisensory Stimulation Program: stimulatory cycles lasting approximately 15 to 20 minutes, repeated every hour for 12 to 14 hours per day, 6 days per week
- Formalized Not-Intensive Stimulation Program: cycles of stimulation of 10 to 60 minutes twice daily
- Sensory Regulation Program: single brief sessions of stimulation in a quiet environment completely free of noise

Whatever program is used, a stimulation schedule should be established. Accurate documentation of the stimulus and response is essential. Coma stimulation programs should be individualized and family members encouraged to participate.

Spinal Cord Injuries

Approximately 12,000 new spinal cord injuries (SCIs) occur annually. Of the new cases of SCI each year, about 4000 patients will die before arrival to the hospital, and 1000 patients will die of complications of their SCI during hospitalization.[11] The diagnosis of SCI begins with a detailed history of events surrounding the incident, precise evaluation of sensory and motor function, and radiographic studies of the spine.

Mechanism of Injury

The type of primary injury sustained depends on the mechanism of injury. Mechanisms of injury can include hyperflexion, hyperextension, rotation, axial loading (vertical compression), and missile or penetrating injuries.

Hyperflexion. Hyperflexion injury most often is seen in the cervical area, especially at the level of C5 to C6, because this is the most mobile portion of the cervical spine. This type of injury most often is caused by sudden deceleration motion, as in head-on collisions. Injury occurs from compression of the cord as a result of fracture fragments or dislocation of the vertebral bodies. Instability of the spinal column occurs because of the rupture or tearing of the posterior muscles and ligaments.

Hyperextension. Hyperextension injuries involve backward and downward motion of the head. With this injury, often seen in rear-end collisions or MVCs, the spinal cord is stretched and distorted. Neurological deficits associated with this injury are often caused by contusion and ischemia of the cord without significant bony involvement. A mild form of hyperextension is the *whiplash* injury.

Rotation. Rotation injuries often occur in conjunction with a flexion or extension injury. Severe rotation of the neck

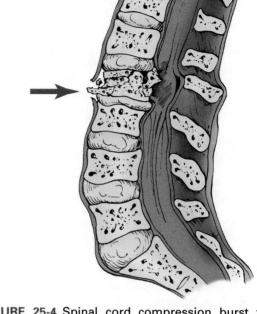

FIGURE 25-4 Spinal cord compression burst fracture. Compression injuries cause burst fractures of the vertebral body that often send bony fragments into the spinal canal or directly into the spinal cord.

or body results in tearing of the posterior ligaments and displacement (rotation) of the spinal column.

Axial Loading. Axial loading—or vertical compression—injuries occur from vertical force along the spinal cord. This most commonly is seen in a fall from a height in which the person lands on the feet or buttocks. Compression injuries cause burst fractures of the vertebral body that often send bony fragments into the spinal canal or directly into the spinal cord (Figure 25-4).

Penetrating Injuries. Injury to the spinal cord can result from a bullet, a knife, or any other object that penetrates the cord. These types of injury cause permanent damage by transection of the spinal cord.

Pathophysiology

SCIs are the result of a mechanical force that disrupts neurological tissue or its vascular supply, or both. Much like the pathophysiology of TBI, the injury process includes primary and secondary injury mechanisms. Primary injury is the neurological damage that occurs at the moment of impact. Secondary injury refers to the complex biochemical processes affecting cellular function. Secondary injury can occur within minutes of injury and can last for days to weeks.[11]

Several events after an SCI lead to spinal cord ischemia and loss of neurological function. A cascade of events is initiated that includes systemic and local vascular changes, electrolyte and biochemical changes, neurotransmitter accumulation, and local edema (Box 25-6). Collectively, these pathophysiological events result in worsening of the injury, potentially extending the level of functional deficit

BOX 25-6 PRIMARY AND SECONDARY MECHANISMS OF ACUTE SPINAL CORD INJURY

Primary Injury Mechanisms
- Acute compression
- Impact
- Missile
- Distraction
- Laceration
- Shear

Secondary Injury Mechanisms
- Systemic effects
- Heart rate: brief increase, then prolonged bradycardia
- Blood pressure: brief hypertension, then prolonged hypotension
- Decreased peripheral resistance
- Decreased cardiac output
- Increased catecholamines, then decreased
- Hypoxia
- Hyperthermia
- Injudicious movement of the unstable spine leading to worsening compression
- Local vascular changes
- Loss of autoregulation
- Systemic hypotension (neurogenic shock)
- Hemorrhage (especially gray matter)
- Loss of microcirculation
- Reduction in blood flow
- Vasospasm
- Thrombosis
- Electrolyte changes
- Increased intracellular calcium
- Increased intracellular sodium
- Increased sodium permeability
- Increased intracellular potassium

Biochemical Changes
- Neurotransmitter accumulation
- Catecholamines (e.g., norepinephrine, dopamine)
- Excitotoxic amino acids (e.g., glutamate)
- Arachidonic acid release
- Free radical production
- Eicosanoid production
- Prostaglandins
- Lipid peroxidation
- Endogenous opioids
- Cytokines
- Edema
- Loss of energy metabolism
- Decreased adenosine triphosphate production
- Apoptosis

Adapted from Sekhon LH, Fehlings MG: Epidemiology, demographics, and pathophysiology of acute spinal cord injury, *Spine* 26(Suppl 24):S2, 2001.

and worsening long-term outcome.[11] Knowledge of the pathophysiology of secondary processes has led to the development of new drugs that target the cellular changes contributing to injury.[11] Despite ongoing research efforts at repairing the primary injury, minimizing damage by reducing secondary injury has shown the most promise.

Functional Injury of the Spinal Cord

Functional injury of the spinal cord refers to the degree of disruption of normal spinal cord function. This depends on what specific sensory and motor structures within the cord are damaged. SCIs are classified as complete or incomplete. SCI cannot be classified until spinal shock has resolved.

Complete Injury. Complete SCI results in a total loss of sensory and motor function below the level of injury. Regardless of the mechanism of injury, the result is a complete dissection of the spinal cord and its neurochemical pathways, resulting in one of two conditions: tetraplegia or paraplegia.

Tetraplegia. With tetraplegia, the injury occurs from the C1 to T1 level. Residual muscle function depends on the specific cervical segments involved. The potential functional status resulting from different neurological levels of injury is described in Table 25-5.

Paraplegia. With paraplegia, the injury occurs in the thoracolumbar region (T2 to L1). Patients with injuries in this area may have full use of the arms but need a wheelchair. Thoracic L1 and L2 injuries produce paraplegia with variable innervation to intercostal and abdominal muscles.

Incomplete Injury. Incomplete SCI results in a mixed loss of voluntary motor activity and sensation below the level of the lesion. Incomplete SCI exists if any function

TABLE 25-5 QUADRIPLEGIA/ TETRAPLEGIA FUNCTIONAL STATUS

NEUROLOGICAL LEVEL (VERTEBRAE) OF COMPLETE INJURY	FUNCTIONAL ABILITY
C1-C4	Requires electric wheelchair with breath, head, or shoulder controls
C5	Needs electric wheelchair with hand control and/or manual wheelchair with rim projections; may require adaptive devices to assist with ADLs
C6	Independent in manual wheelchair on level surface; may need hand controls; adaptive devices may be needed for ADLs
C7	Requires manual wheelchair on most surfaces
C8-T1	May need adaptive devices

ADLs, activities of daily living.

remains below the level of injury. Incomplete injuries can result in a variety of syndromes, which are classified according to the degree of motor and sensory loss below the level of injury.

Spinal Shock. Spinal shock is a condition that can occur shortly after traumatic injury to the spinal cord. Spinal shock is the complete loss of all muscle tone and normal reflex activity below the level of injury.[4] Patients with spinal shock may appear completely without function below the area of the injury, although all of the area may not necessarily be destroyed.

Neurogenic Shock. Neurogenic shock results from injury to the descending sympathetic pathways in the spinal cord. This results from loss of vasomotor tone and sympathetic innervation to the heart. A relative hypovolemia and hypovolemic shock ensues, causing hypotension and decreased systemic vascular resistance. Patients with SCI at T6 or above may have profound neurogenic shock as a result of interruption of the sympathetic nervous system and loss of vasoconstrictor response below the level of the injury. Blood vessels cannot constrict, and the heart rate is slow, which results in hypotension, venous pooling, and decreased cardiac output. Cellular oxygenation is threatened as cardiac output declines because of a decrease in stroke volume (hypovolemia) and heart rate (bradycardia). The duration of this shock state can persist for up to 1 month after injury. Blood pressure support may be required with the use of sympathomimetic drugs (medications that mimic the actions of the sympathetic nervous system). Orthostatic blood pressure changes, leading to hypotension, can occur during change in head-of-bed position, or repositioning in bed.

Autonomic Dysreflexia. Autonomic dysreflexia is a life-threatening complication that may occur with SCI. This condition is caused by a massive sympathetic response to any noxious stimuli (e.g., full bladder, line insertions, fecal impaction), which results in bradycardia, hypertension, facial flushing, and headache. Immediate intervention is needed to prevent cerebral hemorrhage, seizures, and acute pulmonary edema. Treatment is aimed at alleviating the noxious stimuli. A clinical algorithm for treatment of autonomic dysreflexia is provided in Box 25-7.[12] If symptoms persist, antihypertensive agents can be administered to reduce blood pressure. Prevention of autonomic dysreflexia is imperative and can be accomplished through the use of a comprehensive bowel and bladder program.

Assessment

On admission to the ICU, attention to the ABCs is imperative in the patient with known or suspected SCI. Stabilization of the spinal cord is mandatory to prevent further injury, and spinal precautions are maintained until the spine is cleared of injury. Stabilization in the ICU may include the use of bed rest with log-rolling maneuvers and a hard cervical collar until definitive stabilization is achieved. After the ABCs have been evaluated and interventions for life-threatening complications have been initiated, a full physical assessment is made to determine the extent of injury.

BOX 25-7   AUTONOMIC DYSREFLEXIA

- If patient is supine, immediately sit the patient up.
- Begin frequent vital sign monitoring, and perform every 5 minutes.
- Survey for instigating causes; begin with urinary system.
- Loosen clothing, constrictive devices.
- If indwelling catheter is not placed, catheterize the patient. Lidocaine jelly may be instilled 5 minutes before catheter insertion.
- If indwelling catheter is present, do the following: check system for kinks and obstructions to flow.
- Irrigate the bladder with small sterile amount of fluid, utilizing strict aseptic technique.
- If not draining, remove the catheter and replace.
- If systolic blood pressure is greater than 150 mm Hg, consider rapid-onset, short-duration antihypertensive agent.
- If acute symptoms persist, suspect fecal impaction: instill lidocaine jelly into rectum; wait at least 5 minutes.
- Perform digital examination to check for presence of stool; if present, gently remove. If signs of autonomic dysreflexia persist, stop examination; instill additional lidocaine jelly, and wait 20 minutes to re-examine.
- If no stool is found and the abdomen is distended, consider administration of laxative.

Airway. Assessment of ABCs is essential to ensure optimal oxygenation and perfusion to all vital organs, including the spinal cord. Complete cardiovascular and respiratory assessments are essential to the patient's survival and prognosis. The primary assessment begins with an evaluation of airway clearance. In an unresponsive person, an oral airway is inserted while the patient's neck is maintained in a neutral position. The patient must undergo intubation before severe hypoxia can occur, which could further damage the spinal cord.

Breathing. Assessment of breathing patterns and gas exchange is made after an airway has been secured. The level of injury dictates the degree of altered breathing patterns and gas exchange (Table 25-6). Because complete injuries above the C3 level result in paralysis of the diaphragm, patients with these injuries require mechanical ventilatory support.

Circulation. Assessment of cardiac output and tissue perfusion is imperative to detect life-threatening injuries and promote recovery of injured spinal cord tissue. The patient with SCI is at high risk for developing alterations in cardiac output and tissue perfusion because the cardiovascular system is subjected to a variety of serious and potential physiological alterations, including dysrhythmias, cardiac arrest, orthostatic hypotension, emboli, and thrombophlebitis.

The patient with an SCI is assessed for adequate tissue perfusion by means of invasive and noninvasive hemodynamic monitoring techniques. Cardiac monitoring is required to detect bradycardia and other dysrhythmias that occur in response to reflex vagus activity mediated by the dominant parasympathetic nervous system, as well as changes in heart rhythm as a result of hypothermia or hypoxia.

TABLE 25-6	EFFECTS OF SPINAL CORD INJURY ON VENTILATORY FUNCTIONS	
NEUROLOGICAL LEVEL (VERTEBRAE) OF COMPLETE INJURY	RESPIRATORY FUNCTION	COMMENT
C1-C2	Paralysis of diaphragm	Ventilator dependent
C3-C5	Various degrees of diaphragm paralysis	Some diaphragm control; may need ventilatory support; weaning depends on preinjury pulmonary status
C6-T11	Various degrees of impaired intercostal muscles and abdominal muscles	Compromised respiratory function; reduced inspiratory ability; paradoxical breathing patterns; ineffective cough, sneeze

Modified from Moore EE, et al: Organ injury scaling, *Surg Clin North Am* 75(2):293, 1995.

TABLE 25-7	MUSCLE STRENGTH SCALE
ASSESSMENT FINDING	GRADE OF STRENGTH
Active movement against maximal resistance	5
Active movement through range of motion against resistance	4
Active movement through range of motion against gravity	3
Active movement through range of motion with gravity eliminated	2
Flicker or trace of contraction	1
No contraction; total paralysis	0

Neurological Assessment for Spinal Cord Injury. The initial neurological assessment may not be an accurate indication of eventual motor and sensory loss. It focuses on the rapid and accurate identification of present, absent, or impaired functioning of the motor, sensory, and reflex systems that coordinate and regulate vital functions. A detailed motor and sensory examination includes the assessment of all 32 spinal nerves for evidence of dysfunction. Carefully mapped pathways for the sensory portion of the spinal nerves, called *dermatomes,* can assist in localizing the functional sensory level of injury. Motor function may be graded on a 6-point scale (Table 25-7). Initial assessment

must be performed correctly and findings thoroughly documented in detail so that subsequent serial assessments can rapidly identify deterioration. The American Spinal Injury Association (ASIA) has developed a form that outlines the required assessments for initial and ongoing classification of SCIs (Figure 25-5). Ongoing spinal cord assessments must be documented during the critical care phase.

Diagnostic Procedures. Diagnostic radiographic evaluations can identify the severity of damage to the spinal cord. Initial evaluation includes anteroposterior and lateral views for all areas of the spinal cord. A CT scan of all seven cervical vertebrae and the top of T1 must be obtained to rule out cervicothoracic junction injury. Flexion and extension views can identify subtle ligament injuries. Tomography, myelography, and MRI also may be used.

Screening for Spinal Cord Injury. About 15% of trauma patients with an SCI have a cervical spine injury.[10] Screening of the spinal cord for injury becomes an integral part of the assessment for all trauma patients. The degree of trauma, alteration in mentation, intoxication, and distracting injuries dictate the type and extent of examination required to clear the cervical spine. The Eastern Association of Surgeons in Trauma (EAST) developed guidelines for the clearance of the cervical spine (Table 25-8). In these guidelines, CT scan has replaced plain radiography as the principal modality for cervical spine assessment following trauma. On admission, the spine is palpated for obvious deformity, and the patient is assessed for the subjective response of pain to palpation. If the patient is intoxicated, has distracting injuries such as rib fractures, or has received analgesics, examination of the spinal cord may be deferred.[10] MRI may be warranted to definitively diagnose an SCI when the patient is stabilized.

Medical Management

After assessment and diagnosis of the SCI, medical management begins. The primary treatment goal is to preserve remaining neurological function with pharmacological, surgical, and nonsurgical interventions.

Pharmacological Management. Methylprednisolone can improve neurological outcome after SCI, although it has been called into question because of the infection risk in these patients.[12] Current guidelines cite the use of methylprednisolone as an option for the management of acute cervical spine injury.[13] When it is used, patients receive a methylprednisolone bolus followed by a continuous infusion for at least 24 hours (preferably 48 hours) if their treatment began 3 to 8 hours after their injury.[13] Although the exact mechanism is not completely understood, it is thought that methylprednisolone directly affects the changes that occur within the spinal cord after injury, primarily by preventing posttraumatic spinal cord ischemia, improving energy metabolism, restoring extracellular calcium, and improving nerve impulse conduction.

Surgical Management. Surgical intervention provides spinal column stability in the presence of an unstable injury. Unstable injuries include disrupted ligaments and tendons and a vertebral column that cannot maintain normal

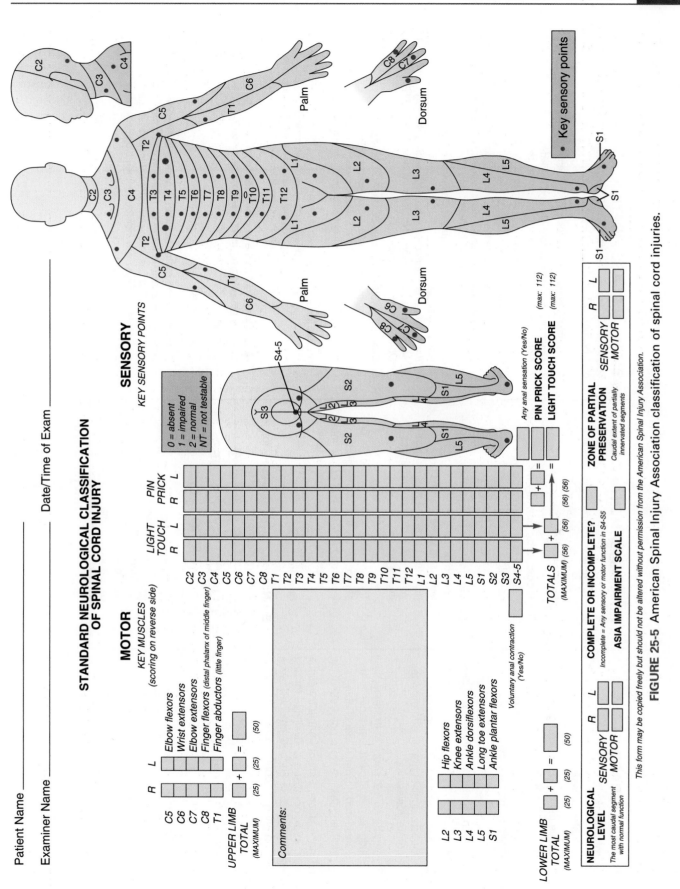

FIGURE 25-5 American Spinal Injury Association classification of spinal cord injuries.

MUSCLE GRADING

0 total paralysis

1 palpable or visible contraction

2 active movement, full range of motion, gravity eliminated

3 active movement, full range of motion, against gravity

4 active movement, full range of motion, against gravity and provides some resistance

5 active movement, full range of motion, against gravity and provides normal resistance

5* muscle able to exert, in examiner's judgment, sufficient resistance to be considered normal if identifiable inhibiting factors were not present

NT not testable. Patient unable to reliably exert effort or muscle unavailable for testing due to factors such as immobilization, pain on effort, or contracture.

ASIA IMPAIRMENT SCALE

☐ **A = Complete**: No motor or sensory function is preserved in the sacral segments S4-S5.

☐ **B = Incomplete**: Sensory but not motor function is preserved below the neurological level and includes the sacral segments S4-S5.

☐ **C = Incomplete**: Motor function is preserved below the neurological level, and more than half of key muscles below the neurological level have a muscle grade less than 3.

☐ **D = Incomplete**: Motor function is preserved below the neurological level, and at least half of key muscles below the neurological level have a muscle grade of 3 or more.

☐ **E = Normal**: Motor and sensory function are normal.

CLINICAL SYNDROMES (OPTIONAL)

☐ Central Cord
☐ Brown-Séquard
☐ Anterior Cord
☐ Conus Medullaris
☐ Cauda Equina

STEPS IN CLASSIFICATION

The following order is recommended in determining the classification of individuals with SCI.

1. Determine sensory levels for right and left sides.

2. Determine motor levels for right and left sides.
   Note: in regions where there is no myotome to test, the motor level is presumed to be the same as the sensory level.

3. Determine the single neurological level.
   This is the lowest segment where motor and sensory function is normal on both sides, and is the most cephalad of the sensory and motor levels determined in steps 1 and 2.

4. Determine whether the injury is Complete or Incomplete. (sacral sparing).
   *If voluntary anal contraction = **No** AND all S4-5 sensory scores = **0** AND any anal sensation = **No**, then injury is COMPLETE. Otherwise injury is incomplete.*

5. Determine ASIA Impairment Scale (AIS) Grade:

Is injury **Complete?**   If **YES**, AIS=A   Record ZPP

    NO ↓   (For ZPP, record lowest dermatome or myotome on each side with some [non-zero score] preservation.)

Is injury
motor incomplete? If **NO**, AIS=B

    YES ↓   (Yes=voluntary anal contraction OR motor function more than three levels below the motor level on a given side.)

Are at least half of the key muscles below the (single) neurological level graded 3 or better?

    NO ↓   YES ↓

    AIS=C   AIS=D

If sensation and motor function is normal in all segments, AIS=E.
Note: AIS E is used in follow up testing when an individual with a documented SCI has recovered normal function. If at initial testing no deficits are found, the individual is neurologically intact; the ASIA Impairment Scale does not apply.

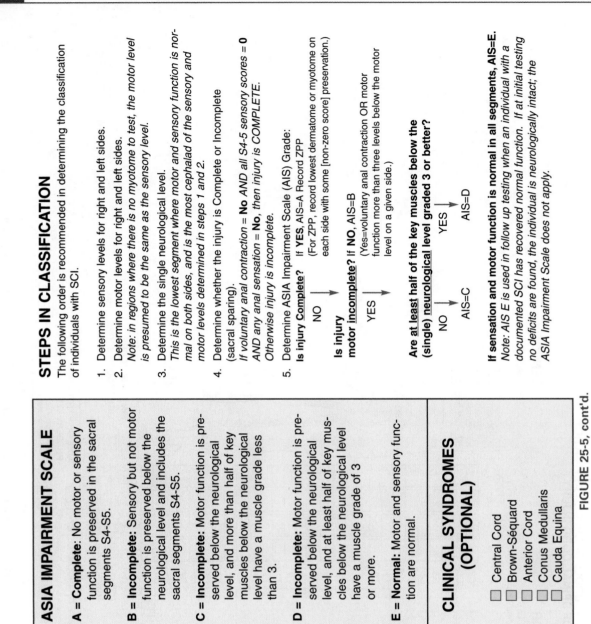

FIGURE 25-5, cont'd.

TABLE 25-8	EAST GUIDELINES FOR CERVICAL SPINE CLEARANCE
TRAUMA PATIENT POPULATION	**RECOMMENDATION**
Trauma patients who are awake, alert, not intoxicated, neurologically normal, and have no complaints of neck pain or tenderness with full range of motion of the cervical spine	Neck is palpated in all directions for tenderness or pain. If physical examination is negative for pain or tenderness, CT imaging of the cervical spine is not required and the cervical collar may be removed.
All other trauma patients with suspected cervical injury must be radiologically evaluated. This includes patients with neck pain or tenderness, whether alert or with altered mental status/neurological deficit, or distracting injury.	Axial CT from occiput to T1 with sagittal and coronal reconstructions If CT is positive for injury, continue cervical collar, obtain spine consultation, and obtain MRI. In the neurologically intact awake patient with neck pain, if the CT is negative (no injury seen), MRI is negative, and adequate flexion/extension films are negative, discontinue cervical collar.
Trauma patients who are obtunded with gross motor function of extremities	Axial CT from occiput to T1 with sagittal and coronal reconstructions If the CT is negative (no injury seen), the risk/benefit of an additional MRI must be determined in each hospital. Options are: A. Continue cervical collar until a clinical exam can be performed. B. Remove the cervical collar on the basis of negative CT alone. C. Obtain MRI. If MRI is negative, collar can be safely removed. Flexion/extension radiography should not be performed.

From Eastern Association for the Surgery of Trauma: *EAST guidelines: determination of cervical spine stability in trauma patients,* Chicago, 2000, Eastern Association for the Surgery of Trauma. Available at www.east.org/tpg/cspine2009.pdf. Accessed October 2010.
CT, computed tomography; *MRI,* magnetic resonance imaging; *EAST,* Eastern Association for the Surgery of Trauma.

alignment. Identification and immobilization of unstable injuries are particularly important for the patient with incomplete neurological deficit. Without adequate stabilization, movement and dislocation of the vertebral column may cause a complete neurological deficit. A variety of surgical procedures may be performed to achieve decompression and stabilization. The question of when surgery should be performed remains controversial.

Nonsurgical Management. If the injury to the spinal cord is stable, nonsurgical management is the treatment of choice. Nonsurgical management for cervical and thoracolumbar injuries is discussed in the following sections.

Cervical Injury. Management of cervical injuries involves the immobilization of the fracture site and realignment of any dislocation. This is accomplished through skeletal traction that involves the use of two-point tongs, which are inserted into the skull through shallow burr holes and are connected to traction weights. Several types of cervical tongs are used. Gardner-Wells and Crutchfield tongs are the most common. These tongs can be applied at the bedside with the use of a local anesthetic.

After the procedure, the patient can be immobilized on a kinetic therapy bed or a regular bed. The kinetic therapy bed is the most popular method used for cervical immobilization because it maintains spinal column alignment while providing constant turning motion to reduce pulmonary and skin breakdown. Use of cervical skeletal traction on a regular bed makes it difficult to provide adequate care to the pulmonary system and skin because of the extensive degree of immobility.

After the spinal column has been adequately realigned by means of skeletal traction, a halo traction brace often is

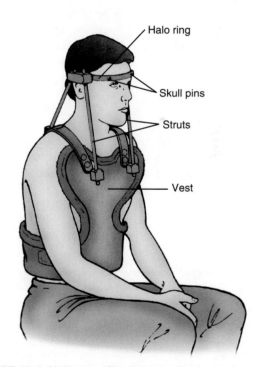

Halo ring

Skull pins

Struts

Vest

FIGURE 25-6 Halo vest. The halo traction brace immobilizes the cervical spine, which allows the patient to ambulate and participate in self-care.

applied. The halo vest consists of a metal ring secured to the skull with two occipital and two temporal screws. Steel bars anchor the screws to the vest to provide cervical immobilization (Figure 25-6). The halo traction brace immobilizes the cervical spine, which allows the patient to ambulate and participate in self-care.

Thoracolumbar Injury. Nonsurgical management of the patient with a thoracolumbar injury also involves immobilization. Skeletal traction may be used in high thoracic injury. For the most part, misalignment of the spinal canal does not occur in stable injuries of the thoracolumbar spine. Immobilization to allow fractures to heal is accomplished by bed rest with the bed in the reverse Trendelenburg position. A plastic or fiberglass jacket, a body cast, or a brace may also be used.

Nursing Management

Nursing priorities for the patient with SCI are aimed at (1) preventing secondary damage to the spinal cord, (2) managing cardiovascular and pulmonary complications, and (3) coaching the patient to overcome the psychosocial challenges associated with severe neurological deficit.

Nursing diagnoses and management for the patient with SCI are summarized in the Nursing Diagnosis Priorities Box on Spinal Cord Injury. The goal during the critical care phase is to prevent life-threatening complications while maximizing the function of all organ systems. Nursing interventions are aimed at preventing secondary damage to the spinal cord and managing the complications of the neurological deficit. Because almost all body systems are affected by SCI, nursing management must include interventions that optimize nutrition, elimination, skin integrity, and mobility. Patients with SCIs have complex psychosocial needs that require a great deal of emotional support from the critical care nurse.

Thoracic Injuries

Thoracic injuries involve trauma to the chest wall, lungs, heart, great vessels, and esophagus. Thoracic trauma most commonly is the result of a violent crime or an MVC.

NURSING DIAGNOSIS PRIORITIES
Spinal Cord Injury

- Decreased Cardiac Output related to lack of sympathetic blockade, p. A-12
- Autonomic Dysreflexia related to excessive autonomic response to noxious stimuli: (e.g., distended bladder, distended bowel, skin irritation), p. A-8
- Impaired Gas Exchange related to alveolar hypoventilation, p. A-22
- Ineffective Breathing Pattern related to musculoskeletal fatigue or neuromuscular impairment, p. A-27
- Disturbed Body Image related to actual change in body structure, function, or appearance, p. A-16
- Ineffective Coping related to situational crisis and personal vulnerability, p. A-30

Mechanism of Injury

Blunt Thoracic Trauma. Blunt trauma to the chest most often is caused by MVCs or falls; thoracic injuries account for 20% of trauma deaths. The underlying mechanism of injury tends to be a combination of acceleration-deceleration injury and direct transfer mechanics, as in a crush injury. Various mechanisms of blunt trauma are associated with specific injury patterns. After head-on collisions, drivers have a higher frequency of injury than do backseat passengers because the driver comes in contact with the steering assembly. Severe thoracic injuries often are seen in patients who are unrestrained.[14,15] Falls from greater than 20 feet are typically associated with thoracic injury.

Penetrating Thoracic Injuries. The penetrating object involved determines the damage sustained from penetrating thoracic trauma. Low-velocity weapons (e.g., .22-caliber gun, knife) usually damage only what is in the weapon's direct path. Of particular concern, however, are stab wounds that involve the anterior chest wall between the midclavicular lines, the angle of Louis, and the epigastric region because of the proximity of the heart and great vessels.

Specific Thoracic Traumatic Injuries
Chest Wall Injuries.

Rib Fractures. Fractures of certain ribs or multiple rib fractures can be serious, even life-threatening, particularly when associated with additional injuries and occurring in older patients.[16] Fractures of the first and second ribs are associated with intrathoracic vascular injuries (e.g., brachial plexus, great vessels), and because they are protected by the scapula, clavicle, humerus, and muscles, they signify a very high degree of force applied to the thorax. Fractures to the lower ribs (7th to 12th) may be associated with abdominal injuries, such as spleen and liver injuries. Fractures to the middle ribs may be associated with lung injury, including pulmonary contusion and pneumothorax. Lack of bone calcification in pediatric trauma patients results in a more compliant chest wall, and rib fractures need not have occurred for a tremendous amount of force to be absorbed, causing injury to the underlying thoracic structures.

The pain associated with rib fractures can be aggravated by respiratory excursion. The patient often splints, takes shallow breaths, and refuses to cough, which can result in atelectasis and pneumonia. Localized pain that increases with respiration or that is elicited by rib compression may indicate rib fractures. A definitive diagnosis can be made with a chest radiograph. Interventions include aggressive pulmonary physiotherapy and pain control to improve chest expansion efforts and gas exchange. Pain management interventions must be tailored to the patient's response to therapy. The primary goal of pain management in patients with rib fractures is prevention of pulmonary complications and patient comfort. Nonsteroidal antiinflammatory drugs (NSAIDs), intercostal nerve blocks, thoracic epidural analgesia, and opiates may be considered to assist with pain control.[17] Epidural analgesia can help increase the functional residual capacity, dynamic lung compliance, and vital capacity; decrease the airway resistance; and increase Pao_2.[17] The patient's preexisting pulmonary status and age may dictate the course of recovery.[16]

Flail Chest. Flail chest, which is caused by blunt trauma, disrupts the continuity of chest wall structures. A flail chest occurs when two or more ribs are fractured in two or more places and are no longer attached to the thoracic cage, producing a free-floating segment of the chest wall. The segment moves independently from the rest of the thorax and causes paradoxical chest wall movement during the respiratory cycle (Figure 25-7). During inspiration, the intact portion of the chest wall expands while the injured part is sucked in. During expiration, the chest wall moves in, and the flail segment moves out. Although the flail segment increases the work of breathing, the main cause of hypoxemia is the underlying pulmonary contusion. The physiological effects of the impaired chest wall motion of a flail chest include decreased

tidal volume and vital capacity and impaired cough, which lead to hypoventilation and atelectasis.

Inspection of the chest reveals paradoxical movement. Palpation of the chest may indicate *crepitus* and tenderness near fractured ribs. A chest radiograph that reveals multiple rib fractures and evidence of hypoxia demonstrated by ABG values aids in the diagnosis.

Interventions focus on ensuring adequate oxygenation, judicious administration of fluids, and analgesia to improve ventilation. Intubation and mechanical ventilation may be required to prevent further hypoxia.

Diaphragmatic Injury. Diagnosis of a diaphragmatic injury is often missed in trauma patients because of the subtle and nonspecific symptoms this injury produces. The mechanism of injury appears to be a rapid rise in intraabdominal pressure as a result of compression force applied to the lower part of the chest or upper region of the abdomen. This injury can occur when a person is thrown forward over the edge of the steering wheel in a high-speed MVC involving deceleration forces. The diaphragm, which offers little resistance to the force, can rupture or tear. Abdominal viscera then can gradually enter the thoracic cavity, moving from the positive pressure of the abdomen to the negative pressure in the

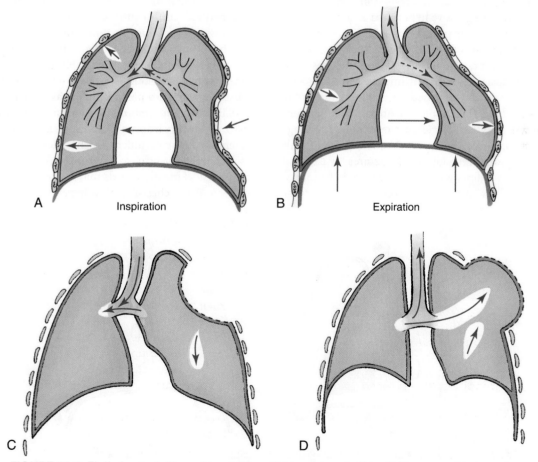

FIGURE 25-7 Flail chest. *A,* Normal inspiration. *B,* Normal expiration. *C,* The area of lung underlying the unstable chest wall sucks in on inspiration. *D,* The same area balloons out on expiration. Notice the movement of mediastinum toward opposite lung on inspiration.

thorax. Diaphragmatic injury can be a life-threatening event. Massive herniation of abdominal contents into the thoracic cavity can compress the lungs and mediastinum, which hampers venous return and decreases cardiac output. Herniated bowel can become strangulated and perforate.

Diaphragmatic herniation may produce significant compromise and changes in respiratory effort. Auscultation of bowel sounds in the chest or unilateral breath sounds may indicate a ruptured diaphragm. The patient may complain of shoulder pain, shortness of breath, or abdominal tenderness. A chest radiograph may reveal the tip of a nasogastric tube above the diaphragm, a unilaterally elevated hemidiaphragm, a hollow or solid mass above the diaphragm, and a shift of the mediastinum away from the affected side. Treatment of a ruptured diaphragm includes its immediate surgical repair.

Pulmonary Injuries

Pulmonary Contusion. A pulmonary contusion is fundamentally a bruise of the lung. Pulmonary contusion often is associated with blunt trauma and other chest injuries, such as rib fractures and flail chest. Pulmonary contusions can occur unilaterally or bilaterally. A contusion manifests initially as a hemorrhage, followed by alveolar and interstitial edema. The edema can remain rather localized in the contused area or can spread to other lung areas. Inflammation affects alveolar-capillary units. This results in a ventilation-perfusion imbalance, progressive hypoxemia and poor ventilation over a 24- to 48-hour period.

Clinical manifestations of pulmonary contusion may take up to 24 to 48 hours to develop. Inspection of the chest wall may reveal ecchymosis at the site of impact. Moist crackles may be auscultated in the contused lung. The patient may have a cough and blood-tinged sputum. Abnormal lung function can manifest as systemic arterial hypoxemia. The diagnosis is made primarily by chest x-ray studies consistent with pulmonary infiltrate corresponding to the area of external chest impact that manifests within 12 to 24 hours of injury. Pulmonary contusions may worsen over a 24- to 48-hour period and then slowly resolve unless complications such as sepsis or acute lung injury occur.

Aggressive respiratory care is the cornerstone for care of non-intubated patients with pulmonary contusion. Interventions include ambulation, deep-breathing exercises, turning, and incentive spirometry. Aggressive removal of airway secretions is important to avoid infection and to improve ventilation. Patients with unilateral contusions and significant hypoxia are placed with the injured side up and uninjured side down ("down with the good lung"). This positioning maximizes the match between pulmonary ventilation and perfusion. Patients with severe contusions may continue to show decompensation despite aggressive nursing management. Respiratory acidosis, increases in peak airway and plateau pressures, and increased work of breathing may require endotracheal intubation and mechanical ventilation with *positive end-expiratory pressure* (PEEP). Adequate pain control is accomplished with administration of NSAIDs, opiates, intercostal nerve blocks, or thoracic epidural analgesia.

Tension Pneumothorax. A tension pneumothorax usually is caused by an injury that perforates the chest wall or pleural space. Air flows into the pleural space with inspiration and becomes trapped. As pressure in the pleural space increases, the lung on the injured side collapses and causes the mediastinum to shift to the opposite side (Figure 25-8). As pressure continues to build, the shift exerts pressure on the heart and thoracic aorta, which results in decreased venous return and decreased cardiac output. Tissue perfusion with oxygenated blood is further hampered because the collapsed lung cannot participate in gas exchange.

Clinical manifestations of a tension pneumothorax include dyspnea, tachycardia, hypotension, and sudden chest pain extending to the shoulders. Tracheal deviation can be observed as the trachea shifts away from the injured side. On the injured side, breath sounds may be decreased or absent. Percussion of the chest reveals a hyperresonant sound over the

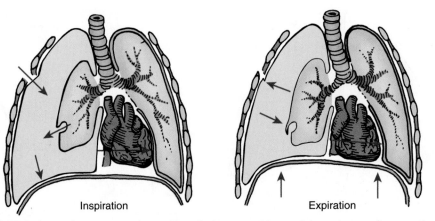

FIGURE 25-8 A tension pneumothorax usually is caused by an injury that perforates the chest wall or pleural space. Air flows into the pleural space with inspiration and becomes trapped. As pressure in the pleural space increases, the lung on the injured side collapses and causes the mediastinum to shift to the opposite side. (From Marx J, et al: *Rosen's Emergency medicine: concepts and clinical practice*, ed 5, St Louis, 2002, Mosby.)

affected side. Diagnosis of a tension pneumothorax is made by clinical assessment.

There is no time for a chest radiograph because this potentially lethal condition must be treated immediately.[4] A large-bore (14-gauge) needle or chest tube is inserted into the affected hemithorax in the second intercostal space, midclavicular line. This procedure allows immediate release of air from the pleural space. A hissing sound is heard as the tension pneumothorax is converted to a simple pneumothorax and a chest tube is then inserted.

Open Pneumothorax. An open pneumothorax ("sucking chest wound") usually is caused by penetrating trauma. Open communication between the atmosphere and intrathoracic pressure results in immediate lung deflation. Air moves in and out of the hole in the chest, producing a sucking sound heard on inspiration. An open pneumothorax produces the same symptoms as a tension pneumothorax. Subcutaneous emphysema may be palpated around the wound.

Initial management of an open pneumothorax is accomplished by promptly closing the wound at end expiration with a sterile occlusive dressing (plastic wrap or petroleum gauze) large enough to overlap the wound's edges.[4] The dressing should be taped securely on three sides. As the patient breathes in, the dressing gets sucked in to occlude the wound and prevent air from entering. A chest tube is placed as soon as possible. Surgical intervention may be required to close the wound.

Hemothorax. Blunt or penetrating thoracic trauma can cause bleeding into the pleural space, resulting in a hemothorax (Figure 25-9). A massive hemothorax results from the accumulation of more than 1500 mL of blood in the chest cavity. The source of bleeding may be the intercostal or internal mammary arteries, lungs, heart, or great vessels. Lacerations to the lung parenchyma are low-pressure bleeds and typically stop bleeding spontaneously. Arterial bleeding from hilar vessels usually requires immediate surgical intervention.[4] In either case, increasing intrapleural pressure results in a decrease in vital capacity. Increasing vascular blood loss into the pleural space causes decreased venous return and decreased cardiac output.

Assessment findings for patients with a hemothorax include hypovolemic shock. Breath sounds may be diminished or absent over the affected lung. With hemothorax, the neck veins are collapsed, and the trachea is at midline. Massive hemothorax can be diagnosed on the basis of clinical manifestations of hypotension associated with the absence of breath sounds or dullness to percussion on one side of the chest.[4]

This life-threatening condition must be treated immediately. Resuscitation with intravenous fluids is initiated to treat the hypovolemic shock. A chest tube is placed on the affected side to allow drainage of blood. An autotransfusion device can be attached to the chest tube collection chamber. Thoracotomy may be necessary for patients who require persistent blood transfusions or who have significant bleeding (200 mL/hr for 2 to 4 hours or more than 1500 mL on initial tube insertion) or when there are injuries to major cardiovascular structures.

Cardiac and Vascular Injuries

Penetrating Cardiac Injuries. Penetrating cardiac trauma can occur from mechanical injuries as a result of bullets, knives, or impalements. The chest wall offers little protection to the heart from penetrating trauma. The most common site of injury is the right ventricle because of its anterior position. The mortality rate from penetrating trauma to the heart is high. The prehospital mortality rate for penetrating cardiac injuries is very high, and most deaths occur within minutes after injury as a result of exsanguination or tamponade.

Cardiac Tamponade. Cardiac tamponade is the progressive accumulation of blood in the pericardial sac (Figure 25-10). With cardiac tamponade, progressive accumulation of 120 to 150 mL of blood increases the intracardiac pressure and compresses the atria and ventricles. An increase in intracardiac pressure leads to decreased venous return and decreased filling pressure, which leads to decreased cardiac output, myocardial hypoxia, cardiac failure, and cardiogenic shock.

Classic assessment findings associated with cardiac tamponade are called *Beck's triad*—presence of elevated central venous pressure with neck vein distention, muffled heart

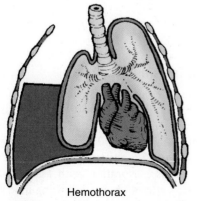

Hemothorax

FIGURE 25-9 Blunt or penetrating thoracic trauma can cause bleeding into the pleural space to form a hemothorax.

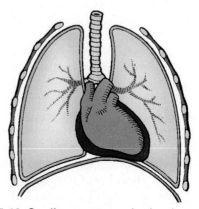

FIGURE 25-10 Cardiac tamponade is the progressive accumulation of blood in the pericardial sac.

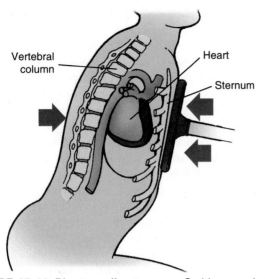

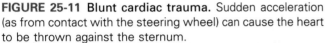

FIGURE 25-11 Blunt cardiac trauma. Sudden acceleration (as from contact with the steering wheel) can cause the heart to be thrown against the sternum.

sounds, and hypotension. Pulsus paradoxus may occur. Pulseless electrical activity (PEA) in the absence of hypovolemia and tension pneumothorax suggests cardiac tamponade.[4] Bedside ultrasound is used to diagnose tamponade.

Immediate treatment is required to remove the accumulation of fluid in the pericardial sac. Pericardiocentesis involves aspiration of fluid from the pericardium by use of a large-bore needle. The inherent risk in this procedure is potential laceration of the coronary artery. Other approaches include surgical procedures such as thoracotomy or median sternotomy. The goal of these procedures is to locate and control the source of bleeding.

Blunt Cardiac Injuries. The most common causes of blunt cardiac trauma include high-speed MVCs, direct blows to the chest, and falls. Because of its mobility and its location between the sternum and thoracic vertebrae, the heart is susceptible to blunt traumatic injury. Sudden acceleration (as from contact with a steering wheel) can cause the heart to be thrown against the sternum (Figure 25-11). Sudden deceleration can cause the heart to be thrown against the thoracic vertebrae by a direct blow to the chest, such as blows caused by a baseball, animal kick, or fall.

Blunt cardiac injury (BCI), formerly called *myocardial contusion*, covers the spectrum of myocardial contusion, concussion, and rupture. Few clinical signs and symptoms are specific for BCI. Evidence of external chest trauma, such as steering wheel imprint or sternal fractures, should raise the suspicion for blunt cardiac injury. However, the presence of a sternal fracture does not predict the incidence of BCI. The patient may complain of chest pain that is similar to angina, but the pain is not relieved with nitroglycerin.[18] The EAST guidelines for screening of BCI are listed in Box 25-8. The 12-lead ECG may reveal dysrhythmias, ST changes, heart block, or unexplained sinus tachycardia.

BOX 25-8   EAST GUIDELINES FOR SCREENING OF BLUNT CARDIAC INJURY

- Obtain an admission ECG for all patients in whom there is suspected BCI.
- If ECG is abnormal, the patient should be admitted for continuous ECG monitoring for 24 to 48 hours.
- If the patient is hemodynamically unstable, an echocardiogram may be performed.
- Cardiac biomarkers such as cardiac troponin T values are not useful in predicting which patients will have complications related to BCI.

BCI, blunt cardiac injury; *EAST,* Eastern Association for the Surgery of Trauma; *ECG,* electrocardiogram.

Nursing Management

Nursing priorities for the patient with traumatic chest or pulmonary injury emphasize delivery of adequate (1) oxygenation, (2) ventilation, (3) pain management, and (4) prevention of complications. Assistance with intubation and monitoring of mechanical ventilation may be required to prevent tissue hypoxia and provide adequate ventilatory support. Judicious administration of IV fluids and analgesia is important to improve patient comfort. Aggressive removal of airway secretions is important to avoid infection and improve ventilation. Hypoxemia is prevented by continuous pulse oximetry monitoring of arterial oxygen saturation (Spo_2) and ABG analysis. See the Nursing Diagnosis Priorities Box on Thoracic Injuries.

NURSING DIAGNOSIS PRIORITIES

Thoracic Injuries

- Impaired Gas Exchange related to alveolar hypoventilation from lung contusion, p. A-22
- Ineffective Breathing Pattern related to pain from rib fractures, p. A-27
- Decreased Cardiac Output related to low preload from tension pneumothorax, hemothorax or cardiac tamponade, p. A-10

Abdominal Injuries

Abdominal injuries often are associated with multisystem trauma. Abdominal injuries are the third leading cause of traumatic death. Injuries to the abdomen are the result of blunt or penetrating trauma. Two major life-threatening conditions that occur after abdominal trauma are hemorrhage and hollow viscus perforation with associated peritonitis. Death occurring after 48 hours following injury is the result of sepsis and its complications. The critical care nurse must pay particular attention to complication-prevention strategies throughout the trauma cycle.

Mechanism of Injury

Blunt Trauma. Blunt abdominal injuries are common. They result most often from MVCs, falls, and assaults. In MVCs, abdominal injury is more likely to occur when a vehicle is struck from the side. In the passenger position of the front seat, hepatic injury is likely when the point of impact is on the same side as the passenger. A driver is likely to sustain injury to the spleen when the impact is on the driver's side. Pedestrians hit by motor vehicles are at risk for serious abdominal injuries. Blunt trauma to the thorax can produce injuries to the liver, spleen, and diaphragm. Deceleration and direct forces can produce retroperitoneal hematomas. Blunt abdominal injuries often are hidden, requiring careful assessment and reassessment. Unrecognized abdominal trauma is a common cause of preventable deaths, and blunt abdominal injury deaths are more likely to be fatal than are penetrating abdominal injuries.

Penetrating Trauma. Penetrating abdominal trauma is often caused by knives or bullets. The danger of penetrating abdominal trauma is that the outside appearance of the wound does not reflect the extent of internal injury. Commonly injured organs from knife wounds are the colon, liver, spleen, and diaphragm. Gunshot wounds to the abdomen usually are more serious than are stab wounds. A bullet destroys tissue along its path. Inside the abdomen, a bullet can travel in erratic paths and ricochet off bone. Death from penetrating injuries depends on the injury to major vascular structures and resultant intraabdominal hemorrhage.

Assessment

The initial assessment of the trauma patient, whether in the emergency department or the critical care unit, follows the primary and secondary survey techniques as outlined by ATLS guidelines.[4] The initial physical assessment may be unreliable given the confounding influences of alcohol, illicit drugs, analgesics, and an altered level of consciousness. Specific assessment findings associated with abdominal trauma are reviewed here.

Physical Assessment. The location of entry and exit sites associated with penetrating trauma are assessed and documented. Inspection of the patient's abdomen may reveal purplish discoloration of the flanks or umbilicus (Cullen's sign), which indicates blood in the abdominal wall. Ecchymosis in the flank area (Turner's sign) may indicate retroperitoneal bleeding or a possible fracture of the pancreas. A hematoma in the flank area suggests kidney injury. A distended abdomen may indicate the accumulation of blood, fluid, or gas resulting from a perforated organ or ruptured blood vessel. Auscultation of the abdomen may reveal friction rubs over the liver or spleen and may indicate rupture. The abdomen is assessed for rebound tenderness and rigidity. These assessment findings indicate peritoneal inflammation. Referred pain to the left shoulder (Kehr's sign) may indicate a ruptured spleen or irritation of the diaphragm from bile or other material in the peritoneum. Subcutaneous emphysema palpated on the abdomen suggests free air as a result of a ruptured bowel.

Diagnostic Procedures. Insertion of a nasogastric tube and urinary catheter serves as a useful diagnostic and therapeutic aid. A nasogastric tube can decompress the stomach, and the contents can be checked for blood. Urine obtained from the urinary catheter can also be tested for the presence of blood, though placement of a urinary catheter is contraindicated if there is noticeable blood at the urethral meatus on initial inspection.

Serial laboratory test results may be nonspecific for the patient with abdominal trauma. A serum amylase determination can detect pancreatic injuries. Because of hemoconcentration, hemoglobin and hematocrit results may not reflect actual values. Serial values are more valuable in diagnosing abdominal injuries.

Because of the unreliability of physical examination alone in the patient suspected of having abdominal trauma, diagnostic testing may occur simultaneously during the primary and secondary surveys. Noninvasive tests include bedside ultrasound, CT, and chest and abdominal radiographs.

The bedside ultrasound, called the focused assessment with sonography for trauma (FAST) examination is done at most trauma centers to evaluate the patient for the presence of intraabdominal blood.[19] This is a quick and noninvasive means of rapid assessment, but success depends on the skill level of the operator.[19] Bedside ultrasonography is used widely in the United States for the detection of abdominal free fluid and hemoperitoneum. Typically, the right and left upper abdominal quadrant areas are examined: the right upper quadrant (Morrison's pouch), the left upper quadrant splenorenal area, the pericardial sac, and the pelvis (Douglas' pouch). The primary disadvantage of FAST is the need for free intraperitoneal fluid to produce a positive study result.[4] An initial negative FAST result may be followed by serial ultrasound examinations or abdominal CT.[19]

Although the FAST test has had good sensitivity and specificity, it is not intended to replace a CT scan. Obese abdomens and patients with ascites may have erroneous results, and further workup for these patients is warranted.[20] Ultrasound is also limited in its ability to diagnose diaphragmatic, intestinal, or pancreas injuries. Abdominal CT provides information about specific organ injury, pelvic injury, and retroperitoneal hemorrhage.

Invasive tests such as the *diagnostic peritoneal lavage* (DPL) can exclude or confirm the presence of intraabdominal injury.[4] DPL is used only when the FAST exam or a CT scan is inconclusive. After the patient's bladder has been emptied, a small incision is made in the abdomen through the skin and into the peritoneum. A small catheter is inserted (Figure 25-12). If frank blood is encountered, intraabdominal injury is evident, and the patient is taken immediately to the operating room. If gross blood is not initially encountered, a liter of fluid (lactated Ringer's or 0.9% normal saline) is infused through the catheter into the abdomen. The intravenous bag is then placed in a dependent position, and abdominal fluid is allowed to drain into the intravenous bag. The drainage

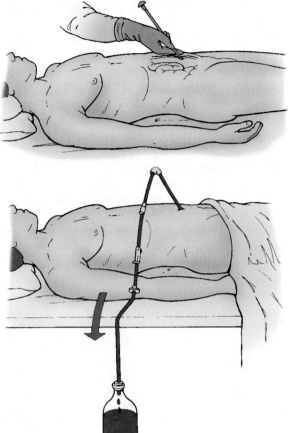

FIGURE 25-12 Diagnostic peritoneal lavage (DPL) can exclude or confirm the presence of intraabdominal injury with a high accuracy rate.

BOX 25-9	POSITIVE PERITONEAL LAVAGE RESULTS

- Red blood cell count: 100,000/mm³
- White blood cell count: 500/mm³
- Amylase: 175 units/dL
- Presence of blood, stool, bile, or bacteria

fluid is sent to the laboratory for analysis. Positive DPL results signal intraabdominal trauma and usually necessitate surgical intervention (Box 25-9). DPL is invasive, has been associated with complications, and cannot exclude retroperitoneal injuries.

Combined Abdominal Organ Injuries

Patients with multiple visceral injuries may require surgical intervention that uses somewhat nontraditional techniques ("damage control" resuscitation). The three phases of this treatment strategy are the *initial operation, ICU resuscitation,* and *definitive reoperation* (Box 25-10).[21] The duration of the initial operation is kept to a minimum. The decision to abbreviate the initial operation is made early during surgery. Factors that may lead the surgeon to choose an abbreviated laparotomy include hypothermia and coagulopathy in a

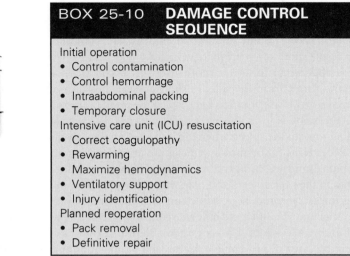

BOX 25-10	DAMAGE CONTROL SEQUENCE

Initial operation
- Control contamination
- Control hemorrhage
- Intraabdominal packing
- Temporary closure

Intensive care unit (ICU) resuscitation
- Correct coagulopathy
- Rewarming
- Maximize hemodynamics
- Ventilatory support
- Injury identification

Planned reoperation
- Pack removal
- Definitive repair

patient who is hemodynamically unstable, an inability to control bleeding by direct pressure, and an inability to close the abdomen because of massive abdominal edema.[21] Hypothermia induced by an open visceral cavity in conjunction with massive blood transfusion can lead to coagulopathy and continued bleeding, which results in shock and metabolic acidosis. The triad of hypothermia, coagulopathy, and acidosis creates a self-propagating cycle that can eventually lead to an irreversible physiological insult.[21] The initial operation must be completed quickly to terminate this self-propagating cycle. Reconstruction and formal closure of the wound may not be completed at this time. The patient is transferred to the ICU.

The goal of the critical care phase of this strategy is to continue resuscitation and correct hypothermia, coagulopathy, and acidosis. Rewarming techniques, described in Box 25-11, are used to correct hypothermia. Coagulation factors and platelets may be administered to correct coagulopathy. Serial lactate and base deficit measurements, as well as a mixed venous oxygen saturation pulmonary artery catheter, may be used to guide fluid resuscitation, inotropic support, and oxygenation to treat and prevent acidosis.

Abdominal Compartment Syndrome. The patient is assessed for additional complications, including ongoing hemorrhage, intraabdominal hypertension, and abdominal compartment syndrome. *Abdominal compartment syndrome* is defined as end-organ dysfunction caused by intraabdominal hypertension.[22] Increased intraabdominal pressure can result from internal bleeding, visceral edema, or a noncompliant abdominal wall. Increased abdominal cavity pressure can impinge on diaphragmatic excursion and can affect ventilation. Clinical manifestations of abdominal compartment syndrome include decreased cardiac output, increased pulmonary vascular resistance, increased peak pulmonary pressures, increased ICP, decreased urine output, and hypoxia.[22] Intraabdominal pressure can be measured through a bladder catheter after the injection of 25 mL of sterile saline.[22]

Surgical decompression of the abdomen may be required for abdominal pressures greater than 20 to 25 mm Hg that

BOX 25-11	**INTERVENTIONS FOR REWARMING THE TRAUMA PATIENT**	
INTERVENTION	**EXTERNAL REWARMING PROCEDURES**	**INTERNAL REWARMING PROCEDURES**
Passive	Maintain a warm room temperature. Remove all wet clothing and linen. Cover the patient with blankets. Avoid bathing patient until normothermia achieved.	Administer warmed, humidified oxygen. Administer warmed intravenous fluids.
Active	Use radiant heat lamps, heating blankets or pads, and hot water bottles.	Perform gastrointestinal irrigation with warmed solutions. Perform extracorporeal rewarming for profound hypothermia. Use esophageal rewarming tubes.

Adapted from Morris J: Environmental emergencies. In Newberry L, editor: *Sheehy's emergency nursing: principles and practice*, ed 5, St Louis, 2003, Mosby.

TABLE 25-9	**LIVER INJURY SCALE**	
GRADE*	**INJURY**	**DESCRIPTION**
I	Hematoma	Subcapsular, <10% surface area
	Laceration	Capsular tear, <1 cm parenchymal depth
II	Hematoma	Subcapsular, 10%-50% surface area; intraparenchymal <10 cm in diameter
	Laceration	Capsular tear, 1-3 cm parenchymal depth, <10 cm long
III	Hematoma	Subcapsular, >50% surface area or expanding; ruptured subcapsular or parenchymal hematoma; intraparenchymal hematoma >10 cm or expanding
	Laceration	>3 cm parenchymal depth
IV	Laceration	Parenchymal disruption involving 25%-75% of hepatic lobe or 1-3 Couinaud's segments within a single lobe
V	Laceration	Parenchymal disruption involving >75% of hepatic lobe or >3 Couinaud's segments within a single lobe
	Vascular	Juxtahepatic venous injuries (retrohepatic vena cava, central major hepatic veins)
VI	Vascular	Hepatic avulsion

Modified from Trunkey DD: Hepatic trauma: contemporary management, *Surg Clin North Am* 84(2):437, 2004.
*Advance one grade for multiple injuries up to grade II.

are associated with other assessment findings such as decreased cardiac output, hypotension, elevated peak inspiratory pressures, and decreased urine output.[23] Surgical decompression involves opening the abdomen and then temporarily closing the abdomen with a sterile perforated plastic sheet, clips, vacuum-assisted techniques, and many other options.[23] The open abdomen is then covered with towels or dressings, and closed suction drains are placed over the top and brought out through a plastic drape over the entire wound. The wound is closed permanently several weeks later, or it is allowed to heal by second intention and eventual skin grafting.

After the patient is hemodynamically stable and the triad of hypothermia, coagulopathy, and acidosis has been corrected, the patient is taken back to the operating room for the definitive surgery, if required. During this phase, definitive repairs and wound closure are performed. Postoperatively, the patient is transported back to the ICU for continued care.

Specific Organ Injuries

Diagnostic studies such as FAST, CT scans, and DPL aid in the detection of specific abdominal organ injuries. The medical and nursing management vary by affected organ: liver, spleen, and bowel injuries, which are seen more commonly, are discussed here.

Liver Injuries. The liver is the primary organ injured in penetrating trauma and the second most often injured organ in blunt trauma. Abdominal CT is considered to be the most reliable diagnostic tool to identify and assess the severity of the injury to the liver.[24] The severity of liver injuries is graded to provide a mechanism for determining the amount of trauma sustained by that organ, the care needed, and the possible outcomes (Table 25-9). Nonoperative management is considered the standard of care for hemodynamically stable patients with liver injury.[24] Patients are admitted to the ICU or a step-down unit and are monitored for signs of hemorrhage. Serial serum hematocrit and hemoglobin levels and vital signs are monitored over several days.

Patients with penetrating or blunt liver trauma who are hemodynamically unstable may require surgical intervention to correct the defect. Resection of the devitalized tissue is required for massive injuries. Hemorrhage is common with liver injuries, and ligation of the hepatic arteries or veins may be required to control hemorrhage. Drains may be placed intraoperatively to drain areas of blood and to prevent hematomas.

Care of the patient with severe liver injuries can be challenging for the critical care nurse. Lack of hemodynamic stability can result from hemorrhage and hypovolemic shock, leading to fluid volume deficit, decreased cardiac output, and decreased tissue perfusion. Combinations of crystalloid and colloid intravenous solutions may be used to correct hypovolemia. Fresh-frozen plasma, platelets, and cryoprecipitate may be administered to correct coagulopathies. A crucial nursing responsibility is to monitor the patient's response to medical therapies. Continued hemodynamic instability (e.g., hypotension, decreased cardiac output) despite aggressive medical intervention may indicate continued hemorrhage, in which case an exploratory laparotomy may be required to determine and correct the source of bleeding. The patient's postoperative ICU course may be complicated by coagulopathy, acidosis, and hypothermia. Jaundice may occur as a sign of hepatic dysfunction, but it may also be caused by reabsorption of hematomas or breakdown of transfused blood.

Spleen Injuries. The spleen is the organ most commonly injured by blunt abdominal trauma and is second to the liver as a source of life-threatening hemorrhage. Spleen injuries, like liver injuries, are graded for the purpose of determining the amount of trauma sustained, the care needed, and the possible outcomes (Table 25-10). Hemodynamically stable patients may be monitored in the critical care unit by means of serial hematocrit values and vital signs. Progressive deterioration may indicate the need for operative management.[24]

Patients who exhibit hemodynamic instability require operative intervention with splenectomy, partial splenectomy, or splenorrhaphy. Patients who have had a splenectomy are at risk for the development of overwhelming postsplenectomy sepsis with streptococcal pneumonia. These patients require polyvalent pneumococcal vaccine (Pneumovax) to help promote immunity against most pneumococcal bacteria. Patients with isolated spleen injuries that require surgical intervention rarely are admitted to the critical care unit. Complications after splenic trauma include wound infection, sepsis, subdiaphragmatic abscess, and fistulas of the colon, pancreas, and stomach.

Intestinal Injuries. Intestinal injuries can result from blunt or penetrating trauma. The diagnosis of small intestinal injuries is difficult. Surgical intervention is usually required in the presence of multiple CT findings (e.g., unexplained free fluid, pneumoperitoneum, bowel wall thickening, mesenteric fat streaking, mesenteric hematoma, intravenous contrast extravasation).[25] Regardless of the mechanism of injury, intestinal contents (e.g., bile, stool, enzymes, bacteria) leak into the peritoneum and cause peritonitis. Surgical resection and repair are required. The patient's postoperative course is dictated by the amount of spillage of intestinal contents. The patient is observed for signs of sepsis and for abscess or fistula formation.

Genitourinary Injuries

Trauma to the genitourinary tract seldom occurs as an isolated injury. A genitourinary injury must be suspected in any patient with penetrating trauma to the torso; pelvic fracture; blunt trauma to the lower chest or flank; contusions, hematoma, tenderness over the flank, lower abdomen, or perineum; genital swelling or discoloration; blood at the urethral meatus; hematuria after Foley catheter placement; or difficulty with micturition.[4]

Mechanism of Injury

Genitourinary injuries, like all other traumatic injuries, can result from blunt or penetrating trauma.

Assessment

Evaluation of genitourinary trauma begins after the primary survey has been conducted and immediate life-threatening conditions have been effectively managed. The conscious patient may complain of flank pain or colic pain. Rebound tenderness can be elicited if intraperitoneal extravasation of urine has occurred. Inspection may reveal blood at the urethral meatus. Bluish discoloration of the flanks may indicate retroperitoneal bleeding, whereas perineal discoloration may indicate a pelvic fracture and possible bladder or urethral injury. Hematuria is the most common assessment finding with genitourinary trauma.[9,26]

Specific Genitourinary Injuries

Kidney Trauma. Most renal trauma is caused by blunt trauma, resulting in contusions or lacerations without urinary extravasation. Injury to the kidneys may be reflected by flank ecchymosis and fracture of inferior ribs or spinous processes. Gross or microscopic hematuria may be present;

TABLE 25-10	SPLEEN INJURY SCALE	
GRADE*	**INJURY**	**DESCRIPTION**
I	Hematoma	Subcapsular, <10% surface area
	Laceration	Capsular tear, <1 cm, parenchymal depth
II	Hematoma	Subcapsular, 10%-50% surface area; intraparenchymal <5 cm in diameter
	Laceration	Capsular tear: 1-3 cm parenchymal depth, which does not involve a trabecular vessel
III	Hematoma	Subcapsular, >50% surface area or expanding; ruptured subcapsular or parenchymal hematoma; intraparenchymal hematoma >5 cm or expanding
IV	Laceration	>3 cm parenchymal depth or involving trabecular vessels
	Laceration	Laceration involving segmental or hilar vessels producing major devascularization (>25% of spleen)
V	Laceration	Completely shattered spleen
	Vascular	Hilar vascular injury that devascularizes spleen

*Advance one grade for multiple injuries up to grade II.

however, the extent of kidney damage is often incongruous with the degree of hematuria.[26] Gross hematuria can exist with minor injuries and usually clears within a few hours. CT is the most accurate modality available for diagnosing kidney injury because it can assess the extent of parenchymal laceration, urine extravasation, hemorrhage, and the presence of vascular injury.[26]

Contusions and minor lacerations can usually be treated with observation. The success of nonoperative management may be enhanced by using angiographic embolization in those who are hemodynamically stable.[27] Operative interventions may be performed in patients with kidney injuries with a devascularized segment of the kidney. Postoperative and postinjury complications can include infection, hemorrhage, infarction, extravasation, calcification, acute tubular necrosis, and hypertension.

Bladder Trauma. A large percentage of bladder injuries result from pelvic fractures.[26] Physical findings may include lower abdominal bruising, distention, and pain. More definitive findings include difficulty voiding or incomplete recovery of irrigation fluids from catheterized patients.[26] Bladder injuries are classified as contusions, extraperitoneal ruptures, intraperitoneal ruptures, or combined injuries. The type of injury depends on the location and strength of the blunt force and volume of urine in the bladder at the time of injury. Extraperitoneal rupture of the bladder may be managed conservatively with catheterization and antibiotics for 7 to 10 days.[27] Unresolved extravasation may require surgical intervention.

Nursing Management

Nursing priorities for the patient with genitourinary trauma include (1) assessment for hemorrhage, (2) maintenance of fluid and electrolyte balance, and (3) maintaining patency of drains and tubes.

After the patient is admitted to the critical care unit, the nurse makes an assessment according to the ATLS guidelines. After the patient's condition has stabilized, nursing management of postoperative kidney trauma is similar to that for genitourinary surgery. The primary nursing interventions include assessment for hemorrhage,[28] maintenance of fluid and electrolyte balance, and maintenance of patency of drains and tubes. Measurement of urinary output includes drainage from the urinary catheter and the nephrostomy or suprapubic tubes. Drainage from these areas is recorded separately. Urine output is measured frequently until bloody drainage and clots have cleared. Gentle irrigation of drainage tubes may be required to clear clots and maintain the patency of the tubes.

COMPLICATIONS OF TRAUMA

Ongoing nursing assessments are imperative for early detection of complications associated with traumatic injuries. A single complication can increase hospital length of stay and the associated costs of treating the complication.

Hypermetabolism

Nutritional support is an essential component in the care of critically ill trauma patients. Within 24 to 48 hours after traumatic injury, a predictable hypermetabolic response occurs. The metabolic response to injury mobilizes amino acids and accelerates protein synthesis to support wound healing and the immunological response to invading organisms. Stress hypermetabolism occurs after any major injury and is characterized by increases in metabolic rate and oxygen consumption. Energy requirements accelerate to promote immune function and tissue repair. The goal of early aggressive nutrition is to maintain host defenses by supporting this hypermetabolism and to preserve lean body mass.[29]

Most nutrition experts advocate beginning enteral nutrition as early as possible. Current guidelines recommend enteral feedings be initiated within 72 hours for patients with blunt and penetrating abdominal injuries and those with severe head injuries.[29] Enteral feeding sites can include the gastric route or any site beyond the pylorus of the stomach, including the duodenum and jejunum. Prompt feeding tube placement by the critical care nurse must be a priority, unless contraindicated. Diminished or absent bowel sounds do not mean the small bowel is not working. Small bowel function and the ability to absorb nutrients remain intact, despite the presence of gastroparesis and absent bowel sounds. Because access to the stomach can be obtained more quickly and easily than the duodenum, early gastric feeding is possible.[29] Patients at risk for pulmonary aspiration due to gastric retention or gastroesophageal reflux should receive enteral feedings into the jejunum.[29] If enteral feeding is not successful, parenteral nutrition should be initiated by day 7.[29]

Infection

Infection remains a major source of mortality and morbidity in critical care units. The trauma patient is at risk for infection because of contaminated wounds, invasive therapeutic and diagnostic catheters, intubation and mechanical ventilation, host susceptibility, and the critical care environment. The patient with multiple trauma injuries is at risk for infection because of host susceptibility (including preexisting medical conditions) and the adverse effect of trauma on the immune system.

Wound contamination poses an infection risk for the trauma patient, especially with injuries resulting from deep or penetrating trauma. Exogenous bacteria (from the external environment) can enter through open wounds. Exogenous bacteria can be introduced by dirt, grass, and debris inoculated into the wound at the time of injury. Endogenous bacteria (from the internal environment) can be released as a result of gastrointestinal or genitourinary perforation, which spills bacteria into the internal environment.

Meticulous wound care is essential. The goals of wound care include minimizing infection risks, removing dead and devitalized tissue, allowing for wound drainage, and promoting wound epithelialization and contraction.

Standard interventions for the prevention of ventilator-associated pneumonia and catheter-related bloodstream infection apply to the trauma patient. Proper hand hygiene, invasive catheter care, patient positioning, sterile technique for all invasive procedures, and tight glucose control are paramount to optimal to patient outcome.

Sepsis

The patient with multiple injuries is at risk for overwhelming infections and sepsis. The source of sepsis in the trauma patient can be invasive therapeutic and diagnostic catheters or wound contamination with exogenous or endogenous bacteria. The source of the sepsis must be promptly identified and treated. Gram stain and cultures of blood, urine, sputum, invasive catheters, and wounds are obtained.

Pulmonary Complications
Respiratory Failure

Posttraumatic respiratory failure often leads to the development of ARDS.[30] ARDS can be caused by direct injury to the lungs or indirect injury (see "Acute Respiratory Failure" in Chapter 15).[30] Primary direct injuries in the trauma patient can include aspiration, inhalation, and pulmonary contusion. The indirect injuries include sepsis, massive transfusion, fat emboli, and missed injury. ARDS in the trauma patient can develop 24 to 72 hours after initial injury. The patient receiving multiple blood products, particularly fresh-frozen plasma, must also be monitored for *transfusion-related acute lung injury* (TRALI).[31] Signs of TRALI are similar to those of ARDS, although there is a temporal relationship between the new onset of respiratory distress and the transfusion of blood products.[31]

Fat Embolism Syndrome

Fat embolism syndrome can occur as a complication of orthopedic trauma. The clinical onset of fat embolism syndrome ranges from 12 to 72 hours after injury, although 90% of patients develop it within 24 hours after injury.[32] Fat embolism syndrome appears to develop as a result of fat droplets that leak from fractured bone and embolize to the lungs. The droplets are broken down into free fatty acids that are toxic to the pulmonary microvascular membranes. Pulmonary fat emboli alter pulmonary hemodynamics and pulmonary vascular permeability. The lung becomes highly edematous and hemorrhagic. The clinical presentation is indistinguishable from that of ARDS. Early stabilization of unstable extremity fractures may limit the seeding of fat droplets into the pulmonary system.[32]

Pain

Pain in the ICU may come from many sources, including surgery, procedures, and trauma. Trauma may contribute to cellular death and inflammation that leads to pain. Relief of pain is a major component in the care of trauma patients.

An issue that often complicates pain management is the high incidence of substance abuse among patients who sustain traumatic injury. The Society of Critical Care Medicine has published guidelines for the optimal use of analgesia and sedatives[33] (see Chapters 8 and 9).

Kidney Complications
Acute Kidney Injury

Assessment and ongoing monitoring of kidney function is critical to the survival of the trauma patient. The cause of posttraumatic renal failure is complex and may involve a variety of factors, as listed in Box 25-12.

Prevention of kidney failure is the best treatment, and it begins with ensuring adequate renal perfusion. Serial assessments of blood urea nitrogen (BUN) and creatinine levels commonly are used to evaluate kidney function. Progressive kidney failure requires prompt diagnosis and treatment (see "Acute Kidney Injury" in Chapter 20).

Myoglobinuria

Patients with a crush injury are susceptible to the development of myoglobinuria, with subsequent secondary kidney failure. Crush injuries can compromise blood flow. Loss of arterial blood flow, particularly to the extremities, results in the loss of oxygen transport to distal tissues and ischemia. This initiates a cascade of events that leads to the necrosis of skeletal muscle cells. As cells die, intracellular contents—particularly potassium and myoglobin—are released. Myoglobin, a muscular pigment, is a large molecule. Dark tea-colored urine suggests myoglobinuria. After myoglobinuria is diagnosed, treatment is aimed at kidney preservation by aggressive administration of intravenous fluids. Nursing management is directed toward achievement of fluid and electrolyte balance. The patient should be assessed for hypernatremia, hyperosmolarity, and volume overload.

Vascular Complications
Compartment Syndrome

Compartment syndrome is a condition in which increased pressure within a limited space compromises circulation, resulting in ischemia and necrosis of tissues within that

---

BOX 25-12 ETIOLOGICAL FACTORS IN POSTTRAUMATIC ACUTE KIDNEY INJURY

- Preexisting disease
  - Hypertension
  - Heart failure
  - Diabetes
  - Chronic kidney disease
  - Chronic liver disease
- Prolonged shock states
- Profound acidosis
- SIRS or reperfusion injury
- Abdominal compartment syndrome
- Muscle ischemia, myoglobinuria
- Microemboli
- Nephrotoxic drugs
- Radiocontrast dye

SIRS, systemic inflammatory response syndrome.

space. Among those at high risk for the development of compartment syndrome are patients with lower extremity trauma, including fractures, penetrating trauma, vascular ruptures, massive tissue injuries, or venous obstruction. Clinical manifestations of compartment syndrome include obvious swelling and tightness of an extremity, paresis, and pain of the affected extremity. Diminished pulses and decreased capillary refill do not reliably identify compartment syndrome because they may be intact until after irreversible changes have occurred. Elevated compartment pressures confirm the diagnosis. The treatment can consist of simple interventions, such as removing an occlusive dressing to fasciotomy.

Venous Thromboembolism

Despite improvements in the care of the trauma patient, venous thromboembolism (VTE) and the attendant risk of pulmonary embolism remain important causes of morbidity and mortality in the multiply injured trauma patient. The factors that form the basis of VTE pathophysiology are blood stasis, injury to the intimal surface of the vessel, and hypercoagulopathy. Trauma patients are at risk for VTE because of endothelial injury, coagulopathy, and immobility.

Trauma patients are at the greatest risk for developing thromboembolism early in their hospitalization. Prevention is key. Practice guidelines for the prevention and management of thromboembolism recommend that trauma patients at high risk for VTE receive sequential compression devices for prophylaxis against VTE.[34] High-risk patients include those with an SCI, lower extremity or pelvic fractures, need for a surgical procedure, increasing age, central venous catheters or venous injury, and prolonged immobility or hospital stay. For patients in whom the lower leg is inaccessible, foot pumps may act as an effective alternative to lower the rate of VTE. Low-molecular-weight heparin (e.g., enoxaparin) is recommended for VTE prophylaxis in trauma patients with the following injury patterns:

- Pelvic fractures requiring operative fixation or prolonged bed rest (longer than 5 days)
- Complex lower extremity fractures requiring operative fixation or prolonged bed rest
- SCI with complete or incomplete motor paralysis

The selection of VTE prophylaxis for trauma patients is often challenging because of the need to achieve balance between VTE risk and bleeding risk. For high-risk trauma patients who cannot receive anticoagulation because of their risk of bleeding, the prophylactic placement of an inferior vena cava filter is considered when the following patterns of injury are present:[34]

- Severe closed head injury with a GCS below 8, intracranial hemorrhage, or intraocular (eye) injury with associated hemorrhage
- Incomplete SCI with paraplegia or quadriplegia
- Complex pelvic fractures with associated long-bone fractures, retroperitoneal hematoma requiring transfusions
- Multiple long-bone fractures

The purpose of inferior vena cava filter placement is to reduce the risk of fatal pulmonary embolism. Filter placement does not negate the requirement to use sequential compression devices and pharmacological prophylaxis against VTE.

Missed Injury

Nursing assessment of the multiply injured patient in the critical care unit may reveal missed diseases or missed injuries. Missed disorders may include preexisting undiagnosed medical illnesses, such as endocrine disorders (diabetes, hypothyroidism), myocardial infarction, hypertension, decreased respiratory reserve, undiagnosed kidney failure, or malnutrition.

Occasionally, injuries may not be diagnosed in the precritical care phases. Missed injuries are commonly discovered in the first 24 to 48 hours of the hospital stay during the routine assessments of the trauma tertiary survey. Injuries are missed for a variety of reasons as summarized in Box 25-13. In the critical care unit, a missed injury may be suspected if the patient fails to show appropriate response to medical or surgical intervention. Nurses play a key role in identifying missed injuries, particularly when patients regain consciousness and begin to increase their activity.

Multiple Organ Dysfunction Syndrome

MODS is a clinical syndrome of progressive dysfunction of organ systems. Trauma patients are at high risk for systemic inflammatory response syndrome (SIRS) and MODS. Organ dysfunction can be the result of primary MODS, which is caused by direct traumatic injury, as may occur with acute lung dysfunction because of pulmonary contusion. Secondary MODS—organ dysfunction that occurs later in the trauma patient's ICU course—results from uncontrolled systemic inflammation with resultant organ dysfunction. Treatment is aimed at controlling or eliminating the source of inflammation, maintenance of oxygen delivery and consumption, and nutritional and metabolic support for individual organs.

BOX 25-13 FACTORS CONTRIBUTING TO MISSED INJURIES

Hemodynamic Instability
- Shock states in the emergency department
- Aggressive resuscitation
- Emergent surgery taking precedence over thorough secondary surveys

Alterations in Consciousness
- Presence of drugs or alcohol intoxication confuses physical assessments and masks physical findings.
- Disoriented patients are challenging to assess.
- Agitation makes diagnostic testing challenging.
- Patients with altered consciousness cannot provide a history of the injury.

SPECIAL CONSIDERATIONS

Meeting the Needs of Family Members and Significant Others

The impact of traumatic injury can be devastating for patients and for family members and significant others. They are faced with a crisis situation for which they have had little time to prepare. Trauma can precipitate a crisis within the family. Families may exhibit physical and sociocultural reactions and a combination of emotional reactions, including anger, fear, powerlessness, confusion, and mistrust. Recovery from traumatic injury can be long and frustrating for families. There may be many peaks and valleys of good days and bad days. During this time, the family may exhaust its social and financial support systems. Nurses should recognize this and facilitate supportive relationships for families. Regardless of the specific system of care delivery, the nurse ensures the family is supported during all aspects of care.

A valuable intervention is to bring families of trauma patients together in support groups. Trauma-related family support groups can offer sharing of experiences, expression of emotions, mutual support, sharing of coping strategies, and education about hospital and community services.

Trauma in Older Adults

Trauma affects people of all ages. Older patients are predisposed to traumatic injuries because of the inevitable consequences of aging. The ability to react to or avoid environmental hazards is impaired because of age-related deterioration of the senses and changes in motor strength, postural stability, balance, and coordination (see Chapter 14).

Older persons experience most of the falls that result in injuries, and these falls are likely to occur from level surfaces or steps.[35] Factors that predispose older persons to falls are summarized in Box 25-14.[35] Because many of the falls may be caused by an underlying medical condition (e.g., syncope, myocardial infarction, dysrhythmias), management of the older patient who has fallen must include an evaluation of events and conditions immediately preceding the fall.

The exposure of older adults to MVC trauma is a consequence of the increasing growth of the older population and the growing number of older drivers and occupants of motor vehicles. Factors that predispose older adults to MVCs are summarized in Box 25-15.[35] A pedestrian struck by a motor vehicle receives one of the most devastating injuries. Many deaths of older individuals occur in crosswalks. Physiological deterioration of cerebral and motor skills and alterations in visual and auditory acuity cause older pedestrians to walk directly into the path of oncoming vehicles.

Trauma in older adults is associated with higher mortality rates, even when the injuries are less severe. Older adults have a higher complication rate and a higher mortality rate, starting at age 40, because of preexisting medical conditions, decreased physiological reserves, and decreased ability to compensate for severe injury. Older patients who do survive traumatic injury are often faced with changes in their preinjury functional status. Relatively minor trauma can be the event that changes the lifestyle of an older person from one of relative independence to one that requires prolonged rehabilitation or skilled nursing care. Discharge planning early in the patient's hospitalization is necessary.

The concept of *limited physiological reserve* in the older trauma patient highlights the key difference between the average younger trauma patient with normal physiological reserve and the older patient with underlying physiological derangements. Age-related changes that occur in virtually every organ system may not produce evidence of organ dysfunction in the resting state. However, the ability of organs to augment function in response to traumatic stress may be greatly compromised. Fluid resuscitation is an integral part of trauma resuscitation. Patients on chronic diuretic therapy may require more volume and potassium supplementation as a result of chronic volume and potassium depletion. The assessment and management of hypovolemic shock is more complex in the older trauma patient. Older adults have limited ability to increase their heart rate in response to blood loss, obscuring one of the earliest signs of hypovolemia—tachycardia.[4] Loss of physiological reserve and the presence of preexisting medical conditions are likely to produce further

---

BOX 25-14   RISK FACTORS FOR FALLS IN OLDER ADULTS

Acute Illness
- Cerebrovascular accidents
- Dysrhythmias
- Syncope
- Diabetes

Cognitive Impairment
- Dementia

Neuromuscular Disorders
- Arthritis
- Lower extremity weakness
- Unstable gait

Medications
- Antidepressants
- Benzodiazepines
- Diuretics
- Phenothiazines

BOX 25-15   FACTORS THAT PREDISPOSE OLDER ADULTS TO MOTOR VEHICLE CRASHES

- Alterations in visual and auditory acuity
- Deterioration in strength and slower reaction times
- Diminution of cerebral skills
- Diminution of motor skills
- Exacerbation of acute or chronic medical conditions
- Medications that may interfere with safe driving

conflicting hemodynamic data. The older patient's lack of physiological reserve makes it imperative that early nutritional support is initiated.

Trauma protocols are well established for the management of young patients after injury. Clinicians increasingly are recognizing that these protocols must be individualized for the older trauma patient. The best outcomes for this patient population have been achieved through early, appropriate, aggressive trauma care, including early hemodynamic monitoring in high-risk older trauma patients (those with a high-risk mechanism of injury, unknown cardiovascular status, or preexisting heart or kidney disease).[36]

CASE STUDY PATIENT WITH TRAUMA

Answers to the Case Study Questions can be found on the Evolve web site at http://evolve.elsevier.com/Urden/priorities/.

Brief Patient History

Mr. G is a 21-year-old man. He was traveling in the back of a pickup truck that collided with another vehicle. He was ejected onto the side of the road and now is not awake and is barely breathing. He was intubated by emergency services, placed in a collar, and immobilized.

Clinical Assessment

Mr. G is admitted to the emergency department with minimal signs of external injury except for some small abrasions to the side of his face.

Diagnostic Procedures

Admission CT scan shows a large subdural hematoma.

Chest x-ray confirms appropriate placement of the endotracheal tube.

Baseline vital signs are blood pressure (BP) 110/60, heart rate (HR) 108 (sinus tachycardia), respiratory rate (RR) 30, temperature (T) 98.3° F, O_2 saturation 88%, Glasgow Coma Scale 7.

Medical Diagnosis

Mr. G is diagnosed with subdural hematoma secondary to trauma.

Questions

1. What major outcomes do you expect to achieve for this patient?
2. What problems or risks must be managed to achieve these outcomes?
3. What interventions must be initiated to monitor, prevent, manage, or eliminate the problems and risks identified above?
4. What interventions should be initiated to promote optimal functioning, safety, and well-being of the patient?
5. What possible learning needs would you anticipate for this patient?
6. What cultural and age-related factors might have a bearing on the patient's plan of care?

REFERENCES

1. American College of Surgeons Committee on Trauma Quick Guide: Available at www.facs.org/trauma/verificationhosp.html. Accessed October 11, 2010.
2. Gentilello LM: Alcohol interventions in trauma centers: the opportunity and the challenge, *J Trauma* 59(Suppl 3):S18, 2005.
3. Field C, Hungerford DW, Dunn C: Brief motivational interventions: an introduction, *J Trauma* 59(Suppl 3):S21, 2005.
4. American College of Surgeons: *Advanced trauma life support*, ed 8, Chicago, 2008, American College of Surgeons.
5. Englehart MS, Schreiber MA: Measurement of acid-base resuscitation endpoints: lactate, base deficit, bicarbonate or what? *Curr Opin Crit Care* 12(6):569, 2006.
6. Tisherman SA, et al: Clinical practice guideline: endpoints of resuscitation, *J Trauma* 57(4):898, 2004.
7. Faul M, et al: Traumatic brain injury in the United States: emergency department visits, hospitalizations, and deaths 2002-2006. Centers for Disease Control and Prevention, National Center for Injury Prevention and Control, 2010. Available at www.cdc.gov/TraumaticBrainInjury/index.html. Accessed October 2010.
8. McQuillan KA, Thurman PA: Traumatic brain injuries. In McQuillan KA, et al, editors: *Trauma nursing: from resuscitation through rehabilitation*, ed 4, Philadelphia, 2009, Saunders.
9. Brain Trauma Foundation, et al: Guidelines for the management of severe traumatic brain injury, *J Neurotrauma* 24(Suppl 1):S1, 2007.
10. Chestnut RM: Management of brain and spine injuries, *Crit Care Clin* 20(1):25, 2004.
11. Sekhon LH, Fehlings MG: Epidemiology, demographics, and pathophysiology of acute spinal cord injury, *Spine* 26(Suppl 24):S2, 2001.
12. Russo-McCourt TA: Spinal cord injuries. In McQuillan KA, et al, editors: *Trauma nursing: from resuscitation through rehabilitation*, ed 4, Philadelphia, 2009, Saunders.
13. Consortium for Spinal Cord Medicine: Early acute management in adults with spinal cord injury: a clinical practice guideline for health-care providers, *J Spinal Cord Med* 31(4): 408, 2008.
14. Inamasu J, Guiot BH: Thoracolumbar junction injuries after rollover crashes: difference between belted and unbelted front seat occupants, *Eur Spine J* 18(10):1464, 2009.
15. Sharma OP, et al: Clinical implications of the seat belt sign in blunt trauma, *Am Surg* 75(9):822, 2009.
16. Winters BA: Older adults with traumatic rib fractures: an evidence-based approach to their care, *J Trauma Nurs* 16(2):93, 2009.
17. Kiraly L, Schreiber M: Management of the crushed chest, *Crit Care Med* 38(Suppl 9):S469, 2010.
18. El-Chami MF, Nicholson W, Helmy T: Blunt cardiac trauma, *J Emerg Med* 35(2):127, 2008.

19. Hoff WS, et al: Practice management guidelines for the evaluation of blunt abdominal trauma: the East practice management guidelines work group, *J Trauma* 53(3):602, 2002.

20. Jones KM: Abdominal injuries. In McQuillan KA, et al, editors: *Trauma nursing: from resuscitation through rehabilitation*, ed 4, Philadelphia, 2009, Saunders.

21. Germanos S, et al: Damage control surgery in the abdomen: an approach for the management of severe injured patients, *Int J Surg* 6(3):246, 2008.

22. Maerz L, Kaplan LJ: Abdominal compartment syndrome, *Crit Care Med* 36(Suppl 4):S212, 2008.

23. Cheatham ML, et al: Results from the International Conference of Experts on Intra-abdominal Hypertension and Abdominal Compartment Syndrome: Recommendations, *Intensive Care Med* 33(6):951, 2007.

24. The EAST Practice Management Guidelines Work Group: *Practice management guidelines for the nonoperative management of blunt injury to the liver and spleen*, 2003, Eastern Association for the Surgery of Trauma. Available at www.east.org. Accessed October 2010.

25. Harris BT, et al: Impact of hollow viscus injuries on outcome of abdominal gunshot wounds, *Am Surg* 75(5):378, 2009.

26. Snyder KA, Veronese V: Genitourinary injuries and renal management. In McQuillan KA, et al, editors: *Trauma nursing: from resuscitation through rehabilitation*, ed 4, Philadelphia, 2009, Saunders.

27. The EAST Practice Management Guidelines Work Group: *Practice management guidelines for the management of genitourinary trauma*, 2004, Eastern Association for the Surgery of Trauma. Available at www.east.org. Accessed October 2010.

28. The EAST Practice Management Guidelines Work Group: Practice management guidelines for hemorrhage in pelvic fracture, 2001, Eastern Association for the Surgery of Trauma. Available at www.east.org. Accessed October 2010.

29. McClave SA, et al: Guidelines for the provision and assessment of nutrition support therapy in the adult critically ill patient: Society of Critical Care Medicine (SCCM) and American Society for Parenteral and Enteral Nutrition (A.S.P.E.N.), *JPEN* 33(3):277, 2009.

30. Shah CV, et al: The impact of development of acute lung injury on hospital mortality in critically ill trauma patients, *Crit Care Med* 36(8):2309, 2008.

31. Jawa RS, Anillo S, Kulaylat MN: Transfusion-related acute lung injury, *J Intensive Care Med* 23(2):109, 2008.

32. Talbot M, Schemitsch EH: Fat embolism syndrome: history, definition, epidemiology, *Injury* 37(Suppl 4):S3, 2006.

33. Jacobi J, et al: Clinical practice guidelines for the sustained use of sedatives and analgesics in the critically ill adult, *Crit Care Med* 30(1):119, 2002.

34. Rogers FB, et al: Practice management guidelines for the prevention of venous thromboembolism in trauma patients: the EAST practice management guidelines work group, *J Trauma* 53(1):142, 2002.

35. Aschkenasy MT, Rothenhaus TC: Trauma and falls in the elderly, *Emerg Med Clin North Am* 24(2):413, 2006.

36. The EAST Practice Management Guidelines Work Group: *Practice management guidelines for geriatric trauma*, 2001, Eastern Association for the Surgery of Trauma. Available at www.east.org. Accessed October 2010.

26

Shock, Sepsis, and Multiple Organ Dysfunction Syndrome

Beverly Carlson, Lorraine Fitzsimmons, Christopher Walker

⊘volve WEBSITE

Be sure to check out the bonus material, including free self-assessment exercises, on the Evolve web site at *http://evolve.elsevier.com/Urden/priorities/*.

OBJECTIVES

- Describe the generalized shock response and systemic inflammatory response.
- List the etiologies of hypovolemic, cardiogenic, and anaphylactic, neurogenic, and septic shock, and multiple organ dysfunction syndrome (MODS).
- Explain the pathophysiology of the five forms of shock and MODS.
- Identify the clinical manifestations of the five forms of shock and MODS.
- Outline the important aspects of the medical management of hypovolemic, cardiogenic, and anaphylactic, neurogenic, and septic shock, and MODS.
- Summarize the nursing priorities for managing a patient with each type of shock or MODS.

Shock is an acute, widespread process of impaired tissue perfusion that results in cellular, metabolic, and hemodynamic alterations. Ineffective tissue perfusion occurs when an imbalance develops between cellular oxygen supply and cellular oxygen demand. This imbalance can occur for a variety of reasons and eventually results in cellular dysfunction and death. This chapter presents an overview of the general shock response, or shock syndrome, followed by a discussion of the various shock states.

SHOCK SYNDROME

Shock is a complex pathophysiological process that often results in multiple organ dysfunction syndrome (MODS) and death. All types of shock eventually result in ineffective tissue perfusion and acute circulatory failure. The shock syndrome is a pathway involving a variety of pathological processes that may be categorized as four stages: initial, compensatory, progressive, and refractory. Progression through each stage varies with the patient's prior condition, duration of initiating event, response to therapy, and correction of underlying cause.

Etiology

Shock can be classified as hypovolemic, cardiogenic, or distributive, depending on the pathophysiological cause and hemodynamic profile. Hypovolemic shock results from a loss of circulating or intravascular volume. Cardiogenic shock results from the impaired ability of the heart to pump. Distributive shock results from maldistribution of circulating blood volume and can be further classified as septic, anaphylactic, or neurogenic. Septic shock is the result of microorganisms entering the body. Anaphylactic shock is the result of a severe antibody-antigen reaction. Neurogenic shock is the result of the loss of sympathetic tone.

Pathophysiology

During the initial stage, cardiac output (CO) is decreased, and tissue perfusion is threatened. Almost immediately, the compensatory stage begins as the body's homeostatic mechanisms attempt to maintain CO, blood pressure, and tissue perfusion. The compensatory mechanisms are mediated by the sympathetic nervous system (SNS) and consist of neural, hormonal, and chemical responses. The neural response includes an increase in heart rate and contractility, arterial and venous vasoconstriction, and shunting of blood to the vital organs. Hormonal compensation includes activation of the renin response and stimulation of the anterior pituitary and adrenal medulla. Activation of the renin response results in the production of angiotensin II, which causes vasoconstriction and the release of aldosterone and antidiuretic hormone (ADH), leading to sodium and water retention. Stimulation of the anterior pituitary results in the secretion of adrenocorticotropic hormone (ACTH), which stimulates the adrenal cortex to produce glucocorticoids, causing a rise in blood glucose levels. Stimulation of the adrenal medulla causes the release of epinephrine and norepinephrine, which further enhance the compensatory mechanisms.

During the progressive stage, the compensatory mechanisms begin failing to meet tissue metabolic needs, and the shock cycle is perpetuated (Concept Map: Shock). As tissue perfusion becomes ineffective, the cells switch from aerobic to anaerobic metabolism to produce energy. Anaerobic metabolism produces small amounts of energy but large amounts of lactic acid, producing lactic acidemia. Increased vascular permeability from endothelial and epithelial hypoxia and inflammatory mediators results in intravascular hypovolemia, tissue edema, and further decline in tissue perfusion.[1,2] A systemic release of inflammatory mediators in response to tissue hypoxia, especially in gut tissue, produces microcirculatory impairment and derangement of cellular metabolism, facilitating progression of the shock cycle.[1-3] The patient is experiencing the systemic inflammatory response syndrome (SIRS), and irreversible damage begins to occur. Some cells die as a result of apoptosis, an injury-activated, preprogrammed cellular suicide. Others die as the sodium-potassium pump in the cell membrane fails, causing the cell and its organelles to swell. Cellular energy production comes to a complete halt as the mitochondria swell and rupture. At this point, the problem becomes one of oxygen use instead of oxygen delivery. Even if the cell were to receive more oxygen, it would be unable to use it because of damage to the mitochondria. The cell's digestive organelles swell and leak destructive enzymes into the cell, accelerating cell death.[3]

Every system in the body is affected by this process (Box 26-1). Cardiac dysfunction develops as a result of the release of myocardial depressant cytokines.[1,2] Ventricular failure eventually occurs, further perpetuating the entire process. Central nervous system (CNS) dysfunction develops as a result of cerebral hypoperfusion, leading to failure of the SNS, cardiac and respiratory depression, and thermoregulatory failure. Endothelial injury from hypoxia and inflammatory cytokines and impaired blood flow result in microvascular thrombosis. Hematological dysfunction occurs as a result of consumption of clotting factors, release of inflammatory cytokines, and dilutional thrombocytopenia. Disseminated intravascular coagulation (DIC) eventually may develop. Pulmonary dysfunction occurs as a result of increased pulmonary capillary membrane permeability, pulmonary microemboli, and pulmonary vasoconstriction. Ventilatory failure and acute lung injury (ALI) develop. Renal dysfunction develops as a result of renal vasoconstriction and renal hypoperfusion, leading to acute tubular necrosis (ATN). Gastrointestinal dysfunction occurs as a result of splanchnic vasoconstriction and hypoperfusion and leads to failure of the gut organs. Disruption of the intestinal epithelium releases gram-negative bacteria into the system, which further perpetuates the entire shock syndrome.[4]

During the refractory stage, shock becomes unresponsive to therapy and is considered irreversible. As the individual

---

BOX 26-1 CONSEQUENCES OF SHOCK

Cardiovascular
- Ventricular failure
- Microvascular thrombosis

Neurological
- Sympathetic nervous system dysfunction
- Cardiac and respiratory depression
- Thermoregulatory failure
- Coma

Pulmonary
- Acute respiratory failure
- Acute lung injury (ALI)

Renal
- Acute tubular necrosis (ATN)

Hematological
- Disseminated intravascular coagulation (DIC)

Gastrointestinal
- Gastrointestinal tract failure
- Hepatic failure
- Pancreatic failure

---

organ systems die, MODS—defined as failure of two or more body systems—occurs. Death is the final outcome. Regardless of the etiological factors, death occurs from ineffective tissue perfusion because of the failure of the circulation to meet the oxygen needs of the cell.[3]

Assessment and Diagnosis

The patient with a mean arterial blood pressure (MAP) less than 60 mm Hg or with evidence of multisystem organ hypoperfusion is considered to be in a shock state.[1,5] Because shock is a dynamic physiological phenomenon, hypotension may occur late in the process.[6] Clinical manifestations vary according to the underlying cause of shock, the stage of the shock, and the patient's response to shock.

Compensatory mechanisms may produce normal hemodynamic values even when tissue perfusion is compromised.[4-7] Global indicators of systemic perfusion and oxygenation include serum lactate, arterial base deficit, serum bicarbonate, and central or mixed venous oxygen saturation levels. Inadequate cellular oxygenation with anaerobic metabolism and increased metabolic lactate production increase the serum lactate level.[8] The level and duration of this hyperlactatemia are predictive of morbidity and mortality.[7-11] The base deficit derived from arterial blood gas (ABG) values also reflects global tissue acidosis and is frequently used to assess the severity of shock.[6,7,9] Studies have demonstrated serum bicarbonate to be an equivalent alternative to arterial base deficit in predicting mortality in surgical and trauma patients.[12,13] The use of mixed venous oxygen saturation (Svo_2) measured by means of a pulmonary artery catheter or central venous oxygen saturation ($Scvo_2$) measured with a central venous

Concept Map: Shock

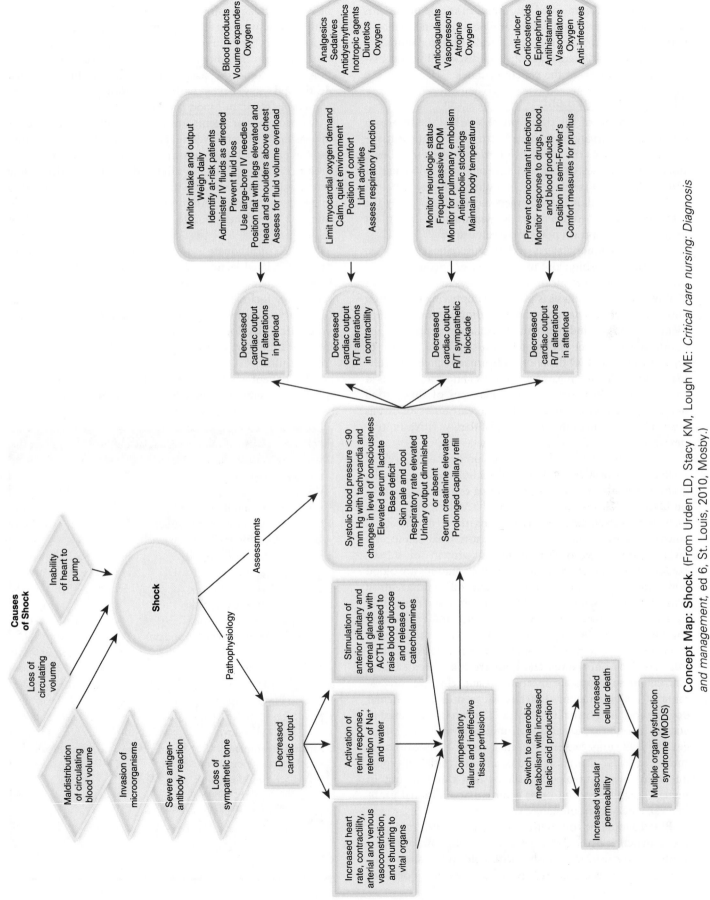

Concept Map: Shock. (From Urden LD, Stacy KM, Lough ME: *Critical care nursing: Diagnosis and management,* ed 6, St. Louis, 2010, Mosby.)

catheter allows assessment of the balance of oxygen delivery and oxygen consumption and the ratio of oxygen extraction.[14-16] After years of recommended use to guide the care of patients with severe sepsis, this measure of global oxygen balance is being evaluated for use in other critically ill populations.[15-21] The sections on different types of shock discuss clinical assessment and diagnosis of the patient in shock.

Medical Management

The major focus of the treatment of shock is the improvement and preservation of tissue perfusion. Adequate tissue perfusion depends on an adequate supply of oxygen being transported to the tissues and the cell's ability to use it. Oxygen transport is influenced by pulmonary gas exchange, CO, and hemoglobin level. Oxygen use is influenced by the internal metabolic environment. Management of the patient in shock focuses on supporting oxygen delivery.[1,22]

Adequate pulmonary gas exchange is critical to oxygen transport. Establishing and maintaining an adequate airway are the first steps in ensuring adequate oxygenation. After the airway is patent, emphasis is placed on improving ventilation and oxygenation. Therapies include administration of supplemental oxygen and mechanical ventilatory support.

An adequate CO and hemoglobin level are crucial to oxygen transport. CO depends on heart rate, preload, afterload, and contractility. A variety of fluids and drugs are used to manipulate these parameters. The types of fluids used include crystalloids and colloids. The categories of drugs used include vasoconstrictors, vasodilators, positive inotropes, and antidysrhythmics.

Fluid administration is indicated for decreased preload related to intravascular volume depletion, and it can be accomplished by use of a crystalloid or colloid solution, or both. Crystalloids are balanced electrolyte solutions that may be hypotonic, isotonic, or hypertonic. Examples of crystalloid solutions used in shock situations are normal saline and lactated Ringer's solution. Colloids are protein- or starch-containing solutions. Examples of colloid solutions are blood and blood components, such as albumin, and pharmaceutical plasma expanders, such as hetastarch, dextran, and mannitol.

The choice of fluid is a subject of debate and depends on the situation.[15,23-25] Fluid resuscitation with normal saline or with albumin produces similar outcomes regardless of baseline serum albumin level, and both are considered safe.[26,27] Crystalloid solutions are inexpensive and effective. Advantages of colloids include faster restoration of intravascular volume and use of smaller amounts. Colloids are believed to stay in the intravascular space, unlike crystalloids, which readily leak into the extravascular space. Disadvantages include expense, allergic reactions, and difficulties in typing and cross-matching blood. Colloids also can leak out of damaged capillaries and cause a variety of additional problems, particularly in the lungs.

Blood should be considered to augment oxygen transport if the patient's hemoglobin level is critically low, although controversy exists about what threshold value should be used.[4,15] Transfusion of stored red blood cells does not

substantially increase oxygen consumption and has been associated with immunosuppression, infection, impairment of microcirculatory flow, coagulopathy, and increased mortality. Restrictive transfusion practice has demonstrated lower mortality.[4,16,28] Transfusion-related acute lung injury (TRALI) resulting from immune and nonimmune neutrophil activation has become the leading cause of transfusion-related death and may occur with transfusion of any plasma-containing blood or blood product.[28-30]

Vasoconstrictor agents are used to increase afterload by increasing the systemic vascular resistance (SVR) and improving the patient's blood pressure level. Vasodilator agents are used to decrease preload or afterload, or both, by decreasing venous return and SVR. Positive inotropic agents are used to increase contractility. Antidysrhythmic agents are used to influence heart rate.[31] Box 26-2 provides examples of each of these agents.

Sodium bicarbonate is not recommended in the treatment of shock-related lactic acidosis.[16,32,33] No overall benefit has been found, and the risks associated with its use are significant. They include shifting of the oxyhemoglobin dissociation curve to the left, rebound increase in lactic acid production, development of hyperosmolar state, fluid overload resulting from excessive sodium, and rapid cellular electrolyte shifts.[11,32,33]

The patient should be started on nutritional support therapy as early as possible. The type of nutritional

---

BOX 26-2 AGENTS USED IN THE TREATMENT OF SHOCK

Vasoconstrictors
- Epinephrine (Adrenalin)
- Norepinephrine (Levophed)
- Alpha-range dopamine (Intropin)
- Phenylephrine (Neo-Synephrine)
- Vasopressin (Pitressin)

Vasodilators
- Nitroprusside (Nipride, Nitropress)
- Nitroglycerin (Nitrol, Tridil)
- Hydralazine (Apresoline)
- Labetalol (Normodyne, Trandate)

Inotropes
- Beta-range dopamine (Intropin)
- Dobutamine (Dobutrex)
- Epinephrine (Adrenalin)
- Norepinephrine (Levophed)

Antidysrhythmics
- Lidocaine (Xylocaine)
- Adenosine (Adenocard)
- Procainamide (Pronestyl)
- Labetalol (Normodyne, Trandate)
- Verapamil (Calan, Isoptin)
- Esmolol (Brevibloc)
- Diltiazem (Cardizem)
- Amiodarone (Cordarone)

supplementation initiated varies according to the cause of shock, and it should be tailored to the individual patient's needs, as indicated by the underlying condition and laboratory data. The enteral route is preferred over the parenteral, although parental nutrition should be considered when enteral feeding is contraindicated.[25,34-37] Supplementation of enteral feeding with parenteral nutrition to increase caloric intake should be considered but has not been shown to improve patient outcomes.[35-37]

Glucose control is recommended for all critically ill patients.[38,39] Benefits of glucose control in the critically ill include lower incidences of infection, renal failure, sepsis, polyneuropathy, need for blood transfusion, prolonged mechanical ventilation, and death.[38-42]

Nursing Management

The nursing management of a patient in shock is a complex and challenging responsibility. It requires an in-depth understanding of the pathophysiology of the disease and the anticipated effects of each intervention, as well as a solid understanding of the nursing process. Later sections discuss specific interventions for the patient in shock.

The psychosocial needs of the patient and family dealing with shock are extremely important. These needs are based on situational, familial, and patient-centered variables. **Nursing priorities in managing the patient in shock are directed toward (1) providing information on patient status, (2) explaining procedures and routines, (3) supporting the family, (4) encouraging the expression of feelings, (5) facilitating problem solving and shared decision making, (6) individualizing visitation schedules, (7) involving the family in the patient's care, and (8) establishing contacts with necessary resources.**[43] Patients and families should be given the option of family presence during invasive procedures and resuscitation.[43-45] Collaborative management of the patient with shock is outlined in the Collaborative Management Box on Shock.

COLLABORATIVE MANAGEMENT

Shock

- Support oxygen transport.
  - Establish a patent airway.
  - Initiate mechanical ventilation.
  - Administer oxygen.
  - Administer fluids (crystalloids, colloids, blood and other blood products).
  - Administer vasoactive medications.
  - Administer positive inotropic medications.
  - Ensure sufficient hemoglobin and hematocrit.
- Support oxygen use.
  - Identify and correct cause of lactic acidosis.
  - Ensure adequate organ and extremity perfusion.
  - Initiate nutritional support therapy.
- Identify underlying cause of shock and treat accordingly.
- Provide comfort and emotional support.
- Maintain surveillance for complications.

HYPOVOLEMIC SHOCK

Hypovolemic shock occurs from inadequate fluid volume in the intravascular space. The lack of adequate circulating volume leads to decreased tissue perfusion and initiation of the general shock response. Hypovolemic shock is the most commonly occurring form of shock.

Etiology

Hypovolemic shock can result from absolute or relative hypovolemia. Absolute hypovolemia occurs when there is a loss of fluid from the intravascular space. This can result from an external loss of fluid from the body or from internal shifting of fluid from the intravascular space to the extravascular space. Fluid shifts can result from a loss of intravascular integrity, increased capillary membrane permeability, or decreased colloidal osmotic pressure. Relative hypovolemia occurs when vasodilation produces an increase in vascular capacitance relative to circulating volume (Box 26-3).

Pathophysiology

Hypovolemia results in a loss of circulating fluid volume. A decrease in circulating volume leads to a decrease in venous return, which results in a decrease in end-diastolic volume or

---

BOX 26-3   ETIOLOGICAL FACTORS IN HYPOVOLEMIC SHOCK

Absolute Factors
- Loss of whole blood
  - Trauma or surgery
  - Gastrointestinal bleeding
- Loss of plasma
  - Thermal injuries
  - Large lesions
- Loss of other body fluids
  - Severe vomiting or diarrhea
  - Massive diuresis
  - Loss of intravascular integrity
  - Ruptured spleen
  - Long bone or pelvic fractures
  - Hemorrhagic pancreatitis
  - Hemothorax or hemoperitoneum
  - Arterial dissection or rupture

Relative Factors
- Vasodilation
  - Sepsis
  - Anaphylaxis
  - Loss of sympathetic stimulation
- Increased capillary membrane permeability
  - Sepsis
  - Anaphylaxis
  - Thermal injuries
- Decreased colloidal osmotic pressure
  - Severe sodium depletion
  - Hypopituitarism
  - Cirrhosis
  - Intestinal obstruction

Relative hypovolemia   Absolute hypovolemia

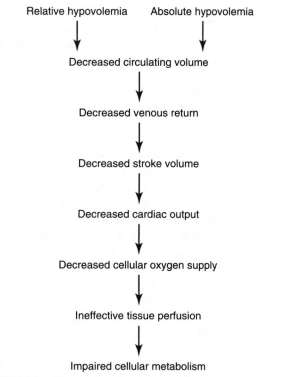

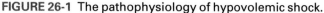

FIGURE 26-1 The pathophysiology of hypovolemic shock.

preload. Preload is a major determinant of stroke volume (SV) and CO. A decrease in preload results in a decrease in SV and CO. The decrease in CO leads to inadequate cellular oxygen supply and ineffective tissue perfusion (Figure 26-1).

Assessment and Diagnosis

The clinical manifestations of hypovolemic shock depend on the severity of fluid loss and the patient's ability to compensate for it. Clinical classes have been developed by the American College of Surgeons to describe the levels of severity of hypovolemic shock. Class I indicates a fluid volume loss up to 15% or an actual volume loss up to 750 mL. Compensatory mechanisms maintain CO, and the patient appears free of symptoms other than slight anxiety.[4,46]

Class II hypovolemia occurs with a fluid volume loss of 15% to 30% or an actual volume loss of 750 to 1500 mL. Falling CO activates more intense compensatory responses. The heart rate increases to more than 100 beats/minute in response to increased SNS stimulation unless blocked by preexisting beta-blocker therapy. The pulse pressure narrows as the diastolic blood pressure increases because of vasoconstriction. The respiratory rate increases to 20 to 30 breaths/minute, and respiratory depth increases in an attempt to improve oxygenation. ABG specimens drawn during this phase reveal respiratory alkalosis and hypoxemia, as evidenced by a low partial pressure of carbon dioxide ($Paco_2$) and a low partial pressure of oxygen (Pao_2), respectively. Urine output starts to decline to 20 to 30 mL/hour as renal perfusion decreases. The urine sodium level decreases, whereas urinary osmolality and specific gravity increase as

the kidneys start to conserve sodium and water. The patient's skin becomes pale and cool with delayed capillary refill because of peripheral vasoconstriction. Jugular veins appear flat as a result of decreased venous return.[4,46]

Hypovolemic shock that is class III occurs with a fluid volume loss of 30% to 40% or an actual volume loss of 1500 to 2000 mL. This level of severity produces the progressive stage of shock as compensatory mechanisms become overwhelmed and ineffective tissue perfusion develops. Blood pressure decreases. The heart rate increases to more than 120 beats/minute, and dysrhythmias develop as myocardial ischemia ensues. Respiratory distress occurs as the pulmonary system deteriorates. ABG values during this phase reveal respiratory and metabolic acidosis and hypoxemia, as evidenced by a high $Paco_2$, low bicarbonate (HCO_3^-), and low Pao_2, respectively. Decreased renal perfusion results in the development of oliguria. Blood urea nitrogen (BUN) and serum creatinine levels start to rise as the kidneys begin to fail. The patient's skin becomes ashen, cold, and clammy, with marked delayed capillary refill. The patient appears confused as cerebral perfusion decreases and the level of consciousness deteriorates.[4,46]

Class IV hypovolemic shock is usually refractory in nature. It occurs with a fluid volume loss of greater than 40% or an actual volume loss of more than 2000 mL. The compensatory mechanisms of the body completely deteriorate, and organ failure occurs.[5] Severe tachycardia and hypotension ensue. Peripheral pulses are absent, and because of marked peripheral vasoconstriction, capillary refill does not occur. The skin appears cyanotic, mottled, and extremely diaphoretic. Urine output ceases. The patient becomes lethargic and unresponsive, and various clinical manifestations associated with failure of the different body systems develop.[4,46]

Assessment of the hemodynamic parameters of a patient in hypovolemic shock varies by stage but commonly reveals a decreased CO and cardiac index (CI). Loss of circulating volume leads to a decrease in venous return to the heart, which results in a decrease in the preload of the right and left ventricles. This is evidenced by a decline in the central venous pressure (CVP) or right atrial pressure (RAP) and pulmonary artery occlusion pressure (PAOP). Vasoconstriction of the arterial system results in an increase in the afterload of the heart, as evidenced by an increase in the SVR. This vasoconstriction may produce a falsely elevated systolic blood pressure when measured by arterial catheter. MAP is more accurate in this low-flow state.[5]

Medical Management

The major goals of therapy for the patient in hypovolemic shock are to correct the cause of the hypovolemia, restore tissue perfusion, and prevent complications. This approach includes identifying and stopping the source of fluid loss and administering fluid to replace circulating volume. Fluid administration can be accomplished with use of a crystalloid solution, a colloid solution, blood products, or a combination of fluids. The type of solution used depends on the type of fluid lost, the degree of hypovolemia, the severity of hypoperfusion, and the cause of hypovolemia.

Aggressive fluid resuscitation in trauma and surgical patients is the subject of great debate. The benefit of limited or hypotensive (systolic blood pressure >80 mm Hg) volume resuscitation in patients with uncontrolled hemorrhage is postulated to lessen bleeding and improve survival.[22,47-49] The type and amount of solutions used for fluid resuscitation and the rate of administration influence immune function, inflammatory mediator release, coagulation, and the incidence of cardiac, pulmonary, and gastrointestinal complications.[23,24,50-52] Consensus on the optimal resuscitative strategy for hypovolemic shock is lacking.[23,24,48]

Nursing Management

Prevention of hypovolemic shock is one of the primary responsibilities of the nurse in the critical care area. Preventive measures include the identification of patients at risk and frequent assessment of the patient's fluid balance. Accurate monitoring of intake and output and daily weights are essential components of preventive nursing care. Early identification and treatment result in decreased mortality.

Management of the patient in hypovolemic shock requires continuous evaluation of intravascular volume, tissue perfusion, and response to therapy. The patient in hypovolemic shock may have any number of nursing diagnoses, depending on the progression of the process (Nursing Diagnosis Priorities Box on Hypovolemic Shock). **Nursing priorities are directed toward (1) minimizing fluid loss, (2) administering volume replacement, (3) providing comfort and emotional support, and (4) maintaining surveillance for complications.**

NURSING DIAGNOSIS PRIORITIES

Hypovolemic Shock

- Deficient Fluid Volume related to active blood loss, p. A-13
- Deficient Fluid Volume related to interstitial fluid shift, p. A-13
- Decreased Cardiac Output related to alterations in preload, p. A-10
- Imbalanced Nutrition: Less Than Body Requirements related to increased metabolic demands or lack of exogenous nutrients, p. A-22
- Risk for Infection, p. A-36
- Anxiety related to threat to biological, psychological, and/or social integrity, p. A-7
- Compromised Family Coping related to a critically ill family member, p. A-9

Measures to minimize fluid loss include limiting blood sampling, observing lines for accidental disconnection, and applying direct pressure to bleeding sites. Measures to facilitate the administration of volume replacement include insertion of large-bore peripheral intravenous catheters, rapid administration of prescribed fluids, and positioning the patient with the legs elevated, trunk flat, and head and shoulders above the chest. Monitoring the patient for clinical manifestations of fluid overload or complications related to fluid and blood product administration is essential for preventing further problems.

CARDIOGENIC SHOCK

Cardiogenic shock is the result of failure of the heart to effectively pump blood forward. It can occur with dysfunction of the right or the left ventricle, or both. The lack of adequate pumping function leads to decreased tissue perfusion and circulatory failure. It occurs in approximately 5% to 8% of the patients with an ST-segment myocardial infarction (MI), and it is the leading cause of death of patients hospitalized with MI.[53,54] The mortality rate for cardiogenic shock has decreased with the advent of early revascularization therapy and is currently about 47% to 60%.[53-56]

Etiology

Cardiogenic shock can result from primary ventricular ischemia, structural problems, and dysrhythmias.[53,54] The most common cause is acute MI resulting in the loss of 40% or more of the functional myocardium. It can occur with ST-elevation or non-ST-elevation MI.[54,57] The damage to the myocardium may occur after one massive MI (usually of the anterior wall), or it may be cumulative as a result of several smaller MIs or a small MI in a patient with preexisting ventricular dysfunction.[53,57] End-stage cardiomyopathy may also cause cardiogenic shock as may structural problems of the cardiopulmonary system and dysrhythmias if they disrupt the forward motion of the blood through the heart (Box 26-4).[53,54,57]

Pathophysiology

Cardiogenic shock results from the impaired ability of the ventricle to pump blood forward, which leads to a decrease in SV and an increase in the blood left in the ventricle at the end of systole. The decrease in SV results in a decrease in CO, which leads to decreased cellular oxygen supply and ineffective tissue perfusion. Typically, myocardial performance spirals downward as compensatory vasoconstriction increases myocardial afterload and low blood pressure worsens myocardial ischemia. Evidence of SIRS has been observed in a substantial number of patients with cardiogenic shock.[55,57-59] Activation of inflammatory cytokines induce systemic vasodilation, defective cellular oxygen use, and occasionally, normalization of the CO. Whether this process contributes to the genesis or the outcome of cardiogenic shock is uncertain, but it is thought to be activated by acute MI and to facilitate development of sepsis.[55,57,58] As left ventricular contractility declines and ventricular compliance decreases, an increase in end-systolic volume results in blood backing up into the pulmonary system and the subsequent development of pulmonary edema. Pulmonary edema causes impaired gas exchange and decreased oxygenation of the arterial blood, which further impair tissue perfusion (Figure 26-2). Death due to cardiogenic shock may result from multiple organ failure or cardiopulmonary collapse.[55,58]

BOX 26-4 ETIOLOGICAL FACTORS IN CARDIOGENIC SHOCK

Primary Ventricular Ischemia
- Acute myocardial infarction
- Cardiopulmonary arrest
- Open heart surgery

Structural Problems
- Septal rupture
- Papillary muscle rupture
- Free wall rupture
- Ventricular aneurysm
- Cardiomyopathies
  - Congestive
  - Hypertrophic
  - Restrictive
- Intracardiac tumor
- Pulmonary embolus
- Atrial thrombus
- Valvular dysfunction
- Acute myocarditis
- Cardiac tamponade
- Myocardial contusion
- Prolonged septic shock
- Recent hemorrhage

Dysrhythmias
- Bradydysrhythmias
- Tachydysrhythmias

Assessment and Diagnosis

A variety of clinical manifestations occur in the patient in cardiogenic shock, depending on etiological factors in pump failure, the patient's underlying medical status, and the severity of the shock state. Some clinical manifestations are caused by failure of the heart as a pump, whereas many are related to the overall shock response (Box 26-5).

BOX 26-5 CLINICAL MANIFESTATIONS OF CARDIOGENIC SHOCK

- Systolic blood pressure <90 mm Hg
- Acute drop in blood pressure >30 mm Hg
- Heart rate >100 beats/min
- Weak, thready pulse
- Diminished heart sounds
- Change in sensorium
- Cool, pale, moist skin
- Urine output <30 mL/hr
- Chest pain
- Dysrhythmias
- Tachypnea
- Crackles
- Decreased cardiac output
- Cardiac index <2.2 L/min/m²
- Increased pulmonary artery occlusion pressure
- Increased right atrial pressure
- Increased systemic vascular resistance

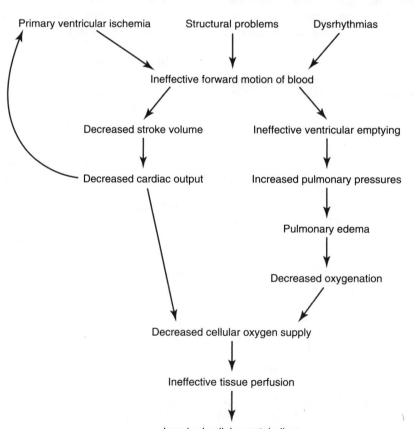

FIGURE 26-2 The pathophysiology of cardiogenic shock.

Initially, clinical manifestations reflect the decline in CO. These signs and symptoms include systolic blood pressure less than 90 mm Hg or an acute drop in systolic or mean blood pressure of 30 mm Hg or more; decreased sensorium; cool, pale, moist skin; and urine output of less than 30 mL/hour.[57,60] The patient also may complain of chest pain. Tachycardia develops to compensate for the decrease in CO. A weak, thready pulse develops, and diminished S_1 and S_2 heart sounds may occur as a result of the decreased contractility. The respiratory rate increases to improve oxygenation. ABG values at this point indicate respiratory alkalosis, as evidenced by a decrease in Pa_{CO_2}. Urinalysis findings demonstrate a decrease in urine sodium level and an increase in urine osmolality and specific gravity as the kidneys start to conserve sodium and water. The patient also may experience a variety of dysrhythmias, depending on the underlying problem.[54]

As the left ventricle fails, auscultation of the lungs may disclose crackles and rhonchi, indicating the development of pulmonary edema. Hypoxemia occurs, as evidenced by a fall in Pa_{O_2} and Sa_{O_2} as measured by ABG values. Heart sounds may reveal an S_3 and S_4. Jugular venous distention is evident with right-sided failure.

Assessment of the hemodynamic parameters of a patient in cardiogenic shock reveals a decreased CO with a CI less than 2.2 L/minute/m^2 in the presence of an elevated PAOP of more than 15 to 18 mm Hg.[53,54,57,59] A proportional pulse pressure (systolic BP/pulse pressure) less than 25% is indicative of left ventricular failure and a CI less than 2.2 and may be useful when direct measurement of CI is unavailable.[61] Increased filling pressures are necessary to rule out hypovolemia as the cause of circulatory failure. The increase in PAOP reflects an increase in the left ventricular end-diastolic pressure (LVEDP) and left ventricular end-diastolic volume (LVEDV) resulting from decreased SV. With right ventricular failure, the RAP also increases. Compensatory vasoconstriction results in an increase in the afterload of the heart, as evidenced by an increase in the SVR. Echocardiography confirms the diagnosis of cardiogenic shock and rules out other causes of circulatory failure.[53,54,57]

As compensatory mechanisms fail and ineffective tissue perfusion develops, other clinical manifestations appear. Myocardial ischemia progresses, as evidenced by continued increases in heart rate, dysrhythmias, and chest pain. Pulmonary function deteriorates, which leads to respiratory distress. ABG values during this phase reveal respiratory and metabolic acidosis and hypoxemia, as indicated by a high Pa_{CO_2}, low HCO_3^-, and low Pa_{O_2}, respectively. Renal failure occurs, as exhibited by the development of anuria and increases in BUN and serum creatinine levels. Cerebral hypoperfusion manifests as a decreasing level of consciousness.

Medical Management

Treatment of the patient in cardiogenic shock requires an aggressive approach. The major goals of therapy are to treat the underlying cause, enhance the effectiveness of the pump, and improve tissue perfusion. This approach includes identifying the etiological factors of pump failure and administering pharmacological agents to enhance CO. Inotropic agents are used to increase contractility and maintain adequate blood pressure and tissue perfusion. A vasopressor may be necessary to maintain blood pressure when hypotension is severe.[57,60] Diuretics are used for preload reduction. After blood pressure has been stabilized, vasodilating agents are used for preload and afterload reduction. Antidysrhythmic agents should be used to suppress or control dysrhythmias that can affect CO.[53] Intubation and mechanical ventilation may be necessary to support oxygenation.

Intraaortic balloon pump (IABP) support should be instituted if drug therapy does not quickly reverse the shock state.[54-57] The IABP is a temporary measure to decrease myocardial workload by improving myocardial supply and decreasing myocardial demand. It achieves this goal by improving coronary artery perfusion and reducing left ventricular afterload. Chapter 13 provides more information about IAPB therapy.

After the cause of pump failure has been identified, measures should be taken to correct the problem if possible. If the problem is related to an acute MI, early revascularization by coronary angioplasty or coronary artery bypass surgery provides significant survival benefit.[53-57,62] Thrombolytic agents may be used in select patients. When conventional therapies fail, a ventricular assist device (VAD) or extracorporeal life support with a membrane oxygenator may be used to support the patient in acute cardiogenic shock.[54,57,63,64] These mechanical circulatory assist devices provide an external means to sustain effective organ perfusion, allowing time for the patient's ventricle to heal or for cardiac transplantation to take place.

Nursing Management

Prevention of cardiogenic shock is one of the primary responsibilities of the nurse in the critical care area. Preventive measures include the identification of patients at risk, facilitation of early reperfusion therapy for acute MI, and frequent assessment and management of the patient's cardiopulmonary status.

The patient in cardiogenic shock may have any number of nursing diagnoses, depending on the progression of the process (Nursing Diagnosis Priorities Box on Cardiogenic Shock). **Nursing priorities are directed toward (1) limiting myocardial oxygen demand, (2) enhancing myocardial oxygen supply, (3) providing comfort and emotional support, and (4) maintaining surveillance for complications.** Measures to limit myocardial oxygen demand include administering analgesics, sedatives, and agents to control afterload and dysrhythmias; positioning the patient for comfort; limiting activities; providing a calm and quiet environment and offering support to reduce anxiety; and teaching the patient about the condition. Measures to enhance myocardial oxygen supply include administering supplemental oxygen, monitoring the patient's respiratory status, and administering prescribed medications.

Cardiogenic Shock

- Ineffective Cardiopulmonary Tissue perfusion related to acute myocardial ischemia, p. A-28
- Decreased Cardiac Output related to alterations in contractility, p. A-11
- Decreased Cardiac Output related to alterations in heart rate, p. A-11
- Imbalanced Nutrition: Less Than Body Requirements related to increased metabolic demands or lack of exogenous nutrients, p. A-22
- Risk for Infection, p. A-36
- Disturbed Body Image related to functional dependence on life-sustaining technology, p. A-16
- Compromised Family Coping related to a critically ill family member, p. A-9

Effective nursing management of cardiogenic shock requires precise monitoring and management of heart rate, preload, afterload, and contractility. This is accomplished through accurate measurement of hemodynamic variables and controlled administration of fluids and inotropic and vasoactive agents. Close assessment and management of respiratory function is also essential to maintain adequate oxygenation. Dysrhythmias are common and require immediate recognition and treatment.

Patients who require IABP therapy need to be observed frequently for complications. Complications include embolus formation, infection, rupture of the aorta, thrombocytopenia, improper balloon placement, bleeding, improper timing of the balloon, balloon rupture, and circulatory compromise of the cannulated extremity.

ANAPHYLACTIC SHOCK

Anaphylactic shock, a type of distributive shock, is the result of an immediate hypersensitivity reaction. It is a life-threatening event that requires prompt intervention. The severe antibody-antigen response leads to decreased tissue perfusion and initiation of the general shock response.[65,66]

Etiology

Anaphylactic shock is caused by an antibody-antigen response. Almost any substance can cause a hypersensitivity reaction. These substances, known as *antigens*, can be introduced by injection or ingestion or through the skin or respiratory tract. A number of antigens have been identified that can cause a reaction in a hypersensitive person. This list includes foods, food additives, diagnostic agents, biological agents, environmental agents, drugs, and venoms (Box 26-6).[66-68] In the hospital environment, latex is an extremely problematic antigen for patients and health care providers (Patient Safety Priorities Box on Latex Allergy).

Latex Allergies

Latex is the milky sap of the rubber tree Hevea brasiliensis. It is treated with preservatives, accelerators, stabilizers, and antioxidants to make a more elastic, stable rubber. Reactions to products containing latex can be triggered by the latex protein or by an additive used in the manufacturing process.

Latex reactions can be classified into three categories: irritation (nonallergic inflammation occurring when the skin is abraded), type IV delayed hypersensitivity (non-IgE-mediated response to the chemical agents added during the manufacturing process), or type I immediate sensitivity (IgE-mediated response to latex proteins). Although the overall prevalence of latex allergy in the general population is only 1%, it is much higher (10% to 55%) in selected groups, such as patients with neural tube defects (e.g., spina bifida, myelomeningocele, lipomyelomeningocele) or congenital urological disorders; those who have undergone multiple operations or who have a history of allergy to anesthetic drugs; and health care, rubber industry, or glove-manufacturing-plant workers.

Five routes of exposure to latex proteins have resulted in systemic reactions: cutaneous (contact with moist skin); mucous membrane (mouth, vagina, urethra, or rectum); internal tissue (during surgery and other invasive procedures); intravascular; and inhalation (exposure to anesthesia equipment or endotracheal tubes or through the aerosolization of glove powder). It has been postulated that the latex allergen adheres to the cornstarch or powder and is released into the air with the manipulation of rubber gloves.

The American Academy of Allergy and Immunology has published guidelines for providing care to persons with latex allergy. All persons at risk for latex allergy should have a careful history and should complete a standardized latex allergy questionnaire. A history suggestive of reactivity to latex includes local swelling or itching after blowing up balloons, dental examinations, contact with rubber gloves, vaginal or rectal examinations, using condoms or diaphragms, and contact with other rubber products. Other historical information that may suggest increased risk of latex allergy includes hand eczema; previous, unexplained anaphylaxis; oral itching after eating bananas, chestnuts, kiwis, or avocados; and multiple surgical procedures in infancy. Patients at high risk should be offered clinical testing for latex allergy.

To minimize the risk of exposure to latex, the use of powder-free latex gloves and non-latex gloves should be adopted when caring for all patients. The patient with a latex allergy should be cared for in a latex-free environment, an environment in which no latex gloves are used and there is no direct patient contact with other latex devices.

From Reines HD, Seifert PC: Patient safety: latex allergy, *Surg Clin North Am* 85(6):1329, 2005.

Anaphylactic reactions can be IgE-mediated or non-IgE-mediated responses. IgE is an antibody that is formed as part of the immune response. The first time an antigen enters the body, an antibody IgE, specific for the antigen, is formed. The antigen-specific IgE antibody is then stored by attachment to mast cells and basophils. This initial contact with the antigen is known as a *primary immune response*. The next time the

BOX 26-6	ETIOLOGICAL FACTORS IN ANAPHYLACTIC SHOCK

Foods
- Eggs and milk
- Fish and shellfish
- Nuts and seeds
- Legumes and cereals
- Soy
- Wheat
- Citrus fruits
- Chocolate
- Strawberries
- Tomatoes
- Avocados
- Bananas
- Kiwi fruit
- Other

Food Additives
- Food coloring
- Preservatives

Diagnostic Agents
- Iodinated contrast dye
- Sulfobromophthalein (Bromsulphalein [BSP])
- Dehydrocholic acid (Decholin)
- Iopanoic acid (Telepaque)

Biological Agents
- Blood and blood components
- Insulin and other hormones
- Gamma globulin
- Seminal plasma
- Enzymes
- Vaccines and antitoxins

Environmental Agents
- Pollens, molds, and spores
- Sunlight
- Animal hair
- Latex

Drugs
- Antibiotics
- Aspirin
- Nonsteroidal antiinflammatory drugs
- Narcotics
- Dextran
- Vitamins
- Local anesthetic agents
- Muscle relaxants
- Neuromuscular blocking agents
- Barbiturates
- Protamine
- Other

Venoms
- Bees, hornets, yellow jackets, and wasps
- Snakes
- Jellyfish
- Spiders
- Deer flies
- Fire ants

antigen enters the body, the preformed IgE antibody reacts with it, and a secondary immune response occurs. This reaction triggers the release of biochemical mediators from the mast cells and basophils and initiates the cascade of events that precipitates anaphylactic shock.[66,69,70]

Some anaphylactic reactions are non-IgE-mediated responses in that they occur in the absence of activation of IgE antibodies. These responses occur as a result of direct activation of the mast cells to release biochemical mediators. Direct activation of mast cells can be triggered by humoral mediators, such as the complement system and the coagulation-fibrinolytic system. Biochemical mediators can be released as a direct or indirect response to many drugs. This type of reaction, formerly known as *anaphylactoid reaction,* is produced in persons not previously sensitized, and it can occur with the first exposure to an antigen.[66,68,70]

Pathophysiology

The antibody-antigen response (immunological stimulation) or the direct triggering (nonimmunological activation) of the mast cells results in the release of biochemical mediators. These mediators include histamine, eosinophil chemotactic factor of anaphylaxis (ECF-A), neutrophil chemotactic factor of anaphylaxis (NCF), platelet-activating factor (PAF), proteinases, heparin, serotonin, leukotrienes (also known as *slow-reacting substance of anaphylaxis*), and prostaglandins. The activation of the biochemical mediators causes vasodilation; increased capillary permeability; laryngeal edema; bronchoconstriction; excessive mucus secretion; coronary vasoconstriction; inflammation; cutaneous reactions; and constriction of the smooth muscle in the intestinal wall, bladder, and uterus. Coronary vasoconstriction causes severe myocardial depression. Cutaneous reactions cause stimulation of nerve endings, followed by itching and pain.[65,66,69]

ECF-A promotes chemotaxis of eosinophils, facilitating the movement of eosinophils into the area. During allergic reactions, eosinophils phagocytose the antibody-antigen complex and other inflammatory debris and release enzymes that inhibit vasoactive mediators, such as histamine and leukotrienes. Secondary mediators such as bradykinin and plasmin are produced that enhance or inhibit the already released biochemical mediators. Peripheral vasodilation results in relative hypovolemia and decreased venous return. Increased capillary membrane permeability results in the loss of intravascular volume, worsening the hypovolemic state. Decreased venous return results in decreased end-diastolic volume and SV. The decline in SV leads to decreased CO and ineffective tissue perfusion. Death may result from airway obstruction or cardiovascular collapse, or both (Figure 26-3).[65,66,69,70]

Assessment and Diagnosis

Anaphylactic shock is a severe systemic reaction that can affect multiple organ systems. A variety of clinical manifestations occur in the patient in anaphylactic shock, depending on the extent of multisystem involvement. The symptoms usually start to appear within minutes of exposure to the

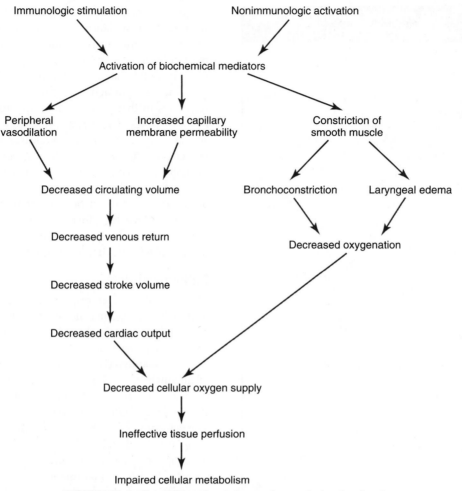

FIGURE 26-3 The pathophysiology of anaphylactic shock.

antigen, but they may not occur for up to 1 hour (Box 26-7).[65] Symptoms may also reappear after a 1- to 72-hour window of resolution. These late-phase reactions may be similar to the initial anaphylactic response, milder, or more severe.[65,71]

The cutaneous effects may appear first and include pruritus, generalized erythema, urticaria, and angioedema. Commonly seen on the face and in the oral cavity and lower pharynx, angioedema develops as a result of fluid leaking into the interstitial space. The patient may appear restless, uneasy, apprehensive, and anxious and may complain of being warm. Respiratory effects include the development of laryngeal edema, bronchoconstriction, and mucous plugs. Clinical manifestations of laryngeal edema include inspiratory stridor, hoarseness, a sensation of fullness or a lump in the throat, and dysphagia. Bronchoconstriction causes dyspnea, wheezing, and chest tightness.[65,66,69] Gastrointestinal and genitourinary manifestations, which may develop as a result of smooth muscle contraction, include vomiting, diarrhea, cramping, and abdominal pain.

As the anaphylactic reaction progresses, hypotension and reflex tachycardia develop. This occurs in response to massive vasodilation and loss of circulating volume. Jugular veins appear flat as right ventricular end-diastolic volume is decreased. The eventual outcome is circulatory failure and ineffective tissue perfusion.[65,66,69] The patient's level of consciousness may deteriorate to unresponsiveness.

Assessment of the hemodynamic parameters of a patient in anaphylactic shock reveals a decreased CO and CI. Venous vasodilation and massive volume loss lead to a decrease in preload, which results in a decline in the RAP and PAOP. Vasodilation of the arterial system results in a decrease in the afterload of the heart, as evidenced by a decrease in the SVR. Box 26-8 outlines the clinical criteria for diagnosing anaphylaxis.

Medical Management

Treatment of anaphylactic shock requires an immediate and direct approach. The goals of therapy are to remove the offending antigen, reverse the effects of the biochemical mediators, and promote adequate tissue perfusion. When the hypersensitivity reaction occurs as a result of administration of medications, dye, blood, or blood products, the infusion should be immediately discontinued. Often, it is not possible to remove the antigen because it is unknown or has already entered the patient's system.

BOX 26-7	CLINICAL MANIFESTATIONS OF ANAPHYLACTIC SHOCK

Cardiovascular
- Hypotension
- Tachycardia

Respiratory
- Lump in throat
- Cough
- Dyspnea
- Dysphagia
- Hoarseness
- Stridor
- Wheezing
- Rales and rhonchi

Cutaneous
- Pruritus
- Erythema
- Urticaria
- Angioedema

Neurological
- Restlessness
- Uneasiness
- Apprehension
- Anxiety
- Dizziness
- Headache
- Decreased level of consciousness

Gastrointestinal
- Nausea
- Vomiting
- Diarrhea
- Abdominal pain

Genitourinary
- Incontinence
- Vaginal bleeding

Subjective Complaints
- Sensation of warmth
- Dyspnea
- Abdominal cramping and pain
- Itching

Hemodynamic Parameters
- Decreased cardiac output (CO)
- Decreased cardiac index (CI)
- Decreased right atrial pressure (RAP)
- Decreased pulmonary occlusion pressure (PAOP)
- Decreased systemic vascular resistance (SVR)

BOX 26-8	CLINICAL CRITERIA FOR DIAGNOSING ANAPHYLAXIS

Anaphylaxis is highly likely when one of the following three criteria is fulfilled:

1. Acute onset of an illness (minutes to several hours) with involvement of the skin or mucosal tissue, or both (e.g., generalized hives; pruritus or flushing; swollen lips, tongue, and uvula) *and at least one of the following:*
   a. Respiratory compromise (e.g., dyspnea, wheeze [bronchospasm], stridor, reduced peak expiratory flow, hypoxemia)
   b. Reduced blood pressure or associated symptoms of end-organ dysfunction (e.g., hypotonia [collapse], syncope, incontinence)
2. Two or more of the following that occur rapidly after exposure *to a likely allergen for that patient* (minutes to several hours):
   a. Involvement of the skin-mucosal tissue (e.g., generalized hives; pruritus or flushing; swollen lips, tongue, and uvula)
   b. Respiratory compromise (e.g., dyspnea, wheeze [bronchospasm], stridor, reduced peak expiratory flow, hypoxemia)
   c. Reduced blood pressure or associated symptoms of end-organ dysfunction (e.g., hypotonia [collapse], syncope, incontinence)
   d. Persistent gastrointestinal symptoms (e.g., crampy abdominal pain, vomiting)
3. Reduced blood pressure after exposure *to known allergen for that patient* (minutes to several hours):
   a. Infants and children: low systolic blood pressure (age-specific) or greater than 30% decrease in systolic blood pressure*
   b. Adults: systolic blood pressure of less than 90 mm Hg or greater than 30% decrease for the person's baseline

From Sampson HA, et al: Second symposium on the definition and management of anaphylaxis: summary report – second National Institute of Allergy and Infectious Disease/Food Allergy and Anaphylaxis Network symposium, *J Allergy Clin Immunol* 117(2):391, 2006.

*Low systolic blood pressure is defined as less than 70 mm Hg for children 1 month to 1 year old, less than (70 mm Hg + [2 × age]) for children 1 to 10 years old, and less than 90 mm Hg for children 11 to 17 years old.

Reversal of the effects of the biochemical mediators involves the preservation and support of the patient's airway, ventilation, and circulation. This is accomplished through oxygen therapy, intubation, mechanical ventilation, and administration of drugs and fluids.

Epinephrine is the first-line treatment of choice for anaphylaxis. It promotes bronchodilation and vasoconstriction and inhibits further release of biochemical mediators. In mild cases of anaphylaxis, 0.3 to 0.5 mg (0.3 to 0.5 mL) of a 1:1000 dilution of epinephrine is administered by intramuscular injection into the anterolateral thigh and repeated every 5 to 15 minutes until anaphylaxis is resolved.[65,66,70-72] Subcutaneous injection is no longer recommended.[71] For anaphylactic shock with hypotension, epinephrine is administered intravenously. The intravenous dose is 0.1 (1 mL) of a 1:10,000 dilution administered over 5 minutes. If hypotension persists, a continuous infusion of epinephrine is recommended, administered at 1 to 4 mcg/min with titration up to 10 mcg/min as needed.[66,67,69,73] Patients receiving beta-blockers may have a limited response to epinephrine. Intravenous glucagon administered as a 20 to 30 mcg/kg bolus over 5 minutes followed by continuous infusion at 5 to 15 mcg/minute is recommended for inotropic and vasoactive support for these patients.[65,66,71,73]

Diphenhydramine (Benadryl), given 1 to 2 mg/kg (25 to 50 mg) by a slow intravenous route every 4 to 8 hours, is a second-line agent used to block the histamine response.[65,66,69,71,73] Corticosteroids also may be given with the goal of preventing a delayed reaction and stabilizing capillary membranes.[65,66,71] Fluid replacement is accomplished by use of a crystalloid or colloid solution. Positive inotropic agents and vasoconstrictor agents may be necessary to reverse the effects of myocardial depression and vasodilation.[65,66,69,71]

Nursing Management

Prevention of anaphylactic shock is one of the primary responsibilities of the nurse in the critical care area. Preventive measures include the identification of patients at risk and cautious assessment of the patient's response to the administration of drugs, blood, and blood products. A complete and accurate history of the patient's allergies is an essential component of preventive nursing care. In addition to a list of the allergies, a detailed description of the type of response for each one should be obtained.

The patient in anaphylactic shock may have any number of nursing diagnoses, depending on the progression of the process (Nursing Diagnosis Priorities Box on Anaphylactic Shock). **Nursing priorities are directed toward (1) facilitating ventilation, (2) administering volume replacement, (3) providing comfort and emotional support, and (4) maintaining surveillance for complications.**

NURSING DIAGNOSIS PRIORITIES

Anaphylactic Shock

- Deficient Fluid Volume related to relative loss, p. A-13
- Decreased Cardiac Output related to alterations in preload, p. A-10
- Decreased Cardiac Output related to alterations in afterload, p. A-10
- Ineffective Breathing Pattern related to decreased lung expansion, p. A-27
- Impaired Gas Exchange related to ventilation/perfusion mismatching or intrapulmonary shunting, p. A-23
- Imbalanced Nutrition: Less Than Body Requirements related to increased metabolic demands or lack of exogenous nutrients, p. A-22
- Risk for Infection, p. A-36
- Ineffective Coping related to situational crisis and personal vulnerability, p. A-30
- Compromised Family Coping related to a critically ill family member, p. A-9

Measures to facilitate ventilation include positioning the patient to assist with breathing and instructing the patient to breathe slowly and deeply. Airway protection through prompt administration of prescribed medications is essential. Measures to facilitate the administration of volume replacement

include inserting large-bore peripheral intravenous catheters; rapidly administering prescribed fluids; and positioning the patient with the legs elevated, trunk flat, and head and shoulders above the chest. Measures to promote comfort include administering medications to relieve itching, applying warm soaks to skin, and if necessary, covering the patient's hands to discourage scratching. Observing the patient for clinical manifestations of a delayed reaction is critical. Patient education about how to avoid the precipitating allergen is essential for preventing future episodes of anaphylaxis.

NEUROGENIC SHOCK

Neurogenic shock, another type of distributive shock, is the result of the loss or suppression of sympathetic tone. The lack of sympathetic tone leads to decreased tissue perfusion and initiation of the general shock response. Neurogenic shock is the most uncommon form of shock.

Etiology

Neurogenic shock can be caused by anything that disrupts the SNS. The problem can occur as the result of interrupted impulse transmission or blockage of sympathetic outflow from the vasomotor center in the brain.[74-76] The most common cause is spinal cord injury. Neurogenic shock may mistakenly be referred to as *spinal shock*. The latter condition refers to loss of neurological activity below the level of spinal cord injury, but it does not necessarily involve ineffective tissue perfusion.[77-79]

Pathophysiology

Loss of sympathetic tone results in massive peripheral vasodilation, inhibition of the baroreceptor response, and impaired thermoregulation. Arterial vasodilation leads to a decrease in SVR and a fall in blood pressure. Venous vasodilation leads to relative hypovolemia and pooling of blood in the venous circuit. The decreased venous return results in a decrease in end-diastolic volume or preload, causing a decrease in SV and CO. The fall in blood pressure and CO leads to inadequate or ineffective tissue perfusion. Loss of sympathetic tone and inhibition of the baroreceptor response result in bradycardia.[74-76,78] The slow heart rate worsens CO, which further compromises tissue perfusion. Impaired thermoregulation occurs because of loss of vasomotor tone in the cutaneous blood vessels that dilate and constrict to maintain body temperature. The patient becomes poikilothermic, or dependent on the environment for temperature regulation (Figure 26-4).

Assessment and Diagnosis

The patient in neurogenic shock characteristically presents with hypotension, bradycardia, and warm, dry skin.[74-76] The decreased blood pressure results from massive peripheral vasodilation. The decreased heart rate is caused by inhibition of the baroreceptor response and unopposed parasympathetic control of the heart.[79] Hypothermia develops from uncontrolled peripheral heat loss. The warm, dry skin occurs

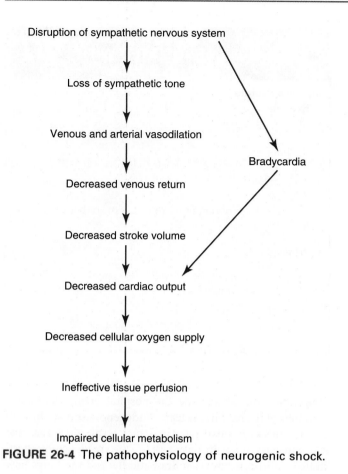

FIGURE 26-4 The pathophysiology of neurogenic shock.

as a consequence of pooling of blood in the extremities and loss of vasomotor control in surface vessels of the skin that control heat loss.

Assessment of the hemodynamic parameters of a patient in neurogenic shock reveals a decreased CO and CI. Venous vasodilation leads to a decrease in preload, which results in a decline in the RAP and PAOP. Vasodilation of the arterial system causes a decrease in the afterload of the heart, as evidenced by a decrease in the SVR.[76]

Medical Management

Treatment of neurogenic shock requires a careful approach. The goals of therapy are to treat or remove the cause, prevent cardiovascular instability, and promote optimal tissue perfusion. Cardiovascular instability can result from hypovolemia, bradycardia, and hypothermia. Specific treatments are aimed at preventing or correcting these problems as they occur.

Hypovolemia is treated with careful fluid resuscitation. The minimal amount of fluid is administered to ensure adequate tissue perfusion. Volume replacement is initiated for systolic blood pressure lower than 90 mm Hg, urine output of less than 30 mL/hour, or changes in mental status that indicate decreased cerebral tissue perfusion. The patient is carefully observed for evidence of fluid overload. Vasopressors are used as necessary to maintain blood pressure and organ perfusion.[74,76,78] The bradycardia associated with neurogenic shock rarely requires specific treatment, but atropine

or electrical pacing can be used when necessary.[69,74] Hypothermia is treated with warming measures and environmental temperature regulation.

Nursing Management

Prevention of neurogenic shock is one of the primary responsibilities of the nurse in the critical care area. This includes the identification of patients at risk and constant assessment of the neurological status. Vigilant immobilization of spinal cord injuries and slight elevation of the head of the patient's bed after spinal anesthesia are essential components of preventive nursing care. Early identification allows for early treatment and decreased mortality.

The patient in neurogenic shock may have any number of nursing diagnoses, depending on the progression of the process (Nursing Diagnosis Priorities Box on Neurogenic Shock). **Nursing priorities are directed toward (1) treating hypovolemia, (2) maintaining normothermia, (3) monitoring for dysrhythmias, (4) providing comfort and emotional support, and (5) maintaining surveillance for complications.**

NURSING DIAGNOSIS PRIORITIES
Neurogenic Shock

- Deficient Fluid Volume related to relative loss, p. A-13
- Decreased Cardiac Output related to sympathetic blockade, p. A-12
- Hypothermia related to exposure to cold environment, trauma, or damage to the hypothalamus, p. A-21
- Imbalanced Nutrition: Less Than Body Requirements related to increased metabolic demands or lack of exogenous nutrients, p. A-22
- Risk for Infection, p. A-36
- Anxiety related to threat to biological, psychological, or social integrity, p. A-7
- Compromised Family Coping related to a critically ill family member, p. A-9

Venous pooling in the lower extremities promotes the formation of deep vein thrombosis (DVT), which can result in a pulmonary embolism. All patients at risk for DVT should be started on prophylaxis therapy. DVT-prophylactic measures include monitoring of calf and thigh measurements, passive range-of-motion exercises, application of sequential pneumatic stockings, and administration of prescribed anticoagulation therapy.

SEVERE SEPSIS AND SEPTIC SHOCK

Sepsis occurs when microorganisms invade the body and initiate a systemic inflammatory response. This host response often results in perfusion abnormalities with organ dysfunction (severe sepsis) and eventually hypotension (septic shock). The primary mechanism of this type of shock is the maldistribution of blood flow to the tissues.[3] Severe sepsis is estimated to occur in more than 750,000 patients annually in

Exogenous sources include the hospital environment and members of the health care team. Endogenous sources include the patient's skin, gastrointestinal tract, respiratory tract, and genitourinary tract. In recent years, the incidence of chest-related infections has risen dramatically, and the lungs have replaced the intraabdominal organs as the most common site of infection producing severe sepsis and septic shock.[83,84] Gram-positive bacteria are responsible for more than one half of the cases of sepsis.[85] Sepsis and septic shock are associated with a wide variety of intrinsic and extrinsic precipitating factors (Box 26-10). All of these factors interfere directly or indirectly with the body's anatomic and physiological defense mechanisms. Several of the intrinsic factors are not modifiable or are very difficult to control. Several of the extrinsic factors may be required for diagnosis and management. All critically ill patients are therefore at risk for septic shock.[80]

Pathophysiology

The syndrome encompassing severe sepsis and septic shock is a complex systemic response that is initiated when a microorganism enters the body and stimulates the inflammatory/immune system. Shed protein fragments and the release of toxins and other substances from the microorganism activate the plasma enzyme cascades (complement, kinin/kallikrein, coagulation, and fibrinolytic factors), as well as platelets, neutrophils, monocytes, and macrophages. On activation, these systems and cells release a variety of mediators, or cytokines, that initiate a chain of complex interactions leading to a maladaptive SIRS.[86-91]

After the mediators are activated, a variety of physiological and pathophysiological events occur that affect clotting, the distribution of blood flow to the tissues and organs, capillary membrane permeability, and the metabolic state of the body.

the United States, with an estimated mortality rate of 30% to 50%.[80] It is the leading cause of death in noncoronary critical care units.[15]

Specific terms are used to describe the continuum of conditions that the patient with an infection may experience. In 1991 at the American College of Chest Physicians/Society of Critical Care Medicine (ACCP/SCCM) Consensus Conference, definitions were developed to describe and differentiate these conditions (Box 26-9).[81] These definitions were clarified and reinforced in subsequent conferences in 2001, 2004, and 2008.[15,16,82] This discussion focuses on severe sepsis and septic shock.

Etiology

Sepsis is caused by a wide variety of microorganisms, including gram-negative and gram-positive aerobes, anaerobes, fungi, and viruses. The source of these microorganisms varies.

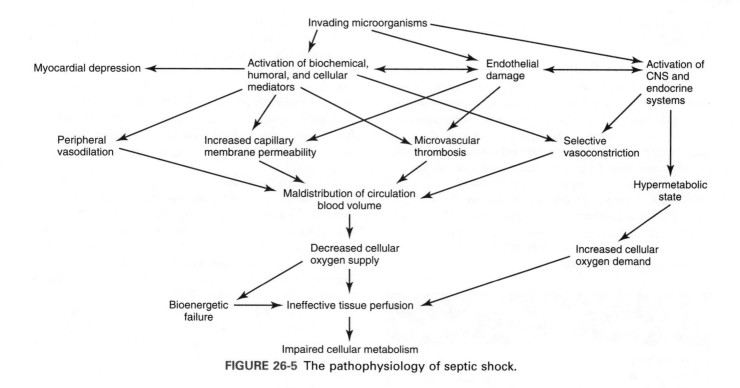

FIGURE 26-5 The pathophysiology of septic shock.

Subsequently, a systemic imbalance between cellular oxygen supply and demand develops that results in cellular hypoxia, damage, hibernation, and death (Figure 26-5).[4,88,90,91]

Hallmarks of severe sepsis are endothelial damage and coagulation dysfunction.[87,88,92,93] Tissue factor is released from endothelial cells and monocytes in response to stimulation by the inflammatory cytokines.[87,88] Release of tissue factor initiates the coagulation cascade, producing widespread microvascular thrombosis and further stimulation of the systemic inflammatory pathways.[88] Diffuse endothelial damage impairs endogenous anticlotting mechanisms.[88] Mediator-induced suppression of fibrinolysis slows clot breakdown. The result is DIC with eventual consumption of coagulation factors, bleeding, and hemorrhage.[92,94]

Significant alterations in cardiovascular hemodynamics are caused by the activation of inflammatory cytokines and endothelial damage.[32,88,93] Massive peripheral vasodilation results in the development of relative hypovolemia. Increased capillary permeability produces a loss of intravascular volume to the interstitium, which accentuates the reduction in preload and CO. These changes, coupled with the microvascular thrombosis, produce maldistribution of circulating blood volume, decreased tissue perfusion, and inadequate oxygen delivery to the cells. Microcirculatory shunting is a key feature of this distributive shock.[88,95,96] Impaired ventricular contractility results from cytokine activity.[4,88]

Activation of the central nervous and endocrine systems also occurs as part of the response to invading microorganisms. This activation leads to stimulation of the SNS and the release of ACTH. These events trigger the release of epinephrine, norepinephrine, glucocorticoids, aldosterone, glucagon, renin, and growth hormone resulting in the development of

a hypermetabolic state and contributing to vasoconstriction of the renal, pulmonary, and splanchnic beds. Selective vasoconstriction in the splanchnic bed may contribute to hypoperfusion of the gastric mucosa. The resulting gut injury propagates the inflammatory response.[2,97]

Several metabolic alterations occur as a result of CNS, endocrine system, and cytokine activation. The hypermetabolic state increases energy expenditure and oxygen demand, and it contributes to cellular hypoxia. Lactic acid is produced as a result of increased metabolic lactate production and hypoxic anaerobic metabolism. Glucocorticoids, ACTH, epinephrine, glucagon, and growth hormone are all catabolic hormones that are released as part of this response. In conjunction with the inflammatory cytokines, these hormones stimulate catabolism of protein stores in the visceral organs and skeletal muscles to fuel glucose production in the liver, hyperglycemia, and insulin resistance.[8] The cytokines also stimulate the use of fats for energy production (lipolysis).[8,91,98]

Metabolic derangements in severe sepsis and septic shock include an inability of the cells to use oxygen even if blood flow is adequate. Mitochondrial dysfunction is thought to be the underlying mechanism.[88,91,98] This bioenergetic failure plays an important role in the development of multiple organ dysfunction.[88,91,98] The exaggerated inflammatory response in severe sepsis results in apoptosis, a programmed cell death or cellular suicide affecting endothelial and immune cells in particular.[88,91,93]

These complex and interrelated pathophysiological changes associated with severe sepsis and septic shock produce a pathological imbalance between cellular oxygen demand and cellular oxygen supply and consumption. If unabated, this situation ultimately results in tissue ischemia, MODS, and death.

Assessment and Diagnosis

Effective treatment of severe sepsis and septic shock depends on timely recognition. The diagnosis of severe sepsis is based on the identification of three conditions: known or suspected infection, two or more of the clinical indications of the systemic inflammatory response, and evidence of at least one organ dysfunction. Clinical indications of systemic inflammatory response and sepsis were included in the original ACCP/SCCM consensus definitions and are listed in Box 26-9. The second consensus conference expanded this list to facilitate prompt clinical recognition (Box 26-11).[82]

Signs of individual organ dysfunction are discussed later in the chapter. The two most common organs to demonstrate

dysfunction in severe sepsis are the cardiovascular system and the lungs. The patient with persistent hypotension requiring vasopressor therapy despite adequate volume resuscitation is demonstrating cardiovascular dysfunction. Pulmonary dysfunction is manifested by a PaO_2/FiO_2 (fraction of oxygen in inspired air) ratio of less than 300, indicating ALI.[87] Signs indicating septic shock are hypotension despite adequate fluid resuscitation and the presence of perfusion abnormalities such as lactic acidosis, oliguria, or acute change in mentation.

The patient in severe sepsis or septic shock may present with a variety of clinical manifestations that may change dynamically as the condition progresses (Box 26-12). During the initial stage, massive vasodilation occurs in the venous and arterial beds. Dilation of the venous system leads to a decrease in venous return to the heart, which results in a decrease in the preload of the right and left ventricles. This is evidenced by a decline in the RAP and PAOP. Dilation of the arterial system results in a decrease in the afterload of the heart, as evidenced by a decrease in the SVR. The patient's skin becomes pink, warm, and flushed as a result of the massive vasodilation. Myocardial contractility is decreased, as evidenced by a decline in the left ventricular stroke work index (LVSWI).

The heart rate rises in response to increased SNS, metabolic, and adrenal gland stimulation. If circulating volume and preload are adequate, this results in a normal-to-high CO and CI despite impaired contractility. The pulse pressure widens as the diastolic blood pressure decreases because of

---

BOX 26-11 EXPANDED LIST OF DIAGNOSTIC CRITERIA FOR SEPSIS

General Variables
- Core temperature >38.3° or <36° C
- Heart rate >90 beats/min
- Tachypnea
- Altered mental status
- Significant edema or positive fluid balance >20 mL/kg over 24 hours
- Hyperglycemia (>120 mg/dL) in absence of diabetes

Inflammatory Variables
- WBC count >12,000, <4000 mm³, or >10% immature forms
- Elevated plasma C-reactive protein level
- Elevated plasma procalcitonin level

Hemodynamic Variables
- Systolic BP <90 mm Hg or decrease >40 mm Hg
- Mean arterial pressure <70 mm Hg
- SvO_2 >70%
- CI >3.5 L/m/m³

Tissue Perfusion Variables
- Serum lactate level >1 mmol/L
- Decreased capillary refill or mottling

Organ Dysfunction Variables
- PaO_2/FiO_2 <300
- Urine output <0.5 mL/kg/hr
- Creatinine increase >0.5 mg/dL
- INR >1.5 or aPTT >60 sec
- Ileus
- Platelet count <100,000 mm³
- Hyperbilirubinemia (plasma total bilirubin >4 mg/dL)

Modified from Levy MM, et al: 2001 SCCM/ESICM/ACCP/ATS/SIS International Sepsis Definitions Conference, *Crit Care Med* 31(4):1250, 2003.
aPTT, activated partial thromboplastin time; *BP*, blood pressure; *CI*, cardiac index; *FiO₂*, fraction of oxygen in inspired air; *INR*, international normalized ratio; *PaO₂*, partial pressure of oxygen; *SvO₂*, mixed venous oxygen saturation; *WBC*, white blood cells.

BOX 26-12 CLINICAL MANIFESTATIONS OF SEPTIC SHOCK

- Increased heart rate
- Decreased blood pressure
- Wide pulse pressure
- Full, bounding pulse
- Pink, warm, flushed skin
- Increased respiratory rate (early) or decreased respiratory rate (late)
- Crackles
- Change in sensorium
- Decreased urine output
- Increased temperature
- Increased cardiac output and cardiac index
- Decreased systemic vascular resistance
- Decreased right atrial pressure
- Decreased pulmonary artery occlusion pressure
- Decreased left ventricular stroke work index
- Decreased PaO_2
- Decreased $PaCO_2$ (early) or increased $PaCO_2$ (late)
- Decreased HCO_3^-
- Increased SvO_2 or $ScvO_2$

PaCO₂, partial pressure of carbon dioxide; *PaO₂*, partial pressure of oxygen; *SvO₂*, mixed venous oxygen saturation; *ScvO₂*, central venous oxygen saturation.

the vasodilation, and the systolic blood pressure increases because of the elevated CO. A full, bounding pulse develops. The net result of these changes is a relatively normal blood pressure in severe sepsis. However, as the reduction in preload and afterload becomes overwhelming and contractility fails, hypotension ensues, resulting in septic shock.

In the lungs, ventilation/perfusion mismatching develops as a result of pulmonary vasoconstriction and the formation of pulmonary microemboli. Hypoxemia occurs, and the respiratory rate increases to compensate for the lack of oxygen. Crackles develop as increased pulmonary capillary membrane permeability leads to pulmonary edema.[79]

The level of consciousness starts to change as a result of decreased cerebral perfusion, immune mediator activation, hyperthermia, and lactic acidosis. This septic encephalopathy is demonstrated by acute onset of impaired cognitive functioning, or delirium, which may fluctuate during its course.[80] The patient may appear disoriented, confused, combative, or lethargic.

ABG values initially reveal hypocarbia, hypoxemia, and metabolic acidosis. This is demonstrated by a low Pa_{O_2}, low Pa_{CO_2}, and low HCO_3^- level, respectively. The respiratory alkalosis is caused by the patient's increased respiratory rate. As pathological pulmonary changes progress and the patient becomes fatigued, the effectiveness of respirations decreases and the Pa_{CO_2} increases, resulting in respiratory acidosis. The metabolic acidosis is the result of a lack of oxygen to the cells and the development of lactic acidemia. Serum lactate levels increase above 2 mmol/L because of anaerobic metabolism. The mixed venous oxygen saturation (Sv_{O_2}) may increase because of microcirculatory shunting or decrease because of inadequate oxygen delivery.[88,96] The white blood cell (WBC) count is elevated as part of the immune response to the invading microorganisms. The WBC differential count reveals an increase in immature neutrophils (shift to the left). This occurs because the body has to mobilize increasing numbers of WBCs to fight the infection. An elevated procalcitonin level is a valuable indicator of significant infection.[88,99] Serum glucose levels increase as part of the hypermetabolic response and the development of insulin resistance. The patient's temperature is elevated in response to pyrogens released from the invading microorganisms, immune mediator activation, and increased metabolic activity. Urine output declines because of decreased perfusion of the kidneys. As impaired tissue perfusion develops, a variety of other clinical manifestations appear that indicate the development of MODS.

Medical Management

Treatment of the patient in severe sepsis or septic shock requires a multifaceted approach. The goals of treatment are to reverse the pathophysiological responses, control the infection, and promote metabolic support. This approach includes supporting the cardiovascular system and enhancing tissue perfusion, identifying and treating the infection, limiting the systemic inflammatory response, restoring metabolic balance, and initiating nutritional therapy. Dysfunction of the individual organ systems must be prevented. Early treatment

---

BOX 26-13   SEVERE SEPSIS BUNDLES

Sepsis Resuscitation Bundle

The goal is to perform all indicated tasks 100% of the time within the first 6 hours of identification of severe sepsis. The tasks are:

1. Measure serum lactate.
2. Obtain blood cultures prior to antibiotic administration.
3. Administer broad-spectrum antibiotic, within 3 hrs of ED admission and within 1 hour of non-ED admission.
4. In the event of hypotension and/or a serum lactate >4 mmol/L:
   a. Deliver an initial minimum of 20 mL/kg of crystalloid or an equivalent.
   b. Apply vasopressors for hypotension not responding to initial fluid resuscitation to maintain mean arterial pressure (MAP) >65 mm Hg.
5. In the event of persistent hypotension despite fluid resuscitation (septic shock) and/or lactate >4 mmol/L:
   a. Achieve a central venous pressure (CVP) of >8 mm Hg.
   b. Achieve a central venous oxygen saturation (Scv_{O_2}) >70% or mixed venous oxygen saturation (Sv_{O_2}) >65%.

Sepsis Management Bundle

Efforts to accomplish these goals should begin immediately, but these items may be completed within 24 hours of presentation for patients with severe sepsis or septic shock.

1. Administer low-dose steroids for septic shock in accordance with a standardized ICU policy. If not administered, document why the patient did not qualify for low-dose steroids based upon the standardized protocol.
2. Maintain glucose control >70, but <150 mg/dL.
3. Maintain a median inspiratory plateau pressure (IPP)* <30 cm H_2O for mechanically ventilated patients.

From Surviving Sepsis Campaign: www.survivingsepsis.org/Bundles/Pages/default.aspx. Reproduced with permission. Copyright 2008. European Society of Intensive Care Medicine, International Sepsis Forum, and Society of Critical Care Medicine.

---

reduces mortality.[16,90,100,101] Guidelines for the management of severe sepsis and septic shock have been developed and updated under the auspices of the Surviving Sepsis Campaign (SSC), an international effort of more than 11 organizations to improve patient outcomes.[15,16] From these guidelines, a group ("bundle") of selected interventions was identified as having the most impact on patient outcomes (Box 26-13). The sepsis resuscitation bundle should be implemented within the first 6 hours, and the sepsis management bundle should be implemented within the first 24 hours. More information regarding these interventions is available at the SSC website (www.survivingsepsis.org).

The patient in severe sepsis or septic shock requires immediate resuscitation of the hypoperfused state. Specific interventions are aimed at increasing cellular oxygen supply and decreasing cellular oxygen demand. These treatments include administration of fluids, vasopressors, and positive inotropic agents. Early goal-directed therapy during the first 6 hours of resuscitation improves survival[100] and is recommended in the

SSC guidelines.[15,16] This therapy includes aggressive fluid resuscitation to augment intravascular volume and increase preload until a CVP of 8 to 12 mm Hg (12 to 15 mm Hg in mechanically ventilated patients) is achieved. Crystalloids or colloids may be used. A fluid challenge for hypovolemia should be initiated with at least 1000 mL of crystalloids or 300 to 500 mL of colloids over 30 minutes. Vasopressors (norepinephrine or dopamine as first-choice agents) should be administered as necessary to maintain a MAP of at least 65 mm Hg. These agents reverse the massive peripheral vasodilation and increase SVR. Epinephrine is recommended as an alternative agent if response to norepinephrine or dopamine is poor.[16] Arterial line placement is recommended for any patient requiring vasopressor therapy. Intermittent or continuous monitoring of central venous or mixed venous oxygen saturation ($Scvo_2$ or Svo_2) allows evaluation of the effectiveness of oxygen delivery. If the $Scvo_2$ is less than 70% or the Svo_2 is less than 65% after the CVP goal is achieved, administration of packed red cells to achieve a hematocrit of at least 30%[16] or inotropic stimulation with dobutamine (administered to a maximum of 20 mcg/kg/minute) to counteract myocardial depression and maintain adequate CO is recommended to obtain this goal.[16,100] The dobutamine infusion should be reduced or discontinued if a tachycardia greater than 120 beats/minute develops.[100]

Intubation and mechanical ventilatory support are usually required to optimize oxygenation and ventilation for the patient in severe sepsis or septic shock. Ventilation with lower than traditional tidal volumes (6 versus 12 mL/kg) in patients with ALI and acute respiratory distress syndrome (ARDS) decreases mortality.[102] SSC guidelines recommend the goals of 6 mL/kg of predicted body weight and plateau pressures no more than 30 cm H_2O for patients with severe sepsis or septic shock with ALI or ARDS.[16] Increased $Paco_2$ may result from this therapy and is acceptable if tolerated as evidenced by hemodynamic stability. Ventilator settings should include positive end-expiratory pressure and be adjusted to provide the patient with a Pao_2 greater than 70 mm Hg. Patients receiving mechanical ventilation should be maintained in a semirecumbent position with the head of the bed raised to 45 degrees to decrease the incidence of ventilator-associated pneumonia.[16] Prone positioning should be considered in the septic patient with ARDS requiring high levels of oxygen.[16] Sedation protocols using intermittent bolus or continuous infusion using a standardized sedation scale and specific goals are recommended for all patients requiring mechanical ventilation. Daily interruption of sedative infusions to allow wakefulness and reevaluation of sedation needs reduces duration of mechanical ventilation and is recommended.[16] Neuromuscular blocking agents should be avoided, if possible, to prevent prolonged blockade after discontinuation.[16]

A key measure in the treatment of septic shock is finding and eradicating the cause of the infection. At least two blood cultures plus urine, sputum, and wound cultures should be obtained to find the location of the infection before antibiotic therapy is initiated.[16] Antibiotic therapy should be started within 1 hour of recognition of severe sepsis without delay for cultures.[16] Each hour of delay is associated with a substantial drop in the survival rate.[101] If the microorganism is unknown, antiinfective therapy with one or more agents known to be effective against likely pathogens should be initiated, with daily reassessment of the regimen. Combination therapy is recommended for known or suspected *Pseudomonas* infection and for neutropenic patients but should be limited to less than 3 to 5 days.[16] A specific source of infection should be established within 6 hours of presentation.[16] Surgical intervention to débride infected or necrotic tissue or to drain abscesses may be necessary to facilitate removal of the septic source.[16] Intravascular devices that may be the source of the infection should be removed after establishment of alternative vascular access.

Intravenous corticosteroids reduce mortality in catecholamine-dependent septic shock patients with relative adrenal insufficiency.[107] Intravenous hydrocortisone is recommended only for the patient in septic shock who is poorly responsive to fluid resuscitation and vasopressor therapy.[16] Doses greater than 300 mg/day may be harmful and should not be used and steroid therapy should be weaned when vasopressors are no longer required.[16]

Continuous infusion of insulin and glucose to maintain a blood glucose level of 150 mg/dL or less improves outcomes[42] and is recommended by SSC guidelines after initial stabilization.[16] Glucose levels should be monitored every 1 to 2 hours until stable and then every 4 hours. Low glucose levels measured by capillary testing may be inaccurate in this population.[16] Platelets should be administered when counts are less than 5000/mm³ and red blood cell transfusions are recommended when the hemoglobin level is less than 7.0 g/dL to obtain a target value of 7 to 9 g/dL.[16] Stress ulcer prophylaxis using histamine₂ (H_2) blockers or proton-pump inhibitors and DVT prophylaxis are recommended for all patients with severe sepsis or septic shock. The SCCM guidelines recommend against the use of sodium bicarbonate for lactic acidemia if the pH is equal to or greater than 7.15.[16] Low-dose dopamine infusion for renal protection is not beneficial and should not be used.[16]

The initiation of nutritional therapy is critical in the management of the patient in severe sepsis or septic shock. The goal is to improve the patient's overall nutritional status, enhance immune function, and promote wound healing. A daily caloric intake of 25 to 30 kcal/kg of usual body weight is recommended. The enteral route is preferred. The ideal nutritional supplement for the patient in septic shock should be high in protein because of the metabolic derangements that develop in the hypermetabolic state. The amount of protein calories given depends on the patient's nitrogen balance. In early sepsis, the mix of nonprotein calories may be divided evenly between carbohydrates and fats. In the later stages, significant alterations in fat metabolism occur, and the lipid content should be limited to 10% to 15% of the total nonprotein calories. Specific nutritional therapies to reduce the inflammatory and hypermetabolic responses associated with sepsis, such as antioxidant supplementation and feeding with long-chain n-3 polyunsaturated fatty acids, are the source of much debate and are being evaluated.[8,108-111] Glutamine is considered by some to be an essential amino acid in critically ill patients and has the most empirical support.[88,108,109,111] Arginine has produced negative outcomes and is not recommended.[110]

Nursing Management

Prevention of severe sepsis and septic shock is one of the primary responsibilities of the nurse in the critical care area. These measures include the identification of patients at risk and reduction of their exposure to invading microorganisms. Hand washing, aseptic technique, and an understanding of how microorganisms can invade the body are essential components of preventive nursing care. Early identification allows for early treatment and decreases mortality.[80] Box 26-14 depicts a simple screening tool for identifying patients with severe sepsis.

The patient in septic shock may have any number of nursing diagnoses, depending on the progression of the

---

NURSING DIAGNOSIS PRIORITIES
Septic Shock

- Deficient Fluid Volume related to relative loss, p. A-13
- Decreased Cardiac Output related to alterations in preload, p. A-10
- Decreased Cardiac Output related to alterations in afterload, p. A-10
- Decreased Cardiac Output related to alterations in contractility, p. A-11
- Impaired Gas Exchange related to ventilation/perfusion mismatching or intrapulmonary shunting, p. A-23
- Imbalanced Nutrition: Less Than Body Requirements related to increased metabolic demands or lack of exogenous nutrients, p. A-22
- Risk for Infection, p. A-36
- Anxiety related to threat to biological, psychological, or social integrity, p. A-7
- Compromised Family Coping related to a critically ill family member, p. A-9

BOX 26-14   EVALUATION FOR SEVERE SEPSIS SCREENING TOOL

Instructions: use this optional tool to screen patients for severe sepsis in the emergency department, on the wards, or in the ICU.

1. Is the patient's history suggestive of a new infection?

☐ Pneumonia, empyema	☐ Skin/soft tissue infection	☐ Endocarditis
☐ Urinary tract infection	☐ Bone/joint infection	☐ Implantable device infection
☐ Acute abdominal infection	☐ Wound infection	☐ Other _____
☐ Meningitis	☐ Bloodstream catheter infection	**___Yes ___No**

2. Are any two of following signs & symptoms of infection both present and new to the patient? *Note*: laboratory values may have been obtained for inpatients but may not be available for outpatients.

☐ Hyperthermia >38.3 °C (101.0 °F)	☐ Acutely altered mental status	☐ Hyperglycemia (plasma glucose
☐ Hypothermia <36 °C (96.8°F)	☐ Leukocytosis (WBC count	>120 mg/dL) in the absence of
☐ Tachycardia >90 bpm	>12,000 mcg–1)	diabetes
☐ Tachypnea >20 bpm	☐ Leukopenia (WBC count <4000 mcg–1)	**___Yes ___No**

If the answer is yes to both either question 1 and 2, *suspicion of infection* is present:

✓ Obtain: **lactic acid**, **blood cultures**, CBC with differential, basic chemistry labs, bilirubin.

✓ At the physician's discretion obtain: UA, chest x-ray, amylase, lipase, ABG, CRP, CT scan.

3. Are any of the following organ dysfunction criteria present at a site remote from the site of the infection that are not considered to be chronic conditions? *Note*: the remote site stipulation is waived in the case of bilateral pulmonary infiltrates.

☐ SBP <90 mmHg or MAP <65 mmHg	☐ Bilateral pulmonary infiltrates with	☐ Platelet count <100,000
☐ SBP decrease >40 mm Hg from	PaO$_2$/FiO$_2$ ratio <300	☐ Coagulopathy (INR >1.5 or aPTT
baseline	☐ Creatinine > 2.0 mg/dl (176.8 mmol/L)	>60 secs)
☐ Bilateral pulmonary infiltrates with a	or Urine Output < 0.5 ml/kg/hour for	☐ Lactate >2 mmol/L (18.0 mg/dl)
new (or increased) oxygen	>2 hours	
requirement to maintain SpO$_2$ >90%	☐ Bilirubin >2 mg/dl (34.2 mmol/L)	**___Yes ___No**

If *suspicion of infection* is present AND *organ dysfunction* is present, the patient meets the criteria for SEVERE SEPSIS and should be entered into the severe sepsis protocol.

Date: ____/____/____ (circle: dd/mm/yy or mm/dd/yy)   Time: ____: ____ (24 hr. clock)

Version 7.12.2005   © 2005 Surviving Sepsis Campaign and the Institute for Healthcare Improvement

From the Institute for Healthcare Improvement, Cambridge, MA.

process (Nursing Diagnosis Priorities Box on Septic Shock). **Nursing priorities are directed toward (1) early identification of sepsis syndrome, (2) administering prescribed fluids and medications, (3) providing comfort and emotional support, and (4) maintaining surveillance for complications.** Continual observation to detect subtle changes

that indicate the progression of the septic process is also very important.

Evidence-based guidelines for the management of the patient with severe sepsis or septic shock are listed in the Evidence-Based Practice box on Severe Sepsis and Septic Shock Management Guidelines.

EVIDENCE-BASED COLLABORATIVE PRACTICE
Severe Sepsis and Septic Shock Management Guidelines

Strength of recommendation and quality of evidence have been assessed using the GRADE criteria, presented in parentheses after each guideline.

Initial Resuscitation (First 6 hrs)
- Begin resuscitation immediately in patients with hypotension or elevated serum lactate >4 mmol/L; do not delay pending ICU admission (1C).
- Resuscitation goals (1C):
  - CVP 8-12 mm Hg[a]
  - Mean arterial pressure ≥65 mm Hg
  - Urine output ≥0.5 mL/kg^{-1}/hr^{-1}
  - Central venous (superior vena cava) oxygen saturation ≥70% or mixed venous ≥65%
- If venous oxygen saturation target is not achieved (2C):
  - Consider further fluid.
  - Transfuse packed red blood cells if required to hematocrit of ≥30%, and/or.
  - Start dobutamine infusion, maximum 20 mcg/kg^{-1}/min^{-1}.
  - A higher target CVP of 12-15 mm Hg is recommended in the presence of mechanical ventilation or preexisting decreased ventricular compliance.

Diagnosis
- Obtain appropriate cultures before starting antibiotics provided this does not significantly delay antimicrobial administration (1C).
  - Obtain two or more BCs.
  - One or more BCs should be percutaneous.
  - One BC from each vascular access device in place >48 hrs.
  - Culture other sites as clinically indicated.
- Perform imaging studies promptly to confirm and sample any source of infection, if safe to do so (1C).

Antibiotic Therapy
- Begin intravenous antibiotics as early as possible and always within the first hour of recognizing severe sepsis (1D) and septic shock (1B).
- Broad-spectrum: one or more agents active against likely bacterial/fungal pathogens and with good penetration into presumed source (1B).
- Reassess antimicrobial regimen daily to optimize efficacy, prevent resistance, avoid toxicity, and minimize costs (1C).
  - Consider combination therapy in *Pseudomonas* infections (2D).
  - Consider combination empiric therapy in neutropenic patients (2D).
  - Combination therapy ≤3-5 days and de-escalation following susceptibilities (2D).

- Duration of therapy typically limited to 7-10 days; longer if response is slow or there are undrainable foci of infection or immunological deficiencies (1D).
- Stop antimicrobial therapy if cause is found to be noninfectious (1D).

Source Identification and Control
- A specific anatomic site of infection should be established as rapidly as possible (1C) and within first 6 hrs of presentation (1D).
- Formally evaluate patient for a focus of infection amenable to source control measures (e.g., abscess drainage, tissue debridement) (1C).
- Implement source control measures as soon as possible following successful initial resuscitation (1C) (exception: infected pancreatic necrosis, where surgical intervention is best delayed) (2B).
- Choose source control measure with maximum efficacy and minimal physiological upset (1D).
- Remove intravascular access devices if potentially infected (1C).

Fluid Therapy
- Fluid-resuscitate using crystalloids or colloids (1B).
- Target a CVP of ≥8 mm Hg (≥12 mm Hg if mechanically ventilated) (1C).
- Use a fluid challenge technique while associated with a hemodynamic improvement (1D).
- Give fluid challenges of 1000 mL of crystalloids or 300-500 mL of colloids over 30 min. More rapid and larger volumes may be required in sepsis-induced tissue hypoperfusion (1D).
- Rate of fluid administration should be reduced if cardiac filling pressures increase without concurrent hemodynamic improvement (1D).

Vasopressors
- Maintain MAP ≥65 mm Hg (1C).
- Norepinephrine and dopamine centrally administered are the initial vasopressors of choice (1C).
- Epinephrine, phenylephrine, or vasopressin should not be administered as the initial vasopressor in septic shock (2C). Vasopressin 0.03 units/min may be subsequently added to norepinephrine with anticipation of an effect equivalent to norepinephrine alone.
- Use epinephrine as the first alternative agent in septic shock when blood pressure is poorly responsive to norepinephrine or dopamine (2B).
- Do not use low-dose dopamine for renal protection (1A).
- In patients requiring vasopressors, insert an arterial catheter as soon as practical (1D).

Severe Sepsis and Septic Shock Management Guidelines

Inotropic Therapy
- Use dobutamine in patients with myocardial dysfunction as supported by elevated cardiac filling pressures and low cardiac output (1C).
- Do not increase cardiac index to predetermined supranormal levels (1B).

Steroids
- Consider intravenous hydrocortisone for adult septic shock when hypotension responds poorly to adequate fluid resuscitation and vasopressors (2C).
- ACTH stimulation test is not recommended to identify the subset of adults with septic shock who should receive hydrocortisone (2B).
- Hydrocortisone is preferred to dexamethasone (2B).
- Fludrocortisone (50 mcg orally once a day) may be included if an alternative to hydrocortisone is being used that lacks significant mineralocorticoid activity. Fludrocortisone if optional if hydrocortisone is used (2C).
- Steroid therapy may be weaned once vasopressors are no longer required (2D).
- Hydrocortisone dose should be ≤300 mg/day (1A).
- Do not use corticosteroids to treat sepsis in the absence of shock unless the patient's endocrine or corticosteroid history warrants it (1D).

Recombinant Human Activated Protein C
- Consider rhAPC in adult patients with sepsis-induced organ dysfunction with clinical assessment of high risk of death (typically APACHE II ≥25 or multiple organ failure) if there are no contraindications (2B, 2C for postoperative patients).
- Adult patients with severe sepsis and low risk of death (typically, APACHE II <20 or one organ failure) should not receive rhAPC (1A).

Blood Product Administration
- Give red blood cells when hemoglobin decreases to <7.0 g/dL (<70 g/L) to target a hemoglobin of 7.0-9.0 g/dL in adults (1B). A higher hemoglobin level may be required in special circumstances (e.g., myocardial ischemia, severe hypoxemia, acute hemorrhage, cyanotic heart disease, or lactic acidosis).
- Do not use erythropoietin to treat sepsis-related anemia. Erythropoietin may be used for other accepted reasons (1B).
- Do not use fresh-frozen plasma to correct laboratory clotting abnormalities unless there is bleeding or planned invasive procedures (2D).
- Do not use antithrombin therapy (1B).
- Administer platelets when (2D):
  - Counts are <5000/mm³ (5 × 109/L) regardless of bleeding.
  - Counts are 5000-30,000/mm³ (5-30 × 109/L) and there is significant bleeding risk.
  - Higher platelet counts (≥50,000/mm³ [50 × 109/L]) are required for surgery or invasive procedures.

Mechanical Ventilation of Sepsis-Induced ALI/ARDS
- Target a tidal volume of 6 mL/kg (predicted) body weight in patients with ALI/ARDS (1B).
- Target an initial upper limit plateau pressure ≤30 cm H_2O. Consider chest wall compliance when assessing plateau pressure (1C).
- Allow $PaCO_2$ to increase above normal, if needed, to minimize plateau pressures and tidal volumes (1C).
- Set PEEP to avoid extensive lung collapse at end-expiration (1C).
- Consider using the prone position for ARDS patients requiring potentially injurious levels of FIO_2 or plateau pressure, provided they are not put at risk from positional changes (2C).
- Maintain mechanically ventilated patients in a semirecumbent position (head of the bed raised to 45°) unless contraindicated (1B), between 30° and 45° (2C).
- Noninvasive ventilation may be considered in the minority of ALI/ARDS patients with mild to moderate hypoxemic respiratory failure. The patients need to be hemodynamically stable, comfortable, easily arousable, able to protect/clear their airway, and expected to recover rapidly (2B).
- Use a weaning protocol and an SBT regularly to evaluate the potential for discontinuing mechanical ventilation (1A).
  - SBT options include a low level of pressure support with continuous positive airway pressure 5 cm H_2O or a T piece.
  - Before the SBT, patients should be arousable, be hemodynamically stable without vasopressors, have no new potentially serious conditions, have low ventilatory and end-expiratory pressure requirement, require FIO_2 levels that can be safely delivered with a face mask or nasal cannula.
- Do not use a pulmonary artery catheter for the routine monitoring of patients with ALI/ARDS (1A).
- Use a conservative fluid strategy for patients with established ALI who do not have evidence of tissue hypoperfusion (1C).

Sedation, Analgesia, and Neuromuscular Blockade in Sepsis
- Use sedation protocols with a sedation goal for critically ill mechanically ventilated patients (1B).
- Use either intermittent bolus sedation or continuous infusion sedation to predetermined end points (sedation scales), with daily interruption/lightening to produce awakening. Re-titrate if necessary (1B).
- Avoid neuromuscular blockers where possible. Monitor depth of block with train-of-four when using continuous infusions (1B).

Glucose Control
- Use intravenous insulin to control hyperglycemia in patients with severe sepsis following stabilization in the ICU (1B).
- Aim to keep blood glucose <150 mg/dL (8.3 mmol/L) using a validated protocol for insulin dose adjustment (2C).
- Provide a glucose calorie source and monitor blood glucose values every 1-2 hrs (4 hrs when stable) in patients receiving intravenous insulin (1C).

Continued

EVIDENCE-BASED COLLABORATIVE PRACTICE—cont'd

Severe Sepsis and Septic Shock Management Guidelines

- Interpret with caution low glucose levels obtained with point-of-care testing, as these techniques may overestimate arterial blood or plasma glucose values (1B).

Renal Replacement
- Intermittent hemodialysis and CVVH are considered equivalent (2B).
- CVVH offers easier management in hemodynamically unstable patients (2D).

Bicarbonate Therapy
- Do not use bicarbonate therapy for the purpose of improving hemodynamics or reducing vasopressor requirements when treating hypoperfusion-induced lactic acidemia with pH ≥7.15 (1B).

Deep Vein Thrombosis Prophylaxis
- Use either low-dose UFH or LMWH, unless contraindicated (1A).

- Use a mechanical prophylactic device, such as compression stockings or an intermittent compression device, when heparin is contraindicated (1A).
- Use a combination of pharmacological and mechanical therapy for patients who are at very high risk for deep vein thrombosis (2C).
- In patients at very high risk, LMWH should be used rather than UFH (2C).

Stress Ulcer Prophylaxis
- Provide stress ulcer prophylaxis using H_2 blocker (1A) or proton pump inhibitor (1B). Benefits of prevention of upper gastrointestinal bleed must be weighed against the potential for development of ventilator-acquired pneumonia.

Consideration for Limitation of Support
- Discuss advance care planning with patients and families. Describe likely outcomes and set realistic expectations (1D).

From Dellinger RP, et al: Surviving Sepsis Campaign: international guidelines for management of severe sepsis and septic shock: 2008, *Crit Care Med* 36(1):296, 2008.
GRADE, Grades of Recommendation, Assessment, Development and Evaluation; *ICU,* intensive care unit; *CVP,* central venous pressure; *BC,* blood culture; *MAP,* mean arterial pressure; *ACTH,* adrenocorticotropic hormone; *rhAPC,* recombinant human activated protein C; *APACHE,* Acute Physiology and Chronic Health Evaluation; *ALI,* acute lung injury; *ARDS,* acute respiratory distress syndrome; *PEEP,* positive end-expiratory pressure; *SBT,* spontaneous breathing trial; *CVVH,* continuous veno-venous hemofiltration; *UFH,* unfractionated heparin; *LMWH,* low-molecular-weight heparin.

MULTIPLE ORGAN DYSFUNCTION SYNDROME

MODS results from progressive physiological failure of two or more separate organ systems. It is defined as the "presence of altered organ function in an acutely ill patient such that homeostasis cannot be maintained without intervention."[81] Dysfunction of one organ may amplify dysfunction in another. Lack of consensus regarding definitions for organ dysfunction, the number of organs involved, and the duration of organ dysfunction have hampered an accurate account of organ dysfunction in critically ill patients. Despite some variations in how previous researchers have defined organ dysfunction, mortality has been closely linked to the number of organ systems involved. Impairment of two or more organs is associated with an estimated mortality rate of 45% to 55%. This may increase to 80% with three or more organ systems and to 100% if three or more organ systems are severely compromised for longer than 4 days.[112]

Although various patient populations are at risk for organ dysfunction, trauma patients are particularly vulnerable because they often experience ischemia-reperfusion events resulting from hemorrhage, blunt trauma, or sympathetic nervous system-induced vasoconstriction.[113] Other high-risk patients include those who have experienced infection, a shock episode, various ischemia-reperfusion events, acute pancreatitis, sepsis, burns, aspiration, multiple blood transfusions, or surgical complications. Patients age 65 years or older

are at increased risk because of their decreased organ reserve and comorbidities.[114]

Etiology

Organ dysfunction may be a direct consequence of the insult (primary MODS) or can manifest latently and involve organs not directly affected in the initial insult (secondary MODS). Patients can experience both primary and secondary MODS (Figure 26-6).

Primary MODS "directly results from a well-defined insult in which organ dysfunction occurs early and is directly attributed to the insult itself"[3] and accounts for only a small fraction of MODS cases. Direct insults initially cause localized inflammatory responses. Examples of primary MODS include the immediate consequences of posttraumatic pulmonary failure, thermal injuries, acute tubular necrosis, or invasive infections.[115] These cellular or microcirculatory events may lead to a loss of critical organ function induced by failure of delivery of oxygen and substrates, coupled with the inability to remove end-products of metabolism.[112,115,116] The inflammatory response in primary MODS has a less apparent presentation and may resolve without long-term implications. This primary dysfunction is thought to set the system up for a more observable inflammatory response leading to secondary MODS.[112]

Secondary MODS is a consequence of widespread systemic inflammation that results in dysfunction of organs not involved in the initial insult.[81,82] Secondary MODS

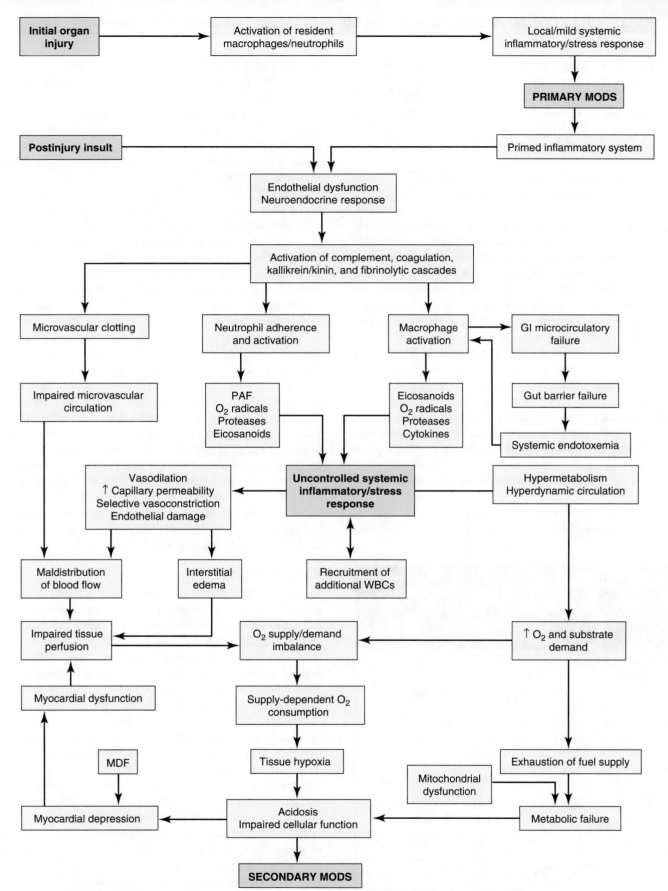

FIGURE 26-6 Pathogenesis of multiple organ dysfunction syndrome. *GI*, gastrointestinal; *MDF*, myocardial depressant factor; *MODS*, multiple organ dysfunction syndrome; *PAF*, platelet activating factor; *WBCs*, white blood cells. (From Cheek DJ, et al: Shock, multiple organ dysfunction syndrome, and burns in adults. In McCance KL, Huether SE, editors: *Pathophysiology: the biologic basis for disease in adults and children*, ed 6, St Louis, 2010, Mosby.)

develops latently after an initial insult. The early impairment of organs normally involved in immunoregulatory function, such as the liver and the GI tract, intensifies the host response to the insult. It is postulated that the initial insult "primes" the inflammatory system in such a way that a mild second insult may perpetuate a hyperinflammatory response.[117]

Systemic inflammatory response syndrome (SIRS) or sepsis is a common initiating event in the development of secondary MODS. The systemic inflammatory response is an abnormal host response characterized by generalized inflammation in organs remote from the initial insult. SIRS is widespread inflammation or clinical responses to inflammation that occurs in patients suffering a variety of insults. Clinical conditions and manifestations associated with SIRS are listed in Box 26-15. These insults produce similar or identical systemic inflammatory responses, even in the absence of infection. SIRS is diagnosed when at least two of four clinical manifestations occur in the high-risk patient. Manifestations of SIRS must represent an acute alteration from the patient's normal baseline and must not be related to other causes (e.g., neutropenia from chemotherapy). Organ dysfunction or failure, such as acute lung injury (ALI), acute renal failure, and MODS, is a complication of SIRS.[81,82,112,115] In epidemiological studies, SIRS was found to occur in one third of all hospitalized patients, in 50% to 93% of all patients in critical care units, and in about 80% of all patients in surgical critical care units.[118,119]

When SIRS is a result of infection, the term *sepsis* is used. Severe sepsis is sepsis with hypoperfusion or systemic manifestations of hypoperfusion. Septic shock is sepsis-induced hypotension despite fluid resuscitation. SIRS, sepsis, severe sepsis, and septic shock represent a hierarchical continuum of the inflammatory response to infection.[16] Although infection and shock remain the most common precipitating factors, any disease that can induce a major inflammatory response is capable of initiating the events that lead to MODS.[115]

When SIRS is not contained locally, several consequences occur that lead to organ dysfunction, including intense, uncontrolled activation of inflammatory cells; direct damage of vascular endothelium; disruption of immune cell function; persistent hypermetabolism; and maldistribution of circulatory volume to organ systems.[112,115] Inflammation becomes a systemic, self-perpetuating process that is inadequately controlled and results in organ dysfunction.[115,120] During hypermetabolism, changes occur in cellular anabolic and catabolic function, resulting in autocatabolism. Autocatabolism manifests as a severe decrease in lean body mass, severe weight loss, anergy, and increased cardiac output and VO_2 resulting from profound alterations in carbohydrate, protein, and fat metabolism.[112,121] Concurrently, GI, hepatic, and immunological dysfunction may occur, which intensifies the SIRS.[122] Clinical consequences may affect gut function, wound healing, muscles wasting, host response, respiratory function, and continued promotion of the hypermetabolic response.[121]

Not all patients develop MODS from SIRS. The development of MODS appears to be associated with failure to control the source of inflammation or infection, persistent hypoperfusion, flow-dependent oxygen consumption (VO_2), or the continued presence of necrotic tissue.[113,115]

Pathophysiology

Secondary MODS results from altered regulation of the patient's acute immune and inflammatory responses. Dysregulation, or failure to control the host inflammatory response, leads to the excessive production of inflammatory cells and biochemical mediators that cause widespread damage to vascular endothelium and organ damage.[112,115,120] The critically ill patient's compromised immune state also fosters an environment conducive to organ failure.

The definitive clinical course of secondary MODS has not been completely identified. One theory suggests that organ dysfunction may occur in a sequential or progressive pattern. This pattern begins with the lungs, the most commonly affected major organ, and then goes on to involve the liver, gut, and kidneys. A late component is cardiac and, sometimes, bone marrow dysfunction. Neurological and autonomic system impairment may occur and propagate the progression of organ failure and is associated with illness severity and mortality.[123] Organs may fail simultaneously; for example, renal dysfunction may take place concurrently with hepatic dysfunction. After the initial insult and resuscitation, patients develop persistent hypermetabolism, a metabolic consequence of sustained systemic inflammation and physiological stress, followed closely by pulmonary dysfunction, manifested as ALI.

BOX 26-15	**CLINICAL CONDITIONS AND MANIFESTATIONS ASSOCIATED WITH SYSTEMIC INFLAMMATORY RESPONSE SYNDROME**

Clinical Conditions
- Infection
- Infection of vascular structures (heart and lungs)
- Pancreatitis
- Tissue ischemia or hypoxia
- Multiple trauma with massive tissue injury
- Hemorrhagic shock
- Immune-mediated organ injury
- Exogenous administration of tumor necrosis factor or other cytokines
- Aspiration of gastric contents
- Massive transfusion
- Host defense abnormalities

Clinical Manifestations
- Temperature >38° C or <36° C
- Heart rate >90 beats/min
- Respiratory rate >20 breaths/min or $PaCO_2$ <32mm Hg
- WBC >12,000 cells/mm^3 or <4000 cells/mm^3 or >10% immature (band) forms

WBC, white blood cell count.

Certain cellular and biochemical activity evoke the inflammatory and immune responses implicated in SIRS and MODS. The mediators associated with SIRS and MODS can be classified as inflammatory cells, biochemical mediators, or plasma protein systems (Box 26-16). Activation of one mediator often leads to activation of another. The biological activity of inflammatory cells, biochemical mediators, and plasma protein systems and how they work in concert to cause SIRS and MODS have not been totally determined.[124]

Assessment and Diagnosis

Secondary MODS is a systemic disease with organ-specific manifestations. Organ dysfunction is influenced by numerous factors, including organ host defense function, response time to the injury, metabolic requirements, organ vasculature response to vasoactive drugs, organ sensitivity to damage, and physiological reserve. The responses of the gastrointestinal, hepatobiliary, cardiovascular, pulmonary, renal, and hematological systems are discussed in the following paragraphs. Clinical manifestations of organ dysfunction are outlined in Box 26-17.

Gastrointestinal Dysfunction

The gastrointestinal tract plays an important role in MODS. Gastrointestinal organs normally have immunoregulatory functions, and the gastrointestinal tract contains about 70% to 80% of the immunological tissue of the entire body. A normally functioning gastrointestinal tract prevents bacteria from entering the systemic circulation.[112] Normal gut flora and gut environment are altered in patients with severe SIRS.[122] With microcirculatory failure to the gastrointestinal tract, the gut's barrier function may be lost. Consequently, gastrointestinal dysfunction amplifies SIRS and gut damage, which may lead to bacterial translocation and endogenous endotoxemia.[112,120]

Three specific mechanisms link the gastrointestinal tract and latent organ dysfunction. First, hypoperfusion and shock-like states damage the normal gastrointestinal mucosa barrier by decreasing mesenteric blood flow, leading to hypoperfusion of the villi, mucosal edema, ischemic necrosis, sloughing of the mucosa, and malabsorption. The gastrointestinal tract is extremely vulnerable to oxygen metabolite-induced reperfusion injury. Endothelial injury and gastrointestinal lesions occur in response to mediator-induced tissue damage. Ischemic events and the absence of feedings can disrupt the normal metabolism of the gastric or intestinal lumen and the normal protective function of the gut barrier.[125,126]

Second, the translocation of normal gastrointestinal bacteria through a "leaky gut" into the systemic circulation initiates and perpetuates an inflammatory focus in the critically ill patient.[126] The gastrointestinal tract harbors organisms that present an inflammatory focus when translocated from the gut into the portal circulation and inadequately cleared by the liver. Healthy probiotics (e.g., *Bifidobacterium, Lactobacillus*) are decreased in a SIRS state, and pathogenic organisms (e.g., *Staphylococcus, Pseudomonas*) proliferate.[122] Hepatic macrophages respond to the presence of enteric organisms by producing tissue-damaging amounts of tumor necrosis factor (TNF), which further propagates the inflammatory mechanisms. The primary mechanism of bacterial translocation has been associated with intestinal bacterial overgrowth.[122]

The third mechanism linking the gastrointestinal tract and organ dysfunction is colonization. The oropharynx of the critically ill patient becomes colonized with potentially pathogenic organisms from the gastrointestinal tract. Pulmonary aspiration of colonized secretions presents an inflammatory focus that can contribute to concomitant pulmonary dysfunction.[127]

BOX 26-16 INFLAMMATORY MEDIATORS ASSOCIATED WITH SYSTEMIC INFLAMMATORY RESPONSE AND MULTIPLE ORGAN DYSFUNCTION SYNDROMES

Inflammatory Cells
- Neutrophils
- Macrophages or monocytes
- Mast
- Lymphocytes
- Endothelial

Biochemical Mediators
- Reactive oxygen species
  - Superoxide radical
  - Hydroxyl radical
  - Hydrogen peroxide
- Tumor necrosis factor
- Interleukins
- Platelet activating factor
- Arachidonic acid metabolites
  - Prostaglandins
  - Leukotrienes
  - Thromboxanes
- Proteases

Plasma Protein Systems
- Complement
- Kinin
- Coagulation

Hepatobiliary Dysfunction

The liver plays a vital role in host homeostasis related to the acute inflammatory response. The liver responds to SIRS by selectively changing carbohydrate, fat, and protein metabolism. Consequently, hepatic dysfunction after a critical insult threatens the patient's survival.[128]

The liver normally controls the inflammatory response by several mechanisms. Kupffer cells, which are hepatic macrophages, detoxify substances that may normally induce systemic inflammation and vasoactive substances that cause

BOX 26-17 CLINICAL MANIFESTATIONS OF ORGAN DYSFUNCTION

Gastrointestinal
- Abdominal distention
- Intolerance to enteral feedings
- Paralytic ileus
- Upper or lower gastrointestinal bleeding
- Diarrhea
- Ischemic colitis
- Mucosal ulceration
- Decreased bowel sounds
- Bacterial overgrowth in stool

Hepatic
- Jaundice
- Increased serum bilirubin (hyperbilirubinemia)
- Increased serum ammonia
- Decreased serum albumin
- Decreased serum transferrin

Gallbladder
- Right upper quadrant tenderness or pain
- Abdominal distention
- Unexplained fever
- Decreased bowel sounds

Metabolic and Nutritional
- Decreased lean body mass
- Muscle wasting
- Severe weight loss
- Negative nitrogen balance
- Hyperglycemia
- Hypertriglyceridemia
- Increased serum lactate
- Decreased serum albumin, serum transferrin, prealbumin
- Decreased retinol-binding protein

Immune
- Infection
- Decreased lymphocyte count
- Anergy

Pulmonary
- Tachypnea
- Acute lung injury pattern of respiratory failure (dyspnea, patchy infiltrates, refractory hypoxemia, respiratory acidosis, abnormal O_2 indexes)
- Pulmonary hypertension

Renal
- Increased serum creatinine, blood urea nitrogen levels
- Oliguria, anuria, or polyuria consistent with prerenal azotemia or acute tubular necrosis
- Urinary indexes consistent with prerenal azotemia or acute tubular necrosis

Cardiovascular
Hyperdynamic
- Decreased pulmonary capillary occlusion pressure
- Decreased systemic vascular resistance
- Decreased right atrial pressure
- Decreased left ventricular stroke work index
- Increased oxygen consumption
- Increased cardiac output, cardiac index, heart rate

Hypodynamic
- Increased systemic vascular resistance
- Increased right atrial pressure
- Increased left ventricular stroke work index
- Decreased oxygen delivery and consumption
- Decreased cardiac output and cardiac index

Central Nervous System
- Lethargy
- Altered level of consciousness
- Fever
- Hepatic encephalopathy

Coagulation Or Hematological
- Thrombocytopenia
- Disseminated intravascular coagulation pattern

hemodynamic instability. Failure to detoxify gram-negative bacteria translocated from the gastrointestinal tract causes endotoxemia, perpetuates SIRS, and may lead to MODS. The liver also produces proteins and antiproteases to control the inflammatory response; however, hepatic dysfunction limits this response.[128]

The liver and gallbladder are extremely vulnerable to ischemic injury. Ischemic hepatitis occurs after a prolonged period of physiological shock and is associated with centrilobular hepatocellular necrosis.[129] The degree of hepatic damage is related directly to the severity and duration of the shock episode. Terms such as *shock liver* and *post-traumatic hepatic insufficiency* have been used to describe ischemic hepatitis. Anoxic and reperfusion injuries damage hepatocytes and the vascular endothelium.[130] Patients at high risk for ischemic hepatitis after a hypotensive event include those with a history of cardiac failure or cardiac dysrhythmias. Clinical manifestations of hepatic insufficiency

are evident 1 to 2 days after the insult. Jaundice and transient elevations in serum transaminase and bilirubin levels occur. Hyperbilirubinemia, possibly the most reliable measure of hepatic dysfunction, results from hepatocyte anoxic injury and an increased production of bilirubin from hemoglobin catabolism.[129] Ischemic hepatitis may resolve spontaneously or progress to acute liver failure. Although ischemic hepatitis is not a life-threatening complication, it can contribute to morbidity and mortality as a component of MODS.[130] Researchers have proposed that serum bilirubin is a valid indicator of hepatic dysfunction in MODS because it significantly differentiates MODS survivors from nonsurvivors.[129] Acute liver failure is discussed further in Chapter 22.

Acalculous cholecystitis manifests 3 to 4 weeks after an insult. Its pathogenesis is unclear, but it may be related to ischemic reperfusion injury, positive end-expiratory pressure (PEEP) greater than 5 cm H_2O, volume depletion, total parenteral nutrition, narcotics, and cystic duct obstruction as a result of hyperviscous bile.[131] Visceral hypotension and vasoactive medication use may decrease perfusion of the gallbladder mucosa contributing to ischemia. Bacterial invasion may stimulate activation of factor XII and initiate the coagulation pathway.[131] Clinical manifestations of acalculous cholecystitis may mimic acute cholecystitis with gallstones. However, patients may demonstrate vague symptoms, including right upper quadrant pain and tenderness. Critical to the detection of acalculous cholecystitis is the recognition of abdominal distention, unexplained fever, loss of bowel sounds, and a sudden deterioration in the patient's condition. About 50% of patients with acalculous cholecystitis have gallbladder gangrene, and 10% have gallbladder perforation, requiring a cholecystectomy.[131]

Pulmonary Dysfunction

The lungs, which are frequent and early target organs for mediator-induced injury, are usually the first organs affected in the progression of SIRS to MODS.[124] Acute lung injury (ALI) is the pulmonary manifestation of the systemic condition of MODS. Patients who develop MODS usually have pulmonary symptoms; however, not all patients with ALI develop secondary MODS. ALI patients who develop SIRS or sepsis concurrently with acute respiratory failure are at the greatest risk for MODS.[132]

ALI associated with MODS usually occurs 24 to 72 hours after the initial insult. Patients initially exhibit a low-grade fever, tachycardia, dyspnea, and mental confusion. As dyspnea, hypoxemia, and the work of breathing increase, intubation and mechanical ventilation are required. Acute pulmonary dysfunction results in refractory hypoxemia caused by intrapulmonary shunting, decreased pulmonary compliance, and altered airway mechanics; there usually is radiographic evidence of noncardiogenic pulmonary edema.[133]

Mediators associated with ALI include inflammatory cells such as polymorphonuclear cells, macrophages, monocytes, endothelial cells, and mast cells; and biochemical mediators such as AA metabolites, toxic oxygen metabolites, proteases, TNF, plate activating factor (PAF), and interleukins. Intense mediator activity damages the pulmonary vascular endothelium and the alveolar epithelium, resulting in surfactant deficiency, mild pulmonary hypertension, and increased pulmonary capillary permeability leading to increased lung water (noncardiogenic pulmonary edema).[133] ALI is discussed further in Chapter 15.

Renal Dysfunction

Acute kidney failure is a common manifestation of MODS. The kidney is highly vulnerable to reperfusion injury. Consequently, renal ischemic-reperfusion injury may be a major cause of renal dysfunction in MODS. The patient may demonstrate oliguria or anuria resulting from decreased renal perfusion and relative hypovolemia. Early oliguria is likely caused by decreases in renal perfusion related to shock-like states; late oliguria is typically a sign of evolving renal injury

and ischemia. The condition may become refractory to diuretics, fluid challenges, and dopamine. Prerenal oliguria may progress to acute tubular necrosis, necessitating hemodialysis or other renal therapies.[121,134] The frequent use of nephrotoxic drugs during critical illness also intensifies the risk of progressive renal impairment. An elevated serum creatinine level is usually a late sign, but it is typically accepted as the index for renal dysfunction.[134] Researchers have proposed that the serum creatinine level is a valid indicator of renal function because it significantly differentiates MODS survivors from nonsurvivors.[135] Additional signs of renal impairment may include decreased erythropoietin-induced anemia, vitamin D malabsorption, and altered fluid and electrolyte balance. Acute renal failure is discussed further in Chapter 20.

Cardiovascular and Hematological System Dysfunction

The initial cardiovascular response in SIRS or sepsis is myocardial depression; decreased right atrial pressure and systemic vascular resistance (SVR); and increased venous capacitance, VO_2, cardiac output (CO), and heart rate. Despite an increased CO, myocardial depression occurs and is accompanied by decreased SVR, increased heart rate, and ventricular dilation. These compensatory mechanisms help maintain CO during the early phase of SIRS or sepsis. An inability to increase CO in response to a low SVR may indicate myocardial failure or inadequate fluid resuscitation, and it is associated with increased mortality. Oxygen consumption may be twice that of normal and may be flow dependent.[136]

As MODS progresses, cardiac failure develops. Cardiac dysfunction is characterized by ventricular dilation, decreased diastolic compliance, and decreased systolic contractile function. Cardiovascular function becomes vasopressor dependent. Cardiac failure may be caused by immune mediators, TNF, acidosis, or myocardial depressant factor, a substance secreted by the pancreas. TNF has a myocardial-depressant effect and is associated with myocardial depression during septic shock. Myocardial depression is exacerbated by myocardial hypoperfusion from a low CO state and persistent lactic acidosis. Cardiogenic shock and biventricular failure occur and lead to death.[136] Cardiac failure is discussed further in Chapter 12, and more information on cardiogenic shock can be found earlier in this chapter.

The most common manifestations of hematological dysfunction in sepsis or MODS are thrombocytopenia, coagulation abnormalities, and anemia.[137] The most severe is coagulation system dysfunction manifesting as DIC. DIC is a complex, consumptive coagulopathy that occurs in patients with a variety of disorders, including sepsis, tissue injury, and shock; it is overstimulation of the normal coagulation process. DIC results simultaneously in microvascular clotting and hemorrhage in organ systems, leading to thrombosis and fibrinolysis in life-threatening proportions. Clotting factor derangement leads to further inflammation and further thrombosis. Microvascular damage leads to further organ injury. Cell injury and damage to the endothelium activate the intrinsic or extrinsic coagulation pathways.[94] Low platelet counts and elevated D-dimer concentrations and fibrinogen degradation products are clinical indicators of DIC. DIC is discussed further in Chapter 27.

Medical Management

The patient with MODS requires multidisciplinary collaboration in clinical management, including fluid resuscitation and hemodynamic support (when appropriate), prevention and treatment of infection, maintenance of tissue oxygenation, nutritional and metabolic support, comfort and emotional support, and support for individual organ function.[81,124] The use of investigational therapies may be part of the patient's clinical management. Collaborative management of the patient with MODS is outlined in the Collaborative Management Box on Multiple Organ Dysfunction Syndrome.

COLLABORATIVE MANAGEMENT
Multiple Organ Dysfunction Syndrome

- Support oxygen transport:
  - Establish a patent airway.
  - Initiate mechanical ventilation.
  - Administer oxygen.
  - Administer fluids (crystalloids, colloids, blood and other blood products).
  - Administer vasoactive medications.
  - Administer positive inotropic medications.
  - Administer antidysrhythmic medications.
  - Ensure sufficient hemoglobin and hematocrit.
- Support oxygen use:
  - Identify and correct cause of lactic acidosis.
  - Ensure adequate organ and extremity perfusion.
- Decrease oxygen demand:
  - Administer sedation or paralytics.
  - Administer antipyretics and external cooling measures.
  - Administer pain medications.
- Identify the underlying cause of inflammation and treat accordingly:
  - Remove infected organs or tissue.
  - Administer antibiotics.
- Initiate nutritional support.
- Treat individual organ dysfunction:
  - Gastrointestinal
  - Hepatobiliary
  - Pulmonary
  - Renal
  - Cardiovascular
  - Coagulation system
- Maintain surveillance for complications, including infection.
- Provide comfort and emotional support.

Identification and Treatment of Infection

Identification and treatment of the underlying source of inflammation or infection are the most important ways to reduce mortality. Medical and surgical intervention to remove sources of infection or contamination may limit the inflammatory response and improve chances of recovery.[124] Surgical procedures such as early fracture stabilization, removal of infected organs or tissue, and burn excision are helpful. Appropriate antibiotics are needed if the cause cannot be removed by surgical débridement or incision and draining.[124] Other timely interventions, such as prevention of skin ulceration and early nutritional support, can improve outcomes.[138] Regardless of the identification of potential risk factors, clinical markers, bacterial contaminants, and investigative approaches for detection and prevention, treatment remains largely supportive and little improvement in the mortality rate has been appreciated.[139]

Maintenance of Tissue Oxygenation

Normally, under steady state conditions, VO_2 is relatively constant and independent of oxygen delivery (DO_2) unless delivery becomes severely impaired. The relationship is called *supply-independent oxygen consumption*. Consequently, a percentage of oxygen is not used (physiological reserve). Patients with SIRS/MODS often develop supply-dependent oxygen consumption in which VO_2 becomes dependent on DO_2, rather than demand, at a normal or high DO_2. When VO_2 does not equal demand, a tissue oxygen debt develops, subjecting organs to failure.[124]

Hypoperfusion and resultant organ hypoxemia often occur in patients at high risk for MODS, subjecting essential organs to failure. Effective fluid resuscitation and early recognition of flow-dependent VO_2 is essential, and patients at risk for MODS require hemodynamic monitoring, frequent measurements or surrogate measurements of DO_2 and VO_2, and serum lactate levels to guide therapy. Serum lactate levels provide information regarding the severity of impaired perfusion and the presence of lactic acidosis and differ significantly in MODS survivors and nonsurvivors.[16,121] Failure to maintain adequate oxygenation to vital organs results in organ dysfunction. Despite adequate DO_2, VO_2 may not meet the needs of the body duringMODS.

Patients with ALI, ARDS, MODS, or sepsis frequently manifest supply-dependent oxygen consumption and are unable to use oxygen appropriately despite normal delivery.[124] Interventions that decrease oxygen demand and increase oxygen delivery are essential. Sedation, mechanical ventilation, rest, and temperature and pain control may be able to decrease oxygen demand.[123] Oxygen delivery may be increased by maintaining normal hematocrit and PaO_2 levels, using PEEP, increasing preload or myocardial contractility to enhance CO, or reducing afterload to increase CO. Various methods of kinetic or prone therapies are available and may enhance alveolar recruitment, improve oxygenation delivery, and decrease other potential complications.

Nutritional and Metabolic Support

Hypermetabolism in SIRS or MODS results in profound weight loss, cachexia, and loss of organ function. The goal of nutritional support is the preservation of organ structure and function. Although nutritional support may not alter the course of organ dysfunction, it prevents generalized nutritional deficiencies and preserves gut integrity. The enteral route is preferable to parenteral support.[35] Enteral feedings are given distal to the pylorus to reduce the risk of pulmonary aspiration. Enteral feedings may limit bacterial translocation. In addition to early nutritional support, the pharmacological properties of enteral feeding formulas may limit SIRS for selected critical care populations. Supplementation of enteral feedings with glutamine may be beneficial;[111,140] however, arginine, a precursor to nitric oxide, should be avoided in critically ill patients.[110] Enteral feedings with omega-3 fatty acids may lessen the development of SIRS and improve outcomes.[110] Nutritional support is discussed further in Chapter 8.

Nursing Management

Preventive measures include a multitude of assessment strategies to detect early organ manifestations of this syndrome. Patients who continue to experience sites of inflammation, septic foci, and inadequate tissue perfusion may be at higher risk. Hand hygiene, aseptic technique, and an understanding of how microorganisms can invade the body are essential components of preventive nursing care.

Nursing management of the patient with MODS incorporates a variety of nursing diagnoses (Nursing Diagnosis Priorities Box on Multiple Organ Dysfunction Syndrome). **Nursing priorities are directed toward (1) preventing development of infection, (2) facilitating oxygen delivery and limiting tissue oxygen demand, (3) facilitating nutritional support, (4) providing comfort and emotional support, and (5) maintaining surveillance for complications.**

NURSING DIAGNOSIS PRIORITIES
Multiple Organ Dysfunction Syndrome

- Decreased Cardiac Output related to alterations in preload, p. A-10
- Decreased Cardiac Output related to alterations in afterload, p. A-10
- Decreased Cardiac Output related to alterations in contractility, p. A-11
- Impaired Gas Exchange related to ventilation/perfusion mismatching or intrapulmonary shunting, p. A-23
- Ineffective Renal Tissue Perfusion related to decreased renal blood flow, p. A-33
- Ineffective Cardiopulmonary Tissue Perfusion related to decreased coronary blood flow, p. A-28
- Imbalanced Nutrition: Less Than Body Requirements related to increased metabolic demands or lack of exogenous nutrients, p. A-22
- Risk for Infection, p. A-36
- Acute Pain related to transmission and perception of cutaneous, visceral, muscular, or ischemic impulses, p. A-5
- Acute Confusion related to sensory overload, sensory deprivation, and sleep pattern disturbance, p. A-2
- Anxiety related to threat to biological, psychological, or social integrity, p. A-7
- Compromised Family Coping related to a critically ill family member, p. A-9

Patients are assessed closely for inflammation and infection. Subtle expressions of infection warrant investigation. Nursing measures include strict adherence to standards of practice to prevent infection. Practices related to infection control with invasive hemodynamic monitoring, urinary catheters, endotracheal tubes, intracranial pressure monitoring devices, total parenteral nutrition (TPN), and wound care must be stringent to prevent further infection. Prevention of a concomitant ventilator-associated pneumonia or aspiration pneumonia is a priority.[16,141]

Measures to limit tissue oxygen consumption include (1) administering analgesics and sedatives, (2) positioning the patient for comfort, (3) limiting activities, (4) offering support to reduce anxiety, (5) providing a calm and quiet environment, and (6) teaching the patient about the condition. Measures to enhance tissue oxygen supply include administering supplemental oxygen, monitoring the patient's respiratory status, and administering prescribed fluids and medications.

CASE STUDY   PATIENT IN SHOCK

Answers to the Case Study Questions can be found on the Evolve web site at http://evolve.elsevier.com/Urden/priorities/.

Brief Patient History
Ms. B is a 76-year-old woman who has been in the surgical intensive care unit for the past 2 days after abdominal surgery for stage III ovarian cancer. Her thrombosed central line needs to be replaced. She has a history of allergy to kiwi and avocados but no known allergy to latex.

Clinical Assessment
Approximately 10 minutes after the central line insertion, Ms. B complains of feeling flushed, and she loses consciousness.

Diagnostic Procedures
Ms. B is unconscious and unresponsive to verbal or physical stimuli. Audible wheezing can be heard at the bedside. Her skin is visibly flushed and clammy to touch. Vital signs include the following: blood pressure of 60 mm Hg (determined by Doppler), heart rate of 160 beats/min (atrial tachycardia), respiratory rate of 30 breaths/min, and temperature of 99° F.

Medical Diagnosis
Ms. B is diagnosed with anaphylactic shock resulting from a latex allergy.

Questions
1. What major outcomes do you expect to achieve for this patient?
2. What problems or risks must be managed to achieve these outcomes?
3. What interventions must be initiated to monitor, prevent, manage, or eliminate the problems and risks identified?
4. What interventions should be initiated to promote optimal functioning, safety, and well-being of the patient?
5. What possible learning needs do you anticipate for this patient?
6. What cultural and age-related factors may have a bearing on the patient's plan of care?

REFERENCES

1. Maier RV: Approach to the patient with shock. In Fauci AS, editor: *Harrison's internal medicine*, ed 17, New York, 2008, McGraw-Hill.
2. Deitch EA, et al: Role of the gut in the development of injury and shock induced SIRS and MODS: The gut-lymph hypothesis, a review, *Front Biosci* 11:520, 2006.
3. Wilmot LA: Shock: early recognition and management, *J Emerg Nurs* 36(2):134, 2010.
4. Hameed SM, et al: Oxygen delivery, *Crit Care Med* 31 (Suppl 12):S658, 2003.
5. Walley KR: Shock. In Hall JB, et al, editors: *Principles of critical care*, ed 3, New York, 2005, McGraw-Hill.
6. Parks JK, et al: Systemic hypotension is a late marker of shock after trauma: A validation study of Advanced Trauma Life Support principles in a large national sample, *Am J Surg* 192(6):727, 2006.
7. Vandromme MJ, et al: Lactate is a better predictor than systolic blood pressure for determining blood requirement and mortality: could prehospital measures improve trauma triage? *J Am Coll Surg* 210(5):861, 2010.
8. Tappy L, Chioléro R: Substrate utilization in sepsis and multiple organ failure, *Crit Care Med* 35(Suppl 9):S531, 2007.
9. Englehart MS, Schreiber MA: Measurement of acid-base resuscitation endpoints: lactate, base deficit, bicarbonate or what? *Curr Opin Crit Care* 12(6):569, 2006.
10. Barbee RW, et al: Assessing shock resuscitation strategies by oxygen debt repayment, *Shock* 33(2):113, 2010.
11. Rachoin JS, et al: Treatment of lactic acidosis: appropriate confusion, *J Hosp Med* 5(4):E1, 2010.
12. FitzSullivan E, et al: Serum bicarbonate may replace the arterial base deficit in the trauma intensive care unit, *Am J Surg* 190(6):941, 2005.
13. Surbatovic M, et al: Predictive value of serum bicarbonate, arterial base deficit/excess and SAPS III score in critically ill patients, *Gen Physiol Biophys* 28 Spec No:271, 2009.
14. Bauer P, et al: Significance of venous oximetry in the critically ill, *Med Intensiva* 32(3):134, 2008.
15. Dellinger RP, et al: Surviving Sepsis Campaign guidelines for management of severe sepsis and septic shock, *Crit Care Med* 32(3):858, 2004.
16. Dellinger RP, et al: Surviving Sepsis Campaign: international guidelines for management of severe sepsis and septic shock: 2008, *Crit Care Med* 36(1):296, 2008.
17. Collaborative Study Group on Perioperative ScvO₂ Monitoring: multicentre study on peri- and postoperative central venous oxygen saturation in high-risk surgical patients, *Crit Care* 10(6):R158, 2006.
18. Ho KM, et al: The impact of arterial oxygen tension on venous oxygen saturation in circulatory failure, *Shock* 29(1):3, 2008.
19. Pinsky MR: Hemodynamic evaluation and monitoring in the ICU, *Chest* 132(6):2020, 2007.
20. Giraud R, et al: ScvO₂ As a Marker to Define Fluid Responsiveness, *J Trauma* 2010 Aug 27. [Epub ahead of print].
21. Vallet B, et al: Physiologic transfusion triggers, *Best Pract Res Clin Anaesthesiol* 21(2):173, 2007.
22. Bunn F, et al: Colloid solutions for fluid resuscitation, *Cochrane Database Syst Rev* Jan 23(1):CD001319, 2008.
23. Alam HB, Rhee P: New developments in fluid resuscitation, *Surg Clin North Am* 87(1):55, 2007.
24. Cotton BA, et al: The cellular, metabolic, and systemic consequences of aggressive fluid resuscitation strategies, *Shock* 26(2):115, 2006.
25. Stapleton RD, et al: Feeding critically ill patients: what is the optimal amount of energy? *Crit Care Med* 35(Suppl 9):S535, 2007.
26. Myburgh JA, Finfer S: Albumin is a blood product too – is it safe for all patients? *Crit Care Resusc* 11(1):67, 2009.
27. SAFE Study Investigators, et al: Effect of baseline serum albumin concentration on outcome of resuscitation with albumin or saline in patients in intensive care units: analysis of data from the saline versus albumin fluid evaluation (SAFE) study, *BMJ* 333(7577):1044, 2006.
28. Dennison CA: Transfusion-related acute lung injury: a clinical challenge, *Dimens Crit Care Nurs* 27(1):1, 2008.
29. Kopko PM: Transfusion-related acute lung injury, *J Infus Nurs* 33(1):32, 2010.
30. Federico A: Transfusion-related acute lung injury, *J Perianesth Nurs* 24(1):35, 2009.
31. Ellender TJ, Skinner JC: The use of vasopressors and inotropes in the emergency medical treatment of shock, *Emerg Med Clin North Am* 26(3):759, 2008.
32. Boyd JH, Walley KR: Is there a role for sodium bicarbonate in treating lactic acidosis from shock? *Curr Opin Crit Care* 14(4):379, 2008.
33. Kwon KT, Tsai VW: Metabolic emergencies, *Emerg Med Clin North Am* 25(4):1041, 2007.
34. McClave SA, Heyland DK: The physiologic response and associated clinical benefits from provision of early enteral nutrition, *Nutr Clin Pract* 24(3):305, 2009.
35. Martindale RG, et al: Guidelines for the provision and assessment of nutrition support therapy in the adult critically ill patient: Society of Critical Care Medicine and American Society for Parenteral and Enteral Nutrition: Executive Summary, *Crit Care Med* 37(5):1757, 2009.
36. Heidegger CP, et al: Enteral vs. parenteral nutrition for the critically ill patient: a combined support should be preferred, *Curr Opin Crit Care* 14(4):408, 2008.
37. Thibault R, Pichard C: Parenteral nutrition in critical illness: can it safely improve outcomes? *Crit Care Clin* 26(3):467, 2010.
38. American Diabetes Association: Standards of medical care in diabetes 2007, *Diabetes Care* 30(Suppl 1):S4, 2007.
39. Blackburn GL, et al: Nutrition support in the intensive care unit: an evolving science, *Arch Surg* 145(6):533, 2010.
40. Schetz M, et al: Tight blood glucose control is renoprotective in critically ill patients, *J Am Soc Nephrol* 19(3):571, 2008.
41. Fahy BG, et al: Glucose control in the intensive care unit, *Crit Care Med* 37(5):1769, 2009.
42. Wiener RS, et al: Benefits and risks of tight glucose control in critically ill adults: a meta-analysis, *JAMA* 300(8):933, 2008.
43. Davidson JE, et al: Clinical practice guidelines for support of the family in the patient-centered intensive care unit: American College of Critical Care Medicine Task force 2004-2005, *Crit Care Med* 35(2):605, 2007.
44. Howlett MS, et al: Health care providers' attitudes regarding family presence during resuscitation of adults: an integrated review of the literature, *Clin Nurse Spec* 24(3):161, 2010.

45. Duran CR, et al: Attitudes toward and beliefs about family presence: a survey of healthcare providers, patients' families, and patients, *Am J Crit Care* 16(3):270, 2007.

46. Hemmila MR, Wahl WL: Management of the injured patient. In Doherty GM, Way LW, editors: *Current surgical diagnosis and treatment*, ed 12, New York, 2006. McGraw-Hill.

47. Kwan I, et al: Timing and volume of fluid administration for patients with bleeding, *Cochrane Database Syst Rev* (3):CD002245, 2003.

48. Roppolo LP, et al: Intravenous fluid resuscitation for the trauma patient, *Curr Opin Crit Care* 16(4):283, 2010.

49. Pepe PE, et al: Preoperative resuscitation of the trauma patient, *Curr Opin Anaesthesiol* 21(2):216, 2008.

50. Bulger EM, et al: Hypertonic resuscitation modulates the inflammatory response in patients with traumatic hemorrhagic shock, *Ann Surg* 245(4):635, 2007.

51. Bulger EM, et al: Hypertonic resuscitation of hypovolemic shock after blunt trauma: a randomized controlled trial, *Arch Surg* 143(2):139, 2008.

52. Mizushima Y, et al: Fluid resuscitation of trauma patients: how fast is the optimal rate? *Am J Emerg Med* 23(7):833, 2005.

53. Josephson L: Cardiogenic shock, *Dimens Crit Care Nurs* 27(4):160, 2008.

54. Topalian S, et al: Cardiogenic shock, *Crit Care Med* 36(Suppl 1):S66, 2008.

55. TRIUMPH Investigators: Effect of tilarginine acetate in patients with acute myocardial infarction and cardiogenic shock: the TRIUMPH randomized controlled trial, *JAMA* 297(15):1657, 2007.

56. Gurm HS, Bates ER: Cardiogenic shock complicating myocardial infarction, *Crit Care Clin* 23(4):759, 2007.

57. Reynolds HR, Hochman JS: Cardiogenic shock: current concepts and improving outcomes, *Circulation* 117(5):686, 2008.

58. Lim N, et al: Do all nonsurvivors of cardiogenic shock die with a low cardiac index? *Chest* 124(5):1885, 2003.

59. Kohsaka S, et al: Systemic inflammatory response syndrome after acute myocardial infarction complicated by cardiogenic shock, *Arch Intern Med* 165(14):1643, 2005.

60. Okuda M: A multidisciplinary overview of cardiogenic shock, *Shock* 25(6):557, 2006.

61. Stevenson LW, Perloff JK: The limited reliability of physical signs for estimating hemodynamics in chronic heart failure, *JAMA* 261(6):884, 1989.

62. Hochman JS, et al: Early revascularization and long-term survival in cardiogenic shock complicating acute myocardial infarction, *JAMA* 295(21):2511, 2006.

63. Aggarwal S, Slaughter MS: Acute myocardial infarction complicated by cardiogenic shock: role of mechanical circulatory support, *Expert Rev Cardiovasc Ther* 6(9):1223, 2008.

64. Hiestand BC: Circulatory assist devices in heart failure patients, *Heart Fail Clin* 5(1):55, 2009.

65. Simons FE: Anaphylaxis, *J Allergy Clin Immunol* 125 (2 Suppl 2):S161, 2010.

66. Lieberman P: Anaphylaxis, *Med Clin North Am* 90(1):77, 2006.

67. Lieberman P, et al: Epidemiology of anaphylaxis: findings of the American College of Allergy, Asthma and Immunology Epidemiology of Anaphylaxis Working Group, *Ann Allergy Asthma Immunol* 97(5):596, 2006.

68. Simons FE: Anaphylaxis, *J Allergy Clin Immunol* 121 (Suppl 2):S402, 2008.

69. American Heart Association: 2005 American Heart Association Guidelines for cardiopulmonary resuscitation and emergency cardiovascular care. Part 10.6: Anaphylaxis, *Circulation* 112(24 Suppl):IV-143, 2005.

70. Kemp SF, et al: Epinephrine: The drug of choice for anaphylaxis. A statement of the World Allergy Organization, *Allergy* 63(8):1061, 2008.

71. Sampson HA, et al: Second symposium on the definition and management of anaphylaxis: summary report – second National Institute of Allergy and Infectious Disease/Food Allergy and Anaphylaxis Network symposium, *J Allergy Clin Immunol* 117(2):391, 2006.

72. Simons FE: Anaphylaxis: Recent advances in assessment and treatment, *J Allergy Clin Immunol* 124(4):625, 2009.

73. Lieberman P, et al: The diagnosis and management of anaphylaxis: an updated practice parameter, *J Allergy Clin Immunol* 115(3 Suppl 2):S483, 2005.

74. Bilello JF, et al: Cervical spinal cord injury and the need for cardiovascular intervention, *Arch Surg* 138(10):1127, 2003.

75. Guly HR, et al: The incidence of neurogenic shock in patients with isolated spinal cord injury in the emergency department, *Resuscitation* 76(1):57, 2008.

76. Stevens RD, et al: Critical care and perioperative management in traumatic spinal cord injury, *J Neurosurg Anesthesiol* 15(3):215, 2003.

77. Ditunno JF, et al: Spinal shock revisited: a four-phase model, *Spinal Cord* 42(7):383, 2004.

78. Krassioukov A, Claydon VE: The clinical problems in cardiovascular control following spinal cord injury: an overview, *Prog Brain Res* 152:223, 2006.

79. Young WF: Shock. In Stone CK, Humphries RL, editors: *Current diagnosis & treatment: emergency medicine*, ed 6, New York, 2008, McGraw-Hill.

80. King JE: Sepsis in critical care, *Crit Care Nurs Clin North Am* 19(1):77, 2007.

81. American College of Chest Physicians/Society of Critical Care Medicine Consensus Conference: Definitions for sepsis and organ failure and guidelines for the use of innovative therapies in sepsis, *Crit Care Med* 20(6):864, 1992.

82. Levy MM, et al: 2001 SCCM/ESICM/ACCP/ATS/SIS International Sepsis Definitions Conference, *Crit Care Med* 31(4):1250, 2003.

83. Guidet B, et al: Incidence and impact of organ dysfunctions associated with sepsis, *Chest* 127(3):942, 2005.

84. Leone M, et al: 2003 Empirical antimicrobial therapy of septic shock patients: adequacy and impact on the outcome, *Crit Care Med* 31(2):462, 2003.

85. Seymour CW: Marital status and the epidemiology and outcomes of sepsis, *Chest* 137(6):1289, 2010.

86. Nduka OO, Parrillo JE: The pathophysiology of septic shock, *Crit Care Clin* 25(4):677, 2009.

87. Ahrens T, Vollman K: Severe sepsis management: are we doing enough? *Crit Care Nurse* 23(Suppl 5):2, 2003.

88. Cinel I, Dellinger RP: Advances in pathogenesis and management of sepsis, *Curr Opin Infect Dis* 20(4):345, 2007.

89. Groeneveld AB, et al: Circulating inflammatory mediators predict shock and mortality in febrile patients with microbial infection, *Clin Immunol* 106(2):106, 2003.

90. Rivers EP, et al: The influence of early hemodynamic optimization on biomarker patterns of severe sepsis and septic shock, *Crit Care Med* 35(9):2016, 2007.

91. Singer M: Mitochondrial function in sepsis: acute phase versus multiple organ failure, *Crit Care Med* 35 (Suppl 9):S441, 2007.

92. Angus DC, Crowther MA: Unraveling severe sepsis: why did OPTIMIST fail and what's next, *JAMA* 290(2):256, 2003.

93. Sharma S, Kumar A: Septic shock, multiple organ failure, and acute respiratory distress syndrome, *Curr Opin Pulm Med* 9(3):199, 2003.

94. Levi M: Disseminated intravascular coagulation, *Crit Care Med* 35(9):2191, 2007.

95. Elbers PW, Ince C: 2006 Bench-to-bedside review: mechanisms of critical illness classifying microcirculatory flow abnormalities in distributive shock, *Crit Care* 10(4):221, 2006.

96. Trzeciak S, et al: Early microcirculatory perfusion derangements in patients with severe sepsis and septic shock: relationship to hemodynamics, oxygen transport, and survival, *Ann Emerg Med* 49(1):88, 2007.

97. Tamion F, et al: Gastric mucosal acidosis and cytokine release in patients with septic shock, *Crit Care Med* 31(8):2137, 2003.

98. Baumgart K, et al: Pathophysiology of tissue acidosis in septic shock: blocked microcirculation or impaired cellular respiration? *Crit Care Med* 36(2):640. 2008.

99. Uzzan B, et al: Procalcitonin as a diagnostic test for sepsis in critically ill adults and after surgery or trauma: a systematic review and meta-analysis, *Crit Care Med* 34(7):1996, 2006.

100. Rivers E, et al: Early goal-directed therapy in the treatment of severe sepsis and septic shock, *N Engl J Med* 345(19):1368, 2001.

101. Kumar A, et al: Duration of hypotension before initiation of effective antimicrobial therapy is the critical determinant of survival in human septic shock, *Crit Care Med* 34(6):1589, 2006.

102. The Acute Respiratory Distress System Network: Ventilation with lower tidal volumes as compared with traditional tidal volumes for acute lung injury and the acute respiratory distress syndrome, *N Engl J Med* 342(18):1301, 2000.

103. Bernard GR, et al: Efficacy and safety of recombinant human activated protein C for severe sepsis, *N Engl J Med* 344(10):699, 2001.

104. Vincent JL, et al: Drotrecogin alfa (activated) treatment in severe sepsis from the global open-label trial ENHANCE: further evidence for survival and safety and implications for early treatment, *Crit Care Med* 33(10):2266, 2005.

105. Powers J, Jacobi J: Treatment of severe sepsis with Xigris: implications for the clinical nurse specialist, *Clin Nurse Spec* 17(3):128, 2003.

106. Dellinger RP, Parrillo JE: Mediator modulation therapy of severe sepsis and septic shock: does it work? *Crit Care Med* 32(1):282, 2004.

107. Annane D, et al: Effect of treatment with low doses of hydrocortisone and fludrocortisone on mortality in patients with septic shock, *JAMA* 288(7):862, 2002.

108. Beale RJ, et al: Early enteral supplementation with key pharmaconutrients improves Sequential Organ Failure Assessment score in critically ill patients with sepsis: outcome of a randomized, controlled, double-blind trial, *Crit Care Med* 36(1):131, 2008.

109. Berger MM, Chioléro RL: Antioxidant supplementation in sepsis and systemic inflammatory response syndrome, *Crit Care Med* 35(Suppl 9):S584, 2007.

110. Bristrian B, McCowen KC: Nutritional and metabolic support in the adult intensive care unit: key controversies, *Crit Care Med* 34(5):1525, 2006.

111. Vincent JL: Metabolic support in sepsis and multiple organ failure: more questions than answers, *Crit Care Med* 35(Suppl 9):S436, 2007.

112. Cheek DJ, et al: Shock, multiple organ dysfunction syndrome, and burns in adults. In McCance KL, Huether SE, editors: *Pathophysiology: the biologic basis for disease in adults and children*, ed 6, St Louis, 2010, Mosby.

113. Cohn SM, et al: Tissue oxygen saturation predicts the development of organ dysfunction during traumatic shock resuscitation, *J Trauma* 62(1):44, 2007.

114. Epstein CD, et al: Oxygen transport and organ dysfunction in the older trauma patient, *Heart Lung* 31(5):315, 2002.

115. Fry DE: Systemic inflammatory response and multiple organ dysfunction syndrome: biologic domino effect. In Baue AE, editor: *Multiple organ failure: pathophysiology, prevention, and therapy*, New York, 2000, Springer-Verlag.

116. Walsh CR: Multiple organ dysfunction syndrome after multiple trauma, *Orthop Nurs* 24(5):324, 2005.

117. Tschoeke SK, et al: The early second hit in trauma management augments the proinflammatory immune response to multiple injuries, *J Trauma* 62(6):1396, 2007.

118. Dulhunty JM, et al: Does severe non-infectious SIRS differ from severe sepsis? Results from a multi-centre Australian and New Zealand intensive care unit study, *Intensive Care Med* 34(9):1654, 2008.

119. Sankoff JD, et al: Validation of the Mortality in Emergency Department Sepsis (MEDS) score in patients with the systemic inflammatory response syndrome (SIRS), *Crit Care Med* 36(2):421, 2008.

120. Rote NS, Huether SE: Innate immunity: inflammation. In McCance KL, Huether SE, editors: *Pathophysiology: the biologic basis for disease in adults and children*, ed 6, St Louis, 2010, Mosby.

121. Majetschak M, Waydhas C: Infection, bacteremia, sepsis, and the sepsis syndrome: metabolic alterations, hypermetabolism, and cellular alterations. In Baue AE, editor: *Multiple organ failure: pathophysiology, prevention, and therapy*, New York, 2000, Springer-Verlag.

122. Shimizu K, et al: Altered gut flora and environment in patients with severe SIRS, *J Trauma* 60(1):126, 2006.

123. Schmidt H, et al: The alteration of autonomic function in multiple organ dysfunction syndrome, *Crit Care Clin* 24(1):149, 2008.

124. Krau SD: Making sense of multiple organ dysfunction syndrome, *Crit Care Nurs Clin North Am* 19(1):87, 2007.

125. Beale RJ, et al: Early enteral supplementation with key pharmaconutrients improves Sequential Organ Failure Assessment score in critically ill patients with sepsis: outcome of a randomized, controlled, double-blind trial, *Crit Care Med* 36(1):131, 2008.

126. Clark JA, Coopersmith CM: Intestinal crosstalk: a new paradigm for understanding the gut as the "motor" of critical illness, *Shock* 28(4):384, 2007.

127. Marshall JC, et al: The gastrointestinal tract. The "undrained abscess" of multiple organ failure, *Ann Surg* 218(2):111, 1993.

128. Dhainaut JF, et al: Hepatic response to sepsis: interaction between coagulation and inflammatory processes, *Crit Care Med* 29(Suppl 7):S42, 2001.

129. Baue A: Liver: multiple organ dysfunction and failure. In Baue AE, editor: *Multiple organ failure: pathophysiology, prevention, and therapy*, New York, 2000, Springer-Verlag.

130. Wong F: Liver and kidney diseases, *Clin Liver Dis* 6(4):981, 2002.

131. Barie PS, Eachempati SR: Acute acalculous cholecystitis, *Gastroenterol Clin North Am* 39(2):343, 2010.

132. Vincent JL, Zambon M: Why do patients who have acute lung injury/acute respiratory distress syndrome die from multiple organ dysfunction syndrome? Implications for management, *Clin Chest Med* 27(4):725, 2006.

133. Crouser ED, Fahy RJ: Acute lung injury, pulmonary edema, and multiple system organ failure. In Wilkins RL, Stoller JK, Kacmarek RM, editors: *Egan's fundamentals of respiratory care*, ed 9, St Louis, 2009, Mosby.

134. Huether SE, Forshee BA: Alterations of renal and urinary tract function. In McCance KL, Huether SE, editors: *Pathophysiology: the biologic basis for disease in adults and children*, ed 6, St Louis, 2010, Mosby.

135. Mullins R: Renal function and dysfunction in multiple organ failure. In Baue AE, editor: *Multiple organ failure: pathophysiology, prevention, and therapy*, New York, 2000, Springer-Verlag.

136. Zanotti-Cavazzoni SL, Hollenberg SM: Cardiac dysfunction in severe sepsis and septic shock, *Curr Opin Crit Care* 15(5):392, 2009.

137. Dhainaut JF, et al: Dynamic evolution of coagulopathy in the first day of severe sepsis: relationship with mortality and organ failure, *Crit Care Med* 33(2):341, 2005.

138. Ely EW, et al: Advances in the understanding of clinical manifestations and therapy of severe sepsis: an update for critical care nurses, *Am J Crit Care* 12(2):120, 2003.

139. Richards M, et al: Epidemiology, prevalence, and sites of infections in intensive care units, *Semin Respir Crit Care Med* 24(1):3, 2003.

140. Weitzel LR, Wischmeyer PE: Glutamine in critical illness: the time has come, the time is now, *Crit Care Clin* 26(3):515, 2010.

141. Villars PS: Multidisciplinary approach to VAP prevention, *Crit Care Nurse* 27(6):12, 2007.

27

Hematological Disorders and Oncological Emergencies

Barbara Mayer

⊖volve WEBSITE

Be sure to check out the bonus material, including free self-assessment exercises, on the Evolve web site at *http://evolve.elsevier.com/Urden/priorities/*.

OBJECTIVES

- Describe the etiology and pathophysiology of disseminated intravascular coagulation, heparin-induced thrombocytopenia, and tumor lysis syndrome.
- Identify the clinical manifestations of disseminated intravascular coagulation, heparin-induced thrombocytopenia, and tumor lysis syndrome.

- Explain the treatment of disseminated intravascular coagulation, heparin-induced thrombocytopenia, and tumor lysis syndrome.
- Discuss the nursing priorities for managing the patient with disseminated intravascular coagulation, heparin-induced thrombocytopenia, and tumor lysis syndrome.

Understanding the pathology of a disease, the areas of assessment on which to focus, and the usual medical management allows the critical care nurse to more accurately anticipate and plan nursing interventions. This chapter focuses on hematological and oncological disorders commonly seen in the critical care environment.

DISSEMINATED INTRAVASCULAR COAGULATION

Disseminated intravascular coagulation (DIC) is a syndrome that arises as a complication of other serious or life-threatening conditions. Although DIC is not seen often, it can seriously hamper diagnostic and treatment efforts for the critically ill patient. An understanding of the etiological and pathophysiological mechanisms of DIC can assist in anticipating the syndrome's occurrence, recognizing its signs and symptoms, and prompting intervention. Also known as consumptive *coagulopathy*, DIC is characterized by bleeding and thrombosis, both of which result from depletion of clotting factors, platelets, and red blood cells (RBCs). If not treated quickly, DIC will progress to multiple organ failure and death.[1]

Etiology

Many clinical events can prompt the development of DIC in the critically ill patient, but the exact underlying trigger may not be identifiable (Box 27-1). There are, however, some

commonly known conditions associated with the development of DIC.

The most common precipitating events for DIC are sepsis and trauma.[1] In sepsis, endotoxins serve as a trigger for activation of tissue factor and the extrinsic coagulation pathway. Metabolic acidosis and hypoperfusion associated with shock syndromes can result in increased formation of free radicals and damage to tissues. Tissue factor is activated, resulting in DIC.[2] Massive trauma or burns are frequently associated with DIC. Direct tissue damage activates the extrinsic coagulation pathway, and damage to endothelial surfaces activates the intrinsic pathway.[2] Obstetric emergencies, such as abruptio placentae, retained placenta, or incomplete abortion, are also associated with the development of DIC. Tissue factor is concentrated in the placenta, and damage or disruption of this structure can activate coagulation pathways, resulting in coagulopathy.[3]

Pathophysiology

Regardless of the cause, the common thread in the development of DIC is damage to the endothelium, which results in activation of the coagulation mechanism (Figure 27-1).[1] The extrinsic coagulation pathway plays a major role in the development of DIC. Direct damage to the endothelium results in the release of tissue factor and activation of this pathway. The secondary surge of thrombin formation as a result of activation of the intrinsic coagulation pathway leads to the massive

---

BOX 27-1   CAUSES OF DISSEMINATED INTRAVASCULAR COAGULATION

Obstetric Complications
- Abruptio placentae
- Placenta previa
- Retained dead fetus
- Septic abortion
- Amniotic fluid embolism
- Toxemia of pregnancy

Infections
- Gram-negative sepsis
- Gram-positive sepsis
- Meningococcemia
- Rocky Mountain spotted fever
- Histoplasmosis
- Aspergillosis
- Malaria

Neoplasms
- Carcinomas of pancreas, prostate, lung, and stomach
- Acute promyelocytic leukemia

- Tumor lysis syndrome
- Chemotherapy

Massive Tissue Injury
- Trauma
- Crush injuries
- Burns
- Extensive surgery
- Heat stroke
- Acute transplant rejection

Miscellaneous
- Acute intravascular hemolysis
- Snakebite
- Giant hemangioma
- Shock
- Vasculitis
- Aortic aneurysm
- Liver disease
- Cardiac arrest

Modified from Cotran RS, Kumar V, Collins T: *Robbins pathologic basis of disease*, ed 6, Philadelphia, 1999, Saunders.

---

disruption of the delicate balance that is hemostasis. Excessive thrombin formation results in rapid consumption of coagulation factors and depletion of regulatory substances—protein C, protein S, and antithrombin.[4] With no checks and balances, thrombi continue to form along damaged epithelial walls, resulting in occlusion of the vessels. As occlusion reaches a critical level, tissue ischemia ensues, leading to further tissue damage and perpetuating the process. Eventually, end-organ function is affected by the ischemia, and failure is evident.[1]

In response to the formation of clots, the fibrinolytic system is activated. As plasmin breaks down the fibrin clots, fibrin split products are released, and they act as anticoagulants.[2,3] Coupled with depletion of circulating clotting factors, activation of fibrinolysis results in excessive bleeding. The end result is shock and further tissue ischemia that aggravate end-organ dysfunction and failure. Death is imminent if this destructive cycle is not interrupted.[5]

Assessment and Diagnosis

Favorable outcomes for patients with DIC depend on accurate and timely diagnosis of the condition. Realization of the role underlying pathology plays, recognition of clinical manifestations, and assessment of appropriate laboratory values are key steps in this process.

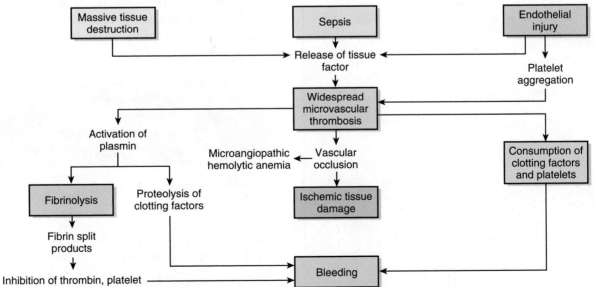

FIGURE 27-1 Pathophysiology of disseminated intravascular coagulation. (From Cotran RS, Kumar V, Collins T: *Robbins pathologic basis of disease*, ed 6, Philadelphia, 1999, Saunders.)

Clinical Manifestations

Clinical manifestations are related to the two primary pathophysiological mechanisms of DIC: the formation of thrombi and bleeding. Thrombi in peripheral capillaries can lead to cyanosis, particularly in the fingers, toes, ears, and nose. In severe, untreated cases, this peripheral ischemia may progress to gangrene.[2,4-6] As the condition progresses, ischemia worsens, and end organs are affected. The result of this more central ischemia can be respiratory insufficiency and failure, acute tubular necrosis, bowel infarction, and ischemic stroke. The tissue damage that results perpetuates the anomalies of DIC.[1]

As coagulation factors are depleted, bleeding from intravenous and other puncture sites is observed. Ecchymoses may result from even routine interventions such as the use of a manual blood pressure cuff, bathing, or turning.[2] Bloody drainage may also occur from surgical sites, drains, and urinary catheters. With progression of DIC, the patient is at risk for severe gastrointestinal or subarachnoid hemorrhage.[2,6] Table 27-1 lists many of the common signs and symptoms of DIC.

Laboratory Findings

Laboratory tests used to diagnose DIC essentially assess the four basic characteristics of this syndrome: (1) increased coagulant activity, (2) increased fibrinolytic activity, (3) impaired regulatory function, and (4) end-organ failure.

Continuous activation of the coagulation pathways results in consumption of coagulation factors. Because of this, the prothrombin time (PT), the activated partial thromboplastin time (aPTT), and the international normalized ratio (INR) values are elevated. Although the platelet count may fall within normal ranges, serial examination reveals a declining trend in values. An unexpected drop of at least 50% in the platelet count, particularly in the presence of known contributing factors and associated signs and symptoms, strongly indicates DIC.[7] Fibrinogen levels drop as more and more clots are formed. Thrombus formation in small vessels narrows the vessel lumen, forcing RBCs to squeeze through. The resulting damage and fragmentation of these cells can be seen on microscopic examination of blood samples. Damaged, fragmented RBCs are called *schistocytes*.[2,6,8]

In response to the excess clotting activity, the fibrinolytic process accelerates, and levels of by-products increase. This is reflected in markedly elevated levels of fibrin degradation products. Another key laboratory test used to evaluate the degree of clot dissolution—and therefore the severity of the coagulopathy—is the D-dimer level.[7] D-dimers exclusively indicate clot degradation because, unlike fibrin degradation products, which also result from the breakdown of free circulating fibrin, D-dimers result only from dissolution of clots.[2] With progression of the coagulopathy, normal regulatory mechanisms are disrupted, as reflected in decreasing levels of inhibitory factors such as protein C, factor V, and antithrombin III.[2,6]

Unchecked DIC resulting in occlusion of vessels and tissue ischemia leads to end-organ dysfunction.[1] Respiratory failure, indicated by abnormal arterial blood gas (ABG) levels; liver failure, indicated by increasing liver enzymes; and renal impairment, indicated by rising blood urea nitrogen (BUN) and creatinine levels, are common findings in advanced DIC.[5]

No single laboratory study can confirm the diagnosis of DIC, but several key results are strong indicators of the condition (Table 27-2). The International Society of Thrombosis and Hemostasis emphasizes early detection of DIC through observation of abnormal trends in laboratory values.[4]

TABLE 27-1	COMMON SIGNS AND SYMPTOMS OF DISSEMINATED INTRAVASCULAR COAGULATION	
SYSTEM	**SIGNS RELATED TO HEMORRHAGE**	**SIGNS RELATED TO THROMBI**
Integumentary	Bleeding from gums, venipunctures, and old surgical sites; epistaxis; ecchymoses	Peripheral cyanosis, gangrene
Cardiopulmonary	Hemoptysis	Dysrhythmias, chest pain, acute myocardial infarction, pulmonary embolus, respiratory failure
Renal	Hematuria	Oliguria, acute tubular necrosis, renal failure
Gastrointestinal	Abdominal distention, hemorrhage	Diarrhea, constipation, bowel infarct
Neurological	Subarachnoid hemorrhage	Altered level of consciousness, ischemic stroke

TABLE 27-2	KEY LABORATORY STUDIES IN DISSEMINATED INTRAVASCULAR COAGULATION
TEST	**VALUE**
Prothrombin time (PT)	>12.5 sec
Platelets	<50,000/mm³, or at least 50% drop from baseline
Activated partial thromboplastin time (aPTT)	>40 sec
D-dimer	>250 ng/mL
Fibrin degradation products (FDP)	>40 mcg/mL
Fibrinogen	<100 mg/dL

Medical Management

Without question, the primary intervention in DIC is prevention. Being aware of the conditions that commonly contribute to the development of DIC and treating them vigorously and without delay provide the best defense against this devastating condition.[2,4,6,8] After DIC is identified, maintaining organ perfusion and slowing consumption of coagulation factors are paramount to achieving a favorable outcome.[1,2]

Multiple organ dysfunction syndrome (MODS) frequently results from DIC and exacerbates the underlying pathology. It is essential to prevent end-organ ischemia and damage by supporting blood pressure and circulating volume. Administration of intravenous fluids and inotropic agents, and, if overt hemorrhaging is evident, infusion of packed RBCs are appropriate interventions to replace blood volume and essential, oxygen-carrying RBCs.

In the presence of severe platelet depletion (<50,000/mm³) and severe hemorrhage, platelet transfusions are often indicated.[4,6] However, caution must be used when administering platelets because antiplatelet antibodies may be formed. These antibodies may become activated during future platelet transfusions and elicit DIC.[2]

Replacement of clotting factors in the patient with DIC is thought by some authorities to perpetuate the coagulopathy; however, there is little scientific evidence to support this theory.[1] Fibrinogen levels less than 100 mg/dL indicate the appropriateness of administering cryoprecipitate. A prolonged PT indicates the need for fresh-frozen plasma.[2,4,6]

Slowing consumption of coagulation factors by inhibiting the processes involved in clot formation is another strategy used in treating DIC. The use of heparin, particularly low-molecular-weight heparin, to prevent formation of future clots is controversial.[5] It is contraindicated in patients with DIC associated with recent surgery or with gastrointestinal or central nervous system (CNS) bleeding. However, heparin has been beneficial in obstetric emergencies such as retained placenta or incomplete abortion, severe arterial occlusions, or MODS caused by microemboli.[2,6]

The use of recombinant activated protein C is gaining popularity in treating DIC, especially in the setting of severe sepsis. Activated protein C acts as an anticoagulant and works to restore normal inhibition of coagulation pathways. However, it has been associated with an increased incidence of intracerebral bleeding and must be used with caution in patients with severely decreased platelets.[2,4]

Thrombin production in DIC surpasses that of antithrombins and other regulatory factors that would normally be present to inactivate thrombin and its subsequent actions. The use of antithrombin III has recently been approved in the United States. Ongoing research is yielding mixed results in the treatment of DIC.[4] One interesting area of research is the use of protease inhibitors. Protease molecules normally inhibit the conversion of fibrinogen to fibrin in the coagulation mechanism, but in DIC, this inhibitory mechanism is impaired. The introduction of protease inhibitors by intravenous infusion may be advantageous in arresting DIC.[2]

Nursing Management

Nursing management of the patient with DIC incorporates a variety of nursing diagnoses (see the Nursing Diagnosis Priorities Box on Disseminated Intravascular Coagulation). Assessment and monitoring are the primary weapons in the critical care nurse's arsenal against DIC. Knowing the diseases and conditions that are most often associated with DIC and understanding the pathophysiological mechanisms involved enables the critical care nurse to anticipate its development and intervene quickly. **Nursing priorities are directed toward (1) supporting the patient's vital functions, (2) initiating bleeding precautions, (3) providing comfort and emotional support, and (4) maintaining surveillance for complications.**

NURSING DIAGNOSIS PRIORITIES

Disseminated Intravascular Coagulation

- Deficient Fluid Volume related to active blood loss, p. A-13
- Decreased Cardiac Output related to alterations in preload, p. A-10
- Risk for Infection, p. A-36
- Anxiety related to threat to biological, psychological, and/or social integrity, p. A-7
- Compromised Family Coping related to a critically ill family member, p. A-9

Supporting Patient's Vital Functions

Frequent assessments should include parameters for neurological status, renal function, cardiopulmonary function, and skin integrity that indicate impaired tissue or organ perfusion. Particular parameters to include are mental status, BUN and creatine levels, urine output, vital signs, hemodynamic values, cardiac rhythm, arterial blood gas and pulse oximetry values, skin breakdown, ecchymoses, or hematomas.[6]

The critical care nurse must recognize and support the patient's vital physiological functions. Administration of intravenous fluids, blood products, and inotropic agents to provide adequate hemodynamic support and tissue oxygenation is essential in preventing or combating end-organ damage. Close monitoring of vital signs, hemodynamic parameters, intake and output, and appropriate laboratory values assists the critical care nurse in administering and titrating appropriate agents.

Initiating Bleeding Precautions

Awareness of the patient's bleeding potential necessitates adjustments to normal nursing interventions. The nurse avoids unnecessary venipunctures that may result in bleeding, bruising, or hematomas by drawing blood from and administering medications through existing arterial or venous lines. The use of manual or automatic blood pressure cuffs is avoided whenever possible. If tracheal or oral suctioning is necessary, the use of low-level suction is recommended.[6] Meticulous skin care is advised, keeping the skin moist and using specialty mattresses and beds as appropriate to prevent breakdown. Gentle care should be used when bathing or turning the patient to prevent bruising or hematoma formation.

Providing Emotional Support

The development of DIC in the already critically ill patient can be stressful for the patient and his or her significant others. It is imperative to provide psychosocial support throughout this crisis. Calm reassurance and uncomplicated explanations of the care the patient is receiving can help to allay much of the anxiety experienced. The critical care nurse must answer all questions and provide information in terms best understood by all parties. The use of an interpreter when English is not the primary language can enhance understanding and help avoid misconceptions. Providing spiritual support as requested may also be of assistance.

Please see the Collaborative Management Box on Disseminated Intravascular Coagulation for more information.

COLLABORATIVE MANAGEMENT
Disseminated Intravascular Coagulation

- Identify and eliminate the underlying cause.
- Provide hemodynamic support to prevent end-organ ischemia.
  - Intravenous fluids
  - Positive inotropic agents
- Administer blood and blood components.
  - Fresh-frozen plasma
  - Platelets
  - Cryoprecipitate
  - Antithrombin III
- Administer medications.
  - Heparin
  - Activated protein C
- Initiate bleeding precautions.
- Maintain surveillance for complications.
  - Hypovolemic shock
  - Peripheral ischemia
  - Central ischemia
  - Multiple organ dysfunction syndrome (MODS)
- Provide comfort and emotional support.

HEPARIN-INDUCED THROMBOCYTOPENIA

One form of thrombocytopenia seen in critical care patients is heparin-induced thrombocytopenia (HIT). There are two distinct types of HIT. The most common form is non-immune-mediated HIT, formally known as type 1 HIT.[9] Seen in up to 30% of patients receiving heparin therapy, this nonautoimmune condition manifests within a few days of initiation of therapy. Platelet depletion is moderate, counts are usually less than 100,000/mm³, and the condition

is transient, often resolving spontaneously. Discontinuation of heparin is not required. The second form is immune-mediated HIT,[9] formally known as type 2 HIT, which is less commonly encountered but has more severe consequences.[10-12] This discussion is limited to immune-mediated HIT.

Etiology

Immune-mediated HIT is a response to the administration of heparin therapy. It has been observed in 1% to 3% of patients treated with unfractionated heparin and has occurred after exposure to low-molecular-weight heparin (LMWH), although to a lesser degree.[9] The disorder is characterized by severe thrombocytopenia during heparin therapy. Diagnostically it is identified by a platelet count less than 50,000/mm³ or at least a 50% decrease from the baseline platelet count from the initiation of therapy. Onset usually occurs 5 to 14 days from the first exposure to heparin, but the onset can occur within hours of a reexposure to heparin.[11-13] Depending on the source of the disorder, reported mortality rates are as high as 30%.[9]

Pathophysiology

The thrombocytopenia that occurs with immune-mediated HIT is related to the formation of heparin-antibody complexes. These complexes release a substance known as platelet factor 4 (PF4). PF4 attracts heparin molecules, forming immunogenic complexes that adhere to platelet and endothelial surfaces (Figure 27-2). Activation of platelets stimulates the release of thrombin and the subsequent formation of platelet clumps.[12]

Patients with immune-mediated HIT are at greater risk for thrombosis than bleeding. Vessel occlusion can result in the need for limb amputation, stroke, acute myocardial infarction, and even death.[10-12] The resultant formation of fibrin-platelet-rich thrombi is the primary characteristic of HIT that distinguishes it from other forms of thrombocytopenia and gives rise to its more descriptive name: white clot syndrome.[10]

Assessment and Diagnosis

HIT can be associated with severe consequences. Rapid recognition of risk factors and subsequent development of signs and symptoms is essential in treating this condition.

Clinical Manifestations

Common signs and symptoms are listed in Table 27-3. The clinical manifestations of HIT are related to the formation of thrombi and subsequent vessel occlusion.[9] Most thrombotic events are venous, although venous and arterial thrombosis can occur. Thrombotic events typically include deep vein thrombosis, pulmonary embolism, limb ischemia thrombosis, thrombotic stroke, and myocardial infarction.[9] The presence of blanching and the loss of peripheral pulses, sensation, or motor function in a limb indicate peripheral vascular thrombi. Neurological signs and symptoms such as

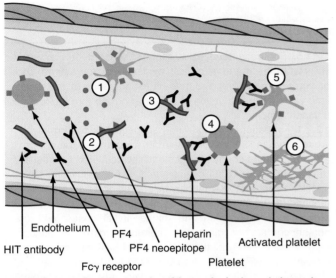

FIGURE 27-2 Pathogenesis of heparin-induced thrombocytopenia (HIT). **(1)** Activated platelets release procoagulant proteins from α-granules, including platelet factor 4 (PF4). Administered heparin binds PF4 **(2)**, which undergoes a conformation change and expresses a new antigen (neoepitope). Individuals with HIT produce an immunoglobulin G (IgG) antibody that specifically reacts **(3)** with multiple identical neoepitopes on the heparin-PF4 complex. The reaction forms heparin-PF4-IgG immune complexes. Platelets express FcγRIIa receptors (Fcγ receptor) that react **(4)** with the Fc portion of IgG in immune complexes. Cross-linking of Fc receptors **(5)** results in FcγRIIa-dependent platelet activation. The activated platelets mediate a series of events that lead to further activation of the coagulation cascade, resulting in thrombin generation. Further release of PF4 from newly activated platelets leads to a cycle of continuing platelet activation and **(6)** formation of a primary clot. The reaction can be enhanced by the release of platelet-derived microparticles that are rich in surface phosphatidylserine and increase activation of coagulation and by the binding of heparin-PF4 complexes and HIT-IgG to the vascular endothelium (not shown.) (From McCance KL, Huether SE, Brashers VL, Rote NS: *Pathophysiology: The biologic basis for disease in adults and children*, ed 6, St Louis, 2010, Mosby.)

confusion, headache, and impaired speech can signal the onset of cerebral artery occlusion and stroke. Acute myocardial infarction may be heralded by dyspnea, chest pain, pallor, and alterations in blood pressure. Thrombi in the pulmonary vasculature may be evidenced by pleuritic pain, rales, and dyspnea.[10,13]

Laboratory Findings

The key indicator for identifying HIT is the platelet count. General consensus in the literature considers a platelet count of less than 100,000/mm³ or a sudden drop of 50% from the patient's baseline after initiation of heparin therapy to strongly indicate HIT.[10-13]

Two types of assays have become available to assist in confirming the diagnosis of HIT: activation assays, based on platelet aggregation or the release of granular contents such as serotonin, and assays that identify the HIT antigen. Activation assays are highly sensitive in detecting the presence of HIT. The most common assay used is heparin-induced platelet aggregation (HIPA). Serotonin release assay (SRA) is used by a few institutions. The enzyme-linked immunosorbent assay (ELISA) identifies the presence of the HIT antigen.[11,12]

Medical Management

Evidenced-based guidelines for the prevention and management of the patient with HIT are listed in the Evidence-Based Collaborative Practice Box on Treatment and Prevention of Heparin-Induced Thrombocytopenia.[14] When a decrease in the platelet count is detected, heparin therapy should be discontinued immediately, and the patient should be tested for the presence of heparin antibodies.[11-14] If the original indication for heparin still exists or new thromboses occur, an alternative form of anticoagulation is usually necessary.[14]

Direct thrombin inhibitors (DTIs) are being used with increasing frequency to treat HIT. DTIs bind directly to the

TABLE 27-3	HEPARIN-INDUCED THROMBOCYTOPENIA: SIGNS, SYMPTOMS, AND LABORATORY DATA
SYSTEM OR STUDY	**SIGNS AND SYMPTOMS**
Cardiac	Chest pain, diaphoresis, pallor, alterations in blood pressure, dysrhythmias
Vascular	Arterial: pain, pallor, pulselessness, paresthesia, paralysis
	Venous: pain, tenderness, unilateral leg swelling, warmth, erythema, a palpable cord, pain on passive dorsiflexion of the foot, and spontaneous maintenance of the relaxed foot in abnormal plantar flexion (Homans' sign)
Pulmonary	Dyspnea, pleuritic pain, rales, chest pain, chest wall tenderness, back pain, shoulder pain, upper abdominal pain, syncope, hemoptysis, shortness of breath, wheezing
Renal	Thirst, decreased urine output, dizziness, orthostatic hypotension
Gastrointestinal	Abdominal pain, vomiting, bloody diarrhea, abnormal bowel sounds
Neurological	Confusion, headache, impaired speech patterns, hemiparesis or hemiplegia, vision disturbances, dysarthria, aphasia, ataxia, vertigo, nystagmus, sudden decrease in consciousness
Laboratory	Platelets <50,000/mm³ or sudden drop of 30% to 50% from baseline; positive results for HIPA, SRA, ELISA

ELISA, enzyme-linked immunosorbent assay; *HIPA*, heparin-induced platelet aggregation; *SRA*, serotonin release assay.

EVIDENCE-BASED COLLABORATIVE PRACTICE
Treatment and Prevention of Heparin-Induced Thrombocytopenia

The following are grade 1 recommendations (unless otherwise specified) from the American College of Chest Physicians. Grade 1 recommendations are strong and indicate that the benefits do, or do not, outweigh risks, burden, and costs.

1.1. For patients receiving heparin for whom the clinician considers the risk of HIT to be >1.0%, we recommend platelet count monitoring over no platelet count monitoring.

1.1.1. For patients who are starting UFH or LMWH treatment and who have received UFH within the past 100 days, or those patients for whom exposure history is uncertain, we recommend obtaining a baseline platelet count and then a repeat platelet count within 24 h of starting heparin over not obtaining a repeat platelet count.

1.1.2. For patients in whom acute inflammatory, cardiorespiratory, neurological, or other unusual symptoms and signs develop within 30 min following an IV UFH bolus, we recommend performing an immediate platelet count measurement, and comparing this value to recent prior platelet counts, over not performing a platelet count.

1.1.7. For patients who are receiving fondaparinux thromboprophylaxis or treatment, we recommend that clinicians do not use routine platelet count monitoring.

1.1.9. In patients who receive heparin, or for whom heparin treatment is planned (e.g., for cardiac or vascular surgery), we recommend against routine HIT antibody testing in the absence of thrombocytopenia, thrombosis, heparin-induced skin lesions, or other signs pointing to a potential diagnosis of HIT.

1.1.10. For patients who are receiving heparin or have received heparin within the previous 2 weeks, we recommend investigating for a diagnosis of HIT if the platelet count falls by ≥50%, and/or a thrombotic event occurs between days 5 and 14 (inclusive) following initiation of heparin, even if the patient is no longer receiving heparin therapy when thrombosis or thrombocytopenia has occurred.

1.2. For postoperative cardiac surgery patients, we recommend investigating for HIT antibodies if the platelet count falls by ≥50%, and/or a thrombotic event occurs, between postoperative days 5 and 14 (inclusive, day of cardiac surgery = day 0).

2.1.1. For patients with strongly suspected (or confirmed) HIT, whether complicated by thrombosis or not, we recommend use of an alternative, non-heparin anticoagulant (danaparoid, lepirudin [Grade 1C], argatroban [Grade 1C], fondaparinux [Grade 2C], bivalirudin [Grade 2C]) over the further use of UFH or LMWH therapy or initiation/continuation of a VKA.

2.1.5. For patients with strongly suspected or confirmed HIT, whether there is clinical evidence of lower-limb DVT or not, we recommend routine ultrasonography of the lower-limb veins for investigation of DVT over not performing routine ultrasonography.

2.2.1. For patients with strongly suspected or confirmed HIT, we recommend against the use of VKA (coumarin) therapy until after the platelet count has substantially recovered (i.e., usually to at least 150×10^9/L) over starting VKA therapy at a lower platelet count; that VKA therapy be started only with low, maintenance doses (maximum, 5 mg of warfarin or 6 mg of phenprocoumon) rather than with higher initial doses; and the non-heparin anticoagulant (e.g., lepirudin, argatroban, danaparoid) be continued until the platelet count has reached a stable plateau, the INR has reached the intended target range, and after a minimum overlap of at least 5 days between non-heparin anticoagulation and VKA therapy rather than a shorter overlap.

2.2.2. For patients receiving a VKA at the time of diagnosis of HIT, we recommend use of vitamin K (10 mg PO or 5-10 mg IV).

2.3.1. For patients with strongly suspected HIT, whether complicated by thrombosis or not, we recommend against use of LMWH.

3.1.1. For patients with a history of HIT who are HIT antibody negative and require cardiac surgery, we recommend the use of UFH over a non-heparin anticoagulant.

3.2.1. For patients with acute HIT (thrombocytopenic, HIT antibody positive) who require cardiac surgery, we recommend one of the following alternative anticoagulant approaches (in descending order): delaying surgery (if possible) until HIT has resolved and antibodies are negative (see 3.1.1.) or weakly positive; using bivalirudin for intraoperative anticoagulation during cardiopulmonary bypass (if techniques of cardiac surgery and anesthesiology have been adapted to the unique features of bivalirudin pharmacology) or during "off-pump" cardiac surgery.

3.2.2. For patients with subacute HIT (platelet count recovery, but continuing HIT antibody positive), we recommend delaying surgery (if possible) until HIT antibodies (washed platelet activation assay) are negative, then using heparin (see Recommendation 3.1.1.) over using a non-heparin anticoagulant.

3.3.1. For patients with strongly suspected (or confirmed) acute HIT who require cardiac catheterization or PCI, we recommend a non-heparin anticoagulant (bivalirudin, argatroban [Grade 1C], lepirudin [Grade 1C], or danaparoid [Grade 1C]) over UFH or LMWH.

Modified from Warkentin TE, et al: Treatment and prevention of heparin-induced thrombocytopenia: American College of Chest Physicians evidence-based clinical practice guidelines, *Chest* 133(Suppl 6):340S, 2008.
DVT, deep vein thrombosis; *HIT*, heparin-induced thrombocytopenia; *IV*, intravenous; *LMWH*, low-molecular-weight heparin; *UFH*, unfractionated heparin; *VKA*, vitamin K antagonist.

thrombin molecule, thereby inhibiting its action.[14] Two such drugs are lepirudin and argatroban.[9] Warfarin, although commonly used to treat deep vein thrombosis, is not indicated as a sole agent in treating HIT because of its prolonged onset of action. Studies have shown that the use of warfarin without concomitant use of DTIs can significantly increase the incidence of thrombosis in patients with

HIT.[9] Comparative information on these medications is provided in Table 27-4.[9,14]

Nursing Management

Nursing management of the patient with HIT incorporates a variety of nursing diagnoses (see the Nursing Diagnosis Priorities Box on Heparin-Induced Thrombocytopenia).

TABLE 27-4 PHARMACOLOGICAL MANAGEMENT: HEPARIN-INDUCED THROMBOCYTOPENIA

DRUG	DOSAGE	ACTIONS	SPECIAL CONSIDERATIONS
Lepirudin (Refludan)	Loading dose: 0.4 mg/ kg IV bolus IV infusion: 0.15 mg/kg/ hr	Used to inhibit free and clot-bound thrombin; a recombinant form of leech-derived hirudin	Monitor aPTT; maintain INR 1.5-2.5 times normal. Reduce dosage in patients with known or suspected renal insufficiency. Side effects include bleeding. Can develop antilepirudin antibodies that enhance anticoagulant effect.
Argatroban	Loading dose: None IV infusion: 2 mcg/kg/min not to exceed 10 mcg/kg/min	Used to inhibit thrombin	Obtain baseline aPTT 2 hr after therapy started. Monitor aPTT; maintain INR 1.5-3.0 times initial baseline. Reduce dosage in patients with known or suspected hepatic impairment.
Bivalirudin	Loading dose: 0.75 mg/ kg IV bolus IV infusion: 1.75 mg/kg/hr	Used to inhibit thrombin	Monitor aPTT; maintain INR 1.5-2.5 times initial baseline. Adjust dose in presence of renal failure.

aPTT, activated partial thromboplastin time; *INR*, international normalized ratio; *IV*, intravenous.

Nursing priorities are directed toward (1) decreasing the incidence of heparin exposure, (2) maintaining surveillance for complications, (3) providing comfort and emotional support, and (4) initiating patient education. The critical care nurse plays a pivotal role in prevention and detection of heparin-induced thrombocytopenia. Initial assessment is crucial to identifying those patients at risk for HIT. Ascertaining a medical history that includes previous heparin therapy, deep vein thrombosis, or cardiovascular surgery that included the use of cardiopulmonary bypass can alert the nurse to potential problems.

NURSING DIAGNOSIS PRIORITIES

Heparin-Induced Thrombocytopenia

- Ineffective Cardiopulmonary Tissue Perfusion related to decreased coronary blood flow, p. A-28
- Ineffective Peripheral Tissue Perfusion related to decreased peripheral blood flow, p. A-32
- Ineffective Renal Tissue Perfusion related to decreased renal blood flow, p. A-33
- Ineffective Gastrointestinal Tissue Perfusion related to decreased gastrointestinal blood flow, p. A-32
- Ineffective Cerebral Tissue Perfusion related to decreased cerebral blood flow, p. A-29
- Powerlessness related to lack of control over the current situation or disease progression, p. A-33
- Deficient Knowledge related to lack of previous exposure to information (see the Patient Education box on Heparin-Induced Thrombocytopenia) , p. A-15

Decreasing the Incidence of Heparin Exposure

Ensuring that all heparin has been removed from the patient's hemodynamic pressure monitoring system, avoiding the use of heparin-coated catheters, and discontinuing heparin flushes to maintain the patency of other intravenous lines are essential elements of nursing management.

Maintaining Surveillance for Complications

Patients with HIT remain at high risk for thrombotic complications for several days or weeks after cessation of heparin. Vigilant monitoring, early recognition of signs and symptoms, deep vein thrombosis prevention strategies, and prompt notification of the physician are key roles of the critical care nurse.

Initiating Patient Education

Prevention of subsequent episodes in patients sensitized to heparin includes education of the patient and family (see the Patient Education Box on Heparin-Induced Thrombocytopenia). Education should include measures to avoid future exposure to heparin. The use of medical alert bracelets and listing heparin allergies in the medical record are necessary to avoid this serious complication in the future.

Please see the Collaborative Management Box on Heparin-Induced Thrombocytopenia for more information.

PATIENT EDUCATION

Heparin-Induced Thrombocytopenia

- Pathophysiology of disease
- Purpose of heparin
- Measures to avoid future exposure to heparin:
  - Identify different types of heparin (unfractionated and low-molecular-weight forms).
  - Encourage purchase of medical alert bracelet or similar type of warning device.
  - Tell any new health care provider about the heparin allergy and previous reaction.

TUMOR LYSIS SYNDROME

Tumor lysis syndrome (TLS) refers to a variety of metabolic disturbances that may be seen with the treatment of cancer. A potentially lethal complication of various forms of cancer treatment, TLS occurs when large numbers of neoplastic cells are rapidly killed, resulting in the release of large amounts of potassium, phosphate, and uric acid into the systemic circulation. It occurs in 5% to 20%[15] of cancer patients and is most commonly seen in patients with lymphoma, leukemia, or multiple metastatic conditions.[15-17]

Etiology

Although most often associated with the use of chemotherapeutic drugs, biological agents, and irradiation used in the treatment of malignant disorders, TLS can in rare instances occur spontaneously. The development of TLS has been linked to other pathophysiological conditions such as elevated WBC counts, large tumors, multiple organ involvement by malignancy, and renal insufficiency.[18]

Pathophysiology

The primary mechanism involved in the development of TLS is the destruction of massive numbers of malignant cells by chemotherapy or radiation therapy (Figure 27-3). Massive destruction of cells releases large amounts of potassium, phosphorus, and nucleic acids, leading to severe metabolic disturbances, such as hyperuricemia, hyperkalemia, hyperphosphatemia, and hypocalcemia (Table 27-5). Vomiting, diarrhea, and other insensible fluid losses from fever or tachypnea also contribute to these electrolyte disturbances.[17] Death of patients with TLS is most often caused by complications of renal failure or cardiac arrest.[18]

Hyperuricemia

Hyperuricemia occurs 48 to 72 hours after the initiation of anticancer therapy.[17] Tumor cells undergo rapid growth and development, and large amounts of nucleic acids are present

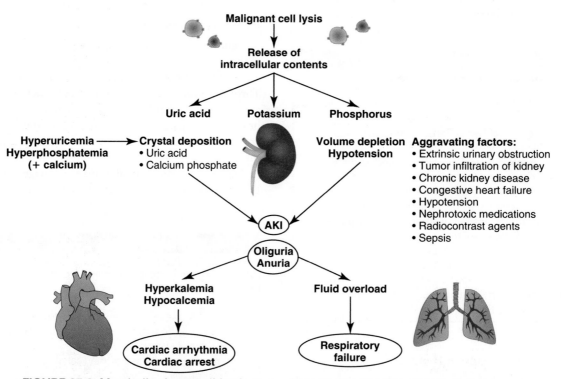

FIGURE 27-3 Metabolic abnormalities in tumor lysis syndrome and clinical consequences. *AKI,* acute kidney injury. (From Abu-Alfa AK, Younes A: Tumor lysis syndrome and acute kidney injury: evaluation, prevention and management, *Am J Kidney Dis* 55[5 Suppl 3]:S1, 2010.)

TABLE 27-5	ELECTROLYTE ABNORMALITIES ENCOUNTERED IN TUMOR LYSIS SYNDROME AND THEIR CLINICAL CONSEQUENCES		
ELECTROLYTE	**PATHOPHYSIOLOGY**	**CLINICAL CONSEQUENCE**	**TREATMENT OPTIONS**
Potassium	Rapid expulsion of intracellular K^+ into the circulation due to cell lysis	Adverse skeletal and cardiac manifestations (e.g., ventricular dysrhythmias, weakness, paresthesias)	Insulin/glucose, sodium bicarbonate, inhaled beta-agonist, K^+-binding resins, dialysis, calcium gluconate
Phosphate	Release of intracellular PO_4^- due to cell lysis May be compounded by renal dysfunction	Muscle cramps, tetany, dysrhythmias, seizures	Dialysis, phosphate binders
Calcium	Precipitation of the calcium phosphate complex because of the rapid increase in the phosphorous concentration	Muscle cramps, tetany, dysrhythmias, seizures, renal failure (acute nephrocalcinosis)	Calcium gluconate (treatment should be reserved for those with neuromuscular irritability)
Uric acid	Cell lysis leads to increased levels of purine nucleic acids into the circulation that are metabolized to uric acid	Renal failure (uric acid nephropathy)	Hydration, dialysis, xanthine oxidase inhibitors, alkalization of urine, urate oxidase

From Davidson MB, et al: Pathophysiology, clinical consequences, and treatment of tumor lysis syndrome, *Am J Med* 116(8):546, 2004.

within them. When therapy is initiated, tumor cell destruction releases nucleic acids, which are metabolized into uric acid. Metabolic acidosis ensues, resulting in crystallization of the uric acid in the distal tubules of the kidney and leading to obstruction of urine flow. Glomerular filtration rates drop as the kidneys are unable to clear the increasing amounts of uric acid. Consequently, renal insufficiency and acute renal failure eventually occur.[19] Acute renal failure is discussed further in Chapter 20.

Hyperuricemia associated with TLS can be potentiated by several other factors, including elevated uric acid levels before the initiation of therapy. Other causes of increased uric acid production are elevated WBC counts, destruction of WBCs, and enlargement of the lymph nodes, spleen, or liver.[17]

Hyperkalemia

Hyperkalemia occurs within 6 to 72 hours after the initiation of chemotherapy. This is the most deleterious of all the manifestations of TLS.[17] In addition to the release of nucleic acids, tumor cell destruction also results in the release of potassium. Renal insufficiency related to hyperuricemia prevents adequate excretion of potassium, and levels rise. The resultant hyperkalemia may have a profound effect on intracellular and extracellular fluid levels.[18] Left untreated, hyperkalemia can have devastating consequences, including cardiac arrest and death.[17]

Hyperphosphatemia and Hypocalcemia

Hyperphosphatemia and hypocalcemia occur 24 to 48 hours after the initiation of therapy.[17] Phosphorus levels also rise as a consequence of tumor cell destruction. Calcium ions then bind with the excess phosphorus, creating calcium phosphate salts and bringing about hypocalcemia. These salts precipitate in the kidney tubules, worsening renal insufficiency. Hypocalcemia causes tetany and cardiac dysrhythmias, which can result in cardiac arrest and death.[17,18]

TABLE 27-6	COMMON FINDINGS IN TUMOR LYSIS SYNDROME
DIAGNOSTIC PARAMETER	**FINDINGS**
Clinical	Weight gain, edema, diarrhea, lethargy, muscle cramps, nausea and vomiting, paresthesia, weakness, oliguria, uremia, seizures
Laboratory	↑Potassium, phosphorus, uric acid, BUN, Cr ↓Calcium, creatinine clearance, pH, bicarbonate, $PaCO_2$
Diagnostic	Positive Chvostek's and Trousseau's signs, hyperactive deep tendon reflexes, dysrhythmias, ECG changes

BUN, blood urea nitrogen; *Cr*, creatinine; *ECG*, electrocardiogram; *PaCO₂*, partial pressure of carbon dioxide; ↑, increased; ↓, decreased.

Assessment and Diagnosis

Detection and recognition of TLS is accomplished through assessment of clinical manifestations, evaluation of laboratory findings, and other diagnostic tests. Table 27-6 summarizes common findings in TLS.[17-19]

Clinical Manifestations

Clinical manifestations are related to the metabolic disturbances associated with TLS.[16] The patient's history reveals an unexplained weight gain after initiation of chemotherapy or radiation therapy. The weight gain is associated with fluid retention due to electrolyte disturbances. Other early signs heralding the onset of TLS include diarrhea, lethargy, muscle cramps, nausea, vomiting, paresthesia, and weakness.[20]

Laboratory Findings

Laboratory findings demonstrate electrolyte disturbances such as elevated potassium and phosphorus levels and a decreased calcium level. Uric acid levels are increased. Elevated levels of BUN and creatinine and a decreased creatinine clearance also indicate TLS. Metabolic acidosis is confirmed by the presence of decreased pH, bicarbonate levels, and partial pressure of carbon dioxide (Pa_{CO_2}) on arterial blood gas measurements.[20]

Other Diagnostic Tests

Physical examination reveals positive Chvostek's and Trousseau's signs related to hypocalcemia. Hyperactive deep tendon reflexes indicate hyperkalemia and hypocalcemia. Potassium and calcium disturbances result in changes that can be seen on the electrocardiogram (ECG), such as peaked or inverted T waves, altered QT intervals, widened QRS complexes, and dysrhythmias.[17]

Medical Management

Medical interventions are aimed at maintaining adequate hydration, treating metabolic imbalances, and preventing life-threatening complications.[15-17] Administration of intravenous fluids may be necessary early in the course of treatment if inadequate hydration exists. The administration of isotonic saline (0.9% normal saline) reduces serum concentrations of uric acid, phosphate, and potassium.[16,17] The use of nonthiazide diuretics to maintain adequate urine output may be required. If renal failure occurs, hemodialysis should be considered.[16-18]

Electrolytes and arterial blood gases are closely monitored. Dietary restrictions of potassium and phosphorus may be necessary. The goals in treating hyperuricemia are to inhibit uric acid formation and to increase renal clearance.[17] This can be accomplished through the administration of sodium bicarbonate to increase the pH of the urine to above 7.0, which increases the solubility of uric acid, preventing subsequent crystallization. Allopurinol administration can also inhibit uric acid formation (see the Priority Medications Box on Allopurinol).[16]

If potassium levels rise dangerously, Kayexalate (sodium polystyrene sulfonate) may be given orally, or if the patient is unable to tolerate oral medications due to nausea and vomiting, rectal instillation may be used. If the patient is oliguric, glucose and insulin infusions may be given to facilitate lowering the potassium levels. A 10% solution of calcium gluconate may be administered to stabilize cardiac tissue membranes to prevent life-threatening dysrhythmias.[21] Phosphorus-binding antacids can be used for treating hyperphosphatemia. Stool softeners may be necessary to treat the constipation often associated with the administration of these antacids. Calcium gluconate may be required to replace calcium, but it should be used judiciously.[17]

Nursing Management

Nursing management of the patient with TLS incorporates a variety of nursing diagnoses (see the Nursing Diagnosis Priorities Box on Tumor Lysis Syndrome). **Nursing priorities are directed toward (1) monitoring fluid and electrolytes, (2) providing comfort and emotional support, (3) maintaining surveillance for complications, and (4) initiating patient education.**

💊 PRIORITY MEDICATIONS

Allopurinol

Drug Class: Antiinflammatory agent

Drug Action: Allopurinol decreases the formation of uric acid by competitively inhibiting xanthine oxidase and thereby blocking the metabolism of hypoxanthine and xanthine to uric acid.

Drug Delivery and Drug Dosage: For the treatment of tumor lysis syndrome, allopurinol may be given orally or intravenously, though the intravenous route is generally reserved for those patient who cannot tolerate oral administration. The oral dose is 600-800 mg/day in 2-3 divided doses. The intravenous dose is 200-400 mg/m^2/day as a single dose or in 2-4 equally divided doses. The maximum dose is 600 mg/day.

Priority Nursing Considerations: Patients receiving allopurinol should have their serum uric acid concentrations closely monitored. When given orally, allopurinol should be administered after meals and with plenty of fluids (unless contraindicated). To prevent kidney stones, the patient's urine output should be maintained at least at 2 L a day.

Clinical Examples: Allopurinol is used for the prevention of acute hyperuricemia during the treatment of leukemia, lymphoma, or solid tumors that may cause tumor lysis syndrome. Allopurinol is also used for the treatment of gout.

NURSING DIAGNOSIS PRIORITIES

Tumor Lysis Syndrome

- Excess Fluid Volume related to renal dysfunction, p. A-19
- Decreased Cardiac Output related to alterations in contractility, p. A-11
- Anxiety related to threat to biological, psychological, and/or social integrity, p. A-7
- Ineffective Coping related to a situational crisis and personal vulnerability, p. A-30

Monitoring Fluid and Electrolytes

Assessment and continued monitoring of the patient is an important role of the critical care nurse when caring for the patient with TLS. Recognizing critical laboratory changes or development of symptoms and notifying the physician in a timely manner are essential.[21] Insertion of a urinary catheter and maintenance of the intravenous line site are necessary to ensure adequate intake and output. Vital signs should be monitored frequently, and weight should be monitored daily.[20]

Maintaining Surveillance for Complications

Nursing interventions are aimed at preventing complications. Seizure precautions should be instituted, especially if calcium levels are disrupted. Insertion of a nasogastric tube is appropriate if nausea or vomiting occurs. Dietary adjustments are necessary, such as potassium and phosphorus restrictions in the presence of elevated serum levels and providing additional fiber to combat the constipation associated with the administration of antacids.

Initiating Patient Education

Education of the patient and family is a primary role of the critical care nurse. All treatments and interventions should be explained before carrying them out, and questions should be answered at a level understandable to the patient and family. Before discharge, potential risk factors and identification of early signs and symptoms should be reviewed.[20]

See the Collaborative Management Box on Tumor Lysis Syndrome for more information.

COLLABORATIVE MANAGEMENT
Tumor Lysis Syndrome

- Facilitate adequate renal function.
  - Volume hydration with 0.9% normal saline
  - Nonthiazide diuretics
- Treat hyperkalemia.
  - Kayexalate
  - Glucose and insulin
- Treat hyperuricemia.
  - Sodium bicarbonate
  - Allopurinol
- Treat hyperphosphatemia.
  - Dietary restrictions
  - Phosphorus-binding antacids
- Treat hypocalcemia.
  - Calcium gluconate
- Maintain surveillance for complications.
  - Acute renal failure
  - Cardiac dysrhythmias
- Provide comfort and emotional support.

CASE STUDY PATIENT WITH HEMATOLOGICAL DISORDERS AND ONCOLOGICAL EMERGENCIES

Answers to the Case Study Questions can be found on the Evolve web site at http://evolve.elsevier.com/Urden/priorities/.

Brief Patient History
Mr. L is an otherwise healthy 23-year-old African American man who presents with a week-long history of diarrhea, nausea, and vomiting after attending a barbecue last weekend.

Clinical Assessment
Mr. L is admitted to the intensive care unit from the emergency department with hypotension, fever, and leukocytosis.

Diagnostic Procedures
His vital signs are as follows: blood pressure of 65/42 mm Hg, heart rate of 145 beats/min (sinus tachycardia), respiratory rate of 35 breaths/min, and temperature of 102.4° F. His white blood cell count is 25,000/mm³ with 15% bands, lactate level is 7 mmol/L, prothrombin time is 25 seconds, and platelet count is 22,000/mm³. Blood cultures reveal gram-negative bacilli.

Medical Diagnosis
Mr. L is diagnosed with severe sepsis and disseminated intravascular coagulation.

Questions
1. What major outcomes do you expect to achieve for this patient?
2. What problems or risks must be managed to achieve these outcomes?
3. What interventions must be initiated to monitor, prevent, manage, or eliminate the problems and risks identified?
4. What interventions should be initiated to promote optimal functioning, safety, and well-being of the patient?
5. What possible learning needs do you anticipate for this patient?
6. What cultural and age-related factors may have a bearing on the patient's plan of care?

REFERENCES

1. Gando S: Microvascular thrombosis and multiple organ dysfunction, *Crit Care Med* 38(Suppl 2):S35, 2010.
2. Geiter H: Disseminated intravascular coagulopathy, *Dimens Crit Care Nurs* 22(3):108, 2003.
3. Levi M: Disseminated intravascular coagulation, *Crit Care Med* 35(9):2191, 2007.
4. Castoldi E, Hackeng TM: Regulation of coagulation by protein S, *Curr Opin Hematol* 15(5):529, 2008.
5. Kitchens CS: Thrombocytopenia and thrombosis in disseminated intravascular coagulation (DIC), *Hematology Am Soc Hematol Educ Program* 240, 2009.
6. Bick RL: Disseminated intravascular coagulation: current concepts of etiology, pathophysiology, diagnosis, and treatment, *Hematol Oncol Clin North Am* 17(1):149, 2003.
7. McCance KL: Structure and function of the hematologic system. In McCance KL, Huether SE, editors: *Pathophysiology: the biologic basis for disease in adults and children*, ed 5, St Louis, 2006, Mosby.
8. Zeerleder S, et al: Disseminated intravascular coagulation in sepsis, *Chest* 128(4):2864, 2005.
9. Shantsila E, Lip GY, Chong BH: Heparin-induced thrombocytopenia. A contemporary clinical approach to diagnosis and management, *Chest* 135(6):1651, 2009.

10. Warkentin TE: Heparin-induced thrombocytopenia, *Hematol Oncol Clin North Am* 21(4):589, 2007.

11. Selleng K, et al: Heparin-induced thrombocytopenia in intensive care patients, *Crit Care Med* 35(4):1165, 2007.

12. Marques MB: Thrombotic thrombocytopenic purpura and heparin-induced thrombocytopenia: two unique causes of life-threatening thrombocytopenia, *Clin Lab Med* 29(2):321, 2009.

13. Battistelli S, Genovese A, Gori T: Heparin-induced thrombocytopenia in surgical patients, *Am J Surg* 199(1):43, 2010.

14. Warkentin TE, et al: Treatment and prevention of heparin-induced thrombocytopenia: American College of Chest Physicians Evidence-Based Clinical Practice Guidelines (8th Edition), *Chest* 133(Suppl 6):340S, 2008.

15. Tosi P, et al: Consensus conference on the management of tumor lysis syndrome, *Haemtologica* 93(12):1877, 2008.

16. Behl D, Hendrickson AW, Moynihan TJ: Oncologic emergencies, *Crit Care Clin* 26(1):181, 2010.

17. Robison J: Metabolic emergencies: tumor lysis syndrome. In Newton S, editor: *Oncology nursing advisor: a comprehensive guide to clinical practice*, St Louis, 2009, Mosby.

18. Abu-Alfa AK, Younes A: Tumor lysis syndrome and acute kidney injury: evaluation, prevention and management, *Am J Kidney Dis* 55(5 Suppl 3):S1, 2010.

19. Shelton BK: Tumor lysis syndrome. In Chernecky CC, Murphy-Ende K, editors: *Acute care oncology*, ed 2, St Louis, 2008, Saunders.

20. Zobec A: Tumor lysis syndrome. In Gates RA, Fink RM, editors: *Oncology nursing secrets*, ed 3, St Louis, 2008, Mosby.

21. Myers JS: Complications of cancer and cancer treatment. In Langhorne ME, editor: *Oncology nursing*, ed 5, St Louis, 2007, Mosby.

Nursing Management Plans of Care

NURSING MANAGEMENT PLAN

Activity Intolerance

Definition: Insufficient physiological or psychological energy to endure or complete required or desired daily activities.

Activity Intolerance Related to Cardiopulmonary Dysfunction

Defining Characteristics
- Chest pain with activity
- Electrocardiographic changes with activity
- Heart rate is >15 beats/min above baseline with activity for patients on beta-blockers or calcium channel blockers
- Heart rate remains elevated above baseline 5 minutes after activity
- Breathlessness with activity
- SpO_2 <92% with activity
- Postural hypotension when moving from supine to upright position
- Patient reports fatigue with activity

Outcome Criteria
- Heart rate is <20 beats/min above baseline with activity and is <10 beats/min above baseline with activity for patients on beta-blockers or calcium channel blockers.
- Heart rate returns to baseline 5 minutes after activity.
- Chest pain with activity is absent.
- Patient reports tolerance to activity.

Nursing Interventions and Rationale
1. Encourage active or passive range-of-motion exercises while the patient is in bed *to keep joints flexible and muscles stretched.*
2. Teach patient to refrain from holding breath while performing exercises and *to avoid the Valsalva maneuver.*
3. Encourage performance of muscle-toning exercises at least three times daily, *because a toned muscle uses less oxygen when performing work than an untoned muscle.*
4. Progress ambulation *to increase tolerance to activity.*
5. Teach patient to take pulse *to determine activity tolerance:* Take pulse for a full minute before exercise and then for 10 seconds and multiply by 6 at exercise peak.

Activity Intolerance Related to Prolonged Immobility or Deconditioning

Defining Characteristics
- Decrease in systolic blood pressure is >20 mm Hg
- Increase in heart rate is >20 beats/min with postural change
- Syncope with postural change
- Patient reports lightheadedness with postural change

Outcome Criteria
- Decrease in systolic blood pressure is <10 mm Hg.
- Increase in heart rate is <10 beats/min with postural change.
- Syncope or lightheadedness is absent with postural change.

Nursing Interventions and Rationale
1. Instruct the patient how to perform straight-leg raises, dorsiflexion or plantar flexion, and quadriceps-setting and gluteal-setting exercises *to increase muscular and vascular tone.*
2. Consult with physician regarding the administration of fluids to ensure that the patient is hydrated to 24-hour fluid requirements per body surface area (BSA) *to increase preload and thereby increase stroke volume and cardiac output.*
3. Reposition patient incrementally *to avoid syncope:*
   a. Head of bed to 45 degrees and hold until symptom-free
   b. Head of bed to 90 degrees and hold until symptom-free
   c. Dangle until symptom-free
   d. Stand until symptom-free and ambulate
4. Collaborate with physician regarding patient's activity level *to ensure patient's safety.*

NURSING MANAGEMENT PLAN
Acute Confusion

Definition: Abrupt onset of reversible disturbances of consciousness, attention, cognition, and perception that develop over a short period of time.

Acute Confusion Related to Sensory Overload, Sensory Deprivation, and Sleep Pattern Disturbance

Defining Characteristics

Early Symptoms

- Sudden onset of global cognitive function impairment (hours to days)
- Restlessness, agitation, and combative behavior
- Drowsiness (can lead to loss of consciousness)
- Slurring of speech, inappropriate statements or "word salad," mumbling, or inappropriate gestures
- Short attention span (needs questions repeated); inability to learn new material
- Disordered sleep-wake cycle
- Disorientation to person, time, place, and situation
- Difficulty in separating dreams from reality (may experience bizarre dreams or nightmares)
- Anger at staff for continued questions about his or her orientation

Later Symptoms

- Symptoms that tend to fluctuate throughout the day and night
- Continuations of early symptoms, which may be more frequent or of longer duration
- Illusions
- Hallucinations
- Extreme agitation (e.g., attempts to climb out of bed, pull out catheters, rip off dressings)
- Calling out in loud voice, swearing, or attempting to bite or hit people who approach patient

Nursing Interventions and Rationale

1. Determine and document the patient's dominant spoken language, his or her literacy, and the languages in which he or she is literate. *Sometimes, people are not literate in their spoken language, or less commonly, they are literate only in their second language.*
2. Determine and document patient's premorbid degree of orientation, cognitive capabilities, and any sensory-perceptual deficits.

For Sensory Overload

1. Initiate each nurse-patient encounter by calling the patient by name and identifying yourself by name. *This fosters reality orientation and assists the patient in filtering irrelevant or impersonal conversation.*
2. Assess the patient's immediate physical environment from his or her viewpoint, and explain equipment, its sounds, and its therapeutic purpose. Demonstrate audible and visual alarms, and explain possible alarm conditions. *This decreases alienation of the patient from the technological environment and reduces the inherent sense of fear and urgency accompanying alarm conditions.*
3. Provide preparatory sensory information by explaining procedures in relation to the sensations the patient will experience, including duration of sensations. *Preparatory sensory information enhances learning and lessens anticipatory anxiety.*
4. Limit noise levels. Audible alarms cannot and must not be silenced, and many critical but noisy activities must take place in the critical care area. It has been shown, however, that noise levels produced by clinical personnel exceed those levels designated as acceptable and are often greater than those generated by technological devices. Keep staff conversations soft enough that they are inaudible to the patient whenever possible. Assume that everything said at or around a patient's bedside is intended for that patient's awareness and that it will be interpreted as pertaining to him or her. *As in the discussion that follows, conversations about the patient but not to him or her foster depersonalization and delusions of reference.*
5. Enforce nighttime noise limits.
6. Readjust alarm limits on physiological monitoring devices as the patient's condition changes (improves or deteriorates) *to lessen unnecessary alarm states.*
7. Consider use of headphones and compact disc or digital music player with patient's favorite music and/or subliminal or classical music. *This can effectively filter out assaultive noise of the critical care environment and supplant it with familiar, soothing sounds and rhythms.*
8. Modify lighting. *Day and night cycles need to be simulated with environmental lighting.* Never turn on overhead fluorescent lights abruptly without warning the patient, assisting him or her out of the supine position, and/or shielding his or her eyes with gauze or a face cloth. *Continuous bright lighting sustains anxiety and promotes circadian rhythm desynchronization.*
9. Shield patients from viewing urgent and emergent events in the critical care unit. Resuscitation efforts, albeit difficult to conceal, engender fear in the patient and a sense of instability and vulnerability (e.g., "I'm next"). When such an event occurs, elicit the patient's cognitive and emotional reaction; thoughts, impressions, and feelings need to be shared and misconceptions clarified. A useful approach in this interchange is that of emphasizing the differences between the patient at hand and the one resuscitated (e.g., "He was considerably older," "he was more unstable," "he had serious lung disease").
10. Ensure patients' privacy, modesty, and dignity. Although they seemingly pale in importance compared with priorities such as physiological assessment and stabilization, physical exposure and nudity are primal indignities for all individuals. Keep the patient minimally exposed. When, in the course of assessment and intervention, it becomes necessary to expose the patient, verbally apologize for this necessity. To be naked is to feel vulnerable; to be vulnerable is to feel fearful. In this regard, fear is an emotion that is preventable through nursing intervention.

NURSING MANAGEMENT PLAN
Acute Confusion—cont'd

For Sensory Deprivation

1. Provide reality orientation in four spheres (personal, place, time, and situation) at more frequent intervals than when testing. Convey this information in the context of routine conversation. *Sample statements:* "Mr. Clark, this is Tuesday morning and you're in University Hospital. Your heart surgery was yesterday morning, and you're doing well. My name is Joe, and I'm your nurse today." *The patient is made to feel patronized by repetitions such as "Do you know where you are?" Given the effects of general anesthesia, opioid analgesics, sedatives, and sleep, it is expected that some degree of disorientation will exist normally.*

2. Ensure the patient's visual access to a calendar.

3. Apprise the patient of daily news events and the weather.

4. Touch patients for the express purpose of communicating caring. Hold their hands, stroke their brows, and rub the skin on an aspect of the arms. *Touch is the universal language of caring. In the setting of critical care, in which there is considerable physical body manipulation, it is useful and important to contrast assaultive touch with comforting touch. Touch can be used as a technique for distraction from painful stimuli when used in conjunction with uncomfortable procedures.* (See later discussion of the use of touch in management of the patient experiencing hallucinations.)

5. Foster liberal visitation by family and significant others. Encourage significant others to touch the patient as consistent with their individual comfort level and cultural norms.

6. Structure and identify opportunities for the patient to exercise decision-making skills, however small. Although not so designated, patients with sensory alterations also experience a type of cognitive deprivation.

7. Assist patients to find meaning in their experiences. Explain the therapeutic purpose of all they are asked to do for themselves and all that is done with them and for them. Avoid statements such as "Will you turn to that side for me?" or "I need you to swallow this medication." *These statements implicitly convey that the maneuver has some value for the nurses instead of the patients.* Similarly, use "thank you" judiciously. *This simple salutation, when used indiscriminately, suggests something was done to benefit the nurses, not the patients. Patients need to find meaning and to identify their roles in the experience of critical illness and critical care. The sensations that constitute this experience and those that do not are made bearable and intelligible when attached to a larger picture of their conditions, treatment, and progress.*

For Hallucinations

1. Approach the patient with a calm, matter-of-fact demeanor. *The goal of this interaction is for the nurse to demonstrate external control. This helps decrease the anxiety and fear that generally accompany hallucinations and allows the patient to feel safe. Anxiety is transferable.*

2. Address the patient by name. *This is a useful presentation of reality because self-identity is the last sphere of orientation to vanish.*

3. In responding to the patient's description of the hallucination, do not deny, argue, or attempt to disprove the existence of the perceived event. *Statements such as "There are no voices coming from that air vent" or "Look, I'm brushing my hand across the wall, and there are no bugs" confuse the patient further, because the hallucination, although frightening, is his or her perceived reality.*

4. Express to the patient that your experiences are dissimilar, and acknowledge how frightening his or hers must be. *Sample statements:* "I don't hear (see, etc.) what you do, but I know how frightening such an experience must be to you. I'm Joe, your nurse, and I'm going to stay with you until the voices (visions, etc.) go away." Remain with any patient who is experiencing a hallucination. *Feelings of fear and anxiety often accelerate when a patient is left alone. He or she needs someone to represent a nonthreatening reality. Validating the patient's feelings demonstrates acceptance and sensitivity to the experience and promotes trust.*

5. Do not explore the content of the hallucination with the patient by asking about its nature or character. *The nurse is the patient's link with reality. Pursuit of a detailed description of a hallucination may signify to the patient that the nurse accepts his or her sensory distortion as factual. This may further confuse the patient and distance him or her more from reality. (An exception is the patient who the nurse suspects is experiencing auditory hallucinations [i.e., hearing voice commands].* Ascertain that the voices are not telling the patient to harm himself or herself, by asking simply and concretely, "What are the voices saying?") *The nurse can help bridge the gap between the patient's misperception and reality by addressing the feelings (e.g., fear, anxiety) and/or meanings (e.g., danger, death) engendered by the hallucination.* Determine how the misperception affects the patient emotionally, acknowledge those feelings, and use a calm, controlled, matter-of-fact approach to provide the trust and comfort the patient needs to tolerate this frightening experience. *In other words, the nurse should deal with the intent more than the content of the hallucination. The resultant decrease in anxiety will enable the patient to focus more accurately on his or her immediate environment.*

6. Talk concretely with the patient about things that are really happening. *Sample statements:* "How does your chest incision feel this afternoon, Mr. Clark?" "Your sister Kate was here to see you, but you were sleeping. She went down to the cafeteria and will be back." "Your secretions are a little easier for you to cough up today." *Interpretation of reality-based stimuli by the nurse encourages the patient to focus on actual circumstances and discourages a preoccupation with sensory misperceptions.*

7. Distract the patient by changing the topic. *This tactic is useful in situations of escalating anxiety and confusion or when all else fails. Topics need to consist of basic themes that are universally understood and culturally congruent, such as music, food, or weather. They may also be topics of special interest to the patient, such as*

Continued

NURSING MANAGEMENT PLAN
Acute Confusion—cont'd

hobbies, crafts, or sports. Topics that evoke strong emotions, such as politics, religion, or sexuality, should be avoided with most patients. This is especially true of the patient with reality distortions; sometimes, hallucinations and delusions are expressions of repressed conflicts associated with religious, sexual, or aggressive issues. Pursuit of such subjects could increase confusion and anxiety.

8. Consider the following regarding the use of touch. ***Touch presents a nonthreatening external reality and can therefore be useful in the management of patients with sensory alterations. However, for the patient experiencing hallucinations (as well as delusions and illusions), touch can be readily misinterpreted as, for instance, aggression or pain, or it can actually provide the basis for a tactile illusion.*** Avoid the use of touch as an intervention strategy for any patient who demonstrates escalating anxiety or paranoid, suspicious, or mistrustful thoughts.

9. For auditory hallucinations:
   a. *Patient behaviors:* Head cocked as if listening to an unseen presence; lips moving.
   b. *Therapeutic nurse responses:* "Mr. Clark, you appear to be listening to something." If the patient acknowledges voices: "I don't hear any voices, but I know this is troubling you. The voices will go away. Nothing is going to harm you. I'm Joe, your nurse, and I'll be here with you."
   c. *Nontherapeutic nurse responses:* "Tell me about your conversations with these voices." "To whom do these voices belong—anyone you know?"

10. For visual hallucinations:
   a. *Patient behaviors:* Staring into space as if focused on an unseen object; startled movements and anxious facial expression.
   b. *Therapeutic nurse responses:* "Mr. Clark, something seems to be troubling you. Tell me what it is." If patient states he visualizes people, images, or the devil in his environment and implies a sense of danger, respond, "There are only nurses and doctors here, Mr. Clark. I know this must be upsetting, but these images will go away. We're here with you in the hospital. Nothing will happen to you."
   c. *Nontherapeutic nurse responses:* "Describe the people you see. What are they wearing?" "What does the devil mean in your life? What about God?"

For Delusions
1. Explain all unseen noises, voices, and activity simply and clearly. ***They readily feed a delusional system.*** *Sample statements:* "That is Dr. Smith. He's come to see you and other patients here in the hospital." "The voices and activity you hear are from the bedside of the patient behind this curtain. He's being helped by one of the nurses."
2. Avoid the "negative challenge" of the patient's delusions (e.g., "Nobody here stole your belongings" or "Doctors and nurses do not harm people"). Similarly, avoid defending the referents of the patient's belief: "Nurses are good" and "Doctors mean well." ***A delusion is a belief, albeit false, that cannot be changed with logic. To attempt this change***

is to challenge the patient's belief system and thereby escalate his or her anxiety, further blurring the boundaries between reality and the patient's internally-based "logic."

3. For the patient with persecutory delusions who refuses food, fluids, or medications because of a belief that they are tainted or have been poisoned, permit the refusal unless it is a life-threatening event. Try again in 20 minutes; allow the patient to choose an alternative selection of food or to read the label on the unit's medication. ***Coercion, show of force, or engagement in complicated, logical justifications will only heighten the patient's suspiciousness and possibly reinforce the delusional belief. When the patient feels more in control, he or she need not rely on the "paradoxical" quality of the delusion to equip him or her with a false sense of power. His or her power instead is derived from making reality-based decisions.***

4. Staff members should be particularly careful not to engage in unnecessary laughter or whispering within view of the delusional patient. ***The delusional patient is hypervigilant, scanning the environment for evidence to corroborate or confirm his or her belief that staff members are colluding against him or her; laughter and whispers easily suggest this belief, this delusion of reference. This rationale also pertains to the patient experiencing hallucinations and/or illusions.***

5. Observe the principles detailed in the third intervention of "For Hallucinations."

For Illusions
1. Interpret a reality-based stimulus for the patient in a calm, matter-of-fact manner. ***Seen and unseen noises, voices, activity, and people can provide the stimulus for a sensory misinterpretation, an illusion.***
2. Minimize stimulation in the patient's immediate environment. ***Nursing interventions detailed previously under "Sensory Overload" are especially relevant here.***
3. Address the feeling and meaning associated with the experience, not the content of the sensory misinterpretation.
   a. *Patient behaviors:* Eyes darting, startled movements, frightened facial expression. "I know who you are. You're the devil come to take me to hell."
   b. *Therapeutic nurse responses:* "I'm Joe, your nurse. I know this experience is troubling for you. You're in the hospital, and no one here will harm you."
   c. *Nontherapeutic nurse responses:* "There are no such things as devils and angels." "Do you think the devil would be dressed in white?" ***The first nontherapeutic nurse response carries a parental tone (i.e., "You know better than that."), infantilizing the patient and adding to his or her feelings of powerlessness over the environment. The second nontherapeutic response reflects obvious logic, which is not in the patient's sensory domain; it cannot be processed and only adds to his or her confused state.***
4. Observe the principles detailed in the fifth intervention of "For Hallucinations."

NURSING MANAGEMENT PLAN
Acute Pain

Definition: Unpleasant sensory and emotional experience arising from actual or potential tissue damage or described in terms of such damage (International Association for the Study of Pain); sudden or slow onset of any intensity—from mild to severe—with an anticipated or predictable end and a duration of less than 6 months.

Acute Pain Related to Transmission of Perception of Cutaneous, Visceral, Muscular, or Ischemic Impulses

Defining Characteristics
Subjective
- Patient verbalizes presence of pain.
- Patient rates pain on a scale of 1 to 10 using a visual analog scale.

Objective
- Increase in blood pressure, heart rate, and respiratory rate
- Pupillary dilation
- Diaphoresis, pallor
- Skeletal muscle reactions (e.g., grimacing, clenching fists, writhing, pacing, guarding or splinting of affected part)
- Apprehension, fearful appearance
- May not exhibit any physiological change

Outcome Criteria
- Patient verbalizes that pain is reduced to a tolerable level or is totally relieved.
- Patient's pain rating is lower on a scale of 1 to 10.
- Blood pressure, heart rate, and respiratory rate return to baseline 5 minutes after administration of an intravenous opioid analgesic or 20 minutes after administration of intramuscular opioid analgesic.

Nursing Interventions and Rationale
1. Modify variables that heighten the patient's experience of pain.
   a. Explain to the patient that frequent, detailed, and seemingly repetitive assessments will be conducted to allow the nurse to better understand the patient's pain experience, not because the existence of pain is in question.
   b. Explain the factors responsible for pain production in the individual. Estimate the expected duration of the pain if possible.
   c. Explain diagnostic and therapeutic procedures to the patient in relation to sensations the patient should expect to feel.
   d. Reduce the patient's fear of addiction by explaining the difference between drug tolerance and drug addiction. ***Drug tolerance is a physiological phenomenon in which a medication begins to lose effectiveness after repeated doses; drug dependence is a psychological phenomenon in which opioids are used regularly for emotional, not medical, reasons.***
   e. Instruct the patient to ask for pain medication when pain is beginning and not to wait until it is intolerable.
   f. Explain that the physician will be consulted if pain relief is inadequate with the present medication.
   g. Instruct patient in the importance of adequate rest, especially when it reduces pain ***to maintain strength and coping abilities and to reduce stress.***
2. Collaborate with physician regarding pharmacological interventions.
   - For postoperative or posttraumatic cutaneous, muscular, or visceral pain, perform the following:

a. Medicate with an opioid analgesic to break the pain cycle as long as level of consciousness and vital signs are stable: check patient's previous response to similar dosage and opioids.
   (1) Given a physician order for a range of doses of an opioid analgesic, start with the lowest dose ***to evaluate the patient's individual response to medication.***
b. Continuous pain requires continuous analgesia.
   (1) Establish optimal analgesic dose that brings optimal pain relief.
   (2) ***To maintain steadier blood levels,*** offer pain medication at prescribed regular intervals rather than making patient ask for it.
   (3) Consider waking patient to avoid loss of opiate blood levels during sleep.
c. If administering medication on an as-necessary (PRN) basis, give it when the patient's pain is just beginning, rather than at its peak. Advise patient to intercept pain, not endure it, or several hours and higher doses of opioid analgesics may be necessary to relieve pain, leading to a cycle of undermedication and pain alternating with overmedication and drug toxicity.
d. Perform rehabilitation exercises (turn, deep breathe, leg exercises, ambulate) shortly before peak of drug effect ***because this will be the optimal time for the patient to increase activity with the least risk of increasing pain.***
e. When making the transition from one drug to another or from intramuscular or intravenous to oral medication, use an equianalgesic chart. ***Equianalgesic means approximately the same pain relief. The patient's response should be closely monitored to determine if the right analgesic choice was made.***
f. To assess effectiveness of pain medication, do the following:
   (1) Reevaluate pain 5 minutes after intravenous and 20 minutes after intramuscular medication administration, observe patient's behavior, and ask patient to rate pain on a scale of 1 to 10.
   (2) Collaborate with the physician to add or delete other medications that potentiate the action of analgesics, such as antiemetics, hypnotics, sedatives, or muscle relaxants.
   (3) Observe for indicators of undertreatment: report of pain not relieved; observed restlessness, sleeplessness, irritability, and anorexia; decreased activity level.
   (4) Observe for indicators of overtreatment: hypotension or bradycardia; respiratory rate <10/min; excessive sedation.
g. If patient-controlled analgesia (PCA) is used, perform the following:
   (1) Instruct the patient on what the drug is, the dose, and how often it can be self-administered by pushing the

Continued

NURSING MANAGEMENT PLAN
Acute Pain—cont'd

button to activate the PCA machine. For example, "When you have pain, instead of asking the nurse to bring medication, push the button that activates the machine and a small dose of the pain medicine will be injected into your IV line. You can keep your pain under control by administering additional medicine as soon as your pain begins to return or increases. Push the button before undertaking a painful activity, such as ambulation. Try to balance your pain relief against sleepiness, and don't activate the machine if you start to feel sleepy. If your pain medicine seems to stop working despite pushing the button several times, call the nurse to check your IV. If you are not receiving adequate pain relief, the nurse will call your doctor."

(2) Monitor vital signs, especially blood pressure and respiratory rate (counted for 30 seconds and if respiratory rate is less than 12/min, then count for a full minute), every 15 minutes for the first hour, then every hour for 4 hours, then every 2 hours.

(3) Assess postural heart rate and blood pressure before initial ambulation.

(4) Initiate capnography if available.

(5) Notify the physician if pulse rate is <50 beats/min or >120 beats/min; SpO_2 <90%; RR <10 breaths/min; $EtCO_2$ >60 mm Hg; apnea >30 seconds.

   (a) Anticipate administration of naloxone.

h. If epidural opioid analgesia is used, do the following:

(1) Keep patient's head elevated 30 to 45 degrees after injection **to prevent respiratory depressant effects.**

(2) Observe closely for respiratory depression up to 24 hours after injection. Monitor respiratory rate every 15 minutes for 1 hour, every 30 minutes for 7 hours, and every hour for the remaining 16 hours.

(3) Assess for adequate cough reflex.

(4) Avoid use of other central nervous system depressants, such as sedatives.

(5) Observe for reports of pruritus, nausea, and vomiting.

(6) Anticipate administration of naloxone for respiratory depression (and smaller doses of naloxone for pruritus).

(7) Assess for and treat urinary retention.

(8) Assess epidural catheter site for local infection. Keep the catheter taped securely **to prevent catheter migration.**

• **For peripheral vascular ischemic pain (hypothetic vascular occlusion of leg),** do the following:

a. Correctly identify and differentiate ischemic pain from other types of pain. **(NOTE: Ischemic pain is usually a** ***burning, aching pain made worse by exercise and lessened or relieved by rest. Eventually, the pain occurs at rest. Coldness and pallor of the extremity may be noted, especially if the limb is elevated above the heart level. Rubor and mottling of the skin may be evident from prolonged tissue anoxia and inability of damaged vessels to constrict. Eventually, cyanosis and gangrenous tissue will be evident. Chronic ischemia leads to visible changes in the limb, such as flaking skin, brittle nails and hair, leg ulcers, and cellulitis).***

b. Administer pain medications, and evaluate their effectiveness as previously described. ***Remember that the pain of ischemia is chronic and continuous and can make the patient irritable and depressed.***

c. Treat the cause of the ischemic pain, and institute measures ***to increase circulation to the affected part.***

3. Initiate nonpharmacological interventions.

a. Treat contributing factors; provide explanations (see intervention no. 2 at beginning of this nursing management plan).

b. Apply comfort measures.

(1) Use relaxation techniques, such as back rubs, massage, warm baths, music, and aromatherapy.

   (a) Use blankets and pillows to support the painful part and reduce muscle tension.

   (b) Encourage slow, rhythmic breathing.

(2) Encourage progressive muscle relaxation techniques.

   (a) Instruct patient to inhale and tense (tighten) specific muscle groups and then relax the muscles as exhalation occurs.

   (b) Suggest an order for performing the tension and relaxation cycle (e.g., start with facial muscles and move down the body, ending with the toes).

(3) Encourage guided imagery.

   (a) Ask patient to recall an experienced image that is very pleasurable and relaxing and involves at least two senses.

   (b) Have patient begin with rhythmic breathing and progressive relaxation and then travel mentally to the scene.

   (c) Have patient slowly experience the scene (e.g., how it looks, sounds, smells, feels).

   (d) Ask patient to practice this imagery in private.

   (e) Instruct patient to end the imagery by counting to three and saying, "Now I'm relaxed." If the person does not end the imagery and falls asleep, the purpose of the technique is defeated.

NURSING MANAGEMENT PLAN
Anxiety

Definition: Vague uneasy feeling of discomfort or dread accompanied by an autonomic response (the source often nonspecific or unknown to the individual); a feeling of apprehension caused by anticipation of danger. It is an alerting signal that warns of impending danger and enables the individual to take measures to deal with threat.

Anxiety Related to Threat to Biological, Psychological, or Social Integrity

Defining Characteristics

Subjective
- Verbalizes increased muscle tension
- Expresses frequent sensation of tingling in hands and feet
- Relates continuous feeling of apprehension
- Expresses preoccupation with a sense of impending doom
- Reports difficulty falling asleep
- Repeatedly expresses concerns about changes in health status and outcome of illness

Objective
- Psychomotor agitation (fidgeting, jitteriness, restlessness)
- Tightened, wrinkled brow
- Strained (worried) facial expression
- Hypervigilance (scans environment)
- Startles easily
- Distractibility
- Sweaty palms
- Fragmented sleep patterns
- Tachycardia
- Tachypnea

Outcome Criteria
- Patient effectively uses learned relaxation strategies.
- Patient demonstrates significant decrease in psychomotor agitation.
- Patient verbalizes reduction in tingling sensations in hands and feet.
- Patient is able to focus on the tasks at hand.
- Patient expresses positive, future-based plans to family and staff.
- Patient's heart rate and rhythm remain within limits commensurate with physiological status.

Nursing Interventions and Rationale
1. Instruct the patient in the following simple, effective relaxation strategies:
   a. If not contraindicated for cardiovascular reasons, tense and relax all muscles progressively from the toes to the head. **Progressive toe-to-head relaxation releases the muscular tension that may be a stress-related effect resulting from the threat or change in the patient's health status and outcome of illness.**
   b. Perform slow deep-breathing exercises. **Deep-breathing exercises provide slow, rhythmic, controlled breathing patterns that relax the patient and distract him or her from the effects of his or her illness and hospitalization.**
   c. Focus on a single object or person in the environment. **Focusing on a single object or person helps the patient dismiss myriad disorienting stimuli from his or her visual-perceptual field, which can have a dizzying, distorted effect. A clear sensorium allows him or her to feel more in control of his or her environment.**
   d. Listen to soothing music or relaxation tapes with eyes closed. **Music or words expressed in soft, low tones tend to produce soothing, relaxing effects that counteract or inhibit escalating anxiety and provide respite from the patient's situational crisis. Closed eyes eliminate distracting visual stimuli and promote a more restful environment.**

2. Actively listen to and accept the patient's concerns regarding the threats from his or her illness, outcome, and hospitalization. **Active listening and unconditional acceptance validate the patient as a worthwhile individual and assure him or her that his or her concerns, no matter how great, will be addressed. Knowledge that he or she has an avenue for ventilation will assuage anxiety.**

3. Help the patient distinguish between realistic concerns and exaggerated fears through clear, simple explanations. *Sample statements:* "Your lab results show that you're doing okay right now." "The shortness of breath you're experiencing is not unusual." "The pain you described is expected, and this medication will relieve it." **A patient who is informed about his or her progress and is reassured about expected symptoms and management of care will be better equipped to maintain a more realistic perspective of his or her illness and its outcome. Anxiety emanating from imagined or exaggerated fears will likely be assuaged or averted.**

4. Provide simple clarification of environmental events and stimuli that are not related to the patient's illness and care. *Sample statements:* "That loud noise is coming from a machine that is helping another patient." "The visitor behind the curtain is crying because she's had an upsetting day." "That gurney is here to take another patient to x-ray." **Clarification of events and stimuli that are unrelated to the patient helps to disengage him or her from the extant anxiety-provoking situations surrounding him or her, avoiding further anxiety and apprehension.**

5. Assist the patient in focusing on building on prior coping strategies to deal with the effects of his or her illness and care. *Sample statements:* "What methods have helped you get through difficult times in the past?" "How can we help you use those methods now?" (See the Nursing Management Plan for Ineffective Coping for interventions that assist patients to use coping strategies effectively.) **Use of previously successful coping strategies in conjunction with newly learned techniques arms the patient with an arsenal of weapons against anxiety, providing him or her with greater control over the situational crisis and decreased feelings of doom and despair.**

6. Give the patient permission to deny or suppress the effects of his or her illness and hospitalization with which he or she cannot cope or control. *Sample statements:* "It's perfectly okay to ignore things you can't handle right now." "How can we help ease your mind during this time?" "What are some things or tasks that may help distract you?" **Adaptive denial can be helpful in reducing feelings of anxiety in patients with life-threatening illness.**

NURSING MANAGEMENT PLAN

Autonomic Dysreflexia

Definition: Life-threatening, uninhibited sympathetic response of the nervous system to a noxious stimulus after a spinal cord injury at T7 or above.

Autonomic Dysreflexia Related to Excessive Autonomic Response to Noxious Stimuli
(e.g., Distended Bladder, Distended Bowel, Skin Irritation)

Defining Characteristics

- Paroxysmal hypertension (sudden increase in both systolic and diastolic blood pressure >20 mm Hg above patient's normal blood pressure); for many spinal cord injury patients, a normal blood pressure may be only 90/60 mm Hg
- Pounding headache
- Bradycardia (may be a relative slowing so the heart rate may still appear within the normal range)
- Profuse sweating (above the level of the injury) especially in the face, neck, and shoulders
- Pilomotor erection (goose bumps) above the level of the injury
- Cardiac dysrhythmias (atrial fibrillation, premature ventricular contractions, and atrioventricular conduction abnormalities)
- Flushing of the skin (above the level of the injury) especially in the face, neck, and shoulders
- Blurred vision
- Appearance of spots in the visual fields
- Nasal congestion
- Feelings of apprehension or anxiety

Outcome Criteria

- Blood pressure returns to patient's baseline level.
- Heart rate and rhythm return to patient's baseline level.
- Absence of headache.
- Absence of sweating, flushing, and piloerection above level of injury.
- Absence of visual disturbances and nasal congestion.
- Absence of feelings of apprehension or anxiety.

Nursing Interventions and Rationale

1. Place the patient on cardiac monitor, and assess for bradycardia or other dysrhythmias. **Disturbances of cardiac rate and rhythm can occur because of autonomic dysfunction associated with dysreflexia.**
2. Check the patient's blood pressure every 3 to 5 minutes **as blood pressure may fluctuate very quickly.**
3. Sit the patient upright and lower his or her legs if possible **to decrease venous return and blood pressure.**
4. Loosen any clothing or constrictive devices **to decrease venous return and blood pressure.**
5. Investigate for and remove instigating cause of dysreflexia:
   a. Bladder
      (1) If indwelling catheter not in place, catheterize patient immediately.

(a) Prior to inserting the catheter, instill 2% lidocaine jelly into the urethra and wait 2 minutes, if possible.
(b) Drain 500 mL of urine, and recheck BP.
(c) If BP still elevated, drain another 500 mL of urine.
(d) If BP declines after the bladder is empty, serial BP must be monitored closely because the bladder can go into severe contractions causing hypertension to recur.
   (2) If indwelling catheter is in place, check the catheter and tubing for kinks, folds, constrictions, or obstructions, and for correct placement. If problem is found, correct it immediately.
   (3) If catheter is plugged, irrigate it gently with no more than 10 to 15 mL of sterile normal saline solution at body temperature.
   (4) If unable to irrigate catheter, remove it and prepare to reinsert a new catheter: proceed with its lubrication, drainage, and observation as outlined above.
   (5) Avoid manually compressing or tapping on the bladder.
   b. Bowel—if systolic blood pressure is ≥150 mm Hg, proceed to #6 prior to checking for a fecal impaction.
      (1) With a gloved hand, instill a topical anesthetic agent (2% lidocaine jelly) generously into the rectum **to decrease flow of impulses from bowel.**
      (2) Wait 2 minutes if possible **for sensation in area to decrease.**
      (3) With a gloved hand, insert a lubricated finger into the rectum and check for the presence of stool.
      (4) If stool is felt, gently remove, if possible.
   c. Skin
      (1) Loosen clothing or bed linens as indicated.
      (2) Inspect skin for pimples, boils, pressure ulcers, and ingrown toenails, and treat as indicated.
6. If symptoms of dysreflexia do not subside, collaborate with physician regarding the administration of antihypertensive medications (e.g., nifedipine [immediate-release form], nitrates [sodium nitroprusside, isosorbide dinitrate, or nitroglycerin ointment], hydralazine, mecamylamine, diazoxide, phenoxybenzamine, captopril, prazosin).
   a. Administer medications, and monitor their effectiveness.
   b. Assess blood pressure and heart rate.
7. Instruct patient about causes, symptoms, treatment, and prevention of dysreflexia.
8. Encourage patient to carry medical bracelet or informational card to present to medical personnel in the event dysreflexia may be developing.

NURSING MANAGEMENT PLAN
Compromised Family Coping

Definition: Usually supportive primary person (family member or close friend) provides insufficient, ineffective, or compromised support, comfort, assistance, or encouragement that may be needed by the patient to manage or master adaptive tasks related to his or her health challenge.

Compromised Family Coping Related to Critically Ill Family Member

Defining Characteristics
- Disruption of usual family functions and roles
- Inability to accept or deal with crisis situation; use of defense mechanisms (e.g., denial, anger); unrealistic expectations of patient's outcome and care provided; judgmental toward health care providers
- Nonrecognition that family is in state of crisis
- Inappropriate emotional outbursts; arguments among family and with others; inability to respond to each other's feelings or support each other
- Misinterpretation of information; short attention span with repeated questions about information already provided; members not sharing information with each other
- Inability to make decisions regarding changes in family structure or about course of care for ill member; noncooperation among family members
- Expressions of grief, hopelessness, powerlessness, and isolation; do not seek or respond to support services
- Hesitancy to spend time with ill person in the critical care unit, or inappropriate behavior when visiting (may upset patient)
- Neglect of own personal health; fatigue, apathy; refusal of offers for respite time

Outcome Criteria
- The family will express an understanding of course/prognosis of illness, therapies, and alternative measures.
- The family will diminish or resolve conflicts and cooperate in decision making.
- The family will develop trust and mutual support for each member and form a cohesive unit.
- The family will support ill person in making decisions (if capable) or respect prior wishes regarding provision of health care.
- Family efforts will be directed toward a purpose and readjust to changes in life patterns and role function. Members will accept responsibility for changes.
- The family will identify and use effective coping strategies.
- The family will identify and use available resources as needed to facilitate resolution of the crisis.
- The family will have a sense of control and confidence in meeting personal and collective needs.

Nursing Interventions and Rationale
1. Identify family's perception of the crisis situation. Determine family structure; role developmental phase; and ethnic, cultural, and belief factors that may affect communication with family and the plan of care. Identify strengths of the family. *All initial nursing interventions should be directed toward resolving the crisis situation. Understanding and using family theory principles will facilitate this process and individualize care.*

2. Provide honest and accurate information in language persons can understand. Give updated information as appropriate. Listen! *This facilitates open communication among family and health care providers, projects a caring attitude and concern for family and patient, and assists family in making decisions and being involved with the plan and goals of care.*
3. Encourage liberal visitation with patient. Before the visit, prepare family members for what they will observe in a technical environment. Inform them about patient's appearance, behaviors, etc. that may be distressing to them. Explain the etiology of patient responses to stimuli (e.g., pain, trauma, surgery, medication), and explain that these behaviors are being monitored and are usually temporary. Encourage them to touch the patient and let the patient know of their presence. *This prevents a strong emotional reaction to an unfamiliar and frightening situation, involves family as support to each other and to the patient, demonstrates the nurse's concern for them as persons, and facilitates satisfaction with care being provided for their loved one.*
4. Identify and support effective coping behaviors. *This aids in the family's sense of control and resolution of helplessness/powerlessness.*
5. Observe for signs of fatigue and the need for emotional/spiritual support and respite from hospital waiting routine. Encourage family to verbalize feelings. Provide information on available resources. Alert interdisciplinary team members (social, psychological, spiritual) to family needs. Provide pager device (if available), or obtain phone numbers when family leaves the hospital premises. *This provides support and comfort, facilitates hope, resolves sense of isolation, gives sense of security, and diminishes guilt feelings for attending to personal needs.*
6. Instruct family in simple caregiving techniques, and encourage participation in patient's care. *This facilitates giving a sense of normalcy to the experience, self-confidence, and assurance that good care is being provided.*
7. Serve as advocate for patient and family. Teach family how to negotiate with the health care delivery system, and include them in health care team conferences when appropriate. *This facilitates informed decision making, promotes control and satisfaction, and permits mutual goal-setting.*
8. Consider nonbiological or nonlegal family relationships. Encourage contact with patient and participation in care. *This facilitates holistic care and support of emotional ties and demonstrates respect for the family unit and relationships.*
9. Provide emotional support and compassion when patient's condition worsens or deteriorates. *The use of touch and expression of concern for the patient and family convey comfort and trust in the health care provider and respect and assurance that the family's loved one will receive appropriate care and attention.*

NURSING MANAGEMENT PLAN
Decreased Cardiac Output

Definition: Inadequate blood pumped by the heart to meet the metabolic demands of the body.

Decreased Cardiac Output Related to Alterations in Preload

Defining Characteristics
- Cardiac output is <4.0 L/min
- Cardiac index is <2.5 L/min/m^2
- Heart rate is >100 beats/min
- Urine output is <30 mL/hr or 0.5 mL/kg/hr
- Decreased mentation, restlessness, agitation, confusion
- Diminished peripheral pulses
- Blue, gray, or dark purple tint to tongue and sublingual area
- Systolic blood pressure is <90 mm Hg
- Subjective complaints of fatigue

Reduced Preload
- Right atrial pressure is <2 mm Hg
- Pulmonary artery occlusion pressure is <6 mm Hg

Excessive Preload
- Right atrial pressure is >8 mm Hg
- Pulmonary artery occlusion pressure is >12 mm Hg

Outcome Criteria
- Cardiac output is 4 to 8 L/min.
- Cardiac index is 2.5 to 4 L/min/m^2.
- Right atrial pressure is 2 to 8 mm Hg.
- Pulmonary artery occlusion pressure is 6 to 12 mg Hg.

Nursing Interventions and Rationale
1. Collaborate with physician regarding the administration of oxygen to maintain an SpO$_2$ >92% **to prevent tissue hypoxia.**
2. Maintain surveillance for signs of decreased tissue perfusion and acidosis **to facilitate the early identification and treatment of complications.**
3. Monitor fluid balance and daily weights **to facilitate regulation of the patient's fluid balance.**

For Reduced Preload Resulting from Volume Loss
1. Collaborate with physician regarding the administration of crystalloids, colloids, blood, and blood products **to increase circulating volume.**
2. Limit blood sampling, observe intravenous lines for accidental disconnection, apply direct pressure to bleeding sites, and maintain normal body temperature **to minimize fluid loss.**
3. Position patient with legs elevated, trunk flat, and head and shoulders above the chest **to enhance venous return.**

4. Encourage oral fluids (as appropriate), administer free water with tube feedings, and replace fluids that are lost through wound or tube drainage **to promote adequate fluid intake.**
5. Maintain surveillance for signs of fluid volume excess and adverse effects of blood and blood product administration **to facilitate the early identification and treatment of complications.**

For Reduced Preload Resulting from Venous Dilation:
1. Collaborate with physician regarding the administration of vasoconstrictors **to increase venous return.**
2. Maintain surveillance for adverse effects of vasoconstrictor therapy **to facilitate the early identification and treatment of complications.**
3. If patient is hyperthermic, administer tepid bath, hypothermia blanket, and/or ice bags to axilla and groin **to decrease temperature and promote vasoconstriction.**

For Excessive Preload Resulting from Volume Overload
1. Collaborate with physician regarding the administration of the following:
   a. Diuretics to remove excessive fluid
   b. Vasodilators to decrease venous return
   c. Inotropes to increase myocardial contractility
2. Restrict fluid intake and double concentrate intravenous drips **to minimize fluid intake.**
3. Position patient in semi-Fowler's or high Fowler's position **to reduce venous return.**
4. Maintain surveillance for signs of fluid volume deficit and adverse effects of diuretic, vasodilator, and inotropic therapies **to facilitate the early identification and treatment of complications.**

For Excessive Preload Resulting from Venous Constriction
1. Collaborate with physician regarding the administration of vasodilators **to promote venous dilation.**
2. Maintain surveillance for adverse effects of vasodilator therapy **to facilitate the early identification and treatment of complications.**
3. If patient is hypothermic, wrap him or her in warm blankets or administer hyperthermia blanket **to increase temperature and promote vasodilation.**

Decreased Cardiac Output Related to Alterations in Afterload

Defining Characteristics
- Cardiac output is <4 L/min
- Cardiac index is <2.5 L/min/m^2
- Heart rate is >100 beats/min
- Urine output is <30 mL/hr
- Decreased mentation, restlessness, agitation, confusion
- Diminished peripheral pulses
- Blue, gray, or dark purple tint to tongue and sublingual area
- Systolic blood pressure is <90 mm Hg
- Subjective complaints of fatigue

Reduced Afterload
- Pulmonary vascular resistance is <100 dyn/sec/cm^{-5}
- Systemic vascular resistance is <800 dyn/sec/cm^{-5}

Excessive Afterload
- Pulmonary vascular resistance is >250 dyn/sec/cm^{-5}
- Systemic vascular resistance is >1200 dyn/sec/cm^{-5}

Outcome Criteria
- Cardiac output is 4 to 8 L/min.
- Cardiac index is 2.5 to 4 L/min/m^2.

NURSING MANAGEMENT PLAN
Decreased Cardiac Output—cont'd

- Pulmonary vascular resistance is 80 to 250 dyn/sec/cm^{-5}.
- Systemic vascular resistance is 800 to 1200 dyn/sec/cm^{-5}.

Nursing Interventions and Rationale
1. Collaborate with physician regarding the administration of oxygen to maintain an SpO$_2$ >92% **to prevent tissue hypoxia.**
2. Maintain surveillance for signs of decreased tissue perfusion and acidosis **to facilitate the early identification and treatment of complications.**

For Reduced Afterload
1. Collaborate with physician regarding the administration of vasoconstrictors **to promote arterial vasoconstriction and prevent relative hypovolemia.** If decreased preload is present, implement Nursing Management Plan for Decreased Cardiac Output Related to Alterations in Preload.
2. Maintain surveillance for adverse effects of vasoconstrictor therapy **to facilitate the early identification and treatment of complications.**

3. If patient is hyperthermic, administer tepid bath, hypothermia blanket, and/or ice bags to axilla and groin **to decrease temperature and promote vasoconstriction.**

For Excessive Afterload
1. Collaborate with physician regarding the administration of vasodilators **to promote arterial vasodilation.**
2. Collaborate with physician regarding initiation of intraaortic balloon pump **to facilitate afterload reduction.**
3. Promote rest and relaxation and decrease environmental stimulation **to minimize sympathetic stimulation.**
4. Maintain surveillance for adverse effects of vasodilator therapy **to facilitate the early identification and treatment of complications.**
5. If patient is hypothermic, wrap patient in warm blankets or administer hyperthermia blanket **to increase temperature and promote vasodilation.**
6. If patient is in pain, treat pain **to reduce sympathetic stimulation.** Implement Nursing Management Plan for Acute Pain Related to Transmission and Perception of Cutaneous, Visceral, Muscular, or Ischemic Impulses.

Decreased Cardiac Output Related to Alterations in Contractility

Defining Characteristics
- Cardiac output is <4 L/min
- Cardiac index is <2.5 L/min/m^2
- Heart rate is >100 beats/min
- Urine output is <30 mL/hr
- Decreased mentation, restlessness, agitation, confusion
- Diminished peripheral pulses
- Blue, gray, or dark purple tint to tongue and sublingual area
- Systolic blood pressure is <90 mm Hg
- Subjective complaints of fatigue
- Right ventricular stroke work index is <7 g/m^2/beat
- Left ventricular stroke work index is <35 g/m^2/beat

Outcome Criteria
- Cardiac output is 4 to 8 L/min.
- Cardiac index is 2.5 to 4 L/min/m^2.
- Right ventricular stroke work index is 7 to 12 g/m^2/beat.
- Left ventricular stroke work index is 35 to 85 g/m^2/beat.

Nursing Interventions and Rationale
1. Collaborate with physician regarding the administration of oxygen to maintain an SpO$_2$ >92% **to prevent tissue hypoxia.**

2. Maintain surveillance for signs of decreased tissue perfusion and acidosis **to facilitate the early identification and treatment of complications.**
3. Ensure preload is optimized. If preload is reduced or excessive, implement Nursing Management Plan for Decreased Cardiac Output Related to Alterations in Preload.
4. Ensure afterload is optimized. If afterload is reduced or excessive, implement Nursing Management Plan for Decreased Cardiac Output Related to Alterations in Afterload.
5. Ensure electrolytes are optimized. Collaborate with physician regarding the administration of electrolyte replacement therapy **to enhance cellular ionic environment.**
6. Collaborate with physician regarding the administration of inotropes **to enhance myocardial contractility.**
7. Monitor ST segment continuously **to determine changes in myocardial tissue perfusion.** If myocardial ischemia is present, implement Nursing Management Plan for Ineffective Cardiopulmonary Tissue Perfusion.

Decreased Cardiac Output Related to Alterations in Heart Rate or Rhythm

Defining Characteristics
- Cardiac output is <4 L/min
- Cardiac index is <2.5 L/min/m^2
- Heart rate is >100 beats/min or <60 beats/min
- Urine output is <30 mL/hr or 0.5 mL/kg/hr
- Decreased mentation, restlessness, agitation, confusion
- Diminished peripheral pulses
- Blue, gray, or dark purple tint to tongue and sublingual area
- Systolic blood pressure is <90 mm Hg
- Subjective complaints of fatigue
- Dysrhythmias

Outcome Criteria
- Cardiac output is 4 to 8 L/min.
- Cardiac index is 2.5 to 4 L/min/m^2.
- Absence of dysrhythmias or return to baseline.
- Heart rate is >60 beats/min or <100 beats/min.

Nursing Interventions and Rationale
1. Collaborate with physician regarding the administration of oxygen to maintain an SpO$_2$ >92% **to prevent tissue hypoxia.**
2. Ensure electrolytes are optimized. Collaborate with physician regarding the administration of electrolyte therapy **to enhance**

NURSING MANAGEMENT PLAN
Decreased Cardiac Output—cont'd

cellular ionic environment and avoid precipitation of dysrhythmias.

3. Collaborate with physician and pharmacist regarding patient's current medications and their effect on heart rate and rhythm *to identify any prodysrhythmic or bradycardic side effects.*

4. Maintain surveillance for signs of decreased tissue perfusion and acidosis *to facilitate the early identification and treatment of complications.*

5. Monitor ST segment continuously *to determine changes in myocardial tissue perfusion.* If myocardial ischemia is present, implement Nursing Management Plan for Altered Cardiopulmonary Tissue Perfusion.

For Lethal Dysrhythmias or Asystole
1. Initiate advanced cardiac life support (ACLS) interventions and notify physician immediately.

For Nonlethal Dysrhythmias
1. Collaborate with physician regarding administration of antidysrhythmic therapy, synchronized cardioversion, and/or overdrive pacing *to control dysrhythmias.*
2. Maintain surveillance for adverse effects of antidysrhythmic therapy *to facilitate the early identification and treatment of complications.*

For Heart Rate <60 Beats/Min
1. Collaborate with physician regarding the initiation of temporary pacing *to increase heart rate.*

Decreased Cardiac Output Related to Sympathetic Blockade

Defining Characteristics
- Decreased cardiac output and cardiac index
- Systolic blood pressure is <90 mm Hg or below patient's baseline
- Decreased right atrial pressure and pulmonary artery occlusion pressure
- Decreased systemic vascular resistance
- Bradycardia
- Cardiac dysrhythmias
- Postural hypotension

Outcome Criteria
- Cardiac output and cardiac index are within normal limits.
- Systolic blood pressure is >90 mm Hg or returns to baseline.
- Right atrial pressure and pulmonary artery occlusion pressure are within normal limits.
- Systemic vascular resistance is within normal limits.
- Sinus rhythm is present.
- Dysrhythmias are absent.
- Fainting or dizziness with position change is absent.

Nursing Interventions and Rationale
1. Implement measures to prevent episodes of postural hypertension:

a. Change patient's position slowly *to allow the cardiovascular system time to compensate.*

b. Apply pneumatic compression stockings *to promote venous return.*

c. Perform range-of-motion exercises every 2 hours *to prevent venous pooling.*

d. Collaborate with the physician and physical therapist regarding the use of a tilt table *to progress the patient from a supine to an upright position.*

2. Collaborate with the physician regarding the administration of the following:

a. Crystalloids and/or colloids to increase the patient's circulating volume, *which increases stroke volume and subsequently cardiac output*

b. Vasopressors if fluids are ineffective to constrict the patient's vascular system, *which increases resistance and subsequently blood pressure*

3. Monitor cardiac rhythm for bradycardia and/or dysrhythmias, *which can further decrease cardiac output.*

4. Avoid any activity that can stimulate the vagal response *because bradycardia can result.*

5. Treat symptomatic bradycardia and symptomatic dysrhythmias according to unit's emergency protocol or advanced cardiac life support guidelines.

NURSING MANAGEMENT PLAN
Decreased Intracranial Adaptive Capacity

Definition: Intracranial fluid dynamic mechanisms that normally compensate for increases in intracranial volumes are compromised, resulting in repeated disproportionate increases in intracranial pressure (ICP) in response to a variety of noxious and non-noxious stimuli.

Decreased Intracranial Adaptive Capacity Related to Failure of Normal Intracranial Compensatory Mechanisms

Defining Characteristics
- Intracranial pressure is >15 mm Hg, sustained for 15 to 30 minutes
- Headache
- Vomiting, with or without nausea
- Seizures
- Decrease in Glasgow Coma Scale score of 2 or more points from baseline
- Alteration in level of consciousness, ranging from restlessness to coma
- Change in orientation: disoriented to time and/or place and/or person
- Difficulty or inability to follow simple commands
- Increasing systolic blood pressure of more than 20 mm Hg with widening pulse pressure
- Bradycardia

NURSING MANAGEMENT PLAN

Decreased Intracranial Adaptive Capacity—cont'd

- Irregular respiratory pattern (e.g., Cheyne-Stokes, central neurogenic hyperventilation, ataxic, apneustic)
- Change in response to painful stimuli (e.g., purposeful to inappropriate or absent response)
- Signs of impending brain herniation:
  - Hemiparesis or hemiplegia
  - Hemisensory changes
  - Unequal pupil size (1 mm or more difference)
  - Failure of pupil to react to light
  - Disconjugate gaze and inability to move one eye beyond midline if third, fourth, or sixth cranial nerves involved
  - Loss of oculocephalic or oculovestibular reflexes
  - Possible decorticate or decerebrate posturing

Outcome Criteria
- Intracranial pressure is ≤15 mm Hg.
- Cerebral perfusion pressure is >60 mm Hg.
- Clinical signs of increased intracranial pressure are absent.

Nursing Interventions and Rationale
1. Maintain adequate cerebral perfusion pressure.
   a. Collaborate with physician regarding the administration of volume expanders, vasopressors, or antihypertensives **to maintain the patient's blood pressure within normal range.**
   b. Implement measures to reduce intracranial pressure.
      (1) Elevate head of bed 30 to 45 degrees **to facilitate venous return.**
      (2) Maintain head and neck in neutral plane (avoid flexion, extension, or lateral rotation) **to enhance venous drainage from the head.**
      (3) Avoid extreme hip flexion.
      (4) Collaborate with the physician regarding the administration of steroids, osmotic agents, and diuretics and need for drainage of cerebrospinal fluid if a ventriculostomy is in place.
      (5) Assist patient to turn and move self in bed (instruct patient to exhale while turning or pushing up in

bed) **to avoid isometric contractions and Valsalva maneuver.**
2. Maintain patent airway and adequate ventilation and supply oxygen **to prevent hypoxemia and hypercarbia.**
3. Monitor arterial blood gas values and maintain PaO_2 >80 mm Hg, $PaCO_2$ >35 mm Hg, and pH at 7.35 to 7.45 **to prevent cerebral vasodilation.**
4. Avoid suctioning beyond 10 seconds at a time; hyperoxygenate and hyperventilate before and after suctioning.
5. Plan patient care activities and nursing interventions around patient's intracranial pressure response. Avoid unnecessary additional disturbances, and allow patient up to 1 hour of rest between activities as frequently as possible. **Studies have shown the direct correlation between nursing care activities and increases in intracranial pressure.**
6. Maintain normothermia with external cooling or heating measures as necessary. Wrap hands, feet, and male genitalia in soft towels before cooling measures **to prevent shivering and frostbite.**
7. With physician's collaboration, control seizures with prophylactic and as-necessary (PRN) anticonvulsants. **Seizures can greatly increase the cerebral metabolic rate.**
8. Collaborate with the physician regarding the administration of sedatives, barbiturates, or paralyzing agents **to reduce cerebral metabolic rate.**
9. Counsel family members to maintain calm atmosphere and avoid disturbing topics of conversation (e.g., patient condition, pain, prognosis, family crisis, financial difficulties).
10. If signs of impending brain herniation are present, implement the following:
    a. Notify the physician at once.
    b. Ensure head of bed is elevated 45 degrees and patient's head is in neutral plane.
    c. Administer mainline intravenous infusion slowly to keep-open rate.
    d. Drain cerebrospinal fluid as ordered if a ventriculostomy is in place.
    e. Prepare to administer osmotic agents and/or diuretics.
    f. Prepare patient for emergency computed tomography head scan and/or emergency surgery.

NURSING MANAGEMENT PLAN

Deficient Fluid Volume

Definition: Decreased intravascular, interstitial, and/or intracellular fluid. This refers to dehydration, water loss alone without a change in sodium concentration.

Deficient Fluid Volume Related to Absolute Loss

Defining Characteristics
- Cardiac output is <4 L/min
- Cardiac index is <2.2 L/min
- Pulmonary artery occlusion pressure is <6 mm Hg
- Right atrial pressure is <2 mm Hg
- Tachycardia
- Narrowed pulse pressure
- Systolic blood pressure is <100 mm Hg
- Urinary output is <30 mL/hr

- Pale, cool, moist skin
- Apprehensiveness

Outcome Criteria
- CO is >4 L/min, and CI is >2.2 L/min.
- Pulmonary artery occlusion pressure is >6 mm Hg or returns to baseline level.
- Right atrial pressure is >2 mm Hg or returns to baseline level.

Continued

NURSING MANAGEMENT PLAN

Deficient Fluid Volume—cont'd

- Heart rate is normal or returns to baseline level.
- Systolic blood pressure is >90 mm Hg.
- Urinary output is >30 mL/hr.

Nursing Interventions and Rationale

1. Secure airway, and administer high-flow oxygen.
2. Place patient in supine position with legs elevated **to increase preload.** For patient with head injury, consider using low Fowler's position with legs elevated.
3. For fluid repletion, use the 3:1 rule, replacing three parts of fluid for every unit of blood lost.
4. Administer crystalloid solutions using the fluid challenge technique: infuse precise boluses of fluid (usually 5 to 20 mL/min) over 10-minute periods; monitor hemodynamic pressures serially **to determine successful challenging.** If the pulmonary artery occlusion pressure elevates more than 7 mm Hg above beginning level, the infusion should be stopped. If the

pulmonary artery occlusion pressure rises only to 3 mm Hg above baseline or falls, another fluid challenge should be administered.

5. Replete fluids first before considering use of vasopressors, **because vasopressors increase myocardial oxygen consumption out of proportion to the reestablishment of coronary perfusion in the early phases of treatment.**
6. When blood replacement is indicated, replace it with fresh-packed red cells and fresh-frozen plasma **to keep clotting factors intact.**
7. Move or reposition patient minimally to decrease or limit tissue oxygen demands.
8. Evaluate patient's anxiety level, and intervene through patient education or sedation **to decrease tissue oxygen demands.**
9. Maintain surveillance for signs and symptoms of fluid overload.

Deficient Fluid Volume Related to Decreased Secretion of Antidiuretic Hormone (ADH)

Defining Characteristics

- Confusion and lethargy
- Decreased skin turgor
- Thirst
- Weight loss over short period
- Decreased pulmonary artery occlusion pressure
- Decreased right atrial pressure
- Urinary output is >6 L/day
- Serum sodium is >148 mEq/L
- Serum osmolality is >295 mOsm/kg
- Urine osmolality is <100 mOsm/kg
- Urine specific gravity is <1.005

Outcome Criteria

- Weight returns to baseline.
- Urinary output is >30 mL/hr and <200 mL/hr.
- Serum osmolality is 280 to 295 mOsm/kg.
- Urine specific gravity is 1.010 to 1.030.

Nursing Interventions and Rationale

1. Record intake and output every hour, noting color and clarity of urine **because color and clarity are an indication of urine concentration.**
2. Monitor cardiac rhythm continuously for dysrhythmias **caused by electrolyte imbalance.**

3. Collaborate with physician regarding administration of vasopressin or desmopressin **to replace ADH.**
   a. Monitor patient for adverse effects of medications (e.g., headache, chest pain, abdominal pain) **caused by vasoconstriction.**
   b. Report adverse effects to physician immediately.
4. Collaborate with physician regarding intravenous fluid and electrolyte replacement therapy **to restore fluid balance, correct dehydration, and maintain electrolyte balance.**
   a. Administer hypotonic saline **to replace free water deficit.**
5. Provide oral fluids low in sodium such as water, coffee, tea, or orange juice **to decrease sodium intake.**
6. Weigh patient daily (at same time, in same amount of clothing, and preferably with same scale) **to ensure accuracy of readings.**
7. Reposition patient every 2 hours to prevent skin integrity issues caused by dehydration.
8. Provide mouth care every 4 hours to prevent breakdown of oral mucous membranes.
9. Collaborate with physician regarding administration of medications to prevent constipation **caused by dehydration.**
10. Maintain surveillance for symptoms of hypernatremia (muscle twitching, irritability, seizures), hypovolemic shock (hypotension, tachycardia, decreased CVP and PAOP), and deep vein thrombosis (calf pain, tenderness, swelling).

Deficient Fluid Volume Related to Relative Loss

Defining Characteristics

- Pulmonary artery occlusion pressure is <6 mm Hg
- Right atrial pressure is <2 mm Hg
- Tachycardia
- Narrowed pulse pressure
- Systolic blood pressure is <100 mm Hg
- Urinary output is <30 mL/hr
- Increased hematocrit level

Outcome Criteria

- Pulmonary artery occlusion pressure is >6 mm Hg or returns to baseline level.
- Right atrial pressure is >2 mm Hg or returns to baseline level.

- Systolic blood pressure is >90 mm Hg.
- Urinary output is >30 mL/hr.
- Hematocrit level is normal.

Nursing Interventions and Rationale

1. Collaborate with the physician regarding the administration of intravenous fluid replacements (usually normal saline solution or lactated Ringer's solution) at a rate sufficient to maintain urinary output >30 mL/hr. Colloid solutions are avoided in the initial phases (but can be used later) because of the possibility of increased edema formation **as a result of the increased capillary permeability.**

NURSING MANAGEMENT PLAN
Deficient Knowledge

Definition: Absence or deficiency of cognitive information related to a specific topic.

Defining Characteristics

- Verbalized statement of inadequate knowledge or skills
- Verbalization of inadequate recall of information
- Verbalization of inadequate understanding of information
- Evidence of inaccurate follow-through of instructions
- Inadequate demonstration of a skill

- New diagnosis or health problem requiring self-management or care
- Lack of prior formal or informal education about the specific health problem
- Demonstration of inappropriate behaviors related to management of health problem

Outcome Criteria

- Patient verbalizes adequate knowledge about or performs skills related to disease process, its causes, factors related to onset of symptoms, and self-management of disease or health problem.

- Patient actively participates in health behaviors required for performance of a procedure or in those behaviors enhancing recovery from illness and preventing recurrence or complications.

Nursing Interventions and Rationale

1. Determine existing level of knowledge or skill.
2. Assess factors that affect the knowledge deficit:
   a. Learning needs, including patient's priorities and the necessary knowledge and skills for safety.
   b. Learning ability of patient, including language skills, level of education, ability to read, preferred learning style.
   c. Physical ability to perform prescribed skills or procedures; consider effect of limitations imposed by treatment such as bed rest, restriction of movement by intravenous or other equipment, or effect of sedatives or analgesics.
   d. Psychological effect of stage of adaptation to disease.
   e. Activity tolerance and ability to concentrate.
   f. Motivation to learn new skills or gain new knowledge.
3. Reduce or limit barriers to learning:
   a. Provide consistent nurse-patient contact to encourage development of trusting and therapeutic relationship.
   b. Structure environment to enhance learning; control unnecessary noise, interruptions.
      (1) Ensure that lights are bright enough to see teaching aids but not too bright.
      (2) Schedule care and medications to allow uninterrupted teaching periods.
      (3) Move patient to quiet, private room for teaching if possible.
   c. Individualize teaching plan to fit patient's current physical and psychological status.
   d. Delay teaching until patient is ready to learn.
   e. Conduct teaching sessions during period of day when patient is most alert and receptive.
   f. Meet patient's immediate learning needs as they arise (e.g., give brief explanation of procedures when they are performed).
4. Promote active participation in the teaching plan by the patient and family:
   a. Solicit input during development of plan.
   b. Develop mutually acceptable goals and outcomes.
   c. Solicit expression of feelings and emotions related to new responsibilities.
   d. Encourage questions.
5. Conduct teaching sessions using the most appropriate teaching methods.
6. Repeat key principles, and provide them in printed form **for reference at a later time.**
7. Give frequent feedback to patient when practicing new skills.
8. Use several teaching sessions when appropriate. New information and skills should be reinforced several times after initial learning.
9. Initiate referrals for follow-up if necessary:
   a. Health educators
   b. Home health care
   c. Rehabilitation programs
   d. Social services
10. Evaluate effectiveness of teaching plan, based on patient's ability to meet preset goals and objectives **to determine need for further teaching.**

NURSING MANAGEMENT PLAN
Disturbed Body Image

Definition: Confusion in mental picture of one's physical self.

Disturbed Body Image Related to Actual Change in Body Structure, Function, or Appearance

Defining Characteristics

- Actual change in appearance, structure, or function
- Avoidance of looking at body part
- Avoidance of touching body part
- Hiding or overexposing body part (intentional or unintentional)
- Trauma to nonfunctioning part
- Change in ability to estimate spatial relationship of body to environment
- Verbalization of the following:
  - Fear of rejection or reaction by others
  - Negative feeling about body
  - Preoccupation with change or loss
  - Refusal to participate in or to accept responsibility for self-care of altered body part
- Personalization of part or loss with a name
- Depersonalization of part or loss by use of impersonal pronouns
- Refusal to verify actual change

Outcome Criteria

- Patient verbalizes the specific meaning of the change to him or her.
- Patient requests appropriate information about self-care.
- Patient completes personal hygiene and grooming daily with or without help.
- Patient interacts freely with family or other visitors.
- Patient participates in the discussions and conferences related to planning his or her medical and nursing management in the critical care unit and transfer from the unit.
- Patient talks with trained visitors (support-group representatives) at least twice about his or her loss.

Nursing Interventions and Rationale

1. Evaluate patient's mental, physical, and emotional state; recognize assets, strengths, response to illness, coping mechanisms, past experience with stress, and support system.
2. Appraise the response of family and significant others. **Body image is derived from the "reflected appraisals" of family and significant others.**
3. Determine the patient's goals and readiness for learning.
4. Provide the necessary information to help the patient and family adapt to the change. Clarify misconceptions about future limitations.
5. Permit and encourage the patient to express the significance of the loss or change; note nonverbal behavior responses.
6. Allow and encourage the patient's expression of anxiety. **Anxiety is the most predominant emotional response to a body image disturbance.**
7. Recognize and accept the use of denial as an adaptive defense mechanism when used early and temporarily.
8. Recognize maladaptive denial as that which interferes with the patient's progress and/or alienates support systems. Use confrontation.
9. Provide an opportunity for the patient to discuss sexual concerns.
10. Touch the affected body part **to provide the patient with sensory information about altered body structure and/or function.**
11. Encourage and provide movement of altered body part **to establish kinesthetic feedback. This enables the person to know his or her body as it now exists.**
12. Prepare the patient to look at the body part. Call the body part by its anatomic name (e.g., stump, stoma, limb) as opposed to "it" or "she." **The use of impersonal pronouns increases a sense of fantasy and depersonalization of the body part.**
13. Allow the patient to experience excellence in some aspect of physical functioning—walking, turning, deep breathing, healing, self-care—and point out progress and accomplishment. **This helps to balance the patient's sense of dysfunction with function.**
14. Avoid false reassurance. Acknowledge the difficulty of incorporating the altered body part or function into one's body image. **This evidences the nurse's sensitivity and promotes trust.**
15. Talk with the patient about his or her life, generativity, and accomplishments. **Patients with disturbances in body image frequently see themselves in a distortedly "narrow" sense. Encouraging a wider focus of themselves and their life reduces this distortion.**
16. Help the patient explore realistic alternatives.
17. Recognize that incorporating a body change into one's body image takes time. Avoid setting unrealistic expectations and **thereby inadvertently reinforcing a low self-esteem.**
18. Suggest the use of additional resources such as trained visitors who have mastered situations similar to those of the patient. Refer the patient to a psychiatric liaison nurse or psychiatrist if needed.

Disturbed Body Image Related to Functional Dependence on Life-Sustaining Technology, Including a Ventilator, Dialysis, IABP, or Halo Traction

Defining Characteristics

- Actual change in function requiring permanent or temporary replacement
- Refusal to verify actual loss
- Verbalization of the following: feelings of helplessness, hopelessness, powerlessness, fear of failure to wean from technology

Outcome Criteria

- Patient verifies actual change in function.
- Patient does not refuse or fight technological intervention.
- Patient verbalizes acceptance of expected change in lifestyle.

NURSING MANAGEMENT PLAN
Disturbed Body Image—cont'd

Nursing Interventions and Rationale

1. Evaluate patient's response to the technological intervention.
2. Assess responses of family and significant others. **Body image is derived from the "reflected appraisals" of family and significant others.**
3. Provide information needed by patient and family.
4. Promote trust, security, comfort, and privacy.
5. Recognize anxiety. Allow and encourage its expression. **Anxiety is the most predominant emotion accompanying body image alterations.** Implement Nursing Management Plan for Anxiety Related to Threat to Biological, Psychological, or Social Integrity.
6. Assist patient to recognize his or her own functioning and performance in the face of technology. For example, assist

patient to distinguish spontaneous breaths from mechanically delivered breaths. **The activity will assist in weaning patient from the ventilator when feasible. To establish realistic, accurate body boundaries, a patient needs help to separate himself or herself from the technology that is supporting his or her functioning. Any participation or function on the part of the patient during periods of dependency is helpful in preventing and/or resolving an alteration in body image.**

7. Plan for discontinuation of the treatment (e.g., weaning from ventilator). Explain procedure that will be followed, and be present during its initiation.
8. Plan for transfer from the critical care environment.
9. Document care, ensuring an up-to-date management plan is available to all involved caregivers.

NURSING MANAGEMENT PLAN
Disturbed Sleep Pattern

Definition: Time-limited disruption of sleep amount and quality due to external factors.

Disturbed Sleep Pattern Related to Fragmented Sleep

Defining Characteristics

- Decreased sleep during one block of sleep time
- Daytime sleepiness
- Decreased sleep
  - Less than one half of normal total sleep time
  - Decreased slow-wave or rapid-eye-movement (REM) sleep
- Anxiety
- Fatigue
- Restlessness
- Disorientation and hallucinations
- Combativeness
- Frequent awakenings

Outcome Criteria

- Patient's total sleep time approximates patient's normal sleep time.
- Patient can complete sleep cycles of 90 minutes without interruption.
- Patient has no delusions or hallucinations.
- Patient has reality-based thought content.

Nursing Interventions and Rationale

1. Assess normal sleep pattern on admission and any history of sleep disturbance or chronic illness that may affect sleep or sedative/hypnotic use. Promote normal sleep activity while patient is in critical care unit. Assess sleep effectiveness by asking patient how his or her sleep in the hospital compares with sleep at home. **The best treatment for sleep pattern disturbance is prevention.**
2. Promote comfort, relaxation, and a sense of well-being. Treat pain; change, smooth, or refresh bed linens at bedtime; and provide oral hygiene. Eliminate stressful situations before bedtime. Use relaxation techniques, imagery, music, massage,

or warm blankets. Have a close family member sit beside the bed and provide the patient with his or her own garments or coverings. Provide quiet or background noise of the television or music (patient preference) **to best promote sleep.** Provide a comfortable room temperature.

3. Minimize noise, particularly that of the staff and noisy equipment. Reduce the level of environmental stimuli. Dim the lights at night.
4. Foods containing tryptophan (e.g., milk, turkey) may be appropriate **because these promote sleep.**
5. Plan nap times to assist in approximating the patient's normal 24-hour sleep time.
6. Minimize awakenings **to allow for at least 90-minute sleep cycles.** Continually assess the need to awaken the patient, particularly at night. Distinguish between essential and nonessential nursing tasks. Organize nursing management to allow for maximal amount of uninterrupted sleep while ensuring close monitoring of the patient's condition. Whenever possible, monitor physiological parameters without waking the patient. Coordinate awakenings with other departments, such as respiratory therapy, laboratory, and radiography, **to minimize sleep interruptions.**
7. Be aware of the effects of commonly used medications on sleep. **Many sedative and hypnotic medications decrease REM sleep.** Sedative and analgesic medications should not be withheld, but rather, medications that minimally disrupt sleep should be used to complement comfort measures, with dosages reduced gradually as the medication is no longer necessary. Do not abruptly withdraw REM-suppressing medications **because this can result in REM rebound.**
8. Document amount of uninterrupted sleep per shift, especially sleep episodes lasting longer than 2 hours. **Sleep pattern disturbance is diagnosed, treated, and resolved more efficiently when formally documented in this manner.**

NURSING MANAGEMENT PLAN
Dysfunctional Ventilatory Weaning Response

Definition: Inability to adjust to lowered levels of mechanical ventilator support that interrupts and prolongs the weaning process.

Dysfunctional Ventilatory Weaning Response (DVWR) Related to Physical, Psychosocial, or Situational Factors

Defining Characteristics

Mild DVWR

- Responds to lowered levels of mechanical ventilator support with:
  - Restlessness
  - Slightly increased respiratory rate from baseline
  - Expressed feelings of increased need for oxygen; breathing discomfort; fatigue; warmth
  - Queries about possible machine malfunction
  - Increased concentration on breathing

Moderate DVWR

- Responds to lowered levels of mechanical ventilator support with:
  - Slight baseline increase in blood pressure is <20 mm Hg
  - Slight baseline increase in heart rate is <20 beats/min
  - Baseline increase in respiratory rate is <5 breaths/min
  - Hypervigilance to activities
  - Inability to respond to coaching
  - Inability to cooperate
  - Apprehension
  - Diaphoresis
  - Eye widening ("wide-eyed look")
  - Decreased air entry on auscultation
  - Color changes: pale, slight cyanosis
  - Slight respiratory accessory muscle use

Severe DVWR

- Responds to lowered levels of mechanical ventilator support with:
  - Agitation
  - Deterioration in arterial blood gases from current baseline
  - Baseline increase in blood pressure is >20 mm Hg
  - Baseline increase in heart rate is >20 beats/min
  - Respiratory rate increases significantly from baseline
  - Profuse diaphoresis
  - Full respiratory accessory muscle use
  - Shallow, gasping breaths
  - Paradoxical abdominal breathing
  - Discoordinated breathing with the ventilator
  - Decreased level of consciousness
  - Adventitious breath sounds, audible airway secretions
  - Cyanosis

Outcome Criteria

- Airway is clear.
- Underlying disorder is resolving.
- Patient is rested, and pain is controlled.
- Nutritional status is adequate.
- Patient has feelings of perceived control, situational security, and trust in the nurses.
- Patient is able to adapt to selected levels of ventilator support without undue fatigue.

Nursing Interventions and Rationale

1. Communicate interest and concern for the patient's well-being, and demonstrate confidence in ability to manage weaning process **to instill trust in the patient.**
2. Use normalizing strategies (e.g., grooming, dressing, mobilizing, social conversation) **to reinforce the patient's self-esteem and feeling of identity.**
3. Identify parameters of the patient's usual functioning before the weaning process begins **to facilitate early identification of problems.**
4. Identify the patient's strengths and resources that can be mobilized **to enhance the patient's coping and maximize weaning effort.**
5. Note concerns that adversely affect the patient's comfort and confidence, and manage them discreetly **to facilitate the patient's ease.**
6. Praise successful activities, encourage a positive outlook, and review the patient's positive progress **to increase the patient's perceived self-efficacy.**
7. Inform the patient of his or her situation and weaning progress **to permit the patient as much control as possible.**
8. Teach the patient about the weaning process and how he or she can participate in the process.
9. Negotiate daily weaning goals with the patient **to gain cooperation.**
10. Position the patient with the head of the bed elevated **to optimize respiratory efforts.**
11. Coach the patient in breath control by regular demonstrations of slow, deep, rhythmic patterns of breathing **to assist with dyspnea.**
12. Remain visible in the room and reassure the patient that help is immediately available if needed **to reduce the patient's anxiety and fearfulness.**
13. Encourage the patient to view weaning trials as a form of training, regardless of whether the weaning goal is achieved **to avoid discouragement.**
14. Encourage the patient to maintain emotional calmness by reassuring, being present, comforting, talking down if emotionally aroused, and reinforcing the idea that he or she can and will succeed.
15. Monitor the patient's status frequently **to avoid undue fatigue and anxiety.**
16. Provide regular periods of rest by reducing activities, maintaining or increasing ventilator support, and providing oxygen as needed before fatigue advances.
17. Provide distraction (e.g., visitors, radio, television, conversation) when the patient's concentration starts to create tension and increases anxiety.
18. Ensure adequate nutritional support, sufficient rest and sleep time, and sedation or pain control **to promote the patient's optimal physical and emotional comfort.**
19. Start weaning early in the day **when the patient is most rested.**

NURSING MANAGEMENT PLAN
Dysfunctional Ventilatory Weaning Response—cont'd

20. Restrict unnecessary activities and visitors who do not cooperate with weaning strategies **to minimize energy demands on the patient during the weaning process.**
21. Coordinate necessary activities to promote adequate time for rest and relaxation.
22. Monitor the patient's underlying disease process **to ensure it is stabilized and under control.**

23. Advocate for additional resources (e.g., sedation, analgesia, rest) needed by the patient **to maximize comfort status.**
24. Develop and adhere to an individualized plan of care **to promote the patient's feelings of control.**

NURSING MANAGEMENT PLAN
Excess Fluid Volume

Definition: Increased isotonic fluid retention.

Excess Fluid Volume Related to Increased Secretion of Antidiuretic Hormone (ADH)

Defining Characteristics
- Headache
- Decreased sensorium
- Weight gain over short period
- Intake greater than output
- Increased pulmonary artery occlusion pressure
- Increased right atrial pressure
- Urine output is <30 mL/hr
- Serum sodium is <120 mEq/L
- Serum osmolality is <275 mOsm/kg
- Urine osmolality greater than serum osmolality
- Urine sodium is >200 mEq/L
- Urine specific gravity is >1.03

Outcome Criteria
- Weight returns to baseline.
- Urine output is >30 mL/hr.
- Serum sodium is 135 to 145 mEq/L.
- Urine specific gravity is 1.005 to 1.030.

Nursing Interventions and Rationale
1. Monitor cardiac rhythm continuously for dysrhythmias **caused by electrolyte imbalance.**
2. Restrict patient's fluids to 500 mL less than output per day **to decrease fluid retention.**
3. Provide patient chilled beverages high in sodium content such as tomato juice or broth **to increase sodium intake.**

4. Collaborate with physician regarding administration of demeclocycline, lithium, and/or opioid agonists **to inhibit renal response to ADH.**
5. Collaborate with physician regarding administration of hypertonic saline and furosemide **for rapid correction of severe sodium deficit and diuresis of free water.**
   a. Administer hypertonic saline at a rate of 1 to 2 mL/kg/hr until the patient's serum sodium is increased no greater than 1 to 2 mEq/L/hr.
6. Weigh patient daily (at same time, in same amount of clothing, and preferably with same scale) **to ensure accuracy of readings.**
7. Provide frequent mouth care to prevent breakdown of oral mucous membranes.
8. Initiate seizure precautions because patient is at high risk as a result of hyponatremia.
   a. Pad side rails of bed to protect patient from injury.
   b. Remove any objects from immediate environment that could injure patient in the event of a seizure.
   c. Keep appropriate-size oral airway at bedside to assist with airway management after the seizure.
9. Collaborate with physician regarding administration of medications to prevent constipation **caused by decreased fluid intake and immobility.**
10. Maintain surveillance for symptoms of hyponatremia (e.g., headache, abdominal cramps, weakness) and congestive heart failure (e.g., dyspnea, rales, increased CVP and PAOP).

Excess Fluid Volume Related to Kidney Dysfunction

Defining Characteristics
- Weight gain that occurs during a 24- to 48-hour period
- Dependent pitting edema
- Ascites in severe cases
- Fluid crackles on lung auscultation
- Exertional dyspnea
- Oliguria or anuria
- Hypertension
- Engorged neck veins
- Decrease in urinary osmolality as renal failure progresses

- Right atrial pressure is >8 mm Hg
- Pulmonary artery occlusion pressure is >12 mm Hg

Outcome Criteria
- Weight returns to baseline.
- Edema or ascites is absent or reduced to baseline.
- Lungs are clear to auscultation.
- Exertional dyspnea is absent.
- Blood pressure returns to baseline.
- Heart rate returns to baseline.

Continued

NURSING MANAGEMENT PLAN
Excess Fluid Volume—cont'd

- Neck veins are flat.
- Mucous membranes are moist.

Nursing Interventions and Rationale

1. Promote skin integrity of edematous areas by frequent repositioning and elevation of areas where possible. Avoid massaging pressure points or reddened areas of skin *because this results in further tissue trauma.*

2. Plan patient care to provide rest periods *to not heighten exertional dyspnea.*
3. Weigh patient daily (at same time, in same amount of clothing, and preferably with same scale).
4. Instruct the patient about the correlation between fluid intake and weight gain, using commonly understood fluid measurements; for example, ingesting 4 cups (1000 mL) of fluid results in an approximate 2-pound weight gain in the anuric patient.

NURSING MANAGEMENT PLAN
Hyperthermia

Definition: Body temperature elevated above normal range.

Hyperthermia Related to Increased Metabolic Rate

Defining Characteristics

- Increased body temperature above normal range
- Seizures
- Flushed skin
- Increased respiratory rate
- Tachycardia
- Skin warm to touch
- Diaphoresis

Outcome Criteria

- Temperature is within normal range.
- Respiratory rate and heart rate are within patient's baseline range.
- Skin is warm and dry.

Nursing Interventions and Rationale

1. Monitor temperature every 15 minutes to 1 hour until within normal range and stable and then every 4 hours *to maintain close surveillance for temperature fluctuations and evaluate effectiveness of interventions.*
   a. Use temperature taken from pulmonary artery catheter or bladder catheter if available *because these methods closely reflect core body temperature.*
   b. Use tympanic membrane temperature if core body temperature devices are unavailable.
   c. Use rectal temperature if none of the methods listed above are available.
2. Collaborate with physician regarding administration of antithyroid medications *to block the synthesis and release of thyroid hormone.*

3. Collaborate with physician regarding the use of cooling blanket *to facilitate heat loss by conduction.*
   a. Wrap hands, feet, and genitalia to protect them from maceration during cooling and to decrease chance of shivering.
   b. Avoid rapidly cooling the patient and overcooling the patient because this initiates the heat-conserving response (i.e., shivering).
4. Place ice packs in patient's groin and axilla *to facilitate heat loss by conduction.*
5. Maintain patient on bed rest *to decrease the effects of activity on the patient's metabolic rate.*
6. Provide tepid sponge baths *to facilitate heat loss by evaporation.*
7. Decrease the patient's room temperature *to facilitate radiant heat loss.*
8. Place fan near patient to circulate cool air *to facilitate heat loss by convection.*
9. Provide patient with nonrestrictive gown and lightweight bed coverings *to allow heat to escape from the patient's trunk.*
10. Collaborate with physician and respiratory therapist on the administration of oxygen to maintain SpO_2 >90% *because patient has increased oxygen consumption resulting from an increased metabolic rate.*
11. Collaborate with physician regarding use of antipyretic medications *to facilitate patient comfort.*
12. Collaborate with physician regarding use of intravenous and oral fluids *to maintain adequate hydration of the patient.*

NURSING MANAGEMENT PLAN

Hypothermia

Definition: Body temperature below normal range.

Hypothermia Related to Decreased Metabolic Rate

Defining Characteristics

- Reduction in body temperature below normal range
- Shivering
- Pallor
- Piloerection
- Hypertension
- Skin cool to touch
- Tachycardia
- Decreased capillary refill

Outcome Criteria

- Temperature is within normal range.
- Heart rate is within patient's baseline range.
- Skin is warm and dry.
- Capillary refill is normal.

Nursing Interventions and Rationale

1. Monitor temperature every 15 minutes to 1 hour until within normal range and stable and then every 4 hours *to maintain close surveillance for temperature fluctuations and evaluate effectiveness of interventions.*

   a. Use temperature taken from pulmonary artery catheter or bladder catheter if available *because these methods closely reflect core body temperature.*

   b. Use tympanic membrane temperature *if core body temperature devices are unavailable.*

   c. Use rectal temperature if none of the methods listed above are available.

2. Collaborate with physician regarding administration of thyroid medications *to replace lacking thyroid hormone.*

3. Collaborate with physician regarding the use of fluid-filled heating blanket *to facilitate rewarming by conduction.*

4. Initiate forced air-warming therapy *to facilitate convective heat gain.*

5. Provide patient with warm blankets *to facilitate heat transfer to the patient.*

6. Increase the patient's room temperature *to decrease radiant heat loss.*

7. Replace wet patient gown and bed linens promptly *to decrease evaporative heat loss.*

8. Warm intravenous fluids and blood products *to facilitate rewarming by conduction.*

Hypothermia Related to Exposure to Cold Environment, Trauma, or Damage to the Hypothalamus

Defining Characteristics

- Core body temperature below 35° C (95° F)
- Skin cold to touch
- Slurred speech, incoordination
- At temperature below 33° C (91.4° F):
  - Cardiac dysrhythmias (atrial fibrillation, bradycardia)
  - Cyanosis
  - Respiratory alkalosis
- At temperatures below 32° C (89.6° F):
  - Shivering replaced by muscle rigidity
  - Hypotension
  - Dilated pupils
- At temperatures below 28° to 29° C (82.4° to 84.2° F):
  - Absent deep tendon reflexes
  - 3 to 4 breaths/min to apnea
  - Ventricular fibrillation possible
- At temperatures below 26° to 27° C (78.8° to 80.6° F):
  - Coma
  - Flaccid muscles
  - Fixed, dilated pupils
  - Ventricular fibrillation to cardiac standstill
  - Apnea

Outcome Criteria

- Core body temperature is greater than 35° C (95° F).
- Patient is alert and oriented.
- Cardiac dysrhythmias are absent.
- Acid-base balance is normal.
- Pupils are normoreactive.

Nursing Interventions and Rationale

1. Monitor core body temperature continuously.

2. Collaborate with the physician regarding the need for intubation and mechanical ventilation.

   a. Heated air or oxygen can be added *to help rewarm the body core.*

   b. Do not hyperventilate the hypothermic patient because carbon dioxide production is low and this action may induce severe alkalosis and precipitate ventricular fibrillation.

3. Maintain cardiopulmonary resuscitation and advanced cardiac life support (ACLS) until core body temperature is up to at least 29.5° C (85.1° F) before determining that patient cannot be resuscitated. *Electrical defibrillation is usually successful in terminating ventricular fibrillation if the temperature is greater than 28° C (82.4° F).*

4. Administer cardiac resuscitation drugs sparingly *because as the body warms, peripheral vasodilation occurs. Drugs that remain in the periphery are suddenly released, leading to a bolus effect that may cause fatal dysrhythmias.*

5. Monitor arterial blood gas values *to direct further therapy,* and ensure that the pH, PaO_2, and $PaCO_2$ are corrected for temperature.

6. Rewarm patient rapidly *because the pathophysiological changes associated with chronic hypothermia have not had time to evolve.*

   a. Institute rapid, active rewarming by immersion in warm water (38° to 43° C; 100.4° to 109.4° F).

   b. Apply thermal blanket at 36.6° to 37.7° C (97.9° to 99.9° F). Some researchers suggest rewarming only the torso or trunk first, leaving the extremities exposed to room temperature. *This is done to prevent early peripheral vasodilation with abrupt redistribution of intravascular volume. This also prevents colder blood trapped in the extremities from returning to the body core before the heart is rewarmed.*

   c. Perform rapid core rewarming with heated (37° to 43° C; 98.6° to 109.4° F) intravenous infusion, hemodialysis, peritoneal dialysis, and colonic or gastric irrigation fluids.

7. Monitor peripheral circulation because gangrene of the fingers and toes is a common complication of accidental hypothermia.

NURSING MANAGEMENT PLAN

Imbalanced Nutrition: Less than Body Requirements

Definition: Intake of nutrients insufficient to meet metabolic needs.

Imbalanced Nutrition: Less than Body Requirements Related to Lack of Exogenous Nutrients and Increased Metabolic Demand

Defining Characteristics

- Unplanned weight loss of 20% of body weight within the past 6 months
- Serum albumin is <3.5 g/dL
- Total lymphocytes are <1500/mm³
- Anergy
- Negative nitrogen balance
- Fatigue; lack of energy and endurance
- Nonhealing wounds
- Daily caloric intake less than estimated nutritional requirements
- Presence of factors known to increase nutritional requirements (e.g., sepsis, trauma, multiple organ dysfunction syndrome)
- Maintenance of nothing by mouth (NPO) status for >7 to 10 days
- Long-term use of 5% dextrose intravenously
- Documentation of suboptimal calorie counts
- Drug or nutrient interaction that might decrease oral intake (e.g., chronic use of bronchodilators, laxatives, anticonvulsives, diuretics, antacids, opioids)
- Physical problems with chewing, swallowing, choking, and salivation and presence of altered taste, anorexia, nausea, vomiting, diarrhea, or constipation

Outcome Criteria

- Patient exhibits stabilization of weight loss or weight gain of one-half pound daily.

- Serum albumin is >3.5 g/dL.
- Total lymphocytes are <1500/mm³.
- Patient has positive response to cutaneous skin antigen testing.
- Patient is in positive nitrogen balance.
- Wound healing is evident.
- Daily caloric intake equals estimated nutritional requirements.
- Increased ambulation and endurance are evident.

Nursing Interventions and Rationale

1. Inquire if patient has any food allergies and food preferences **to ensure the food provided to the patient is not contraindicated.**
2. Monitor patient's caloric intake and weight daily **to ensure adequacy of nutritional interventions.**
3. Collaborate with dietitian regarding patient's nutritional and caloric needs **to determine the appropriateness of the patient's diet to meet those needs.**
4. Monitor patient for signs of nutritional deficiencies **to facilitate evaluation of extent of nutritional deficit.**
5. Provide patient with oral care before eating **to ensure optimal consumption of diet.**
6. Assist patient to eat as appropriate **to ensure optimal consumption of diet.**
7. Collaborate with physician regarding the administration of parenteral and enteral nutrition as needed.

NURSING MANAGEMENT PLAN

Impaired Gas Exchange

Definition: Excess or deficit in oxygenation and/or carbon dioxide elimination at the alveolar-capillary membrane.

Impaired Gas Exchange Related to Alveolar Hypoventilation

Defining Characteristics

- Abnormal arterial blood gas values (decreased PaO_2, increased $PaCO_2$, decreased pH, decreased SaO_2)
- Somnolence
- Neurobehavioral changes (e.g., restlessness, irritability, confusion)
- Tachycardia or dysrhythmias
- Central cyanosis

Outcome Criteria

- Arterial blood gas values are within patient's baseline.
- Central cyanosis is absent.

Nursing Interventions and Rationale

1. Initiate continuous pulse oximetry or monitor SpO_2 every hour.
2. Collaborate with physician on the administration of oxygen to maintain an SpO_2 >90%.

a. Administer supplemental oxygen by an appropriate oxygen-delivery device **to increase driving pressure of oxygen in the alveoli.**
b. If supplemental oxygen alone is not effective, administer continuous positive airway pressure (CPAP) by noninvasive positive pressure ventilation (NPPV) or positive end-expiratory pressure (PEEP) by invasive positive pressure mechanical ventilation **to open collapsed alveoli and increase the surface area for gas exchange.**

3. Prevent hypoventilation.

a. Position patient in high Fowler's or semi-Fowler's position **to promote diaphragmatic descent and maximal inhalation.**
b. Assist with deep-breathing exercises and/or incentive spirometry with sustained maximal inspiration 5 to 10 times/hr **to help reinflate collapsed portions of the lung.** See the Nursing Management Plan for Ineffective Breathing

NURSING MANAGEMENT PLAN

Impaired Gas Exchange—cont'd

Pattern Related to Decreased Lung Expansion for further instructions.

c. Treat pain, if present, **to prevent hypoventilation and atelectasis.** Implement the Nursing Management Plan for

Acute Pain Related to Transmission and Perception of Cutaneous, Visceral, Muscular, or Ischemic Impulses.

4. Assist physician with intubation and initiation of mechanical ventilation as indicated.

Impaired Gas Exchange Related to Ventilation/Perfusion Mismatching or Intrapulmonary Shunting

Defining Characteristics
- Abnormal arterial blood gas values (decreased PaO_2, decreased SaO_2)
- Somnolence
- Neurobehavioral changes (restlessness, irritability, confusion)
- Central cyanosis

Outcome Criteria
- ABG values are within patient's baseline.
- Central cyanosis is absent.

Nursing Interventions and Rationale
1. Initiate continuous pulse oximetry, or monitor SpO_2 every hour.
2. Collaborate with physician on the administration of oxygen to maintain an SpO_2 >90%.
   a. Administer supplemental oxygen by an appropriate oxygen-delivery device **to increase driving pressure of oxygen in the alveoli.**
   b. If supplemental oxygen alone is not effective, administer continuous positive airway pressure (CPAP) by noninvasive positive pressure ventilation (NPPV) or positive end-expiratory pressure (PEEP) by invasive positive pressure mechanical ventilation **to open collapsed alveoli and increase the surface area for gas exchange.**
3. Position patient to optimize ventilation/perfusion matching.
   a. For patient with unilateral lung disease, position with the good lung down **because gravity will improve perfusion to this area, and this will best match ventilation with perfusion.**

   b. For patient with bilateral lung disease, position with the right lung down **because this lung is larger than the left and affords a greater area for ventilation and perfusion,** or change position every 2 hours, favoring positions that improve oxygenation.
   c. For patient with diffuse bilateral disease, collaborate with the physician regarding the use of prone positioning **to encourage perfusion to the anterior region of the lungs, which are usually less damaged than the posterior region.**
   d. Avoid any position that seriously compromises oxygenation status.
4. Perform procedures only as needed and provide adequate rest and recovery time in between **to prevent desaturation.**
5. Collaborate with the physician regarding the administration of the following:
   a. Sedatives **to decrease ventilator asynchrony and facilitate patient's sense of control.**
   b. Neuromuscular blocking agents **to prevent ventilator asynchrony and decrease oxygen demand.**
   c. Analgesics **to treat pain if present.** Implement the Nursing Management Pan for Acute Pain Related to Transmission and Perception of Cutaneous, Visceral, Muscular, or Ischemic Impulses.
6. Evaluate patient for the presence of secretions. If present, implement the Nursing Management Plan for Ineffective Airway Clearance Related to Excessive Secretions or Abnormal Viscosity of Mucus.

NURSING MANAGEMENT PLAN

Impaired Spontaneous Ventilation

Definition: Decreased energy reserves results in an individual's inability to maintain breathing adequate to support life.

Impaired Spontaneous Ventilation Related to Respiratory Muscle Fatigue or Metabolic Factors

Defining Characteristics
- Dyspnea and apprehension
- Increased metabolic rate
- Increased restlessness
- Increased use of accessory muscles
- Decreased tidal volume
- Increased heart rate
- Abnormal arterial blood gas (ABG) values (decreased PaO_2, increased $PaCO_2$, decreased pH, decreased SaO_2)
- Decreased cooperation

Outcome Criteria
- Metabolic rate and heart rate are within patient's baseline.
- Patient experiences eupnea.
- ABG values are within patient's baseline.

Nursing Interventions and Rationale
1. Collaborate with the physician regarding the application of pressure support to the ventilator **to assist patient in overcoming the work of breathing imposed by the ventilator and endotracheal tube.**
2. Carefully snip excess length from the proximal end of the endotracheal **tube to decrease dead space and thereby decrease the work of breathing.**
3. Collaborate with the physician and dietitian to ensure that at least 50% of the diet's nonprotein caloric source is in the form of fat rather than carbohydrates **to prevent excess carbon dioxide production.**
4. Collaborate with the physician and respiratory therapist regarding the best method of weaning for individual **patients**

Continued

NURSING MANAGEMENT PLAN
Impaired Spontaneous Ventilation—cont'd

because each situation is different and a variety of weaning options are available.

5. Collaborate with the physician and physical therapist regarding a progressive ambulation and conditioning plan *to promote overall muscle conditioning and respiratory muscle functioning.*
6. Determine the most effective means of communication for the patient *to promote independence and reduce anxiety.*
7. Develop a daily schedule and post it in patient's room *to coordinate care and facilitate patient's involvement in the plan.*
8. Treat pain, if present, *to prevent respiratory splinting and hypoventilation.* Implement the Nursing Management Plan for Acute Pain Related to Transmission and Perception of Cutaneous, Visceral, Muscular, or Ischemic Impulses.
9. Ensure that patient receives at least 2- to 4-hr intervals of uninterrupted sleep in a quiet, dark room. Collaborate with the physician and respiratory therapist regarding the use of full ventilatory support at night *to provide respiratory muscle rest.*
10. Place patient in semi-Fowler's position or in a chair at the bedside *for best use of ventilatory muscles and to facilitate diaphragmatic descent.*
11. Explain the weaning procedure to the patient before the trial *so that patient will understand what to expect and how to participate.*
12. Monitor patient during the weaning trial for evidence of respiratory muscle fatigue *to avoid overtiring the patient.*
13. Provide diversional activity during the weaning trial *to reduce the patient's anxiety.*
14. Collaborate with physician and respiratory therapist regarding the removal of the ventilator and artificial airway *when patient has been successfully weaned.*

NURSING MANAGEMENT PLAN
Impaired Swallowing

Definition: Abnormal functioning of the swallowing mechanism associated with deficits in oral, pharyngeal, or esophageal structure or function.

Impaired Swallowing Related to Neuromuscular Impairment, Fatigue, and Limited Awareness

Defining Characteristics
Evidence of difficulty swallowing
- Drooling
- Difficulty handling oral secretions
- Absence of gag, cough, and/or swallow reflex
- Moist, wet, gurgling voice quality
- Decreased tongue and mouth movements
- Presence of dysarthria
- Difficulty handling solid foods:
  - Uncoordinated chewing or swallowing
  - Stasis of food in the oral cavity
  - Wet-sounding voice or change in voice quality
  - Sneezing, coughing, or choking with eating
  - Delay in swallowing of more than 5 seconds
  - Change in respiratory patterns
- Difficulty handling liquids:
  - Momentary loss of voice or change in voice quality
  - Nasal regurgitation of liquids
  - Coughing with drinking

Evidence of aspiration
- Hypoxemia
- Productive cough
- Frothy sputum
- Wheezing, crackles, or rhonchi
- Temperature elevation

Outcome Criteria
- Evidence of swallowing difficulties is absent.
- Evidence of aspiration is absent.

Nursing Interventions and Rationale
1. Collaborate with physician and speech therapist regarding swallowing evaluation and rehabilitation program *to decrease the incidence of aspiration.*
2. Collaborate with physician and dietitian regarding a nutritional assessment and nutritional plan *to ensure that the patient is receiving enough nutrition.*
3. Place the patient in an upright position with the head midline and the chin slightly down *to keep food in the anterior portion of the mouth and to prevent it from falling over the base of the tongue into the open airway.*
4. Provide patient with single-textured soft foods (e.g., cream cereals) that maintain their shape *because these foods require minimal oral manipulation.*
5. Avoid particulate foods (e.g., hamburger) and foods containing more than one texture (e.g., stew) *because these foods require more chewing and oral manipulation.*
6. Avoid dry foods (e.g., popcorn, rice, crackers) and sticky foods (e.g., peanut butter, bananas) *because these foods are difficult to manipulate orally.*
7. Provide patient with thick liquids (e.g., fruit nectar, yogurt) *because thick liquids are more easily controlled in the mouth.*
8. Thicken thin liquids (e.g., water, juice) with a thickening preparation or avoid them *because thin liquids are easily aspirated.*
9. Place foods in the uninvolved side of the mouth *because oral sensitivity and function are greatest in this area.*
10. Avoid the use of straws *because they can deposit the liquid too far back in the mouth for the patient to handle.*

NURSING MANAGEMENT PLAN

Impaired Swallowing—cont'd

11. Serve foods and liquids at room temperature **because the patient may be overly sensitive to heat or cold.**
12. Offer solids and liquids at different times **to avoid patient swallowing solids before they are properly chewed.**
13. Provide oral hygiene after meals **to clear food particles from the mouth that could be aspirated.**
14. Collaborate with physician and pharmacist regarding oral medication administration **to adjust medication regimen to prevent aspiration and choking and to ensure all prescribed medications are swallowed.**

15. Crush tablets (if appropriate) and mix with food that is easily formed into a bolus, use thickened liquid medications (if available), and/or embed small capsules into food **to facilitate oral medication administration.**
16. Inspect mouth for residue after all medication administration **to ensure medication has been swallowed.**
17. Educate patient and family on the swallowing problem, rehabilitation program, and emergency measures for choking.

NURSING MANAGEMENT PLAN

Impaired Verbal Communication

Definition: Decreased, delayed, or absent ability to receive, process, transmit, and use a system of symbols.

Impaired Verbal Communication Related to Cerebral Speech Center Injury

Defining Characteristics
- Inappropriate or absent speech or responses to questions
- Inability to speak spontaneously
- Inability to understand spoken words
- Inability to follow commands appropriately through gestures
- Difficulty or inability to understand written language
- Difficulty or inability to express ideas in writing
- Difficulty or inability to name objects

Outcome Criterion
- Patient is able to make basic needs known.

Nursing Interventions and Rationale
1. Consult with physician and speech pathologist **to determine the extent of the patient's communication deficit (e.g., whether fluent, nonfluent, or global aphasia is involved).**
2. Have the speech therapist post a list of appropriate ways to communicate with the patient in the patient's room **so that all nursing personnel can be consistent in their efforts.**
3. Assess the patient's ability to comprehend, speak, read, and write.
   a. Ask questions that can be answered with "yes" or "no." If a patient answers "yes" to a question, ask the opposite (e.g., "Are you hot?" "Yes." "Are you cold?" "Yes."). **This may help determine whether the patient understands what is being said.**
   b. Ask simple, short questions, and use gestures, pantomime, and facial expressions to give the patient additional clues.
   c. Stand in the patient's line of vision, giving a good view of your face and hands.
   d. Have the patient try to write with a pad and pencil. Offer pictures and alphabet letters at which to point.
   e. Make flash cards with pictures or words depicting frequently used phrases (e.g., glass of water, bedpan).
4. Maintain an uncluttered environment, and decrease external distractions **that could hinder communication.**

5. Maintain a relaxed and calm manner, and explain all diagnostic, therapeutic, and comfort measures before initiating them.
6. Do not shout or speak in a loud voice. **Hearing loss is not a factor in aphasia, and shouting will not help.**
7. Have only one person talk at a time. **It is more difficult for the patient to follow a multisided conversation.**
8. Use direct eye contact, and speak directly to the patient in unhurried, short phrases.
9. Give one-step commands and directions, and provide cues through pictures and gestures.
10. Try to ask questions that can be answered with a "yes" or a "no," and avoid topics that are controversial, emotional, abstract, or lengthy.
11. Listen to the patient in an unhurried manner, and wait for his or her attempt to communicate.
   a. Expect a time lag from when you ask the patient something until the patient responds.
   b. Accept the patient's statement of essential words without expecting complete sentences.
   c. Avoid finishing the sentence for the patient if possible.
   d. Wait approximately 30 seconds before providing the word the patient may be attempting to find (except when the patient is very frustrated and needs something quickly, such as a bedpan).
   e. Rephrase the patient's message aloud **to validate it.**
   f. Do not pretend to understand the patient's message if you do not.
12. Encourage the patient to speak slowly in short phrases and to say each word clearly.
13. Ask the patient to write the message, if able, or draw pictures if only verbal communication is affected.
14. Observe the patient's nonverbal clues for validation (e.g., answers "yes" but shakes head "no").
15. When handing an object to the patient, state what it is **because hearing language spoken is necessary to stimulate language development.**
16. Explain what has happened to the patient, and offer reassurance about the plan of care.

Continued

NURSING MANAGEMENT PLAN
Impaired Verbal Communication—cont'd

17. Verbally address the problem of frustration over the inability to communicate, and explain that both the nurse and the patient need patience.
18. Maintain a calm, positive manner, and offer reassurance (e.g., "I know this is very hard for you, but it will get better if we work on it together").
19. Talk to the patient as an adult. Be respectful, and avoid talking down to the patient.
20. Do not discuss the patient's condition or hold conversations in the patient's presence without including him or her in the discussion. *This may be the reason some aphasic patients develop paranoid thoughts.*
21. Do not exhibit disapproval of emotional utterances or spontaneous use of profanity; instead, offer calm, quiet reassurance.

22. If the patient makes an error in speech, do not reprimand or scold but try to compliment the patient by saying, "That was a good try."
23. Delay conversation if the patient is tired. *The symptoms of aphasia worsen if the patient is fatigued, anxious, or upset.*
24. Be prepared for emotional outbursts and tears from patients who have more difficulty in expressing themselves than with understanding. *The patient may become depressed, refuse treatment and food, ignore relatives, and push objects away.* Comfort the patient with statements such as, "I know it's frustrating and you feel sad, but you are not alone. Other people who have had strokes have felt the way you do. We will be here to help you get through this."

NURSING MANAGEMENT PLAN
Ineffective Airway Clearance

Definition: Inability to clear secretions or obstructions from the respiratory tract to maintain a clear airway.

Ineffective Airway Clearance Related to Excessive Secretions or Abnormal Viscosity of Mucus

Defining Characteristics
- Abnormal breath sounds (displaced normal sounds, adventitious sounds, diminished or absent sounds)
- Ineffective cough with or without sputum
- Tachypnea, dyspnea
- Verbal reports of inability to clear airway

Outcome Criteria
- Cough produces thin mucus.
- Lungs are clear to auscultation.
- Respiratory rate, depth, and rhythm return to baseline.

Nursing Interventions and Rationale
1. Assess sputum for color, consistency, and amount.
2. Assess for clinical manifestations of pneumonia.
3. Provide for maximal thoracic expansion by repositioning, deep breathing, splinting, and pain management **to avoid hypoventilation and atelectasis.** If hypoventilation is present, implement the Nursing Management Plan for Ineffective Breathing Pattern Related to Decreased Lung Expansion.
4. Maintain adequate hydration by administering oral and intravenous fluids (as ordered) **to thin secretions and facilitate airway clearance.**
5. Provide humidification to airways by an oxygen-delivery device or artificial airway **to thin secretions and facilitate airway clearance.**
6. Administer bland aerosol every 4 hours **to facilitate expectoration of sputum.**
7. Collaborate with the physician regarding the administration of the following:
   a. Bronchodilators **to treat or prevent bronchospasms and facilitate expectoration of mucus**

   b. Mucolytics and expectorants **to enhance mobilization and removal of secretions**
   c. Antibiotics **to treat infection**
8. Assist with directed coughing exercises **to facilitate expectoration of secretions.** If patient is unable to perform cascade cough, consider using huff cough (patients with hyperactive airways), end-expiratory cough (patient with secretions in distal airway), or augmented cough (patient with weakened abdominal muscle).
   a. Cascade cough—instruct patient to do the following:
      (1) Take a deep breath, and hold it for 1 to 3 seconds.
      (2) Cough out forcefully several times until all air is exhaled.
      (3) Inhale slowly through the nose.
      (4) Repeat once.
      (5) Rest, and then repeat as necessary.
   b. Huff cough—instruct patient to do the following:
      (1) Take a deep breath, and hold it for 1 to 3 seconds.
      (2) Say the word "huff" while coughing out several times until air is exhaled.
      (3) Inhale slowly through the nose.
      (4) Repeat as necessary.
   c. End-expiratory cough—instruct patient to do the following:
      (1) Take a deep breath, and hold it for 1 to 3 seconds.
      (2) Exhale slowly.
      (3) At the end of exhalation, cough once.
      (4) Inhale slowly through the nose.
      (5) Repeat as necessary, or follow with cascade cough.
   d. Augmented cough—instruct patient to do the following:
      (1) Take a deep breath, and hold it for 1 to 3 seconds.
      (2) Perform one or more of the following maneuvers to increase intraabdominal pressure:
         (a) Tighten knees and buttocks.
         (b) Bend forward at the waist.

NURSING MANAGEMENT PLAN
Ineffective Airway Clearance—cont'd

(c) Place a hand flat on the upper abdomen just under the xiphoid process and press in and up abruptly during coughing.

(d) Keep hands on the chest wall and press inward with each cough.

(3) Inhale slowly through the nose.

(4) Rest and repeat as necessary.

9. Suction nasotracheally or endotracheally as necessary **to assist with secretion removal.**

10. Reposition patient at least every 2 hours or use kinetic therapy **to mobilize and prevent stasis of secretions.**

11. Allow rest periods between coughing sessions, suctioning, or any other demanding activities **to promote energy conservation.**

NURSING MANAGEMENT PLAN
Ineffective Breathing Pattern

Definition: Inspiration and/or expiration that does not provide adequate ventilation.

Ineffective Breathing Pattern Related to Decreased Lung Expansion

Defining Characteristics
- Abnormal respiratory patterns (hypoventilation, hyperventilation, tachypnea, bradypnea, obstructive breathing)
- Abnormal arterial blood gas values (increased $PaCO_2$, decreased pH)
- Unequal chest movement
- Shortness of breath, dyspnea

Outcome Criteria
- Respiratory rate, rhythm, and depth return to baseline.
- Minimal or absent use of accessory muscles.
- Chest expands symmetrically.
- Arterial blood gas values return to baseline.

Nursing Interventions and Rationale
1. Treat pain, if present, **to prevent hypoventilation and atelectasis.** Implement the Nursing Management Plan for Acute Pain Related to Transmission and Perception of Cutaneous, Visceral, Muscular, or Ischemic Impulses.
2. Position patient in high Fowler's or semi-Fowler's position **to promote diaphragmatic descent and maximal inhalation.**

3. Assist with deep-breathing exercises and incentive spirometry with sustained maximal inspiration 5 to 10 times/hr **to help reinflate collapsed portions of the lung.**
   a. Deep breathing—instruct patient to do the following:
      (1) Sit up straight or lean forward slightly while sitting on edge of bed or chair (if possible).
      (2) Take in a slow, deep breath.
      (3) Pause slightly, or hold breath for at least 3 seconds.
      (4) Exhale slowly.
      (5) Rest, and repeat.
   b. Incentive spirometry—instruct patient to do the following:
      (1) Exhale normally.
      (2) Place lips around the mouthpiece, and close mouth tightly around it.
      (3) Inhale slowly and as deeply as possible, noting the maximal volume of air inspired.
      (4) Hold maximal inhalation for 3 seconds.
      (5) Take the mouthpiece out of mouth, and slowly exhale.
      (6) Rest, and repeat.
4. Assist physician with intubation and initiation of mechanical ventilation as indicated.

Ineffective Breathing Pattern Related to Musculoskeletal Fatigue or Neuromuscular Impairment

Defining Characteristics
- Unequal chest movement
- Shortness of breath, dyspnea
- Use of accessory muscles
- Tachypnea
- Thoracoabdominal asynchrony
- Abnormal arterial blood gas values (increased $PaCO_2$, decreased pH)
- Nasal flaring
- Assumption of 3-point position

Outcome Criteria
- Respiratory rate, rhythm, and depth return to baseline.
- Use of accessory muscles is minimal or absent.
- Chest expands symmetrically.
- Arterial blood gas values return to baseline.

Nursing Interventions and Rationale
1. Prevent unnecessary exertion **to limit drain on patient's ventilatory reserve.**

2. Instruct patient in energy-saving techniques **to conserve patient's ventilatory reserve.**
3. Assist with pursed-lip and diaphragmatic breathing techniques **to facilitate diaphragmatic descent and improved ventilation.**
   a. Diaphragmatic breathing—instruct the patient to do the following:
      (1) Sit in the upright position.
      (2) Place one hand on the abdomen just above the waist and the other on the upper chest.
      (3) Breathe in through the nose, and feel the lower hand push out; the upper hand should not move.
      (4) Breathe out through pursed lips, and feel the lower hand move in.
4. Position patient in high Fowler's or semi-Fowler's position **to promote diaphragmatic descent and maximal inhalation.**
5. Assist physician with intubation and initiation of mechanical ventilation as indicated.

NURSING MANAGEMENT PLAN

Ineffective Cardiopulmonary Tissue Perfusion

Definition: Decrease in oxygen resulting in the failure to nourish the tissues at the capillary level.

Ineffective Cardiopulmonary Tissue Perfusion Related to Decreased Coronary Blood Flow

Defining Characteristics

- Chest discomfort with or without radiation to the arms, back, neck, jaw, or epigastrium
- Shortness of breath
- Weakness
- Diaphoresis
- Nausea
- Lightheadedness
- ST-segment elevation on 12-lead electrocardiogram (ECG)
- Elevated troponin I
- Elevated CK-MB enzymes
- Elevated myoglobin

Outcome Criteria

- Systolic blood pressure is >90 mm Hg.
- Mean arterial pressure is >60 mm Hg.
- Heart rate is <100 beats/min.
- Pulmonary artery pressures are within normal limits or back to baseline.
- Cardiac index is >2.2 $L/min/m^2$.
- Urine output is >0.5 mL/kg/hr or >30 mL/hr.
- 12-lead ECG is normalized without new Q waves.
- Chest pain is absent.
- CK-MB enzymes, troponin I, and myoglobin levels are within normal range.

Nursing Interventions and Rationale

1. Collaborate with the physician regarding the administration of fibrinolytic therapy or the preparation of the patient for percutaneous coronary intervention (PCI) *to restore myocardial blood flow.*
2. Collaborate with physician regarding the administration of oxygen at 2 L/min to achieve SpO_2 >90% *to maximize myocardial oxygen supply.*
3. Collaborate with physician regarding the administration of sublingual nitroglycerin and/or intravenous nitroglycerine infusion *to augment coronary blood flow and reduce cardiac work by decreasing preload and afterload.*
   a. Do not administer nitrates to patients who have taken phosphodiesterase inhibitors for erectile dysfunction within

the last 24 to 48 hours (depending on the medication) *as severe hypotension may occur.*
4. Collaborate with physician regarding the administration of morphine *to control pain.*
5. Collaborate with the physician regarding the administration of aspirin, antiplatelet therapy, and heparin *to prevent recurrent thrombosis and inhibit platelet function.*
6. Collaborate with the physician regarding the administration of beta-blockers *to decrease myocardial oxygen demand and prevent recurrent ischemia.*
7. Collaborate with the physician regarding the administration of angiotensin-converting enzyme (ACE) inhibitors *to block the conversion of angiotensin I to angiotensin II, a potent vasoconstrictor.*
8. Maintain the patient on bed rest with bedside commode privileges *to minimize myocardial oxygen demand.*
9. Monitor patient's hemodynamic and cardiac rhythm status:
   a. Select cardiac monitoring leads based on infarct location and rhythm to obtain the best rhythm for monitoring.
   b. Evaluate cardiac rhythm for presence of dysrhythmias, which are common complications of myocardial ischemia.
   c. Collaborate with physician regarding the administration of antidysrhythmic medications.
   d. Assess serum electrolytes (potassium and magnesium) and arterial blood gases.
   e. Collaborate with physician regarding the administration of electrolytes to correct any imbalances.
   f. Monitor ST segment continuously to determine changes in myocardial tissue perfusion.
   g. Monitor patient's blood pressure at least every hour as many conditions (e.g., drugs, dysrhythmias, myocardial ischemia) may cause hypotension (systolic blood pressure <90 mm Hg).
   h. Treat symptomatic dysrhythmias according to unit's emergency protocol or advanced cardiac life support (ACLS) guidelines.
10. Instruct patient to avoid the Valsalva maneuver as forced expiration against a closed glottis causes sudden and intense changes in systolic blood pressure and heart rate.

NURSING MANAGEMENT PLAN

Ineffective Cerebral Tissue Perfusion

Definition: Decrease in oxygen resulting in the failure to nourish the tissues at the capillary level.

Ineffective Cerebral Tissue Perfusion Related to Decreased Blood Flow

Defining Characteristics

- Decreased level of consciousness
- Hemiparesis or hemiplegia
- Visual changes
- Aphasia
- Dysphagia
- Facial droop
- Cognitive deficits
- Ataxia

Outcome Criteria

- Absence of neurological deficits.
- Blood pressure within ordered parameters.

Nursing Interventions and Rationale

1. Collaborate with physician regarding the administration of fibrinolytic therapy **to facilitate lysis of the clot and restoration of blood flow to affected area.**
2. Monitor the patient for alterations in blood pressure, oxygenation, temperature, rhythm, and glucose levels.
3. Collaborate with physician regarding the administration of vasodilators for hypertension **to maintain the patient's blood pressure within desired range.** Use caution in lowering blood pressure **as hypotension decreases cerebral blood flow.**
   a. Patients receiving fibrinolytic therapy: keep systolic blood pressure <185 mm Hg and diastolic blood pressure <110 mm Hg.
   b. Patients not receiving fibrinolytic therapy: keep systolic blood pressure <220 mm Hg and diastolic blood pressure <120 mm Hg.
4. Collaborate with physician regarding the administration of intravenous fluids and vasoconstrictors for hypotension **as hypotension decreases cerebral blood flow.**
5. Collaborate with physician regarding the administration of oxygen to maintain SpO_2 >95% **to prevent hypoxemia and potential worsening of the neurological injury.**
6. Collaborate with physician regarding administration of acetaminophen for elevated temperature **because hyperthermia is associated with increased morbidity in the stroke patient.**
7. Collaborate with the physician regarding the treatment of dysrhythmias **due to increased sympathetic nervous system stimulation.**
8. Collaborate with the physician regarding the administration of insulin for hyperglycemia **as elevated blood glucose has been linked to an increase in the area of infarct.**
9. Collaborate with the speech therapist regarding the patient's ability to swallow before initiating oral feedings **to ensure patient is not at risk for aspirating.**
10. Collaborate with the physical therapist to assess the patient's ability to ambulate safely **to ensure the patient is not at risk for falling** and ability to perform activities of daily living **to facilitate discharge home.**
11. Maintain surveillance for complications such as increased intracranial pressure, seizures, and acute respiratory failure.
12. Collaborate with the physician and rehabilitation specialist regarding the patient's need for rehabilitation **to maximize the patient's independence.**

Ineffective Cerebral Tissue Perfusion Related to Hemorrhage

Defining Characteristics

Intracerebral Hemorrhage
- Alteration in level of consciousness
- Nausea and vomiting
- Headache
- Seizures
- Hypertension
- Focal neurological deficits

Subarachnoid Hemorrhage
- Sudden onset of severe headache, nausea, and/or vomiting
- Symptoms of meningeal irritation:
  - Nuchal rigidity and pain
  - Back pain
  - Bilateral leg pain
  - Kernig's sign: resistance to full extension of the leg at the knee when the hip is flexed
  - Brudzinski's sign: flexion of the hip and knee during passive neck flexion
- Photophobia and visual changes
- Sudden loss of consciousness
- Altered level of consciousness
- Seizures
- Focal neurological deficits

Outcome Criteria

- Patient is oriented to time, place, person, and situation.
- Pupils are equal and normoreactive.
- Blood pressure is within baseline.
- Motor function is bilaterally equal.
- Headache, nausea, and vomiting are absent.
- Patient verbalizes importance of and displays compliance with reduced activity.

Nursing Interventions and Rationale

1. Assess for indicators of increased intracranial pressure and brain herniation (see the Nursing Management Plan for Decreased Intracranial Adaptive Capacity Related to Failure of Normal Intracranial Compensatory Mechanisms).
2. Collaborate with the physician regarding the administration of anticonvulsant medications **to prevent the onset of seizures or to control seizures.**
3. Collaborate with physician regarding the administration of vasodilators for hypertension **to avoid further bleeding.** Use

NURSING MANAGEMENT PLAN

Ineffective Cerebral Tissue Perfusion—cont'd

caution in lowering blood pressure *as hypotension decreases cerebral blood flow.*

a. If systolic blood pressure is >200 mm Hg or mean arterial pressure is >150 mm Hg, aggressive reduction in blood pressure is indicated.

b. If systolic blood pressure is >180 mm Hg or mean arterial pressure is >130 mm Hg in the presence of increased intracranial pressure, cautious reduction in pressure is indicated maintaining cerebral perfusion pressure >60 to 80 mm Hg.

c. If systolic blood pressure is >180 mm Hg or mean arterial pressure is >130 mm Hg in the absence of elevated intracranial pressure, reduction in blood pressure is indicated with a target of 160/90 mm Hg.

4. Collaborate with the physician regarding the administration of insulin for hyperglycemia *as elevated blood glucose has been linked to an increase in the area of infarct.*

5. Collaborate with the physician regarding administration of acetaminophen for elevated temperature *because hyperthermia is associated with increased morbidity in the stroke patient.*

6. Initiate precautions *to prevent rebleeding.*

a. Ensure bed rest in a quiet environment *to lessen external stimuli.*

b. Maintain a darkened room to lessen symptoms of photophobia.

c. Restrict visitors, and instruct them to keep conversation as nonstressful as possible.

d. Administer sedatives as prescribed *to reduce anxiety and to promote rest.*

e. Administer analgesics as prescribed *to relieve or lessen headache.*

f. Provide a soft, high-fiber diet and stool softeners to prevent constipation, which can lead to straining and increased risk of rebleeding.

g. Assist with activities of daily living (feeding, bathing, dressing, toileting).

h. Avoid any activity that could lead to increased intracranial pressure; ensure that patient does not flex hips beyond 90 degrees and avoids neck hyperflexion, hyperextension, or lateral hyperrotation *that could impede jugular venous return.*

7. Collaborate with the physical therapist to assess the patient's ability to ambulate safely *to ensure the patient is not at risk for falling* and ability to perform activities of daily living *to facilitate discharge home.*

8. Collaborate with the physician and rehabilitation specialist regarding the patient's need for rehabilitation *to maximize the patient's independence.*

NURSING MANAGEMENT PLAN

Ineffective Coping

Definition: Inability to form a valid appraisal of the stressors, inadequate choices of practiced responses, and/or inability to use available resources.

Ineffective Coping Related to Situational Crisis and Personal Vulnerability

Defining Characteristics

- Verbalization of inability to cope. *Sample statements:* "I can't take this anymore." "I don't know how to deal with this."
- Ineffective problem solving (problem lumping). *Sample statements:* "I have to eliminate salt from my diet. They tell me I can no longer mow the lawn. This hospitalization is costing a mint. What about my kids' future? Who's going to change the oil in the car? This is an incredible amount of time away from work."
- Ineffective use of coping mechanisms
  - Projection: blames others for illness or pain
  - Displacement: directs anger and/or aggression toward family. *Sample statements:* "Get out of here. Leave me alone." Cursing, shouting, or demanding attention; striking out or throwing objects
  - Denial: of severity of illness and need for treatment
- Noncompliance. *Examples:* activity restriction; refusal to allow treatment or to take medications
- Suicidal thoughts (verbalizes desire to end life)
- Self-directed aggression. *Examples:* disconnects or attempts to disconnect life-sustaining equipment; deliberately tries to harm self
- Failure to progress from dependent to more independent state (refusal or resistance to care for self)

Outcome Criteria

- Patient verbalizes beginning ability to cope with illness, pain, and hospitalization. *Sample statements:* "I'm trying to do the best I can." "I want to help myself get better."
- Patient demonstrates effective problem solving (lists and prioritizes problems from most to least urgent).
- Patient uses effective behavioral strategies to manage the stress of illness and care.
- Patient demonstrates interest or involvement in illness or environment. *Examples:* patient does the following:
  - Requests medications when anticipating pain
  - Questions course of treatment, progress, and prognosis
  - Asks for clarification of environmental stimuli and events
  - Seeks out supportive individuals in his or her environment
  - Uses coping mechanisms and strategies more effectively to manage situational crisis
  - Demonstrates significant reduction in impulsive, angry, or aggressive outbursts (projection, shouting, cursing) directed toward family
  - Verbalizes future-based plans, with cessation of self-directed aggressive acts and suicidal thoughts
  - Willingly complies with treatment regimen
  - Begins to participate in self-care

NURSING MANAGEMENT PLAN
Ineffective Coping—cont'd

Nursing Interventions and Rationale

1. Actively listen and respond to patient's verbal and behavioral expressions. *Active listening signifies unconditional respect and acceptance for the patient as a worthwhile individual. It builds trust and rapport, guides the nurse toward problem areas, encourages the patient to express concerns, and promotes compliance.*

2. Offer effective coping strategies to help the patient better tolerate the stressors related to his or her illness and care. Give permission to vent feelings in a safe setting. *Sample statements*: "I don't blame you for feeling angry or frustrated." "Others who are ill like you have expressed similar feelings." "I will listen to anything you want to share with me." "We don't have to talk; I'd like to sit here with you." "It's perfectly okay to cry." *Individuals who are provided with opportunities to express their feelings will be better able to release pent-up emotions and derive a greater sense of relief and comfort. They are less likely to resort to overly impulsive, aggressive acts, which may harm self or others.*

3. Inform the family of the patient's need to displace anger occasionally but that you will be working with the patient to help him or her release his or her feelings in a more constructive, effective way. *Family members who are well informed are better equipped to cope with their loved one's emotional anguish and outbursts. They are less likely to waste energy on feelings of guilt, fear, anger, or despair and can use their strength to help the patient in more constructive ways. The knowledge that their loved one is being cared for emotionally as well as physically provides family members with a greater sense of comfort and understanding. They will feel nurtured and respected by the nurse's attempt to include them in the process.*

4. With the patient, list and number problems from the most to least urgent. Assist him or her in finding immediate solutions for most urgent problems; postpone those that can wait; delegate some to family members; and help him or her to acknowledge problems that are beyond his or her control. *Listing and numbering problems in an organized fashion helps to break them down into more manageable "pieces" so that the patient is better able to identify solutions for those that are solvable and to suppress those that are less relevant or not amenable to interventions.*

5. Identify individuals in the patient's environment who best help him or her to cope, and identify those who do not. Validate your observations with the patient. *Sample statements*: "I notice you seemed more relaxed during your daughter's visit." "After the clergy left, you were able to sleep a bit longer than usual; would you like to see him more often?" "Your grandson was a bit upset today; I'll be glad to talk to him if you like." *Supportive persons can invoke a calming effect on the patient's physiological and psychological states.*

Conversely, well-meaning but nonsupportive individuals can have a deleterious effect on the patient's ability to cope and must be carefully screened and counseled by the nurse.

6. Teach the patient effective cognitive strategies to help him or her better manage the stress of critical illness and care. Help him or her construct pleasant thoughts, situations, or images that can simultaneously inhibit unpleasant realities. *Examples*: a day at the beach, a walk in the park, drinking a glass of wine, or being with a loved one. *Pleasant thoughts and images constructed during critical illness and care tend to inhibit or reduce the intensity of the unpleasant, stressful effects of the experience.*

7. Assist the patient in using coping mechanisms more effectively so he or she can better manage his or her situational crisis.
   a. Suppression of problems beyond his or her control
   b. Compensation for illness and its effects; focusing on his or her strengths, interests, family, and spiritual beliefs
   c. Adaptive displacement of anger, fear, or frustration through healthy, verbal expressions to staff. *Effective use of coping mechanisms helps to assuage the patient's painful feelings in a safe setting. The patient is strengthened and need not resort to the use of more ineffective defenses to eliminate anxiety.*

8. Initiate a suicidal assessment if the patient verbalizes the desire to die, states that life is not worth living, or exhibits self-directed aggression. *Sample statement:* "We know that this is a bad time for you. You're saying repeatedly that you want to die. Are you planning to harm yourself?" If the response is "yes," remain with the patient, alert staff members, and provide for psychiatric consultation as soon as possible. Continue to express concern to the patient and protect him or her from harm. *Suicidal thoughts as a result of ineffective coping or exhaustion of coping devices are not an uncommon occurrence in critically ill patients. If the mood state is distressing enough, a patient may seek relief by attempting a self-destructive act. Although the patient may not imminently have the energy to succeed in his or her attempt, voicing a specific plan signifies a depressed mood state and depletion of coping strategies. Immediate intervention is needed, because the attempt may be successful when the patient's energy is restored.*

9. Encourage the patient to participate in self-care activities and treatment regimen in accordance with his or her level of progress. Offer praise for his or her efforts toward self-care. *Patients who take an active role in their own treatment and progress are less apt to feel like helpless or powerless victims. This greater sense of control over their illness and environment will guide them more swiftly toward becoming as independent as possible.*

NURSING MANAGEMENT PLAN
Ineffective Gastrointestinal Tissue Perfusion

Definition: Decrease in oxygen resulting in the failure to nourish the tissues at the capillary level.

Ineffective Gastrointestinal Tissue Perfusion Related to Decreased Gastrointestinal Blood Flow

Defining Characteristics
- Abdominal pain
- Melena
- Abdominal distention
- Bowel sounds range from hyperactive to absent
- Guarding
- Fever
- Hypotension
- Tachycardia
- Altered mental status
- Urine output is <30 mL/hr

Outcome Criteria
- Normal bowel sounds.
- Absence of abdominal pain, distention, and guarding.
- Urinary output is >30 mL/hr.
- Vital signs at baseline.
- Normal mentation.

Nursing Interventions and Rationales
1. Collaborate with physician regarding the administration of crystalloids, colloids, blood, and blood products **to maintain adequate circulating volume.** Implement the Nursing Management Plan for Deficit Fluid Volume Related to Absolute Loss.
2. Collaborate with physician regarding pain management. Implement the Nursing Management Plan for Acute Pain Related to Transmission and Perception of Cutaneous, Visceral, Muscular, or Ischemic Impulses.
3. Collaborate with physician regarding the administration of oxygen to maintain SpO$_2$ >92% **to prevent hypoxemia and potential worsening of the gastrointestinal injury.**
4. Collaborate with physician regarding the administration of electrolyte replacement therapy **to maintain adequate electrolyte balance.**
5. Collaborate with dietitian regarding administration of nutrition **because patient will be unable to eat.** Implement the Nursing Management Plan for Imbalanced Nutrition: Less than Body Requirements.
6. Maintain surveillance for complications such as gastrointestinal hemorrhage, hypovolemic shock, and septic shock.
7. Collaborate with physician regarding preparation for surgery **to remove infarcted bowel.**

NURSING MANAGEMENT PLAN
Ineffective Peripheral Tissue Perfusion

Definition: Decrease in blood circulation to the periphery that may compromise health.

Ineffective Peripheral Tissue Perfusion Related to Decreased Peripheral Blood Flow

Defining Characteristics
- Weak and/or unequal peripheral pulses
- Delayed capillary refill
- Ischemic pain from extremity
- Cool skin on extremity
- Pale extremity
- Paresthesias from extremity

Outcome Criteria
- Peripheral pulses are full and equal bilaterally.
- Capillary refill is equal bilaterally.
- Ischemic pain is absent.
- Skin temperature is equal in both extremities.
- Skin is pink and warm in both extremities.
- Paresthesias are absent.

Nursing Interventions and Rationale
1. Collaborate with physician regarding the administration of antiplatelet, anticoagulant, and/or fibrinolytic therapy.
2. Collaborate with physician regarding pain management. Implement the Nursing Management Plan for Acute Pain Related to Transmission and Perception of Cutaneous, Visceral, Muscular, or Ischemic Impulses.
3. Ensure patient is adequately hydrated **to decrease blood viscosity.**
4. Maintain affected extremity in dependent position if possible **to enhance blood flow.**
5. Keep affected extremity warm and protect it from injury. **Do not apply heat directly to the affected extremity because this can result in injury.**
6. Maintain surveillance for pain, pallor, pulselessness, paresthesia, paralysis, and poikilothermia **as indicators of abrupt change in blood flow.**
7. Maintain surveillance for tissue breakdown and arterial ulcers **as indicators of injury.**
8. Prepare patient for possible surgery or interventional procedure to restore blood flow.

NURSING MANAGEMENT PLAN

Ineffective Renal Tissue Perfusion

Definition: At risk for a decrease in blood circulation to the kidney that may compromise health.

Ineffective Renal Tissue Perfusion Related to Decreased Renal Blood Flow

Defining Characteristics
- Anuria or oliguria
- Decreased urinary creatinine clearance
- Increased serum creatinine
- Increased blood urea nitrogen (BUN)
- Electrolyte abnormalities: potassium, sodium
- Increased mean arterial pressure, pulmonary artery occlusion pressure, and right atrial pressure
- Sinus tachycardia
- Metabolic acidosis
- Crackles on lung auscultation
- Engorged neck veins
- Fluid weight gain
- Pitting edema
- Mental status changes
- Anemia

Outcome Criteria
- CO is >4.0 L/min.
- CI is >2.2 L/min/m^2.
- Mean arterial pressure, pulmonary artery occlusion pressure, and right atrial pressure are within normal limits for patient.
- Electrolytes are within normal range.
- Serum creatinine and BUN are within normal range.
- Normal acid-base balance.
- Level of consciousness is normal.
- Lungs are clear on auscultation.
- Urinary output is within normal limits, or patient is stable on dialysis.
- Hemoglobin and hematocrit values are stable.

Nursing Interventions and Rationale
1. Monitor intake and output, urine output, and patient weight.
2. Collaborate with physician regarding the administration of crystalloids, colloids, blood, and blood products **to increase circulating volume and maintain mean arterial pressure >70 mm Hg.**
3. Collaborate with physician regarding the administration of inotropes **to enhance myocardial contractility and increase cardiac index to >2.5 L/min.**
4. Collaborate with physician regarding the administration of diuretics to the oliguric patient **to flush out cellular debris and increase urine output.**
5. Minimize the patient's exposure to nephrotoxic drugs **to decrease damage to kidneys.**
6. Monitor blood levels of drugs cleared by kidneys **to avoid accumulation.**
7. Monitor patient for signs of electrolyte imbalance **due to impaired electrolyte regulation.**
8. Maintain surveillance for signs and symptoms of fluid overload.
9. Monitor patient's clinical status and response to dialysis therapy to ensure the patient is receiving safe and effective dialytic therapy.

NURSING MANAGEMENT PLAN

Powerlessness

Definition: Perception that one's own action cannot significantly affect an outcome; a perceived lack of control over a current situation or immediate happening.

Powerlessness Related to Lack of Control over Current Situation or Disease Progression

Defining Characteristics

Severe
- Verbal expressions of having no control or influence over situation
- Verbal expressions of having no control or influence over outcome
- Verbal expressions of having no control over self-care
- Depression over physical deterioration that occurs despite patient's compliance with regimens
- Apathy

Moderate
- Nonparticipation in care or decision making when opportunities are provided
- Expressions of dissatisfaction and frustration about inability to perform previous tasks and/or activities
- Lack of progress monitoring
- Expressions of doubt about role performance
- Reluctance to express true feelings, fearing alienation from caregivers
- Passivity
- Inability to seek information about care
- Dependence on others that may result in irritability, resentment, anger, and guilt
- No defense of self-care practices when challenged

Low
- Passivity

Outcome Criteria
- Patient verbalizes increased control over situation by wanting to do things his or her way.
- Patient actively participates in planning care.
- Patient requests needed information.
- Patient chooses to participate in self-care activities.
- Patient monitors progress.

Continued

NURSING MANAGEMENT PLAN
Powerlessness—cont'd

Nursing Interventions and Rationale

1. Evaluate the patient's feelings and perception of the reasons for lack of power and sense of helplessness.
2. Determine as far as possible the patient's usual response to limited-control situations. Determine through ongoing assessment the patient's usual locus of control (i.e., believes that influence over his or her life is exerted by luck, fate, powerful persons [external locus of control] or that influence is exerted through personal choices, self-effort, self-determination [internal locus of control]).
3. Support patient's physical control of the environment by involving him or her in care activities; knock before entering room if appropriate; ask permission before moving personal belongings. Inform the patient that, although an activity may not be to his or her liking, it is necessary. *This gives the patient permission to express dissatisfaction with the environment and the regimen.*
4. Personalize the patient's care using his or her preferred name. *This supports the patient's psychological control.*
5. Provide therapeutic rationale for all the patient is asked to do for himself or herself and for all that is being done for and with him or her. Reinforce the physician's explanations; clarify misconceptions about the illness situation and treatment plans. *This supports the patient's cognitive control.*
6. Include the patient in care planning by encouraging participation and allowing choices wherever possible (e.g., timing of personal care activities; deciding when pain medicines are needed). Point out situations in which no choices exist.

7. Provide opportunities for the patient to exert influence over himself or herself and his or her body, thereby affecting an outcome. For example, share with the patient the nurse's assessment of his or her breath sounds and explain that they can be improved by self-initiated deep-breathing exercises. *Feedback that the patient has been successful in helping clear his or her lungs reinforces the influence he or she does retain.*
8. Encourage family to permit patient to do as much independently as possible *to foster perception of personal power.*
9. Assist the patient to establish realistic short-term and long-term goals. *Setting unrealistic or unattainable goals inadvertently reinforces the patient's perception of powerlessness.*
10. Document care to provide for continuity *so that the patient can maintain appropriate control over the environment.*
11. Assist the patient to regain strength and activity tolerance as appropriate, *increasing a sense of control and self-reliance.*
12. Increase the sensitivity of the health team members and significant others to the patient's sense of powerlessness. Use power over the patient carefully. Use the words *must*, *should*, and *have to* with caution *because they communicate coercive powers and imply that the objects of "musts" and "shoulds" are of benefit to the nurse instead of the patient.*
13. Plan with the patient for transfer from the critical care unit to the intermediate unit and eventually to home.

NURSING MANAGEMENT PLAN
Relocation Stress Syndrome

Definition: Physiological and/or psychological disturbances after transfer from one environment to another.

Relocation Stress Syndrome Related to Transfer out of the Intensive Care Unit

Defining Characteristics

- Alienation
- Aloneness
- Anger
- Anxiety
- Concern over relocation
- Dependency
- Depression
- Fear of an unknown environment
- Frustration
- Increased illness
- Increased physical symptoms
- Increased verbalization of needs
- Insecurity
- Loneliness
- Loss of identify
- Loss of self-esteem
- Loss of self-worth
- Move from intensive care unit to another environment
- Pessimism
- Sleep disturbance
- Unwillingness to move
- Withdrawal
- Worry

Outcome Criteria

- Patient will express willingness to move to new environment.
- Absence of anxiety.

Nursing Interventions and Rationale

1. Initiate pretransfer teaching as soon as appropriate during the patient's stay in the intensive care unit *to ease the transition from the intensive care unit to the next environment*. Teaching should focus on the differences in the environment and the care patient will receive.
2. Provide the patient and family written information regarding the transfer (if available) *to enhance effectiveness of teaching.*
3. Help the patient see that progress is being made *in preparation for transfer*. Each time a tube is removed or a treatment frequency is decreased, reinforce with the patient and family that the patient is progressing.

NURSING MANAGEMENT PLAN
Relocation Stress Syndrome—cont'd

4. Remove monitoring and supportive equipment from the patient's room when no longer needed **to allow the patient to experience the loss of technology while still in the intensive care unit.**
5. Encourage patient and family to discuss concerns regarding relocation.

6. Assist patient and family members to develop and maintain a positive perception of the transfer.
7. Arrange for the patient's family to have a tour of the new unit **as a means of familiarizing them with the unit before the patient's transfer.**

NURSING MANAGEMENT PLAN
Risk for Aspiration

Definition: At risk for entry of gastrointestinal secretions, oropharyngeal secretions, solids, or fluids into tracheobronchial passages.

Risk Factors

- Impaired laryngeal sensation or reflex
- Reduced level of consciousness
- Extubation
- Impaired pharyngeal peristalsis or tongue function
  - Neuromuscular dysfunction
  - Central nervous system dysfunction
  - Head or neck injury
- Impaired laryngeal closure or elevation
  - Laryngeal nerve dysfunction
  - Artificial airways
  - Gastrointestinal tubes
- Increased gastric volume
  - Delayed gastric emptying
  - Enteral feedings
  - Medication administration

- Increased intragastric pressure
  - Upper abdominal surgery
  - Obesity
  - Pregnancy
  - Ascites
- Decreased lower esophageal sphincter pressure
  - Increased gastric acidity
  - Gastrointestinal tubes
- Decreased antegrade esophageal propulsion
  - Trendelenburg or supine position
  - Esophageal dysmotility
  - Esophageal structural defects or lesions

Outcome Criteria

- Breath sounds are normal, or there is no change in patient's baseline breath sounds.
- Arterial blood gas values remain within patient's baseline.

- There is no evidence of gastric contents in lung secretions.

Nursing Interventions and Rationale

1. Assess gastrointestinal function **to rule out hypoactive peristalsis and abdominal distention.**
2. Position patient with head of bed elevated 30 degrees **to prevent gastric reflux through gravity.** If head elevation is contraindicated, position patient in right lateral decubitus position **to facilitate passage of gastric contents across the pylorus.**
3. Maintain patency and functioning of nasogastric suction apparatus **to prevent accumulation of gastric contents.**
4. Provide frequent and scrupulous mouth care **to prevent colonization of the oropharynx with bacteria and inoculation of the lower airways.**
5. Ensure that the endotracheal or tracheostomy cuff is properly inflated **to limit aspiration of oropharyngeal secretions.**
6. Treat nausea promptly; collaborate with physician on an order for antiemetic **to prevent vomiting and resultant aspiration.**

Additional Interventions for Patient Receiving Continuous or Intermittent Enteral Tube Feedings

7. Position patient with head of bed elevated 45 degrees **to prevent gastric reflux.** If a head-down position becomes

necessary at any time, interrupt the feeding 30 minutes before the position change.
8. Check placement of feeding tube by auscultation or radiographically at regular intervals (e.g., before administering intermittent feedings and after position changes, suctioning, coughing episodes, or vomiting) **to ensure proper placement of the tube.**
9. Monitor patient for signs of delayed gastric emptying **to decrease potential for vomiting and aspiration.**
   a. For large-bore tubes, check residuals of tube feedings before intermittent feedings and every 4 hours during continuous feedings. Consider withholding feedings for residuals greater than 150% of the hourly rate (continuous feeding) or greater than 50% of the previous feeding (intermittent feeding).
   b. For small-bore tubes, observe abdomen for distention, palpate abdomen for hardness or tautness, and auscultate abdomen for bowel sounds.

NURSING MANAGEMENT PLAN

Risk for Infection

Definition: At increased risk for being invaded by pathogenic organisms.

Risk Factors

- Inadequate primary defenses (e.g., broken skin, traumatized tissue, decreased ciliary action, stasis of body fluids, change in pH secretions, altered peristalsis)
- Inadequate secondary defenses (e.g., decreased hemoglobin, leukopenia, suppressed inflammatory or immune response)
- Immunocompromise

- Inadequate acquired immunity
- Tissue destruction and increased environmental exposure
- Chronic disease
- Invasive procedures
- Malnutrition
- Pharmacological agents (e.g., antibiotics, steroids)

Outcome Criteria

- Total lymphocyte count is >1000/mm^3.
- White blood cell count is within normal limits.
- Temperature is within normal limits.

- Blood, urine, wound, and sputum culture results are negative.

Nursing Interventions and Rationale

1. Perform proper hand hygiene before and after patient care *to reduce the transmission of microorganisms.*
2. Use appropriate personal protective equipment in accordance with CDC guidelines.
   a. Ensure physician uses maximum barrier precautions when inserting lines.
      (1) Ensure sterile gloves, gown, and mask are worn.
      (2) Drape patient completely with a sterile sheet.
3. Use aseptic technique for insertion and manipulation of invasive monitoring devices, intravenous (IV) lines, and urinary drainage catheters *to maintain sterility of environment.*
   a. Swab all ports with chlorhexidine for 15 to 30 seconds using friction in a twisting motion prior to using.
   b. Consult with physician daily to remove all lines and catheters when no longer needed.
4. Stabilize all invasive lines and catheters *to avoid unintentional manipulation and contamination.*
5. Use aseptic technique for dressing changes *to prevent contamination of wounds or insertion sites.*
6. Change any line placed under emergent conditions within 24 hours *because aseptic technique is usually breached during an emergency.*
7. Collaborate with the physician to change any dressing that is saturated with blood or drainage *because these are mediums for microorganism growth.*
8. Minimize use of stopcocks and maintain caps on all stopcock ports *to reduce the ports of entry for microorganisms.*
9. Avoid the use of nasogastric tubes, nasotracheal tubes, and nasopharyngeal suctioning in the patient with a suspected cerebrospinal fluid leak *to decrease the incidence of central nervous system infection.*
10. Change ventilator circuits with humidifiers no more often than every 48 hours *to avoid introducing microorganisms into the system.*
11. Provide the patient with a clean manual resuscitation bag *to avoid cross-contamination between patients.*
12. Provide oral care to patient with artificial airway or unresponsive patient every 2 to 4 hours and as necessary (PRN) *to decrease the incidence of hospital-acquired pulmonary infections.*

a. Swab mouth and moisten lips every 4 hours.
b. Brush teeth with chlorhexidine oral rinse using inline suction toothbrush every 12 hours.
c. Suction subglottic secretions (secretions pooling above the cuff of the endotracheal [ET] or tracheostomy tube) every 12 hours and before repositioning the tube or deflation of the cuff.
d. Provide lip moistener to keep patient's lips moistened PRN during each shift.

13. Cleanse in-line suction catheters with sterile saline according to the manufacturer's instructions *to avoid accumulation of secretions within the catheter.*
14. Maintain the head of the bed elevated at 30 to 45 degrees in patients with an artificial airway *to decrease the incidence of aspiration.*
15. Use disposable sterile scissors, forceps, and hemostats *to reduce the transmission of microorganisms.*
16. Maintain a closed urinary drainage system *to decrease incidence of urinary infections.*
17. Keep the urinary drainage tubing and bag below the level of the patient's bladder *to prevent the backflow of urine.*
18. Assess the urinary drainage tubing for kinks *to prevent stasis of urine.*
19. Protect all access device sites from potential sources of contamination (nasogastric reflux, draining wounds, ostomies, sputum).
20. Refrigerate parenteral nutrition solutions and opened enteral nutrition formulas *to inhibit bacterial growth.*
21. Maintain daily surveillance of invasive devices for signs and symptoms of infection.
22. Notify physician of elevated temperature or if any signs or symptoms of infection are present.

Additional Interventions for Patient Receiving Immunosuppressive Drugs

23. Obtain blood, urine, and sputum cultures for temperature elevations >38° C (100.4° F) *inasmuch as elevation likely is caused by bacteremia or bladder or pulmonary infection.*

NURSING MANAGEMENT PLAN
Risk for Infection—cont'd

24. Auscultate breath sounds at least every 6 hours. ***Pulmonary infection is the most common type of infection, and changes in breath sounds might be an early indication.***

25. Inspect wounds at least every 8 hours for redness, swelling, and/or drainage, ***which may indicate infection.***

26. Inspect overall skin integrity and oral mucosa for signs of breakdown, ***which place the patient at risk for infection.***

27. Notify physician of new-onset cough. ***Even a nonproductive cough may indicate pulmonary infection.***

28. Monitor white blood cell count daily, and report leukocytosis or sudden development of leukopenia, ***which may indicate an infectious process.***

29. Protect patient from exposure to any staff or family member with contagious lesion (e.g., herpes simplex) or respiratory infections.

30. Collaborate with dietitian regarding the patient's nutritional status and need for augmentation of nutritional intake as necessary ***to prevent debilitation and increased susceptibility to infection.***

31. Collaborate with physician to remove invasive lines and catheters as soon as possible ***to decrease potential portals of entry.***

32. Teach patient the clinical manifestations of infection. ***A knowledgeable patient will seek medical attention promptly, which will result in earlier treatment and a decreased risk that infection will become life threatening.***

NURSING MANAGEMENT PLAN
Unilateral Neglect

Definition: Impairment in sensory and motor response, metal representation and spatial attention of the body, and the corresponding environment characterized by inattention to one side and over-attention to the opposite side. Left side neglect is more severe and persistent than right side neglect.

Unilateral Neglect Related to Perceptual Disruption

Defining Characteristics
- Neglect of involved body parts and/or extrapersonal space
- Denial of existence of the affected limb or side of body
- Denial of hemiplegia or other motor and sensory deficits
- Left homonymous hemianopia
- Difficulty with spatial-perceptual tasks
- Left hemiplegia

Outcome Criteria
- Patient is safe and free from injury.
- Patient is able to identify safety hazards in the environment.
- Patient recognizes disability and describes physical deficits present (e.g., paralysis, weakness, numbness).
- Patient demonstrates ability to scan the visual field to compensate for loss of function or sensation in affected limbs.

Nursing Interventions and Rationale
1. Adapt environment to patient's deficits ***to maintain patient safety.***
   a. Position the patient's bed with the unaffected side facing the door.
   b. Approach and speak to the patient from the unaffected side. If the patient must be approached from the affected side, announce your presence as soon as entering the room ***to avoid startling the patient.***
   c. Position the call light, bedside stand, and personal items on the patient's unaffected side.
   d. If the patient will be assisted out of bed, simplify the environment ***to eliminate hazards*** by removing unnecessary furniture and equipment.
   e. Provide frequent reorientation of the patient to the environment.
   f. Observe the patient closely, and anticipate his or her needs. ***In spite of repeated explanation, the patient may have difficulty retaining information about the deficits.***
   g. When patient is in bed, elevate his or her affected arm on a pillow ***to prevent dependent edema and support the hand in a position of function.***
2. Assist the patient to recognize the perceptual defect.
   a. Encourage the patient to wear any prescriptive corrective glasses or hearing aids ***to facilitate communication.***
   b. Instruct the patient to turn the head past midline ***to view the environment on the affected side.***
   c. Encourage patient to look at the affected side and to stroke the limbs with the unaffected hand. Encourage handling of the affected limbs ***to reinforce awareness of the affected side.***
   d. Instruct the patient to look for the affected extremity when performing simple tasks ***to know where it is at all times.***
   e. After pointing to them, have the patient name the affected parts.
   f. Encourage the patient to use self-exercises (e.g., lifting the affected arm with the unaffected hand).
   g. If the patient is unable to discriminate between the concepts of *right* and *left*, use descriptive adjectives such as "the weak arm," "the affected leg," or "the good arm" to refer to the body. Use gestures, not just words, to indicate right and left.
3. Collaborate with the patient, physician, and rehabilitation team ***to design and implement a beginning rehabilitation program for use during the critical care unit stay.***

Continued

NURSING MANAGEMENT PLAN
Unilateral Neglect—cont'd

a. Use adaptive equipment (braces, splints, slings) as appropriate.

b. Teach the patient the individual components of any activity separately, and then proceed to integrate the component parts into a completed activity.

c. Instruct the patient to attend to the affected side, if able, and to assist with the bath or other tasks.

d. Use tactile stimulation to reintroduce the arm or leg to the patient. Rub the affected parts with different textured materials to stimulate sensations (e.g., warm, cold, rough, soft).

e. Encourage activities that require the patient to turn the head toward the affected side, and retrain the patient to scan the affected side and environment visually.

f. If the patient is allowed out of bed, cue him or her with reminders to scan visually when ambulating. Assist and remain in constant attendance *because the patient may have difficulty maintaining correct posture, balance, and locomotion.* There may be vertical-horizontal perceptual problems, with the patient leaning to the affected side to align with the perceived vertical. Provide sitting, standing, and balancing exercises before getting the patient out of bed.

4. Assist patient with oral feedings.

a. Avoid giving patient any very hot food items that could cause injury.

b. Place the patient in an upright sitting position if possible.

c. Encourage the patient to feed himself or herself; if necessary, guide the patient's hand to the mouth.

d. If the patient is able to feed himself or herself, place one dish at a time in front of the patient. When the patient is finished with the first, add another dish. Tell the patient what he or she is eating.

e. Initially, place food in patient's visual field; then gradually move the food out of the field of vision and teach the patient to scan the entire visual field.

f. When the patient has learned to visually scan the environment, offer a tray of food with various dishes.

g. Instruct the patient to take small bites of food and to place the food in the unaffected side of the mouth.

h. Teach the patient to sweep out pockets of food with the tongue after every bite *to eliminate retained food in the affected side of the mouth.*

i. After meals or oral medications, check the patient's oral cavity for pockets of retained material.

5. Initiate patient and family health teaching.

a. Assess to ensure that the patient and the family understand the nature of the neurological deficits and the purpose of the rehabilitation plan.

b. Teach the proper application and use of any adaptive equipment.

c. Teach the importance of maintaining a safe environment, and point out potential environmental hazards.

d. Instruct family members how to facilitate relearning techniques (e.g., cueing, scanning visual fields).

Physiological Formulas for Critical Care

HEMODYNAMIC FORMULAS

Mean Arterial Pressure (MAP)

$$MAP = \frac{SBP + (2 \times DBP)}{3}$$

SBP = Systolic blood pressure (measured via arterial line or blood pressure cuff)
DBP = Diastolic blood pressure (measured via arterial line or blood pressure cuff)
Normal range: 70 to 100 mm Hg

Cardiac Index (CI)

$$CI = \frac{CO}{BSA}$$

CO = Cardiac output (measured via pulmonary artery catheter)
BSA = Body surface area (calculated value)
Normal range: 2.5 to 4.0 L/min/m^2

Stroke Volume (SV)

$$SV = \frac{CO \times 1000}{HR}$$

CO = Cardiac output (measured via pulmonary artery catheter)
HR = Heart rate (measured via bedside electrocardiogram)
Normal range: 60 to 100 mL/beat

Stroke Volume Index (SVI)

$$SVI = \frac{CI \times 1000}{HR}$$

CI = Cardiac index (calculated value)
HR = Heart rate (measured via bedside electrocardiogram)
Normal range: 33 to 47 mL/m^2/beat

Systemic Vascular Resistance (SVR)

$$SVR = \frac{MAP - RAP}{CO} \times 80$$

MAP = Mean arterial pressure (measured via arterial line or calculated value)

RAP = Right atrial mean pressure (measured via pulmonary artery catheter)
CO = Cardiac output (measured via pulmonary artery catheter)
Normal range: 800 to 1200 dynes/sec/cm^{-5}

Pulmonary Vascular Resistance (PVR)

$$PVR = \frac{PAMP - PAOP}{CO} \times 80$$

PAMP = Pulmonary artery mean pressure (measured via pulmonary artery catheter)
PAOP = Pulmonary artery occlusion pressure or "wedge" pressure (measured via pulmonary artery catheter)
CO = Cardiac output (measured via pulmonary artery catheter)
Normal range: less than 250 dynes/sec/cm^{-5}

Left Ventricular Stroke Work Index (LVSWI)

$$LVSWI = (MAP - PAOP) \times SVI \times 0.0136$$

MAP = Mean arterial pressure (measured via arterial line or calculated value)
PAOP = Pulmonary artery occlusion pressure or "wedge" pressure (measured via pulmonary artery catheter)
SVI = Stroke volume index (calculated value)
Normal range: 50 to 62 g-m/m^2/beat

Right Ventricular Stroke Work Index (RVSWI)

$$RVSWI = (PAMP - RAP) \times SVI \times 0.0136$$

PAMP = Pulmonary artery mean pressure (measured via pulmonary artery catheter)
RAP = Right atrial mean pressure (measured via pulmonary artery catheter)
SVI = Stroke volume index (calculated value)
Normal range: 7.9 to 9.7 g-m/m^2/beat

Corrected QT Interval (QTc)

$$QTc = \frac{QT}{\sqrt{RR}}$$

QT = QT interval
RR = R-to-R interval
Upper limit: 0.44 second

Body Mass Index (BMI)

$$\text{Body Mass Index} = \text{Weight (kg)}/\text{Height (m)}^2$$

Body Surface Area (BSA)

To calculate (Figure A-1):
1. Obtain patient's height and weight.
2. Mark height on the left scale and weight on the right scale.
3. Draw a straight line between the two points marked on each scale.

The number where the line crosses the middle scale is the BSA value.

PULMONARY FORMULAS

Shunt Equation (Qs/Qt)

$$Qs = Cco_2 - Cao_2$$
$$Qt = Cco_2 - Cvo_2$$

Cco_2 = Pulmonary capillary oxygen content (calculated value)
Cao_2 = Arterial oxygen content (calculated value)
Cvo_2 = Venous oxygen content (calculated value)
Normal range: less than 5%

Pulmonary Capillary Oxygen Content (Cco₂)

$$Cco_2 = (Hgb \times 1.34 \times Sco_2) + (Pco_2 \times 0.003)$$

Hgb = hemoglobin (measured via laboratory sample or arterial blood gas)
Sco_2 = Pulmonary capillary oxygen saturation
Pco_2 = Partial pressure of oxygen in capillary blood

Arterial Oxygen Content (Co₂)

$$Cao_2 = (Hgb \times 1.34 \times Sao_2) + (0.003 \times Pao_2)$$

Hgb = Hemoglobin (measured via laboratory sample or arterial blood gas)
Sao_2 = arterial oxygen saturation (measured via arterial blood gas)
Pao_2 = Partial pressure of oxygen in arterial blood (measured via arterial blood gas)
Normal range: 17 to 20 mL/dL

Venous Oxygen Content (Cvo₂)

$$Cvo_2 = (Hgb \times 1.34 \times Svo_2) + (0.003 \times Pvo_2)$$

Hgb = Hemoglobin (measured via laboratory sample or arterial blood gas)
Svo_2 = Mixed venous oxygen saturation (measured via mixed venous blood gas)

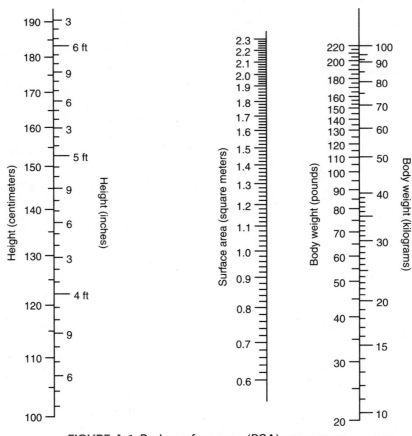

FIGURE A-1 Body surface area (BSA) nomogram.

P_{vO_2} = Partial pressure of oxygen in mixed venous blood (measured via mixed venous blood gas)
Normal range: 12 to 15 mL/dL

Alveolar Pressure of Oxygen (P$_{AO_2}$)

$$P_{AO_2} = F_{IO_2} \times (P_b - P_{H_2O}) - P_{aCO_2}/RQ$$

F_{IO_2} = Fraction of inspired oxygen (obtained from oxygen settings)
P_b = Barometric pressure (assumed to be 760 mm Hg at sea level)
P_{H_2O} = Water pressure in the lungs (assumed to be 47 mm Hg)
P_{aCO_2} = Partial pressure of carbon dioxide in arterial blood (measured via arterial blood gas)
RQ = Respiratory quotient (assumed to be 0.8)
Normal range: 60 to 100 mm Hg

Arterial/Inspired Oxygen Ratio

$$P_{aO_2}/F_{IO_2} \text{ ratio} = \frac{P_{aO_2}}{F_{IO_2}}$$

P_{aO_2} = Partial pressure of oxygen in arterial blood (measured via arterial blood gas)
F_{IO_2} = Fraction of inspired oxygen (obtained from oxygen settings)
Normal range: greater than 300

Arterial/Alveolar Oxygen Ratio

$$P_{aO_2}/P_{AO_2} = \frac{P_{aO_2}}{P_{AO_2}}$$

P_{aO_2} = Partial pressure of oxygen in arterial blood (measured via arterial blood gas)
P_{AO_2} = Partial pressure of oxygen in alveoli (calculated value)
Normal range: greater than 0.75 (75%)

Alveolar-Arterial Gradient

$$P(A\text{-}a)O_2 = P_{AO_2} - P_{aO_2}$$

P_{AO_2} = Partial pressure of oxygen in alveoli (calculated value)
P_{aO_2} = Partial pressure of oxygen in arterial blood (measured via arterial blood gas)
Normal range: 25 to 65 mm Hg

Dead Space Equation (Vd/Vt)

$$V_d = \frac{P_{aCO_2} - P_{etCO_2}}{V_t \, P_{aCO_2}}$$

P_{aCO_2} = Partial pressure of carbon dioxide in arterial blood (measured via arterial blood gas)
P_{etCO_2} = Partial pressure of carbon dioxide in exhaled gas (measured via end-tidal CO_2 monitor)
Normal range: 0.2 to 0.4 (20% to 40%)

Static Compliance (C$_{ST}$)

This value is calculated for mechanically ventilated patients.

$$C_{ST} = \frac{V_t}{PP} - PEEP$$

V_t = Tidal volume (obtained from ventilator)
PP = Plateau pressure (measured via ventilator)
PEEP = Positive end-expiratory pressure (obtained from ventilator)
Normal value: 60 to 100 mL/cm H_2O

Dynamic Compliance (C$_{DY}$)

Also called *characteristic*, this value is calculated for mechanically ventilated patients.

$$C_{DY} = \frac{V_t}{PIP} - PEEP$$

V_t = Tidal volume (obtained from ventilator)
PIP = Peak inspiratory pressure (obtained from ventilator)
PEEP = Positive end-expiratory pressure (obtained from ventilator)
Normal value: 40 to 80 mL/cm H_2O

NEUROLOGICAL FORMULAS

Cerebral Perfusion Pressure (CPP)

$$CCP = MAP - ICP$$

MAP = Mean arterial pressure (measured via arterial line or blood pressure cuff)
ICP = Intracranial pressure (measured via ICP monitoring device)
Normal range: 60 to 150 mm Hg

Arteriojugular Oxygen Difference (AjDO$_2$)

$$AjDO_2 = (S_{aO_2} - S_{jvO_2}) \times 1.34 \times Hgb$$

S_{aO_2} = arterial oxygen saturation (measured via arterial blood gas)
S_{jvO_2} = jugular venous oxygen saturation (measured via jugular blood gas or jugular venous catheter)
Hgb = hemoglobin (measured via laboratory sample or arterial blood gas)
Normal range: 5 to 7.5 mL/dL

ENDOCRINE FORMULA

Serum Osmolality

$$\text{Serum Osmolality} = 2\,(Na^+ + K^+) + \frac{Glucose}{18} + \frac{BUN}{2.8}$$

Na^+ = Sodium
K^+ = Potassium
BUN = Blood urea nitrogen
Normal range: 275 to 295 mOsm/kg of water

RENAL FORMULA

Renal Clearance

$$\text{Clearance} = [U] \times \frac{V}{[P]}$$

[U] = Concentration of substance in urine
V = Time
[P] = Concentration of substance in plasma
Normal range: dependent on substance measured

NUTRITIONAL FORMULAS*

Estimate of Caloric Needs

Step 1. Calculate basal energy expenditure (BEE). This is the energy needed for basic life processes, such as respiratory function and maintenance of body temperature.

$$\text{Women: BEE} = 795 + 7.18 \times \text{Weight (kg)}$$

$$\text{Men: BEE} = 879 + 10.20 \times \text{Weight (kg)}$$

TYPE OF STRESS	MULTIPLY VALUE FROM STEP 2 BY:
Fever	1 + 0.13/° C elevation above normal (or 0.07/° F)
Pneumonia	1.2
Major injury	1.3
Severe sepsis	1.5
Burn 15%-30% BSA	1.5
Burn 31%-49% BSA	1.5-2.0
Burn 50% or greater BSA	1.8-2.1

BSA, Body surface area.

*Data from Deitch EA: *Crit Care Clin* 11:735, 1995; Owen OE, et al: *Am J Clin Nutr* 44:1, 1986; Owen OE, et al: *Am J Clin Nutr* 46:875, 1987; and Garrel DR, Jobin N, de Jonge LH: *Nutr Clin Pract* 11:99, 1996.

Step 2. Multiply by an appropriate stress factor to meet needs of ill or injured patients (see the above table). If patient has more than one stress present (e.g., burn and pneumonia), use only the stress factor for the *highest level* of stress.

Estimate of Protein Needs

Protein needs vary with degree of malnutrition and stress (see the following table).

Example of Calculation of Caloric and Protein Needs

A 28-year-old female patient has a fracture of the left femur and burns on 40% of her body surface area (BSA) after a motor vehicle crash. Her height is 1.65 m (5 ft 5 in), and her weight is 59.1 kg (130 lb).

Energy needs
1. BEE = 795 + 7.18 × 59.1 = 1219 calories/day
2. Energy needs for injury = 1219 calories × 1.75 = 2133 calories/day
Protein needs
Protein needs = 59.1 kg × 1.75 g = 103 g/day

CONDITION	MULTIPLY DESIRABLE BODY WEIGHT (KG) BY:
Healthy individual	0.8-1.0 g protein
Well-nourished elective surgery patient	
Malnourished or catabolic state	1.2-2+ g protein
• Sepsis	
• Major injury	
Burns	
• 15%-30% BSA	1.5 g protein
• 31%-49% BSA	1.5-2.0 g protein
• 50% or greater BSA	2.0-2.5 g protein

BSA, Body surface area.

Page numbers followed by "f" indicate figures, "t" indicate tables, and "b" indicate boxes.

E

SPECIAL FEATURES